Medical

Rehabilitation

of Traumatic

Brain Injury

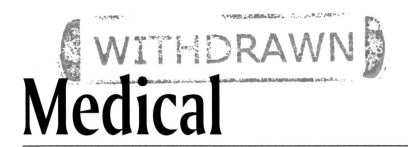

Medical

Rehabilitation

of Traumatic

Brain Injury

Edited by

Lawrence J. Horn, MD

Coghlin Chair and Professor
Department of Physical Medicine and Rehabilitation
Medical College of Ohio
Toledo, Ohio

Nathan D. Zasler, MD, FAADEP

CEO and Executive Medical Director
National NeuroRehabilitation Consortium, Inc.
Medical Director, Concussion Care Centres of America, Inc.
Director, Brain Injury Rehabilitation Programs
Sheltering Arms Hospital
Richmond, Virginia

HANLEY & BELFUS, INC. / Philadelphia
MOSBY / St. Louis Baltimore Berlin Boston Carlsbad Chicago London Madrid
Naples New York Philadelphia Sydney Tokyo Toronto

Publisher: HANLEY & BELFUS, INC.
Medical Publishers
210 S. 13th Street
Philadelphia, PA 19107
(215) 546-7293
FAX (215) 790-9330

North American and worldwide sales and distribution:

MOSBY
11830 Westline Industrial Drive
St. Louis, MO 63146

In Canada: Times Mirror Professional Publishing, Ltd.
130 Flaska Drive
Markham, Ontario L6G 1B8
Canada

Library of Congress Cataloging-in-Publication Data

Medical rehabilitation of traumatic brain injury / [edited by]
Lawrence J. Horn, Nathan D. Zasler.
     p.   cm.
   Includes bibliographical references and index.
   ISBN 1-56053-070-7 (hard : alk. paper)
   1. Brain—Wounds and injuries—Patients—Rehabilitation.
2. Brain—Wounds and injuries—Complications.   I. Horn, Lawrence,
J., 1954–   .   II. Zasler, Nathan D, 1958–   .
   [DNLM: 1. Brain Injuries—rehabilitation.   2. Brain Injuries—
complications.   WL 354 M4893 1995]
RD594.M43   1995
617.4′81044-dc20
DNLM/DLC
for Library of Congress   95-39446
                                           CIP

MEDICAL REHABILITATION OF TRAUMATIC BRAIN INJURY   ISBN 1-56053-070-7

Library of Congress catalog card number 95-39446

Last digit is the print number: 9 8 7 6 5 4 3 2 1

Dedication

To Roxanne, the person who inaugurated my career in brain injury rehabilitation, now consummated in this text.

To my family, for giving me a gift of empathy which has quietly benefited my patients and their loved ones.

To the authors, for putting up with delays and annoyances from the publisher.

To our publisher, for putting up with delays and annoyances from the authors.

To all of the above, for putting up with me.

LJH

From a professional standpoint, I would like to dedicate this book to the professionals who most guided my entry into the field as well as my continued professional development. I would like to particularly remember Dr. Sheldon Berrol, a man whose knowledge, style, and empathy I will always strive to emulate.

I would also like to acknowledge the support, friendship, and wisdom of Drs. Jeffrey Kreutzer, Henry Stonnington, and Larry Horn, all of whom have shaped me as a professional and allowed me to hone my clinical skills.

On a personal note, I would like to thank my wife Carol for her patience, understanding, and love as it related to the birth of this "second child" in our family.

NZ

Contents

Contributors

TERRI ANTOINETTE, MHSA, RNC, CRRN
Director of Nursing, Horizon Health Care Corporation D.B.A. Greenery Rehabilitation Center, Canonsburg, Pennsylvania

KERTIA L. BLACK, MD
Assistant Professor, Department of Physical Medicine and Rehabilitation, and Staff Physiatrist, Traumatic Brain Injury Unit, Rehabilitation Institute of Michigan, Wayne State University, Detroit, Michigan

CORWIN BOAKE, PhD
Assistant Professor, Department of Physical Medicine and Rehabilitation, University of Texas–Houston Medical School, Houston, Texas

CATHERINE F. BONTKE, MD
System Medical Director of Rehabilitation Services, The Rehabilitation Hospital of Connecticut, Hartford, Connecticut

MICHAEL GEORGE BOYESON, PhD
Associate Professor, Department of Communicative Disorders, Texas Women's University, Denton, Texas

GEORGE J. CARNEVALE, PhD
Assistant Director, Department of Psychology and Neuropsychology, Kessler Institute for Rehabilitation, East Orange, New Jersey; Assistant Professor, University of Medicine and Dentistry of New Jersey, New Jersey Medical School, Newark, New Jersey

DANIEL M. CLINCHOT, MD
Assistant Professor, Department of Physical Medicine and Rehabilitation, The Ohio State University College of Medicine, Columbus, Ohio

JANICE L. COCKRELL, MD
Clinical Associate Professor, Department of Pediatrics, Oregon Health Sciences University, Portland; Medical Director of Pediatric Rehabilitation, Legacy Emanuel Children's Hospital, Portland, Oregon

D. NATHAN COPE, MD
Chief Medical Officer, Paradigm Health Corporation, Concord, California

ROBERT STEVEN DJERGAIAN, MD
Medical Director, Department of Rehabilitation Services, Southwest Washington Medical Center, Vancouver, Washington

ELIE ELOVIC, MD
Associate Medical Director, Center for Head Injuries, JFK Johnson Rehabilitation Institute, Edison, New Jersey; Clinical Assistant Professor, Department of Physical Medicine and Rehabilitation, University of Medicine and Dentistry of New Jersey, Robert Wood Johnson Medical School, New Brunswick, New Jersey

ALBERTO ESQUENAZI, MD
Director, Gait and Motion Analysis Laboratory, Moss Rehabilitation Hospital, Philadelphia; Associate Professor of Rehabilitation Medicine, Temple University School of Medicine, Philadelphia, Pennsylvania

LISA P. FUGATE, MD
Department of Rehabilitation Medicine, The Ohio State University College of Medicine, Columbus, Ohio

KARYL MAUREEN HALL, EdD
Clinical Assistant Professor, Department of Functional Restoration, Stanford University Medical School, Stanford, California

LAWRENCE J. HORN, MD
Coghlin Chair and Professor of Clinical Physical Medicine and Rehabilitation, Department of Physical Medicine and Rehabilitation, Medical College of Ohio, Toledo, Ohio

CINDY B. IVANHOE, MD
Co-Director of Brain Injury Program, The Institute for Rehabilitation and Research; Assistant Professor, Department of Physical Medicine and Rehabilitation, Baylor College of Medicine, Houston, Texas

MARK V. JOHNSTON, PhD
Assistant Professor, Department of Physical Medicine and Rehabilitation, University of Medicine and Dentistry of New Jersey, New Jersey Medical School, Newark, New Jersey; Director of Outcomes Research, Kessler Institute for Rehabilitation, Inc., East Orange, New Jersey

JENNIFER L. JONES, MS
Department of Neurology, Medical College of Wisconsin, Milwaukee, Wisconsin

MARY ANN KEENAN, MD
Professor, Department of Orthopaedic Surgery, Temple University School of Medicine; Chairman, Department of Orthopaedic Surgery, Albert Einstein Medical Center, Philadelphia, Pennsylvania

MARIA L.C. LABI, MD, PhD
Assistant Professor, Department of Rehabilitation Medicine, State University of New York at Buffalo, Buffalo, New York

DAVID FULLERTON LONG, MD
Clinical Director, Brain Injury Program, Bryn Mawr Rehabilitation Hospital, Malvern, Pennsylvania

NANCY R. MANN, MD
Associate Chair and Assistant Professor, Department of Physical Medicine and Rehabilitation, Wayne State University School of Medicine, Detroit, Michigan

DONALD W. MARION, MD
Associate Professor, Department of Neurological Surgery, University of Pittsburgh School of Medicine, Pittsburgh, Pennsylvania

NATHANIEL H. MAYER, MD
Professor, Department of Physical Medicine and Rehabilitation, Temple University School of Medicine; Director, Drucker Brain Injury Center and Motor Control Analysis Laboratory, Moss Rehabilitation Hospital, Philadelphia, Pennsylvania

JAMES T. McDEAVITT, MD
Medical Director and Clinical Assistant Professor, Department of Physical Medicine and Rehabilitation, Charlotte Institute of Rehabilitation, Charlotte, North Carolina

MARY ANN MYERS, MD
Assistant Professor, Department of Physical Medicine and Rehabilitation, Medical College of Ohio, Toledo, Ohio

W. JERRY MYSIW, MD
Associate Professor, Department of Physical Medicine and Rehabilitation Medicine, The Ohio State University College of Medicine, Columbus, Ohio

MICHAEL W. O'DELL, MD
Associate Professor, Department of Physical Medicine and Rehabilitation, University of Cincinnati College of Medicine; Director, Brain Injury Rehabilitation Programs, Drake Center, Inc., Cincinnati, Ohio

LOUIS E. PENROD, MD
Assistant Professor, Departments of Orthopaedics and Physical Medicine and Rehabilitation, University of Pittsburgh School of Medicine, Pittsburgh, Pennsylvania

MAURICE RAPPAPORT, MD, PhD
Former Head, Brain Function Study Unit at Agnews, San Jose, California; Department of Psychiatry, University of California, San Francisco, San Francisco, California

RICHARD VINCENT RIGGS, MD
Medical Director, HealthSouth Rehabilitation Hospital, Dothan, Alabama

M. ELIZABETH SANDEL, MD
Associate Professor, Department of Rehabilitation Medicine, and Director, Division of Neurorehabilitation, University of Pennsylvania School of Medicine, Philadelphia, Pennsylvania

MILTON D. THOMAS, MD
Medical Director, Mid-America Rehabilitation Hospital, Overland Park, Kansas

STUART A. YABLON, MD
Assistant Professor, Department of Physical Medicine and Rehabilitation, Baylor College of Medicine, Houston; Co-Director, Brain Injury Program, The Institute for Rehabilitation and Research, Houston, Texas

ROSS D. ZAFONTE, DO
Assistant Professor, Department of Physical Medicine and Rehabilitation, Wayne State University School of Medicine; Medical Director, Traumatic Brain Injury Unit, Rehabilitation Institute of Michigan; Chief, Department of Physical Medicine and Rehabilitation, Detroit Receiving Hospital, Detroit, Michigan

NATHAN D. ZASLER, MD, FAAPM&R, FAADEP, BCFE
CEO and Executive Medical Director, National NeuroRehabilitation Consortium, Inc.; Medical Director, Concussion Care Centres of America, Inc.; and Director, Brain Injury Rehabilitation Programs, Sheltering Arms Hospital, Richmond, Virginia

Preface

Dramatic changes in the care of persons with traumatic brain injury (TBI) have occurred in the past two decades. These changes have affected the entire spectrum of TBI care from acute medical/surgical management to the development of novel post-acute rehabilitation programs. While many people with TBI have benefited from this plethora of TBI programs and improved professional knowledge and skills, others continue to have difficulty accessing appropriate services, and some have been exploited by unethical organizations. New threats to consumers of TBI services may be emerging as many in the health care industry focus on *cost* rather than on cost/outcome, especially since outcomes have been difficult to define and measure in this population using "standard" techniques.

In the past decade there has been an extraordinary increase in the scientific literature germane to brain injury care. The intent of this text is to complement the existing body of literature by addressing medical issues pertinent to the care of people with TBI over their lifetimes. It will provide, for the first time, a medical reference text with a global and in-depth summary of current state-of-the-art practice of TBI rehabilitative medicine. While this text focuses on the medical aspects of rehabilitation, it is not our intent to minimize the importance of the contributions of other health care professionals or other medical specialists in the care of people with TBI. Indeed, we would hope that this volume will serve as a consolidated reference tool for colleagues in other disciplines. In each clinical chapter, reference is made to the practice of other rehabilitation team members; we hope that a clear message pervades this text that any attempt to "correct" the multifactorial problems posed by TBI through implementation of a single practitioner, a single drug, or a single treatment technique is likely doomed to failure or will not be of lasting benefit to the person with a TBI or his or her nuclear social system. The impairments, disabilities, and handicaps associated with TBI are invariably intertwined with preexisting psychological, social, cultural, and intellectual factors. A coordinated interdisciplinary team approach provided across a continuum of clinical services will best serve this population and society at large.

The definition of interdisciplinary practice is also undergoing revision. Given the changes affecting and afflicting the health care system, it is important to recognize that interdisciplinary care has evolved to include participation of multiple agencies and organizations as well as specific rehabilitation providers outside the context of the immediate acute (traditional) healthcare system. If interfaced appropriately, these entities may help to optimize provision of services to manage the multiple social, economic, and environmental issues confronting persons with TBI and their families.

TBI may encompass a spectrum of conditions that will affect an individual's general health status. The resultant implications for primary and preventive medicine are not always recognized. The differential diagnosis for a given complaint becomes expanded, often incorporating possibilities that would be unusual in the general population. Furthermore, the primary care physician for someone with TBI needs to have considerable insight into the psychological and behavioral consequences of the injury: patient compliance may become a significant issue and alternative strategies to learn medication or treatment regimens may need to be employed. Whether as a rehabilitation team leader in acute settings, or as a team member in "post-acute" settings, the physiatrist (physical medicine and rehabilitation specialist) with special expertise in TBI medical rehabilitation is optimally qualified to serve as the primary care physician for this patient population and as the integrative member of a team of medical specialists working with the patient. While this position may not be endorsed by every reader of (or even all contributors to) this text, the fact remains that of all medical specialties, it is PM&R that articulates interdisciplinary practice and requires specific training in it. A model of a primary care clinic for people with disabilities currently being introduced in some rehabilitation centers, incorporating medical and PM&R services at a single site, may prove the most effective mechanism to manage all of the health care needs of a person with TBI.

Finally, we hope most of all that if we have been even moderately effective in achieving the goals of this text that our collective work will ultimately have a beneficial effect on the *standard* of medical care that persons with TBI and their families can expect to receive in both the acute and chronic phases of recovery.

Lawrence J. Horn, MD
Nathan D. Zasler, MD

PART ONE

Issues in the Continuum of Care

ELIE ELOVIC M.D.

TERRI ANTOINETTE MHSA, RNC, CRRN

1

Epidemiology and Primary Prevention of Traumatic Brain Injury

The impact of traumatic brain injury (TBI) on humankind and society has been known since Biblical times. The course of history itself has been changed by the devastating ramifications of its sequelae:

> And David put his hand in his bag, and took thence a stone, and slang it, and smote the Philistine forehead that the stone sunk into his forehead; and he fell upon his face to the earth. So David prevailed over the Philistine with a sling and with a stone, and smote the Philistine, and slew him; but there was no sword in the hand of David.
>
> *I Samuel 17:49–50*

Given the enormous personal suffering, morbidity, mortality, and societal and financial impact, the need for the study of TBI becomes self-evident. This chapter first reviews past epidemiologic studies, emphasizing the differences among the varying subpopulations as well as discussing the shortcomings and unanswered questions. The second major focus is the nature and effect of primary prevention. Finally, future legislative initiatives, prevention programs, and registry issues are discussed.

GENERAL OVERVIEW

Data from the 1989 Department of Health and Human Services Interagency Head Injury Task Force Report estimated that in the United States over two million head injuries occur each year with 500,000 requiring hospital admissions.[38] In 1985 Frankowski et al. reported that of these 500,000, approximately 30–50% were moderate, severe, or fatal injuries.[49] The Interagency Head Injury Task Force Report also states that up to 100,000 deaths can be attributed to TBI each year. TBI is the leading cause of death and disability in children and young adults. Yearly economic costs approach twenty-five billion dollars for medical treatment, rehabilitative and support services, and lost income.[38]

The first epidemiologic studies of TBI in the United States were not published until 1980 when Annegers et al. described the epidemiology of TBI in Olmsted County, Minnesota,[5] and Anderson and McLaurins[4] reported on the National Head and Spinal Cord Injury Survey (HSCI Survey). There have been numerous other studies since that time; however, what becomes obvious is that TBI is not a homogeneous diagnosis. Before addressing the many factors that influence diagnosis, classification, and treatment, it is first necessary to establish a working definition of TBI.

DEFINITION OF TRAUMATIC BRAIN INJURY

Unfortunately, many of the past discussions of the epidemiology of TBI used diverse definitions for data collection. Exacerbating the problem was the confusion between inclusion criteria and a working definition for TBI. Researchers introduced selection bias, obtaining information about select subsections of the brain-injured population. This bias has greatly complicated the comparison of results among the different studies. Criteria for inclusion in a database for the purposes of research should not be confused with an actual definition, as the discriminating reader must understand to draw correct conclusions from reviewing these studies.

As a review of the epidemiologic literature indicates, certain definitions are noteworthy because of their respective historical and/or practical significance. In the first major American-based epidemiologic study, Annegers et al.[5] defined head trauma as a head injury with evidence of presumed brain involvement, i.e., concussion with loss of consciousness, posttraumatic amnesia, or neurologic signs of brain injury. The National Head and Spinal Cord Injury Survey,[4] which was the first national attempt to quantify traumatic neurologic injury, defined head and spinal cord injury as trauma to the brain or spinal cord. In this survey, trauma referred to physical injury to living tissue caused by an external (mechanical) force, excluding birth trauma.

Frankowski[48] was more generalized in his definition, which included all injuries to the head. He defined head injury as acute physical damage to the face, scalp, skull, dura, or brain caused by external mechanical (kinetic) energy. Field[43a] defined injury as "trauma which carried some risk of damage to the brain." The application of this criterion depends on the treating physician's judgment as to what type of injury carried such risk.

Definitions of TBI are almost as numerous as the papers written on the subject. The diversity and inconsistencies clearly exacerbate the difficulty in analyzing data related to head injury and weaken conclusions. This problem is unavoidable when leaders in the field are unable to come to a unified consensus on what constitutes TBI.

One of the best functional definitions of TBI was developed by the National Head Injury Foundation (NHIF)[59]:

Traumatic head injury is an insult to the brain, not of a degenerative or congenital nature but caused by an external physical force, that may produce a diminished or altered state of consciousness, which results in impairment of cognitive abilities or physical functioning. It can also result in the disturbance of behavioral or emotional functioning. These impairments may be either temporary or permanent and cause partial or total functional disability or psychosocial maladjustment.

This definition has many strengths. First is its comprehensiveness. A patient whose initial clinical examination shows complete resolution of symptoms and impairments is not excluded. The conditions of many boxers, such as Muhammed Ali, are an excellent example. Despite the absence of overt early symptoms, the eventual outcomes speak for themselves. A second advantage is that the patient's eventual outcome in no way affects application of the term TBI. This approach facilitates data collection for future studies. Finally, the NHIF definition allows ease of understanding by the lay public. Only if TBI is presented in a simple, understandable fashion can the public respond to education and prevention messages.

This definition, however, is not perfect. Failure to include a system for grading injuries by severity and extent, outcome, and impairment sacrifices valuable information for the sake of simplicity. Although this approach may be excellent for data surveillance, it may lead to inappropriate targeting of resources with a failure to emphasize the more severe range of the injury spectrum. The NHIF definition, used by itself, gives only limited information. It must be used in coordination with more clinically based criteria. For example, the trauma registries of Utah and Arkansas[59] define a case of traumatic brain injury as a person:

(1) admitted to a hospital with a history of trauma to the head and at least one of the following: (a) observed or self-reported loss of consciousness due to head trauma; (b) observed or self-reported retrograde amnesia and/or posttraumatic amnesia attributed to head trauma; (c) skull fracture; (d) objective neurological signs that can be reasonably attributed to head injury; (e) traumatic intracranial hemorrhage or cerebral contusion or laceration based on radiographic or neurosurgical findings; or

(2) dying as a result of trauma with head injury listed on the death certificate in the sequence of conditions that resulted in death.

The first complicating factor is the requirement that the injury must cause either death or hospital admission. The requirement of amnesia eliminates clinical grade I injuries, as mentioned by Ommaya and Gennarelli.[113] In addition, subtle behavioral or cognitive changes may easily go unnoticed by the diagnostician. Such an approach clearly biases data collection to the more severe end of the injury spectrum. The softness of some of the clinical signs, furthermore, complicates the attempt to formulate an objective diagnosis of TBI. Finally, the definition is in fact part of the inclusion criteria for the state trauma registry. Unfortunately, the lack of uniformity among such registries is typical of state-based health care proposals in the United States. The need for a federally based, uniform approach to such issues becomes apparent.

The magnitude of the problem caused by neurotrauma has been recognized by the CDC, and since 1988 it has been investigating a means of providing appropriate surveillance. It created a task force with the mission of forming a working definition; Thurman et al.[155c] have recently published the results of these efforts. What may be more important than the actual inclusion and exclusion criteria is its potential national significance. The definition is similar to that of previously mentioned state registries, with traumatic brain injury defined as follows:

> an occurrence of injury to the head that is documented in a medical record, with one of the following conditions attributed to head injury:
> 1. observed or self-reported decreased level of consciousness
> 2. amnesia
> 3. skull fracture
> 4. objective neurological or neuropsychological abnormality

The definition excludes (1) lacerations or contusions of the face, eye, ear, or scalp without the other criteria listed above; (2) fractures of facial bones without other criteria listed above; (3) birth trauma; (4) primary anoxic, inflammatory, infectious, toxic, or metabolic encephalopathies that are not complications of head trauma; (5) cancer; and (6) brain infarction (ischemic stroke) and intracranial hemorrhage (hemorrhagic stroke) without associated trauma.

No definition of TBI meets the need for both inclusiveness and practicality. Although the NHIF definition is the most accurate, practical application is difficult. Eventually the state registries will have to use some derivative of the clinically based definition. It may be impossible to count accurately the most trivial injuries, but the number of injuries that require intervention may be obtainable. For the moment, the words of Jennett seem most pertinent:

> No universal definition of practical value can be proposed to cover the many minor injuries known only to general practitioners, traffic police, or officials at sporting events and those that are never reported unless complications develop. The actual incidence of head injury is therefore an abstraction. It is, however, reasonable for those concerned with preventing head injuries and planning health services for their care to focus on injuries that lead to death, hospital admissions, or attendance at accident departments.

EPIDEMIOLOGY OF TRAUMATIC BRAIN INJURY

Now that the question of definition has been explored, it is appropriate to create a profile of who sustains TBI. The important questions are who, what, how, when, where, and why. Substantial controversy surrounds the answers.

Incidence

Numerous attempts have been made in the last 20 years to quantify the incidence and total number of traumatic brain injuries within the United States and the rest of the world.[5,32,39,45,66,69,71,75,77,95,156] Table 1 reviews some of the more recent data.

The first attempt at defining the problem was the National Health Interview Survey.[4,71] Approximately 41,000 households and 111,000 people were surveyed every year in an attempt to estimate the annual number of head injuries in the United States. For the purpose of the survey, anyone who, as a result of an accident or act of violence, was either medically attended or limited in activity for

TABLE 1. Incidence per 100,000 by Study Male/Female Ratio

Author	Incidence	M/F Ratio
Annegers, 1980[5] Olmsted County	270 Male 116 Female	2.3
Kalsbeek, 1980[71] NHSCIS USA	272 Male 132 Female 200 Total	2.1
Klauber, 1981[77] San Diego	295 Total	1.3–2.8
Cooper, 1983[32] Bronx	391 Male 142 Female 249 Total	2.8
Jagger, 1984[66] Northern Virginia	208 Total	2.4
Whitman, 1984[164] Chicago	403 Inner city 394 Suburban black 196 Suburban white	2.5 2.8 2.3
Kraus, 1984[30] San Diego	247 Male 111 Female 180 Total	2.2
Missouri Trauma Registry, 1988[95]	135 Male 71 Female	1.9
Tiret, 1990[156] Aquitane, France	384 Male 185 Female 281 Total	2.1

1 day was considered injured. Using these data, Caveness[21] estimated that 4% of the population sustained some sort of head injury each year and that more than one million people sustained a "major" head injury each year from 1970–1976. For the purpose of the survey, a "major" injury was defined as involving the potential for brain injury.

There were numerous problems with the study. First, because population surveys depend on self-reports there was no clinical verification of injury. Compounding this problem was the survey's loose definition of head injury, which included lacerations and contusions to the face and head. Still, this was the first work in the United States that pointed to the magnitude of the problem.

Since that time numerous attempts have been made to obtain a better profile of the traumatically brain-injured patient. The problem has been greatly complicated by inconsistencies and differences among the studies. Table 2 compares some of the studies and highlights differences in inclusion criteria, sample size, and time frame over which data were collected.

The differences in inclusion data are more than academic. The decision about which cases to include directly affects the number of traumatic brain injuries identified by the study team. Whereas some studies required physician documentation of a head injury in addition to clinical criteria,[80] others included patients solely on the basis of a review of the International Classification of Diseases adapted. Some studies restricted their focus to hospital admissions, excluding cases seen in the emergency department and prehospital deaths. Some studies were even more specific, requiring admissions of certain lengths.[66,95] The Missouri Trauma Registry, for example, requires that a patient must be admitted for at least 24 hours to become a reportable case. Any attempt to compare results among these studies requires knowledge of their structural differences.

Most studies report the incidence of TBI at approximately 200 cases/100,000 population per year. This figure was quoted most recently by Kraus[79] in 1993. Extrapolating to the entire United States population, this places the estimate of total cases of TBI per year at 500,000 per year.

Examination of past inquiries gives a better understanding of Kraus's calculations. The reported incidence ranges between 152 and 367/100,000.[5,32,39,45,66,71,77,80,164] The major discrepancies between these values can be explained by a critical review of the studies. The exclusion by Fife et al.[45] of prehospital deaths accounts to some extent for their relatively low estimate of 152 cases/100,000 in Rhode Island between 1979 and 1980. On the other hand, the estimate of 376 cases/100,000 by Whitman et al.[164] is based on an inner city population with a high rate of interpersonal violence and lower socioeconomic status.

The work of Willer et al.,[166] based on data from the Missouri Trauma Registry in 1988, is not as easy to explain. They estimate the total incidence of moderate and severe disability upon discharge from the hospital at 12.4/100,000. This estimate is misleading for several reasons. First, the data specifying the degree of disability were missing in 925 of 4877 cases (19%).[95] No correction was made in determining the incidence for the general population. Second, data were collected at the end of rehabilitation, perhaps many months

TABLE 2. Inclusion Criteria for Recent Studies

Author	Time Frame	Population Location	No. of Cases	Inclusion Criteria
Annegers, 1980[5]	1935 1974	Olmsted, county	3,587	Head injury with evidence of presumed brain involvement.
Kalsbeek, NHSCIS 1980[71]	1974	U.S.	1,310	Head injuries admitted for inpatient care; prehospital deaths excluded.
Klauber, 1981[77]	1978	San Diego, county	5,055	Hospital admissions and deaths with diagnosis of head injury by ICDA. Gunshots, bruises and lacerations excluded.
Cooper, 1983[32]	1980 1981	Bronx, N.Y., urban	1,209	Residency, onset of injury < 24 hours. Loss of consciousness > 10 min, skull fracture, neurologic sign or seizure.
Jagger, 1984[66]	1978	Virginia, rural	735	Residency, hospitalized for > 15 hours; 99% had loss of consciousness, skull fracture or posttraumatic amnesia. Prehospital death excluded.
Desai, 1983[39]	1979 1980	Chicago, urban	702	Injury < 7 days old; blow to head or blow to face with change in consciousness or facial laceration. Hospital admissions only.
Kraus, 1984[80]	1981	San Diego	3,358	Physician diagnosed brain injury; blunt and penetrating included; facial and skull fractures without brain injury excluded.
Jennett, 1981[69]	1974	England, Scotland, and Wales	Not reported	ICDA codes for death and admissions.
Tiret and Cohadon, 1991[156]	1986	Aquitaine, France	8,172	Head injuries including contusions, lacerations, skull fractures, brain injuries and loss of consciousness; admissions and immediate deaths.
Wong, 1993[168]	1978 1991	Toronto, Canada	498	Consecutive rehabilitative admissions to brain injury rehabilitation unit. Over 18 with diagnosis of "TBI" with rehabilitative potential.

ICDA = International Classification of Diseases, Adapted.

after injury. Even in severe cases, only approximately 50% have moderate or severe deficits 6 months after injury.[70,165] Third, closer examination of the actual data from 1988 reveals an incidence of 102/100,000. The lower estimate in the registry can be explained by its inclusion criteria. Patients with TBI who were seen in the emergency department or had only an overnight stay were not included. Therefore, many minor head injuries, which comprise the largest component of TBI incidence, were excluded. The lower incidence may well be explained by the use of stricter inclusion criteria than any of the previously published literature.

Mortality

Kraus[79] estimated that in 1990 75,000 deaths resulted from TBI, accounting for 52% of the 148,480 injury-related deaths in the same year. His estimate was based on an annual incidence of 30 TBI-related deaths per 100,000 population. The mortality rate, however, varies among different population studies[5,32,77,80,147,164] (Table 3). Despite such variation, depending on location and socioeconomic class studied, the mortality numbers are substantially higher for males than for females (by a factor of 2.5–5).

Equally apparent is the difference in the numbers produced by population studies versus the work done by Sosin et al.,[147,147a] who reviewed death certificates using the Multiple Cause-of-Death Public Use Data Tapes. The incidence of TBI mortality reported by Sosin et al. was substantially lower than that of the other studies. Sosin himself raised questions about his work, conceding the potential for severe undercounting because of the lack of clinical information to back up the data. The work of Gennarelli et al.,[54] which showed the major impact of TBI on trauma center mortality,

TABLE 3. Mortality Incidence in Various Studies

Author	Time Frame	Population Location	Mortality Incidence per 100,000	M/F Ratio
Annegers, 1980[5]	1935–1974	Olmsted, county	35 Male, 10 Female	3.5
Klauber, 1981[77]	1978	San Diego, county	32 Male, 12 Female, 22 Total	2.7
Cooper, 1983[32]	1980–1981	Bronx, N.Y., urban	50 Male, 10 Female, 28 Total	5.0
Whitman, 1984[164]	1978	Chicago Inner city Suburb	32 Inner city 19 Suburban blacks 11 Suburban whites	4.6 2.6 2.3
Kraus, 1984[80]	1981	San Diego	45 Male, 15 Female, 30 Total	3.0
Sosin, 1989[146]	1979–1986	Multiple cause of death tapes	26, Male, 9 Female, 17 Total	3.0
Sosin, 1995[147a]	1992	MC death tapes	19 Total	3.4

further supports the contention of under-counting in the estimate by Sosin et al. Even with the lower figures, however, TBI accounts for 26% of injury-related deaths and is the number-one cause of preventable deaths in the United States.

The annual incidence of TBI fatalities is a somewhat controversial subject. Although the differing inclusion criteria for epidemiologic studies affect all incidence data, mortality rate is affected more dramatically. Gennarelli et al.[54] reported that 60–75% of vehicular head injury deaths occurred before hospital admission. Because motor vehicles are the most common cause of TBI, studies that look only at hospital admissions have limited value for estimating the incidence of TBI mortality.

A further complication is the combination of head injury and extracranial trauma. How should the death of the patient with multiple trauma be classified? Classifying the death of all patients who sustain a brain injury as TBI-induced grossly overestimates the incidence.

Gennarelli et al. tried to answer such questions by reviewing the data collected from numerous trauma centers around the country. They found that TBI plays an extremely critical role in patient mortality. Two-thirds of the deaths in patients with multiple trauma were related to TBI. Only 1 of 16 patients with multiple trauma succumbed to an extracranial injury. In the remaining 25% death was attributed to a combination of TBI and extracranial trauma. Only with minor-to-moderate TBIs did extracranial injury play a significant role in increasing patient mortality. Therefore it is reasonable to include

all deaths associated with brain injury as part of the TBI statistics.

Severity of Injury

In discussing the epidemiology of injury severity, it is critical to determine the measurement scale used to compare results. A minor head injury based on the Glasgow Coma Score (GCS) often differs from minor injury based on the Abbreviated Injury Scale (AIS). Clearly, the method used for determining severity of injury directly affects its distribution. An appreciation of the different methods is critical to understand the terms in common use. Grading of severity is more than an academic exercise; to some extent it determines prognosis and treatment decisions.

Glasgow Coma Score and Glasgow Liege Scale

Numerous methods have been used, but none is as well known as the GCS.[152] First published in 1974, the GCS has gained wide popularity because of its ease of use, interrater reliability, and value as a prognosticator of patient outcome. The GCS is based on the scoring of three separate items: eye opening, best motor response, and verbal response. The scores of each subscale are added together to give the total score. The perfect score is 15, whereas a totally unresponsive patient receives a score of 3. Based on their GCS, patients are assigned to different categories. A GCS of 13–15 is associated with a minor injury; a score of 9–12 with moderate injury; and a score of 8 or less with severe brain injury. Intubation is a minor problem in the scoring of the severely injured patient, as the motor subscore is the most critical factor for these patients.

Research in the 1980s demonstrated two facts: (1) brainstem reflexes are important prognosticators in the first 24 hours after injury, and (2) in severely injured patients with TBI the motor component is the most critical factor in determining the GCS. As an outgrowth of this research, the Glasgow-Liege Scale (GLS) was developed in 1982.[13] The GLS consists of the GCS with an additional section for brainstem reflexes, which were organized in a hierarchy based on their order of disappearance during deterioration in a caudal fashion. In 1988 Born demonstrated that the combined data were a more accurate predictor of recovery than motor or brainstem reflex alone. Although not a replacement for the GCS, the GLS is an adjunct for determining patient outcome

Grading of Injury

Donald Becker's *Textbook of Head Injury*[101] described a system for rating severity of injury based on the patient's level of consciousness upon presentation at the emergency department. Patients are given a grade from I through IV. Grade I patients are alert and oriented with no focal neurologic lesion. Grade II includes patients who demonstrate a decreased level of consciousness, with the ability to follow simple commands, or who are awake with a focal neurologic lesion. Grade III patients are characterized by an inability to follow a simple one-step command. Patients with grade IV injuries show no evidence of brain function or are brain-dead. The two purposes of this classification are triage and determination of the appropriate level of care.

In 1974, Ommaya and Gennarelli[113] developed a scale for grading TBI based on the level of brain disturbance. They hypothesized that the diffuse axonal injury caused by the mechanically induced strain occurs in a centripetal pattern. As a result, higher cortical centers are affected long before the subcortical area and brainstem, and memory disturbance from cortical injury precedes loss of consciousness. The grading system based on this pattern depends on clinical presentation. With grades I, II, and III, the patient sustains a blow that results in confusion without loss of consciousness. The three grades are differentiated by

the presence or absence of amnesia. In grade I injuries no amnesia is noted, whereas grade II injuries are characterized by post-traumatic amnesia and grade III injuries by retrograde amnesia. In grade IV injuries the brainstem is affected with concomitant loss of consciousness. In grades V and VI the lesions are more severe, and more extensive structural injury results in extended coma, persistent vegetative state (PVS), and death.

The previous discussion of grading of injury severity is based totally on clinical presentation. In 1982 Gennarelli et al.[55] published the results of their work with traumatic coma in primates. Brain injury was graded on the basis of neuropathologic findings found after the animals were sacrificed. These data were then correlated with clinical information, and a grading system of 0, 1, 2, and 3 was used to describe the severity of diffuse axonal injury (DAI). Grade 0 was assigned to animals that showed no evidence of DAI on examination and had suffered a concussion or mild coma. Grade 1 DAI was defined as axonal abnormalities restricted primarily to the parasaggital white matter. The primates in this group have suffered mild-to-moderate coma. Grade 2 DAI involved the corpus callosum in addition to the parasagittal white matter in the cerebral hemispheres. The primates in this group have more severe injury with longer coma and more extensive long-term disability. Grade 3 DAI involved the superior cerebellar peduncle. Animals in this group had much more severe injury, as demonstrated by longer duration of coma and worse outcome.

Length of Coma

In the past the length of coma was one of the means used to assess severity of injury. Jennett and Teasedale[68–70] defined an injury with a 6-hour duration of coma as severe. However, "coma" or loss of consciousness, even of very short duration, may have long-term neuropsychological effects.

The majority of such data predates the development of computed tomography (CT); health care providers evaluated patients only on the basis of clinical examination. Several authors have discussed the relationship between length of coma and severity of injury. In 1968 Carlson et al.[20] reported on 320 patients who suffered coma of greater than 12 hours' duration without surgical complications. They defined restitution time as the time needed for the patient to return to work. They also reported a direct relationship between length of coma and the patient's age.

APACHE II

The APACHE II[78,169] (Acute Physiological and Chronic Health Evaluation), published by Knaus et al. in 1985, was developed in an attempt to predict outcome and risk of hospital death for acutely injured patients by measuring and quantifying the derangement of physiologic function. The APACHE II includes three separate scores. The most critical is the acute physiologic score, which consists of 11 physiologic measures graded from 0 to 4 on the basis of level of abnormality. In addition, the points lost from the GCS are added to the score. Unlike the GCS, the APACHE II uses the worst values from the first 24 hours. In the two remaining sections, points are added for the patient's age and chronic health. With a possible total of 71 points, the APACHE II was used to predict the risk of in-hospital death.

Abbreviated Injury Scale and Injury Severity Score

The Abbreviated Injury Scale[28,31,90] (AIS) was first developed in 1971 and has undergone several revisions. It has become one of the most widely used scales for the rating of severity of trauma; many countries use it for national crash investigation teams. The severity of individual injuries is graded on a scale from 1 to 6. An AIS score of 1 is assigned to minor injuries, whereas 6 is assigned to fatal injuries.

The AIS is designed for individual organ systems; the Injury Severity Scores (ISS) was developed to summarize the total picture for the multiply traumatized patient. The ISS is the sum of the squares of the three highest AIS scores. A major problem with the ISS is that injuries to all organ systems are considered equal, even though the ramifications of injury are more important in some systems than others.

Revised Trauma Score

The Revised Trauma Score[28,29] (RTS), published in 1989, considers three different parameters: the GCS, systolic blood pressure, and respiratory rate. Each of these is given a 0–4 value. Their sum gives the triage revised trauma score, but the values also can be used as an outcome predictor when each factor is multiplied by weighting coefficients.

Posttraumatic Amnesia

Russell[132,133] was among the first to recognize the relationship between severity of injury and length of posttraumatic amnesia (PTA). PTA ends when the patient is able to integrate new information and to form new memories. It is important to differentiate between the end of PTA and the patient's ability to interact and talk. The latter often occurs long before PTA ends. It is often difficult to determine the end point of PTA; interrater reliability may be poor. In an attempt to define objectively the length of PTA, Levin et al.[86] developed the Galveston Orientation and Amnesia Test (GOAT), a quick, easy-to-perform bedside examination that allows objective measurement of orientation. When a patient consistently scores higher than 75 of 100 points, the period of PTA is considered to be over.

The original work by Russell was expanded by numerous authors to clarify the relationship between PTA and severity of injuries.

Distribution of Injury Severity

Different researchers who studied TBI have used various methods to assign injury severity.[5,39,54,80,95,156,164] Table 4 shows the different methods, and Table 5 shows the distribution of severity by incidence of TBI in past studies. The majority of TBIs seen are minor. In Anneger's study roughly 55–60% of survivors sustained minor injuries, compared with 80% in the more recent study by Tiret et al.[156] Part of the difference between the two studies may be diverse definitions of minor injury. PTA of greater than 30 minutes duration qualifies as moderate TBI in Anneger's work but constitutes a mild TBI in Tiret's study as long as loss of consciousness is less than 15 minutes. Another explanation is that increased use of safety devices, such as seat belts, may be lowering the severity of injury. Kraus's work in 1981 and Whitman's in 1980 also reported a 75-80% incidence of minor head injury, lending credence to the idea that minor head injury is becoming even more prevalent.

Moderate TBI is the second most common category among survivors (9–30% of hospital admissions), whereas severe injury accounts for roughly 10% of hospital admissions for TBI and 5–10% of all TBIs. Kraus estimates that 80% of all hospital admissions involve minor injuries, with the remaining 20% equally divided between moderate and severe. Although Kraus's estimate is a slight over-simplification, it is not far from the truth, according to recent epidemiologic studies.

Gender and Traumatic Brain Injury

Review of all epidemiologic data reflects a significant difference between the genders, both in incidence and mortality. Men are far more like both to suffer TBI and to die from the injury. This finding has been consistently reported in all of the major U.S. epidemiologic studies to date (see Tables 1 and 3). Although differing somewhat among different age groups, the overall male-to-female ratio is almost always 2–3 to 1. For mortality data, the overall ratio appears to be about 3 to 1. The exception is the inner city; because of the high prevalence of interpersonal violence,

TABLE 4. Severity Determination by Study

Author	Method of Severity Determination
Annegers, 1980[5] Olmsted County	Combination of clinical findings, length of posttraumatic amnesia and period of unconsciousness
Desai, 1983[39] Chicago	Combination of Gennarelli's and length of posttraumatic amnesia
Whitman, 1984[164] Chicago	Length of posttraumatic amnesia, period of unconsciousness and clinical findings
Kraus, 1984[80] San Diego	Primarily Glasgow Coma Score with some clinical findings
Gennarelli, 1989[54] 95 trauma centers	Abbreviated Injury Scale
Tiret, 1990[156]	Length of loss of consciousness determined severity. Data on Index-Injury Severity Score and Abbreviated Injury Scale also reported
MacKenzie, 1989[90] Maryland	Abbreviated Injury Scale
Missouri, 1989[90] Maryland	Patient's severity determined by Glasgow Coma Scale and Abbreviated Injury Scale

TABLE 5. Distribution of Severity by Study Incidence per 100,000

Author	Fatal	Severe	Moderate	Minor/ Trivial
Annegers, 1980[5] Olmsted County	M 35 F 10	17 6	69 29	149 71
Whitman, 1984[164] Chicago	ICB 32 SB 19 SW 11	14 32 15	34 6 20	328 303 118
Kraus, 1984[80] San Diego	30	14	15	131
Tiret, 1991[156]	M 33 F 12 T 22	23†	28†	227†

M = male, F = female, ICB = inner city black, SB = suburban black, SW = suburban white, T = total.
* Includes hospital admissions with minor head injury and TBIs not admitted to hospital.
† Estimate calculated by using the percent of each injury group reported multiplied by the (total incidence – fatalities).

the male-to-female ratio of mortality approaches 5 to 1.

Socioeconomic Influences and Race

Several studies have examined the influence of socioeconomic variables on the epidemiology of TBI. An inverse relationship between median family income and TBI incidence has been reported consistently.[81,123] Kraus et al.[81] attributed the increased incidence in the lower income group to interpersonal violence. The incidence of TBI-related mortality shows a similar inverse relationship with income, as demonstrated by Whitman et al.[164]

The relationship between race and incidence of TBI is not totally clear. Some studies have shown a much higher incidence of TBI for blacks versus whites, whereas others have shown an almost one-to-one ratio. Table 1 reviews some of the data about the relationship of TBI incidence to race. The relationship between mortality due to TBI and race is equally unclear. Whitman et al.[164] reported a higher mortality rate for blacks, while the original work published by Sosin[147] found the same rates for blacks and whites. More recently, Sosin et al.[147a] reported a divergence between the black and white male mortality data since 1984. They reported that in 1992 there was a drop in the rate of

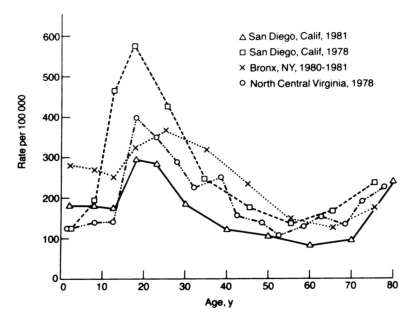

FIGURE 1. Age-specific brain injury incidence rates per 100,000 population, selected U.S. studies.

white male TBI mortality to 29/100,000, while at the same time the rate for blacks increased to 42/100,000. This change resulted from a greater decrease in white MVA mortality and significant increase in black male firearm-related deaths.

Previous Injury

The relationship between incidence and previous TBI has been addressed in several studies. Rimel et al.[123] reported that 31% of all patients in Charlottesville, Virginia had a previous history of hospitalization for TBI. Annegers et al.[5] reported a significant increase in the risk of TBI with a history of previous brain injury. They estimated that the risk increased threefold after one injury and eightfold after two. Neither study offered an explanation for the increased risk of repeat injury, which may be due to selection, premorbid patterns of behavior, or perhaps sequelae of the earlier injury. This question has not yet been answered satisfactorily.

Age and its Influence on Traumatic Brain Injury

Age is one of the most important variables for determining subpopulations of patients with TBI. Age affects not only the rate of TBI but also its etiology. Numerous studies have

pointed out that the highest incidence for TBI has been noted for the young adult between 15 and 24 years of age; other peaks have been noted in infants, children, and the elderly. Figure 1 summarizes the data from several U.S. studies.

Age also has a significant influence on the etiology of TBI. Past work[79] has shown that during the first few years of life, falls are the most prominent cause of injury. With maturity falls become less pervasive, and motor vehicle accidents become the most common cause of injury. Finally, in later life (after 70–75 years of age) falls again become responsible for the majority of TBIs.

In the inner city, violence is a critically important cause of injury.[32,39] For the adult aged 20–50 years, it is the most common cause of TBI; however, its incidence declines rapidly on both sides of the 20–50 year age range.

Finally, mortality due to TBI demonstrates a relationship with age.[146] As expected, incidence rate for TBI-related mortality is high in the young adult. However, because of the higher incidence of lethal injuries among the elderly, the highest rate of TBI-related mortality is found in persons older than 75 years.

Cause of Injury

One of the final important epidemiologic points that must be addressed to deal with the important issue of TBI prevention is cause. A thorough review of the data shows that the cause of TBI is almost as varied as the different populations studied.

Table 6 is a representative sampling of the distribution of cause as reported in the literature. In the majority of studies, motor vehicle accidents are the leading cause of TBI (approximately 50% of all injuries). The higher incidence in Gennarelli's work may well result from the pattern of referral to tertiary care trauma centers for severe injuries.

In most studies, vehicular causes, including pedestrian, car, motorcycle, and sometimes bicycle accidents, are grouped together. Because different studies use different means of classification, it is often difficult to divide the subsections; however, a review of the literature shows that 62–78% of vehicular accidents involve automobiles; 8–21% involve motorcycles; and 12–15% involve pedestrians. The information regarding bicycles is unclear. Motorcycles are used much less commonly than automobiles, which accounts for the relatively high ratio of automobile-to-motorcycle injury. Mile for mile, motorcycle usage involves a 15-fold increase in risk of death compared with cars.

After vehicular accidents, falls are the second most common source of injury (roughly 20–30% of all TBIs). The lower incidence in the works of Sosin and Gennarelli can be explained by selection bias. Sosin's work was taken from mortality data, and falls often result in less severe TBIs. In a similar fashion, Gennarelli's work was based on data from a major trauma center and also has a selection bias against less damaging injuries.

Interpersonal violence is normally a distant third as a cause of TBI; however, the data from inner cities show a reversal of trends. In the inner city interpersonal violence may be the number-one cause of injury. The work of Cooper and Whitman clearly points out the different etiologic agents of TBI in the inner cities. Efforts to reduce the incidence of TBI obviously have different target behaviors in different subpopulations.

Sports and recreational injuries are not as common as the above causes but still account for a significant number of injuries (10–20%). Appropriate preventive measures may have a significant impact on these numbers.

TABLE 6.　Distribution of TBI Causes Among Various Studies

Author	Vehicle (%)	Falls (%)	Violence (%)	Recreation (%)	Others (%)
Annegers, 1980[5]	46	29	6	9	9
Cooper, 1983[32]	28	32	34	NR	7
Kraus, 1984[80]	49	21	18	10	4
Whitman, 1984[164]	31	20	40	3	6
	32	21	26	11	10
	39	31	10	14	6
Jagger, 1984[66]	55	20	11	NR	14*
Sosin, 1989[147]	57	12	15	NR	13
Gennarelli, 1989[54]	66	15	19	NR	0
Tiret, 1990[156]	60	33	7	NR	1
Missouri Trauma Registry, 1988[95]	48	29	7	NR	17

ICB = inner city blacks, SB = suburban blacks, SW = suburban whites, NR = not reported.
* Other includes some pedestrian accidents. Other studies include them as vehicle accidents.

Relative Lethality

The final point that needs to be discussed in reference to causes of TBI is the lethality of different types of injuries. The most lethal TBI injury is the gunshot wound. Gennarelli et al.[54] reported that gunshot wounds accounted for 10.5% of all trauma-related deaths but only for 1.6% of patients. In Olmsted County,[5] only 2.6% of TBIs were due to gunshot wounds, which, however, accounted for 20% of fatalities. Data from the Bronx also support the lethality of violence in general and gunshot wounds in particular. Siccardi et al.[140a] published the results of their series of 314 cases of penetrating missile injuries, reporting a mortality rate of 92%, with the majority (264) dying within 3 hours of injury. No other injury has such a high mortality rate.[140a] Sosin has also reported that since 1990 firearms have passed MVAs as the leading cause of TBI-related deaths.[147a]

Vehicular injuries are the second most lethal cause of TBI. They may account for the largest number of fatalities, because of their high incidence. Gennarelli[53] reported that the highest percentage of trauma-related deaths was due to vehicular injury. Other literature also supports the severe morbidity and mortality of the vehicular injury.

Falls, in contrast, show a relatively low morbidity and mortality relative to their incidence.

The issues of incidence by cause and lethality are critical in directing prevention programs. Only with an extensive knowledge of epidemiologic information can effectively targeted prevention programs be created and implemented.

Traumatic Brain Injury and the Military

A review of the TBI-related military literature reveals substantial differences in incidence, causality, lethality, and other epidemiologic features compared with the civilian population. Such differences, of course, are not unexpected because of the nature of the military lifestyle and purpose. During wartime especially, a substantial number of open-head injuries result from gunshots and other projectiles. Levi et al.[84,85] reported that over 60% of the head injuries seen at Rambam Medical Center during the Lebanese hostilities between 1982 and 1985 were of the open variety. Lethality of TBI during military conflict also is much higher than in the civilian population; Levi reported a mortality rate of 19% for closed injury and 26% for open injury. These figures have not changed much since the Vietnam studies 58 years earlier. The improved technology of health care delivery during military conflict has made only minimal improvement in outcome, because the technology of destruction has kept pace.

McCarroll and Gunderson[92] studied the military population from 1983–1987, a time when the army was not involved in military conflict. Even then the differences in epidemiologic information were substantial compared with the civilian population. Not surprisingly, the overall incidence of TBI was higher and the relationship with alcohol use was lower. In addition, the male-to-female ratio was lower than that found in civilian studies. Perhaps the most unexpected finding was the higher rate of TBI in the white population when compared with the black. Such differences may be explained by the removal of numerous other sociologic issues, such as employment and financial status.

Alcohol and Drugs

Although not a direct cause of TBI, the use of both licit and illicit drugs has a significant effect. The association of alcohol and TBI has been well documented. Rimel et al.[123] stated that alcohol was the most significant contributing factor to accidents in Western countries. They further reported that 72% of accident victims had a blood alcohol level > 0.1%. Other studies support the strong correlation between alcohol and TBI. The association with other drugs is not as well documented, but according to Lindenbaum et al.,[87] almost three-fourths of patients in an urban trauma center tested positive for drugs. Clearly prevention efforts must deal with this issue.

PRIMARY PREVENTION

TBI often has been attributed to "accidental causes," with the historical implication that all persons have the same random, unpredictable likelihood of sustaining an injury.[57] The previous epidemiologic discussion refutes this implication by clearly identifying specific predisposing risk factors and a typical profile of individuals most likely to sustain a TBI. The goal of primary prevention is to diminish the causative factors that lead to injury.[154]

The epidemiologic model of injury can be compared with that of disease if one defines an etiologic agent impacting negatively on a host in a specific environment.[7] The scientific analysis of phases of injury and the subsequent interruption of critical components provide the basis for the development of theoretically sound preventive approaches.[57]

Motor Vehicle Accidents

Motor vehicle accidents (MVAs) are the cause of approximately 50% of all TBIs.[5,54,66,80,95,147,156] Factors in the precrash phase determine whether a crash will occur, including driver attributes and deficits (e.g., alcohol or physiologic impairment, inexperience, legal noncompliance), vehicle design and equipment (e.g., brake dysfunction, condition of tires, speed capacity, safety-related mechanical defects), and socioeconomic and environmental factors (e.g., road surface or traffic discontinuities, drunk driving laws).[30]

The crash phase includes the injury itself and factors that determine whether actual injury occurs. Factors that affect the degree of injury include use of restraint systems, physical attributes of occupants, safety modifications to the vehicle, highway safety designs, and mandatory use laws (MULs) for safety belts. The postcrash or tertiary prevention phase involves emergency personnel response time and outcome potential.[30]

Preventive countermeasures have had a dramatic effect on MVA occupant fatalities, which have progressively decreased in the United States from 39,170 in 1988 to 34,293 in 1994.[24,106,106a]

Air Bags

Jagger strongly supported the efficacy of air bags: "Air bags, if provided as standard equipment in front seat positions in all passenger vehicles, have the potential to prevent more brain trauma than any other prevention measure."[65] She estimated that nearly 25% of patients admitted to hospitals with TBI sustained injuries that air bags are specifically designed to protect against.[67] By allowing the occupant's head and brain to decelerate more gradually and by protecting the head from impact, air bags provide some degree of protection in frontal crashes, particularly for high-risk individuals not wearing safety belts.[65] Because air bags inflate early in a frontal crash, do not remain inflated, and provide minimal side protection,[30] there is an estimated 41–43% greater risk of fatality if a lap/shoulder belt system is not used in conjunction with air bags.[42] Air bags are supplemental protection designed for moderate-to-severe frontal crashes. Because air bags will not deploy in all crashes, lap/shoulder belts should be worn at all times.[106]

After more than two decades of public controversy and regulatory complications, the Intermodal Surface Transportation Efficiency Act of 1991 (ISTEA) was passed which requires auto makers to provide lap/shoulder safety belts plus air bags by model year 1997 in passenger cars and by model year 1999 in cars, light trucks and vans. An actual delay of full compliance in all vehicles can be anticipated, however, due to the 10-year vehicle turnover rate.[65]

Safety Belts

The use of lap/shoulder safety belts by front-seat motor vehicle occupants reduces the risk of fatal injury by 45% and of moderate-to-critical injury by 50%. When lap/shoulder belts are used in conjunction with air bags, risk is reduced by 55–60%.[106,110]

During the crash phase, a proper fitting lap/shoulder belt allows the body to decelerate at a slower speed and distributes the energy force more diffusely, thus lessening the severity and probability of a diffuse axonal injury. Safety belts also reduce the likelihood of the head striking a hard surface inside the vehicle as well as the possibility of ejection from the vehicle.[30]

The 1987–1988 Iowa Safety Restraint Assessment (ISRA) study noted a threefold increase in the risk of hospitalization and a hospital stay 2.6 times longer in unbelted persons, who also had an 8.4 times greater likelihood of sustaining TBI with loss of consciousness. The risk of TBI was increased both at low-impact speeds of less than 30 mph (7.8% vs. 1.1%) and at high-impact speeds of over 30 mph (20.3% vs. 2.5%). In addition, average AIS scores for head injuries were higher in unbelted persons (2.6 vs. 1.6).[22] The ISRA study also found an increased incidence of fractures and lacerations in unbelted persons, with more severe AIS scores in all anatomic regions.[22]

In comparing ISS and AIS scores for restrained versus unrestrained crash victims, Breath et al.[14] found an increased frequency and severity of head, neck, chest, extremity, and skin injuries in unrestrained persons. Mean ISS scores of unrestrained victims were 8.28 vs. 4.44 for restrained victims; in addition, 20% of unrestrained victims had ISS scores > 15 compared with 7% of restrained victims. Particularly noteworthy was a 64% reduction in mean hospital charges for restrained vs. unrestrained patients. This finding becomes controversial from a societal standpoint, because unrestrained patients were more than twice as likely to receive Medicaid as restrained patients.[14]

Belted persons in the ISRA study demonstrated an increased incidence of strains and sprains; however, such relatively minor injuries may have been underreported by unbelted persons because of the serious injuries that many of them sustained.[22] In the study by Breath et al.[14] an increased number of minor abdominal wall injuries occurred in belted persons. As in the ISRA study, these injuries are certainly minor compared with the catastrophic injuries previously described.

From 1975–1984, only 10–18% of drivers wore safety belts.[103] Public awareness and educational campaigns and economic, insurance, and employer-sponsored incentives were only minimally effective at increasing compliance; consequently, a series of legislative actions was initiated, beginning with the implementation of the first mandatory use law in 1984.[30] As of December 1994, 47 states and the District of Columbia have passed such laws, and safety-belt compliance in these jurisdictions is nearly twice as high as in states without laws.[61,106]

From 1980–1994, safety belt use in the United States increased from 11% to 67%.[106,109] From 1982–1994, an estimated 65,290 lives were saved by safety belts and 1.5 million moderate-to-critical injuries prevented.[106] Even with safety belt use laws, however, compliance typically increases initially but over time decreases and finally stabilizes at 40–50%.[103] When New York became the first state to enforce mandatory use laws in 1984, belt use increased immediately from 16% to 57% but declined to 46% within 9 months.[131]

The initial and ongoing enforcement of mandatory use laws, combined with public education, has been demonstrated to be critically important if the laws are to remain efficacious. Pilot programs in the North Carolina safety belt initiative, the first multiyear enforcement and publicity program in the United States, demonstrated an increase in belt use by 10–38 percentage points.[62]

Injury prevention is further supported by Section 153 of the previously discussed ISTEA law, which includes a federal financial incentive program to encourage states to pass safety belt and motorcycle helmet laws and to enforce compliance. Conversely, if states fail to enact safety belt and motorcycle helmet laws by October 1, 1993, 1.5% of their funding for federal highway programs must be transferred to highway safety programs.

The transfer penalty increases to 3% by October 1, 1994.[110]

The National Highway Traffic Safety Administration (NHTSA) has been instrumental in the establishment and ongoing management of prevention programs. From inception of NHTSA in 1966 to 1990, an estimated 243,000 lives have been saved, largely because of the success of the agency's programs. For 1997 NHTSA has established the goal of increasing safety belt use from 66% to 75%, with an anticipated saving of an additional 1,700 lives per year at an economic cost estimated at $3.6 billion a year.[109]

Speed Limit

In 1984, in response to the oil crisis, Congress enacted a 55-mph speed limit, which has been credited with saving 2,000-4,000 lives per year and reducing serious or critical injuries by 2,500-4,500 annually.[104] Federal legislation in 1987, however, allowed states to increase speed limits on rural interstate highways to 65 mph.[50]

New Mexico, the first state to adopt the 65-mph speed limit on rural interstate highways, demonstrated that after 1 year (1987–1988), with all non–speed-related variables controlled, fatal crashes increased from the predicted rate of 1.5 to 2.9 per 100 million vehicle miles traveled.[50] In 1990 the Insurance Institute for Highway Safety reported a 32% increase in death rates on U.S. rural interstate highways with 65-mph speed limits.[65]

Reinstatement and enforcement of the 55-mph speed limit are critically important preventive interventions. Of interest, a Gallup poll conducted in Great Britain reported 69% of respondents favored the use of speed-limiting devices in cars.[63]

Teenage Drivers

It is critically important that preventive interventions be aimed at altering the high-risk driving behaviors of teenagers, the group with the highest rates of MVA fatalities. Teenagers (15–19 years) have an MVA fatality rate 10 times that of children under the age of 10 years,[1] and 62% of teenage passengers who die in MVAs were occupants of cars driven by other teenagers.[46,72,167] Overall, 23% of all passenger fatalities occur when a teenager is driving.[46]

Prevention strategies must target reducing the number of high-risk teenage drivers. Raising universal licensure to age 17 years, for example, could result in an estimated 65–85% reduction in MVA fatalities among 16-year-olds[167a] as well as decreased public exposure to this high-risk group.

In a four-state study, implementation of curfew laws restricting nighttime driving reduced the rate of nighttime crashes.[118] Surprisingly, studies also have confirmed that elimination of driver education classes results in licensing of fewer 16-and 17-year-olds, with a subsequent decrease in the per-capita rate of MVAs.[128,129] (The impact of alcohol and other drugs is discussed in the alcohol section of this chapter.)

Prevention Countermeasures

The numerous preventive strategies focusing on vehicle design and environmental countermeasures (e.g., antilock brakes, head rests, structural and interior features, energy-attenuating design and construction, improved curve delineation, breakaway signs, edgelines, wrong-way signs), while certainly beneficial, are beyond the scope of this chapter. The interested reader is referred to *Injury Control* by Waller,[159] NHTSA, and the Federal Highway Administration.

Correct use of prevention countermeasures is imperative, because improper use of devices meant to protect lives can contribute to increased risk of injury and, in some instances, even death. In vehicles with passenger air bags, for example, rear-facing seats for children must be placed in the back seat, because an inflating air bag can severely injure a child.[60] An unrestrained child standing in the passenger side footwell also can be severely injured by an inflating bag.[158]

Integral headrests have proved highly effective in reducing injuries (31.6%) when used correctly, with the center of the headrest even with the user's ear.[150] Incorrect use of adjustable headrests, however, has resulted in neck injuries.[60]

Pedestrian Injury

Gennarelli et al.[53] reported that of all persons injured in MVAs, pedestrians were most likely to sustain a head injury. Pedestrian injuries are most prevalent in persons over the age of 70 years and in young children, particularly from ages 5–9 years.[159] (Pediatric TBI is discussed more extensively in the pediatric section of this chapter.)

Pedestrian behavior significantly contributes to susceptibility to injury, as demonstrated by findings that in 75% of fatalities in 1992 the pedestrian was "improperly crossing the roadway or intersection (40%) and walking, playing, working, or standing in the roadway (30%)." The use of alcohol by either the driver or the pedestrian was reported in nearly one-half of MVA/pedestrian fatalities.[108]

Preventive countermeasures include public education, selective conversion of two-way to one-way streets, effective lighting, sidewalks and roadway barriers, pedestrian crossing signs, rescinding of right-on-red laws, and use of reflective materials and devices for nighttime activities. Flashlights or bicyclist leg lamps have been shown to be more effective devices for enhancing conspicuity than retroreflective disks, head- and wristbands, belts, anklebands, and fluorescent vests.[158]

Motorcycle Injury

In the United States from 1979–1986, 15,194 motorcycle deaths were associated with head injury.[146] Precrash factors in motorcycle accidents include failure of another motor vehicle driver to either see or perceive the motorcycle, inexperience of the operator, and operator error. Operator error was a contributing factor in 76% of fatal crashes in 1994, with excessive speed being the contributing factor most often noted. Operators in fatal crashes in 1994 had higher blood alcohol concentrations (0.1 g/dl or more) than any other motor vehicle drivers, and 22% did not even have a valid license. In addition, 43% of fatally injured operators did not wear a helmet.[106a,106b] The size and instability of motorcycles as well as their susceptibility to environmental hazards also contribute to the probability of injury, because the rider is often catapulted over the machine or dragged along the ground.[159] Motorcycle riders in fatal crashes have a five-to sixfold higher risk of TBI than persons in other fatal MVAs.[146]

Well-designed, appropriately worn helmets can reduce the severity of TBI by absorption of energy and distribution of impact. Riders without helmets sustain a 2–3 times greater rate of TBI injury and a 3–9 times greater rate of fatal TBI than helmeted riders.[161,162] Ofner et al.[112] reported that helmet use reduced the risk of TBI by 41% and acute care costs by 40%.

Findings in the literature confirm that legislative initiatives increase helmet use. A 1966 law that withheld federal funds for highway construction from states without compulsory motorcycle helmet laws resulted in the implementation of such laws in 47 states by 1975.[125] The use of helmets subsequently increased from 40–50% to almost 100%, and mortality rates dropped by about 30%.[102,112,161] In 1976, in reaction to strong pressure from motorcyclist groups, helmet laws in 26 states were either repealed or modified, and fatalities increased by a corresponding 44%.[112,125]

A 1988 study in Illinois of the efficacy of helmet use reported that nonhelmeted patients had higher injury severity scores (11.9 vs. 7.02), an increased incidence of head and neck injuries (41.7% vs. 24.1%), and lower Glasgow Coma Scores (13.73 vs. 14.51). Twenty-five of the 26 fatalities were nonhelmeted patients. The study not only demonstrated a reduction in overall incidence and severity of TBI with helmet use, but also cited a 23% increase in health care costs for non-helmeted patients. The study concluded that helmet use may reduce the overall incidence and severity of TBI from motorcycle crashes.[76]

Helmet laws are often regarded as an abridgement of civil liberties and personal freedom, but the question that must be answered is who pays for the cost of care? In 1985 2,714 fatalities occurred in states without helmet laws. In 1989 Rice et al.[120] predicted that if helmet laws produced even a 24% reduction in death and injuries, an estimated 651 fewer deaths and 1,953 fewer TBIs would have occurred, with an estimated cost reduction of $393 million dollars in human capital terms or $1.5 billion by willingness-to-pay estimates. The impact on society becomes even more apparent if one considers the Seattle study by Rivera et al.,[125] which noted that 63.4% of costs were paid by public funds.

A giant step toward injury prevention is anticipated as a result of the previously mentioned ISTEA Act of 1991, which mandates motorcycle helmet laws. California, the state in which one-fifth of all motorcycles are registered, reported an increase in helmet use from under 50% to greater than 99% throughout 1992.[81b] Fatalities decreased by 37.5% and head injuries decreased significantly among fatally and nonfatally injured cyclists.[81a]

Head Injuries to Adult Bicyclists

Sacks et al.[136] reported an estimated 2,985 TBI deaths and 905,752 bicycle-associated head injuries in the United States from 1984–1988. In fact, fatalities secondary to TBI were responsible for 62% of all bicycle-related deaths and 32% of bicycle-related injuries treated at one emergency department.

The proportion of 25–64 year-old pedal-cyclist fatalities increased twofold from 21% to 41% in the past 10 years. In 1994 the average age of bicyclist fatalities rose to 28.8 years.[107] In his analysis of fatality risk patterns, Rodgers adjusted fatality rates by including estimates of riding exposure and found a high relative risk for males, for bicyclists over 44, and for bicyclists who ride after dark. Relative risk tended to increase with age secondary to cognitive, visual, and perceptual deterioration, delayed reaction time, alcohol intake, and adverse medical outcomes.[16a]

Helmet use for bicyclists of all ages is the most critical preventive countermeasure in reducing bicycle-related TBI morbidity, mortality, and economic costs. Bicycle helmets reduce the incidence of TBI by 74–85%.[155] Sacks et al. predicted that from 1984–1988 as many as 2,500 deaths and 757,000 TBIs (1 death per day and a head injury every 4 minutes) may have been prevented by universal helmet use.[136] Concussion, the injury that is most responsive to the protective benefits of helmet use, is found in 11–14% of bicycle injuries across all age groups.[11] It is a sad commentary that, despite the known efficacy of helmet usage, only approximately 10% of bicyclists wear helmets all or most of the time.[129a]

Mandatory helmet laws combined with education, mass media publicity, and enforcement have proved efficacious in increasing compliance rates among bicyclists. In Victoria, Australia, a 10-year comprehensive prevention campaign preceded the enactment and subsequent enforcement of a statewide law passed on July 1, 1990, mandating helmet use by all bicyclists. Compliance increased from 31% to 75% among all age groups (teenage rates were lowest), with a corresponding decrease of 51% in TBI fatalities and hospital admissions.[27]

Gunshot Wounds

In 1990, firearm-related injuries surpassed MVAs as the leading cause of death from injuries in both Louisiana and Texas.[25] Gunshot wounds to the head are extremely lethal, with an estimated mortality rate of 75–80%.[73] The total cost of gunshot wounds in 1988 was estimated at $16.2 billion per year, with most victims being uninsured.[73] In a 1984 study in San Francisco, taxpayers paid 86% of the hospital costs incurred by victims of gunshot wounds.[36]

Of the over 250 million guns in the United States, 60–70 million are handguns and 1–3 million are assault weapons.[37,73] A 1991 national Gallup survey revealed that guns are present in almost one-half of households and that handguns are present in approximately one-fourth of households. Over 50% of the handgun owners reported that the guns were loaded.[51] According to Patterson and Smith,[115] 10% of the gun owners in their study reported that guns were "loaded, unlocked and within reach of children."[115]

In 1991 the Centers for Disease Control and Prevention reported 38,317 firearm deaths in the United States. Of these deaths, 18,526 were suicides, 17,746 were homicides, 1,441 were accidents, and 604 were attributed to unknown reasons. According to the Uniform Crime Report of the Federal Bureau of Investigation (FBI), in 1992 handguns were used in 12,489 of the 22,540 reported homicides. In 1983 Kaufman reported that in Houston, gunshot wounds to the head occurred in 46% of homicides and 50% of suicides.[73]

The FBI Uniform Crime Report also indicated that for children under the age of 18 years, homicide by firearms rose 143% from 602 in 1986 to 1,468 in 1992. Adult homicide by firearms rose 30% during the same period. Firearms are the second leading cause of death for children 10–19 years of age. Among young black males (10–19 years of age) firearms are the leading cause of death.

A study conducted in Seattle reported that 34% of public high school students have access to handguns and 6.4% own guns. Of even greater concern is the finding that one-third of high school gun owners had fired at someone.[19]

Despite these staggering statistics, the national debate about how to most effectively reduce firearm injuries and deaths continues to rage, with gun violence having clearly become a public health emergency. Whether or not accessibility to firearms precipitates violent behavior will be the subject of debate for years to come. One unarguable fact remains, however. The use of firearms significantly increases the probability of serious injury and/or death.

Opponents of gun control attempt to refute research and maintain that the Second Amendment guarantees the right of every American "to bear arms." The strength of their commitment, as reported by the Federal Election Commission, is evidenced by the $3,015,659 spent for gun lobbying. It is interesting to note that anti-gun lobbying totaled only $287,185.

Opponents of gun control argue that guns are necessary in the home to protect the safety of the family. The validity of this argument is highly questionable. Studies clearly demonstrate that guns purchased for self-protection are more likely to be involved in suicide, homicide, and domestic violence than as a mean of self-protection.[15,16,36,74,151]

Brent et al.,[16] for example, confirmed that availability of guns in the home increases the risk of adolescent suicide. Saltzman et al.[137] confirmed that the availability of guns increases twelvefold the rate of death from violent domestic arguments. According to the FBI Uniform Crime Reports, of the 15,377 firearm-related homicides in 1992, only 308 were considered justifiable for reasons of self-defense. Kellerman and Reay[74] reported that suicides, homicides, and accidental deaths were 40 times more likely than deaths for reasons of self-defense.

From 1982–1988, 3,607 youth under the age of 19 years died in unintentional firearm-related injuries. Children are particularly at risk because of their impulsivity, curiosity, thrill-seeking behaviors, and feelings of immortality.[26] In a North Carolina study, 16% of unintentional fatal incidents involved children playing with guns.[97]

Gun violence has created a social, political, and medical crisis. It is a national disgrace that in 1990 10,567 handgun fatalities occurred in the United States compared with

22 in Great Britain, 68 in Canada, and 87 in Japan.[47] As a nation we must support interventions that not only decrease but also prevent firearm-related deaths and injuries.

A public health approach as previously described would facilitate the collection of objective, reliable, epidemiologic information. Once the magnitude of the problem is clearly defined and the risk of injury has been accurately quantified, interventions can be developed, implemented, and evaluated. The development of a Firearm Fatality Reporting System similar to NHTSA's Fatal Accident Reporting System would facilitate a systematic, uniform collection of data from which informed decisions could be made.[5a,153]

Certainly one point on which both sides of the gun control issue agree is the importance of educational programs that focus on gun safety and the necessity of safe gun storage. The CDC's National Center for Injury Prevention and Control and the Department of Health and Human Services are mandating the development of interventions to reduce the health consequences of violence.[73] A 20% reduction in the proportion of households with inappropriately stored weapons is targeted as a national health objective of the Department of Health and Human Services for the year 2000.

The right to own a firearm should incur specific responsibilities, such as the knowledge and skill required for safe use and storage. The issue of liability insurance is now under debate as a way to demand responsibility from gun owners and to recover damages for victims. Twelve states currently have parental responsibility laws that hold parents liable if a child is injured by the firearm.[117]

Certainly the most controversial intervention is restrictive and permissive licensing. Gun control opponents argue that because criminals obtain guns illegally, gun control laws will affect only honest citizens who are trying to protect themselves. One nationwide survey of state prison inmates, however, found that criminals get guns from retail outlets (27%), on the streets (28%), from family and friends (31%), by theft (9%), and from other sources.[1a] Although the illegal obtaining of firearms cannot be eliminated totally, closing off the legal market entirely, except for individuals who can demonstrate a legitimate need, eventually would decrease the number of available guns.

The efficacy of a restrictive gun control law was demonstrated in a study contrasting Seattle and Vancouver. Despite comparable rates of law enforcement, demographic profiles, and criminal activities, the rate of handgun homicides was five times higher and the rate of handgun suicide among young adults six times higher in Seattle than in Vancouver. The purchase of guns was minimally restricted in Seattle, whereas in Vancouver a restrictive licensing policy required special permits to own a gun.[143,144]

Loftin et al.[88] reported an abrupt decline of nearly 25% in firearm homicides and suicides after a 1976 District of Columbia law restricted the purchase, sale, transfer, and possession of handguns by civilians unless the guns were previously owned and registered.

Restrictive licensing must be considered to prohibit the manufacture, importation, and sale of handguns except in special circumstances. Individuals applying for licenses should be subjected to a mandatory criminal record check, a mandatory waiting period, and a certification of competence. In addition, possession should be prohibited without clearly demonstrated need, such as law enforcement or security.[139,158]

Other preventive measures related to gun design need to be considered, including gun safety modifications, such as load indicators and safety catches to prevent accidental shooting; limitations of bullet velocity; restrictions in caliber; and increases in the amount of trigger pressure needed for discharge. At the same time, weapon detectors must become more prevalent to eliminate firearms from high-risk areas such as amusement parks, schools, and bars.[36,158]

In the political arena the February 1994 passage of the Brady Bill, with its 5-day waiting period for handgun purchases, background checks, and $200 licensing fee, has prohibited the sale of handguns to up to 45,000 convicted felons. In addition, the number of federally licensed dealers has dropped from 284,000 to 224,000.[18a] In the "crime bill" currently under negotiation, proposals include funding for 100,000 new police, a ban on designated assault weapons, and life imprisonment for three-time violent and drug felons.[160] Commitment and coordination at the national, state, and local level are imperative if a comprehensive approach is to be successful in decreasing the epidemic of gun violence.

Falls

Falls, the second leading cause of TBI, account for 20%–30% of injuries across all populations; the greatest number occur in children under 5 years of age and in the elderly over age 75 years.[5,32,48,66,79,80,95] More than half of all fatal falls involve persons over 75.[8] (See the pediatric section for a discussion of falls in children.)

Factors in the preinjury phase include alcohol use, health problems, and age. Health problems, particularly dizzy spells, visuo-perceptual disorders, postural instability, confusion, orthostatic hypotension, and systemic impairments, contribute to 34% of falls in the elderly.[159]

The National Bureau of Standards reported that 18–50% of falls in homes are due to environmental factors, including highly polished or wet and slippery floors; patterned stairs and falls; uneven risers; broken, unavailable, or short banisters; unsafe placement of light switches; sharp edges on furniture; inappropriate bed heights; inappropriately bright or inadequate lighting; slippery tubs and showers; and edges of rugs. Pets can be a hazard if they tangle themselves around their owner's legs.[158,159]

Public education about the need for inspection and correction of environmental hazards as well as installation of residential safety equipment (e.g., grab bars in tubs or nonskid showers) is critically important. Teaching by the medical community about ways to minimize the physiologic changes of aging, including the benefits of exercise to increase muscle tone and balance, the role of fluoride, calcium and vitamin D supplements as well as hormonal replacement, and the effect of medication in increasing the predisposition toward falls in the elderly, are critical elements of a preventive approach.[158]

Alcohol and Drug Abuse in Traumatic Brain Injury

In head injury programs throughout the United States, approximately 55% of patients had premorbid problems with substance abuse. The NHIF Substance Abuse Task Force reported that "neither age, nor occupation, nor any other factors place an individual at a greater risk of a TBI than does alcohol."[111] Alcohol use is a predisposing factor in 35–72% of all TBIs, with blood alcohol concentrations being highest in MVAs (66%), followed by assaults (60%), falls (44%), firearms (35%), and other causes (42%).[81c,123,148] The role of drugs (prescribed, over-the-counter, or illicit) in relation to TBI has been much less firmly established.

The first step in any prevention program is identification of the problem. Despite the etiologic role of alcohol in MVAs, only 55.2% of surveyed trauma centers across the country routinely obtained blood alcohol levels.[145]

Lindenbaum et al.[87] studied patterns of alcohol and drug abuse in a random sample of patients admitted to an urban trauma center and reported that 74.5% of all tested patients were positive for illicit or prescription drugs. Cocaine (54.4%) and cannabinoids (37.2%) were found even more frequently than alcohol (35.5%). Illicit drugs were found in 80.3% of cases related to violent crime. The study by Sloan et al.[142] of toxicology screening in urban trauma patients similarly revealed positive toxicology screens in 86%. Further research is needed to determine specifically the etiologic role of drug use in TBI as well as the effect of substance abuse in complicating diagnosis and potentiating the severity of the injury.

Nearly one-half of all TBIs result from MVAs. The impact of alcohol on MVAs is particularly noteworthy; studies in the past decade demonstrated that 54–86% of patients had positive blood alcohol concentrations (BACs).[39,41,111,123,148]

Preventive programs, however, have significantly affected alcohol-related traffic fatalities, which reached the lowest point in a decade in 1994 when the total number of reported deaths was 16,589—a 30% decrease since 1984. Alcohol-related MVAs decreased from 57% of the total MVA fatalities in 1982 to 40.8% in 1994,[24,107a] with intoxication rates decreasing most dramatically in drivers 65 and older (38% decline) and 16–20 years of age (47% decline).

A major contributing factor to fatal MVAs among adolescents is alcohol use. According to the Fatal Accident Reporting System, 48.7% (1990) and 46.8% (1991) of 15- to 20-year-old victims of fatal MVAs had elevated blood alcohol levels.[24]

Mothers Against Drunk Driving (MADD) has been instrumental in leading a nationwide effort to reduce drunk driving deaths. All 50 states and the District of Columbia now have raised the legal drinking age to 21 years, a major victory for MADD, which led the crusade to change state drinking age laws. MADD is also soliciting legislative support for lowering the legal threshold for intoxication to a BAC of 0.08% for adult drivers and 0.00% for drivers under 21 years of age, with administrative revocation of license for any any driver with a BAC exceeding legal levels. MADD reported that during a 1-year period in California in which the BAC limit was reduced from 0.10% to 0.08% with corresponding license revocation, alcohol-related traffic fatalities were reduced by 12%.[24,158]

Additional preventive interventions include strict enforcement of minimum drinking age laws, mandatory sentencing, license suspension, compulsory BAC testing in MVAs, sobriety checkpoints, dram shop laws, educational programs, and DWI enforcement program costs paid by DWI offenders.[24,158]

Sports-Related Traumatic Brain Injuries

Epidemiologic data on sports-related injuries are inadequate because of the diversity of activities as well as the lack of scientific, objective reporting of information by individuals involved in recreational activities. In competitive organized sports, overall injury rates are typically underestimated.[158] According to the NHIF, sports and recreational activities account for 10% of TBIs; boxing, football, and other higher-risk contact sports lead to serious injury with the greatest frequency.

TBI occurs in only 5% of all football injuries[12] but accounts for approximately 70% of all football fatalities; 75% of fatal TBIs occur during tackling.[98] Football also has the highest rate of concussive injuries of all contact sports.[134] A dramatic decrease in TBIs was noted from 1975 through 1984 after significant rule changes were enforced. For example, the 1976 rule prohibiting head butting and face tackling and the 1978 helmet standard implemented by the National Operating Committee on Standards for Athletic Equipment (NOCSAE) had a major effect on reducing TBI fatalities.[99]

Other preventive countermeasures include improved helmet fit and construction,[135] emphasis by coaches on tackling techniques,[40] comprehensive preseason medical examinations,[83] educational programs aimed at injury prevention, and physician evaluation immediately after every head injury, with specific return-to-play criteria and medical follow-up.[83,134,135] Physician follow-up is critically important, because a history of previous TBI correlates with increased morbidity and mortality if a second injury occurs.[138]

Boxing

Boxing deserves particular mention, because no other sport involves the deliberate delivery of multiple blows to the head with the intention of injuring the opponent by rendering him unconscious.[96] The study by Atha et al.[6] concluded that the impact delivered by a top-ranked heavyweight boxer is equal to that of a "13-pound wooden mallet swung at 20 miles per hour."

Since 1928, when Martland first identified the punch-drunk syndrome, various studies have identified numerous neuroanatomic changes (e.g., fenestrated cavum septi pellucidi,[91] neurofibrillary tangles without senile plaques[33]) that are pathognomonic for injuries sustained in boxers.

The medical community has recommended unequivocally the abolition of boxing through legislation. Controversy continues, however. Supporters of boxing argue for freedom of choice and applaud the positive physical conditioning and personal development that boxing encourages, particularly among poor and minority youths.[96]

Various recommendations have been made to decrease the risk of injury, including increasing ring safety and equipment, establishing a federal regulatory body, shortening professional bouts, disqualifying blows to the head, and mandating intensive medical screening.[96] The medical community, at a minimum, must advocate appropriate safety measures accompanied by strict medical supervision until the ultimate goal of a legislative ban can be achieved.

Pediatric Traumatic Brain Injury

Each year an estimated 1 million children sustain TBIs.[41a] Falls are a leading cause of pediatric TBI, a trend even more pronounced in the extremely young.[82] The actual frequency of falls and the location and circumstances of their occurrence are often age-related. Children under the age of 3 years more commonly fall in the home, whereas older children typically fall outdoors.[64] Pediatric falls from heights account for the most serious TBIs and the largest number of fall-related deaths in children.[9] Nonwhite children less than 5 years old have one of the highest national death rates from falls.[100]

Preventive interventions include enforcement of public building codes that require design changes for domestic and child safety. A 96% decrease in falls from windows was noted after the implementation of the "Children Can't Fly" program in New York City. Window guards are required by law in apartments with children 10 years of age or younger.[149]

As one would expect, frequent injuries occur on stairways. One study demonstrated that 30% of homes with young children did not have toddler gates.[51a] This statistic is even more disturbing if one considers the widespread (55–86%) use of baby walkers.[121] The American Academy of Pediatrics has recommended that safety gates be firmly attached and equipped with double closures that children cannot open. Toddler gates with accordion tops have been associated with strangulation and should not be used. Considering the high risk of injury vs. the almost negligible benefit of baby walkers, the American Academy of Pediatrics recommends parent counseling by pediatricians,[3] and many health care providers recommend that baby walkers be banned.[91a,126]

MVAs are the cause of approximately 32–37% of all TBIs in children.[82] The fallacy that an infant can be held safely on an adult's lap was demonstrated by a study that examined the impact of a 30-mph crash on a 10-pound infant. To hold on to the infant, an adult wearing a seat belt would need the strength required for lifting 300 pounds one foot off the ground.[127]

From 1982–1994 child safety booster seats saved the lives of an estimated 2,655 children.

The correct use of safety seats reduced fatality risk by an estimated 69% for infants and 47% for toddlers. In the United States from 1982–1990 use of child safety seats for infants increased from 60% to 83% and for toddlers from 38% to 84%.[23] Even with this increased utilization, 682 children under 5 years of age died in MVAs in 1994, 55% of whom were not restrained.[23,106a]

By 1985 all 50 states and the District of Columbia had passed laws mandating the use of safety seats, most of which cover children up to the age of 4 years. However, the restrictiveness of the regulation varies by state.[105] The immediate benefit of child restraint laws is typically a 9% reduction in fatalities.[114]

Hospital-based child safety seat loaner programs have proved efficacious in achieving a 90% correct safety use rate for mothers being discharged with their infants. Even 12 months later an 80% correct use rate was maintained.[30a] The importance of public education, particularly by physicians, must be emphasized since studies report a sustained increase in restraint use upon physician recommendation as opposed to a less successful patient compliance response to nonphysician health educators.[118a] Further research into the development of child safety seats that ensure the safety of low-birthweight infants and children with disabilities should also be prioritized.[18]

As many as two-thirds of MVA-related TBIs occur when the child is a pedestrian.[64] Children ages 5–9 years are most at risk for impulsively running into traffic,[157] whereas children under 5 years of age are more likely to be injured in their own driveways as parents back out the car.[17] Children from low-income families are at particularly high risk for pedestrian injuries because of the unavailability of safe play areas.[124] Preventive measures include simulation and model-training educational programs at school and in the home,[119] installation of sidewalks, construction of safe play areas, police enforcement of traffic laws that protect pedestrians, and mass media public education campaigns.[158]

Bicycle—Child

In 1993, 310 child bicyclists between the ages of 0 and 15 were killed in traffic/bicycle crashes.[107b] Although helmets reduce the chance of head injury by 74–85%,[155] it is estimated that only 2–15% of children actually wear helmets.[129b,163]

Helmet programs that combine community campaigns and helmet legislation have proved most efficacious in increasing helmet-use rates. In Victoria, Australia a community campaign increased the helmet-use rate from 6% to 36%. Upon introduction of a statewide law requiring that all bicyclists wear an approved safety helmet, compliance increased from 36% to 73% and hospitalizations for bicycle-related head injuries decreased by 37%.[158a]

In Howard County, Maryland, helmet compliance increased from 4% to 47% after the enactment of the nation's first helmet use law for bicyclists under the age of 16 years.[34] The Seattle children's helmet campaign increased compliance from 5% in 1987 to 60% in 1993. Bicycle-related head injuries decreased approximately 67% among children 5–14 years old of age who were members of a health maintenance organization.[126a,130]

A cost-effective analysis of a bicycle helmet subsidy program was conducted at an HMO in Washington state in conjunction with the Seattle campaign. Thompson reported that $5–$10 helmet subsidies to achieve a cost of $14 to $20 per helmet would be cost effective in 5–9 year olds if 40–50% use rates are achieved.[155a]

Regulatory action and enforcement are the most effective means of ensuring that bicyclists wear helmets. As of September 1994, nine states and 19 counties and cities have age-specific helmet laws. In addition, the Child Safety Protection Act of 1994 required the Consumer Product Safety Commission to develop a mandatory helmet standard and authorized NHTSA to make discretionary grants for programs requiring children under the age of 16 to wear helmets. ISTEA requires states to establish and fund a Bicycle and Pedestrian Coordinator position to facilitate the use of nonmotorized modes of transportation and to develop facilities to promote public education and safety programs.[107b]

Child Abuse

The NHIF reports that nearly 1.6 million children experience some form of abuse or neglect; 89% of children suffering physical abuse are under 4 years of age. Of physically abused children, 50%–60% sustain head and neck injuries. Diagnostically, it is difficult to ascertain the actual prevalence rate of abuse-related TBI. McClelland and Heiple suggested that nearly one-half of head injuries in children under 6 years of age may be caused by abuse.[93] Billmire and Myer reported that 64% of all infant admissions to their hospital for TBI were secondary to child abuse.[10]

The most common TBIs secondary to child abuse involve skull fractures and concussions. Such injuries occur when children are struck in the head with fists or blunt objects, have their heads banged against a wall or floor, or strike their heads during a fall.[52] In a study of 24 children with acute head trauma from child abuse, Sinal and Ball[141] reported that 70% were victims of whiplash shaken infant syndrome (WSIS), 12% died, and 50% suffered serious neurologic consequences.

According to Alexander et al.,[2] "shaking in and of itself" has been found to be sufficient to cause severe or fatal TBI. Merten and Osborne[94] describe such injury as secondary to repeated acceleration and deceleration. Brain parenchyma undergoes shearing, and bridging veins between the cortex and venous sinuses rupture. In a two-decade review of fatal child abuse, Showers et al.[140] reported that severe shaking was the cause of 13% of deaths.

Early identification of abused children is critical. The study by Sinal et al.[141] confirmed the efficacy of serial CT scans, combined with clinical findings, to support a reliable diagnosis of WSIS. From a preventive standpoint, an accurate diagnosis is critical, because it allows the physician to provide accurate, objective, reliable testimony, which can facilitate appropriate decisions in regard to placement disposition and interventions with parents.[141]

PREVENTION STRATEGIES

According to the Interagency Head Injury Task Force Report, "Every fifteen seconds someone receives a head injury in the United States; every five minutes, one of those people will die and another will become permanently disabled."[38] The Think First prevention program (formerly the National Head and Spinal Cord Injury Prevention Program) is coordinated with "Healthy People 2000," a national program with the objective of reducing hospitalizations for nonfatal head injuries from the current rate of 124/100,000 persons to 106/100,000 persons.[43]

The Think First program targets teenagers primarily through the public school systems and focuses on increasing awareness of the types and causes of TBI and spinal cord injury, the consequences of risk-taking behaviors, the influence of peer pressure, and action strategies to avoid risks. Supplementing the educational programs are community awareness programs, media support of preventive education, advocacy for state and federal initiatives for prevention and research efforts, and establishment of a national TBI registry.[43]

Since 1986 more than 3.3 million students in 47 states, the District of Columbia, Canada, Brazil, Mexico, and Chile have received the program. Long-term modification of risk-taking behaviors has been demonstrated. A multifaceted elementary curriculum, "Think First for Kids," has also been developed and will be presented to 100,000 elementary students for the 1995–96 school year.[154a]

The 1989 Interagency Head Injury Task Force recommended that prevention efforts be coordinated by a federal agency in cooperation with state and private sector programs. Emphasis was placed on advocacy of passive restraints and helmets, behavioral intervention strategies, and research into the technologic and biomechanic aspects of injury prevention.[38]

At a national level, the 1989 Interagency Head Injury Task Force also recommended the establishment of TBI as a reportable condition or disability in federal, state, and local systems. Such specific epidemiologic information can be used to identify high-risk groups, to facilitate health care planning, and to determine the societal impact and cost-effectiveness of prevention programs.[59,89,116]

Some states had statewide registries for TBI with legislative mandates for reporting; however, standardized definitions, inclusion criteria, definitions of severity of injury, case-finding codes (ICD-9), and reporting requirements were inconsistent.[38]

In response to the recommendations of the Federal Interagency Head Injury Task Force Report, the CDC was designated to be the lead federal agency for planning and coordinating central nervous system injury prevention programs. In order to design and implement effective prevention programs, it was necessary first to clearly define TBI and then to develop uniform injury surveillance standards that would ensure the systematic collection, analysis, and interpretation of data that can be compared across time and between jurisdictions. The 1995 release of Guidelines for Surveillance of Central Nervous System Injury defines TBI and specifies core variables that are considered to be the minimum data set necessary to describe the incidence, demographics, nature, and cause of injury. Once accurate, reliable data are obtained, public health needs can be identified, priorities established for prevention programs, and interventions objectively evaluated.[155b]

In the political arena, several bills (Traumatic Brain Injury Act of 1993 [S725] and Brain Injury Rehabilitation Quality Act of 1993 [S1098]), were proposed over the past few years which would have directly supported TBI prevention efforts. Unfortunately, they were not successfully acted upon. As of September 1995, the Traumatic Brain Injury Act still sits in committee on the House side. In the Senate, [S555], which contains the TBI act, still waits to see action on the full Senate floor. Other bills pertinent to TBI include [S96] and [HR248], which would provide for the conduction of expanded studies and the establishment of innovative TBI programs. [HR1539] would provide a minimum level of funding for bicycle transportation facilities and pedestrian walkways.

A particularly disturbing trend is the introduction of several bills that seek to reverse previous gains made in TBI prevention. The States Rights Empowerment Act of 1995 [HR607] proposes the elimination of penalties for noncompliance by states with requirement relating to the use of safety belts, motorcycle helmets, the national maximum speed limit, and the national minimum drinking age. Bills [S234], [HR899], and [S388] also support these ideas.

Rehabilitation, the process aimed at minimizing complications and maximizing functional recovery, is the topic of the remainder of this text. The catastrophic problems associated with the medical rehabilitation of TBI have no simple solutions. Perhaps the greatest contribution of rehabilitation professionals is to make the prevention of TBI their highest priority.

APPENDIX 1
Glasgow Coma and Glasgow Liege Scale

Eye Opening		Verbal Response	
Spontaneously	4	Oriented	5
To speech	3	Confused	4
To pain	2	Inappropriate	3
No response	1	Incomprehensible	2
		No response	1

Motor Response		Brain Stem Reflexes (GLS Only)	
Obeys	6	Frontoobicular	5
Localizes	5	Vertical oculovestibular	4
Withdraws	4	Pupillary light	3
Flexion	3	Horizontal oculovestibular	2
Extension	2	Oculocardiovascular	1
No Response	1	No response	0

APPENDIX 2
Abbreviated Injury Scale (AIS)

1. Minor
2. Moderate
3. Severe: Not life threatening
4. Severe: Life threatening
5. Critical: Survival uncertain
6. Fatal

Injury Severity Score (I.S.S.)

The sum of the squares of the three highest Abbreviated Injury Score.

The ISS is 75 automatically if any AIS = 6

APPENDIX 3
Grading of Injury

Ommaya and Gennarelli (1974)

Grade 1	Confusion, no amnesia
Grade 2	Confusion + posttraumatic amnesia
Grade 3	Confusion + antegrade amnesia
Grade 4	Loss of consciousness
Grade 5	Coma > persistent vegetative state
Grade 6	Coma > death

Gennarelli (1982)

Grade 1	Diffuse axonal injury in parasagittal white matter
Grade 2	Diffuse axonal injury in corpus callosum
Grade 3	Diffuse axonal injury also in superior cerebellar peduncle

Becker

Grade 1	Awake and alert, nonfocal neurologic examination
Grade 2	Awake with focal neurologic examination or decreased level of consciousness but follows commands
Grade 3	Unable to follow one-step commands
Grade 4	Without evidence of brain function or brain dead

REFERENCES

1. Agran P, Castillo D, Winn D: Childhood motor vehicle occupant injury. Am J Dis Child 144:653–662, 1990.
1a. Albert JL: Where criminals get guns: Survey of state prison inmates. USA Today, Dec 29,1993.
2. Alexander R, Sato Y, Smith W, et al: Incidence of impact trauma with cranial injuries ascribed to shaking. Am J Dis Child 144:724–726, 1990.
3. American Academy of Pediatrics: Injury control for children and youths. Elk Grove Village, IL, American Academy of Pediatrics, 1987.
4. Anderson DW, McLaurins RL: Report on the National Head and Spinal Cord Survey. Neurosurg 53(Suppl): S1–S43, 1980.
5. Annegers JF, Grabow JD, Kurland LT, et al: The incidence, causes and secular trends of head trauma in Olmsted County, Minnesota, 1935–1974. Neurology 30:919–929. 1980.
5a. Annest JL, Mercy JA. Gibson DR, et al: National estimates of nonfatal firearm-related injuries. JAMA 273:1749–1754, 1995.
6. Atha J, Yeadon MR, Sandover J, Parsons KC: The damaging punch. BMJ 291:21–28. 1985.
7. Baker SP: Determinants of injury and opportunities for intervention. Am J Epidemiol 101:98–102. 1975.
8. Baker SP, O'Neill B, Karpf RS, et al (eds): The Injury Fact Book. Lexington, MA, Lexington Books, 1984.
9. Bergner L, Mayer S, Harris D: Falls from heights: A childhood epidemic in an urban area. Am J Public Health 61:90, 1971.
10. Billmire ME, Myers PA: Serious head injury in infants: Accidents or abuse? Pediatrics 75:340–342, 1985.
11. Bjornstig U, Ostrom M, Eriksson A, et al: Head and face injuries in bicyclists with special reference to possible effects of helmet use. J Trauma 33:887– 893, 1992.
12. Blyth CS, Mueller F: Football injury survey: Part 1 When and where players get hurt. Physician Sportsmed Sept:45–52, 1974.
13. Born JD: The Glasgow-Liege Scale. Acta Neurochir 91:1–11, 1988.
14. Breath DB, Kirby J, Lynch M, et al: Injury cost comparison of restrained and unrestrained motor vehicle crash victims. Trauma 29:1173–1177, 1989.
15. Brent DA, Perper JA: In reply: Firearm access and suicide. JAMA 267:3026–3027, 1992.

16. Brent DA, Perper JA, Allman CJ, et al: The presence and accessibility of firearms in the homes of adolescent suicides. A case-control study. JAMA 266:2989–2995, 1991.

16a. Brewer RD, Fenley MA, Protzel PI, et al: Injury-control recommendations: Bicycle helmets. MMWR 44: 1–17, Feb. 17, 1995.

17. Brison RJ, Wicklund K, Mueller BA: Fatal pedestrian injuries to young children: A different pattern of injury. Am J Public Health 78:793–795, 1988.

18. Bull MJ, Breener K: Premature infants in car seats. Pediatrics 75:336–339, 1985.

18a. Butterfield F: Studies say Brady law checks working. Pittsburgh Post-Gazette, March 12, 1995.

19. Callahan CM, Rivara FP: Urban high school youth and handguns. A school-based survey. JAMA 267:3038–3042, 1992.

20. Carlson C, Essen C, Lofgen J: Clinical factors in severe head injuries. J Neurosurg 29:242–251, 1968.

21. Caveness WF: Incidence of craniocerebral trauma in the United States in 1976 with trends from 1970 to 1975. In Thompson RA, Green JR (eds): Advances in Neurology. New York, Raven Press, 1979, pp 1–3.

22. Center for Disease Control and Prevention: Safety restraint assessment—Iowa, 1987–1988. MMWR 38:735–738, 1989.

23. Center for Disease Control and Prevention: Child passenger restraint use and motor vehicle related fatalities among children, United States, 1982–1990. MMWR 40:600–602, 1991.

24. Center for Disease Control and Prevention: Factors potentially associated with reductions in alcohol related traffic fatalities—United States, 1990–1991. MMWR 41:893–899, 1992.

25. Center for Disease Control and Prevention: Firearm related deaths, Louisiana and Texas, 1970–1990. MMWR 41:213–215, 1992.

26. Center for Disease Control and Prevention: Unintentional firearm related fatalities among children, teenagers—United States 1982–1988. MMWR 41:442–445, 1992.

27. Center for Disease Control and Prevention: Mandatory bicycle helmet use in Victoria, Australia. MMWR 42:359–363, 1993.

28. Champion HR, Copes WS, Sacko WJ, et al: Injury severity scoring. In Border JR (ed): Blunt Multiple Trauma: Comprehensive Pathophysiology and Care. New York, Marcel Dekker, 1990, pp 261–278.

29. Champion HR, Sacco WJ, Copes WS, et al: A revision of the Trauma Score. J Trauma 29:623–629, 1989.

30. Chorba T: Assessing technologies for preventing injuries in motor vehicle crashes. Int J Technol Assess Health Care 7:296–314, 1992.

30a. Christopherson ER, Sosland-Edelman D, LeClaire S: Evaluation of two comprehensive infant car seat loaner programs with 1 year follow-up. Pediatrics 76:36–42, 1985.

31. Committee on Injury Scaling: The Abbreviated Injury Scale-Revision. American Association for Automobiles, 1980.

32. Cooper K, Tabaddor K, Hauser WA, et al: The epidemiology of head injury in the Bronx. Neuroepidemiology 2:70–88, 1983.

33. Corsellis JAN, Bruton CJ, Freeman-Brown D: The aftermath of boxing. Psychol Med 3:270–303, 1973.

34. Cote TR, Sacks JJ, Lambert-Huber DA, et al: Bicycle helmet use among Maryland children: Effect of legislation and education. Pediatrics 89:1216–1220, 1992.

35. Cotton P: Highway fund threat is no easy ride for motorcycle helmet law opponents. JAMA 268:311–312, 1992.

36. Cotton P: Gun-associated violence increasingly viewed as a public health challenge. JAMA 267:1171–1174, 1992.

37. Council on Scientific Affairs American Medical Association: Assault weapons as a public health hazard in the United States. JAMA 267:3067–3070, 1992.

38. Department of Health and Human Services: Interagency Head Injury Task Force Report. Washington, DC, Department of Health and Human Services, 1989.

39. Desai B, Whitman S, Coonly-Hoganson R, et al: Urban head injury. J Natl Med Assoc 75:875–881, 1983.

40. Duff J: Spearing: Clinical consequences in the adolescent. J Sports Med 2:175–177, 1974.

41. Edna T: Alcohol influence and head injury. ACTA Chir Scand 148:209–212, 1982.

41a. Eiben CF, Anderson TP, Lockman C, et al: Functional outcome of closed head injury in children and young adults. Arch Phys Med Rehabil 65:168–170, 1984.

42. Evans J: Restraint effectiveness, occupant ejection from cars and fatality reductions. Accident Anal Prevent 22:167–175, 1990.

43. Eyster EF, Kelker DB, Porter RW: Think First. The national head injury and spinal cord injury prevention program. February, 1993.

43a. Field JR: Epidemiology of head injuries in England and Wales—with particular application to rehabilitation. London, Her Majesty's Stationery Office, Department of Health and Social Security, 1975.

44. Fife D, David J, Tate L, et al: Fatal injuries to bicyclists: The experience of Dade County, Florida. J Trauma 23:745–755, 1983.

45. Fife D, Faich G, Hollingshead E, et al: Incidence and outcome of hospital treated head injury in Rhode Island. Am J Public Health 76:773–778, 1986.

46. Fleming A (ed): Teenagers. Washington, DC, Insurance Institute for Highway Safety, 1988.

47. Frankel B: USA in its own league when it comes to firearms. USA Today, December 29, 1993.

48. Frankowski RF: Descriptive epidemiologic studies of head injury in the United States, 1974–1984. Adv Psychosom Med 16:153–172, 1986.

49. Frankowski RF, Annegers J, Whitman S: Epidemiological and descriptive studies: Part 1. The descriptive epidemiology of head trauma in the United States. Central Nervous System Data Report, 1985, pp 33–43.

50. Gallagher MM, Sewell M, Flint S, et al: Effects of the 65-mph speed limit on rural interstate fatalities in New Mexico. JAMA 262:2243–2245, 1989.

51. Gallup Organization: Hand gun ownership in America. Los Angeles Times Syndicate, May 29, 1991.

51a. Garrettson LK, Gallagher SS: Falls in children and youth. Pediatr Clin North Am 32:153–162, 1985.

52. Geffner R, Rosenbaum A: Brain impairment and family violence. In Templer DI, Hartlage LC, Cannon WG (eds): Preventable Brain Damage, Brain Vulnerability and Brain Health. New York, Springer Publishing, 1992, pp 58–71.

53. Gennarelli TA, Champion HR, Copes WS: Importance of mortality from head injury in immediate survivors of vehicular injuries. International Research Council on Biokinetics of Impact, 1992, pp 167–178.

54. Gennarelli TA, Champion HR, Sacco W, et al: Mortality of patients with head injury and extracranial injury treated in trauma centers. J Trauma 29:1193–1202, 1989.

55. Gennarelli TA, Thibault LE, Adams JH, et al: Diffuse axonal injury and traumatic coma in the primate. Ann Neurol 12:564–574, 1982.

56. Goldsmith MF: Campaigns focus on helmets as safety experts warn bicycle riders to use and preserve heads. JAMA 268:308–310, 1992.

57. Guyer B, Gallagher S: An approach to the epidemiology of childhood injuries. Pediatr Clin North Am 32: 5–15, 1985.

58. Hammon WM: Analysis of 2187 consecutive penetrating wounds of the brain from Vietnam. J Neurosurg 34:127–131, 1971.

59. Harrison CL, Dijkers M: Traumatic brain injury registries in the United States: An overview. Brain Injury 6:203–212, 1992.

60. Hartford C: Safety features should be used with right care. Pittsburgh Post Gazette, July 10, 1994.

61. Insurance Institute for Highway Safety: Two states become no. 43 and no. 44 to enact safety belt use laws. Status Report 28(6):6, 1993.

62. Insurance Institute for Highway Safety: First North Carolina results show mix of publicity, enforcement sends belt use up to about 80 percent. Status Report 28(10):1, 4–5, 1993.

63. Insurance Institute for Highway Safety: Gallup finds supports for devices to limit speed in Great Britain. Status Report 28(10):7, 1993.

64. Ivan LP, Choo SH, Ventureyra EC: Head injuries in childhood: A two-year study. Can Med Assoc 128:281–284, 1983.

65. Jagger J: Prevention of brain trauma by legislation, regulation and improved technology: A focus on motor vehicles. Neurotrauma 9S:313–316, 1992.

66. Jagger J, Levine J, Jane J, et al: Epidemiological features of head injury in a predominantly rural population. J Trauma 24:40–44, 1984.

67. Jagger J, Vernberg K, Jane J: Air bags, reducing the toll of brain trauma. Neurosurgery 20:815–817, 1987.

68. Jennett B, Bond M: Assessment of outcome after severe brain injury: A practical scale. Lancet 1:480–484, 1975.

69. Jennett B, Macmillan R: Epidemiology of head injury. BMJ 282:101–104, 1981.

70. Jennett B, Teasedale G: Assessment of outcome. In Jennett B (ed): Management of Head Injuries. Philadelphia, F.A .Davis, 1981, pp 301–306.

71. Kalsbeek WD, Mclaurin RL, Harris BS, et al: The National Head and Spinal Cord Injury Survey: Major findings. Neurosurgery 53:S19–S31, 1980.

72. Karpf RS, Williams AF: Teenage drivers and motor vehicle deaths. Accident Anal Prevent 15:55–63, 1983.

73. Kaufman H: Civilian gunshot wounds to the head. Neurosurgery 32:962–964, 1993.

74. Kellerman AL, Reay DT: Protection or peril? An analysis of firearm related deaths in the home. N Engl J Med 314:1557–1560, 1986.

75. Reference deleted.

76. Kelly P, Sansin T, Strange G, et al: A prospective study of the impact of helmet usage on motorcycle trauma. Ann Emerg Med 20:852–856, 1991.

77. Klauber RK, Barrett-Connor E, Marshall LF, et al: The epidemiology of head injury: A prospective study of an entire community, San Diego County, California 1978. Am J Epidemiol 113:500–509, 1981.

78. Knaus WA, Draper EA, Wagner DP, et al: Apache II: A severity of disease classification system. Crit Care Med 13:818–828, 1985.

79. Kraus JF: Epidemiology of Head Injury. In Cooper PR (ed): Head Injury. Baltimore, Williams & Wilkins, 1993, pp 1–24.

80. Kraus JF, Black MA, Hessol N, et al: The incidence of acute brain injury and serious impairment of a defined population. Am J Epidemiol 119:186–201, 1984.

81. Kraus JF, Fife D, Ramsein K, et al: The relationship of family income to the incidence, external causes and outcomes of serious brain injury. Public Health 76: 1345–1347, 1986.

81a. Kraus JF, Peck C, McArthur DL, et al: The effect of the 1992 California motorcycle helmet use law on motorcycle crash fatalities and injuries. JAMA 272: 1506–1511, 1994.

81b. Kraus JF, Peck C, Williams A: Compliance with the 1992 California motorcycle helmet use law. Am J Public Health 85:96–99, 1995.

81c. Kraus JF, Morgenstern H, Fife D, et al: Blood alcohol tests, prevalence of involvement and outcome following brain injury. Am J Public Health 79:294–299, 1989.

82. Kraus JF, Rock A, Hemyari P: Brain injuries among infants children, adolescents and young adults. Am J Dis Child 144:684–691, 1990.

83. Lehman LB, Ravich SJ: Closed head injuries in athletes. Clin Sports Med 9:247–261, 1990.

84. Levi L, Borovich B, Guilburd JN, et al: Wartime neurosurgical experience in Lebanon, 1982–1985: I. Penetrating craniocerebral injuries. Isr J Med Sci 26:548–554, 1990.

85. Levi L, Borovich B, Guilburd JN, et al: Wartime neurosurgical experience in Lebanon, 1982–1985: II: Closed craniocerebral injuries. Isr J Med Sci 26:555–558. 1990.

86. Levin HS, O'Donnell VM, Grossman RG: The Galveston orientation and amnesia test: A practical scale to assess cognition after head injury. J Nerv Ment Dis 167:675–684, 1979.

87. Lindenbaum GA, Carroll SF, Daskel I, et al: Patterns of alcohol and drug abuse in an urban trauma center: The increasing role of abuse. J Trauma 29:1654–1658, 1989.

88. Loftin C, McDowall D, Wiersem AB, et al: Effects of restrictive licensing of hand guns on homicide and suicide in the District of Columbia. N Engl J Med 325:1615–1620, 1991.

89. Loyd LE, Graitcer PL: The potential for using a trauma registry for injury surveillance and prevention. Am J Prevent Med 5:34–37, 1989.

90. MacKenzie E, Shapiro S, Eastham J: Rating AIS severity using emergency department sheets vs inpatient charts. Trauma 25:984–988, 1985.

91. Mawdsley C, Ferguson FR: Neurological disease in boxers. Lancet 1:795–801, 1963.

91a. Mayr J, Gais IM, Purtscher K, et al: Baby walkers— an underestimated hazard for our children? Eur J Pediatr 153:531–534, 1994.

92. McCarroll JE, Gunderson C: 5-year study of incidence rates of hospitalized cases of head injuries in the US Army. Neuroepidemiology 9:296–305, 1990.

93. McClelland CQ, Heiple KG: Fractures in the first year of life: A diagnostic dilemma? Am J Dis Child 136:26–29, 1982.

94. Merten DF, Osborne DRS: Craniocerebral trauma in the child abuse syndrome. Pediatr Ann 12: 882–887, 1983.

95. Missouri Head and Spinal Cord Injury Registry. 1988 [unpublished].

96. Morrison RG: Medical and public health aspects of boxing. JAMA 255:2475–2480, 1986.

97. Morrow L, Hudson P: Accidental firearm fatalities in North Carolina, 1976–1980. Am J Public Health 76:1120–1123, 1986.

98. Mueller FO, Blyth CS: Fatalities and catastrophic injuries in football. Physician Sportsmed 10:135–138, 1982.

99. Mueller FO, Blyth CS: Fatalities from head and cervical spine injuries occurring in tackle football: 40 years experience. Clin Sports Med 6:185–196, 1987.

100. Musemeche CA, Barthel M, Consentino C, et al: Pediatric falls from heights. J Trauma 31:1347–1349, 1991.

101. Najaryan R: Emergency room management of the head injured patient. In Becker DP, Gudeman SK (eds): Textbook of Head Injury. Philadelphia, W.B. Saunders, 1989 pp 24–26.

102. National Highway Traffic Safety Administration, U.S. Department of Transportation: A Report to Congress on the Effect of Motorcycle Helmet Use Law Repeal: A Case for Helmet Use. Washington, DC, U.S. Department of Transportation, 1980.

103. National Highway Traffic Safety Administration, U.S. Department of Transportation: Final Regulatory Impact Analysis: Amendment to FMVSS 208; Passenger Car Front Seat Occupant Protection. Washington, DC, U.S. Department of Transportation, 1984.

104. National Highway Traffic Safety Administration, U.S. Department of Transportation: Report to Congress on the Effects of the 65-mph Speed Limit during 1987. Washington, DC, U.S. Department of Transportation, 1989.

105. National Highway Traffic Safety Administration, U.S. Department of Transportation: Buckle Up for Love. Report Number DOT-HF-807-650. Washington, DC, U.S. Department of Transportation, 1990.

106. National Highway Traffic Safety Administration, National Center for Statistics and Analysis: Traffic Safety Facts 1994: Occupant Protection Washington, DC, U.S. Department of Transportation, 1994.

106a. National Highway Traffic Safety Administration, U.S. Department of Transportation: Traffic Safety Facts—TSF-1994. Washington, DC, U.S. Department of Transportation, 1994.

106b. National Highway Traffic Safety Administration, U.S. Department of Transportation: Traffic Safety Facts 1994: Motorcycles. Washington, DC, U.S. Department of Transportation, 1994.

107. National Highway Traffic Safety Administration, U.S. Department of Transportation: Traffic Safety Facts 1994: Pedalcyclists. Washington, DC, U.S. Department of Transportation, 1994.

107a. National Highway Traffic Safety Administration, U.S. Department of Transportation: Traffic SAfety Facts 1994: Alcohol. Washington, DC, U.S. Department of Transportation, 1994.

107b. National Highway Traffic Safety Administration, U.S. Department of Transportation: Bicycle Helmet Use Laws. Washington, DC, U.S. Department of Transportation, 1994.

108. National Highway Traffic Safety Administration, National Center for Statistic and Analysis: Traffic Safety Facts 1992: Pedestrians. Washington, DC, U.S. Department of Transportation, 1992.

109. National Highway Traffic Safety Administration, U.S. Department of Transportation: Saving lives and Dollars: Highway Safety Contribution to Health Care Reform and Deficit Reduction. Washington, DC, U.S. Department of Transportation, 1993.

110. National Highway Traffic Safety Administration, U.S. Department of Transportation: Safety Belt and Motorcycle Helmet Use Incentive Grant program. Washington, DC, U.S. Department of Transportation, 1993.

111. NHIF Professional Council Substance Abuse Task Force. White Paper. Washington, DC, National Head Injury Foundation, 1988.

112. Offner P, Rivara FP, Maier R: The impact of motorcycle helmet use. J Trauma 32:636–642, 1992.

113. Ommaya AK, Gennarelli TA: Cerebral concussion and traumatic unconsciousness: Correlation of experimental and clinical observations on blunt head injuries. Brain 97:633–654, 1974.

114. Partyka SC: Effect of child occupant protection laws on fatalities. Washington, DC, U.S. Department of Transportation, 1989.

115. Patterson PJ, Smith LR: Firearms in the home and child safety. Am J Dis Child 141:221–223, 1987.

116. Pollock DA, McClain PW: Trauma registries: Current status and future prospects. JAMA 262:2280–2283, 1989.

117. Ponticel P: Gun control foes agree: Kids and guns don't mix. Observer Reporter, July 23, 1994.

118. Preusser DF, Williams AF, Zador PL: The effects of curfew laws on motor vehicle crashes. Law Policy 6:115–128, 1984.

118a. Reisinger KS, Williams AF, Wells JA: The effect of pediatricians counseling on infant restraint use. Pediatrics 67:201–206, 1981.

119. Renaud L, Suissa S: Evaluation of the efficacy of simulation games in traffic safety education of kindergarten children. Am J Public Health 79:307–309, 1989.

120. Rice DP, MacKenzie EJ, et al: Cost of injury in the United States: A Report to Congress. San Francisco, Institute for Health and Aging, University of California, and Injury Prevention Center, The Johns Hopkins University, 1989.

121. Rieder MJ, Schwartz C, Newman J: Pattern of walker use and walker injury. Pediatrics 78:488–493, 1986.

122. Reference deleted.

123. Rimel RW, Jane JA, Bond MR: Characteristics of the head injured patient. In Rosenthal M, Griffith ER, Bond MR, Miller JD (eds): Rehabilitation of the Adult and Child with Traumatic Brain Injury. Philadelphia, FA Davis, 1990, pp 8–16.

124. Rivara FP, Barba M: Demographic analysis of childhood pedestrian injuries. Pediatrics 76:375–381, 1985.

125. Rivara FP, Dicker BG, Bergman AB, et al: The public cost of motorcycle trauma. JAMA 260:221–223, 1988.

126. Rivara FP, Kamitsuka MS, Quan L: Injuries to children younger than one year of age. Pediatrics 81:93–97, 1988.

126a. Rivara FP, Thompson DC, Thompson RS, et al: The Seattle children's bicycle helmet campaign: Changes in helmet use and head injury admissions. Pediatrics 93:567–569, 1994.

127. Robertson LS: Motor vehicles. Pediatr Clin North Am 32:97–94, 1985.

128. Robertson LS, Zador PL: Driver education and fatal crash involvement of teenaged drivers. Am J Public Health 68:959–965, 1979.

129. Robertson LS, Zador PL: Crash involvement of teenaged drivers when driver education is eliminated from high school. Am J Public Health 70:599–605, 1980.

129a. Rodgers GB: Bicyclist deaths and fatality risk patterns. Accid Anal Prev 27:215–223, 1995.

129b. Rodgers GB: Bicycle and Bicycle Helmet Use Patterns in the United States: A Description and Analysis of National Survey Data. Washington, DC, U.S. Consumer Product Safety Commission, 1993.

130. Rogers LW, Bergman AB, Rivara FP: Promoting bicycle helmets to children: A campaign that worked. J Musculoskel Dis 8:64–67, 1991.

131. Rood DH, Kraichy PP, Carubia J: Evaluation of New York State's mandatory occupant restraint law: Observational survey of safety restraint use in New York State. Albany, NY, Institute for Traffic Safety Management and Research, 1985.

132. Russell WR: Cerebral involvement in head injury. Brain 55:549–603, 1932.

133. Russell WR, Nathan PW: Traumatic amnesia. Brain 69:183–187, 1946.

134. Rutherford G, Miles R: Overview of Sports Related Injuries to Persons 5–14 years of Age. Washington, DC, U.S. Consumer Product Safety Commission, 1981.

135. Saal JA, Sontag MJ: Head injuries in contact sports: Sideline decision making. Phys Med Rehabil State Art Rev 4:649–658, 1987.

136. Sacks J, Holmgreen P, Smith SM, et al: Bicycle associated head injuries and deaths in the United States from 1984 through 1988. How many deaths are preventable? JAMA 266:3016–3018, 1991.

137. Saltzman LE, Mercy JA, O'Carrol PW, et al: Weapon involvement and injury outcomes in family and intimate assaults. JAMA 267:3043– 3047, 1992.

138. Saunders R, Harbaugh R: The second impact in catastrophic contact—sports, head trauma. JAMA 252:538–539, 1984.

139. Second World Conference on Injury Control: Injury Control in the 1990's: A National Plan for Action. Association for the Advancement of Automotive Medicine, 1993.

140. Showers J, Apolo J, Thomas J, et al: Fatal child abuse: A two decade review. Pediatr Emerg Care 1:66–70, 1985.

140a. Siccardi D, Cavaliere R, Pau A, et al: Penetrating craniocerebral missle injuries in civilians: A retrospective analysis of 314 cases. Surg Neurol 35: 455–460, 1991.

141. Sinal SH, Ball MR: Head trauma due to child abuse. Serial computerized tomography in diagnosis and management. South Med J 80:1505–1512, 1987.

142. Sloan EP, Zalenski RJ, Smith RF, et al: Toxicology screening in urban trauma patients: Drug prevalence and its relationship in trauma severity and management. J Trauma 29:1647–1653, 1989.

143. Sloan JH, Kellerman AL, Reay DT, et al: Handgun regulations, crime assault and homicide: A tale of two cities. N Engl J Med 319:1256–1262, 1988.

144. Sloan JH, Rivara FP, Reay DT, et al: Firearm regulations and rates of suicide: A comparison of two metropolitan areas. N Engl J Med 322:369–373, 1990.

145. Soderstrom C, Cowley A: A national alcohol and trauma center survey: Missed opportunities, failure of responsibility. Arch Surg 122:1067–1071, 1987.

146. Sosin DM, Sacks JJ: Motorcylce helmet use laws and head injury prevention. JAMA 267:1649–1650, 1992.

147. Sosin DM, Sacks JJ, Smith S: Head injury associated deaths in the United States from 1979 to 1986. JAMA 262:2251–2255, 1989.

147a. Sosin DM, Sniezek JE, Waxweiler RJ: Trands in death associated with traumatic brain injury. JAMA 273:1778–1780, 1995.

148. Sparadeo FR, Gill D: Effects of prior alcohol use on head injury recovery. J Head Trauma Rehabil 4:72–82, 1989.

149. Spiegel CN, Lindaman FC: Children can't fly. A program to prevent childhood morbidity and mortality from window falls. Am J Public Health 67:1143, 1977.

150. Stewart JR, U.S. Department of Transportation: Statistical Evaluation of the Effectiveness of FMVSS 202; Head Restraints. Washington, DC, National Highway Traffic Safety Administration, 1980.

151. Taubes G: Violence epidemiologists test the hazards of gun ownership. Science 258:213–215, 1992.

152. Teasdale G, Jennett B: Assessment of coma and impaired consciousness: A practical scale. Lancet 2: 81–84, 1974.

153. Teret SP, Wintemute GJ, Beilenson P: The firearm fatality reporting system. JAMA 267:3073–3074, 1992.

154. Teutsch SM: A framework for assessing the effectiveness of disease and injury prevention. MMWR 4:1–12, 1992.

154a. Think First for Kids—Elementary Education Program [pamphlet]. Washington, DC, National Brain and Spinal Cord Injury Prevention Program, 1995.

155. Thompson RS, Rivara FP, et al: A case control study of the effectiveness of bicycle safety helmets. N Engl J Med 320:1361–1367, 1989.

155a. Thompson RS, Thompson DC, Rivara FP, et al: Cost-effectiveness analysis of bicycle helmet subsidies in a defined population. Pediatrics 91:902–907, 1993.

155b. Thurman DJ, Sniezek JE, Johnson D, et al: Guidelines for Surveillance of Central Nervous System Injury. Atlanta, Centers for Disease Control and Prevention, 1995.

156. Tiret L, Hausherr E, Thicoipe M, et al: The epidemiology of head trauma in Aquitaine (France) 1986: A community based study of hospital admissions and deaths. Int J Epidemiol 19:133–140, 1990.

157. University of Virginia: For Kids Sake, vol. 7. Charlottesville, VA, University of Virginia, 1989.

158. US Department of Health and Human Services: Injury Prevention, Meeting the Challenge. Am J Prevent Med 5 (Suppl): 1–289, 1989.

158a. Vulcan AP, Cameron MH, Heiman L: Evaluation of mandatory bicycle helmet use in Victoria, Australia. Portland, OR, Association for the Advancement of Automotive Medicine, 36th Annual Proceedings.

159. Waller JA (ed): Injury Control: A Guide to the Causes and Prevention of Trauma. Lexington, MA, D.C. Heath, 1985.

160. Washington AP: House nears crime bill compromise. Observer Reporter, August 21, 1994.

161. Watson G, Zador P, Wilks M: Helmet use, helmet use laws and motorcycle fatalities. Am J Public Health 71:297–300, 1981.

162. Watson GS, Zador PL, Wilks A: The repeal of the helmet use laws and increased motorcyclist mortality in the United States, 1975–1978. Am J Public Health 70:579–585, 1980.

163. Weiss BD: Bicycle helmet use by children. Pediatrics 77:677–679, 1986.

164. Whitman S, Coonley-Hogason R, Desai B: Comparative head trauma experience in two socioeconomically different Chicago area communities: A population study. Am J Epidemiol 119:570–580, 1984.

165. Whyte J, Rosenthal M: Rehabilitation of the patient with head injury. In Delisa JA (eds): Rehabilitation Medicine: Principles and Practice. Philadelphia, J.B. Lippincott, 1988 pp 585–611.

166. Willer B, Abosh S, Dalmer E: Epidemiology of disability from traumatic brain injury. In Wood R (ed): Neurobehavioral Sequalae of TBI. London, Taylor & Francis, 1990.

167. Williams AF, Karpf RS: Death of teenagers as passengers in motor vehicles. Accident Anal Prevent 15: 49–54, 1983.

167a. Williams AF, Karpf RS, Zador PL: Variations in minimum licensing age and fatal motor vehicle crashes. Am J Public Health 73:1401–1402, 1983.

168. Wong PP, Dornan J, Schentag CT: Statistical profile of traumatic brain injury: A Canadian rehabilitation population. Brain Injury 7:283–294, 1993.

169. Zagara G, Scaravilli P, Mastorgio P, et al: Validation of a prognostic system in severe brain injured patients. J Neurolog Sci 35:77–81, 1991.

2

Pathophysiology and Initial
Neurosurgical Care: Future Directions

Thirty years ago, the outcome for most cases of traumatic brain injury (TBI) was thought to be determined at the time of impact. All injuries to the brain were considered instantaneous and irreversible. In 1965 Lundberg reported that brain swelling was an important concomitant of severe TBI based on a series of patients in whom he systematically monitored intracranial pressure (ICP).[90] During the next decade, severe or uncontrollable brain swelling became recognized as the most common cause of death in victims of severe TBI who were not brain dead upon arrival at the emergency department.[5,102]

Thus, the cornerstone of acute care for patients with severe TBI became prophylaxis against brain swelling. Prophylactic measures included aggressive hyperventilation, which was considered beneficial because it led to a rapid and sustained reduction of ICP by inducing cerebral vasoconstriction and reducing cerebral blood flow (CBF).[89] Reducing the intravascular volume and increasing serum osmolality with osmotic diuretics, such as urea or mannitol, also were thought to prevent swelling by decreasing the amount of free water in the edematous brain.[71,168]

Optimal acute care during the late 1970s included controlled ventilation and early evacuation of intracranial mass lesions such as hematomas. However, no study had clearly demonstrated that the pharmacologic reduction of elevated ICP improved outcome, and many neurosurgeons did not consider ICP monitoring necessary for all comatose patients with TBI. In 1978 Langfitt reviewed all available studies of severe TBI outcome and found that patients who had ICP monitoring fared no better than patients treated without the use of ICP monitoring.[83] Results of a prospective study in Australia, published in 1983, also showed little effect on outcome with the use of ICP monitoring.[156]

Such observations seemed to support the notion that severe TBI was not treatable. Consequently, many neurosurgeons lost interest in TBI research. In general, the care of patients with severe TBI was a frustrating experience, particularly because mortality rates averaged 50% for patients who remained in a coma for 6 hours or more after injury.[74] However, in 1980, Marshall and colleagues reported a 15–20% reduction in mortality and similar improvement in the rate of good outcome in a group of 200 patients with severe TBI compared with prior reports.[12] They attributed their improved results to high-quality prehospital care and to better in-hospital acute care, which included the routine use of ICP monitoring.[102] Theirs was the first study clearly showing that damage to the brain also occurred after impact and that this secondary damage could be diminished with appropriate treatment.

From 1984–1987 the National Institutes of Health (NIH) sponsored a prospective multicenter study of outcome after severe TBI.[99] All four participating trauma centers used the principles of pre- and intrahospital care described by Marshall, including ICP monitoring. This study involved over 700 patients with closed head injuries who were comatose at the time of admission to the trauma centers. Their outcomes also were better than in previous reports: mortality was reduced from 50% to 35–40%, and good recovery increased from 20% to 30%.[100]

The recognition that changes in acute care can improve outcome after TBI has stimulated basic science investigators to define the cellular and molecular mechanisms through which trauma not only causes immediate damage but also leads to secondary brain injury. The genesis of secondary brain injury may be ischemia in brain tissue surrounding cerebral contusions or hematomas.[19,113,147] Ischemia causes a cascade of deleterious cellular and molecular events that ultimately damage cell membranes and vessel walls, causing brain swelling.[157] Research suggests that the biochemical events resulting in secondary injury do not occur instantaneously but rather over several hours or days.[33] Thus, there is a temporal window of opportunity during which treatment that inhibits deleterious reactions can be effective. Such findings have prompted the clinical trial of several promising treatments for TBI, which, based on preliminary results, may lead to a substantial improvement in outcome during the next few years.[4,46,119,170]

PATHOPHYSIOLOGY OF TRAUMATIC BRAIN INJURY

Damage to the brain following trauma includes both the immediate, or primary, injury and the secondary injury that develops during the first few days after the impact. Primary brain injury is defined as the physiologic and anatomic damage to the brain that results from an impact to the cranium or from rapid translational or angular acceleration or deceleration of the head. It is the direct result of mechanical deformation of the brain. Primary brain injuries are classified as either closed or penetrating, depending on the mechanism of injury, and as mild, moderate, or severe, depending on the neurologic status of the patient soon after impact.

Penetrating Head Injuries

The severity of a penetrating brain injury is associated most closely with the velocity of the missile at impact.[77] The importance of velocity to subsequent brain damage is best described by the kinetic energy equation (KE = ½ mass × velocity²), which indicates that the energy imparted to the brain is directly related to the square of the velocity of the missile.[36] Thus, the most severe injuries are caused by high-velocity gunshot wounds. High-velocity bullets cause a percussion injury to the brain adjacent to the bullet tract, leaving a cylinder of damaged brain tissue up to 30 times the diameter of the bullet.[36,67] In addition, bullets frequently fragment when passing through the rigid skull, thereby penetrating the brain in multiple locations.[77] Fragments of bone driven into the brain cause further destruction, and contaminated fragments of skin or hair that are driven into the brain are a potential source for infection.

In addition to the velocity of a missile, the extent of neurologic injury depends on the location of the missile tract. Thus, even low-velocity penetrating injuries, such as those caused by an ice pick or knife, may result in severe neurologic disability if the missile penetrates the brainstem or basal ganglia or damages a large artery. Conversely, high-velocity bullet wounds may not cause permanent neurologic deficits if confined to the anterior frontal or temporal lobes. The extent of permanent injury caused by missile wounds is closely related to the patient's neurologic status soon after the injury. In one study of 100 persons rendered comatose by a gunshot wound to the head, all but 3 died or were left with severe disabilities.[44] Other studies have found that a victim who is conscious after the injury has a greater than 80% chance of surviving with mild or no neurologic impairment.[51,66]

Severe and Moderate Closed Head Injuries

Closed head injuries usually are caused by motor vehicle accidents, assaults, or falls and by definition do not involve penetration of the brain by foreign objects.[100] However, they may include skull fractures, either depressed or nondepressed. The types of brain injury depend on the velocity and vector of the forces applied to the head. High-speed motor vehicle accidents usually include high-velocity translational and rotational vectors of force. Rotational forces cause shearing of brain tissue at the border between the cortical gray matter and the underlying white matter.[47] Because gray matter is denser than white matter, rotational forces have a greater effect on the gray matter. High-velocity translational forces cause bulk movement of the brain within the skull. Because most of the inner surface of the skull is smooth, the outer surface of the brain can glide along it without being damaged during such translational movements. However, because of significant irregularities in the floor of the anterior and middle cranial fossae, rapid acceleration of the head typically causes contusions of the brain surfaces that glide along these areas—specifically, in the inferior frontal and temporal lobes.

Focal brain contusions may occur anywhere over the convexities of the brain when the head is struck with a blunt object. With increasing force, the blow is more likely to cause a skull fracture, and the most severe injuries cause a depressed skull fracture (Fig. 1). When the head is stationary and struck by a blunt object, the most severe brain injury is in the area underlying the point of impact.[72] However, if the head is in motion and strikes a stationary object or surface (as in a fall), the most severe brain damage usually is on the hemisphere contralateral to the impact.[58] This injury, called a "contrecoup," results from rebound translation of the brain with sudden deceleration. The more severe the force to the head, the more likely vessels will be torn, causing a hematoma to develop within the contused brain tissue or on the surface of the brain. Very severe injuries may cause large intracerebral hematomas, which can rupture into the ventricles, causing intraventricular hemorrhage. Relatively minor trauma may cause disruption of bridging vessels in the subarachnoid space, leading to hemorrhage confined to the subarachnoid space (post-traumatic subarachnoid hemorrhage).

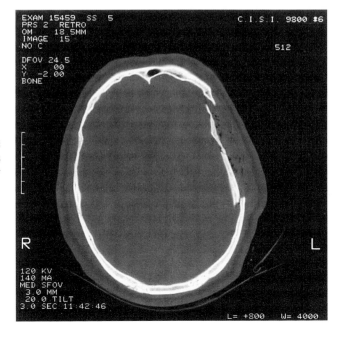

FIGURE 1. Computerized tomographic image of the head in a patient with a left convexity depressed skull fracture caused by impact with a baseball bat.

Posttraumatic intracranial hematomas are classified according to their relationship to the meninges. Epidural hematomas, which occur in about 6% of patients, are located between the inner table of the skull and dura mater. They are commonly associated with a fracture through the temporal bone, which lacerates the middle meningeal artery and causes the hematoma.[44] Because epidural hematomas result from high-pressure arterial bleeding, they expand rapidly and classically lead to neurologic deterioration within minutes to a few hours. However, the surface of the brain is protected by the dura, and neurologic deterioration usually is caused only by the expanding mass. Thus, rapid evacuation of an epidural hematoma often leads to complete neurologic recovery.

Subdural hematomas are much more common than epidural hematomas, occurring in 24% of comatose patients with TBI.[44] Located between the dura mater and the brain, they are caused by the tearing of bridging vessels in the subdural space or vessels on the surface of the brain. The damaged vessels are low-pressure medium or small veins or arterioles. Thus, subdural hematomas typically do not expand rapidly, and neurologic deterioration often results not from the hematoma but from the brain injury underlying the clot. Therefore, evacuation of a subdural hematoma often does little to change the patient's neurologic status.

Posttraumatic hematomas, either epidural or subdural, are most likely to occur in the elderly, as a result of a fall, or in association with a skull fracture.[59] They are much less common in patients under 20 years of age and are less often due to motor vehicle accidents.

Contusions within the temporal lobes as well as mass lesions adjacent to the temporal lobes, such as epidural and subdural hematomas, may cause transtentorial herniation of the medial part of the temporal lobe, which also may lead to neurologic deterioration. The foramen transtentorium, through which the midbrain passes, lies adjacent to the medial temporal lobe (uncus). Masses that develop lateral to the uncus may push it into the foramen and compress the midbrain. This syndrome of uncal herniation may result in coma, pupil dilation, and/or hemiparesis. A portion of the reticular activating system—the neural network responsible for maintaining consciousness—resides in the midbrain. Damage to this system from midbrain compression results in coma. The third cranial nerves, including the parasympathetic fibers responsible for pupil constriction, exit the brainstem at the base of the midbrain en route to the orbits. Distortion of the midbrain from herniation stretches the third cranial nerves and damages the parasympathetic fibers, causing pupil dilation, usually on the side of the mass. Hemiparesis may result from damage to the cerebral peduncles at the base of the midbrain, which are compressed against the edge of the tentorial notch opposite the side of herniation. The neurologic injury caused by midbrain compression from uncal herniation may be reversible, but only if the causative mass lesion is removed soon after herniation occurs.[164]

Epidural and subdural hematomas are best diagnosed with computerized tomography (CT). Epidural hematomas appear as lenticular, hyperdense masses along the inner surface of the skull (Fig. 2). They have a smooth medial border, which is the dura mater that has been stripped from the skull. Subdural hematomas are hyperdense masses that extend over the convexity of the brain and have an irregular inner surface, conforming to the gyri and sulci of the surface of the brain (Fig. 3). Because the CT density of both types of hematomas depends somewhat on the hematocrit, they may appear isodense with brain tissue if the hematocrit is less than 20%. Magnetic resonance imaging (MRI) is not as useful as CT in the early detection of epidural and subdural hematomas, because the blood clot may have the same density as brain on early MR images. Detection of blood clots on MRI requires that the hemoglobin be transformed to deoxyhemoglobin; this process takes 24–36 hours.

Skull fractures, which usually result from blunt trauma to the head, are classified as linear, depressed, or basilar. The most common location of linear fractures is over the lateral convexity of the skull. Linear fractures almost always heal without surgical intervention, but the presence of a fracture may increase the risk of intracranial hematoma. In one study of mild TBI (Glasgow Coma

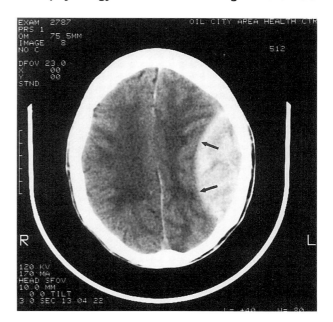

FIGURE 2. On computerized tomography, epidural hematomas appear as lenticular hyperdense intracranial lesions based along the inner surface of the skull. Note the smooth medial surface (*arrows*) caused by stretching the dura mater into the brain.

Scale [GCS] score of 13–15), hematomas were seen in 10% of patients with skull fractures but in only 0.3% of patients without fractures.[40] However, two recent studies found no significant association between surgical intracranial mass lesions and skull fractures.[88,141] CT rather than plain skull radiography is recommended when a skull fracture is suspected, because plain radiography does not reveal intracranial hematomas.

Depressed skull fractures result from trauma to the head with an object of relatively small surface area. Typically, one or more leaves of the skull are fractured inward, hinged on one surface. The jagged border of the fracture surface may lacerate the dura and underlying brain tissue, causing a focal contusion or intracerebral hematoma. If the dura is violated, cerebrospinal fluid (CSF) may leak from the wound, posing

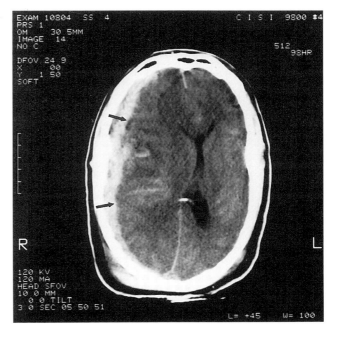

FIGURE 3. Acute subdural hematomas are hyperdense lesions on the surface of the brain that follow the convexity of the brain and have an irregular inner surface (*arrows*), as seen on this CT scan of the head.

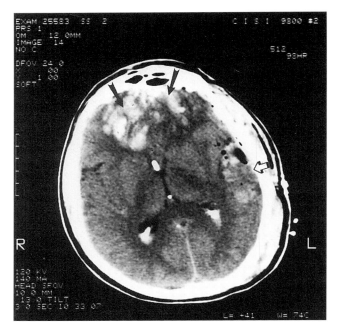

FIGURE 4. Computerized tomographic image of the head in a patient with extensive hemorrhagic contusions of both frontal lobes (*closed arrows*) and the left temporal lobe (*open arrow*). Despite extensive contusions, the patient made a full recovery and returned to work, demonstrating that the location of brain injuries can be more important to recovery than the size of the lesions.

a high risk for meningitis because the CSF spaces are contaminated.

Basilar skull fractures are caused by blunt trauma to the head over a larger surface area. They most commonly occur in the ethmoid bone—a part of the floor of the anterior cranial fossa—or through the petrous portion of the temporal bone.[15] Ethmoid fractures often are associated with hemorrhage into the soft tissues surrounding the orbits (periorbital ecchymoses). The hemorrhage gives the appearance of raccoon eyes, a physical sign of the possibility of an anterior basilar skull fracture. Likewise, fractures through the petrous bone may cause hemorrhage in the scalp overlying the mastoid eminence; ecchymosis in this area is called Battles sign. Basilar skull fractures usually heal without medical or surgical intervention.[15] However, they frequently violate adjacent paracranial sinuses, which are normally contaminated with bacteria. Thus, if the fracture also is associated with a laceration of the dura mater and CSF leak, the patient is at high risk for contamination of the CSF spaces and meningitis.

The mortality and permanent neurologic disability that results from severe closed head injuries are related to both the size and the location of the lesion. Small contusions or intracerebral hematomas within the brainstem or basal ganglia may cause severe neurologic

disability, whereas large epidural hematomas that are evacuated quickly or large cerebral contusions confined to one frontal lobe may cause no permanent disability (Fig. 4). The brain is normally compliant and, to some extent, can accommodate a mass lesion by reducing its content of blood or CSF.[73] However, when the volume of hematoma or contused, edematous brain tissue reaches 100–150 cc, any further increase in mass results in an increase in ICP because the intracranial contents are confined within the rigid skull.[76] With larger hematoma volumes, the ICP reaches the level of the blood pressure and becomes a hydrostatic barrier to perfusion of the brain, resulting in death.

Mild Closed Head Injuries

Patients who suffer relatively low-velocity head trauma, which commonly occurs during contact sports, or motor vehicle accidents, may transiently lose consciousness and /or recall of the events immediately before or after the trauma. A detailed neurologic assessment soon after the injury may show normal findings or may reveal subtle dysfunction in carrying out complex tasks under pressure.[68] CT findings are usually normal, although MRI may show focal punctate densities near the cortical gray-white junction on long TR images.[172] The term "concussion" is used to describe this type of closed head injury and classically implies a transient physiologic disturbance without anatomic injury, although sensitive imaging techniques such as MRI frequently demonstrate subtle damage. A classification system for various grades of concussion, devised by Ommaya and Gennarelli, is useful in determining the need for hospitalization and the subsequent risk of permanent neurologic deficit.[131]

Some victims of mild head injury are incapable of returning to their former occupation for months or years after the injury. Disability is usually due to posttraumatic headaches, inability to concentrate, dizziness, or sleep disturbances. If prolonged such symptoms lead to anxiety, depression, or other psychological or social problems.[8] This complex of symptoms is called postconcussion syndrome, but many of the components in fact may be due to trauma to the scalp or cervical spine. Through improved understanding of its components, effective treatment is being developed for postconcussion syndrome. Most such treatments, however are directed toward the symptoms. Little is known about the pathophysiology, in part because mild head injury rarely causes death; thus postmortem studies are not available. Nonetheless, the effects of mild closed head injury are cumulative; concussions occur more frequently and with greater severity in patients who have suffered at least one prior head injury.[48] Concussion also tends to affect the ability to carry out complex tasks much more than it affects other cognitive abilities.[55]

The evaluation and initial management of patients with mild TBI must include a careful determination of the events surrounding the accident. Did the patient lose consciousness? If so, did some other disease or drug intoxication cause loss of consciousness, which led to the motor vehicle accident or fall? The duration of antegrade and retrograde amnesia also should be determined, because prolonged amnesia, particularly retrograde, is associated with an increased risk for skull fractures and hematomas.[122] A careful neurologic evaluation and CT images are mandatory for patients with persistent confusion, severe headaches, or focal neurologic deficits, and for patients who cannot be adequately examined because of drug intoxication. In one study of 75 patients with normal or near-normal GCS scores (14–15), CT revealed contusions or hematomas in 17%, although only one patient required surgery.[88] If, however, the patient is truly asymptomatic, with no prolonged loss of consciousness or amnesia, CT may not be necessary. Such patients often can be discharged with observation by family members. The decision to admit the patient to the hospital for observation is made after careful assessment of neurologic status, circumstances surrounding the accident, and family support.

Secondary Brain Injury

Secondary brain injury refers to damage that occurs after the initial trauma. Several physiologic autoregulatory mechanisms are disrupted after impact. In addition, the initial damage to brain tissue causes the release of several potentially neurotoxic compounds.[57] These two events initiate a series of complex biochemical cascades, producing high levels of reactive oxygen species (oxygen free radicals) and the cellular inflammatory response.[154,157,173] Oxygen free radicals have an extremely toxic effect on the brain by degrading cell membranes and damaging vessel walls.[82,154] Most secondary injury occurs during the first 12–24 hours after trauma, but it may occur at any time during the first 5–10 days in patients with very severe primary brain injury.[33]

Using various head injury models, investigations during the last decade have defined many of the metabolic, physiologic, and biochemical events that occur soon after mechanical impact to the brain.[57,82,134,135,154] Such studies have found that focal areas of cerebral ischemia are common after brain injury and that ischemia initiates many of the most toxic biochemical cascades.[157] Graham and colleagues studied the incidence of ischemic cell change in several brain regions of patients who died from severe TBI.[50,146] They found histologic evidence of focal cerebral ischemia in almost 90%.

To define the prevalence of posttraumatic ischemia, cerebral blood flow (CBF) has been studied extensively with techniques that use xenon as a marker. Serial xenon studies obtained early after injury reveal that global or even regional CBF is typically low during the first 24–36 hours and then increases.[10,11,94,128] In areas of the brain surrounding subdural hematomas or cerebral contusions, blood flow in fact may be quite low and remain so for up to several days after injury.[19,147]

Local variation in CBF is consistent with findings of substantial local variation in cerebrovascular responsiveness to changes in the arterial partial pressure of carbon dioxide (pCO_2). Such variation indicates that trauma has disrupted the normal cerebrovascular regulatory mechanisms.[91]

The degree of oxygen extracted from cerebral venous blood also can be measured to estimate the adequacy of cerebral perfusion and the prevalence of ischemia. Cerebral oxygen extraction is measured by comparing the oxygen content in arterial blood with the oxygen content in jugular venous blood ($AVdO_2$)[95,139] Such studies show that the level of oxygen extraction typically is exaggerated during the first 24 hours after injury, a finding that supports the presence of early cerebral ischemia. Robertson and colleagues measured the incidence and severity of jugular venous oxygen desaturations during the first week after severe TBI and found a strong correlation with neurologic outcome: such occurrences were most common in patients who died or were left in a vegetative state.[32,140]

Both the appropriate level of regional or global CBF after TBI and the threshold value for ischemia depend on the metabolic requirements of the brain, since ischemia is defined as blood flow that is insufficient to meet the metabolic demands of the tissue. Obrist showed that cerebral metabolism is normally depressed after severe TBI and suggested that low CBF in fact may be appropriate for the metabolic demands of the posttraumatic brain.[127] At the University of Pittsburgh both CBF and metabolic requirements of focal areas of the brain were measured by combining a local technique of monitoring CBF (thermodiffusion probes) with in vivo microdialysis in two patients with TBI. The combined techniques enabled the determination of the CBF level associated with ischemia by directly measuring the metabolites of ischemia in the brain

tissue adjacent to the monitor. At 24 and 36 hours after injury, local CBF fell to 16–20 ml/100 gm/min, with a sharp increase in extracellular levels of ischemic byproducts, including glutamate and malondialdehyde (a metabolite of free radicals). These events occurred at 24 and 36 hours after injury, indicating that ischemia may occur at various times during the first few days.

The prevalence of posttraumatic cerebral ischemia has important implications for the clinical management of patients with severe TBI, because many traditional treatment modalities reduce CBF even further. One such treatment is aggressive diuretic therapy, which may lead to hypovolemia and reduced blood pressure.[112] The Traumatic Coma Databank and other studies show that sustained hypotension (systolic blood pressure < 90 mmHg) immediately or in the first several days after injury is associated with a doubling of the incidence of poor outcomes.[25,98,136,166] Bouma and associates provided a physiologic perspective on how hypotension is likely to cause ischemia, regardless of the state of cerebral autoregulation.[9] Rosner demonstrated, both experimentally and clinically, that when cerebral perfusion pressure (CPP) drops below 70 mmHg, there is an increased incidence of sudden elevations in ICP, known as plateau waves.[142,144] CPP is calculated as the difference between the mean arterial pressure (MAP) and the ICP. Patients with severe TBI often have an ICP of 20 mmHg or higher; thus a reduction of the MAP below 90 mmHg usually causes the CPP to fall below 70 mmHg.

Prophylactic hyperventilation therapy also has been advocated for the treatment of severe TBI,[89] but hypocapnia is a potent stimulant of cerebral vasoconstriction, potentially aggravating preexisting cerebral ischemia. Muizelaar and associates prospectively randomized patients with severe TBI to hyperventilation therapy ($pCO_2 = 25$ mmHg) or relative normoventilation ($pCO_2 = 35$ mmHg) and found significantly worse outcomes at 3 and 6 months in the group with the lower pCO_2.[118]

The discovery of specific components of the biochemical and cellular responses to ischemia has led to the development of novel therapies by which they can be retarded or blocked. The cellular inflammatory response to TBI, mediated by polymorphonuclear leukocytes (PMNs), is an important component of secondary brain injury. Studies of cerebral freeze and cortical contusion injuries have found significant correlation between the local accumulation of PMNs and both ICP and brain water content.[6,150,173] Cytokines, such as interleukin-1 and 6, which are released into the extracellular space after trauma, are responsible for attracting PMNs.[81,171] Thus therapy that suppresses the release of cytokines or blocks their chemotactic effect may reduce both the cellular inflammatory response and brain swelling.

Among the more important biochemical responses to ischemia are inactivation of ion exchange systems that maintain low levels of extracellular potassium and abnormal stimulation of membrane receptors that control influx of calcium into the cell.[157] This response may be summarized as follows: inactivation of the sodium-potassium-adenosine triphosphatase system (due to ischemia) → increased afflux of excitatory amino acids (glutamate and aspartate) → supranormal activation of membrane-associated, enzyme-linked calcium channels (NMDA receptor, AMPA receptor) → influx of calcium into the cell → increased cellular phospholipase activity → high levels of reactive oxygen species (free radicals).

The onset and duration of these processes is of obvious therapeutic relevance, because most head-injured patients do not reach the trauma center until 1 hour or more after injury. There is reason to believe that the biochemical pathway described above occurs over several hours. In models of ischemia using radiolabeled calcium as a metabolic tracer, abnormal uptake of calcium into the cell continues for up to 24 hours after the injury.

Table 1 lists most of the major biochemical events that are currently known to contribute to secondary brain injury as well as therapies

TABLE 1. Secondary Brain Injury: Proposed Mechanisms and Potential Treatment

Secondary Injury	Toxicity	Potential Treatment
Ischemia	Lactic acidosis ↑ Excitatory amino acids (EAAs) ↑ Extracellular K$^+$	CPP > 70 mmHg[144] Normovolemia[144] pCO$_2$ > 32 mmHg[118] Avoid hypotension[9]
↑ EAAs (glutamate, aspartate)	Free radicals	Hypothermia[22,28,95,152]
↑ Cytokines (interleukins)	Inflammation	Hypothermia[28,81,95,153]
↑ Acetylcholine	↑ Sensitivity to ischemia	Scopolamine[65]
↑ Opioids	↓ Cerebral perfusion	Naloxone[108] Thyrotropin-releasing hormone[41,137]
↑ Catecholamines	Ischemia	Amphetamines[42]
↑ Free radicals	Edema, hyperemia	Alpha tocopherol[29] Ascorbic acid[60] Superoxide dismutase[87] Dimethylsulfoxide[30]
↑ Lipid peroxides	Edema, hyperemia	Methylprednisolone[14,60,62] 21-Aminosteroids[62,109]
↑ Extracellular potassium	Edema, seizures	Ethacrynic acid[123,124] Indacrinone[124]
↑ Arachidonic acid metabolism	Leukotrienes, free fatty acids	Ibuprofen[54,63] Meclofenamic acid[54,63] U63447A[54,63]

↑ Calcium entry into cells:
  NMDA receptors
  Voltage-gated channels
	Free radicals
	↑ Arachidonic acid metabolism
		NMDA receptor antagonists:[26]
		  Magnesium[155]
		  MK-801[106,110]
		  Ketamine[155]
		Calcium-channel blockers:
		  Nimodipine[84]
		  (S)-emopamil[148]

↓ Magnesium	↑ Calcium entry into cells	Magnesium chloride[107,111]

that have shown promise for blocking the reactions. All of the biochemical events cause cerebral edema or hyperemia and a subsequent increase in ICP. The association between high ICP and poor outcome is well established, as is the correlation between outcome and the ability to control or reduce ICP.[5,102] Therefore, mortality and neurologic morbidity after TBI are expected to decline with the early use of therapies that retard or inhibit the biochemical cascades responsible for secondary brain injury. Treatment that alleviates cerebral ischemia, such as enhancement of cerebral perfusion and elimination of prophylactic hyperventilation therapy, already has been shown to improve outcome.[91,118,144] Several of the most promising therapies intended to retard or inhibit the damaging biochemical consequences of secondary injury have been studied in prospective randomized clinical trials, including tromethamine (THAM), superoxide dismutase conjugated to polyethylene glycol (PEG-SOD), 21-amino steroid, nimodipine, and moderate hypothermia.[4,28,46,95,119,153,170] The results of these studies are described in the discussion of the clinical trials.

CONTEMPORARY TREATMENT OF SEVERE TRAUMATIC BRAIN INJURY

To avoid or reduce the severity of secondary brain injury, the management of patients with severe TBI must account for the aforementioned metabolic and physiologic derangements. Consequently, many traditional standards of care must be critically reviewed and, in some cases, rejected. Diuretic therapy must be used cautiously, and hypotension must be aggressively avoid. Hyperventilation should be used only as a last resort or when an expanding intracranial mass lesion is likely. Dextrose intravenous solutions should be avoided during the first few days after injury, because increased levels of dextrose have been shown to drive anaerobic glycolysis and the production of lactate in ischemic brain tissue.[125] These and other principles aimed at avoiding secondary brain injury are incorporated into management protocols for all phases of care of the patient with severe TBI. Because most secondary brain injury occurs during the first few hours after injury, contemporary management protocols must focus on this interval including the period before the patient arrives at the trauma center.

Prehospital Care

Because paramedics are usually the first medical responders to a victim of severe TBI, they must be educated about contemporary principles of TBI management. In an effort to avoid cerebral ischemia immediately after injury, most comatose patients are endotracheally intubated soon after paramedics arrive and mechanically ventilated at a rate of approximately 12 breaths/minute, which results in a near-normal arterial pCO_2 (35–40 mmHg). Peripheral O_2 saturation is monitored, and O_2 saturations of greater than 94% are maintained by administering supplemental oxygen, if necessary. Several large-bore intravenous catheters are inserted and isoosmotic crystalloid or colloid is infused as necessary to maintain an MAP of greater than 90 mmHg. Once the paramedics have ensured an adequate airway and stabilized the blood pressure (a goal that is not always possible in the field), the patient is immobilized on a rigid back board, with the neck immobilized separately in a rigid cervical spine collar, and transported to a trauma center capable of definitive neurosurgical intervention. En route to the trauma center, the patient's vital signs are checked frequently, and any deterioration is addressed immediately. Occasionally it is necessary to stop at a primary care hospital to intubate a patient with a difficult airway or to obtain venous access for the administration of fluids or blood.

Emergency Department

In the emergency department of the trauma center, evaluation and treatment of the head-injured patient follows the Advanced Trauma Life Support Guidelines published by the American College of Surgeons.[1] Protection of the airway and adequacy of breathing and blood pressure remain the primary concerns. Once the patient's vital signs are stabilized, a general assessment of injuries is performed, including a summary of the patient's neurologic status in terms of the GCS.[158] This 15-point system was developed by Jennett and Teasdale in 1974 to test motor, eye-opening, and speech capabilities of the neurologically impaired patient (Table 2).[158] It was intended to be an easily determined, objective assessment that could be used to communicate the patient's neurologic status to nurses and physicians. Since its inception the GCS has gained international recognition, and its validity has been established in numerous studies.[13,43] The GCS is most useful for assessment of moderate or severe TBI and is relatively insensitive to subtle neuropsychological deficits that may occur in patients with mild TBI, especially children and infants, in whom a determination of the verbal score is not possible. For comatose patients with severe injuries, several investigators have found that the GCS motor score correlates best with the severity of brain injury and with outcome.[27,31] This applies to children as well as adults.

A CT scan of the head is obtained as soon as possible, usually within the first 30 minutes after the patient arrives. CT is the most reliable and convenient test available for determining the presence and location of surgical intracranial mass lesions. Risk factors for surgical intracranial mass lesions include neurologic deterioration since the time of the accident, advanced age, blunt or low-velocity head injury, and skull fractures. Young children (less than 2 years of age) also have an increased incidence of intracranial hematomas compared with older children or young adults. It is important to identify and remove such lesions as rapidly as possible. In one study, patients with an acute subdural hematoma that was evacuated within 2 hours after injury had a 60% lower mortality rate than patients whose clots were not evacuated for at least 4 hours.[151]

The safest and most effective method for removing posttraumatic intracranial mass lesions is to perform a large craniotomy in a fully equipped operating room. Most trauma centers in the United States maintain an operating room and support personnel 24 hours a day for immediate surgery when necessary. In the past, burr holes were placed in victims of trauma who suffered rapid neurologic deterioration or who had lateralizing neurologic

TABLE 2. The Glasgow Coma Scale

		Score
Eye opening:	Spontaneously	4
	To voice	3
	To painful stimuli	2
	Nil	1
Verbalization:	Normal, conversant	5
	Confused, conversant	4
	Intelligible words, not conversant	3
	Unintelligible sounds	2
	Nil	1
Motor (upper extremities):	Follows commands	6
	Localizes painful stimuli	5
	Withdraws from painful stimuli	4
	Flexion posturing	3
	Extension posturing	2
	Nil	1

Total Score (eye opening + verbal + motor) = 3–15

deficits. In such patients this procedure was considered the quickest way to relieve intracranial pressure caused by the blood clot. Now, however, it is discouraged for several reasons: (1) acute posttraumatic blood clots such as subdural hematomas are solid, not liquid, and cannot be effectively drained through a burr hole; (2) significant hemorrhage may occur because of the high risk of damage to large arteries and the lack of efficient hemostatic devices in most emergency departments; and (3) the procedure is likely to delay the transfer of the patient to an operating room for craniotomy. In elderly patients with lateralizing neurologic signs, in whom a CT scan of the head cannot be rapidly obtained, the placement of diagnostic burr holes has been advocated.[3] However, intracerebral hematomas were missed by this approach, and CT remains the diagnostic procedure of choice.

If hemodynamic or respiratory instability persists despite aggressive resuscitative efforts, the patient usually requires an emergent laparotomy or thoracotomy and is taken to the operating room before a CT scan of the head is obtained. A recent study found that victims of multiple trauma who require emergent surgery to stop internal hemorrhage are not likely to suffer permanent neurologic impairment from the delay in obtaining a CT scan.[169] This approach also is supported by reports implicating prolonged hypotension as a major cause of secondary brain injury.[98]

Proper assessment of the patient's neurologic status in the emergency department is critical for determining the severity of the primary brain injury and the likelihood of brain swelling. The clinical neurologic examination is a sensitive indicator of general cerebral functioning and helps to detect damage to critical brain regions that may appear normal on the initial CT scan. In some cases, however, alcohol or other drug intoxication, pharmacologic paralysis, or sedation prevents an accurate neurologic assessment immediately after the patient arrives. Although agitated or combative patients may require sedative medications for safe transport from the field to the trauma center, an accurate neurologic assessment can be obtained soon after arrival if short-acting medications are used. Drug intoxications usually can be reversed pharmacologically, but alcohol intoxication may necessitate a delay of several hours to obtain a reliable examination.

An additional problem, identified through a national survey, is widespread misunderstanding and ineptitude among neurosurgical residents and nonneurosurgical trauma staff about the proper methods for determining the GCS score.[92] The GCS is an internationally recognized standard scale for the rapid assessment of brain-injury severity, but its correct use requires training. Unfortunately, this fact is frequently overlooked in many residency training programs. Without an accurate and objective assessment of the patient's initial neurologic status, however, it is impossible to audit the quality of TBI care provided by trauma centers or to conduct meaningful clinical trials.

Intensive Care Unit

After appropriate evaluation and treatment of life-threatening injuries, the patient is taken to the intensive care unit (ICU). The ICU is equipped for continuous monitoring of ICP, blood pressure, and other physiologic parameters and staffed by specially trained nurses who are familiar with all aspects of neurotrauma care. The goals are to optimize cerebral perfusion and brain tissue oxygenation, to minimize brain swelling, and to maintain all other physiologic variables within normal range. Abnormalities of glucose, electrolytes, and body temperature are rapidly identified and corrected. The CPP is maintained above 70 mmHg and arterial pO_2 above 98 mmHg. Body temperature is maintained between 37° and 38° C, and hyperthermia is rigorously avoided. Studies using animal models of cerebral ischemia have found a logarithmic increase in neuronal injury for each degree above 39° C.[20,21] Nutritional supplementation is provided within 48 hours after injury, preferably via an enteral feeding tube. If the patient does no tolerate enteral nutrition, parenteral intravenous hyperalimentation is used. Early nutritional support has not been shown to improve outcome but may reduce the degree of protein wasting after severe TBI. In one study, daily nitrogen loss was reduced form 9.2 gm to 5.7 gm when feeding was begun within the first 2–3 days.[80]

The optimal care of patients with severe TBI requires monitoring of several physiologic variables, including ICP, blood pressure, and central venous pressure. In some centers CBF is determined several times each day with the xenon technique. $AVdO_2$ also is measured several times each day with blood samples obtained from a catheter placed in the jugular bulb. Measurements of CBF and $AVdO_2$ provide an estimate of the adequacy of cerebral perfusion. In addition, the product of the CBF and $AVdO_2$ provides an estimate of the cerebral metabolic rate for oxygen.[79]

Control of brain swelling in patients with severe TBI is often difficult and may require the administration of one or more of the following: narcotic sedation, systemic neuromuscular paralysis, osmotic or loop diuretics, moderate hyperventilation, or barbiturates. Most authorities advocate a stepwise approach that begins with sedation and paralysis, and adds each subsequent measure only when the prior measure has failed to control the swelling. Steroids have not been shown to be efficacious in the management of posttraumatic brain swelling and should not be used.[96]

The length of stay in the ICU is determined primarily by the ability to manage the patient's brain swelling. Aggressive monitoring and treatment in the ICU are always required when swelling is difficult to control. Usually, however, swelling subsides within 4–5 days, and the invasive monitors are then removed. Patients who regain consciousness are extubated and transferred from the ICU. Those who remain comatose require placement of a tracheostomy for adequate pulmonary toilet and a gastrostomy tube for feeding prior to transfer.

A physiatrist is consulted on the day the patient is admitted to the ICU and follows the patient throughout the hospital stay. Early involvement of the physiatrist and the rehabilitation team gives a better understanding of the patient's injuries and should optimize neurologic recovery and minimize neuromedical and functional morbidity associated with the acute phase of care. The well-trained physiatrist should be familiar with physical management of problems germane to severe brain injury, such as spasticity, neurogenic heterotopic ossification, central dysautonomia, bowel and bladder dysfunction, and skin care. The physiatrist can also assist the acute care team by providing input about appropriate pharmacologic choices. Among the many choices for treating a problem such as posttraumatic seizures, for example, some may expedite, whereas others may suppress the process of recovery. Because most neurosurgeons have little or no training in dealing with such problems, it is important to include rehabilitation specialists as part of the acute-care team.

Anticonvulsant prophylaxis is used only for patients with contusions or subdural hematomas and for victims of penetrating wounds. Phenytoin is used initially, because it is one of the least sedating anticonvulsants and can be administered intravenously. Despite potential sedating effects, phenobarbital is a good alternative. It has not been shown to cause the idiopathic febrile response induced by phenytoin in some patients. If the patient has no seizures during the first week after injury, the anticonvulsant is discontinued. In a randomized clinical trial, Temkin and colleagues found that phenytoin does not decrease the risk of posttraumatic seizures after the first week.[160] A subsequent study showed that phenytoin significantly impaired cognitive abilities in patients tested 1 month after a severe TBI compared with a similar group of patients who did not receive the drug.[59] Patients who have one or more seizures beyond the first 24 hours after injury are given anticonvulsants for 6 months. When the patient can tolerate enteral medications, the anticonvulsant is changed to carbamazepine, which may have fewer cognitive and visuomotor side effects than phenytoin.[163] The recommendations for anticonvulsant prophylaxis are evolving and remain somewhat controversial. For example, the most appropriate time for discontinuation of anticonvulsant therapy has not been established, and the 6-month guideline has been determined arbitrarily by the author on the basis of his own experience and the existing literature. The chapter on posttraumatic epilepsy contains a comprehensive discussion of this topic.

Once the patient is discharged from the ICU to the general neurosurgical unit, the goals are to maximize recovery of neurologic function, to teach compensatory functional strategies using impaired and unimpaired limbs, and to minimize medical complications. Patients who are comatose after TBI are at high risk for infections, deep venous thrombosis, pulmonary complications, and decubitus ulcers. Prevention of such problems requires that the patient be mobilized frequently and receive daily physical therapy. Pulmonary complications are minimized with aggressive pulmonary toilet several times each day, and the incidence for deep venous thrombosis may be reduced by administering low-dose warfarin sodium to maintain prothrombin times of 15–16 seconds, as demonstrated by several orthopedic studies of patients with hip fractures.[132,133] Pneumatic compression stockings and subcutaneous heparin (5,000 units every 8 hours) are alternative measures but may not be as effective as warfarin.[45,115] Recently, low-molecular-weight heparin has been introduced as an easier-to-use alternative to warfarin, but a large prospective trial comparing the two drugs found that the rate of hemorrhagic complications was more than twice as high for the group treated with low-molecular-weight heparin.[69] Patients requiring further rehabilitation are transferred to specialized rehabilitation programs for brain injury.

Patients who have suffered from severe TBI are also at risk for hydrocephalus, which may not become symptomatic until weeks or months after injury. At greatest risk are patients who had a posttraumatic hematoma, subarachnoid hemorrhage, craniotomy, or meningitis.[23] Hydrocephalus should be considered in awake patients who complain of headaches, gait problems, or incontinence or who develop problems with mentation. Obtunded patients with hydrocephalus may have a plateau in neurologic recovery. A CT scan of the head usually reveals dilated ventricles, and an MRI may reveal transependymal edema, which is most prominent adjacent to the frontal horns of the lateral ventricles. However, the radiologic diagnosis of hydrocephalus may be difficult, because patients with the most severe brain injuries are also the most likely to have progressive encephalomalacia and ex-vacuo dilation of the ventricles. Thus, although up to 72% of patients admitted to rehabilitation hospitals after severe TBI may have dilated ventricles, less than 20% are likely to benefit from a CSF diversion procedure (shunt).[56,85] The diagnosis of hydrocephalus is best accomplished by careful consideration of both the patient's clinical course and the CT images. In some cases serial spinal taps and withdrawal of 30–40 cc of CSF lead to neurologic improvement and confirm the diagnosis.

CONTROVERSIES IN ACUTE CARE FOR SEVERE TBI

High-quality prehospital care, use of the Advanced Trauma Life Support Program (ATLS), rapid evacuation of intracranial mass lesions, and aggressive intensive care are now commonly accepted standards that have helped to reduce the mortality rate of TBI. However, several acute-care issues generate a great deal of debate among neurosurgeons. The need for ICP monitoring in all comatose patients with TBI is one such issue. Given the invasive nature of this technique and the potential for serious complications, such as infection and hemorrhage, many authorities advocate monitoring only patients at highest risk for elevated ICP. Certain characteristics defined on CT images, such as absence of basilar cisterns or small ventricles, are associated with elevated ICP.[121,162] Most neurosurgeons agree that ICP monitoring is beneficial

for patients who have CT evidence of brain swelling or large intracranial mass lesions.[149] Until recently, many also believed that without such CT evidence of brain swelling, the likelihood of elevated ICP was low and that the use of ICP monitoring was not indicated.[121] However, O'Sullivan and coworkers reported significant ICP elevations in 7 of 8 patients with severe TBI who had no evidence of brain swelling on CT.[126] In 5 of these patients ICP increased to 30 mmHg or more at various times after injury, despite aggressive treatment. Thus ICP monitoring for all comatose patients with TBI may still be necessary, regardless of the appearance of the CT scans.

The best type of ICP monitor is also somewhat controversial. The ventriculostomy system designed by Lundberg more than 40 years ago continues to offer several advantages and is generally considered the most reliable.[89] A Silastic catheter is inserted into the lateral ventricle through a burr hole in the skull and connected to a transducer. Pressure waves transmitted by a column of CSF in the tubing are thereby transformed into an analog display that indicates both the absolute ICP and the ICP wave-form. With this system CSF can be drained periodically to help to reduce elevated intracranial pressure. Because the pressure throughout the ventricles of the brain is theoretically monitored, this system is most likely to detect immediate changes in ICP. Disadvantages of the ventriculostomy include difficulty in inserting the catheter into small ventricles, infection (1–9%), and hemorrhage (1–2%).[103,121] An alternative that avoids most of these problems is the fiberoptic ICP monitor, which can be placed into the white matter of the brain and provides reliable ICP measurements.[35] Although the infection and hemorrhage risks are minimal, the fiberoptic monitor does not allow drainage of CSF for control of elevated ICP.

At some trauma centers, neurosurgeons interested in TBI research use various monitoring techniques to clarify the pathophysiology of brain injury. In the future, some of these techniques may be considered essential to high-quality acute care. Data obtained by monitoring CBF values,[11,19,70,94,147] $AVdO_2$,[70,94,139] CBF velocity (transcranial Doppler),[24,167] and various electrophysiologic events with electroencephalograms (EEG),[117,159,161] brainstem auditory evoked potentials,[2,86] and somatosensory evoked potentials[52,53,86] have provided new insights into the location and extent of primary brain injury, as well as possible mechanisms of secondary brain injury. CBF monitoring, for example, has defined typical changes in regional CBF that occur after TBI and has demonstrated the heterogeneity of the cerebrovascular response to therapeutic interventions.[91,91,128] This information has led to a more conservative use of hyperventilation therapy. Transcranial Doppler analysis has led to a better understanding of the incidence and severity of posttraumatic vasospasm.[24,167] Electrophysiologic monitoring has been most useful in characterizing the severity of brain injury, particularly for patients who are nearly brain dead or remain in a vegetative state.[18,152] Although single measurements of brainstem evoked potentials or somatosensory evoked potentials have limited value, serial or continuous measurements provide useful prognostic information.[75,116] Sudden changes in a continuously monitored EEG may predict impending clinical deterioration.[16] EEG data can be analyzed quantitatively if recordings collected over hours or days are converted to a compressed array of tracings that illustrate a spectrum of frequencies and relative power; this conversion is known as compressed spectral array (CSA). Moulton and colleagues found a close correlation between the GCS score and quantitative CSA.[117] They also found that spectral analysis was slightly more accurate than neurologic examination in predicting 6-month outcome.

Such monitoring techniques have provided valuable insights into the pathophysiology of brain injury, but many are also very expensive. However, centers currently using these techniques are obtaining information that applies to most patients with severe TBI. Thus, some of the more expensive techniques, such as CBF monitoring, will not be necessary for high-quality acute care at other centers.

Another area of controversy is which specialty group should have primary responsibility for the acute care of patients with TBI. A recent national survey of response times and availability of trauma specialists found that neurosurgeons were the most difficult to contact when trauma patients arrived in the emergency department.[129] In some communities, general surgeons have responded to the problem by assuming primary responsibility for all trauma patients, including those with isolated TBI. In some cases, they diagnose the type of injury, determine candidacy for craniotomy, and prepare the patient for surgery. Although general surgeons usually are not permitted to perform the craniotomy, they may take primary responsibility for the postoperative care of patients with TBI, including the treatment of brain swelling. This trend raises concern, because general surgeons usually do not have a specific research interest in TBI, nor do they have the neurosurgeon's extensive training in neurologic disease. A multispecialty approach is optimal for the patient with TBI, wherein the neurosurgeon is directly involved from the emergency department evaluation until discharge. Through professional journals and meetings, neurosurgeons are most likely to be familiar with contemporary treatment of TBI that will provide the greatest opportunity for functional recovery. However, because of the relatively small number of neurosurgeons, this recommendation may not be practical for all communities and may require a nationwide restructuring of trauma programs so that all patients with severe TBI are admitted to designated regional trauma centers.

CLINICAL TRIALS

Controlled, randomized clinical trials are essential for determining the efficacy of new treatments for TBI. However, such trials are much more difficult to design and execute than those for other neurologic diseases because of the small numbers of patients with TBI at any single trauma center, the heterogeneity of injury even among patients with similar GCS scores, and the obstacles to obtaining an accurate initial neurologic evaluation. In addition, a high percentage of patients with TBI are indigent and/or homeless, making follow-up very difficult. For all of these reasons, a high-quality clinical trial that can be completed in less than 3–5 years is very expensive and requires collaboration among a number of trauma centers. The United States Public Health Service has provided the resources for some of the studies, but others have had to rely on the sponsorship of pharmaceutical companies, a situation with inescapable potential for bias.

During the last decade, clinical trials of four treatments for severe TBI have been completed: tromethamine (THAM), an alkalizing agent; nimodipine, a calcium channel blocker; superoxide dismutase conjugated to polyethylene glycol (PEG-SOD), a free-radical scavenger; and moderate hypothermia, which is believed to reduce the posttraumatic levels of extracellular excitatory amino acids. In Europe, THAM was studied in 80 patients with severe TBI, and its efficacy in reducing brain swelling was compared with that of mannitol and sorbitol.[46] THAM was found to cause a more sustained reduction in ICP than the other two drugs. In the United States, the efficacy of THAM was studied in a controlled, randomized multicenter trial of 149 patients with severe TBI.[170] Neurologic outcome measured 3, 6, and 12 months after injury was no better in the THAM-treated group than in the placebo group, but the patients who received THAM had a lower ICP during the first 48 hours after injury. In Ireland, nimodipine was investigated in a series of 356 patients with TBI who were randomized to receive either the drug or placebo.[4] Six months after injury, the rate of moderate or good recovery was slightly higher in the nimodipine-treated group than in the placebo group, but the differences did not reach statistical significance. A recently completed multicenter trial compared the effects of PEG-SOD at different doses with those of a placebo.[119] In this study of 104 patients, the group that received high-dose PEG-SOD (10,000 U/kg) had a significantly lower rate of death ($p < 0.03$) or vegetative state ($p = 0.04$) at both 3 and 6 months after injury. The rate of mild or no disability, however, was not significantly different from that of the placebo group.

The results of three independent clinical trials of therapeutic moderate hypothermia in patients with severe TBI were reported during the autumn of 1993. In a Japanese study, 33 patients who had ICP elevations refractory to barbiturate therapy were randomized to receive at least 2 days of hypothermic therapy (surface cooling to 34° C) or to be kept normothermic.[153] The hypothermic group had significantly reduced ICP and significantly higher cerebral perfusion pressures compared with the normothermic group, as well as a trend toward improved outcome. At the University of Pittsburgh, 40 patients with severe TBI were randomized to hypothermia (32–33° C) for 24 hours or to normothermia immediately after stabilization in the emergency department.[95] The study found a significant reduction in ICP and a trend toward improved outcome in the hypothermia group as compared with the normothermic group. A University of Texas study of 46 patients with TBI—of similar design except that the experimental group was cooled for 48 instead of 24 hours—also noted a trend toward improved outcome in the hypothermic patients.[28] A multicenter study of moderate hypothermia has been initiated based on the hypothesis that statistically significant differences in outcome will emerge if a larger number of patients is studied.

Tirilazad, a synthetic 21-amino steroid, is currently under evaluation in an international multicenter study sponsored by Upjohn Corporation. In animal models, the drug has been more effective than conventional steroids in retarding or inhibiting membrane lipid peroxidation, an important component of secondary brain injury.[61] Studies also have found that Tirilazad-treated animals have a significantly better behavioral and functional outcome after TBI than control animals.[109] Results of the clinical multicenter trial are expected within the next 1–2 years.

EARLY PROGNOSTICATION

The results of a large epidemiologic study of patients with severe TBI were published in late 1991, providing a relatively recent database from which early prognostic indicators can be distilled.[44] This prospective NIH-supported study, the Traumatic Coma Databank, included more than 1,000 patients admitted to four participating trauma centers from 1984–1987. Data from the study indicate that the likelihood of death or severe disability can be predicted for most patients with TBI within hours or days after injury. In their review of the data, Choi et al. found that the presence of a fixed and dilated pupil, low motor score on the Glasgow Coma Scale, and age greater than 60 years strongly predicted death or severe disability.[27] When considered independently, however, the predictive accuracy of these clinical findings was substantially reduced.

Kaufman et al. studied 100 patients with severe TBI to determine the reliability of combined findings from the neurologic examination and radiologic studies during the first 24 hours after injury in predicting outcome.[78] Ultimate neurologic outcome was estimated correctly in only 56–59% of the cases. The authors concluded that even with sophisticated clinical and radiologic techniques, it was not possible to predict outcome during the first day with sufficient accuracy to guide early treatment or to justify withholding of treatment. Others have suggested that MRI may be used during the first several days to predict outcome. MRI is more sensitive than CT for detecting posttraumatic lesions, but MRI scans obtained within 30 days after injury reveal many small and temporary lesions that do not correlate with functional outcome.[130] MRI obtained several months after injury, however, may be useful for defining the extent of permanent anatomic injury.[7]

Analysis of the ventricular or lumbar CSF after TBI reveals high levels of a number of compounds not normally found. Both the concentration and rate of decline of CSF creatine kinase BB,[34] lactate,[138] catecholamines,[97] and cytokines[104,105] have been correlated with outcome. In one study, the isoenzyme activity of creatine kinase BB was more closely associated with outcome at 6 months than four other risk factors, including GCS and age.[64] However, most of these studies found that CSF analysis was best for predicting death or good outcome and not highly sensitive for predicting in-between categories.

Exposure to models of outcome prediction has been shown to affect the acute care provided to patients with severe TBI. Murray et al. prospectively studied over 1,000 patients with TBI admitted to 4 neurosurgical units in Great Britain from 1986 to 1989.[120] The study was divided into three phases: a baseline period of at least 1 year before the introduction of a computer-based model for outcome prediction, 1 year when outcome predictions were provided to the attending physicians, and the final 7 months when prediction models were withdrawn. During the period when outcome predictions were provided, the use of osmotic diuretics, ICP monitors, and intubation and/or controlled ventilation increased for patients predicted to have a good outcome and decreased by 39% for patients predicted to have a poor outcome.

During the last several years, the prognostic utility of several other clinical findings and monitoring techniques has been investigated, but the value of many remains inconclusive. The following list summarizes the reliability of clinical signs or tests that can be used in the first few days after injury to determine the ultimate functional outcome:

Very Reliable

> Glasgow Coma Scale Score, particularly the motor subscore*[27]
> Pupil abnormalities*[27]
> Age*[165]
> Intracranial pressure†[98,114,145]
> Cerebral blood flow (absence of flow)[49]
> Electroencephalogram (no electrical activity even at high gain)[17]

* When all three are considered together, they are a very powerful predictive tool.
† Strong negative predictor when sustained above 30 mmHg for several hours, despite aggressive treatment.

Probably Reliable

> CT scan[100,101]
> Evoked potentials (repeated studies)[75,116]
> Continuous EEG (compressed spectral array)[117,159]
> Levels of creatine kinase BB isoenzyme in the cerebrospinal fluid[64]

Not Reliable

> MRI[130]
> CBF (other than absent flow)[70]
> AVdO$_2$ studies[70]
> Transcranial Doppler[167]
> Evoked potentials (single study)[86]

Most of these studies are much more accurate for predicting who will die or remain severely disabled than for determining who will recover with minimal or no disabilities. Serial observations of neurologic recovery over weeks or months remain the best means to predict complete or near-complete recovery.

Early prognostication requires careful consideration of several issues. First, for obvious humanitarian and economic reasons, the patient's family should be given prognostic information that is fairly certain. Particularly when the prognosis is poor, the physician and family can arrive at a consensus about withholding or withdrawing inappropriate surgery or medications. With increasingly scarce health care resources, care should not be diverted from patients who may benefit to preserve vegetative survival. However, models of outcome prediction must take into account the most recent findings regarding outcome-improving therapy and must be updated carefully and rapidly. In addition, clinicians must remember that predictive models are based on the statistical analysis of a large number of patients and may not apply to specific individuals. In analyzing the literature to identify reliable early predictors of outcome, it also is important to interpret the data correctly with particular care to distinguish between "associations" vs. "cause and effect." For example, in a study of 102 patients with severe TBI, Robertson et al. found that the mortality rate at 3 months was 32% in the subgroup of patients with a mean CBF of 29 ml/100gm/min and 20% in the subgroup with a mean CBF of 62 ml/100gm/min.[139] Despite the association between low CBF and poor outcome, the study was not designed to test the hypothesis that low CBF causes a poor outcome or that all patients with a low CBF have a poor outcome; nor do the results validate either hypothesis. In addition, the study did not determine whether outcome could be improved by artificially elevating the CBF when it was low.

ROLE OF THE NEUROSURGEON IN LONG-TERM CARE OF PERSONS WITH TRAUMATIC BRAIN INJURY

After the period of acute hospitalization most patients with TBI are unlikely to develop neurosurgical diseases, and involvement of neurosurgeons becomes less important than the care provided by physiatrists, neuropsychologists, and therapists. This is particularly true for patients with mild or moderate TBI, in whom the most likely long-term disabilities are elements of postconcussion syndrome. Patients who suffer severe TBI are at greatest risk for developing hydrocephalus or chronic subdural hematomas and therefore should be reevaluated by the neurosurgeon every 3–6 months for several years after their injury. Because the neurosurgeon is the first physician with whom the patient and family have closely interacted regarding the TBI, long-term follow-up is of great emotional benefit.

Neurosurgical consultation should be requested for persons with a history of TBI who initially improve and then develop headaches, visual blurring, diplopia, cranial nerve or peripheral motor or sensory deficits, gait difficulties, or incontinence. Such symptoms and signs may indicate the development of hydrocephalus or chronic subdural hematoma.

Most neurosurgical training programs, however, do not prepare the neurosurgeon for contemporary long-term rehabilitation of patients with TBI. Typically, the neurosurgeon knows little about proper physical therapy for comatose patients, heterotopic ossification, central neurostimulants, or many other issues related to long-term TBI rehabilitation. Thus, neurosurgeons should not attempt to direct rehabilitation. This role is best filled by a physiatrist or neurologist with physiatric training.

CONCLUSION

Innovations in the treatment of secondary brain injury undoubtedly will lead to continued improvement in outcome, and new therapeutic options will be discovered as the biochemical and cellular mechanisms for secondary injury are better defined. Together with improved prevention, including the widespread use of air bags and seat belts and improved motor vehicle design to lessen the damage caused by side collisions, a dramatic decline in mortality and morbidity from TBI can be expected during the next 10 years. There is an urgent need for carefully conducted and well-financed multicenter clinical trials to establish the efficacy of promising new treatments. However, the initiation of such trials will require substantial commitment from the federal government as well as from pharmaceutical companies. Clinicians must resist the temptation to act on anecdotal reports of the efficacy of new therapies. Another important avenue for improving care is the more appropriate use of traditional therapies such as hyperventilation and mannitol. In the past, the inappropriate use of hyperventilation therapy may in fact have jeopardized neurologic outcome. If hyperventilation and other therapies are used only when appropriate for the physiologic requirements of the damaged brain, outcome can be improved substantially. The current decade will be an exciting era for the acute care of patients with TBI, and rapid advances in effective treatment are anticipated.

REFERENCES

1. American College of Surgeons, Subcommittee on Advanced Trauma Life Support of the Committee on Trauma: Advanced Trauma Life Support. Chicago, American College of Surgeons, 1993.
2. Anderson DC, Bundie S, Rockswold GL: Multimodality evoked potentials in closed head trauma. Arch Neurol 41:369–374, 1984.
3. Andrews BT, Pitts LH, Lovely MP, et al: Is computed tomographic scanning necessary in patients with tentorial herniation? Results of immediate surgical exploration without computed tomography in 100 patients. Neurosurgery 19:408–414, 1986.
4. Bailey I, Bell A, Gray J, Gullan R: A trial of the effect of nimodipine on outcome after head injury. Acta Neurochir (Wien) 110:97–105, 1991.
5. Becker DP, Miller JD, Ward JD, et al: The outcome from severe head injury with early diagnosis and intensive management. J Neurosurg 47:491–502, 1977.
6. Biagas KV, Uhl MW, Schiding JK, et al: Assessment of posttraumatic polymorphonuclear leukocyte accumulation in rat brain using tissue myeloperoxidase assay and vinblastine treatment. J Neurotrauma 9:363–371, 1992.
7. Biglere ED, Kurth SM, Blatter D, Abildskov TJ: Degenerative changes in traumatic brain injury: Post-injury magnetic resonance identified ventricular expansion compared to pre-injury levels. Brain Res Bull 28:651–653, 1992.
8. Bornstein RA, Miller HB, Van Schoor JT: Neuropsychological deficit and emotional disturbance in head-injured patients. J Neurosurg 70:509–513, 1989.
9. Bouma GJ, Muizelaar JP, Bandoh K, Marmarou A: Blood pressure and intracranial pressure-volume dynamics in severe head injury: Relationship with cerebral blood flow. J Neurosurg 77:15–19, 1992.
10. Bouma GJ, Muizelaar JP, Choi SC, et al: Cerebral circulation and metabolism after severe traumatic brain injury: The elusive role of ischemia. J Neurosurg 75:685–693, 1991.
11. Bouma GJ Muizelaar JP, Stringer WA, et al: Ultra early evaluation of regional cerebral blood flow in severely head injured patients using xenon enhanced computed tomography. J Neurosurg 77:360–368, 1992
12. Bowers SA, Marshall LF: Outcome in 200 consecutive cases of severe head injury treated in San Diego County: A prospective analysis. Neurosurgery 6:237–242, 1980.
13. Braakman R, Avezaat CJ, Maas AI, and et al: Interobserver agreement in the assessment of the motor response of the Glasgow 'coma' scale. Clin Neurol Neurosurg 80:100–106, 1977.
14. Bracken MB, Shepard MJ, Collins WF, et al: Methyl-prednisolone or naloxone treatment after acute spinal cord injury: 1-year follow-up data. J Neurosurg 76:23–31, 1992
15. Brawley BW, Kelly WA: Treatment of basal skull fractures with and without cerebrospinal fluid fistulae. J Neurosurg 26:57–61, 1967.
16. Bricolo A: Electoencephalography in neurotraumatology. Clin Electroencephalography 7:184–197, 1976.
17. Buchner H, Schuchardt, V: Reliability of the electroencephalogram in the diagnosis of brain death. Eur Neurol 30: 138–141, 1990.
18. Buckley P, Stack JP, Madigan C, et al: Magnetic resonance imaging of schizophrenia-like psychoses associated with cerebral trauma: Clinicopathological correlates. Am J Psychiatry 150:146–148, 1993.
19. Bullock R, Sakas D, Patterson J, et al: Early posttraumatic cerebral blood flow mapping: Correlation with structural damage after focal injury. Acta Neurochir Suppl (Wien) 55:14–17, 1992.
20. Busto R, Dietrich WD, Globus MYT, Ginsberg MD: The importance of brain temperature in cerebral ischemic injury. Stroke 20:1113–1114, 1989.
21. Busto R, Dietrich WD, Globus MYT, et al: Small differences in intraischemic brain temperature critically determine the extent of ischemic neuronal injury. J Cereb Blood Flow Metab 7:729–738, 1993.
22. Busto R, Globus MYT, Dietrich WD, et al: Effect of mild hypothermia on ischemia-induced release of neurotransmitters and free fatty acids in rat brain. Stroke 7:904–910, 1989.
23. Cardoso ER Galbraith S: Posttraumatic hydrocephalus: A retrospective review. Surg Neurol 23:261–268, 1985.
24. Chan KH, Miller JD, Dearden NM: Intracranial blood flow velocity after head injury: Relationship to severity of injury, time, neurological status and outcome. J Neurol Neurosurg Psychiatry 55:787–791, 1992.
25. Chestnut RM, Marshall LF, Klauber MR, et al: The role of secondary brain injury in determining outcome from severe head injury. J Trauma 34:216–222, 1993.
26. Choi D: Methods for antagonizing glutamate neurotoxicity. Cerebrovasc Brain Metab 2:105–147, 1990.
27. Choi SC, Narayan RK, Anderson RL, Ward JD: Enhanced specificity of prognosis in severe head injury. J Neurosurg 69:381–385, 1988.

28. Clifton GL, Allen S, Barrodale P, et al: A phase II study of moderate hypothermia in severe brain injury. J Neurotrauma 10:263–271, 1993.

29. Clifton GL, Lyeth BG, Jenkins LW, et al: Effect of D1 α-tocopherol succinate and polyethylene glycol on performance tests after fluid percussion brain injury. Neurotrauma 6:71–81, 1989.

30. Coles JC, Ahmed SM, Mehta ITU, Kaufman JC: Role of radical scavenger in protection of spinal cord during ischemia. Ann Thorac Surg 41:555–556, 1986.

31. Colohan ART, Alves WM, Gross CR, et al: Head injury mortality in two centers with different emergency medical services and intensive care. J Neurosurg 71:202–207, 1989.

32. Contant CF, Robertson CS, Gopinath SP, et al: Determination of clinically important thresholds in continuously monitored patients with head injury (abstract). Glasgow, Scotland, Second International Neurotrauma Symposium, July 4–9, 1993, p 4.

33. Cooper PR: Delayed brain injury: Secondary insults. In Becker DP, Povlishock J (eds): Central Nervous System Trauma Status Report. Bethesda, MD, National Institute of Neurological and Communicative Disorders and Stroke, National Institutes of Health, 1985, pp 217–228.

34. Cooper PR, Chalif DJ, Ramsey JF Moore RJ: Radioimmunoassay of the brain type isoenzyme of creatine phosphokinase (CK-BB): A new diagnostic tool in the evaluation of patients with head injury. Neurosurgery 12:536–541, 1983.

35. Crutchfield JS, Narayan RK, Robertson CS, et al: Evaluation of a fiberoptic intracranial pressure monitor. J Neurosurg 71:482–487, 1990.

36. DeMuth WE: Bullet velocity as applied to military rifle wounding capacity. J Trauma 9:27–38, 1969.

37. Derosier C, Brinquin L, Bonsignour JP, Cosnard G: MRI and cranial traumas in the acute phase. J Neuroradiol 18:309–319, 1991.

38. Dienel GA: Regional accumulation of calcium in postischemic rat brain. J Neurochem 43:913–925, 1984.

39. Dikmen SS, Temkin NR, Miller B, et al: Neurobehavioral effects of phenytoin prophylaxis of posttraumatic seizures [see comments]. JAMA 265:1271–1277, 1991.

40. Edna TH: Acute traumatic intracranial hematoma and skull fractures. Acta Chir Scand 149:449–451, 1983.

41. Faden AI: TRH analog YM-14673 improves outcome following traumatic brain and spinal cord injury. Brain Res 486:229–235, 1989.

42. Feeney DM, Gonzalez A, Law WA: Amphetamine, heloperidol and experience interact to affect rate of recovery after motor cortex injury. Science 217:855–857, 1982.

43. Fielding K, Rowley G: Reliability of assessments by skilled observers using the Glasgow Coma Scale. Aust J Adv Nurs 7:12–21, 1990.

44. Foulkes MA, Eisenberg HM, Jane JA, et al: the traumatic coma data bank: Design, methods, and baseline characteristics. J Neurosurg 75:S8–S13, 1991.

45. Francis CW, Pellegrini VD Jr, Marder VJ, et al: Comparison of warfarin and external pneumatic compression in prevention of venous thrombosis after total hip replacement [see comments]. JAMA 267:2911–2915, 1992.

46. Gaab MR, Seegers, Smedema RJ, et al: A comparative analysis of THAM (tris-buffer) in traumatic brain edema. Acta Neurochir Suppl (Wien) 51:320–323, 1990.

47. Gennarelli TA, Thibault LE, Adams JH, et al: Diffuse axonal injury and traumatic coma in the primate. Ann Neurol 12:564–574, 1982.

48. Gerberich SG, Priest JD, Boen JR: Concussion incidences and severity in secondary school varsity football players. Am J Public Health 73:1370–1375, 1983.

49. Goodman JM, Heck LL, Moore BD: Confirmation of brain death with portable isotope angiography: A review of 204 consecutive cases. Neurosurgery 16:492–497, 1985.

50. Graham DI, Ford I, Adama JH, et al: Ischaemic brain damage is still common in fatal non-missile head injury. J Neurol Neurosurg Psychiatry 52:346–350, 1989

51. Grahm TW, Williams FC, Harrington T, Spetzler RF: Civilian gunshot wounds to the head: A prospective study. Neurosurgery 27:695–700, 1990.

52. Greenberg RP, Becker DP, Miller JD, et al: Evaluation of brain function in severe human head trauma with multimodality evoked potentials: Part 2: Localization of brain dysfunction and correlation with posttraumatic neurological conditions. J Neurosurg 47:163–177, 1977.

53. Greenberg RP, Mayer DJ, Becker DP: Evaluation of brain function in severe human head trauma with multimodality evoked potentials: Part 1: Evoked brain injury potentials: Methods and analysis. J Neurosurg 47:150–162, 1977.

54. Grice S, Chappell E, Prough D, et al: Ibuprofen improves cerebral blood flow after global cerebral ischemia in dogs. Stroke 18:787–791, 1987.

55. Gronwall D, Wrightson P: Delayed recovery of intellectual function after minor head injury. Lancet 2:605–609, 1974.

56. Gudeman SK, Kishore PRS, Becker DP: Computed tomography in the evaluation of the incidence and significance of posttraumatic hydrocephalus. Neuroradiology 141:397–341, 1981.

57. Gurdijian ES, Webster JG, Stone WE: Experimental head injury with specific reference to certain chemical factors in acute trauma. Surg Gynecol Obstet 78:618–626, 1944.

58. Gurdjian ES: Cerebral contusions: Re-evaluation of the mechanisms of their development. J Trauma 16:35–51, 1976.

59. Gutman MB, Moulton RJ, Sullivan I, et al: Risk factors predicting operable intracranial hematomas in head injury. J Neurosurg 77:9–14, 1992.

60. Hall E, Braughler J: Role of lipid peroxidation in post-traumatic spinal cord degeneration—a review. J Neurotrauma 3:281–294, 1986.

61. Hall ED: Lipid antioxidants in acute central nervous system injury. Ann Emerg Med 22:1022–1027, 1993.

62. Hall ED, Yonkers PA, Andrus PK, et al: Biochemistry and pharmacology of lipid antioxidants in acute brain and spinal cord injury. J Neurotrauma 9:S425–S442, 1992.

63. Hallenbeck JT, Jacobs TP, Faden AI: Combined PGI2, indomethacin and heparin improve recovery after spinal trauma in cats. J Neurosurg 58:749–754, 1983.

64. Hans P, Albert A, Franssen C, Born J: Improved outcome prediction based on CSF extrapolated creatine kinase BB isoenzyme activity and other risk factors in severe head injury [see comments]. J Neurosurg 71:54–58, 1989.

65. Hayes R, Stonnington H, Lyeth B, et al: Metabolic and neurophysiologic sequelae of brain injury: A cholinergic hypothesis. J Neurotrauma 3:163–173, 1986.

66. Hernesniemi J: Penetrating craniocerebral gunshot wounds in civilians. Acta Neurochir 49:199–205, 1979.

67. Hopkinson DAW, Marshall TK: Firearm injuries. Br J Surg 54:344–353, 1967.

68. Hugenholtz H, Stuss DT, Stethem LL, Richard MT: How long does it take to recover from a mild concussion. Neurosurgery 22:853–858, 1988.

69. Hull R, Raskob G, Pineo G, et al: A comparison of subcutaneous low-molecular-weight heparin with warfarin sodium for prophylaxis against deep-vein thrombosis after hip or knee implantation [see comments]. N Engl J Med 329: 1370–1376, 1993.

70. Jaggi JL, Obrist WD, Gennarelli TA, Lanfitt TW: Relationship of early cerebral blood flow and metabolism to outcome in acute head injury. J Neurosurg 72:176–182, 1990.

71. Javid M, Settlage P: Effect of urea on cerebrospinal fluid pressure in human subjects. Preliminary report. JAMA 160:943–949, 1956.

72. Jennett B, Teasdale G: Management of Head Injuries, 20th ed. Philadelphia FA Davis, 1981, pp 19–43.

73. Jennett B, Teasdale G: Management of Head Injuries, 20th ed. Philadelphia, FA Davis, 1981, pp. 45–75.

74. Jennett B, Teasdale G, Galbraith S, et al: Severe head injuries in three countries. J Neurol Neurosurg Psychiatry 40:291–298, 1977.

75. Kamath MV, Reddy SN, Ghista DN, et al: Power spectral analysis of normal and pathological brainstem auditory evoked potentials. Int J Biomed Comput 21:33–54, 1987.

76. Kanter MJ, Narayan RK: Intracranial pressure monitoring. In Eisenberg HM, Aldrich EF (eds): Neurosurgery Clinics of North America, 2nd ed. Philadelphia, WB Saunders, 1991, pp 387–397.

78. Kaufmann MA, Buchmann B, Scheidegger D, et al: Severe head injury: Should expected outcome influence resuscitation and first-day decisions. Resuscitation 23:199–206, 1992.

79. Kety SS, Schmidt CF: The nitrous oxide method for the quantitative determination of cerebral blood flow in man: Theory, procedure and normal values. J Clin Invest 27:476–483, 1948.

80. Kirby DF Clifton GL, Turner H, et al: Early enteral nutrition after brain injury by percutaneous endoscopic gastrojejunostomy. J Parent Ent Nutrit 15:298–302, 1991.

81. Kochanek PM, Hallenbeck JM: Polymorphonuclear leukocytes and monocytes/macrophages in the pathogenesis of cerebral ischemia and stroke. Stroke 23:1367–1379, 1992.

82. Kontos, HA: Oxygen radicals in central nervous system damage. Chem Biol Int 72:229–255, 1989.

83. Langfitt TW: Measuring the outcome from head injuries. J Neurosurg 48:673–678, 1978.

84. LeVere TE, Brugler T, Sandin M, Gray-Silva S: Recovery of function after brain damage: Facilitation by the calcium entry blocker nimodipine. Behav Neurosci 103:500–511, 1989.

85. Levin HS, Meyers CA, Grossman RG: Ventricular enlargement after closed head injury. Arch Neurol 38:623–628, 1981.

86. Lindsay K, Pasaoglu A, Hirst D, et al: Somatosensory and auditory brain stem conduction after head injury: A comparison with clinical features in predictions of outcome. Neurosurgery 26:278–285, 1990.

87. Liu TH, Beckman JS, Freeman BA, et al: Polyethylene-glycol-conjugated superoxide dismutase and catalase reduce ischemic brain injury. Am J Physiol 256:H589–H592, 1989.

88. Livingston, DH, Loder PA, Hunt, CD: Minimal head injury: Is admission necessary? Am Surg 57:14–17, 1991.

89. Lundberg N, Kjallquist A, Bien C: Reduction of increased intracranial pressure by hyperventilation. Acta Psychiatr Scand 34:4–64, 1959.

90. Lundberg N, Troupp H, Lorin H: Continuous recording of the ventricular fluid pressure in patients with severe acute traumatic brain damage. A preliminary report. J Neurosurg 22:581–590, 1965.

91. Marion DW, Bouma GJ: The use of stable xenon-enhanced computed tomographic studies of cerebral blood flow to define changes in cerebral blood flow to define changes in cerebral carbon dioxide vasoresponsivity caused by a severe head injury. Neurosurgery 29:869–873, 1991.

92. Marion DW, Carlier PM: Problems with initial glasgow coma score assessment caused by the prehospital treatment of head-injured patients: Results of a national survey. J Trauma 36:89–95, 1994.

93. Marion DW, Carlier PM, Obrist WD, Darby JM: Treatment of cerebral ischemia improves outcome following severe traumatic brain injury (abstract). INS 2nd: O72, 1993.

94. Marion DW Darby J, Yonas H: Acute regional cerebral blood flow changes caused by severe head injuries. J Neurosurg 74:407–414, 1991.

95. Marion DW, Obrist WD, Carlier PM, et al: The use of moderate therapeutic hypothermia for patients with severe head injuries: A preliminary report. J Neurosurg 79:354–362, 1993.

96. Marion DW, Ward JD: Steroids in closed-head injury. In Cerra FB (ed): Perspectives in Critical Care. St. Louis, Quality Medical Publishing, 1990, pp 19–39.

97. Markianos M, Seretis A, Kotsou S, et al: CSF neurotransmitter metabolites and short-term outcome of patients in coma after head injury. Acta Neurol Scand 86:190–193, 1992.

98. Marmarou A, Anderson RL, Ward JD, et al: Impact of ICP instability and hypotension on outcome with severe head trauma. J Neurosurg 75:S59–S66, 1991.

99. Marshall LF, Becker DP, Bowers SA, et al: The national traumatic coma data bank. J Neurosurg 59:276–284, 1983.

100. Marshall LF, Gautille T, Klauber MR, et al: The outcome of severe closed head injury. J Neurosurg 75:S28–S36, 1991.

101. Marshal LF, Marshall SB, Klauber MR, et al: The diagnosis of head injury requires a classification based on computed axial tomography. J Neurotrauma 9:S287–S292, 1992.

102. Marshall LF, Smith RW, Shapiro HM: The outcome with aggressive treatment in severe head injuries:I. The significance of intracranial pressure monitoring. J Neurosurg 50:20–25, 1979.

103. Mayhall CG, Archer NH, Lamb VA, et al: Ventriculostomy - related infections. N Engl J Med 311:553–559, 1984.

104. McClain C, Cohen D, Phillips R, et al: Increased plasma and ventricular fluid interleukin-6 levels in patients with head injury [see comments]. J Lab Clin Med 118:225–231, 1991.

105. McClain CJ, Cohen D, Ott L, et al: Ventricular fluid interleukin-1 activity in patients with head injury. J Lab Clin Med 110:48–54, 1987.

106. McIntosh T, Soares H, Hayes R, Simon R: The NMDA receptor antagonist MK-801 prevents edema and restores magnesium homeostasis after traumatic brain injury in the rat. In Cavaliero J, Lehman J (eds): Frontiers in Excitatory Amino Acid Research. New York, Alan Liss, 1988.

107. McIntosh TK, Faden AI, Yamakami I, Vink R: Magnesium deficiency exacerbates and pretreatment improves outcome following traumatic brain injury in rats: 31P magnetic resonance spectroscopy and behavioral studies. J Neurotrauma 5:17–31, 1988.

108. McIntosh TK, Fernyak S, Faden AI: The effects of naloxone hydrochloride treatment after experimental traumatic brain injury. J Cereb Blood Flow Metab 11 (Suppl 2):S734, 1991.

109. McIntosh TK, Thomas M, Smith DF, Banbury M: The novel 21-aminosteroid U74006F attenuates cerebral edema and improves survival after brain injury in the rat. J Neurotrauma 9:33–46, 1992.

110. McIntosh TK, Vink R, Soares H, et al: Effects of the N-methyl-D-aspartate receptor blocker MK-801 on neurologic function after experimental brain injury. J Neurotrauma 6:247–259, 1989.

112. Mendelow AD, Teasdale, GM, Russell T, et al: Effect of mannitol on cerebral blood flow and cerebral perfusion pressure in human head injury. J Neurosurg 63:43–48, 1985.

113. Miller JD, Bullock R, Graham DI, et al: Ischemic brain damage in a model of acute subdural hematoma. Neurosurgery 27:433–439, 1990.

114. Miller JD, Dearden NM, Piper IR, Chan KH: Control of intracranial pressure in patients with severe head injury. J Neurotrauma 9 (Suppl 1): S317–S326, 1992.

115. Mohr DN, Silverstein MD, Ilstrup et al: Venous thromboembolism associated with hip and knee arthroplasty: Current prophylactic practices and outcomes. Mayo Clin Proc 67:861–870, 1992

116. Moulton R, Kresta P, Ramirez M, Tucker W: Continuous automated monitoring of somatosensory evoked potentials in posttraumatic coma. J Trauma 31:676–685, 1991.

117. Moulton RJ, Marmarou A, Ronen J, et al: Spectral analysis of the EEG in craniocerebral trauma. Can J Neurol Sci 15:82–86, 1988.

118. Muizelaar JP, Marmarou A, Ward JD, et al: Adverse effects of prolonged hyperventilation in patients with severe head injury: A randomized clinical trial. J Neurosurg 75:731–739, 1991.

119. Muizelaar JP, Marmarou A, Young HF, et al: Improving the outcome of severe head injury with the oxygen radical scavenger polyethylene glycol-conjugated superoxide dismutase: A phase II trial. J Neurosurg 78:375–382, 1993.

120. Murray LS, Teasdale GM, Murray GD, et al: Does prediction of outcome alter patient management. Lancet 341:1487–1491, 1993

121. Narayan RK, Kishore PRS, Becker DP, et al: Intracranial pressure: To monitor or not to monitor. J Neurosurg 46:650–659, 1982

122. Nee PA, Hadfield JM, Yates DW: Biomechanical factors in patient selection for radiography after head injury. Injury 24:471–475, 1993

123. Nelson LR, Auen E, Bourke R, et al: A comparison of animal head injury models developed for treatment modality evaluation. In Grossman RG, Gildenberg P (eds): Head Injury: Basic and Clinical Aspects. New York, Raven Press, 1982, pp 117–127.

124. Nelson LR, Bourke RS, Popp AJ: A comparison of animal head injury models developed for treatment modality evaluation. In Popp AJ, Bourke LR, Nelson LR, Kimelberg HK (eds): Neural Trauma. New York, Raven Press, 1979, pp 291–311.

125. Nemoto EM, Shiu GK, Bleyaert AL: Efficacy of therapies and attenuation of brain free fatty acid liberation during global ischemia. Crit Care Med 9:397–398, 1981.

126. O'Sullivan MG, Statham PF, Jones PA, et al: Role of intracranial pressure monitoring in severely head-injured patients without signs of intracranial hypertension on initial computerized tomography. J Neurosurg 80:46–50, 1994.

127. Obrist WD, Langfitt TW, Jaggi JL, et al: Cerebral blood flow and metabolism in comatose patients with acute head injury. J Neurosurg 61:241–253, 1984.

128. Obrist WD, Marion DW, Aggarwal S: Time course of cerebral blood flow and metabolism in comatose patients with acute head injury [abstract]. J Cereb Blood Flow Metab 1993.

129. Office of the Inspector General: Specialty Coverage in Hospital Departments. Washington DC, Department of Health and Human Services, No OEI-01-91-007771, 1992.

130. Ogawa T, Sekino H, Uzura M, et al: Comparative study of magnetic resonance and CT scan imaging in cases of severe head injury. Acta Neurochir Suppl (Wien) 55:8–10, 1992.

131. Ommaya AK, Gennarelli TA: Cerebral concussion and traumatic unconsciousness. Correlation of experimental and clinical observations on blunt head injuries. Brain 97:638–642, 1974.

132. Paiement GD, Schutzer SF, Wessinger SJ, Harris WH: Influence of prophylaxis on proximal venous thrombus formation after total arthroplasty. J Arthroplasty 7:471–475, 1992.

133. Paiement GD, Wessinger SJ, Hughes R, Harris WH: Routine use of adjusted low-dose warfarin to prevent venous thromboembolism after total hip replacement. J Bone Joint Surg 75A:893–898, 1993.

134. Palmer AM, Marion DW, Botscheller ML, Redd EE: Traumatic brain injury-induced elevations in interstitial concentrations of aspartate and glutamate: Influence of therapeutic hypothermia, [abstract]. J Neurochem S284B, 1993.

135. Palmer AM, Marion DW, Botscheller ML, et al: Traumatic brain injury induced excitotoxicity assessed in a controlled cortical impact model. J Neurochem 61:2015–2024, 1993.

136. Piek J, Chesnut RM, Marshall LF, et al: Extracranial complications of severe head injury. J Neurosurg 77:901–907, 1992

137. Puniak MA, Freeman GM, Agresta CA, Salzman S: Comparison of serotonin antagonist, opioid antagonist and TRH analog for the acute treatment of experimental spinal cord trauma. J Neurotrauma 8:193–203, 1991.

138. Rabow L, DeSalles AF, Becker DP, et al: CSF brain creatine kinase levels and lactic acidosis in severe head injury. J Neurosurg 65:625–629, 1986.

139. Robertson CS, Contant CF, Gokaslan ZL, et al: Cerebral blood flow, arteriovenous oxygen difference, and outcome in head injured patients. J Neurol Neurosurg Psychiatry 55:594–603, 1992.

140. Robertson CS, Contant CF, Narayan RK, Grossman RG: Cerebral blood flow, AVDO2, and neurologic outcome in head-injured patients. J Neurotrauma 9:S349–S358, 1992.

141. Rosenorn J, Duus B, Nielsen K, et al: Is a skull X-ray necessary after milder head trauma? [see comments]. Br J Neurosurg 5:135–139, 1991.

142. Rosner MJ, Becker DP: Origin and evolution of plateau waves: experimental observations and a theoretical model. J Neurosurg 60:312–324, 1984.

143. Rosner MJ, Coley I: Cerebral perfusion pressure, the ICP and head elevation. J Neurosurg 65:636–641, 1986.

144. Rosner MJ, Daughton S: Cerebral perfusion pressure management in head injury. J Trauma 30: 933–941, 1990.

145. Ross AM, Pitts LH, Kobayashi S: Prognosticators of outcome after major head injury in the elderly. J Neurosci Nurs 24:88–93, 1992.

146. Ross DT, Graham KI, Adams JH: Selective loss of neurons from the thalamic reticular nucleus following severe human head injury. J Neurotrauma 10:151–165, 1993.

147. Salvant JB, Muizelaar JP: Changes in cerebral blood flow and metabolism related to the presence of subdural hematoma. Neurosurgery 33:387–393, 1993.

148. Salzman SK, Chaum JM, Wang L, et al: S-Emopamil improves functional recovery from experimental spinal trauma. J Neurotrauma 9:69, 1992.

149. Saul TG, Ducker TB: Effect of intracranial pressure monitoring and aggressive treatment on mortality in severe head injury. J Neurosurg 56: 498–503, 1982.

150. Schoettle RJ, Kochanek PM, Magargee MJ, et al: Early polymorphonuclear leukocyte accumulation correlates with the development of posttraumatic cerebral edema in rats. J Neurotrauma 7:207–217, 1990.

151. Seelig JM, Becker DP, Miller JD, et al: Traumatic acute subdural hematoma. Major mortality reduction in comatose patients treated within four hours. N Engl J Med 304:1511–1512, 1982.

152. Shin DY, Ehrenberg B, Whyte J, et al: Evoked potential assessment: Utility in prognosis of chronic head injury. Arch Phys Med Rehabil 70:189–193, 1989.

153. Shiozaki T, Hisashi S, Taneda M, et al; Effect of mild hypothermia uncontrollable intracranial hypertension after severe head injury. J Neurosurg 79:363–368, 1993.

154. Siesjo BJ, Wieloch T: Brain injury: Neurochemical aspects. In Becker DP, Povlishock J (eds): Central Nervous System Status Report. Bethesda, MD, National Institute of Neurological and Communication Disorders and Stroke, National Institutes of Health, 1985, pp 5133–532.

155. Smith DH, Okiyama K, McIntosh TK: Magnesium and ketamine attenuate cognitive dysfunction following experimental brain injury. Neurosci Lett 1993 (in press).

156. Stuart GG, Merry GS, Smith JA, Yelland JDN: Severe head injury managed without intracranial pressure monitoring. J Neurosurg 59:601–605, 1983.

157. Teasdale G. The treatment of head trauma: Implications for the future. J Neurotrauma 8 (Suppl 1): S53–S58, 1991.

158. Teasdale G, Jennett B: Assessment of coma and impaired consciousness. A practical scale. Lancet 2:81–84, 19974.

159. Tebano MT, Cameroni M, Gallozzi G, et al: EEG spectral analysis after minor head injury in man. Electroencephalogr Clin Neurophysiol 70:185–189, 1988.

160. Temkin NR, Dikmen SS, Wilensky AJ, et al: A randomized double-blind study of phenytoin for the prevention of post-traumatic seizures. N Engl J Med 323:497–502, 1990.

161. Thatcher RW, Walker RA, Gerson I, et al: EEG discriminant analyses of mild head trauma. Electroencephalogr Clin Neurophysiol 73:94–106, 1989.

162. Tomei, G, Sganzerla E, Spagnoli D, et al: Posttraumatic diffuse cerebral lesions. Relationship between clinical course, CT findings and ICP. J Neurosurg Sci 35:61–75, 1991.

163. Trimble MR: Anticonvulsant drugs and cognitive function: A review of the literature. Epilepsia 28:537–545, 1987.

164. Tseng SH: Reduction of herniated temporal lobe in patients with severe head injury and uncal herniation. J Formos Med Assoc 91:24–28, 1992.

165. Vollmer, DG, Torner JC, Jane JA, et al: Age and outcome following traumatic coma: Why do older patients fare worse? J Neurosurg 75:S37–S49, 1991.

166. Wald SL, Shackford SR, Fenwich J: The effect of secondary insults on mortality and long-term disability after severe head injury in a rural region without a trauma system. J Trauma 34:377–381, 1993.

167. Weber M, Grolimund P, Seiler RW: Evaluation of posttraumatic cerebral blood flow velocities by transcranial doppler ultrasonography. J Neurosurgery 27:106–112, 1990.

168. Wise BL, Chater N: The value of hypertonic mannitol solution in decreasing brain mass and lowering cerebrospinal-fluid pressure. J Neurosurg 19:1038–1043, 1962.

169. Wisner DH, Victor NS, Holcroft JW: Priorities in the management of multiple trauma: Intracranial versus intra-abdominal injury. J Trauma 35:271–278, 1993.

170. Wolf AL, Levi L, Marmarou A, et al: Effect of THAM upon outcome in severe head injury: A randomized prospective clinical trial. J Neurosurg 78:54–59, 1993.

171. Woodroofe MN, Sarna GS, Wadhwa M, et al: Detection of interleukin-1 and interleukin-6 in adult rat brain, following mechanical injury, by in vivo microdialysis: Evidence of a role for microglia in cytokine production. J Neuroimmunol 33:227–236, 1991.

172. Yokota H, Kurokawa A, Otsuka T, et al: Significance of magnetic resonance imaging in acute head injury. J Trauma 31:351–357, 1991.

173. Zhuang J, Shackford SR, Schmoker JD, Anderson ML: The association of leukocytes with secondary brain injury. J Trauma 35:415–422, 1993.

W. JERRY MYSIW   M.D.

LISA P. FUGATE   M.D.

DANIEL M. CLINCHOT   M.D.

3

Assessment, Early Rehabilitation Intervention, and Tertiary Prevention

The initial physiatric evaluation of the patient who survives traumatic brain injury ideally should occur within the first 24 hours of the event. Rehabilitation no longer should be considered the final stage of the recovery process; instead rehabilitative assessment and intervention should be implemented in the acute recovery period and continue through the subacute and chronic stages for a comprehensive approach that maximizes functional outcome. Indeed, a small yet compelling body of evidence is evolving to support the concept that the early application of rehabilitation strategies shortens the length of hospitalization and enhances the quality of outcome.

The issues that a physiatrist must consider during the initial evaluation of a patient with moderate-to-severe traumatic brain injury include (1) assessment of residual impairments; (2) estimation of prognosis; (3) initiation of early rehabilitation intervention, emphasizing preparation for ongoing rehabilitation needs and prevention of complications; and (4) formulation of a long-term treatment plan that addresses the rehabilitation and reintegration needs of the patient. This chapter reviews the issues that are most germane to the physiatrist during the phase of intervention after traumatic brain injury.

ASSESSMENT

Residual Impairments

The impairments incurred secondary to a severe traumatic brain injury can be broadly categorized as physical, cognitive and neurobehavioral. Specific potential impairments are numerous and have been comprehensively reviewed elsewhere.[1] A thorough documentation of all impairments and deficits during the initial physiatric evaluation is neither practical nor possible, but attention certainly should be directed to impairments that affect prognosis or immediate rehabilitation strategies.

Because the majority of traumatic brain injuries result from motor vehicle accidents,[2] it is not unusual to find other organ systems primarily or secondarily affected by the blunt trauma (Table 1).[1] Hence, the rehabilitation team must be cognizant of medical issues, such as fractures, that may have been undetected during the acute stabilization. Similarly, team members ideally should use objective measures of recovery that are also

TABLE 1. Medical Complications of Traumatic Brain Injury with Early Rehabilitation Implications

Gastrointestinal system
  Nutrition
  Hemorrhage
Respiratory system
  Hypoxia
    Trauma—pulmonary/chest wall
    Infection
    Neurogenic pulmonary edema
Endocrine–metabolic system
  Fluid-electrolyte imbalance
  Hypothalamic–pituitary dysfunction
Hematologic system
  Anemia
  Bleeding diathesis
  Thromboembolic disease
Genitourinary system
  Neurogenic bladder
  Infection
  Stricture
Musculoskeletal
  Fracture
  Joint instability
  Heterotopic ossification
Cardiovascular system
  Arrhythmia
  Ischemia
  Contusion
  Hypotension
  Hypertension

TABLE 2. Neurologic Impairments*

Spasticity	Autonomic dysfunction
Rigidity	Causalgia
Monoparesis-plegia	Entrapment neuropathy
Hemiparesis-plegia	Field cuts
Triparesis-plegia	Diplopia
Quadraparesis-plegia	Dysphagia
Ataxia	Hearing loss
Tremor	

* Partial list emphasizing impairments that are important to note during the early assessment.

TABLE 3. Cognitive Impairments in the Coma-emerging Patient

Arousal	Orientation	Apraxia	Aphasia
Attention	Memory	Agnosia	Abstraction

TABLE 4. Common Neurobehavioral Deficits in the Coma-emerging Patient

Apathy	Aggressiveness	Emotional lability
Impulsivity	Anxiety	Lack of initiative
Irritability	Depression	Restlessness

sensitive to declines in function and thus may provide the first indication of medical complications.

The physical consequences of neurotrauma most critical for assessment and early intervention are those that affect swallowing, communication, mobility, and location (Table 2). Preliminary evaluation of swallowing and recommendations for treatment can be started at bedside while the patient is still in the intensive care unit and completed as the patient becomes more alert. The establishment of a consistent communication system is a prerequisite for determining the extent of cognitive deficits and thus appropriate rehabilitation interventions. Disorders affecting mobility and locomotion are often the primary focus of the family and render the survivor at risk for secondary complications.

Long-term follow-up studies suggest that the broad category of cognitive deficits has a greater impact on functional outcome than residual physical deficits.[3] However, the specific cognitive deficits with the most profound effect on long-term outcome remain to be determined. Thus, the cognitive skills most appropriate for screening during the initial assessment are those that affect communication and the ability to learn basic functional skills (Table 3).

Potential neurobehavioral consequences of severe traumatic brain injury are similarly comprehensive and often present the most challenging management problems (Table 4).[1] Agitation, the most dramatic behavioral consequence of severe TBI, has significant impact on the initial type of rehabilitation services. Both the presence and presentation of agitation have long-term prognostic implications.[4]

Prognosis

Predicting the outcome after a traumatic brain injury permits the development of a more meaningful individualized rehabilitation plan (Table 5). This information is also important to the family, who need to adjust to the catastrophic event. Finally, the ability to predict outcome accurately is important for program evaluation and in designing studies targeted to influence functional outcome. This section reviews the premorbid

TABLE 5. Indicators of Functional Prognosis after Traumatic Brain Injury

Indicator	Good Outcome	Poor Outcome
Increased premorbid intelligence	Missile injury	
Higher education	Higher verbal intelligence quotient	
Age	< 40 yr	> 50 yr
Recurrent traumatic brain injury	No	Yes
Coma duration	< 2 wks	> 4 wks
Glasgow Coma Scale (> 24 hrs)	> 5	≤ 5
Posttraumatic amnesia	< 2 wks	> 12 wks
Mass lesion		+
Subdural hematoma		+
Diffuse axonal injury	+	
3rd ventricle/basal cistern	Normal	Obliteration
Midline shift (> 4 mm)		+
Intracranial pressure	Normal	Increased
Hypotension (< 90 mmHg)		+
Hypoxia		+
Cerebral ischemia		+
Systemic injury	None	> 1 organ
Evoked potentials	Grade I	Grade IV
Catecholamines	Normal	Increased
Glucose	Normal	Increased
Cortisol	Normal	Increased
Thyroid	Normal	Decreased
Cerebrospinal fluid	Normal	Increased
Hydrocephalus ex vacuo		+
Early rehabilitation intervention	+	

characteristics and the factors of acute injury severity and status at presentation to rehabilitation that predict outcome.

Intelligence is one of the several premorbid characteristics that is predictive of outcome. It seems logical to assume that greater premorbid intelligence implies greater residual functional outcome after a traumatic brain injury of given severity. Pre- and post-injury intelligence scores do in fact correlate after a missile injury.[5] Severe blunt injuries, however, appear to have an equalizing affect; that is, blunt injuries matched for severity appear to result in uniform cognitive defects, regardless of premorbid intelligence. Lower premorbid intelligence, however, appears to lessen the potential for returning to work after a blunt injury. A survivor's premorbid educational level appears to have no impact on subsequent performance, IQ scores, or functional classification on the Glasgow Outcome Scale. There is, however, some correlation with premorbid level of education and the subsequent verbal IQ score.[5]

Age at the time of injury appears to be the most powerful premorbid prognostic indicator of both mortality and functional outcome.

Studies stratifying patients with severe TBI at 50, 60, 65, and 70 years of age have shown consistently that mortality dramatically increases with increasing age. This prognostic indicator remains significant even when the severity of the injury is controlled by using the Glasgow Coma Scale, the Injury Severity Scale, or other measures of trauma severity.[6] For example, one study compared outcome for survivors of a severe traumatic brain injury who were either over 60 or less than 40 years of age. The mortality rate was 79% in patients older than 60 years and 33% in those younger than 40 years.[6] The same study compared outcome at 6 months. Good outcome was limited to 2% of patients older than 60 years compared with 38% of patients younger than 40 years. Finally, age remained a significant prognostic indicator even after controlling for past medical history.[7] The reason for the age-based discrepancy in functional outcome is presumably due to the negative impact of age on motor recovery.[8,9] Impact of age on cognitive recovery[10] appears to be minimal.

Recurrent traumatic brain injury has recently received some attention as a premorbid prognostic indicator.[11] Most authorities believe that the consequences of a second traumatic brain injury are disproportionate to its severity. However, a recent review of the literature has documented the difficulty of supporting this hypothesis with existing studies that characteristically have no precise description of the initial injury, lack comparison groups, and fail to take into account the frequency of mild traumatic brain injury.[11]

The majority of purported prognostic indicators are related to the severity of injury. Both duration and depth of coma are markers of severity of injury with powerful prognostic implications. Prolonged coma has been associated with greater residual impairments in both motor and cognitive function.[10,12] When the primary mechanism of injury is diffuse axonal injury, the relationship between duration of coma and recovery time is almost linear.[13] When the duration of coma exceeds 1 month, functional outcome is classified as vegetative or severely disabled in approximately 20.5% of survivors, whereas it is classified as good or moderately disabled in 58.5%. Another study found that functional outcome was proportionately worse at 1 year after injury with increasing periods of coma. No patients who remained comatose for longer than 2 weeks achieved a good recovery.[13]

Studies looking at brief periods of coma also have documented significant impairments. Even 1 hour of coma had a significant impact on subsequent employment.[13] Overall the literature suggests that the duration of coma is more closely related to outcome in patients who suffer diffuse axonal injury without focal or extracerebral lesions.[13]

Depth of coma, as measured by the Glasgow Coma Scale, appears to be an important prognostic indicator of both mortality and outcome. Glasgow Coma Scale scores during the first 24 hours after injury appear to be better predictors of survival than scores after the first 24 hours, but Glasgow Coma Scale scores 2–3 days after injury are better predictors of functional outcome. For example, patients with initial Glasgow Coma Scale scores less than 8 have a mortality rate of 30.8%, whereas patients with initial Glasgow Coma Scale scores greater than 8 demonstrate

a mortality rate of only 0.9%.[14] It is estimated that 33% of survivors will die or remain in a prolonged vegetative state if their worst Glasgow Coma Scale score at 24 hours after injury is less than 7. On the other hand, 53% of patients whose best Glasgow Coma Scale score at 24 hours after injury is less than 7 will die or remain in a vegetative state.[15] Glasgow Coma Scale scores less than 7 up to 1 week after injury imply less than a 12% probability of achieving a favorable functional outcome.[16]

The depth of coma has been explored as an indicator of more specific aspects of outcome such as motor and cognitive recovery. However, it appears that motor recovery and cognitive recovery are more profoundly affected by duration than by depth of coma.[9,10] The relationship between recovery and duration appears to be somewhat linear; no clear cut-off point on the Glasgow Coma Scale predicts recovery.[8]

Glasgow Coma Scale scores also have been explored as a means of predicting quality of life, productivity, and subsequent living arrangements. In conjunction with other variables, the Glasgow Coma Scale scores can help to predict quality of life and productivity but are poor predictors of subsequent living arrangements, which are influenced significantly by other social forces.[17,18]

The duration of posttraumatic amnesia (PTA) is thought to have an even stronger relationship with outcome than depth or duration of coma. Periods of posttraumatic amnesia ranging from 1 hour to several days have resulted in impairments of divided attention, as determined by the Paced Auditory Serial Addition Task (PASAT), that persist for 15 and 40 days after injury, respectively.[8] Data from the International Data Coma Bank indicate that 80% of patients with less than 2 weeks of PTA achieve a good recovery and that 0% remain in the functional outcome category of severe disability, whereas only 27% of patients with more than 4 weeks of PTA achieve a good recovery and 30% remain severely disabled.[13] Others have indicated that virtually no patients with more than 4 weeks of PTA achieve a good recovery. Clearly, after 12 weeks of PTA cognitive deficits are severe, and the prognosis for functional independence at 1 year is poor.[8] As a caveat, duration of PTA affects functional prognosis most directly in patients with primarily diffuse axonal injury. The relationship between duration of PTA and outcome in patients with predominantly focal pathology is less clear.[13]

The type of central nervous system lesion incurred at the time of trauma has been correlated with survival and functional outcome. For example, the presence of a mass lesion implies a higher mortality rate and a poorer functional outcome. However, mass lesions convey a paradoxical "protective effect" on motor recovery and "invalidate" the motor scores of the Glasgow Coma Scale[8]—that is, unusually poor motor subscale scores on the Glasgow Coma Scale are not valid indicators of motor recovery in the presence of a mass lesion.

Most studies agree that the injury with the highest mortality rate and the poorest functional outcome is the subdural hematoma. One study compared the effects of focal versus diffuse injuries, Glasgow Coma Scale scores, and duration of coma on survival and outcome. The injury with the highest mortality and the poorest functional outcome was the subdural hematoma with Glasgow Coma Scale scores of 3–5 and coma duration greater than 6 hours; the mortality rate was 74%, and only 14% of patients achieved a good or moderate functional outcome.[19] On the other hand, the injury with the lowest mortality and the best functional outcome was diffuse axonal injury with Glasgow Coma Scale scores of 6–8 and coma limited to less than 24 hours; the mortality rate was 9%, and 68% of patients achieved a good recovery.[19] However, the mortality rate with diffuse axonal injury may be high (1) when the Glasgow Coma Scale score is less than 5; pupil abnormalities are present; and the mechanism of injury involves sagittal forces or (2) when perimesencephalic or subarachnoid hemorrhage, intrapeduncular contusion, or intraventricular hemorrhage is present.[20]

Other acute changes imaged by computed tomography (CT) that carry prognostic implications include the presence of third ventricle or basal cistern abnormalities. Obliteration of these structures, which implies raised intracranial pressure in excess of 20 mm, may occur after unilateral or bilateral contusion

or with diffuse axonal injury. The functional outcome of survivors with these acute CT findings remains poor at 6 months after injury.[21]

Temporal lobe lesions with a resulting midline shift of more than 4 mm carry negative prognostic implications for both survival and functional outcome.[16] The survivor who "talks and deteriorates" carries a worse prognosis; in 75% of cases, this phenomenon is secondary to delayed intracranial hematoma with poor prognosis for both survival and functional outcome.[22]

Basal ganglion hemorrhages are fairly rare CT abnormalities after a severe traumatic brain injury. Typically this lesion results in contralateral hemiparesis; depending on the laterality of the lesion, other typical subsequent findings include apraxia, aphasia, and visual spatial deficits. As a primary lesion, basal ganglion hemorrhages carry a fairly good prognosis; the majority of patients achieve a moderate or good functional outcome.[23] Overall functional prognosis in such patients is then determined by the extent of associated injuries.

The relative importance of location versus size of the lesion has engendered considerable debate. TBI studies have shown that location and type of lesion have little significant impact on Glasgow Outcome Scale level 6–12 months after injury, whereas size may have a significant impact on functional outcome. In one study survivors with a lesion volume greater than 4100 mm^3 universally demonstrated a poor outcome, whereas less than half of survivors with a lesion volume less than 4100 mm^3 had a poor functional outcome.[24]

Several studies have attempted to correlate magnetic resonance imaging (MRI) findings with neurobehavioral outcome, but to date results have been disappointing. One study found that acute MRI findings classified according to lesion type, location, and severity did in fact correlate with neurobehavioral testing results several months after injury.[25] However, most studies indicate that chronic MRI findings more accurately predict neurobehavioral testing results.

Raised intracranial pressure has been evaluated as a mechanism of secondary brain injury. Although the effect of raised intracranial pressure on neuropsychological function and Glasgow Outcome Scale score is controversial, most authorities believe that the presence of raised intracranial pressure has a negative effect on functional outcome.[13] Both initial and maximal intracranial pressures have prognostic significance, but maximal pressure predicts outcome more accurately.[26] The effect of intracranial pressure on outcome is unrelated to age, Glasgow Coma Scale scores, or type of central nervous system lesion.

Perhaps the most ominous type of secondary brain injury in terms of survival and functional outcome is the presence of hypotension. Systolic pressures of less than 90 mmHg at the time of resuscitation double the mortality rate and significantly decrease functional outcome.[27] Although hypoxia is certainly more prevalent than hypotension at resuscitation, it results in only a slight increase in mortality and appears to have little effect on long-term outcome.[27]

The relative importance of cerebral ischemia as a mechanism of secondary brain injury has been debated. A recent study of posttraumatic cerebral ischemia below infarct threshold has shed some light on this mechanism of secondary brain injury. As one would intuitively expect, cerebral ischemia below infarct threshold has a negative impact on functional outcome as measured by the Glasgow Outcome Scale.[28]

Associated injuries at the time of brain trauma influence mortality and functional outcome. The incidence of systemic injury with severe traumatic brain injury approaches 60%.[29] Brain injury accompanied by injury to one other organ system doubles mortality from 11% to 22%. Traumatic brain injury accompanied by hypovolemia results in a greater preponderance of deficits. Hypovolemia after TBI has been shown to increase the requirement for acute comprehensive inpatient rehabilitation service from 40% to 60%.[29]

Injury severity scores at the time of trauma have been examined as predictors of functional prognosis.[30] Of the two most common scales, the Abbreviated Injury Scale has some predictive ability for functional outcome at discharge from acute stabilization and at 6 months after injury; extremity scores and scores suggesting spine injury have the most predictive potential.[30] The Injury Severity Scale score is a poor predictor of functional outcome.

Evoked potentials, particularly somatosensory evoked potentials, have been used effectively as prognostic indicators after severe traumatic brain injury. Graded multimodality evoked potential performed within the first week of injury strongly correlates with Glasgow Outcome Scale level at 1 year.[31] Grade 1 (normal) evoked potentials imply a 71% probability of good recovery at 1 year, whereas grade 4 (profoundly abnormal) evoked potentials imply a 0% probability of a good recovery at 1 year. Multimodality evoked potentials add to the prognostic information gained from clinical findings and CT scan abnormalities. However, evoked potentials performed on survivors of chronic TBI add little prognostic information.[32]

Significant elevations of norepinephrine and catecholamines in general correlate with profound central nervous systems injuries as measured by the initial Glasgow Coma Scale scores.[33,34] Persistent catecholamine elevations at day 2 predict that Glasgow Coma Scale scores will improve slowly throughout the following week. The elevation in catecholamines correlates with increased lesion size and a lower Glasgow Outcome Scale level at discharge from acute care. The exact mechanism for the increase in catecholamines is not known, but it does not appear to be related directly to elevations of intracranial pressure. Animal studies have demonstrated that graded increases in intracranial pressure do not correlate with increases in systemic catecholamines.[35]

Other endocrine parameters that have been explored as potential prognostic indicators include levels of glucose and cortisol. One study stratified initial glucose as greater than or less than 250 mg/100 m and found that elevations in glucose correlated with lower Glasgow Coma Scale scores, higher Abbreviated Injury Scores, and abnormal pupillary responses.[36] Patients with elevated glucose also demonstrated a lower Glasgow Outcome Scale level at discharge from acute hospitalization. Similarly, cortisol levels at admission correlate with Glasgow Outcome Scale level. Lower levels of cortisol imply a better functional prognosis, whereas higher levels imply a worse prognosis and longer hospitalization for acute care.[37]

Thyroid function tests also appear to carry functional prognostic implications. Thyroid function tests tend to reach their lowest level approximately 4 days after injury. Lower thyroid function tests correlate with lower acute Glasgow Coma Scale scores and a lower Glasgow Outcome Scale level at discharge from acute care. The mechanism for thyroid suppression is probably secondary to the elevated norepinephrine.[38]

A number of cerebral metabolites released at the time of injury or shortly thereafter have been explored as potential prognostic indicators.[39,40] For example, CK-BB bands have been correlated with both Glasgow Coma Scale scores and functional outcome as measured by the Glasgow Outcome Scale.[39] Perhaps some of the more exciting work currently in progress is related to excitatory neurotransmitters.[41] Known to be neurotoxic in high concentrations, excitatory neurotransmitters are believed to mediate their toxicity by agonist activity at the N-methyl-D-aspartate (NMDA) receptor. Excitatory neurotransmitters have been implicated in the pathophysiology of other neuronal injury such as ischemia, hypoglycemia, seizure disorders, and Alzheimer's disease.[41] Glutamate, an excitatory neurotransmitter, has been serially monitored in the cerebral spinal fluid after TBI, and elevations appear to correlate with a poorer outcome.[41] NMDA antagonists appear to exert a protective effect after brain injury.

Few studies to date have explored the relationship between functional outcome and clinical features at the time of presentation to rehabilitation. One study looked at CT scan abnormalities at the time of admission to acute rehabilitation; correlation was noted with functional outcome and disposition at discharge from rehabilitation.[42] Normal CT scans implied an 83% chance of achieving independent living skills and mobility and returning to home. On the other hand, large ventricles implied a poor prognosis for independence in self-care skills and mobility. Only half of the patients with large ventricles were able to return home.[42]

The effect of early and more aggressive rehabilitation on functional outcome is an area

of critical ongoing research. Cope et al. stratified patients at admission to acute rehabilitation; the early group was admitted less than 35 days after injury, whereas the late group was admitted more than 35 days after injury. Admission to rehabilitation more than 35 days after injury resulted in more prolonged hospitalization, but functional outcome in the early and the late admission groups was comparable at 2 years.[43] Another study examined early intervention at a neurotrauma center while the patient was still on a ventilator.[44] Early intervention resulted in shorter rehabilitation stays, higher Rancho Los Amigos levels at discharge from rehabilitation, improvement in the percentage of subsequent patients requiring institution placement after acute rehabilitation, and, perhaps most remarkably, shorter durations of coma. Studies such as these are of enormous significance, because the role of rehabilitation in decreasing impairments, disability, and handicap as well as long-term health care expenditures has not been directly proved. These studies, however, are part of a growing body of evidence to support the important role of early rehabilitation intervention.

In summary, the overwhelming preponderance of studies exploring the impact of premorbid, acute injury and postinjury indicators on functional outcome have used the Glasgow Outcome Scale as a primary measure of outcome. The Glasgow Outcome Scale, however, provides limited information about functional skills and limited insight into the comprehensive cognitive, behavioral, and physical deficits common after a traumatic brain injury. Few studies have looked at the prognostic information available at the time of presentation to rehabilitation. Hence, the physiatrist is capable only of broad generalizations about prognosis when formulating the initial rehabilitation plan.

EARLY REHABILITATION INTERVENTION

Coma Stages

Definable stages of recovery for patients emerging from traumatic coma have been outlined most lucidly by Hagen, Malkmus,

TABLE 6. *Rancho Los Amigos Levels of Cognitive Function*

I	No response
II	Generalized response
III	Localized response
IV	Confused—agitated
V	Confused—inappropriate
VI	Confused—appropriate
VII	Automatic—appropriate
VIII	Purposeful—appropriate

and Durham, who developed the Rancho Los Amigos Scale of Cognitive Functioning (Table 6).[45] This scale uses behavioral observation to categorize a patient's level of cognitive functioning; it works well as a simple means by which clinicians can communicate an individual's level of cognitive functioning and develop appropriate rehabilitation strategies.

The initial three Rancho stages represent the low-level survivor of brain injury. Patients emerging into level III begin to demonstrate localized responses such as tracking, pulling their tubes, restlessness, and following commands. Responses are initially inconsistent but become more reliable as the patient progresses through level IV. Recovery through levels I, II, and III may be protracted. Therefore, objective means to document progress, to monitor cognitive status, and to determine the therapeutic efficacy of intervention become essential. The two most widely used scales for monitoring low-level survivors of brain injury are the Western Neurosensory Stimulation Profile and the Coma/Near Coma Scale.

The Coma/Near Coma Scale recently has been advocated for use with low-level brain-injured patients, including those in the vegetative state.[46] It consists of eight parameters, each with a specified number of stimuli and trials. Based on the numerical scoring system, patients are stratified into 1 of 5 categories: no coma, near coma, moderate coma, marked coma, and extreme coma. Because this scale is relatively new, its practical utility in the rehabilitation of the traumatically brain-injured patient remains to be determined.

The Western Neurosensory Stimulation Profile has been advocated for use in head-injured patients who are slow to recover.[47] The battery consists of 32 items that assess arousal, attention, response to stimuli, and expressive communication. The profile is divided into six subscales that allow for the assessment of individual patterns of responses.

Coma rehabilitation awareness stimulation programs designed for patients in coma and the vegetative state have as a primary goal the prevention of complications associated with prolonged immobilization and the creation of an environment in which the patient has the maximal chance to emerge. This goal is accomplished by means of a well-defined program involving medical and nursing interventions, sensory stimulation, regular exercise, and family education.[48] It is believed that in this environment central nervous system pathways will begin to process information with increasing complexity. Advocates of such programs profess that they potentiate the maximal chance of recovery, allow close monitoring of cortical function, and facilitate the development of the best overall care plan for the patient.

Sensory stimulation programs are individualized according to the patient's current level of physical and cognitive functioning. It is necessary to obtain a baseline level of cognitive function in the low-level brain-injured patient through multiple periods of observation and detailed discussion with caregivers, because patient responsiveness may fluctuate over the course of the day. Once a baseline has been determined, the clinician can tailor the sensory stimulation program for the specific patient and use the baseline as a means to monitor progress during the course of intervention.

In sensory stimulation programs, the five senses are directly stimulated and patient responses are carefully recorded and assessed using a graded scale.[48] The optimal frequency of direct sensory stimulation has not been determined. LeWinn and Dimancescu[49] and Wilson et al.[50] have advocated performing at least 36 repetitions of the sensory stimulation procedure per day. Conversely, DeYoung and Grass[48] suggest using sensory stimulations every hour for 11 successive hours per day.

Physical exercise, including range of motion exercises and a daily sitting program, are central components of awareness stimulation intervention. The daily sitting program helps to minimize the effects of prolonged bedrest (i.e, contractures, pressure sores, disrupted calcium homeostasis), to inhibit interfering primitive reflexes, and to facilitate arousal by stimulating the visual and vestibular systems.[51] Finally, the amount of range of motion obtained during exercise and the amount of individual patient participation are used as evaluation criteria.[48]

In summary, the early application of awareness stimulation techniques has a beneficial role that extends beyond the potential benefits of sensory stimulation. Although rehabilitation for comatose patients may not result in a return to independent living, it offers the opportunity to maximize the postaccident level of functioning by reducing support care needs and maintaining the patient as free of complications as possible. Also, as previously mentioned, compelling data suggest that the early application (in intensive and acute care settings) of sensory stimulation, in fact, leads to a better functional outcome.[44]

Posttraumatic Amnesia

Traumatic brain injury survivors emerging from the coma stages remain amnestic. The period of posttraumatic amnesia has considerable clinical significance. As mentioned previously, prognostic information may be gained from this stage of recovery. In addition, the cognitive and behavioral characteristics of posttraumatic amnesia have an impact on rehabilitation intervention strategies.

In 1882 Ribot proposed a classification of amnesia that included both anterograde and retrograde amnesias.[52] In 1928 Symonds was the first to identify length of coma as a prognostic indicator after brain injury.[53] The concept and clinical significance of posttraumatic amnesia, however, were first suggested in 1932 by Russell.[54]

Retrograde amnesia implies an inability to retrieve information that was acquired before the onset of a specific pathologic event.[55] Typically retrograde amnesia involves a gradient; events closer to the injury are less likely to be recalled than events occurring earlier before the injury. As the patient improves and confusion clears, the duration of retrograde amnesia shrinks from perhaps years to approximately 30 minutes or so preceding the pathologic event. After the posttraumatic amnesia clears, remote memory remains impaired, but there is no longer a temporal gradient; that is, the oldest memories are not selectively spared.[55,56]

Retrograde amnesia is rarely an isolated event.[57] Posttraumatic amnesia typically lasts significantly longer than retrograde amnesia. Largely because of this relationship, it has been speculated that both retrograde amnesia and posttraumatic amnesia are mediated by similar mechanisms; however, more recent neuroautonomic data suggest that they have independent mechanisms.

The ventral/tegmental region of the mesencephalon or bilateral, anterior, lateral, temporal lobes has been suggested as the neuroanatomic basis for retrograde amnesia.[57] Relevant studies primarily implicate medial temporal lobe or midline diencephalic structures.[58] The amnesia secondary to injury of diencephalic structures is typically characterized as a deficit involving initial learning, whereas forgetting occurs over a normal rate, implying faulty encoding.[59] On the other hand, the amnesia typical of temporal lobe lesions is characterized by the accelerated rate of forgetting new information, implying faulty storage mechanisms. Levin et al. found that during posttraumatic amnesia, initial learning and accelerated forgetting are both problematic; however, forgetting is particularly accelerated, whereas acquisition of new information is less impaired.[59]

The duration of posttraumatic amnesia is a marker of injury severity and carries significant prognostic implications. By 1961 the duration of posttraumatic amnesia was thought to represent "the best yardstick we have"[60] to measure the severity of blunt head injury. Over the decades, it has been demonstrated that the length of posttraumatic amnesia is predictive of functional outcome, return to work, posttraumatic epilepsy, and cognitive recovery.[61]

The definition of posttraumatic amnesia has evolved over time. Initially it was described as indicating a period of impaired consciousness after head injury.[54] Later, posttraumatic amnesia was defined as "ending" at the time from which the patient can give a clear and consecutive account of what is happening around him.[62] Others have described posttraumatic amnesia as an absence of continuous memory or an inability to retain new information. Today posttraumatic amnesia suggests the broader syndrome of disorientation to time, place, and person; confusion; diminished memory; and reduced capabilities for attending and responding to environmental cues.[61]

It is important to note that posttraumatic amnesia is rarely if ever complete[63]; that is, patients during posttraumatic amnesia may demonstrate long-term learning, especially of tasks that require limited attention. For example, a patient may demonstrate learning during posttraumatic amnesia in situations in which the probability of response is increased with repetition.[64] A patient also may learn during posttraumatic amnesia through stimulus response training such as acquisition of motor skills.[64] The concept of learning during posttraumatic amnesia is salient to the rehabilitation professional in that issues of self-care, mobility, and locomotion can be successfully addressed during this stage. Similarly, problem behaviors can be addressed with behavioral interventions that are consistent and repetitious.

Predicting the resolution of posttraumatic amnesia carries significant therapeutic implications. Resolution of posttraumatic amnesia is often associated with marked improvement in behavior, reduction in agitation, improvement in attention, readiness to tolerate the demands of a more comprehensive neuropsychological assessment, and increased capacity to participate more fully in a comprehensive rehabilitation program.[65] Predicting whether and when posttraumatic amnesia will resolve is therefore useful in establishing the patient's programming needs. It has been speculated that the duration of posttraumatic amnesia is approximately four times the duration of coma.[66] However, more recent studies fail to support the length of coma as a reliable predictor of the resolution of posttraumatic amnesia.[65] A younger age implies a greater likelihood of resolution, but age does not accurately predict when it will occur. Finally, the length of time after injury is significantly correlated with the duration and cessation of posttraumatic amnesia.[65]

Traditionally, the duration of posttraumatic amnesia has been estimated retrospectively. This approach is potentially problematic; islands of intact memory may develop when the patient otherwise is unable to sustain continuous memory.[67,68] Therefore, retrospective inquiry as to the time of the first intact memory after injury may underestimate the duration result in an underestimation of posttraumatic amnesia. Similarly, retrospective inquiry as to the interval when orientation normalized may lead to a misleading estimate of duration; 10–20% of survivors may be oriented before posttraumatic amnesia resolves.[67,69]

The first instrument developed to assess prospectively the duration of posttraumatic amnesia was the Galveston Orientation and Amnesia Test (GOAT),[68] which has proved to be reliable (Kendell correlation coefficient of 0.99). Its core application is the assessment of temporal orientation. The GOAT can be administered daily at bedside during the course of a brief interview. Its construct validity has been demonstrated through correlation with Glasgow Outcome Scale level, severity of computed tomography findings, and functional outcome. Finally, the brevity of the GOAT renders it more useful in monitoring recovery from PTA in the acute care setting than more extensive instruments such as the Orientation Group Monitoring System.[70–72]

Thus, the duration of posttraumatic amnesia has tremendous clinical significance and carries prognostic implications for long-term outcome. During PTA, acquisition and storage of memory are impaired, but under proper circumstances new functional skills can be acquired. Finally, the behavioral and cognitive abnormalities characteristic of PTA carry significant therapeutic implications about the patient's needs for formalized programming.

Perhaps the most compelling behavioral change during posttraumatic amnesia is agitation. In 1945 Denny-Brown first described restlessness as a natural sequela of traumatic brain injury.[73] The classic example of agitation is the patient at level IV of the Rancho Los Amigos Level of Functioning, who is "confused-agitated" and functions in a heightened state of activity and diminished capability for processing new information or responding to events in the environment. Estimates of the incidence of agitation have ranged from 11% and 33% to over 50%.[74,75] In part this disparity is related to the lack of a consistent definition. Invariably any definition agreed upon in the future will have to consider the fact that agitation occurs during posttraumatic amnesia and involves some combination of excessive behaviors consistent with aggression, restlessness, and emotional lability.

The initial approach to the agitated patient should include a comprehensive examination with emphasis on potential noxious stimuli such as fractures, peripheral nerve injuries and skin lesions and an evaluation of jejunostomy or gastrotomy and tracheostomy sites for potential problems. Other medical etiologies for agitation include seizure disorders, infection of the central nervous system, and deterioration in neurologic status. The past medical history should be reviewed for indications of substance withdrawal. All pharmacologic intervention should be reviewed for evidence of toxicity or adverse reactions. Finally, the evaluation should include screening for cardiopulmonary, endocrine, hepatic, renal, or other metabolic etiologies for altered mental status.[76]

Management strategies used in treating agitated behavior include one-to-one monitoring, behavioral modification, physical restraints, environmental modification, and pharmacologic intervention.[77] As rehabilitation stays shorten, the prompt resolution of agitation becomes increasingly important to avoid interference with other treatment goals.[77] Therefore, pharmacologic intervention also has become increasingly important as an adjunct in the treatment of the survivor of traumatic brain injury.

Unfortunately, there is little consensus regarding specific pharmacologic agents effective in the management of agitation. In part, the optimal management of agitation has not been defined because of the lack of consensus in defining agitation. Secondly, before the relatively recent development of the Agitated Behavior Scale,[78] no instrument for measuring agitation had been validated for a TBI population. Thirdly, the studies describing

pharmacologic intervention for posttraumatic agitation are typically nonrandomized and noncontrolled.[77] Finally, there are persistent concerns about the effect of pharmacologic intervention on long-term outcome. To date, the posttraumatic pathophysiologic cascade causing secondary brain damage remains too poorly understood, and the critical window for the pharmacologic treatment of trauma to the central nervous system is uncertain.[79] Therefore, it is premature to imply that certain pharmacologic interventions are either indicated or contraindicated during this acute posttraumatic period.

The pharmacologic strategies used by physicians appear to vary considerably.[80] Interventions intended to diminish the extent and severity of agitation include stimulating agents, such as amantadine or methylphenidate[78,81]; antidepressants, such as amitriptyline[74] or trazodone[82]; and agents that presumably reduce excitatory or augment inhibitory affects, such as beta blockers,[83] lithium,[84] carbamazepine,[80] and buspirone.[85] During episodes of extreme agitation, abortive agents that are sedating in nature and have a short half-life (e.g., lorazepam) are used.

In addition, to monitor objectively the efficacy of intervention strategies with the Agitated Behavior Scale, it is important to monitor simultaneously cognitive recovery. Data suggest that as patients emerge from coma, improvement in cognition precedes resolution of agitation.[71] Such data supports the clinical observation that management strategies that diminish cognition may prolong and exacerbate agitation. Two instruments that lend themselves to monitoring cognitive recovery during pharmacologic management of agitation include the previously mentioned Galveston Orientation and Amnesia Test and the Orientation Group Monitoring System.[68,70] In the rehabilitation setting, the Orientation Group Monitoring System offers a distinct advantage over the GOAT because of its increased sensitivity in detecting medical complications, such as adverse drug effects, infections, and hydrocephalus.[72] Although the brevity of the GOAT renders it more useful in the acute care setting, its sensitivity to medical complications has not been validated.

In summary, multiple pharmacologic treatments have been proposed for the management of posttraumatic agitation; the efficacy and indications remain largely unproved. The optimal medication should (1) control behavior without sedation; (2) augment or at least not delay or interfere with recovery of cognition; and (3) maintain a low profile of side effects. Given the heterogeneity of primary and secondary brain injury mechanisms, injury severity, preexisting conditions, and clinical presentation of posttraumatic agitation, it is unlikely that one pharmacologic agent will evolve as effective for all or even a majority of patients.

Cardiovascular Disorders

Cardiovascular disorders associated with TBI include rhythm disturbances, ischemic changes, contusion, hypotension, and hypertension. Of these, hypertension is the most common and immediate cardiovascular disorder associated with severe head injury.[86] Excessive catecholamine, increased cardiac output, and tachycardia usually dominate the acute physiologic state of patients who are hypertensive immediately after brain injury.[87] Animal studies of severe brain injury demonstrate a graded increase in release of catecholamine from the adrenal glands and vasoconstrictor sympathetic postganglionic neurons proportionate to severity of injury.[88] Rise in systolic blood pressure is closely coupled with the initial release of catecholamines.

Although hypertension is often seen immediately after severe brain injury, in the rehabilitation setting the incidence is estimated at 10–15%, and the prevalence diminishes rapidly to less than 3% after discharge.[86,88] In Labi and Horn's retrospective study of 74 patients with no premorbid history of hypertension who were discharged from a rehabilitation hospital after their first TBI, 11 (15%) developed hypertension during admission. Five patients (7%) were discharged on antihypertension medication, of whom 3 discontinued or reduced medication at 1 month after discharge and 2 were lost to follow-up.

Because brain injury can disrupt reabsorption of cerebrospinal fluid and injure central blood pressure control centers, hypertension that occurs de novo or persists after discharge from the acute medical care admission warrants a thorough evaluation. In rare cases, hypertension is the presenting symptom of normal-pressure hydrocephalus after TBI.[89] Centers involved in regulation of blood pressure include the ambiguous and solitary nuclei, hypothalamus, thalamus, amygdala, and orbital-frontal cortex.[90–93] Hypertension that first presents in the rehabilitation setting merits computerized axial tomography or magnetic resonance imaging (MRI) to rule out increased intracranial pressure. MRI has the advantage of allowing the clinician to assess the brainstem.[94]

Autonomic dysfunction associated with brain injury has been reported in the absence of identifiable secondary causes.[90] Episodic hypertension associated with hyperhidrosis, headaches, and facial flushing, however, warrants evaluation for an occult spinal cord lesion. Pheochromocytoma, although uncommon, may be unmasked by trauma and therefore should be considered in the differential diagnosis.[90] Laboratory evaluation should be performed to rule out neuroendocrine etiologies such as hypothalamic or pituitary disorders.[95] In the immediate postinjury period, additional laboratory and imaging studies may be appropriate to rule out renal or adrenal hemorrhage.

Medication should be evaluated for possible contribution to hypertension. Steroids are commonly known to predispose to elevated blood pressure. Infrequently nonsteroidal antiinflammatory drugs, such as indomethacin, may reduce prostaglandin-dependent renal profusion, causing a secondary pressor effect.

Treatment of hypertension in the patient with TBI is directed toward lowering blood pressure, identifying the causes and minimizing side effects that interfere with recovery and rehabilitation. Beta blockers are the mainstay of treatment for hypertension secondary to increased adrenergic tone.[96] The choice of beta blockers may be critical in the setting of cognitive recovery. Propranolol, the standard beta blocker, easily crosses the brain barrier because of its high lipid solubility and has been associated with depression, impairments of attention and memory, and impotence.[97] Thus, when beta blockers are considered, a more polar compound such as atenolol or nadolol may provide effective control of blood pressure and reduce cognitive side effects. Alpha-methyldopa, which is associated with depression, confusion, and other cognitive changes in the elderly, is not recommended for use after brain injury because sensitivity to cognitive impairment is increased.[97] Clonidine, another alpha-adrenergic agonist, also may suppress cognition. Diuretics are not associated with cognitive suppression but require monitoring of serum electrolyte concentrations. Hypokalemia is adjusted routinely to avoid potentiating dysrhythmia. In patients with motor impairment, attention also should be directed to repletion of calcium, magnesium, and phosphate, all of which may affect muscle function. Diuretics are best avoided when restoration of urinary continence is an active rehabilitation goal. Calcium channel blockers and angiotensin-converting enzyme inhibitors are rarely associated with cognitive impairment.

Hypotension in the rehabilitation setting is frequently associated with prolonged bedrest or side effects of medications. The most common medications that cause orthostatic hypotension are antihypertensive agents, in particular diuretics, alpha blockers, and vasodilators. When hypotension persists or is precipitous, the increased likelihood of cardiac or autonomic dysfunction necessitates a thorough evaluation. Volume loss secondary to hemorrhage or neuroendocrine imbalance should be considered initially in the early recovery period.

Electrocardiographic abnormalities commonly accompany early recovery from TBI. The incidence after severe head injury varies from greater than 80% during the acute medical admission[98] to approximately 20% during inpatient rehabilitation.[86] EKG evidence of myocardial ischemia, including prolonged QT interval, inverted T waves, and ST segment elevation, has been well documented in the neurosurgical literature.[98–100] Myocardial injury has been corroborated through laboratory medicine and at autopsy. CK-MB activity may remain elevated at least 3 days after injury.[99] Histologic evidence of myocardial necrosis at autopsy has confirmed the presence of myocardial injury after head injury.[101] In the absence of direct cardiac trauma, myocardial damage may be secondary to massive release of catecholamine from sympathetic nerve endings during the adrenergic surge that follows severe TBI.[87]

Dysrhythmias appear to occur less commonly after TBI, although the incidence has not been studied. Case reports include life-threatening torsade de pointes, concomitant pulsus alternans and U-wave alternans, and transient heart block ranging from prolonged PR intervals to high-grade atrioventricular block with ventricular escape rhythm.[102–105] Most commonly seen in the rehabilitation setting are nonspecific ST and T wave changes.[86] Given the potential for underlying myocardial damage, baseline EKG at the time of rehabilitation admission is a valuable screening exam and an important adjunct to a thoughtful cardiopulmonary evaluation.

Respiratory Disorders

The most common medical complication after TBI is hypoxemia and respiratory failure.[106] Painstaking monitoring of respiratory function during the acute rehabilitation period is critical to the prevention of secondary brain injury from hypoxia and the reduction of preventable mortality. In a British analysis of mortality after pediatric TBI, 93% of potentially preventable deaths prior to hospital admission were of respiratory etiology, predominantly aspiration.[107] After admission one-fourth of all deaths were attributable to pulmonary abnormalities. Of those considered to be preventable, nearly 60% were secondary to respiratory arrest or airway obstruction.

Acute respiratory complications may include central depression of respiratory drive from brainstem injury or pharmacologic sedation, aspiration, pulmonary and chest wall injury, neurogenic pulmonary edema, infection, or fat embolus.[106,108–111] Pulmonary embolus, aspiration, complications related to endotracheal respiration or tracheostomy, and reduced strength and coordination of respiratory musculature are frequent complications encountered in the rehabilitation hospital.[110,112–116]

Alcohol intoxication, a significant risk factor for respiratory complications, is frequently associated with TBI. In a study of 520 patients, nearly 40% were intoxicated at the time of admission.[111] Although injuries appeared equally severe in the nonintoxicated cohort, intoxicated patients were 30% more likely to require intubation before admission and 80% more likely to have respiratory distress requiring artificial ventilation during acute care. Potential factors contributing to a 40% greater risk of pneumonia included enthanol-related immune suppression, higher likelihood of aspiration, and/or a higher prevalence of pneumonia before the TBI. Of note, when alcohol intoxication was documented on admission, length of hospital stay was not extended unless pulmonary complications developed, specifically respiratory distress or pneumonia. Given the frequency of such complications, alcohol intoxication associated with TBI has obvious economic and public health ramifications.

Patients with TBI frequently require prolonged endotracheal intubation, mechanical ventilation, and eventual tracheostomy. Such techniques of airway management are associated with colonization of the upper respiratory track by bacteria commonly found in the posterior nasopharynx. Not uncommonly, a shift toward more pathologic flora follows. Prophylactic antibiotics neither alter the rate of aberrant colonization nor prevent infection, but they facilitate the appearance of gram-negative pathogens, especially *Pseudomonas aeruginosa*, that are associated with more severe infections.[109] Clear evidence of respiratory tract infections should be documented before use of antibiotics.

The majority of patients who undergo tracheostomy recover sufficient neurologic integrity to consider decannulation. Usually the patient is decannulated in a stepwise fashion: incremental decreases in cannula diameter are followed by a trial of plugging the tube; finally the tube is removed, and an occlusive dressing is applied. Decannulation always should be attempted on a week-day morning when optimal staff are available to observe the patient closely.

Prospective studies of patients with long-term tracheostomy, using direct laryngeal visualization before decannulation, have demonstrated an incidence of serious abnormalities that exceeds 30% in both the acute and subacute settings.[113–115] Tracheal stenosis, subglottic stenosis, glottic stenosis, tracheomalacia, and tracheal granuloma with varying degrees of clinical symptoms are seen most frequently. When patients are stratified by cognitive level, morbidity and mortality, as expected, are much higher for decannulation at Rancho levels II and III.[113] Central respiratory lability and poor pulmonary toilet with resultant pneumonia that leads to sepsis contribute significantly to the increased mortality in the vegetative and coma-emerging patient.

Predictors of successful decannulation include (1) traumatic mechanism of brain injury; (2) younger age; and (3) alert cognitive status.[114] However, among patients in whom adequate cough and swallowing reflexes are documented, no correlation is observed with age, diagnosis, Rancho scale, or duration of tracheostomy.[115] Female patients with a smaller tracheal diameter may have an increased likelihood of a clinically significant obstructive lesion.[115]

Several factors may predispose to increased laryngotracheal mucosal reaction after traumatic brain injury.[113] Emergent intubation frequently occurs under less than optimal circumstances. The peri-injury and acute stabilization period are frequently complicated by hypotension and resultant tissue hypoxia.[113] Cervical hyperextension associated with decerebrate or decorticate posturing may cause the posterior pharyngeal tissues to act as a fulcrum for the rigid endotracheal tube.[116] Head movement, which may be marked with agitation, potentially creates a seesaw movement of the tube.[116]

Prolonged tracheal intubation is known to result in a number of complications. Such complications can be diminished by proper attention to factors that increase the risk of tissue injury: choice of tube; meticulous airway management to prevent excessive movement of the tube during turning, suctioning, and ventilator connection or disconnection; adequate sedation to prevent coughing, agitation, and decerebrate or decorticate posturing; adequate humidification;

use of soft nasogastric tubes; and prevention of tissue hypoxia, anemia, and infection.

Fever

A common acute complication after severe traumatic brain injury is fever. Frank fever of unknown origin, defined as temperature elevation of greater than 38.2° C on several occasions over at least a 3-week period and inability to diagnose the underlying cause after at least 1 week of intensive investigation,[117] is unusual, but a systematic approach to diagnosis is often warranted. The differential diagnosis for fever of unknown origin is extensive and includes infectious, neoplastic, autoimmune, granulomatous, metabolic, inherited, psychogenic, periodic, and thermoregulatory disorders.[117] The list of likely sources of fever after a severe traumatic brain injury is less extensive, but the same framework is often useful for accurate diagnosis.[118]

Urinary tract infections affect approximately 40% of traumatic brain injury survivors during the rehabilitation phase of recovery.[86] Ureteral obstruction is seen in approximately 1% of patients after traumatic brain injury. Other potential genitourinary sources of fever include pyelonephritis, perinephric abscess, and prostatic abscess.

Approximately 34% of traumatic brain injury survivors develop respiratory complications that predispose to pulmonary infections.[86] Poor ventilation with secondary atelectasis is thought to be the most common pulmonary complication of trauma and a potential forerunner of pneumonia. Tissue necrosis secondary to lung trauma with subsequent formation of a pulmonary cavity also may predispose the patient to secondary lung infections.[119] Endotracheal or tracheostomy tubes predispose patients to bacterial colonization and a greater risk of secondary lung infection. Finally, tubes used for enteral feeding increase the probability of aspiration pneumonia by as much as 25%.[120,121]

The head and neck area includes several other potential sources of fever after a traumatic brain injury. For example, perinasal sinusitis after nasotracheal intubation has been estimated to occur in approximately 26% of patients.[122,123] Nasogastric intubation

has been reported to cause a similar rate of sinusitis and fever in trauma survivors. Finally, dental abscess secondary to teeth rendered nonviable by trauma is a potential cause.[124]

Cardiovascular etiologies for fever include subacute and acute endocarditis,[125] dissecting aortic aneurysm,[126] intravenous line sepsis,[127] and thromboembolic disease.[128] The incidence of thromboembolic disease after traumatic brain injury has been reported to be as low as 4% during the rehabilitation course. However, the low incidence may be due to the nonspecific clinical presentation of thromboembolic disorders and concomitant impairment of arousal and cognition.

Other sources of fever include musculoskeletal disorders such as heterotopic ossification,[129] which may mimic deep venous thrombosis in presentation, and osteomyelitis from either hematogenous or contiguous spread.[86] Perisplenic, pericardial, and retroperitoneal cryptic hematomas have been associated with prolonged fever after trauma.[86,130] Adverse reactions to medications include drug fever; an important and potentially life-threatening example is the neuroleptic malignant syndrome.[131,132] Finally, neurologic causes of fever after trauma include bacterial meningitis, infected intraventricular shunts, hyperthermic reactions to acute hydrocephalus, neurogenic hypothermia, and the postictal period.[133–137]

Bladder and Bowel Function

Traumatic brain injury often results in injury to the frontal lobes and resultant loss of cortical control over urination and defecation.[138] In addition, injury to the subcortical structures may result in the development of bladder dyssynergia.[77] In one large study, 38% of brain-injured patients developed urinary tract infections. Although the majority of patients had indwelling Foley catheters, 37% did not. Bladder dysfunction was seen in 8% of the cohort.[86]

Symptoms of urgency and incontinence are commonly seen in the bladder after brain injury.[138] When dealing with patients who are incontinent, the clinician must be diligent in monitoring for skin integrity, fungal infections, and urinary tract infections. In addition, all predisposing factors to urinary tract infections, such as Foley catheters, fecal incontinence, and inadequate hydration, should be removed or treated.

Initiating a timed voiding schedule often retrains the bladder to empty at regular intervals and allows the patient to achieve continence. A timed voiding program begins with frequent toileting, followed by gradual increases in interval length. For the patient who voids frequently in small amounts with low postvoid residual volumes, anticholinergic agents may be considered as an adjunct.[139] It is important, however, to monitor for the possible affects of anticholinergic agents on cognitive recovery.

Bowel dysfunction after traumatic brain injury often results from a loss of cortical control over the defecation reflex, which causes incontinence. In addition, constipation due to lack of mobility, use of potentially constipating medication, and alteration in normal diet is frequent in the acute care setting. Stool softeners, stimulant suppositories, and adequate hydration are often helpful initially to maintain bowel regularity. As the patient recovers, the bowel program should be tailored to utilize both the gastrocolic reflex (approximately 30 minutes after eating) and gravity (by having the patient sit in an upright position to defecate).

Diarrhea, which is common in low-level-brain-injured patients on enteral feedings, may lead to loss of skin integrity, infected pressure sores and other wounds, and severe dehydration. Formulas high in fiber and isosmotic formulas are often helpful. Supplementing the enteral feeding with fiber compounds such as psyllium mucilloid also may be helpful in forming stool. Antidiarrheal medications are not necessary, and some (e.g., loperamide) are potentially sedating. Patients with severe traumatic brain injury often require antibiotic treatment for various infections. They are debilitated and in the hospital, and thus they are at significant risk for the development of bowel infections. In the patient with persistent diarrhea, an infectious cause should be sought.

Swallowing and Nutrition

Swallowing disorders are estimated to occur in 25-30% of brain injury survivors.[140,141]

After traumatic brain injury, patients have a significant increase in their caloric requirements.[142] The early use of parenteral feedings to correct a negative nutritional balance has been shown to improve outcome significantly. When the patient is stable, enteral feedings are begun, initially by means of nasogastric tube; early placement of a gastrostomy or jejunostomy tube is warranted in severely brain-injured patients in whom recovery is projected to be prolonged. As arousal improves, swallowing evaluations involving a combination of bedside swallowing assessments or video fluoroscopy are performed by a speech-language pathologist or occupational therapist. The video fluoroscopic evaluation is often an essential adjunct to evaluation, because physical findings alone are not sufficiently sensitive to predict the ability to swallow safely. In a study by Winstein,[141] 12% of patients with swallowing disorders had normal gag reflexes and 77% had a good voluntary cough reflex. Thus, the information provided by a comprehensive assessment helps the clinician to make important judgments about the patient's ability to begin oral feeding and which strategies will most facilitate safe swallowing.

Safe swallowing obviously refers to swallowing with the least risk of aspiration. At first, oral feeding is often restricted to therapeutic purposes and requires direct supervision and intervention by a speech-language pathologist or occupational therapist. Safe therapeutic feeding is predicated on the patient's behavior. The patient should be monitored for behavioral sequelae such as agitation, impulsivity, lack of initiation, and hyperphagia; when present, such sequelae should be treated with appropriate behavioral management interventions.

After oral feeding has begun, it is sometimes difficult for the patient to maintain adequate caloric intake; thus close monitoring of nutritional status is necessary. Many patients complain of having no appetite. In such instances a specific cause should be sought; for example, the patient should be evaluated for taste and smell disorders which may result in decreased food craving. Cranial nerve or cortical dysfunction as well as local trauma may lead to anosmia and/or gustatory dysfunction, which may play a significant role in the patient's desire to eat. Depression in the postinjury period, along with neuroendocrine sources for lack of appetite, also should be considered.

Spasticity

After traumatic brain injury, spasticity is believed to develop as a result of the loss of cortical control over spinal reflex centers. This loss often results in a greater increase in flexor tone in the upper limbs, which causes the arm to fold in toward the trunk. The lower limbs show a tendency toward extensor tone, which acts to keep the lower limb away from the trunk. Hypertonicity is not limited to the limbs but also may present in the torsal, facial, and oral pharyngeal musculature.

Interventions are warranted when spasticity significantly interferes with achievement of rehabilitation goals. The first stage of treatment for spasticity involves physical modalities, range of motion and exercise. Cryotherapy has been found to be helpful in temporarily reducing spasticity for 1–3 hours after application.[143] This interval is often sufficient to allow therapeutic interventions, including serial casting, ambulation, or range-of-motion exercises. Application of casts to preserve or increase range of motion has been shown to have a secondary beneficial affect on reducing spasticity.[144] Thus, serial casting early in the care of brain-injured patients can foster improvements in tone and maintenance of joint range of motion.

If spasticity continues despite such interventions, pharmacologic therapy is indicated. Unfortunately, antispasticity medications may have negative effects on cognition.[72] In traumatically brain-injured patients, dantrolene sodium is an attractive pharmacologic agent, primarily because of its low potential for cognitive side effects; however, routine blood monitoring is required because of potential toxic effects on the liver. Other antispasticity medications include clonidine, baclofen, and the benzodiapines; although these medications may help with tone reduction, they also require close monitoring because of the significant potential for impairing cognition.

If pharmacotherapeutic interventions fail to reduce spasticity, motor point blocks and nerve blocks are effective in reducing tone in a specific group of muscles, such as lower limb adductors or plantar flexors.[145] Neurectomies and intrathecal infusion of antispasticity medications have been shown to help with persistent hypertonicity.[146] However, during the early rehabilitation assessment and intervention after TBI, the more invasive interventions are rarely indicated.

TERTIARY PREVENTION

Thrombophlebitis

Deep venous thrombosis (DVT) represents a significant source of morbidity and potential mortality for patients with head trauma. Pulmonary embolism from DVT is apparently increasing in importance as a cause of death among inpatients with traumatic brain injury.[147] The National Institutes of Health Consensus Conference estimated the incidence of DVT after severe traumatic brain injury to be approximately 40%. The incidence of fatal pulmonary embolus is approximately 1%.[148] The incidence of DVT may be significantly reduced using a specialized approach of prophylactic intervention in conjunction with routine monitoring in high-risk patients. High-risk factors include (1) advanced age; (2) severe injury; (3) prolonged immobilization; (4) number of transfusions; and (5) elevated thromboplastin time on admission.[147,149–153]

For prophylaxis against DVT, Dennis et al.[147] recommend the use of full-length lower extremity sequential compression stockings or subcutaneous heparin, 5000 U twice daily. They also recommend routine monitoring with noninvasive Doppler ultrasound or duplex scanning. In patients who are unable to receive such forms of prophylaxis, placement of a prophylactic Greenfield filter deserves strong consideration.

Contractures

Contractures of the limbs as well as the axial skeleton may have devastating implications for self-care mobility, and even vocalization. Persons at greatest risk for contractures are those with (1) a long period of coma and immobilization; (2) severe brain injury; and (3) altered muscle tone. The best treatment of joint contractures is prevention by an ongoing program of range-of-motion exercises and maintenance of postural adaptation (i.e., sitting, lying prone or supine, and standing). Serial casting has been shown to be useful in the prevention and treatment of contractures.[144,154,155] The therapeutic benefit of continual casting versus casting and bi-valve splinting has been debated, but the current literature suggests that continuous casting has a slight therapeutic advantage.[155]

Once contractures develop, treatment depends on their severity. Treatment options include an aggressive stretching program in association with physical modalities, serial casting, and dynamic bracing. In extreme cases surgical release of the contracted tissue may be warranted to increase function. Surgical release of contracted tissue improves skin care and hygiene, prevents the development and fosters the healing of pressure sores, reduces pain, and improves transfers and ambulation.[149] However, such aggressive intervention for contractures is limited to the more chronic survivor who has failed conservative measures.

Fractures

The incidence of concurrent fractures in patients with traumatic brain injury is approximately 30%[157]; approximately 11% of fractures are initially undetected.[158] In brain-injured patients, fractures are associated with a high risk of heterotopic ossification,[159] especially forearm[160] and hip fractures.[157] In a cohort of patients with hip fractures after traumatic brain injury, 100% developed heterotopic ossification.[150] Conventional treatment of fractures, including splints and casting, often results in less than desirable results. Uncontrolled limb motion is common in the brain-injured patient, especially early in the recovery as the patient emerges from coma.[157] Early definitive fixation of upper and lower limb fractures allows for a shorter period of immobilization, early range-of-motion activity, and less overall nursing care.[160] Early mobilization and range-of-motion activities reduce the likelihood of developing severe spasticity, contractures, and ankylosing heterotopic ossification. In addition, early definitive fixation diminishes the need for casting of limbs, which often interferes with rehabilitation intervention.

Peripheral Nerve Injuries

An estimated 34% of patients admitted to one rehabilitation unit were diagnosed with previously undetected peripheral nerve injuries.[161] A large majority of the patients were involved in high-speed collisions. Ulnar nerve entrapment in the cubital tunnel was found most frequently; brachial plexus injury and common peroneal compression neuropathies were slightly less frequent.[161] Median nerve compression at the wrist has been reported in brain-injured patients with wrist and finger flexor spasticity.[162] Factors believed to contribute to compression neuropathies in brain-injured patients include (1) extrinsic pressure from a hematoma or heterotopic ossification; (2) prolonged coma; (3) severe spasticity; (4) improper positioning; (5) fractures; and (6) improperly applied casts.[161–163]

An estimated 50% of such neuropathies are preventable;[161] thus, in the acute care setting, it is essential to incorporate into the overall rehabilitation plan preventive measures such as proper positioning, monitoring of cast application, and early treatment of spasticity and heterotopic ossification.

Heterotopic Ossification

The brain-injured patient's risk of developing heterotopic ossification increases as the severity of injury, length of immobilization, and duration of coma increase.[164] Heterotopic ossification usually involves the large joints of the body (hips, elbows, shoulder, and knees). Excessive bone formation may result in significant disability by severely limiting the range of motion of a joint. Progressive loss of joint mobility and markers of increased osteoblastic activity, such as an elevated fractionated alkaline phosphatase level, warrant a comprehensive musculoskeletal examination with three-phased bone scan and radiographs to confirm the presence, distribution, and extent of heterotopic ossification.[165] Osteocalcin, another marker of osteoblastic activity, does not appear to be useful in the early detection of heterotopic ossification or in assessing its maturity.[167]

Diphosphonates have been shown to prevent heterotopic bone formation,[161] and a recent study suggests that warfarin therapy may afford the same protection.[167] Diphosphonates also may minimize the extent of heterotopic ossification formation after its onset, but their role in this setting remains controversial.

The treatment of heterotopic ossification also includes physical modalities such as aggressive range-of-motion exercises, which may reduce the likelihood of bony ankylosis, and indomethacin, which reduces tissue inflammation.[168,169] As heterotopic ossification significantly impedes functional recovery, surgery is usually performed in combination with radiation of the involved area in an attempt to arrest further bone development.

INDIVIDUALIZED REHABILITATION PLAN

After documenting the extent of impairment and estimating functional outcome, the physiatrist is charged with determining the most appropriate rehabilitation interventions. Early rehabilitation is initiated while the patient remains on the trauma or neurosurgical service. Rehabilitation options after this early stage are predicated on the nature of residual impairments.[170] In the unlikely event that a patient with severe traumatic brain injury recovers sufficiently during acute care to permit rehabilitation management on an outpatient basis, individual outpatient services or a day-treatment program may be recommended. Day-treatment rehabilitation typically offers integrated programs of physical therapy, occupational therapy, speech therapy, cognitive remediation, and psychological services up to 8 hours/day, 5 days/week.

If at discharge from acute care the residual impairments are of such severity that the patient remains dependent, options include either an acute or subacute rehabilitation program. The typical candidate for a traumatic brain injury acute rehabilitation unit is the patient who is able to follow consistently a one-step command, but is often confused, disoriented, and restless, if not overtly agitated; many have a combination of physical limitations or medical complications. The ideal goal of this phase of rehabilitation is to assist the patient from the late stages of unconsciousness through the clearing of posttraumatic amnesia, resolution of agitation, and at least minimal independence in activities of daily living. For both patient and family, the most salient goal of the acute rehabilitation phase is to regain optimal independence in activities of daily living. To remain in this rehabilitation environment, the patient must be able to tolerate and benefit from a minimum of 3 hours of therapy, 5 days/week.

Subacute rehabilitation programs are largely based in nursing homes. Such programs do not require that the patient tolerate 3 hours of therapy per day. Consequently, subacute rehabilitation programs are most appropriate for patients who remain in the coma stages, respond to simple commands inconsistently, or show a low rate of progress. The typical length of stay is considerably longer than the present national average of approximately 30 days in acute rehabilitation. Largely because of staffing and overhead, subacute rehabilitation offers health care providers a less expensive form of specialized intervention. Although data support the importance of early rehabilitation interventions to outcome,[43,44] virtually no data compare the outcomes of acute versus subacute intervention.

After inpatient rehabilitation, a number of postacute management strategies are available. If the patient can be managed at home, then rehabilitation options include individual in-home or outpatient therapy or comprehensive day-treatment services. If the patient in an acute rehabilitation setting fails to achieve basic functional independence in a timely fashion, transfer to a subacute rehabilitation program may be warranted. In the event that behavioral problems such as agitation preclude discharge to the home, more specialized inpatient behavioral treatment programs are indicated.

Another level in the continuum of rehabilitation includes transitional living programs, which typically are residential, community-based alternatives for patients with primarily cognitive and neurobehavioral deficits that preclude independent living. The length of stay in a transitional living program may be as long as 12 months; the ultimate goal is independent living.

The final stage in the rehabilitation continuum includes vocational rehabilitation. This stage is initiated several months after acute injury. Hence, vocational rehabilitation, transitional living, and even specialized behavioral programs are rarely relevant or pressing program options to consider during the initial physiatric evaluation.

REFERENCES

1. Griffith ER: Types of disability. In Rosenthal M, Griffith ER, Bond MR, Miller JD (eds): Rehabilitation of the Head Injured Adult. Philadelphia, F.A. Davis, 1983, pp 23–32.
2. Frankowski RF: The demography of head injury in the United States. In Miner M, Wagner KA (eds): Neurotrauma, vol 1. Boston, Butterworths, 1986, pp 1–17.
3. Jennett B, Teasdale G: Management of Head Injuries. Philadelphia, F.A. Davis, 1981, pp 301–316.
4. Reyes RL, Bhattacharyya AK, Heler D: Traumatic head injury: Restlessness and agitation as prognosticators of physical and psychologic improvements in patients. Arch Phys Med Rehabil 62:20– 23, 1981.
5. Mayes, SD, Pelco LE, Campbell CJ: Relationships among pre- and post-injury intelligence, length of coma and age in individuals with severe closed-head injuries. Brain Inj 3:301–313, 1989.
6. Pennings JL, Bachulis BL, Simon CT, Slazinski T: Survival after severe brain injury in the aged. Arch Surg 128:787–794, 1993.
7. Broas PL, Stappaerts KH, Rommens PM, et al: Polytrauma in patients of 65 and over. Injury patterns and outcome. Int Surg 73:119–122, 1988.
8. Mack H, Horn LJ: Functional prognosis in traumatic brain injury. Phys Med Rehabil State Art Rev 3:13–26, 1989.
9. MacPherson V, Sullivan SJ, Lambert J: Prediction of motor status 3 and 6 months post severe traumatic brain injury: A preliminary study. Brain Inj 6:489–498, 1992.
10. Wilson B, Vizor A, Bryant T: Predicting severity of cognitive impairment after severe head injury. Brain Inj 5:189–197, 1991.
11. Salcido R, Costich JF: Subject review: Recurrent traumatic brain injury. Brain Inj 6:293–298, 1992.
12. Vogenthaler DR, Smith KR Jr, Goldfader P: Head injury, a multivariate study: Predicting long-term productivity and independent living outcome. Brain Inj 3:369–385, 1989.
13. Katz DI: Neuropathology and neurobehavioral recovery from closed head injury. J Head Trauma Rehabil 7(2):1–15, 1992.
14. Baxt WG, Moody P: The differential survival of trauma patients. J Trauma 27:602–606, 1987.
15. Jennett B, Teasdale G, Braakman R et al: Prognosis of patients with severe head injury. Neurosurgery 4:283–289, 1979.
16. Young B, Rapp RP, Norton JA, et al: Early prediction of outcome in head-injured patients. J Neurosurg 54:300–303, 1981.
17. Stambrook M, Moore AD, Kowalchuk S, et al: Early metabolic and neurologic predictors of long-term quality of life after closed head injury. Can J Surg 33:115–118, 1990.
18. Vogenthaler DR, Smith KR, Goldfader P: Head injury, an empirical study: Describing long-term productivity and independent living outcome. Brain Inj 3:355–368, 1989.
19. Gennarelli TA, Spielman GM, Langfitt TW, et al: Influence of the type of intracranial lesion on outcome from severe head injury. J Neurosurg 56: 26–32, 1982.
20. Takenaka N, Mine T, Sugu S, et al: Interpeduncular high-density spot in severe shearing injury. Surg Neurol 34:30–38, 1990.
21. Colquhoun IR, Burrows EH: The prognostic significance of the third ventricle and basal cisterns in severe closed head injury. Clin Radiol 40:13–16, 1989.
22. Rockswold GL, Pheley PJ: Patients who talk and deteriorate. Ann Emerg Med 22:1004–1007, 1993.
23. Katz DI, Alexander MP, Seliger GM, Bellas DN: Traumatic basal ganglion hemorrhage: Clinicopathologic features and outcome. Neurology 39: 798–904, 1989.
24. Kido DK, Cox C, Hamill RW, et al: Traumatic brain injuries: Predictive usefulness of CT. Radiology 182:777–781, 1992.
25. Godersky JC, Gentry LR, Travel D, et al: Magnetic resonance imaging and neurobehavioral outcome in traumatic brain injury. Acta Neurochir 51:311–314, 1990.
26. Nordby KH, Gunnerod N: Epidural monitoring of the intracranial pressure in severe head injury characterized by non-localizing motor response. Acta Neurochir 74:21–26, 1985.
27. Chestnut RM, Marshall LF, Klauber MR, et al: The role of secondary brain injury in determining outcome from severe head injury. J Trauma 34:216–222, 1993.
28. Bouma GJ, Muizelaar JP, Choi SC, et al: Cerebral circulation and metabolism after severe traumatic brain injury: The elusive role of ischemia. J Neurosurg 75:685–693, 1991.
29. Siegel JH, Gens DR, Mamanto T, et al: Effect of associated injuries and blood volume replacement on death, rehabilitation needs, and disability in blunt traumatic brain injury. Crit Care Med 19: 1252–1265, 1991.
30. Mackenzie EJ, Shapiro S, Moody M, et al: Predicting post-traumatic functional disability for individuals without severe brain injury. Med Care 24:377–387, 1986.
31. Greenberg RP, Newlon PG, Hyatt MS, et al: Prognostic implications of early multimodality evoked potentials in severely head-injured patients. J Neurosurg 55:227-236, 1981.

32. Shin DY, Ehrenberg B, Whyte J, et al: Evoked potential assessment: Utility in prognosis of chronic head injury. Arch Phys Med Rehabil 70:189–193, 1989.

33. Woolf PD, Hamill RW, Lee LA, et al: The predictive value of catecholamines in assessing outcome in traumatic brain injury. J Neurosurg 66:875–882, 1987.

34. Hamill RW, Woolf PD, McDonald JV, et al: Catecholamines predict outcome in traumatic brain injury. Ann Neurol 21:438–443, 1987.

35. van Loon J, Shivalker B, Plets C, et al: Catecholamine response to a gradual increase of intracranial pressure. J. Neurosurg 79:705–709, 1993.

36. Michaud LJ, Rivara FP, Longstreth WJ, Grady MS: Elevated initial blood glucose levels and poor outcome following severe brain injuries in children. J Trauma 31:1356–1362, 1991.

37. Woolf PD, Cox C, Kelly M, et al: The adrenocortical response to brain injury: Correlation with the severity of neurologic dysfunction, effects of intoxication and patient outcome. Alcoholism 14:917–921, 1990.

38. Woolf PD, Lee LA, Hammill RW, McDonald JV: Thyroid test abnormalities in traumatic brain injury: Correlation with neurologic impairment and sympathetic nervous system activation. Am J Med 84:201–208, 1988.

39. Passaoglu A, Passaoglu H: Enzymatic changes in the cerebrospinal fluid as indices of pathologic change. Acta Neurochir 97:71–76, 1989.

40. Viallard JL, Gaulme J, Dalens B, Dastugue B: Cerebral spinal fluid enzymology: Creatine kinase, lactate dehydrogenase activity and isozyme pattern as a brain change index. Clin Chim Acta 89:405–409, 1978.

41. Baker AJ, Moulton RJ, MacMillan VH, Shedden PM: Excitatory amino acids in cerebrospinal fluid following traumatic brain injury in humans. J Neurosurg 79:369–372, 1993.

42. Timming R, Orrison WW, Mikula JA: Computerized tomography and rehabilitation outcome after severe head trauma. Arch Phys Med Rehabil 63:154–159, 1982.

43. Cope N, Hall K: Head injury rehabilitation: Benefit of early intervention. Arch Phys Med Rehabil 63:433–437, 1982.

44. Mackay LE, Bernstein BA, Chapman PE, et al: Early intervention in severe head injury: Long-term benefits of a formalized program. Arch Phys Med Rehabil 73:635–641, 1992.

45. Hagen C, Malkmus D, Durham P: Levels of cognitive functioning: In Rehabilitation of the Head Injured Adult: Comprehensive Physical Management. Downey, CA, Professional Staff Association of Rancho Los Amigos Hospital, 1979.

46. Rappaport M, Dougherty A, Kelting D: Evaluation of coma and vegetative states. Arch Phys Med Rehabil 73:628–634, 1992.

47. Ansell BJ, Keenan JE: The Western Neuro Sensory Stimulation Profile: A tool for assessing slow-to-recover head injured patients. Arch Phys Med Rehabil 70:104–108, 1989.

48. DeYoung S, Gross R: Coma recovery program. J Rehabil Nursing 12:121–123, 1991.

49. LeWinn EB, Dimancescu MP: Environmental deprivation and enrichment in coma. Lancet 1: 156–157, 1978.

50. Wilson SL, Powell GE, Elliott K, Thwaites H: Sensory stimulation in prolonged coma: Four single case studies. Brain Inj 5:393–400, 1991.

51. Shaw R: Persistent vegetative state: Principles and techniques for seating and positioning. J Head Trauma Rehabil 1:31–37, 1986.

52. Levin HS, Peters BH, Hulkonen DA: Early concepts of anterograde and retrograde amnesia. Cortex 19:427–440, 1983.

53. Symonds CP: Observations on the differential diagnosis and treatment of cerebral states consequent upon head injuries. BMJ 2:828–832, 1928.

54. Russell WR: Cerebral involvement in head injury. Brain 55:549–603, 1932.

55. High WM, Levin HS, Gary HE: Recovery of orientation following closed head injury. J Clin Exp Neuropsychol 12:703–714, 1990.

56. Levin HS, High WM, Meyers CA, et al: Impairment of remote memory after closed head injury. J Neurol Neurosurg Psychiatry 48:556–563, 1985.

57. Kapur N, Ellison D, Smith MP, et al: Focal retrograde amnesia following bilateral temporal lobe pathology: A neuropsychological and magnetic resonance study. Brain 115:73–85, 1992.

58. Squire LR: Mechanisms of memory. Science 232:1612–1619, 1986.

59. Levin HS, High WM Jr, Eisenberg HM: Learning and forgetting during post-traumatic amnesia in head injured patients. J Neurol Neurosurg Psychiatry 51:14–20, 1988.

60. Jennett B: Assessment of the severity of head injury. J Neurol Neurosurg Psychiatry 39:647–655, 1976.

61. Mysiw WJ, Corrigan JD, Carpenter D, Chock SKL: Prospective assessment of posttraumatic amnesia: A comparison of the GOAT and OGMS. J Head Trauma Rehabil 5:65–72, 1990.

62. Symonds CP, Russell RW: Accidental head injuries. Lancet 187, 1943.

63. Hirst W. Volpe BT: Memory strategies with brain damage. Brain Cogn 8:379–408, 1988.

64. Warrington EK, Weiskrantz L: Amnesia: A disconnection syndrome: Neuropsychologia 20:233–243, 1982.

65. Saneda DL, Corrigan JD: Predicting clearing of post-traumatic amnesia following closed head injury. Brain Inj 6:167–174, 1992.

66. Jennett B, Teasdale G: Management of Head Injuries. Philadelphia, F.A. Davis, 1981, p 90.

67. Crovitz HF: Techniques to investigate post-traumatic and retrograde amnesia after head injury. In Levin HS, Grafman J, Eisenburg HM (eds): Neurobehavioral Recovery from Head Injury. New York, Oxford University Press, 1987, pp 330–340.

68. Levin HS, O'Donnell VM, Grossman RG: The Galveston Orientation and Amnesia Test: A practical scale to assess cognition after head injury. J Nerv Ment Dis 167:675–684, 1979.

69. Gronwall D, Wrightson P: Duration of post-traumatic amnesia after mild head injury. J Clin Neuropsychol 1:51–60, 1980.

70. Corrigan JD, Arnett JA, Houck LJ, Jackson RD: Reality orientation for brain injured patients: Group treatment and monitoring of recovery. Arch Phys Med Rehabil 66:675–684, 1984.

71. Corrigan JD, Mysiw WJ: Agitation following traumatic head injury: Equivocal evidence for a discrete stage of cognitive recovery. Arch Phys Med Rehabil 69:487–492, 1988.

72. Jackson RD, Mysiw WJ, Corrigan JD: Orientation Group Monitoring System: An indicator for reversible impairments in cognition during post-traumatic amnesia. Arch Phys Med Rehabil 70:33–36, 1989.

73. Denny-Brown D: Disability arising from closed head injury. JAMA 127:429–436, 1945.

74. Mysiw WJ, Jackson RD, Corrigan JD: Ami–triptyline for post-traumatic agitation. Am J Phys Med Rehabil 67:29–33, 1988.

75. Brooke MM, Questad KA, Patterson DR, Bashak KJ: Agitation and restlessness after closed head injury: A prospective study of 100 consecutive admissions. Arch Phys Med Rehabil 73:320–323, 1992.

76. Young GP: The agitated patient in the emergency department. Emerg Med Clin North Am 5:765–781, 1987.

77. Whyte J, Rosenthal M: Rehabilitation of the patient with traumatic brain injury. In DeLisa JA (ed): Rehabilitation Medicine: Principles and Practice. Philadelphia, J.B. Lippincott, 1993, pp 825–860.

78. Corrigan JD: Development of a scale for assessment of agitation following traumatic brain injury. J Clin Exp Neuropsychol 11:261–277, 1989.

79. McIntosh T: Novel pharmacologic therapies in the treatment of experimental traumatic brain injury. J Clin Exp Neuropsychol 11:261-277, 1989.

80. Gualtieri CT: Pharmacotherapy and the neurobehavioral sequelae of traumatic brain injury. Brain Inj 2:101–129, 1988.

81. Chandler MC, Barnhill JL, Gualtieri CT: Amantadine for the agitated head-injury patient. Brain Inj 2:309–3111, 1988.

82. Rowland T, Mysiw WJ, Bogner JA, Corrigan JD: Trazodone for post-traumatic agitation. Arch Phys Med Rehabil 73:963, 1992.

83. Brooke MM, Patterson DR, Questad KA, et al: The treatment of agitation during initial hospitalization after traumatic brain injury. Arch Phys Med Rehabil 73:917–921, 1992.

84. Hale MS, Donaldson JO: Lithium carbonate in the treatment of organic brain syndrome. J Nerv Ment Dis 170:362–365, 1982.

85. Levine AM: Buspirone and agitation in head injury. Brain Inj 2:165–167, 1988.

86. Kalisky Z, Morrison DP, Meyers CA, von Laufen AO: Medical problems encountered during rehabilitation of patients with head injury. Arch Phys Med Rehabil 66:25–29, 1985.

87. Clifton GL, Ziegler MG, Grossman RG: Circulating catecholamines and sympathetic activity after head injury. Neurosurgery 8:10-14, 1981.

88. Labi ML, Horn LJ: Hypertension in traumatic brain injury. Brain Inj 4:365–370, 1990.

89. Mysiw WJ, Jackson RD: Relationship of new-onset systemic hypertension and normal pressure hydrocephalus. Brain Inj 4:233–238, 1990.

90. Sandel ME, Abrams PL, Horn LJ: Hypertension after brain injury: Case report. Arch Phys Med Rehabil 67:469–472, 1986.

91. Panzatelli MR, Pavlakis SG, Gould RJ, DeVivo DC: Hypothalamic-midbrain dysregulation syndrome: Hypertension, hyperthermia, and decerebration. J Child Neurol 6:115–122, 1991.

92. Ferrario CM, Barnes KL, Bohonek S: Neurogenic hypertension produced by lesions of nucleus tractus solitarii alone or with sinoaortic denervation in dog. Hypertension 3:112–118, 1981.

93. Cromptom MR: Hypothalamic lesions following closed head injury. Brain 94:165–172, 1971.

94. Birbamer GG, Buchberger W, Aichner FT: Management of head injury (letter). N Engl J Med 328:1125, 1993.

95. Ziegler MG, Morrissey EC, Marshall LF: Catecholamine and thyroid hormones in traumatic injury. Crit Care Med 18:253–258, 1990.

96. Robertson CS, Clifton GL, Taylor AA, Grossman RG: Treatment of hypertension associated with head injury. J Neurosurg 59:455–560, 1983.

97. Solomon S, Hotchkiss E, Saravay SM, et al: Impairment of memory function by antihypertensive medication. Arch Gen Psychiatry 40:1109–1112, 1983.

98. Miner ME: Systemic effects of brain injury. Trauma 2:75–83, 1985.

99. Hackenberry LE, Miner ME, Rea GL, et al: Biochemical evidence of myocardial injury after severe head trauma. Crit Care Med 10:641–644, 1982.

100. McLeod AA, Neil-Dwyer CH, Meyer CH, et al: Cardiac sequelae of acute head injury. Br Heart J 47:221–229, 1982.

101. Rose AG, Novitsky D, Cooper DK: Myocardial and pulmonary histopathologic changes. Transplant Proc 20(suppl):29–32, 1988.

102. Rotem M, Constantini S, Shir Y, Corteu S: Life-threatening torsade de pointes arrhythmia associated with head injury. Neurosurgery 23:89–92, 1982.

103. Lee YC, Sutton FJ: Concomitant pulses and U-wave alternans after head trauma. Am J Cardiol 55:851–852, 1985.

104. Wirth R, Fenster PE, Marcus FI: Transient heart block associated with head trauma. J Trauma 28:262–264, 1988.

105. Dire DJ, Patterson R: Transient first-degree AV block and sixth nerve palsy in a patient with closed head injury. J Emerg Med 5:393–397, 1987.

106. Fink ME: Emergency management of the head-injured patient. Emerg Med Clin North Am 5:783–795, 1987.

107. Sharples PM, Storey A, Aynsley-Green A, Eyre JA: Avoidable factors contributing to death of children with head injury. BMJ 300:87–91, 1990.

108. Dettbarn CL, Davidson LJ: Pulmonary complications in the patient with acute head injury: Neurogenic pulmonary edema. Heart Lung 18:583–589, 1989.

109. Goodpasture HC, Romig DA, Voth DW, et al: Prospective study of tracheobronchial bacterial flora in acutely brain-injured patients with and without antibiotic prophylaxis. J Neurosurg 47: 228–235, 1977.

110. Akers SM, Bartter TC, Pratter MR: Respiratory car. Phys Med Rehabil State Art Rev 4:527–542, 1990.

111. Gurney JG, Rivara FP, Mueller BA, et al: The effects of alcohol intoxication on the initial treatment and hospital course of patients with acute brain injury. J Trauma 33:709–713, 1992.

112. Becker E, Bar-Or O, Mendelson L, Najenson T: Pulmonary functions and responses to exercise of patients following craniocerebral injury. Scand J Rehabil Med 10:47–50, 1978.

113. Nowak P, Cohn AM, Guidice MA: Airway complications in patients with closed head injuries. Am J Otolaryngol 8:91–96, 1987.

114. Woo P, Kelly G, Kirshner P: Airway complications in the head injured. Laryngoscope 99:725–731, 1989.

115. Law JH, Barnhart K, Rowlett W, et al: Increased frequency of obstructive airway abnormalities with long-term tracheostomy. Chest 104:136–138, 1993.

116. Klinbeil GE: Airway problems in patients with traumatic brain injury. Arch Phys Med Rehabil 69:493–495, 1988.

117. Petersdorf RR: Chills and fever. In Petersdorf RG, Adams RD, Braunwald E, et al (eds): Harrison's Principles of Internal Medicine. New York, McGraw-Hill, 1983 pp 57–65.

118. Jackson RD, Mysiw WJ: Fever of unknown origin following traumatic brain injury. Brain Inj 5:93–100, 1991.

119. Carrol K, Cheeseman SH, Fink MP, et al: Secondary infection of posttraumatic pulmonary cavitary lesions in adolescents and young adults: Role of computed tomography and operative debridement and drainage. J Trauma 29:601–604, 1984.

120. Craven DE: Nosocomial pneumonia: New concepts on an old disease. Infect Control Hosp Epidemiol 9:57–58, 1988.

121. Watts C, Pulliam M: Problems associated with multiple trauma, In Youcnau JR (ed): Neurologic Surgery. Philadelphia, W.B. Saunders, 1982, pp 2475–2530.

122. O'Reilly MJ, Reddick EJ, et al: Sepsis from sinusitis in nasotracheally intubated patients. Am J Med 66:463–467, 1979.

123. Bell RM, Page GV, Bynoe RP, et al: Post-traumatic sinusitis. J Trauma 28:923–930, 1988.

124. Levinson SL, Barondess JA: Occult dental infection as a cause of fever of obscure origin. Am J Med 66:463–467, 1979.

125. Douglas A, Moore-Gillon J, Eykyn S: Fever during treatment of infective endocarditis. Lancet i:1341–1343, 1986.

126. Murray HW, Mann JJ, Genecin A, McKusick VA: Fever with dissecting aneurysm of the aorta. Am J Med 61:140–144, 1976.

127. Cunha BA, Tu RP: Fever in the neurosurgical patient. Heart Lung 17:608–611, 1988.

128. Sasahara AA, Sharma GVRK, Barsamian EM, et al: Pulmonary thromboembolism: Diagnosis and treatment. Clin Cardiol 249:2945–2950, 1983.

129. Ragone DJ Jr, Kellerman WC, Bonner FJ Jr: Heterotopic ossification masquerading as deep venous thrombosis in head injured adult: Complication of anticoagulation. Arch Phys Med Rehabil 67:339–341, 1986.

130. Scott CM, Grasberger RC, Heeran TF, et al: Intra-abdominal sepsis after hepatic trauma. Am J Surg 155:284–288, 1988.

131. Mackowiak PA, Le Maistre CF: Drug fever: A critical appraisal of conventional concepts. Ann Intern Med 106:728–733, 1987.

132. Cohen BM, Baldessarini RJ, Pope HG, et al: Neuroleptic malignant syndrome. N Engl J Med 313:1293, 1985.

133. Buckwald FJ, Haud R, Hanselbout RR: Hospital acquired bacterial meningitis in neurosurgical patients. J Neurosurg 46:494–500, 1977.

134. Mancebo J, Domingo P, Blanch L, et al: Post-neurosurgical and spontaneous gram-negative bacillary meningitis in adults. Scand J Infect Dis 18:533–538, 1986.

135. Talman WT, Florek G, Bullard DE: A hyperthermic syndrome in two subjects with acute hydro-cephalus. Arch Neurol 45:1037–1040, 1988.

136. Benedek G, Toth-Daru P, Janaky J, et al: Indomethacin is effective against neurogenic hyperthermia following cranial trauma or brain surgery. Can J Neurol Sci 14:145–148, 1987.

137. Semel JD: Complex partial status epilepticus presenting as fever of unknown origin. Arch Intern Med 147: 1571–1572, 1987.

138. Zasler ND, Horn LJ: Rehabilitative management of sexual dysfunction. J Head Trauma Rehabil 5(2):14–24, 1990.

139. Whyte J, Glenn MB: The care and rehabilitation of the patient in a persistent vegetative state. J Head Trauma Rehabil 1(1):39–53, 1986.

140. Field LH, Weiss CJ: Dysphagia with head injury. Brain Inj 3:19–26, 1989.

141. Winstein CJ: Neurogenic dysphasia: Frequency, progression, and outcome in adults following head injury. Phys Ther 63:1992–1997, 1983.

142. Rapp RP, Young B, Twyman D, et al: The favorable effect of early parenteral feeding on survival in head-injured patients. J Neurosurg 58:906–912, 1983.

143. Price R, Lehmann JF, Boswell-Bessette S, et al: Influence of cryotherapy on spasticity at the human ankle. Arch Phys Med Rehabil 74:300–304, 1993.

144. Barnard P, Dill H, Eldredge P, et al: Reduction of hypertonicity by early casting in a comatose head-injured individual. Phys Ther 64:1540–1542, 1984.

145. Easton JKM, Ozel T, Halpern D: Intramuscular neurolysis for spasticity in children. Arch Phys Med Rehabil 60:155–158, 1979.

146. Garland DE, Thompson R, Waters RL: Musculo-cutaneous neurectomy for spastic elbow flexion in non-functional upper extremities in adults. J Bone Joint Surg 62:108–112, 1980.

147. Dennis JW, Menawat S, Von Thron J, et al: Efficacy of deep venous thrombosis prophylaxis in trauma patients and identification of high-risk groups. J Trauma 35:132–139, 1993.

148. Consensus Conference: Prevention of venous thrombosis and pulmonary embolism. JAMA 25: 744–749, 1986.

149. Shackford SR, Davis JW, Hollingsworth-Fridlund P, et al: Venous thromboembolism in patients with major trauma. Am J Surg 159:365–369, 1990.

150. Ruiz AJ, Hill SL, Berry RE: Heparin, deep venous thrombosis and trauma patients. Am J Surg 162: 159–162, 1991.

151. Knudson MM, Collins JA, Goodman SB, McCory DW: Thromboembolism following multiple trauma. J Trauma 32:2–11, 1992.

152. O'Malley KF, Ross SE: Pulmonary embolism in major trauma patients. J Trauma 30:748–750, 1990.

153. Kudsk KA, Fabian TC, Baum S, et al: Silent deep venous thrombosis in immobilized multiple trauma patients. Am J Surg 158:515–519, 1989.

154. Conine TA, Sullivan T, Mackie T, Goodman M: Effect of serial casting for the prevention of equi-nus in patients with acute head injury. Arch Phys Med Rehabil 71:310–312, 1990.

155. Imie PC, Eppinhous CE, Boughton AC: Efficacy of non-bivalved and bivalved serial casting on head injured patients in intensive care. Phys Ther 66:748, 1986.

156. Keenan MA, Ure K, Smith CW, Jordan C: Hamstring release for knee flexion contracture in spastic adults. Clin Orthop Rel Res 236:221–226, 1988.

157. Garland DE, Bailey S, Rhoades ME: Orthopedic management of brain injured adults. Part II. Clin Orthop Rel Res 131:111–122, 1978.

158. Garland DE, Bailey S: Undetected injuries in head-injured adults. Clin Orthop Rel Res 155: 162–165, 1981.

159. Garland DE, Keenan ME: Orthopedic strategies in the management of the adult head-injured patient. Phys Ther 63:2004–2009, 1983.

160. Garland, DE, Dowling V: Forearm fractures in the head-injured adult. Clin Orthop Rel Res 176:190–196, 1983.

161. Stone L, Keenan MA: Peripheral nerve injuries in the adult with traumatic brain injury. Clin Orthop Rel Res 233:136–144, 1988.

162. Orcutt SA, Kramer WG, Howard MW, et al: Carpal tunnel syndrome secondary to wrist and finger flexor spasticity. J Hand Surg 15:940–944, 1990.

163. Philip PA, Philip M: Peripheral nerve injuries in children with traumatic brain injuries. Brain Inj 6:53–58, 1992.

164. Varghese G: Heterotopic ossification. Rehabil Clin North Am 3:407–415, 1992.

165. Mysiw WJ, Tan J, Jackson RD: Heterotopic ossification: The utility of osteocalcin in diagnosis and management. Am J Phys Med Rehabil 72:184–187, 1993.

166. Lindholm TS, Bauer FC, Rindell K: High doses of the disphosphonate EHDP for the prevention of heterotopic ossification. Scand J Rheum 16:33–39, 1987.

167. Buschbacher R, McKinley W, Buschbacher L, et al: Warfarin in prevention of heterotopic ossification. Am J Phys Med Rehabil 71:86–91, 1992.

168. Garland DE, Razza BE, Waters RL: Forceful joint manipulation in head-injured adults with heterotopic ossification. Clin Orthop Rel Res 169:133–138, 1982.

169. Ritter MA, Gioe TJ: The effect of indomethacin on para-articular ectopic ossification following total hip arthroplasty. Clin Orthop Rel Res 167:113–117, 1982.

170. Commission for the Accreditation of Rehabilitation Facilities. Standards Manual. Tucson, AZ, CARF, 1991.

MICHAEL G. BOYESON Ph.D.

JENNIFER L. JONES M.S.

4

Theoretical Mechanisms of Brain Plasticity and Therapeutic Implications

The observation that a significant amount of spontaneous behavioral recovery occurs over time after traumatic brain injury—without significant regrowth of tissue—has spawned much speculation about possible underlying mechanisms. Some of the mechanisms proposed, while intuitively plausible, have little empirical support or explanatory power. Although many physiologic events have been shown to correlate with spontaneous recovery, it has been much more difficult to verify causality. It is likely that recovery of function after brain injury represents a complex interaction of many processes; no current single theory can be offered as the sole explanation. This chapter reviews and critiques the major hypotheses that attempt to explain functional recovery and places them in appropriate perspective with regard to current prospects for rehabilitation in the brain-injured patient.

A major focus is to dispel the notion that functional recovery is a consequence of some genetically controlled, a priori plan of functional brain reorganization designed to accommodate a potential injury. Although arguments against such an interpretation are not new,[74,155] recent information has focused empirical data more clearly within the conceptional framework. What we term "functional recovery" is more likely related to (1) the lack of direct involvement of the lost tissue in observed spontaneous recovery, and (2) when different from true recovery, the result of genetically driven activation of developmental and growth processes[19,60,153,154] that later in life do *not* function as in normal early development. Normal sprouting and growth of neurons and supporting cells in early development are quite distinct from the process that occurs in the mature organism after injury. This is perhaps illustrated by the fact lesions occurring very early in development are associated with more sparing of function. Such functional sparing may be related to the more appropriate development-oriented milieu of injuries during early maturation. However, even during this phase functional sparing may be as maladaptive as later in development.[153,154]

Finger[19] has provided persuasive arguments against the likelihood of a mechanism(s) specifically designed to enhance functional recovery. He suggests that the only designed protection from injury has been the evolutionary development of cranial and spinal bone encasement and isolation of the brain (via the blood-brain barrier) from the rest of the body. From an evolutionary point of view, most of the physiologic consequences of brain injury should be maladaptive because, in the wild, a brain-injured animal is likely to be easy prey. If an injury early in life leads to the animal's death, the result is loss of contribution to the gene pool rather than selective advantage. Even if the animal survives the brain injury, any resulting behavioral abnormality is likely to place the animal at a selective disadvantage in the mating process, further limiting access to the gene pool. Consistent with this argument is the observation that many physiologic changes following brain injury are correlated with maladaptive behaviors, such as spasticity[164,177] and epilepsy,[18] rather than with beneficial behaviors.

This chapter provides examples demonstrating the possible relationships between spontaneous recovery of function and modifications in intact tissue. Arguments are made that, to date, the only realistic expectation is to increase the rate and, perhaps to a lesser extent, the level of recovery; in general, the actual incidence of recovery is unaffected. To avoid a fatalistic view of the efficacy of therapeutic intervention, the rehabilitation professional must realize that it is possible to affect, either beneficially or negatively, the rate of recovery. However, hastening the rate at which functional recovery occurs may hasten the onset of associated consequences, such as later evolving maladaptive behavior. Empirical evidence indicates that recovery from brain injury is a continuously evolving process that parallels certain neurochemical and neuroanatomic modifications of the brain. Many behavioral deficits that have recovered spontaneously can be pharmacologically reinstated long after recovery by partially mimicking the neurochemical events that occurred during the primary injury. Although in some cases the underlying residual deficit does not pragmatically interfere with day-to-day functioning, simply ignoring the deficit does not increase understanding of the mechanisms of recovery. Only in rare instances[213,214] is it possible to prevent permanently the recovery of one's behavior through normal pharmacologic treatment of other symptoms associated with a brain injury. Moreover, the interventional procedures

that are likely to affect spontaneous recovery generally affect systems that were involved only marginally in the primary injury. The extent to which remote, transiently affected areas can control a particular behavior independently of the injured area primarily determines the effectiveness of a given therapeutic intervention (and in large part whether or not recovery occurs independently of therapy). All of these issues are addressed within the context of rehabilitation after brain injury.

THEORETICAL MECHANISMS

From a certain perspective, our theoretical explanations for functional recovery reflect what we were taught constitutes an "adequate" explanation; the result is a wide range of hypotheses, varying from those based on molecular processes to those based on more global behavioral mechanisms. In general, all hypotheses attempt to explain the same empirical events and represent variations on a central theme. They share the view that all functional recovery after brain injury represents compensation on some behavioral, structural, and/or biochemical level. Clearly some type of compensation occurs after traumatic brain injury, as demonstrated by significant spontaneous recovery of function without significant regrowth of lost tissue. Hypotheses differ in their approach to the question of *how* the compensation occurs after injury.

Examples of the different ways in which the brain may "accommodate" an injury have been offered somewhat arbitrarily as distinct, although the processes most likely occur simultaneously or sequentially. For example, denervation supersensitivity has been proposed as a possible mechanism underlying spontaneous recovery of function.[43] In essence, after an injury that results in partial denervation of some inputs to a particular location, the receptive area changes its sensitivity characteristics (through various mechanisms of neurotransmitter reuptake and release, receptor upregulation, and increased sprouting[235] to compensate for the partially lost input. As such changes in sensitivity are completed, there are presumably parallel recoveries of some behavior. Sprouting into the area which occurs after increases in receptor upregulation, in turn may lead to downregulation and decreases in the sensitivity of other mechanisms if the sprouts become viable.

This section begins with a discussion of two partially related hypotheses to explain recovery of function: (1) vicariation, which proposes that systems not originally involved in the lost function come to assume the responsibility, and (2) redundancy or unmasking, which suggests that the circuitry that assumes the lost function is always present but unused until injury occurs. Other topics to be explored include diaschisis and compensation hypotheses.

Vicariation

Hypotheses of vicariation are related conceptually to hypotheses of physiologic compensation but exemplify the most extreme form of reorganization. Based on their interpretation of early data about the recovery of voluntary motor control after a cortical injury, Flourens and colleagues[81] suggested that, because the loss of cortical tissue was permanent other parts of the brain must have taken over the lost function for behavioral recovery to occur. In contrast, Ferrier[74] suggested that it was unlikely that, for instance, the organ of sight could take over for hearing or that motor systems could take over for sensory systems if one or the other was lost. At that time it was not clear how a structure (cells or systems) could assume another function, in addition to its normal one, within the brain.

Formalized by Hermann Munk in the 1800s,[181] the concept of vicariation suggests that after a brain injury structures not originally involved in the mediation of the affected behavior come to control its expression. Since then persuasive arguments have suggested that, although intuitively plausible, the concept ultimately may be theoretically untestable,[75] because it is difficult to prove that a structure is *not* involved in the control of a particular behavior. Nevertheless, attempts have been made to test the hypothesis that adjacent or homotypical cortex reorganizes to take over lost functions after various cortical injuries.

In general support of the hypothesis, Spear and colleagues[229] have shown that neurons in the lateral suprasylvian gyrus normally unresponsive to specific visual input can become responsive to such stimuli if normal visual cortical areas are impaired. Although these findings are suggestive, it is not clear whether functional recovery is related causally to the ability of a neuron to be driven by visual stimulus (see below).

Glees and Cole[98] found that after undercutting the cortical thumb area in the monkey, which results in loss of pinch strength that recovers with 3 weeks, microstimulation in the vicinity of the injury evoked movements of the thumb from areas in which no such movements could be obtained before the injury. More recent studies[96,97] using chronic indwelling electrodes have found no qualitative changes in movements elicited by stimulation in the vicinity of an injury, exploratory capacity afforded by a fixed electrode array is limited.

To avoid some of these difficulties, Boyeson et al.[26] conducted systematic microstimulation of rat cortex after unilateral contusion, laceration, or suction ablation to a portion of the sensorimotor cortex representing the hindlimb. They found that no new responses could be evoked (from hours up to 475 days after injury). In addition, they found no changes in stimulation threshold at the level of the cortex that could be reasonably correlated with functional recovery. For example, although contusion and laceration induced widespread elevation of thresholds that recovered by 9–15 days after injury (when motor behavior recovered), suction ablation revealed no threshold changes up to the leading edge of the ablation at any time (hours to days) after injury. Animals injured by suction ablation recovered in the same time period as animals injured by contusion and/or laceration, indicating that changes in microstimulation thresholds of adjacent cortex cannot be considered correlates of functional motor recovery.

Although the above findings provide strong evidence against the likelihood of cortically mediated vicariation, they do not rule out the possibility that a form of vicariation may occur at some other hierarchical level in the brain. For example, the results of one study[69] showed that cats with bilateral ablation of areas 17, 18, and 19 and the lateral suprasylvian gyrus can permanently recover depth perception if given visual experience while under the influence of amphetamine. One animal with a particularly large bilateral lesion of all cortical visual areas recovered visual ability, indicating that visual recovery can be achieved pharmacologically at noncortical levels.

The utility of the vicariation hypothesis is diminished when recovery continues, even as the burden on other tissue to take over the function increases. For example, if an animal recovers from some behavioral deficit after cortical injury and the adjacent tissue is lesioned, the animal reveals the same deficit. If the animal subsequently recovers from this deficit, the burden then is placed on the remaining available tissue, and so on. This problem is also a general argument for behavioral compensation hypotheses (see below), which, like vicariation hypotheses, exhibit little explanatory power.

Redundancy/Unmasking

One possible explanation for spontaneous recovery of function without significant regrowth of tissue is that some normally quiescent circuitry in the brain is activated (unmasked) after injury. Conceptually, this hypothesis is similar to the concept of vicariation. The main difference is that the brain does not significantly reorganize itself to realize functional recovery; instead, multiple back-up systems already in place are released after injury.

As the most thoroughly studied example of this concept, Wall and colleagues[63,252] examined changes in the receptive fields of the thalamus after surgical removal of the nucleus gracilis in the medulla of rats. Normally, somatotopic representation of the hindlimb is in the lateral one-third of the ventralis posterolateralis nucleus of the thalamus, whereas the forelimb area is represented in the medial two-thirds of the nucleus. After damage to the representation of the hindlimb area at the level of the medulla, the forelimb receptive field of the thalamus expands into the vacated hindlimb area within minutes after the lesion (too soon for sprouting to occur). The authors postulate the existence of latent synapses that

normally are unused but are expressed after the injury. However, it is possible that the fibers involved in the expanded forelimb representation are remnant forelimb components of the trunk region. Cortical motor representation provides a conceptual example: after removal of the cortical hindlimb area in the rat, the forelimb area "appears" to move into the trunk region (which is located between the forelimb and hindlimb areas).[26,116,185] In the normal trunk region, stimulation at low intensity primarily activates trunk behaviors, whereas stimulation at a slightly higher intensity recruits a rotary-type movement that involves the forelimb, trunk, and hindlimb (much like a stepping movement). The forelimb response in this rotary movement is quite distinct from the various wrist, supination, pronation, and digit responses obtained in the forelimb area anterior to the trunk region , but it is the same forelimb response that appears to move into the trunk region after a hindlimb injury.[26] As others have demonstrated,[63,252] the forelimb component of the trunk response can also be detected immediately after focal suction ablation of the hindlimb area.[26] Such data indicate that the response was always present as a component of the synergistic trunk response. After removal of the hindlimb component, the only component that can be expressed is the residual forelimb response; thus, many examples of redundancy and unmasking after injury may be due to the release from transcortical control of intact homunculi representations that are remnants of a larger behavioral response. In fact, observations of "disinhibited" behaviors are a frequent sequelae of cortical injuries in humans (e.g., exaggerated reflex activity).[220] In addition, what appears to be redundancy may arise from the complexity of the neural substrates for the behavior; thus, if the neural substrate for a particular behavior is broadly represented in the brain, the behavior may recover after injury because of extensive neural controls that are left intact rather than because of redundant or repeated systems.

In general, it perhaps makes no biologic or energetic sense for a species to maintain normally unused circuitry for long periods of time, unless brain injuries were a frequent occurrence. From an evolutionary standpoint, disuse atrophy would be expected to remove systems that were maintained without functional use. Given this caveat and its implications for rehabilitation medicine, it is important to realize that, whatever the mechanisms, events such as those described above occur after brain trauma. Currently, such events (e.g., spasticity) usually can be managed with appropriate pharmacologic agents or treated as peripherally manifested symptoms and manipulated surgically for relief, with or without a sound theoretical explanation.

Diaschisis

Any brain injury that destroys a particular collection of neurons is likely to produce more generalized disturbances that transiently affect the responsiveness of other neurons. In 1905, the term *diaschisis* was coined by the anatomist Constantin von Monakow[247,248] to describe the distant effects of brain lesions that seemed to be reversible. Von Monakow believed that the temporary behavioral deficits following focal brain injury were due partly to disturbances in tissue remote from, but anatomically connected to, the primary site of injury. Morphologically intact brain regions, he believed, were functionally depressed by deprivation of some level of "excitation" from the injured area. Dissipation of this remote functional depression was proposed as a basis for spontaneous behavioral recovery after brain injury. The concept of diaschisis has its origins in Galen's concept of "sympathy," according to which damage to a particular organ of the body may sympathetically (secondarily) affect other connected structures.[75] In addition, before the turn of the century, Gower[105] distinguished between symptoms that were a "direct" result of ischemic stroke and symptoms that resulted from interference with function in structures outside the primary injury site. Although von Monakow proposed no physiologic mechanism through which diaschisis might operate, over time use of the term has expanded to include a host of potentially reversible, nonspecific effects that make the immediate consequences of a brain lesion more intense than persistent deficits.[59] These ideas have been cogently summarized by Feeney.[66,67]

Clearly, elements of the vicariation and redundancy hypotheses can be integrated into the concept of diaschisis. Remote structures may come to perform the lost function through reactivation of phylogenetically older circuits that were involved in the behavior before evolution of new anatomic structures. Refinement of techniques capable of measuring the functional state of specific brain regions has enabled experimental study of diaschisis. In the 1940s, Kempinski[141] found remote electrophysiologic changes that recovered over time in brain regions contralateral to cortical injury. Using positron emission tomography, Baron[9] was the first to show significant reduction in metabolic activity and blood flow in the cerebral hemisphere contralateral to the lesion (termed "crossed cerebellar diaschisis"). More recently, a change in neurotransmitter functioning after brain injury has been offered as a possible mechanism through which diaschisis may operate.[19,20,30] Numerous studies have shown a positive correlation between behavioral outcome after critical injury and pharmacologic manipulation of various neurotransmitter systems, particularly with agents that increase noradrenergic activity.[24,27,28,31,70-73,103,104,130,250,251] Amelioration of depressed neurotransmitter activity in brain areas that are otherwise morphologically intact may well underlie the restoration of many behaviors. Most currently available intervention strategies involve such pharmacologic manipulation of functionally depressed regions, primarily because they provide symptomatic relief from the behavioral deficit. Only recently, however, have the mechanisms been elucidated through the use of effective animal models. With increased understanding of the temporal course of the changes that follow brain injury and the possible mechanisms involved in diaschisis, future pharmacologic treatment may be more effectively focused on modifying behavioral recovery at the appropriate time.

Compensation Hypotheses

Behavioral Compensation

Explanations of functional recovery based on behavior compensation in many respects are outgrowths of constructs advocated by B.F.

Skinner. According to Skinner,[225] behavior can be controlled largely by manipulating variables external to the brain. By regulating what the brain receives, it is possible to regulate what the brain does, regardless of the neural mechanism. In a similar "black box" fashion, hypotheses based on behavioral compensation do not require an underlying explanation for change in behavior; instead, they simply state that the behavior changed in response to some externally supplied manipulation or simply with the passage of time. Thus, there is no need to understand the changes in internal physiologic brain mechanisms after brain injury and during the recovery process. If a behavioral deficit appears to recover after injury, one simply concludes that the brain was able to compensate; conversely, if no recovery occurs, compensation was not possible.

Obviously such a tautologic hypothesis has no real explanatory power, but it has been used to rationalize the use of various therapeutic strategies based on the symptoms of the injury. For example, after certain brain injuries physical therapists may attempt to achieve normal range of limb motion (which also decreases contractures), because it enhances functional use. If function is enhanced compared with untreated and similarly injured patients, the procedure is judged effective without knowledge of the underlying mechanisms. Likewise, most forms of speech therapy after brain injury are improvisations supported by some degree of clinical success rather than protocols based on knowledge of the brain mechanisms of speech (e.g., repetition exercises, auditory stimulation). Such procedures may result in poorly understood and inappropriately applied techniques that clearly need a more sound theoretical basis.

Physiologic Compensation

Compensatory hypotheses tied to an underlying physiologic event have greater explanatory power than those based on behavioral compensation. By tying the behavioral deficit to some physiologic change, it is theoretically possible to link elements of recovery with changes in brain functioning. Experimental analysis of posttraumatic physiologic changes to determine their relative importance in the recovery process becomes possible. For example, if behavioral recovery is determined to coincide with a particular functional sprouting event, it can be argued that the two events are at least temporally correlated (but not necessarily causally related). A stronger argument can be made if subsequent destruction of the new sprouts reinstates the original deficit. If destruction is not followed by additional sprouting and the deficit becomes permanent, spouting would appear to be directly involved in the recovery process. If behavioral recovery occurs with no subsequent increase in sprouts, it can be argued only that the initial sprouting event was related indirectly to or coincident with recovery.

The process of sprouting during early development has some parallel to the sprouting that occurs after injury, although it is clearly not as genetically ordered after injury in an adult.[21,60,153,154] During normal development, sprouting is genetically driven by multiple protooncogenes (e.g., fos, jun) involved in instructions for mitosis, receptive sites, process outgrowth, and a host of other protein-based regulatory processes.[120,236] In contrast, after injury to the brain c-fos activates transcription factors involved in producing neurotrophic factors, thus allowing for process outgrowth as well as coding for increases in receptor sites.[126] However, the basic genetic plan necessary for de novo cell regeneration (mitosis) is unable to cause sufficient regrowth of neurons and support cells to constitute total tissue replacement.[15] Understanding of the relationships between such processes and functional recovery requires an understanding of the basic neurotrophic factors and their probable functional relationship, which leads to sprouting after brain injury.

Neurotrophic Factors. More than 45 years ago, Buecker[38] reported the results of an experiment in which a mouse sarcoma was transplanted into 3-day-old chick embryos. Histologic analysis of the embryos a few days later revealed a slight but consistent increase in sensory and sympathetic ganglia. Levi-Montalcini et al.[158] replicated and confirmed Buecker's findings a few years later and postulated that the tumor contained a substance that affected neural growth. The substance was eventually isolated and termed *nerve growth factor* (NGF); its discovery eventually earned Levi-Montalcini and Cohen (discovered epidermal growth factor) a Nobel Prize in 1986. Conceptually, of course, the existence of such a trophic factor predated their work by many years.[197,255]

NGF was the first of many subsequently discovered but less well-characterized molecules to exhibit properties of regulating cell growth and survival.[123,156] The GM-1 gangliosides, although not involved in facilitating normal neuronal outgrowth in some transplanted cell lines, stimulate growth of cell projections after certain types of injury, and to some degree also seem to prevent degeneration.[50,86] Most other subsequently discovered factors (e.g., acidic and basic fibroblast growth factor, insulin and insulin growth factor fragments, triiodothyronine) have been characterized as mitotic; that is, they are involved in cellular division and intermediary metabolism. Although NGF apparently is not involved in mitosis,[92] some evidence suggests that the subsequently discovered factors are involved, much like NGF, in cell survival.[124] Presumably, these factors act in concert with NGF to regulate cell numbers, cell survival, and process outgrowth from individual cells.[15]

After an injury (and during normal development) neurotrophic molecules are released from cells to aid in the directional regrowth (and growth) and eventual synaptic formation necessary for normal transmission of neuronal information.[153] With respect to brain injury, such processes may be termed "genetically-driven reactive synaptogenesis,"[60] because the injury leads to a cascading sequence of cellular events that are involved in neurotrophic production and culminate in some level of process outgrowth.[120,236] For example, after brain injury the protooncogene c-fos encodes for activator proteins involved in transcription factors,[120] which in turn regulate the expression of genes that activate NGF.[236] Of course, c-fos encodes for many different proteins and is activated for many purposes; for example, it is elevated immediately after depolarization of a neuron as well as in response to drug manipulations.[120,126,236] "Reactive" is a good descriptor for the process, because there appears to be no

preprogrammed design that activates NGF to aid any particular functional recovery. The reactive process is more likely related to the genetic circumstances and cellular milieu involved in normal early development. In the injured adult, such reactive sprouting is superimposed on a clearly different biochemical and anatomic environment.

NGF is synthesized in targets of responsive neurons and plays a critical role in regulating their survival.[156,157] If NGF is not present at the target, growth is not maintained and the connection is lost. For example, treatment of neonatal mice or rats with anti-NGF antiserum results in degeneration of neurons in the sympathetic nervous system.[157] Recent studies indicate that cholinergic neurons of the basal forebrain and the caudate putamen also responded to NGF,[99,178] which supports their growth, differentiation, and maintenance. The distribution and ontogenesis of NGF and its receptor in the central nervous systems (CNS) are consistent with such studies.[221] Cholinergic neurons in the CNS apparently depend on a given level of NGF in the normal state[11,114] as well as in the acutely[112,113,115,123] or chronically[79] injured state. It is not clear whether similar conditions exist for systems other than the highly "plastic" septohippocampal structures that are involved in short-term memory.

Given the above caveat, it is also appropriate to question whether or not NGF, when administered to a brain-injured animal, causes additional stimulus-induced growth in uninjured systems. For example, the administration of NGF to normal adults results in hypertrophy characterized by an increase in protein synthesis and neurotransmitter production.[42,122] Such findings suggest the potential for some type of neural growth in the brain of the mature animal; however, they also suggest that normal levels of NGF in the developmentally mature adult maintain a specific level of chemical stability and growth in existing neuronal systems, and thus, the nonspecific application of additional NGF after trauma may interfere with this process in the remaining normal tissue. Therefore, any potential therapeutic strategy involving NGF must ensure that process outgrowth is functionally focused. Moreover, the activation of NGF is just as likely (perhaps even more likely) to result in deleterious errors in sprouting effects. In the normal course of recovery, sprouting activity may exceed optimal levels because of the genetically driven characteristics of "conservation of arborization"[21,60] and NGF may hasten the spontaneous onset of maladaptive behaviors. For example, one possible long-term consequence of certain cortical injuries is the advent of sprouting that increases spasticity.[164,177,212] Initial benefits obtained by pharmacologically increasing the activity of NGF and thereby facilitating certain sprouting events (for example, an initial alleviation of hypotonus) may not prove worthwhile if the eventual result is an earlier or more severe onset of spasticity. In addition, an increase in NGF activation may also have untoward effects on tissue that remains intact after the injury. For example, the administration of NGF to normal neonates or mature animals results in profound hyperalgesias.[159] In the future it may be possible to administer antibodies to NGF that halt the expected onset of maladaptive behaviors, but such agents must act specifically on the affected area to avoid possible undesirable side effects on normal tissue.

From a rehabilitation standpoint, it is mandatory to understand more clearly the effects of possible NGF-like therapies before they are clinically used in brain-injured patients. Because antibodies to NGF have been shown to decrease process outgrowth,[12,186] such therapy may prove to be specifically useful in preventing the development of spasticity. In some cases, compounds like the GM-1 gangliosides (glycosophingolipids) may prevent greater degeneration of existing neurons (their effects on process outgrowth seem less important to functional recovery), although the relative benefits and risks have not been clearly established.[50,86] Beneficial effects in the brain-injured patients have been reported with GM-1 gangliosides, but the results do not differ greatly from controls and reach statistical significance only with extremely large sample sizes,[21] suggesting that in humans the GM-1 gangliosides are not as critical to functional recovery as other agents may be. Currently it has been proposed that GM-1 acts as a neuroprotectant acutely and is involved

in facilitating release of other neurotrophic factors at longer intervals.[224]

Sprouting.   The cellular events that begin after an injury are genetically driven to maintain, for example, a given number of neuronal arborizations (dendritic or axonal).[60] Although such outgrowth may replace the function of the structure that was lost, this perhaps is possible only if one small, bundle-specific lesion is induced independently of other injury and if some appropriate scaffold or bridge is present for the regrowth.[113] Such conditions may be met under extreme experimental control[174] but they rarely accompany brain trauma in real life. The many sprouting errors that may be induced with (or even without) additional NGF are less likely to result in beneficial outcomes because of the greater probability of a large area of primary tissue loss and subsequent loss of terminal fields of systems communicating with the area of primary injury.[45]

After the release of NGF and subsequent process outgrowth, several conditions must be met if a sprout is to function successfully. A newly formed sprout may (1) reach a location with no receptive areas, then prune back; (2) inappropriately synapse on a target; or (3) overinnervate an area. Three conceptually distinct forms of posttraumatic sprouting have been observed: regenerative sprouting, homotypical collateralization, and heterotypical collateralization.

Regenerative Sprouting.   Severing axonal processes in the peripheral nervous system (PNS) often results in regrowth of new processes that functionally and specifically reinnervate the area denervated by injury.[218,238] For such processes to become functional, two major consequences of the injury must be overcome:

1. The new fibers must have access through or around the build-up of connective tissue (scar formation). Minimizing the amount of scar tissue improves the success of regrowth through the area.[113]

2. Successful regeneration in the PNS requires the remyelinization of injury-induced demyelinated fibers (accomplished by reattachment of Schwann cells).[91]

In the PNS these consequences of injury are frequently and successfully overcome, but in the CNS the same consequences are major obstacles to successful regeneration. In general, oligodendrocytes (the CNS equivalent of the Schwann cell) do not remyelinate the regrowing axon.[218] The few notable exceptions include diffuse axonal injury induced by fluid percussion in animals.[193] In this case, it is not clear whether the remyelinization occurs only in slightly injured axons (with only a brief separation between the oligodendrocyte and the axonal membrane) or in completely damaged axons.

Homotypical and Heterotypical Collateralization. In homotypical collateralization, axons from intact fibers of the system that was partially damaged branch off and take over synaptic locations vacated by the degenerated fibers. In heterotypical collateralization, fibers from a system originally unrelated to the damaged area take over the vacant synaptic locations. In some cases this may occur by means of a functionally distinct neurotransmitter system (e.g., an inhibitory system replacing an excitatory one).[179] In general, such reactive sprouting conditions occur in response to injury-induced release of various growth factors that lead to process outgrowth. The processes are related to the injury itself and are not part of a specific compensatory mechanism designed to improve functional outcome. Indeed, many of these processes may result in deleterious or minimal effects on behavioral function, depending on the location and type of sprouting. Often new sprouts are pruned back after accessing the damaged area because of incompatibility or simple lack of available receptive sites.[60]

Synaptic Mechanisms. Once sprouting has occurred, functional synapses must be formed that presynaptically synthesize and release the appropriate neurotransmitter, have mechanisms for neurotransmitter deactivation (reuptake, degradation), and postsynaptically provide functional receptive actions.[235] Such presynaptic and postsynaptic changes in the regulation of neurotransmitter formation, activation, and degradation are probably the most important mechanisms through which compensation for lost function occurs.

In response to a slow-growing injury (e.g., certain tumors) functional behavioral deficits probably will not be detectable until sufficiently large amounts of tissue are lost. This phenomenon has been appropriately described by Jackson[137] as the "momentum" of a lesion, which refers to its immediate size displaced over a certain time interval. An immediately large lesion is associated with a greater momentum than an extremely slow-growing lesion in the same area. In general, the greater the momentum of a lesion, the more severe the behavioral consequences; conversely, the slower the momentum, the less severe the behavioral deficits. For example, functional sparing by reducing the momentum of a lesion is observed in animal models in which two "half-sized" lesions are spaced by at least 7 days and compared with one immediate "full-sized" lesion of the same tissue.[76,234] Because effective sparing of function decreases quickly when the time interval between lesions is less than 7 days, this interval must represent the time required for complete compensatory reorganization within this particular model. A delay of more than 7 days confers no additional functional benefit to the animal.

The lack of behavioral symptoms with a slow-growing lesion may be due to the ability of the brain to make subtle adjustments in remaining tissue. Stricker and Zigmond[235] used the brain's catecholamine system as a model of such adjustments. They found that, after a 50-60% loss of catecholamines, the brain compensates exclusively through a decrease in inactivation (decreases in monoamine oxidase and catechol-O-methyltransferase). After a 60-85% loss of catecholamines, in addition to the decrease in inactivation, synthesis and release of catecholamines increase. After a greater than 85% loss of catecholamines, in addition to the above mechanisms, there is an exponential increase in postsynaptic receptors. The first two compensatory processes are rapidly induced after injury, whereas an increase in the number of postsynaptic receptors is a slow process. It is likely that during a slow-growing injury, these mechanisms maintain a homeostatic balance until some critical volume of tissue is lost.

At a superficial glance such changes in synaptic functioning may not appear to be significant factors in traumatic brain injury. However, intact systems that previously communicated with or received input from the injured area may undergo subtle changes to adjust for the loss of input or output and may aid in the maintenance of recovery (particularly when a recovery "plateau" has been reached). Often these processes are revealed pharmacologically when it is demonstrated that certain drugs reinstate original deficits in recovered animals.[22,27-29,34,133] Such effects are generally drug-dependent, but continuous administrations of certain drugs may be contraindicated after certain cortical as well as subcortical injuries.[25] Nevertheless, such findings underscore that, even when compensation has occurred and the individual has "recovered" from a brain injury, the brain remains in a vulnerable state.

Transplantation. Transplantation techniques clearly involve neurotrophic factors to the extent that the graft favorable attaches to the host brain. In principle, the early hopes for transplantation of neural tissue were based on the realization that perhaps for total, true recovery to occur, much of the lost tissue would have to be replaced.[14] The demonstration that grafted tissue could interact with the host brain anatomically gave rise to the somewhat naive assumption that the interaction was somehow normal. Adding to the confusion of such studies were the occasional demonstrations that some functional improvement was obtained in both experimental animals[13,45] and in the clinical population (particularly in patients with Parkinson's symptoms).[196] Although grafted tissue supplies the needed neurotransmitter (e.g., dopamine in patients with Parkinson's disease), the anatomic graft/host connections are aberrant in appearance. Technically many of the same benefits could be provided by drugs, thereby avoiding complications associated with an invasive neurosurgical procedure.

Numerous studies of transplantation have indicated a complete range of functional outcomes from favorable[160,161] to maladaptive,[170,171] and in large part such studies have precisely the same variability and difficulties associated with studies of sprouting. Recently greater attention has been focused on replacement of stem cells (developmental precursor cells) in the hope that they may approximate more closely a normally developing system.[55,64,65,231] The full import of such studies will not be realized soon, because federal legislation barring the use of fetal tissue for research has been rescinded only recently by presidential decree. Even so, the obtaining of the appropriate "fetal-age" donor is beset with ethical considerations.

Some of the same issues that confront the administration of neurotrophic factors will have to be addressed with transplantation procedures. One technique currently under investigation is the possible encasement of precursor cells in a matrix that is temporarily or partially isolated from the host brain during the developmental growth period.[21] This procedure may help to restrict growth to the intended area as well as avoid complications[159,170,171] associated with growth factors on normal host tissue.

IMMEDIATE AND LONG-TERM INTERVENTION STRATEGIES

Acute Stage After Injury

Recent research has indicated that, despite the direct tissue damage incurred at the time of injury, marginal/penumbral areas of tissue can be saved from some of the devastating effects of excitatory neurotransmitter-induced calcium loading into cells, which initiates the biochemical cascade of events leading to cell death.[217] Such penumbral areas are more extensive after injuries related to changes in oxygen or blood flow (e.g., strokes),[125] but they are present to some extent in all brain injuries. Current therapeutic areas of interest include (1) prevention of the effects of the massive release of excitatory neurotransmitters, (2) prevention of the massive influx of calcium into the cells caused by the excitation, (3) prevention of the formation of free radicals, and (4) scavenging of the free radicals once they have formed in an effort to prevent cell membrane lysis.

Blocking Receptor-activated Channels after the Release of Excitotoxic Neurotransmitters

After a brain injury the release of a large number of excitatory and inhibitory neurotransmitters results in a net excess of excitatory neurotransmitters (e.g., glutamate and acetylcholine). This massive release initiates a cascade of events that causes the opening of multiple cellular access channels to various molecules, especially to calcium. Homeostatically the concentration of calcium is maintained at a much higher level extracellularly than intracellularly.[147] The massive extracellular influx of calcium reaches neurotoxic levels (approximately 10 times normal and higher) and is beyond what the cell can reasonably extrude through active pumping mechanisms.[163,172,173] The subsequent formation of certain radical compounds (see below) causes the cell membrane to lyse, and the cell dies.[48,49,244,260] Of interest for the rehabilitation of brain-injured patients is where and when one may reasonably intercede in this series of events to prevent the end result of cell death. In general, treatment beginning too late (in some cases within 30 minutes after injury) is not likely to benefit the patient[49,173] by blocking calcium entry. However, recent findings indicate that possibly preventable forms of slower degeneration in the hippocampal area take hours to days[190,195]; preventing this degeneration may have some cognitive therapeutic benefit.

Therapeutic interventions that reduce excessive excitotoxicity will have a greater functional benefit after injuries such as ischemia and strokes than after traumatic injuries that involve primary tissue loss. Greater protective effects from excitatory neurotransmitter antagonists have been found with focal ischemia[189,194] than with global ischemia.[17,93] In patients with traumatic brain injury, reductions in the excitotoxic death of tissue that is penumbral to the area of primary injury may prevent secondary injury,[125] although the functional benefits of such sparing have not been clearly established.

Of great concern to the clinical management of patients with brain trauma is the optimal time to treat the excitotoxic cascade after injury. Unfortunately, some of the most effective treatments of calcium loading entail administration before the onset of injury. Indeed, intracellular calcium loading is rapidly induced within 30 minutes[49]; thus, excitatory antagonists to glutamate, acetylcholine, or aspartate (or certain inhibitory agonist drugs or neurotransmitters) are unlikely to be delivered within a reasonable therapeutic window if the patient is not immediately available for treatment. To the extent that the injury is slowly expanding (e.g., delayed hippocampal damage),[190,195] such procedures may have greater utility.

Blocking Voltage-activated Calcium Channels

Preventing excessive calcium entry into the cell is one way to attenuate cell death and to promote recovery.[6,128,203,245] The two general types of calcium entry points are the voltage-activated (low-threshold and high-threshold)[147,242,258] and receptor-activated channels (discussed above). The receptor-activated channels are opened by the extracellular release of excitatory neurotransmitters, and blocking drugs can interfere with this process.[49,259] The greater functional effectiveness of blocking the N-methyl-D-aspartate (NMDA) receptor compared with the kainate and quisqualate receptor may be related to the fact that the former receptor is 70 times more permeable to calcium entry.[176] However, there still remain alternate pathways for the entry of calcium that are uniquely distinct from one another. To date, we know of four different voltage-activated calcium channels,[147] but we do not know whether the majority of entry points have to be blocked to achieve total protection (not all cells have all types of calcium channels). Clearly, however, blocking both receptor-activated and voltage-activated channels is more effective functionally and anatomically than blocking only one type of channel.[128,203] No currently available clinical compounds have been demonstrated to block all calcium channels, but this goal is not necessarily desirable. Because normal calcium metabolism is necessary for life-sustaining functions, generalized blocking of all calcium channels would be life-threatening. Intracellular stores of calcium[241] also may be released in high glutamate mediums, even in the absence of external calcium, but external calcium appears more toxic.[49] In vitro studies indicate that the neurotoxic consequences of calcium entry can be prevented if extracellular calcium is removed during glutamate application within 30 minutes.[173] It is not the entry of calcium per se that results in cell death, but rather the formation of toxic byproducts (free radicals) initiated by the high levels of calcium. Levels of these toxic compounds are normally kept in check primarily by metabolic factors arising from diet and secondarily by activity of various enzymes.

Preventing the Formation of Free Radicals: Role of Nutritional Factors

The internally or externally induced formation of free radicals is a normal byproduct of biologic systems, and in noninjured systems the brief appearance of radicals is modulated by various cellular processes.[52,88,89,106-108] Many of the primary biochemical defenses against oxidation within the nervous system arise from dietary sources; therefore, nutrition is likely to play an important role in maintaining appropriate biologic antioxidant properties after an injury. This may explain in large part the devastating consequences of malnutrition on the CNS in the very young, in whom free radicals induce permanent damage[256] as well as the deleterious effects of malnutrition coupled with aging.[118]

Among the normal defenses against free radical damage are appropriate levels of vitamins E, C, A, and glutathione, which protect against different types of free radical damage. For example, at concentrations less than 1 mM, ascorbic acid is a beneficial antioxidant,[10,11,39] but higher concentrations enhance the formation of free oxygen radicals.[7,8,95] Vitamin E (the lipophilic tocopherol) is an effective antioxidant against membrane lipid peroxidation through reactions with lipid peroxyl and alkoxyl radicals.[41] Vitamin C (the hydrophilic ascorbic acid) protects most effectively against plasma lipid peroxidation[87,138] and also can reduce already oxidized vitamin E, thereby revitalizing its effectiveness as an antioxidant.[257] Vitamin A (carotenoids, particularly the metabolic precursor beta-carotene) also protects against lipid peroxidation[82,83,148-151]; like vitamin C, it exhibits good antioxidant properties but also can exhibit prooxidation under conditions of greater oxygen partial pressures.[40] Glutathione, an effective antioxidant against hydrogen peroxide, hydroxyl, and reduced oxygen formations,[2,3] appears to be diminished in the elderly, in whom high

levels of peroxides are found.[2] It is not clear, however, whether the high peroxides forced depletion of glutathione or whether reduced levels of glutathione allowed increased formation of peroxides. Such findings suggest that, if other factors are constant, the elderly are at risk for greater than normal levels of excitotoxic damage after an injury. Uric acid, although less extensively investigated, also has antioxidant properties.[5,58]

Scavenging of Free Radicals after Trauma-induced Release

The second line of defense against excitotoxic damage occurs after calcium has entered the cell. Once inside, the calcium ions bind to mitochrondria, block electron transfer, and subsequently release excessive hydrogen into the now acidic cytosol.[47,222] Greater than normal amounts of oxygen are reduced to superoxides, which then are converted into hydrogen peroxide. Whereas normally the generation of radicals is controlled within the mitochrondria by various enzymes,[47] after injury excessive amounts may be released into the cytosol, producing deleterious effects on cellular membranes. In the presence of iron or additional superoxide, hydrogen peroxide forms OH^-.[111] The formation of free radicals through the breakdown of hydrogen peroxide or reduction of oxygen destroys the cellular member by peroxidation of membrane polyunsaturated fatty acids.[95,244,260] Therefore, reduction in such metabolic processes through administration of greater amounts of mitochrondrial enzymes may offer some benefit to cell survival and perhaps functional recovery.

For example, superoxide dismutase removes the superoxide radical,[52,106,107] whereas glutathione peroxidase[3] and catalase remove peroxide.[84,165] Efforts directed toward scavenging free radicals have demonstrated some efficacy in reducing cell loss and improving functional outcome.[46,84,146,165] The lipolytic[246,260] and proteolytic[56,57,199,200] enzymes also affect free radicals. These enzymes are involved in repairing the damage to cellular membranes and in removing free radical-induced oxidized proteins within the cell before they cause further damage.

A related consequence of calcium entry after membrane depolarization is passive influx of chloride, which leads to further cation increases and entry of water into the cell. Under severe conditions the entry of water, which occurs within minutes and under certain conditions is reversible, can lyse the cell through excessive osmotic pressure.[206] Perhaps some level of edema reduction may reduce water-induced damage, although a certain amount of edema may serve to dilute and eliminate some of the free radicals. Reduction of water entry alone, however, is not sufficient to prevent cell death.[49]

Postacute Stage After Injury

Apart from possible therapeutic manipulations in the acute stage, what are the realistic hopes of facilitating recovery at later times and what are the likely mechanisms?

Recent research indicates that the rate of recovery after traumatic brain injury is significantly affected by administration of various pharmacologic agents at longer times after injury.[19,20,30,66,70,73,104,237] In general, such manipulations involve changing the status of certain neurotransmitters. Feeney has summarized many of the effects of various drugs on functional recovery.[70-73] To avoid duplication of his work, this section provides a brief overview of the agents that appear to have some effect (either beneficial or deleterious) on functional recovery, with emphasis on understanding the mechanisms.

Cholinergic and Anticholinergic Drugs

An early study by Sachs[208] demonstrated that high levels of acetylcholine were associated with higher magnitudes of injury, suggesting that acute excitation of cholinergic receptors may contribute to the pathophysiology of brain injury through excitotoxic mechanisms similar to those observed with glutamate. Several studies have shown that preinjury treatment or immediate postinjury treatment with anticholinergic drugs (e.g., scopolamine) reduces behavioral deficits after traumatic brain injury, presumably through modulation of the brief and transient period of excessive neuronal excitation.[119,168,169,201,209]

Although such a treatment regimen is promising, the temporal effectiveness of

receptor antagonist intervention appears to be quite brief. For example, treatment with scopolamine 15 minutes after injury significantly reduced motor deficits associated with fluid percussion injury in rats. However, treatment with the same drug at 30 or 60 minutes after injury was ineffective.[169] In addition, the extent of cell loss after various forms of injury involves an as yet unspecified level of "net" excitation (i.e., the amount of excitatory and inhibitory neurotransmitters released); thus the relative ineffectiveness of anticholinergic therapy may be due to its inability to block other more abundant excitatory neurotransmitters (e.g., glutamate).

At later points (days after the acute stage) in functional recovery, when levels of acetylcholine decrease below normal,[119] administration of cholinergic agonists may provide some therapeutic benefit. Over 50 years ago, Sciclounoff[219] found that use of a cholinergic agonist 30–40 days after injury had beneficial effects on recovery of function in patients with hemiplegic stroke. Sciclounoff's undercited study provided the first controlled clinical test of such therapy in patients with stroke. The often cited study by Ward and Kennard[253] also found positive effects on motor recovery in primates, but the study is difficult to evaluate because of methodologic problems.

Gamma-Aminobutyric Acid and Benzodiazepines

Chronic administration of the benzodiazepine diazepam, an indirect agonist of gamma-aminobutyric acid (GABA), significantly enhances subcortical degeneration produced by unilateral lesions of the anteromedial cortex (AMC) in rats.[223] Behavioral deficits caused by unilateral AMC lesions (somatosensorimotor asymmetries) are generally transient, with recovery in less than 2 weeks, whereas deficits caused by direct damage to subcortical tissue may be chronic. Therefore, Schallert and colleagues[127,213,214] predicted that benzodiazepines would have an adverse effect on behavioral recovery after cortical injury. Using a bilateral cutaneous stimulation paradigm, they demonstrated that administration of diazepam over a period of 1–2 weeks after unilateral AMC lesions permanently disrupted behavioral recovery.[213,223] Coadministration of a benzodiazepine antagonist prevents the diazepam-induced retardation of recovery.[127] When subjects with AMC lesions were allowed to recover for at least 3 weeks before exposure to diazepam, they showed only a transient (2-day) reinstatement of the deficit despite continuous drug treatment.[213] Others have reported that infusions of GABA directly into the sensorimotor cortex of unrestrained rats results in contralateral hemiparesis.[36,37] In the experience of the authors, drugs such as the GABA-B presynaptic inhibitor baclofen appear to exert minimal effects on recovery from motor deficits.

The clinical crossover of the benzodiazepine effect to sensory recovery in humans has not been reported (nor thoroughly tested to our knowledge). Permanent sensory deficits may be restricted to animals, but caution in using such drugs in patients with brain injury is warranted until more conclusive clinical studies are performed.

Catecholaminergic and Anticatecholaminergic Drugs

Historically, research into the beneficial effects of the catechol dopamine on brain injury began in patients with Parkinson's disease,[145,262] some of whom showed marked improvement in motor capacity. Intriguing experimental evidence suggests that it is possible to either facilitate or retard recovery of motor function after injury to the sensorimotor cortex with a single injection of catecholamine agonist (e.g., amphetamine) or antagonist (e.g., haloperidol), respectively. Given early after the injury and before any significant reorganization was expected, such drugs were effective only if the animals received appropriate motor experience while under the influence of the drug.[68,131–133] The therapeutic effect of amphetamine may involve stimulation of functionally depressed catecholaminergic systems, although the drug has other CNS effects.[94] That specific environmental and task-relevant stimulation is required for drug-induced recovery has clear clinical applicability and suggests that normal rehabilitation procedures can be made more effective. In the presence of the

appropriate drug and appropriate environmental stimulation, apparently permanent changes can be made in remaining neural systems similar to those that underlie learning and memory.[16,72]

The study of catecholaminergic facilitation of recovery was originally based on the assumption that restoration of some biochemical parameter should parallel the recovery process. Initially, through the use of intraventricular infusions, an attempt was made to tease out which of the major catechols, norepinephrine (NE) or dopamine (DA), was involved in the recovery process.[23,24] Infusion of NE alone and infusion of DA with a DA-beta-hydroxylase inhibitor were tested in animals with an injury to the unilateral sensorimotor cortex. Only NE facilitated functional motor recovery in animals in a manner similar to amphetamine, suggesting its greater involvement in the recovery process. Further studies showed that NE antagonists or depletion of NE[22,33,100,101,132,192] not only slows recovery of function after brain injury but also reinstates the same motor deficits in animals that have long since recovered from brain injury.[34,133,233]

Two additional pieces of information suggest that the cerebellum contralateral to the injury may be critically involved in the manifestation of hemiparesis after cortical injury:

1. Cerebellar ablations that include the deep cerebellar nuclei result in a permanent motor deficit on the same behavioral task used in assessing the cortical injury.[25] In this type of injury, catecholamine agonists interfere with recovery.[25] Moreover, whereas the cerebellum appears able to compensate for injury to the sensorimotor cortex, the reverse does not appear to be true.[261]

2. A single infusion of NE into the contralateral, but not ipsilateral, cerebellum 24 hours after injury to the sensorimotor cortex markedly facilitates functional recovery.[31,35] The cerebellum appears to be involved in the maintenance of functional recovery once it occurs; infusion of phenoxybenzamine (an alpha-adrenergic antagonist) into the contralateral, but not ipsilateral, cerebellum reinstates a unilateral motor deficit in recovered animals.[34] In addition, peripheral administration of clonidine (an alpha-2 adrenergic agonist) reinstates a unilateral

deficit in recovered animals,[233] as does a unilateral 6-OHDA lesion of the locus ceruleus (LC),[34] the major noradrenergic projection in the brain.[166,167]

After injury to the sensorimotor cortex, perturbations in NE functioning are observed in the contralateral cerebellum.[23,102,152] The mechanism most likely involves the observation that the same LC fibers that project to the ipsilateral sensorimotor cortex bifurcate and travel to the contralateral cerebellum to inhibit Purkinje cell output.[129] Infusions of NE into the contralateral, but not ipsilateral, cerebellum facilitate functional recovery and provide strong evidence for this interpretation.[31,35] Dissimilar dyes injected into each area (e.g., cerebellum and sensorimotor cortex) are transported retrogradely to the same LC neurons.[1,54,182,204,230] In addition, electrophysiologic studies have demonstrated that antidromic stimulation in each terminal area directly fires the same LC cell.[183] After injury to the sensorimotor cortex, the projection arm that remains intact (i.e., the one that projects to the cerebellum) is transiently rendered dysfunctional, while the LC soma engages in protein synthesis for repair of the damaged arm to the sensorimotor cortex.[205] Infusion of NE into the contralateral cerebellum seems to restore functional inhibition of Purkinje cell output,[31,35] although the mechanism is not clear. The volume bolus infusion may restore normal synaptic functioning by way of some biochemical feedback mechanism[5] between the NE terminal and the Purkinje cell. As reported for other NE-innervated areas, the NE fiber may recede beyond an optimal synaptic distance from the receptive site while repair mechanisms are in progress,[205] thus allowing degrading enzymes to exert greater influence on NE before protective reuptake.

Such findings are significant when one considers the widespread simultaneous bifurcations of the NE system to multiple structures in the brain other than sensorimotor cortex.[166,167,182,204] It may be possible, therefore, to facilitate recovery of function from a host of other behavioral deficits in addition to motor deficits[53,130,175] For example, it is possible to facilitate[69,140] or retard[132,140] recovery from visual deficits in animals as well as from speech deficits in humans[130,250,251]

with the same NE agonist that facilitates motor recovery. Clearly the NE system serves only a modulatory role in controlling the rate of recovery; animals in fact recover motor function (although it is significantly delayed) after complete removal of ascending LC projections with 6-OHDA[33] or DSP-4 neurotoxic[22,100] lesions. Furthermore, if only the dorsal bundle connection between the LC neuron and sensorimotor cortex is unilaterally removed 2 weeks before unilateral injury to the sensorimotor cortex, compensatory LC sprouting and/or increases in NE turnover occur in the cerebellum.[32] Because this results in a heightened cerebellar NE response before the injury,[35] the animals do not exhibit significant hemiparesis after the injury.

The results from the above studies of the NE system incorporate both physiologic compensation models and the concept of diaschisis; they also supply a mechanism for the resolution of diaschisis. It is unclear whether such findings represent a phenomenon similar to the crossed cerebellar diaschisis observed in metabolic studies after parietal brain injury in humans.[9,61,67,207] The decreases in metabolic activity in humans may result from the loss of corticopontocerebellar input or from an increase in inhibition of Purkinje cells[129] caused by increased NE sprouting in the region.[35,60,191] Because all cerebellar output is from Purkinje cells,[136] the increase in NE-induced inhibition may be reflected in a decreased metabolic need for Purkinje cells. In all likelihood both processes operate simultaneously to decrease metabolic demand. Strong correlations of this metabolic anomaly with behavioral changes are rarely tested or manipulated; thus the functional significance of the metabolic disturbance in crossed cerebellar diaschisis remains unknown.

Although early administration (10–30 days after injury) of an NE agonist may be useful after most cortical injuries in humans,[53,250,251] such drugs may have deleterious effects in patients with damage to the cerebellum[25] or brainstem when hemorrhage is a potential problem. In addition, although many psychostimulant drugs (which generally affect NE) may prove clinically beneficial, it may be wise first to use less addictive and more specifically acting NE agonists (e.g., desipramine).[28,109,110] Dopaminergic drugs, such as L-dopa combined with carbidopa[262] and rehabilitative therapy (see below), also may have beneficial effects on depressed NE systems, because dopamine is taken up by noradrenergic cells before its conversion into NE within the vesicle. Because side effects are associated with all drugs, shifting to similarly acting drugs and using the rehabilitation strategy described below may be necessary for some patients. For example, if spasticity arises long after the brain injury,[177] antidepressant drugs such as desipramine (and other NE agonists) may be contraindicated[212]; a shift to an antidepressant with largely serotonergic actions may be indicated (e.g., trazodone[28] or fluoxetine).[29]

Serotonergic Drugs

In general, serotonergic drugs have produced transient effects on motor recovery in animal models.[28,29,51,184,188] For example, an infusion of serotonin shortly after injury into the ventricle only transiently disrupts motor behavior; recovery to normal levels occurs within 1 hour after infusion.[29] This effect is mimicked by a single intraperitoneal injection of trazodone.[28] If serotonin is infused into the cerebellum contralateral to an injury to the motor cortex after the animal has recovered, an extremely brief reinstatement of the motor deficit peaks at 2 minutes and resolves within 15 minutes (unpublished observation). Nevertheless, some clinical success has been achieved with the serotonin precursor L-tryptophan in the treatment of cerebellar ataxia,[211,243] with methysergide in the treatment of stroke,[254] and with mianserin in the treatment of spinal trauma[210] and appetite disorders following brain injury.[180]

The Role of Task-relevant Experience in Drug Therapy

Perhaps the most important aspect of drug therapies is the necessity of relevant physical rehabilitation (which is actively, not passively, induced) while the drug is active in the system.[68] For example, if a patient has a speech deficit, active speech therapy coupled with drug therapy[250,251] is necessary; likewise,

if a patient is hemiplegic, active use of the limb (even if initially it involves only thinking about trying to move the limb) should be coupled with the drug therapy[53] to realize greater functional benefits.

In an unpublished study of patients with stroke, a group in France waited 3 hours after oral delivery of d-amphetamine (10–15 mg) before beginning active rehabilitation and found no significant effects on motor recovery. This is not surprising, because rehabilitation should have been instigated at 30 minutes after delivery of the drug and repeated through at least 3 hours (but no longer) since peak drug activity is approximately 1.5 hours.[94] It is also important to space each drug administration by 72–96 hours to prevent build-up of tolerance and to avoid exhausting stores of the neurotransmitters that the program is designed to stimulate. Spacing, of course, is more important with drugs like amphetamine, which act by releasing stores of neurotransmitters, than with drugs like desipramine, which act to prevent reuptake deactivation of already released neurotransmitters. Because of the incidence of poststroke depression,[78,162,198,202] appropriate task-relevant experience combined with certain antidepressants may prove beneficial.

It is difficult to control for the interaction between amphetamine and motor experience in experimental protocols based on motor tasks. In the original study of this phenomenon, Feeney et al.[68] placed control animals with amphetamine injections into small boxes with lids to prevent ambulatory motion. However, it was not possible to prevent all motor experience; for example, the animal could actively strain with limb movements within the box. An often overlooked but important study,[69] however, totally controlled for the experience of functional deficit under the influence of amphetamine in cats by using a visual modality confirmed the results of the drug-experience interaction. Cats with large bilateral ablations of visual cortex permanently lose depth perception as measured on a visual cliff apparatus. However, cats given amphetamine and allowed to experience normal room lighting permanently recovered depth perception in the bilateral absence of areas 17, 18, and 19 and lateral suprasylvian gyrus. Cats given amphetamine and placed in total darkness for 8 hours did not recover depth perception. Perhaps this finding could have been predicted; species such as the falcon, which have great stereoscopic depth perception, do not have a well-developed visual cortex.[85] Nevertheless, this rather novel experiment allowed excellent control over visual stimulation and also confirmed the general role of amphetamine in facilitating the rate (and, in this case, apparently the absolute occurrence) of recovery from more than speech and motor deficits. Amphetamine may act through the NE system in facilitating recovery from visual deficits, given NE's modulatory role in visual cortical development[140]; in addition, its action may be modulated through activation of cerebellar areas involved in vision.[62,90,232]

The mechanism(s) through which amphetamine can facilitate recovery only if appropriate experience is given is unclear and represents a valuable area for future research by neurotraumatologists. By interaction with experience amphetamine may well alter permanently the postsynaptic functioning, for example, of pyramidal cells in the cerebellum (either through changes in sensory input and/or motor output) along some measurable physiologic parameter.

Developmental Considerations in the Postacute Treatment of Brain Injury

Since the early studies by Kennard,[142–144] which showed considerable sparing of function in young compared with older primates with presumably comparable lesions, much research indicated that it was indeed "better" to have a brain injury early in life.[117,134,135,215,216] Of course, the observation of greater sparing of function in perinatal injuries has a longer history than Kennard's studies,[228,249] but her work generated the most attention, perhaps because of the greater acceptance of the ability of the brain to exhibit some level of neural plasticity. However, as more appropriate and rigorous control groups were added, results indicated that brain damage early in life can be at least as deleterious as among the older population[4,77,134,215,226,227] and occasionally much worse.[239,240,256] Finger and

Almi summarized in detail the developmental effects.[4,77]

Nevertheless, there are differences in recovery between developmentally immature and adult organisms, and such differences are likely to indicate differences in therapeutic approaches. Much of the genetically induced sprouting during early development occurs in a more appropriate biological milieu than sprouting after developmental growth has waned.[153,154] It is tempting to posit this difference as the reason for the instances of sparing observed after perinatal injuries,[80] but numerous other factors mitigate against such a simple interpretation:

1. In certain postnatal developmental periods, axon severing at terminal projection sites, which in adults results in cell body survival, causes cell body loss in younger people.

2. Some of the sparing of function observed in younger children may be related more to the fact that cortical tissue has not yet been functionally committed (for example, to language acquisition).[44]

3. Some brain regions are more susceptible to behavioral deficits than others.[139,187] The different effects on various types of learning may confound deficit assessments.[121,139]

Age per se does not constitute an appropriate explanation for sparing of function in old vs. young populations. Age simply reflects different developmental periods.

Presently, no data are available about pharmacologic manipulations designed to enhance functional recovery in the perinatal stage other than manipulations designed to halt spread of damage. Although not tested, treatments designed to limit neuronal death following injury—for example, early treatment of excitotoxic-induced damage—may be entertained as a first line of treatment. Developmental differences aside, protection against more extensive damage due to calcium loading is likely to be similar in adults and infants to the extent that the excitatory neurotransmitters are developmentally available. It has not been established experimentally or clinically whether the anatomic mechanisms are mature enough during early perinatal periods for pharmacologic treatments designed to enhance specific neurotransmitter activity to have the same effect as in older children. Such studies (in particular, appropriate animal models) are desperately needed because of the increasing reports of incidents of brain damage due to "excessive shaking" in children, which can have severe and permanent developmental consequences.

CONCLUSION

Although it is clear that substantial recovery of function occurs following a traumatic brain injury involving permanent tissue loss, it is not entirely clear how the recovery can occur in the absence of significant regrowth of tissue. Conceptually, because true point-to-point regeneration of neurons and supporting glia does not occur after brain injury that involves primary tissue loss, "true" functional recovery is unlikely: that is, whatever unique function that was associated specifically with the lost tissue is also lost.

Presently, either we have insufficient knowledge of the exact function of any given portion of tissue (whether dependent on or independent of the rest of the brain and environmental interactions), or we simply circumvent the problem by generalizing our definition of recovery. Many of our preferences for explanations reside in a "comfort zone" initiated by individual training. Although nothing is inherently wrong with individual preferences, concepts such as behavioral compensation and vicariation reveal little about underlying mechanisms and indicate only what we already observe—that patients can compensate for many deficits, sometimes in unique ways.

Compensatory explanations tied to physiologic events that can be manipulated or controlled offer strong explanations for functional recovery if tested in an appropriate and rigorous fashion. In examining physiologic compensation hypotheses, great caution must be exercised to rule out physiologic events that are merely correlated with recovery rather than causally related. For example, it is not enough to show that sprouting occurs at the same time as the recovery of a certain behavior. Experimentally we must destroy the new sprouts to see whether the behavioral deficit reemerges, and if no new sprouting occurs, the behavioral deficit must remain for the life of the organism. Such animal models allow us to devise appropriate strategies of clinical intervention to help the patient through the long-term evolving process of brain injury.

In view of research suggesting that specific neurotransmitter systems influence functional recovery, investigation of the potential impact of certain drugs on the recovery process must take into account the continuously evolving nature of the injury over long periods of time. Unfortunately, we do not have adequate models of drug-induced facilitation of recovery at various developmental periods after injury. Currently we can realistically expect only to hasten or slow a patient's progress through the phases of recovery. The particular characteristics of the recovery process are determined in large part by the type, magnitude, and location of the injury. The most effective therapy for certain brain-injured patients appears to include three components: (1) very early treatment with drugs that counteract the acute excitotoxic effects associated with calcium loading; (2) late pharmacologic intervention with certain drugs (in particular NE agonists); and (3) concomitant deficit-related physical therapy. Caution should be exercised in prescribing certain treatment regiments at longer intervals after injury; recovery is a long-term, evolving process (for example, the slow development of spasticity) that reflects changes in the anatomic substrate.

In conclusion, behavioral recovery after brain injury in which primary tissue is lost must represent some functional change in portions of the brain that remain intact. Changes in physiologic (and subsequent behavioral) functioning in areas remote from the site of primary injury are more likely a direct reaction to the actual loss of tissue than to any mechanism of anatomic reorganization designed to enhance functional recovery.

REFERENCES

1. Ader J-P, Room P, Postrema F, et al: Bilateral diverging axon collaterals and contralateral projections from rat locus coeruleus neurons. J Neural Trans 49:207–218, 1980.
2. Al-Turk WA, Stohs SJ: Hepatic glutathione content and aryl hydrocarbon hydroxylase activity of acetaminophen-treated mice as a function of age. Drug Chem Toxicol 4:37–48, 1981.

3. Al-Turk WA, Stohs SJ, El-Rashidy FH, et al: Changes in glutathione, glutathione reductase, and glutathione-S-transferase as a function of cell concentration and age. Pharmacology 34:1–8, 1987.

4. Almi CR, Finger S: Early Brain Damage, Vol. 1. New York, Academic Press, 1984.

5. Ames BNR, Cathcart R, Schwiers E, Hochstein P: Uric acid provides an antioxidant defense in humans against oxidant- and radical-caused aging and cancer: A hypothesis. Proc Natl Acad Sci 78: 6858–6862, 1981.

6. Andersen AB, Finger S, Andersen CS, et al: Sensorimotor cortical lesion effects and treatment with nimodipine. Physiol Behav 47:1045–1052, 1990.

7. Aust SD, Morehouse LA, Thomas CE: Role of metals in oxygen radical reactions. Free Radic Biol Med 1:3–25, 1985.

8. Aust SD, Svingen BA: The role of iron in enzymatic lipid peroxidation. In Pryor WA (ed): Free Radicals in Biology, Vol. 5. New York, Academic Press, 1982, pp 1–28.

9. Baron JC, Bousser MG, Comar D, et al: "Crossed cerebellar diaschisis" in human supratentorial brain infarction. Trans Am Neurol Assoc 8:120–135, 1980.

10. Bendich A, D'Apolito P, Gabriel E, Machlin LJ: Interaction of dietary vitamin C and vitamin E on guinea pig immune responses to mitogens. J Nutr 114:1588–1593, 1984.

11. Bendich A, Machlin AJ, Scandurra O: The antioxidant role of vitamin C. Adv Free Radic Biol Med 2:419–444, 1986.

12. Bjerre B, Bjorklund A, Stenevi U: Inhibition of the regenerative growth of central noradrenergic neurons by intracerebrally administered anti-NGF serum. Brain Res 74:1–18.

13. Bjorklund A, Brundin P, Isacson O: Neuronal replacement by intracerebral neural implants in animal models of neurodegenerative disease. Adv Neurol 47:455–492, 1988.

14. Bjorklund A, Stenevi U: Intracerebral neural grafting: A historical perspective. In Bjorklund A, Stenevi U (eds): Neural Grafting in the Mammalian CNS. Amsterdam, Elsevier, 1985, pp 3–14.

15. Black IB, DiCicco-Bloom E, Dreyfus CF: Nerve growth factor and the issue of mitosis in the nervous system. Curr Top Dev Biol 24:161–193.

16. Bliss DK: Dissociated learning and state-dependent retention induced by pentobarbitol in rhesus monkeys. J Comp Physiol Psychol 84:149–161, 1972.

17. Boast CA, Gerhardt SC, Pastor G, et al: The N-methyl-D-aspartate antagonists CGS 19755 and CPP reduce ischemic brain damage in gerbils. Brain Res 442:345–348, 1988.

18. Bowen FP, Demirjian C, Karpiak SE, et al: Sprouting of noradrenergic nerve terminals subsequent to freeze lesions of rabbit cerebral cortex. Proceedings of the Society for Neuroscience Third Annual Meeting, San Diego, California, November 1973, p 112.

19. Boyeson MG: Neurotransmitter aspects of traumatic brain injury. In Bach-y-Rita P (ed): Traumatic Brain Injury. New York, Demos Publications, 1989, pp 97–104.

20. Boyeson MG: Neurochemical alterations after brain injury: Clinical implications for pharmacologic rehabilitation. Neurorehabilitation 1:33–43, 1991.

21. Boyeson MG, Bach-y-Rita P: Determinants of brain plasticity. J Neurol Rehabil 3:35–57, 1989.

22. Boyeson MG, Callister T, Cavozos J: Biochemical and behavioral effects of a sensorimotor cortex injury in rats pretreated with the neurotoxin DSP-4. Behav Neurosci 106:964–973, 1992.

23. Boyeson MG, Feeney DM: The role of norepinephrine in recovery from brain injury. Neurosci Abst 10:68, 1884.

24. Boyeson MG, Feeney DM: Intraventricular norepinephrine facilitates motor recovery following sensorimotor cortex injury. Pharmacol Biochem Behav 35:497–501, 1990.

25. Boyeson MG, Feeney DM: Adverse effects of catecholaminergic drugs following unilateral cerebellar ablations. Restor Neurol Neurosci 3:227–233, 1991.

26. Boyeson MG, Feeney DM, Dial WG: Cortical microstimulation adjacent to a sensorimotor cortex injury. J Neurotrauma 8:205–217, 1991.

27. Boyeson MG, Harmon RL: Effects of trazodone and desipramine on motor recovery in brain-injured rats [abstract]. Arch Phys Med Rehabil 73:994, 1992.

28. Boyeson MG, Harmon RL: Effects of trazadone and desipramine on motor recovery in brain-injured rats. Am J Phys Med Rehabil 72:286–293, 1993.

29. Boyeson MG, Harmon RL, Jones JL: Differential effects of fluoxetine, amitriptyline, and serotonin on functional motor recovery after sensorimotor cortex injury. Am J Phys Med Rehabil 73:76–83, 1994.

30. Boyeson MG, Jones JL, Harmon RL; Sparing of motor function after cortical injury: A new perspective on underlying mechanisms. Arch Neurol 51: 405–414, 1994.

31. Boyeson MG, Krobert KA: Cerebellar norepinephrine infusions facilitate recovery after sensorimotor cortex injury. Brain Res Bull 29:435–439, 1992.

32. Boyeson MG, Krobert KA: Cortical norepinephrine depletion protects animals from hemiparesis induced by sensorimotor cortex injury. Soc Neurosci Abstr 13:1665, 1987.

33. Boyeson MG, Krobert KA, Grade CM, et al: Unilateral but not bilateral locus ceruleus lesions facilitate recovery from sensorimotor cortex injury. Pharmacol Biochem Behav 43:771–777, 1992.

34. Boyeson MG, Krobert KA, Scherer PJ, et al: Reinstatement of motor deficits in brain-injured animals: The role of cerebellar norepinephrine. Restor Neurol Neurosci 5:283–290, 1993.

35. Boyeson MG, Scherer PJ, Grade CM, et al: Unilateral locus ceruleus lesions facilitate motor recovery from cortical injury through supersensitivity mechanisms. Pharmacol Biochem Behav 44:297–305, 1993.

36. Brailowski S, Knight RT, Blood K, et al: Gamma-aminobutyric acid-induced potentiation of cortical hemiplegia. Brain Res 362:322–330, 1986.

37. Brailowski S, Knight RT, Efron R: Phenytoin increases the severity of cortical hemiplegia in rats. Brain Res 376:71–77, 1986.

38. Buecker ED: Implantation of tumors in the hind limb field of the embryonic chick and in the developmental response of the lumbosacral nervous system. Anat Rec 102:369–390, 1948.

39. Buettner GR: Ascorbate autooxidation in the presence of iron and copper chelates. Free Radic Res Commun 1:349–353, 1986.

40. Burton GW, Ingold KU: Beta-carotene is an unusual type of lipid antioxidant. Science 224:569–573, 1984.

41. Burton GW, Royce A, Ingold KU: First proof that vitamin E is a major lipid-soluble, chain-breaking antioxidant in human blood plasma. Lancet 2:327, 1982.

42. Butcher LL, Wolff NJ: Neurotrophic agents may exacerbate the pathologic cascade of Alzheimers disease. Neurobiol Aging 10:557–570, 1989.

43. Cannon WB, Rosenbluth A: The supersensitivity of denervated structures. New York, Macmillan, 1949.

44. Carter RL, Hohenegger MK, Satz P: Aphasia and speech organization in children. Science 218:797–799, 1982.

45. Cassel JC, Kelche C, Majchrazak M, Will BE: Factors influencing structure and function of intracerebral grafts in the mammalian brain: A review. Restor Neurol Neurosci 4:65–96, 1992.

46. Chan PH, Longar S, Fishman RA: Protective effects of liposome-entrapped superoxide dismutase on posttraumatic brain edema. Ann Neurol 21:540–547, 1987.

47. Chance B: The energy-linked reaction of calcium with mitochrondria. J Biol Chem 240:2729–2748, 1965.

48. Choi DW: Glutamate neurotoxicity in cortical cell culture is calcium dependent. Neurosci Lett 58:293–297, 1985.

49. Choi DW: Glutamate neurotoxicity and diseases of the nervous system. Neuron 1:623–634, 1988.

50. Commissiong JW, Toffano G: The effect of GM-1 ganglioside on coerulospinal, noradrenergic, adult neurons and fetal monoaminergic neurons transplanted into the transected spinal cord of the adult rat. Brain Res 380:205–215, 1986.

51. Costa JL, Ito U, Spatz M, et al: 5–Hydroxy–tryptamine accumulation in cerebrovascular injury. Nature 249:135, 1974.

52. Crapo JD, Tierney DF: Superoxide dismutase and pulmonary oxygen toxicity. Am J Physiol 226:1401–1507, 1974.

53. Chrisostomo EA, Duncan PW, Propst M, et al: Evidence that amphetamine with physical therapy promotes recovery of motor function in stroke patients. Ann Neurol 23:94–97, 1988.

54. Crowley JN, Maas JW, Roth RH: Biochemical evidence for simultaneous activation of multiple locus coeruleus efferents. Life Sci 26:1373–1378, 1980.

55. Das DG, Hallas B, Das KG: Transplantation of brain tissue on the brain of the rat: Growth characteristics of neocortical transplants from embryos at different ages. Am J Anat 158:135–145, 1980.

56. Davies KJA: Intracellular proteolytic systems may function as secondary antioxidant defenses: A hypothesis. Free Radic Biol Med 2:155–173, 1986.

57. Davies KJA: Proteolytic systems as secondary antioxidant defenses. In Chow EK (ed): Cellular Antioxidant Defense Mechanisms. Boca Raton, CRC Press, 1988, pp 25–67.

58. Davies KJA, Sevanian A, Muakkassah-Kelly SF, Hochstein P: Uric acid-iron complexes: A new aspect of the antioxidant function of uric acid. Biochem J 235:747–754, 1986.

59. Demeurisse G, Verhas M, Capon A: Remote dysfunction in aphasic stroke patients. Stroke 22:1015–1020, 1991.

60. Devor M, Schneider GE: Neuroanatomical plasticity: The principle of conservation of total axonal arborization. In Vital-Durand, Jeannerod (eds): Aspects of Neural Plasticity/Plasticite Nerveuse, vol. 166. INSERM, 1975, pp 49–72.

61. Di Peiro V, Chollet F, Dolan RJ, et al: The functional nature of diaschisis. Stroke 21:1365–1369, 1990.

62. Donald IML, Hawthorne ME: Coding of visual information by units of the cat cerebellar vermis. Exp Brain Res 34:27–48, 1979.

63. Dostrovsky JO, Millar J, Wall PD: The immediate shift of afferent drive of dorsal column nucleus cells following deafferentation: A comparison of acute and chronic deafferentation in gracile nucleus and spinal cord. Exp Neurol 52:480–495, 1976.

64. Dunnet SB, Bjorklund A, Schmidt RH, et al: Intracerebral grafting of neuronal cell suspensions. IV: Behavioral recovery in rats with unilateral 6-OHDA lesions following implantation of nigral cell suspensions in different brain sites. Acta Physiol Scand Suppl 572:29–39, 1983.

65. Dunnet SB, Richards SJ: Neural transplantation: From molecular basis to clinical application. Prog Brain Res 82:1–11, 1990.

66. Feeney DM: Pharmacologic modulation of recovery after brain injury: A reconsideration of diaschisis. J Neurol Rehabil 5:113–128, 1991.

67. Feeney DM, Baron JC: Diaschisis. Stroke 17:817–830, 1986.

68. Feeney DM, Gonzalez A, Law WA: Amphetamine, haloperidol, and experience interact to affect rate of recovery after motor cortex injury. Science 217:855–857, 1982.

69. Feeney DM, Hovda DA: Reinstatement of binocular depth perception by amphetamine and visual experience after visual cortex ablation. Brain Res 342:352–356, 1985.

70. Feeney DM, Sutton RL: Pharmacotherapy for recovery of function after brain injury. CRC Crit Rev Neurol 13:135–197, 1987.

71. Feeney DM, Sutton RL, Boyeson MG, et al: The locus coeruleus and cerebral metabolism: Recovery of function after cortical injury. Physiol Psychol 13:197–203, 1985.

72. Feeney DM, Weisend MP, Kline AE: Noradrenergic pharmacotherapy, intracerebral infusions and adrenal transplants promote functional recovery after cortical damage. J Neural Transplant Plast 1994.

73. Feeney DM, Westerberg VS: Norepinephrine and brain damage: Alpha noradrenergic pharmacology alters functional recovery after cortical trauma. Can J Psychol 44:233–252, 1990.

74. Ferrier D: The functions of the brain. London, Smith, Elder, 1886.

75. Finger S, Stein D (eds): Brain Damage and Recovery: Research and Clinical Perspectives. New York, Academic Press, 1982.

76. Finger S, Walbran B, Stein DG: Brain damage and behavioral recovery: Serial lesion phenomena. Brain Res 63:1–18, 1973.

77. Finger S, Almi CR: Early Brain Damage, vol 2. New York, Academic Press, 1984.

78. Finklestein SP, Weintraub RJ, Karmouz N, et al: Antidepressant drug treatment for post-stroke depression: Retrospective study. Arch Phys Med Rehabil 68:772–776, 1987.

79. Fischer W, Wictorin K, Bjorklund A, et al: Intracerebral infusion of nerve growth factor ameliorates cholinergic neuron atrophy and spatial memory impairments in aged rats. Nature 329:65–68, 1987.

80. Fletcher JM, Satz P: Age, plasticity, and equipotentiality: A reply to Smith. J Consult Clin Psychol 51:763–767, 1983.

81. Flourens JPM: Recherches experimentales sur les proprietes et les fonctions du systeme nerveau dans les animaux vertebres, 2nd ed. Paris, Balliere, 1842.

82. Foote CS: Quenching of singlet oxygen. In Wassermann HH, Murray RW (eds): Singlet Oxygen. New York, Academic Press, 1979, pp 139–171.

83. Foote CS, Denny RW: Chemistry of singlet oxygen: Quenching by beta-carotene. J Am Chem Soc 90:6233–6235, 1988.

84. Forsman M, Fleischer JE, Milde JH, et al: Superoxide dismutase and catalase failed to improve neurologic outcome after complete cerebral ischemia in the dog. Acta Anaesth Scand 32:152–155, 1988.

85. Fox R, Lehmkuhle SW, Bush RC: Stereopsis in the falcon. Science 197:79–81, 1977.

86. Freed WJ: GM-1 ganglioside does not stimulate reinnervation of the striatum by substantia nigra grafts. Brain Res Bull 14:91–95, 1985.

87. Frei B: Ascorbic acid protects lipid in human plasma and LDL against oxidative damage. Am J Clin Nutr 54(Supp) 113S–1118S, 1991.

88. Fridovich I: Superoxide dismutases. Ann Rev Biochem 44:147–159, 1975.

89. Fridovich I: The biology of oxygen radicals. Science 201:875–880, 1978.

90. Frisby JP: An old illusion and a new theory of stereoscopic depth perception. Nature 307:592–593, 1984.

91. Friede RL, Bischhausen R: The five structures of stumps of transected nerve fibers in subserial sections. J Neurol Sci 44:181–192, 1980.

92. Gage FH, Tuszynski M, Yoshida K, Higgins G: nerve growth factor expression and function in the CNS. In Hefti F, Brachet P, Will B, and Christen Y (eds): Growth Factors and Alzheimers Disease. Heidelberg, Springer, 1991.

93 Gill R, Foster AC, Woodruff GN: Systemic administration of MD-801 protects against ischemia-induced hippocampal neurodegeneration in the gerbil. J Neurosci 7:3343–3349, 1987.

94. Gilman AG, Goodman LS, Rall TW, et al: The Pharmacological Basis of Therapeutics, 8th ed. 1990, pp 210–213.

95. Girotti AW: Mechanisms of lipid perioxidation. Free Radic Biol Med 1:87–95, 1985.

96. Glassman RB: Recovery following sensorimotor cortical damage: Evoked potentials, brain stimulation and motor control. Exp Neurol 33:16–29, 1971.

97. Glassman RB, Malamut BL: Recovery from electroencephalographic slowing and reduced evoked potentials after somatosensory cortical damage in cats. Behav Biol 17:333–354, 1976.

98. Glees P, Cole J: Recovery of skilled motor functions after small repeated lesions of motor cortex in macaque. J Neurophysiol 13:137–148, 1950.

99. Gnahn H, Hefti F, Heumann R, et al: NGF-mediated increase of choline acetyltransferase (ChAT) in the neonatal rat forebrain: Evidence for a physiological role of NGF in the brain? Dev Brain Res 9:45–52, 1983.

100. Goldstein LB, Coviello A, Miller GD, et al: Norepinephrine depletion impairs motor recovery following sensorimotor cortex injury in the rat. Restor Neurol Neurosci 3:41–47, 1991.

101. Goldstein LB, Davis JN: Clonidine impairs recovery of beam walking after a sensorimotor cortex lesion in the rat. Brain Res 508:305–309, 1990.

102. Goldstein LB, MacMillan V: Acute unilateral sensorimotor cortex injury in rats blocks d-amphetamine induced norepinephrine release in the cerebellum. Soc Neurosci Abstr 17(2):1575, 1991.

103. Goldstein LB, Matchar DB, Morgenlander JC, et al: Influence of drugs on the recovery of sensory-motor function after stroke. J Neuro Rehab 4:137–144, 1990.

104. Goldstein LB, Matchar DB, Morgenlander JC, et al: Drugs influence the recovery of function after stroke. Stroke 21:179, 1990.

105. Gower WR: Diseases of the Nervous System, vol II. Philadelphia, Blakiston, 1898.

106. Gregory EM, Fridovich I: Oxygen toxicity and superoxide dismutase. J Bacteriol 114:1193–1197, 1973.

107. Gregory EM, Yost FJ, Fridovich I: Superoxide dismutases of E-coli: Intracellular localization and functions. J Bacteriol 115:987–991, 1973.

108. Griffiths HR, Unsworth J, Blake DR, Lunec J: Free Radicals in Chemistry, Pathology and Medicine. London, Richelieu, 1988, pp 439–454.

109. Gustafson I, Westerberg E, Wieloch T: Protection against ischemia-induced neuronal damage by the a-2 adrenoceptor antagonist idazoxan: Influence of time of administration and possible mechanisms of action. J Cereb Blood Flow Metabol 10:885–894, 1990.

110. Gustafson I, Westerberg E, Weiloch T: Extracellular brain cortical levels of noradrenaline in ischemia: Effects of desipramine and postischemic administration of idazoxan. Exp Brain Res 86:555–561, 1991.

111. Haber F, Weiss JJ: The catalytic decomposition of hydrogen peroxide by iron salts. Proc R Soc Lond Ser, A147: 332–351, 1934.

112. Hagg T, Fass-Holmes B, Vahlsing HL, et al: Nerve growth factor (NGF) reverses axotomy-induced decreases in choline acetyltransferase, NGF-receptor and size of medial septum cholinergic neurons. Brain Res 505:29–38, 1989.

113. Hagg T, Gulati AK, Behzadian MA, et al: Nerve growth factor promotes CNS axonal regeneration into acellular peripheral nerve grafts. Exp Neurol 112(1):79–88.

114. Hagg T, Hagg F, Vahlsing HL, et al: Nerve growth factor effects on cholinergic neurons of the neostriatum and nucleus accumbens in the adult rat. Neuroscience 30:95–103, 1989.

115. Hagg T, Vahlsing HL, Manthorpe M, et al: Delayed treatment with nerve growth factor reverses the apparent loss of cholinergic medial septal neurons after brain damage. Exp Neurol 101:303–312, 1988.

116. Hall RD, Lindholm EP: Organization of motor and somatosensory neocortex in the albino rat. Brain Res 66:23–28, 1974.

117. Hamm RJ, White-Gbadebo DM, Leyth BG, et al: The effect of age on motor and cognitive deficits after traumatic brain injury in rats. Neurosurgery 31:1072–1078, 1992.

118. Harman D: Free radical theory of aging: Nutritional implications. Age:143–150, 1978.

119. Hayes RL, Jenkins LW, Lyeth BG: Neurotransmitter-mediated mechanisms of traumatic brain injury: Acetylcholine and excitatory amino acids. J Neurotrauma 9(1):173–187, 1992.

120. He X, Rosenfeld MG: Mechanisms of complex transcriptional regulation: Implications for brain development. Neuron 7:183–196, 1991.

121. Hecaen H, Albert ML: Human Neuropsychology. New York, Wiley, 1978.

122. Hefti F: Detrimental actions of neurotrophic agents. Neurobiol Aging 10:571–583, 1989.

123. Hefti F, Hartikka J, Knusel B: Functions of neurotrophic facts in the adult and aging brain and their treatment of neurodegenerative diseases. Neurobiol Aging 10:515–533, 1989.

124. Hefti F, Knusel B: Neurotrophic factors and neurodegenerative disorders. In Hefti F, Brachet P, Will B, Christen Y (eds): Growth Factors and Alzheimers Disease. Heidelberg, Springer, 1991.

125. Heiss W-D, Huber M, Fink GR, et al: Progressive derangement of periinfarct viable tissue in ischemic stroke. J Cereb Blood Flow Metab 12:193–203, 1992.

126. Hengerer B, Lindholm D, Heumann R, et al: Lesion-induced increase in nerve growth factor mRNA is mediated by c-fos. Proc Natl Acad Sci USA 87:3899–3903, 1990.

127. Hernandez TD, Jones GH, Schallert T: Co-administration of Ro 15-1788 prevents diazepam-induced retardation of recovery of function. Brain Res 487(1):89–95, 1989.

128. Hewlitt K, Corbett D: Combined treatment with MK-801 and nicardipine reduces global ischemic damage in the gerbil. Stroke 23:82–86, 1992.

129. Hoffer BJ, Siggins GR, Oliver AP, et al: Activation of the pathway from locus coeruleus to rat Purkinje neurons: Pharmacological evidence of noradrenergic central inhibition. Exp Ther 184:553–569, 1973.

130. Homan R, Panksepp J, McSeweeny J, et al: d-Amphetamine effects on language and motor behaviors in a chronic stroke patient. Soc Neurosci Abstr 16:439, 1990.

131. Hovda DA, Feeney DM: Amphetamine with experience promotes recovery of locomotor function after unilateral frontal cortex injury in the cat. P West Pharm Soc 29:209–211.

132. Hovda DA, Feeney DM: Haloperidol blocks amphetamine-induced recovery of binocular depth perception after bilateral visual cortex ablation in the cat. P West Pharm Soc 28:209–211, 1985.

133. Hovda DA, Feeney DM, Salo AA, et al: Phenoxybenzamine but not haloperidol reinstates all motor and sensory deficits in cats fully recovered from sensorimotor cortex ablations. Soc Neurosci Abstr 9:1001, 1983.

134. Isaacson RL: The myth of recovery from early brain damage. In NR Ellis (ed): Aberrant Development in Infancy. Potomac, NJ, Erlbaum, 1975.

135. Isaacson RL, Nonneman AJ, Schmaltz LW: Behavioral and anatomical sequelae of damage to the infant limbic system. In Isaacson RL (ed): The Neuropsychology of Development. New York, Wiley, 1968.

136. Ito M: The Cerebellum and Neural Control. New York, Raven Press, 1984.

137. Jackson JH: Lectures on the diagnosis of tumors in the brain. Medical Times and Gazette 2:139ff, 1883.

138. Jialal I, Vega GL, Grundy SM: Physiologic levels of ascorbate inhibit oxidative modification of LDL. Atherosclerosis 82:185–191, 1990.

139. Johnson D, Almi CR: Age, brain damage, and performance. In Finger S (ed): Recovery from Brain Damage. New York, Plenum, 1978.

140. Kasamatsu T, Pettigrew JD, Ary M: Cortical recovery from effects of monocular deprivation: Acceleration with norepinephrine and suppression with 6-hydroxydropamine. J Neurophysiol 45:254–266, 1981.

141. Kempinski WH: Experimental study of distal effects of acute focal injury. Arch Neurol Psychria 79:376–389, 1958.

142. Kennard MA: Age and other factors in motor recovery from precentrallesions in monkeys. Am J Physiol 115:138–146, 1936.

143. Kennard MA: Reorganization of motor function in the cerebral cortex of monkeys deprived of motor and premotor areas in infancy. J Neurophysiol 1:477–496, 1938.

144. Kennard MA: Cortical reorganization of motor function: Studies on a series of monkeys at various ages from infancy to maturity. Arch Neurol Psychria 47:227–240, 1942.

145. Koller WC, Wong GF, Lang A: Post-traumatic movement disorders: A review. Mov Disord 4:20–36, 1989.
146. Kontos HA, Wei EP: Superoxide production in experimental brain injury. J Neurosurg 64:803–807, 1986.
147. Kostyuk PG, Tepikin AV: Calcium signals in nerve cells. Physiol Sci 6:6–10, 1991.
148. Krinsky NI: Biological roles of singlet oxygen. In Wasserman HH, Murray RW (eds): Singlet Oxygen. New York, Academic Press, 1979, pp 597–641.
149. Krinsky NI: Carotenoid protection against oxidation. Pure App/Chem 512:649–660, 1979.
150. Krinsky NI: Photobiology of carotenoid protection. In Regan JD, Parrish JA (eds): The Science of Photomedicine. New York, Plenum, 1982, pp 397–403.
151. Krinsky NI, Deneke SM: Interaction of oxygen and oxyradicals with carotenoid. J Natl Cancer Inst 69:205–209, 1982.
152. Krobert KA, Sutton RL, Feeney DM: Spontaneous and amphetamine-evoked release of cerebellar noradrenaline after sensorimotor cortex contusion: An in vivo microdialysis study in the awake rat. J Neurochem 62:2233–2240, 1994.
153. La Velle A: Levels of maturation and reactions to injury during neuronal development. Prog Brain Res 40:161–166, 1973.
154. LaVelle A, LaVelle FW: Neuronal reaction to injury during development. In Finger S, Almi CR (eds): Early Brain Injury, vol. 2, New York, Academic Press, 1984, pp 3–16.
155. LeVere TE: Neural stability, sparing, and behavioral recovery following brain damage. Psychiatry Rev 82:344–358, 1975.
156. Levi-Montalcini R: The nerve growth factor: Thirty-five years later. Biosci Rep 7:681–699, 1987.
157. Levi-Montalcini R, Booker B: Excessive growth of the sympathetic ganglia evoked by a protein isolated from mouse salivary glands. Proc Natl Acad Sci USA 46:373–384, 1960.
158. Levi-Montalcini R, Hamburger V: Selective growth stimulating effects of mouse sarcoma on the sensory and sympathetic nervous system of the chick embryo. J Exp Zool 116:321–362, 1951.
159. Lewin GR, Ritter AM, Mendell LM: Nerve growth factor-induced hyperalgesia in the neonatal and adult rat. J Neurosci 13:2136–2148, 1993.
160. Lindvall O: Transplantation into the human brain: Present status and future possibilities. J Neurol Neurosurg Psychia Spec Suppl:39–54, 1989.
161. Lindvall O, Brundin P, Widner H, et al: Grafts of fetal dopamine neurons survive and improve motor function in Parkinson's Disease. Science 247:574–577, 1990.
162. Lipsey JR, Robinson RG, Pearlson GD, et al: Nortriptyline treatment of post-stroke depression: A double-blind study. Lancet 1:297–300, 1984.
163. Lipton P, Lobner D: Mechanisms of intracellular calcium accumulation in the CA1 region of rat hippocampus during anoxia in vitro. Stroke 21 (Suppl III):60–64, 1990.
164. Liu CN, Chambers WW: Intraspinal sprouting of dorsal root axons. Arch Neurol Psychiatry 79:46–61, 1958.
165. Liu TH, Beckman JS, Freeman BA, et al: Polyethylene glycol-conjugated superoxide dismutase and catalase reduce ischemic brain injury. Am J Physiol 256:H589–H593, 1989.
166. Loughlin SE, Foote SL, Fallon JH: Locus coeruleus projections to cortex: Topography, morphology and collateralization. Brain Res Bull 9:287–294, 1982.
167. Loughlin SE, Foote SL, Grzanna R: Efferent projections of nucleus locus coeruleus: Morphologic subpopulations have different efferent targets. Neuroscience 18:307–319, 1986.
168. Lyeth BG, Dixon CR, Jenkins LW, et al: Effects of scopolamine treatment on long-term behavioral deficits following concussive brain injury to the rat. Brain Res 452:39–48, 1988.
169. Lyeth BG, Ray M, Hamm RJ, et al: Post-injury scopolamine administration in experimental traumatic brain injury. Brain Res 569:281–286, 1992.
170. Macias AE, Valencia A, Vilana M: Long-lasting dementia following brain grafting for the treatment of Parkinsons disease. Transplantation 48:348, 1989.
171. Madrazo I, Francobourland R, Ostroskysolis F, et al: Dementia following brain grafting. Transplantation 49:1026–1027, 1990.
172. Manev H, Favaron M, DeErausquin G: Destabilization of ionized Ca2+ homeostasis in excitatory amino acid neurotoxicity: Antagonism by glycosphingolipids. Cell Biol Int Rep 14:3–14, 1990.
173. Manev H, Favaron M, Guidotti A, Costa E: Delayed increase in Ca2+ influx elicited by glutamate: Role in neuronal death. Mol Pharmacol 36:379–387, 1989.
174. Marks AF: Regenerative reconstruction of a tract in a rat's brain. Exp Neurol 34:455–464, 1972.
175. Marotta RF, Logan N, Potegal M, et al: Dopamine agonists induce recovery from surgically-induced septal rage. Nature 269:513–515, 1977.
176. Mayer ML, Vylkicky L, Sernagor E: A physiologist's view of the NMDA receptor: An allosteric ion channel with multiple regulatory sites. Drug Dev Res 17:263–280, 1989.
177. McCouch GP, Austin GM, Liu CN, et al: Sprouting as a cause of spasticity. Neurophysiol 21:205–216, 1958.
178. Mobley WC, Rutkowski JL, Tennekoon GI, et al: Nerve growth factor increase choline acetyltransferase activity in developing basal forebrain neurons. Mol Brain Res 1:53–62, 1986.
179. Moore RY, Bjorklund A, Stenevi U: Plastic changes in the adrenergic innervation of the rat septal area in response to denervation. Brain Res 33:13–35, 1971.
180. Morley JE: An approach to the development of drugs for appetite disorders. Neuropsychobiology 21:22–30, 1989.
181. Munk H: Zur physiologie der grosshirnrinde. Berl Klin Wochenschr 14:505–506, 1877.
182. Nagai T, Satoh K, Imamoto K, et al: Divergent projections of catecholamine neurons of the locus coeruleus as revealed by fluorescent retrograde double labeling technique. Neurosci Lett 23:117–123, 1981.

183. Nakamura K, Iwama K: Antidromic activation of the rat locus coeruleus neurons from hippocampus, cerebral, and cerebellar cortex. Brain Res 62:115–133, 1975.

184. Nakayama H, Ginsberg MD, Deitrich WD: S-Emopamil, a novel calcium channel blocker and serotonin S2 antagonist, markedly reduces infarct size following middle cerebral artery occlusion in the rat. Neurology 38:1667–1673, 1988.

185. Neafsey EJ, Bold EL, Haas G, et al: The organization of rat motor cortex: A microstimulation mapping study. Brain Res Rev 11:77–96, 1986.

186. Nitta A, Murase Y, Furukawa K, et al: Memory impairment and neural dysfunction after continuous infusion of anti-NGF antibody into the septum of adult rats. Neuroscience 57:495–499, 1993.

187. Nonneman AJ, Isaacson RL: Task dependent recovery after early brain injury. Behav Biol 8:143–172, 1973.

188. Osterholm JL, Bell J, Meyer R: Experimental effects of free serotonin on the brain and its relationship to brain injury. J Neurosurg 31:408–421, 1969.

189. Ozyurt E, Graham DI, Woodruff GN, McCulloch J: Protective effect of the glutamate antagonist MK-801 in focal cerebral ischemia in the cat. J Cereb Blood Flow Metab 8:138–143, 1988.

190. Petito CK, Feldman E, Pulsinelli WA, Plum F: Delayed hippocampal damage in humans following cardiorespiratory arrest. Neurology 37:1281–1286, 1987.

191. Pickel VM, Krebs H, Bloom FE: Proliferation of norepinephrine-containing axons in rat cerebellar cortex after peduncle lesions. Brain Res 59:169–179, 1973.

192. Porch B, Wyckes J, Feeney DM: Haloperidol, thiazides and some antihypertensives slow recovery from aphasia. Soc Neurosci Abstr 11:52, 1985.

193. Povlishock JT, Becker DP, Miller JD, et al: Axonal changes in minor had injury. J Neuropathol Exp Neurol 42:225–242, 1983.

194. Prince DA, Feeser HR: Dextromethorphan protects against cerebral infarction in a rat model of hypoxia-ischemia. Neurosci Lett, 85:291–296, 1988.

195. Pulsinelli WA, Brierley JB, Plum F: Temporal profile of neuronal damage in model of transient forebrain ischemia. Ann Neurol 11:491–498, 1982.

196. Quinn NP: The clinical application of cell grafting techniques in patients with Parkinson's disease. In Dunnet SB, Richards SJ (eds): Neural Transplantation: From Molecular Basis to Clinical Application. Prog Brain Res 82:619–625, 1990.

197. Ramon y Cajal S: Degeneration and Regeneration of the Nervous System, vol 2. May RM (ed. and trans). New York, Hafner, 1959 (originally published 1928).

198. Reding MJ, Orto LA, Winter SE, et al: Antidepressant therapy after stroke: A double-blind trial. Arch Neurol 43:763–765, 1986.

199. Rivett AJ: Purification of a liver alkaline protease which degrades oxidatively modified glutamine synthetase. Characterization as a high molecular weight cysteine proteinase. J Biol Chem 260:12600–12606, 1985.

200. Rivett, AJ: High molecular mass intracellular proteases. Biochem J 263:25–633, 1989.

201. Robinson SE, Fox SD, Posner MG, et al: The effect of MI muscarinic blockade on behavior following traumatic brain injury in the rat. Brain Res 511:141–148, 1990.

202. Robinson RG, Price TR: Post-stroke depressive disorders: A follow-up study of 103 patients. Stroke 13:635–641, 1982.

203. Rod MR, Auer RN: Combination therapy with nimodipine and dizocilpine in a rat model of transient forebrain ischemia. Stroke 23:725–732, 1992.

204. Room P, Postrema F, Korf J: Divergent axon collaterals of rat locus coeruleus neurons: Demonstration by a fluorescent double labeling technique. Brain Res 221:219–230, 1981.

205. Ross RA, Joh TH, Reis DJ: Reversible changes in the accumulation and activities of tyrosine hydroxylase and dopamine-beta-hydroxylase in neurons of nucleus locus coeruleus during the retrograde reaction. Brain Res 92:57–72, 1975.

206. Rothman SM, Olney JW: Excitotoxicity and the NMDA receptor. TINS 10:299–302, 1987.

207. Rousseaux M, Steinling M: Crossed hemispheric dischisis in unilateral cerebellar lesions. Stroke 23:511–514, 1992.

208. Sachs E Jr: Acetylcholine and serotonin in the spinal fluid. J Neurosurg 14:22–27, 1957.

209. Saija A, Robinson SE, Lyeth BG, et al: The effects of scopolamine and traumatic brain injury on central cholinergic neurons. Neurotrauma 5:161–170, 1988.

210. Salzman SK, Puniak MA, Liu Z, et al: The serotonin antagonist mianserin improves functional recovery following experimental spinal trauma. Ann Neurol 30:533–541, 1991.

211. Sandyk R, Lacona RP: Post-traumatic cerebellar syndrome: response to L-tryptophan. Int J Neurosci 47:301–302, 1989.

212. Sanford PR, Spengler SE, Sawasky KB: Clonidine in the treatment of brainstem spasticity: Case report. Am J Phys Med Rehabil 71;301–303, 1992.

213. Schallert T, Hernandez TD, Barth TM: Recovery of function after brain damage: Severe and chronic disruption by diazepam. Brain Res 379:104–111, 1986.

214. Schallert T, Jones TA, Lindner MD: Multilevel transneuronal degeneration after brain damage. Stroke 21(11):143–146, 1990.

215. Schneider G: Is it really better to have your brain lesion early? A revision of the "Kennard Principle". Neuropsychologia 17:557–583, 1979.

216. Schneider G, Jhaveri SR: Neuroanatomical correlates of spared or altered function after brain lesion in the hamster. In Stein DJ, Rosen JJ, Butters N (eds): Plasticity and Recovery of Function in the Central Nervous System. New York, Academic Press, 1974, pp 65–110.

217. Schanne FA, Kane AB, Young EE, Farber JL: Calcium dependence of toxic cell death: A common pathway. Science 206:700–702, 1979.

218. Schoenfeld TA, Hamilton LW: Secondary brain changes following lesions: A new paradigm for lesion experimentation. Physiol Behav 18:951–967, 1977.

219. Sciclounoff S: L'acetylcholine dans le traitement de L'ictus hemiplegique. La Presse Medicale 56:1140–1142, 1934.

220. Seyffarth H, Denny-Brown D: The grasp reflex and instinctive grasp reaction. Brain 73:109–183, 1948.

221. Shelton DS, Reichardt LF: Studies on the expression of the nerve growth factor (NGF) gene in the central nervous system: level and regional distribution of NGF mRNA suggest that NGF functions as a trophic factor for several distinct populations of neurons. Proc Natl Acad Sci USA 83:2714–2718, 1986.

222. Siesjo BK, Bendek G, Koide T, et al: Influence of acidosis on lipid peroxidation in brain tissues in vitro. J Cereb Blood Flow Metab 5:253–258, 1985.

223. Sims JS, Jones TA, Fulton RL, et al: Benzodiazepine effects on recovery of function linked to trans-neuronal morphological events. Soc Neurosci Abstr 16:342, 1990.

224. Skaper SD, Mazzari S, Vantini, et al: Monosialoganglioside GM1 and modulation of neuronal plasticity in CNS repair processes. In Timiras PS, et al (eds): New York, Plenum Press, 1991.

225. Skinner BF: The Behavior of Organisms: An Experimental Analysis. New York, Appleton-Century, 1938.

226. Smith A: Overview or underview? Comment on Satz and Fletcher "Emergent trends in neuropsychology: An overview. J Consult Clin Psychol 51:768–775, 1983.

227. Smith A: Early and long term recovery from brain damage in children and adults: Evolution of concepts of localization, plasticity and recovery. In Almi CR, Finger S (eds): Early Brain Damage, vol 1. New York, Academic Press, 1984.

228. Soltmann O: Experimentelle Studien uber die Functionen des Grosshirns der Neugeborenen. Jahrbuck fur Kinderherkunde 9:106–148, 1876.

229. Spear PD: Behavioral and neurophysiological consequences of visual cortex damage. In Sprague JM, Epstein AN (eds): Progress in Psychobiology and Physiological Psychology, vol. 8. New York, Academic Press, 1977, pp 45–83.

230. Steindler D: Locus coeruleus neurons have axons that branch to forebrain and cerebellum. Brain Res 223:367–373, 1981.

231. Stenevi U, Bjorklund A, Svendgaard NA: Transplantation of central and peripheral monoamine neurons to the adult rat brain: Techniques and conditions for survival. Brain Res 114:1–20, 1976.

232. Stenton SP, Frisby JP, Mayhew JEW: Vertical disparity pooling and the induced effect. Nature 309:622–623, 1984.

233. Stephens J, Goldberg G, Demopoulos JT: Clonidine reinstates deficits following recovery from sensorimotor cortex lesion in rats. Arch Phys Med Rehabil 67:666–667, 1986.

234. Stewart JW, Ades HW: The time factor in reintegration of a learned habit after frontal lobe lesions in the monkey (Macaca mulatta). J Comp Physiol Psychol 44:479–486, 1951.

235. Stricker EM, Zigmond MJ: Brain monoamines, homeostasis, and adaptive behavior. In Mountcastle VB, Bloom FE, Geiger SR (eds): Handbook of Physiology—the Nervous System, vol 4. Baltimore, Waverly Press, 1986, pp 677–700.

236. Struhl K: Mechanisms for diversity in gene expression patterns. Neuron 7:177–181, 1991.

237. Sutton RL, Feeney DM: Alpha-adrenergic agonists and antagonists affect recovery and maintenance of beam-walking ability after sensorimotor cortex ablation in the rat. Restor Neurol Neurosci 4:1–11, 1992.

238. Svengaardt N-A, Bjorkjund A, Stenevi U: Regeneration of central cholinergic neurones in the adult rat brain. Brain Res 102:1–22, 1976.

239. Teuber HL, Rudel RG: Behavior after cerebral lesions in children and adults. Dev Med Child Neurol 4:3–20, 1962.

240. Teuber HL: Mental retardation after early trauma to the brain. Some issues in search of facts. In Angle CR, Bering EA (eds): Physical Trauma as an Etiological Agent in Mental Retardation. Published conference proceedings. Bethesda, MD, U.S. Department of Education, 1970.

241. Thayer SA, Miller RJ: Regulation of the intracellular free calcium concentration in single rat dorsal root ganglion neurones in vitro. J Physiol 425:85–115, 1990.

242. Triggle DJ: Calcium antagonists. Stroke 21:iv49–iv58, 1990.

243. Trouillas P, Brudon F, Adeleine P: Improvement of cerebellar ataxia with levoratory form of 5-hydroxytryptophan. A double-blind study with quantified data processing. Arch Neurol 45:1217–1222, 1988.

244. Tyler DD: Role of superoxide radicals in the lipid peroxidation of cellular membranes. FEBS Lett 51d:180–183, 1975.

245. Uematsu D, Araki N, Greenberg JH, et al: Combined therapy with MD-801 and nimodipine for protection of ischemic brain damage. Neurology 41:88–94, 1991.

246. Van Deenen LLM: Phospholipids and membranes. In Holman RT (ed) Progress in the Chemistry of Fats and Other Lipids. New York, Pergamon, 1985, p 102.

247. Von Monakow C: Gehirpathologie. Wien A., Holder, 1905, pp 240–248.

248. Von Monakow C: Die lokalistion'im Grosshirn und der Funktion durch Kortikale Herde. Wiesbaden: JF Bergman, 1914 (excerpted and translated by G. Harris) In Pribram KH (ed): Brain and Behavior I: Mood States and Mind. Baltimore, Penguin, 1969, pp 27–36.

249. Vulpian A: Lecons sur la physiologie generale et comparee du systeme nerveux (1866). In Kennard MA, Fulton JF (eds): Age and Reorganization of the Central Nervous System. J Mount Sinai Hosp 9:594–605, 1942.

250. Walker-Batson D, Devous MD, Curtis SS, et al: Response to amphetamine to facilitate recovery from aphasia subsequent to stroke. In Prescott TE (ed): Clinical Aphasiology. Austin, TX, pro-ed, 1991, p 20.

251. Walker-Batson D, Unwin H, Curtis S, et al: Use of amphetamine in the treatment of aphasia. Restor Neurol Neurosci 4:47–50, 1992.

252. Wall PD, Egger MD: Formation of new connections in adult rat brains after partial deafferentation. Nature 232:542–545, 1971.

253. Ward AA, Kennard MA: The effect of cholinergic drugs on recovery of function following lesions of the central nervous system. Yale J Biol Med 15:189–228, 1942.

254. Weintraub MI: Methysergide (Sansert) treatment in acute stroke: Community pilot study. Angiology 36:137, 1985.

255. Weiss P: Selectivity controlling the central-peripheral relations in the nervous system. Biol Rev 11:494–531, 1936.

256. Winick M: Malnutrition and Brain Development. New York, Oxford University Press, 1976.

257. Witting LA, Horwitt MK: Effect of degree of fatty acid unsaturation in tocopherol deficiency-induced creatinuria. J Nutr 82:19–23, 1964.

258. Wong MCW, Haley EC Jr: Calcium antagonists: Stroke therapy coming of age. Stroke 21:494–501, 1990.

259. Young W: The post-injury responses in trauma and ischemia: Secondary injury or protective mechanisms? Centr Nerv Sys Trauma 4:27–51, 1987.

260. Yu BP, Suescun EA, Yang SY: Effect of age-related lipid peroxidation on membrane fluidity and phospholipase A2: Modulation by dietary restriction. Mech Ageing Dev 65:17–33, 1992.

261. Yu J, Eidelberg E: Recovery of locomotor function in cats after localized cerebellar lesions. Brain Res 273:121–131, 1983.

262. Zasler ND: Advances in neuropharmacological rehabilitation for brain dysfunction. Brain Inj 6:1–14, 1992.

MICHAEL W. O'DELL   M.D.

RICHARD V. RIGGS   M.D.

5

Management of the Minimally Responsive Patient

The care and management of the minimally responsive adult patient represent a unique and somewhat specialized aspect of brain injury rehabilitation.[16,25,143,172] Technologic advances in the specialties of trauma surgery, neurosurgery, and critical care medicine have substantially reduced mortality rates in patients with severe brain injury.[13,34,35,129,187] Whether the widespread use of air bags will enhance the effect of advanced technology is uncertain[123]; most patients with prolonged unconsciousness are injured in motor vehicle accidents.[32,34,103,147]

Many rehabilitation centers that provide excellent clinical care for patients at Rancho levels (RL) 4 and higher[77] avoid caring for the low-level patient at RL 3 and below. Reasons may include the complicated medical problems seen in this population,[5,143] difficulty with documentation of progress for third-party payers,[7] dealing with family members under extraordinary stress,[66,89,156] potentially problematic long-term placement, or the sheer physical effort required by the staff, especially nurses. In a recent report from the Traumatic Coma Data Bank,[103] one explanation offered for the longer length of acute hospital stay for low-level patients was the "unavailability of suitable rehabilitation."

Medical and surgical advances combined with poor access to acute and subacute rehabilitation have resulted in a group of "unwanted children of technology."[34] Addressing concerns in Europe, Bricolo[34] stated that outcome in many severely brain-injured patients is worse than may be expected on the basis of the neurologic insult because of the "inadequacy of rehabilitation therapy." In addition to obvious human cost, the economic ramifications of prolonged unconsciousness are considerable. In 1990 Deutsch[51] estimated that the cost of 24-hour, at-home attendant care by a licensed practical nurse ranged from $70,000–105,000/year. The costs of institutional care and other medical and durable equipment needs are also substantial.[51]

Characterization of minimally responsive patients is difficult, because they are not usually distinguished in studies examining severe brain injury as a whole.[151] The distinction is justified, however, because patients with prolonged unconsciousness have the potential for a more complicated and protracted medical course,[5] are severely limited in their ability to articulate complaints, may progress at a much slower rate, and often require a management approach resembling a blend of rehabilitation and internal medicine.[143,172]

Despite these differences, a significant minority of minimally responsive patients managed *acutely* (within 1–6 months after injury) regain a degree of cognitive awareness, and some progress to surprisingly functional levels.[74,147]

TERMINOLOGY

Several terms germane to this discussion, which addresses only issues related to adults, must be defined. Although minimally responsive patients are often considered "coma patients," this is usually not the case.[172] **Coma** is a specific diagnosis defined as "a pathologic state in which arousal and awareness are not present; without eyes opening or evidence of a sleep/wake cycle."[3,18,187,188] Coma is only one stage in the recovery from severe brain injury and rarely lasts longer than a few weeks.[3,17,187] **Vegetative state**, originally described by Jennett,[91] is also a specific diagnosis; it is applied to patients who are "wakeful, but devoid of conscious content; without cognitive or affective mental function."[3,16,18,188] In contrast to coma, the patient in vegetative state demonstrates eye opening and sleep/wake cycles.[3,16,18,188] The term **minimally responsive patient** is not a diagnosis; it denotes a syndrome of severe cognitive and motoric limitation due to brain injury.[187] It also includes persons functioning at a somewhat higher level than coma and vegetative state with voluntary movement and behavior.

The diagnosis of vegetative state is based on serial evaluation and cannot be made at a single bedside examination.[16,183] Recent evidence suggests that vegetative state is quite often misdiagnosed (especially 3 months or longer after traumatic injury), perhaps because of confusion in terminology or lack of extended, serial observation.[38] The American Neurologic Association[3] has indicated that "the presence of voluntary movements or behavior, no matter how rudimentary, is a sign of cognition and incompatible with the diagnosis of vegetative state." There is no universal agreement on the duration required for diagnosis of **persistent vegetative state**; opinions range from 1[3,188] to 3[83,84] to 12 months[34,183] to avoiding the term altogether.[187] The term "persistent" probably

should be reserved for durations of 12 months or longer, at which time significant recovery is highly unlikely and intensive rehabilitation efforts are not appropriate.[183] This interpretation of "persistent" is not universal, however.[3,187,188]

Coma, vegetative state, and persistent vegetative state should be distinguished from **brain death**, which is characterized by a flat electroencephalogram indicating no brain activity.[18,23,58,188] Various authors have suggested that persistent vegetative state be distinguished from akinetic mutism,[35,140,187,188] a condition characterized by severely diminished neurologic drive with intact visual tracking.[187] **Locked-in syndrome**[126] is a distinct diagnosis applied to patients who demonstrate "alert wakefulness with paralysis of the body and inability to speak" but are relatively intact cognitively.[3,188] Locked-in syndrome is far more likely to be due to vascular rather than traumatic causes.[126]

In this discussion, vegetative state is used in describing natural history and outcome, because it represents a discrete category in the Glasgow Outcome Scale. The term minimally responsive patient is used in discussions of assessment and management, in which the rehabilitation and medical approaches apply to a broader range of patients. These interventions also apply to patients in coma and vegetative state

An interdisciplinary approach to the care of the minimally responsive patient is ideal.[183] Crucial components include superb rehabilitation nursing (with particular attention to skin care, bowel, and bladder); occupational and/or cognitively based therapists with training in the use of standardized assessment instruments; physical therapists with expertise in serial casting, positioning, and seating techniques[143]; and patient, compassionate social workers and psychologists aggressive in family counseling and intervention. Health care reform in the United States eventually may require the use of specially trained, less expensive rehabilitation "technicians" within subacute or long-term care facilities.[85] The basic medical and rehabilitation principles discussed below remain the same, however. **Intensive rehabilitation** refers to the provision of ongoing, daily treatment of at least a few hours' duration and does not denote a particular location (e.g., inpatient hospital, rehabilitation unit, nursing home).

This chapter considers (1) natural history and prognosis, (2) behaviorally based assessments, (3) medical management, (4) arousal-specific management, and (5) psychosocial considerations related to the care and rehabilitation of the minimally responsive adult patient. The focus is assessment and intervention for the traumatically brain-injured patient from the time of medical stability to approximately 6 months after injury, the period during which intensive rehabilitation efforts are most likely to be cost-effective.[85,144] The reader is referred to chapter 3 for a discussion of acute management, to chapter 7 for pediatric issues, and to other sources for information about nontraumatic injury.[22,105,106,188,189]

NATURAL HISTORY AND PROGNOSIS

Anatomy

In general, attempts to provide a precise anatomic localization for either coma or vegetative state have not been successful.[112,126,149,187] The reticular activating system (RAS) is the primary anatomic structure responsible for arousal,[126,173] but conscious behavior is cortically mediated.[126] This difference distinguishes arousal from awareness.[180] The RAS projects widely to the cortex, with the projections determined primarily by the class of neurotransmitter.[173] In addition, extensive reciprocal projections from the cortex to the RAS suggest that arousal is also consciously influenced.[173] Levin et al.[104] examined the relationship between length of unconsciousness and depth of acute brain lesions with magnetic resonance imaging (MRI). They found that the longest duration of impaired consciousness (mean = 28.8 days) was associated with lesions of the deep central gray matter and the brainstem. The association of increased length of coma with acute rostral damage was also noted by Bricolo et al.[34] Although coma may occur in patients with damage to large areas of the cerebral hemispheres (especially the forebrain and neocortical structures[34,187]), with or without

involvement of the diencephalon or brainstem,[3,17,112,126,187,188] brain lesions in patients with prolonged coma and vegetative state "tend to be multifocal and inconsistent."[149]

Outcome Measurement in Severe Brain Injury

Estimating prognosis and predicting outcome are among the most professionally and emotionally difficult aspects of caring for persons in coma and vegetative state. As Sandel and Labi[145] pointed out, rehabilitation physicians are generally more skeptical than other medical specialists about the clinician's ability to predict outcome early after injury.[3,12,33] It is appropriate to distinguish between neurologic recovery (e.g., increased arousal, attention, or voluntary motor movement) and functional recovery (e.g., increased communicative, locomotor, or self-care skills), because the former often occurs without significant improvement in the latter.[189] Familiarity with the natural history of recovery after severe brain injury is helpful in counseling family members and planning rehabilitation strategies, but the available research generally has addressed neurologic[32-35,83,84,103] rather than functional[74,147] recovery. In addition, little is known about the factors that influence outcome and prognosis in coma and vegetative state, including rehabilitation intervention. The prognostic value of premorbid factors, traumatic factors, and posttraumatic factors has been inconsistently addressed[145] (Table 1).

Outcome after brain injury of any severity has been traditionally measured in terms of the Glasgow Outcome Scale (GOS), which is considered a "social outcome scale" by its authors.[92] Despite its importance and widespread use, the GOS has broad categories that complicate clinically meaningful predictions. Even within the "good recovery" category, considerable cognitive disability may be present, and a substantial variability of physical and cognitive disability may be present in the "moderate disability (conscious but disabled)" category.[144] The clinical utility of the scale is further compromised when the five GOS categories are collapsed into only two: "good outcome" (good recovery or moderate disability) and "poor

TABLE 1. **Natural History of Persons in Vegetative State**

Study/ Location	Years of Study	No. of Patients	Duration of VS at Entry	Methodology/ Etiology	Age (yr)	M:F	Incidence of VS
Levin et al.[103] United States	Not specified (1980s)	93	Median: 1 mo (75% < 2 mo)	GCS ≤ 8 Evaluation within 48 hr Gunshot wounds and age > 16 excluded Study pool = 650 (Original pool = 1030)	Median = 27 (range: 16–89)	Not Specified	14% at 1 mo; 2.3% at 1 year (of study pool)
Sazbon and Groswasser[147,148] Israel	1974–1983	134	At least 30 days	Original sample 148 patients admitted to rehabilitation 14 patients excluded because of insufficient data 68.7% = MVA 11.9% = Penetrating injury 5.2% = Work-related injury 14.2% = Other	Median = 27 (range: 3–79)	4:1	Not specified
Braakman et al.[32] Europe and United States	Before 1980	140	1 mo	Coma > 6 hr VS at 1 mo (? included coma) 140 patients "with available data"; number of records excluded not specified Total pool = 1373 "Trauma"; cause not specified	Not specified	Not specified	10% at 1 mo; 1% at 12 mo
Bricolo[34] Italy	1967–1976	135	2 wk	94 cases admitted to author's institution, 41 transferred from outside Retrospective study Total pool = 2300 800 consecutive patients with TBI used as comparison group	Mean = 29	Not specified	4% at 2 wk
Choi et al.[191] United States (Medical College of Virginia)	1976	91	Mean 76.5 days	GCS < 9 Not following commands Admitted to neurosurgical service GSW excluded Original pool = 786 subjects	Not specified	Not specified	N/A

GCS = Glasgow Coma Score, GSW = gunshot wound, M:F = male-to-female ratio, MVA = motor vehicle accident, TBI = traumatic brain injury, VS = vegetative state.

(Columns continued on opposite page.)

outcome" (severe disability, vegetative state, or death).[133,145,191] Outcome in severe brain injury has been examined extensively in the literature, but relative few studies have focused specifically on the natural history and prognosis of patients in coma or vegetative state (see Table 1). Because these studies differ substantially in methodology and years of study, one should draw only broad conclusions.

Natural History

Of patients who initially survive severe brain injury (variably defined as an initial score on the Glasgow Coma Scale [GCS] ≤ 8 or loss of

TABLE 1. *(Columns continued)*

Outcome Prediction		Outcome		Comments
Recovery was not predicted by Age GCS Pupillary status Shock Hypoxia Intracranial diagnosis		**At study completion** (mean follow-up: at least 1.3 yr) 	With follow-up 20/84(24%) 15/84 (18%) 49/84 (58%) 9/93	"Slight chance" of regaining consciousness > 1 yr after injury No predictors of recovery Follow-up: 6 mo, n = 18; 1 yr, n = 35; 2 yr, n = 24; 3 yr, n = 6
		Dead Vegetative Severe or mod- erate disability or good recovery Lost to follow-up		
Predictors of **nonrecovery** Late epilepsy Late hydrocephalus Motor activity (see comments) Diffuse body sweating Central fever Associated injuries Abnormal ADH secretion Respiratory disturbance	**Recovery not** **correlated with** Age ICP Intracranial mass Skull fracture Shunt placement Surgical inter- vention Duration of coma Early epilepsy	**At least 1 yr** Dead Vegetative Severe or mod- erate disability or good recovery Incomplete data	With follow-up 43/134 (32%) 19/134 (14%) 72/134 (54%) 14/148 (9%)	"Most" of those recovering consciousness did so during 2nd or 3rd mo after injury Mean time to recovery: 11.3 wk (SD = 8.9) Motor activity: flaccid, decerebrate, decor- ticate in order of worsening prognosis 50% of recovery group independent in ADL; 14/72 (20%) partially independent 8/72 (11.1%) resumed competitive and 35/72 (48.6%) sheltered employment 52/72 (72%) returned to live with family members
Predictors for recovery Age Eye opening Pupillary reactivity Eye movement (spontaneous and conjugate)		**At 1 yr** Dead Vegetative Severe disability Moderate disability or good recovery Lost to follow-up	71/140 (51%) 15/140 (11%) 37/140 (26%) 14/140 (10%) 3/140 (2%)	No patient > 40 yr achieved independence 83% of those regaining consciousness did so by 3 mo; 93% by 6 mo after injury Of 12 patients with nonreactive pupils at 1 mo, 10 died and 2 were VS at 1 yr Of 41 patients without spontaneous eye movement, only 1 became independent
Predictors for nonrecovery Age Rostral brain damage (Not statistically analyzed)	Intracranial mass Premorbid disease	**At 1 yr** Dead Vegetative Severe disability Moderate disability Good recovery Lost to follow-up	40/135 (29.6%) 11/135 (8.1%) 42/135 (31.1%) 24/135 (13.3%) 18/135 (13.3%) 0 (0%)	Study is descriptive in nature, with little formal statistical analysis Mortality and morbidity increased with increasing age
Recovery (at 3 mo) not correlated with Intracranial diagnosis Age GCS Location of hematoma Pupillary status		**At 1 yr** Dead Vegetative Severe disability Moderate disability Good recovery	10/65 (15.4%) 8/65 (12,3%) 29/65 (44.6%) 11/65 (44.6%) 7/65 (10.9%)	Study examined severe injury; all data in table refers *only* to subjects in VS Majority of "improvement" from 3–12 mo was VS to severe disability Slightly better outcome than Levin et al. probably due to

ADH = antidiuretic hormone, ADL = activities of daily living, GCS = Glasgow Coma Score, ICP = intracranial pressure, SD = standard deviation, TBI = traumatic brain injury, VS = vegetative state.

consciousness for longer than 6 hours), approximately 10–14% remain in vegetative state at 1 month and 1–2% at 1 year.[32,34,103] Moreover, 25–50% of patients in vegetative state 2–4 weeks after injury die during the first year. The most recent data (from the 1980s)[103,191] indicate a mortality rate of 15–24% between approximately 1 month and 1 year and are probably a better reflection of recent advances in surgical and medical care. Other studies were completed before 1980 and in other countries.[32,34,74,147] Of patients in vegetative state at 2–4 weeks after injury (a fairly common scenario at admission to rehabilitation), 8–18% remain so at 1 year. On the basis of such data, therefore, "some recovery" can be expected at 1 year in up to 50% of patients who have been in vegetative state for approximately 1 month. Caution must be exercised, however, because "some recovery" does not necessarily imply functionally significant recovery, and may progress from vegetative state to severe disability.[191]

Studies by Bricolo et al.[34] and Levin et al[103] do not distinguish between the two highest GOS categories, resulting in an extremely broad clinical outcome category. Sazbon and Groswasser,[74,147] however, provide details about functional outcome, indicating that 50% of their sample of 134 patients achieved independence in activities of daily living and 11% returned to unsupported employment. Patients survived long enough to be identified for, admitted to, and followed in a specialized rehabilitation unit; thus, these results are perhaps overly optimistic.

Several smaller studies (not included in Table 1), conducted mostly in rehabilitation units, also shed light on the natural history of vegetative state, although they do not address outcome per se. Because these studies focus primarily on patients who received rehabilitation intervention, results may not be representative of all patients in vegetative state. Sandel and O'Dell[146] reviewed 295 patients admitted to a brain injury rehabilitation hospital, of whom 68 (23%) were in coma or vegetative state (i.e., RL 1 or 2) at admission. The majority were traumatic injuries admitted at least several weeks after injury. Over a mean follow-up longer than 15 months, 40% progressed to RL ≥ 4 and 15% to RL ≥ 5. Whitlock[171] reported the outcomes of 23 patients with a score on the Functional Independence measure of < 19 (18 is the lowest possible score) admitted to a rehabilitation facility at a mean of 44 days (range = 13–92 days) after injury. At 6 months, 35% of the 23 patients were classified, according to the GOS, as "good recovery" or "moderate disability"; 52% as "severe disability"; and 13% as "vegetative." Ansell[7] analyzed 116 patients at RL 2 or 3 (mean time from injury at admission = 93 days; range = 25–364 days) in a long-term rehabilitation facility. Of the 116 patients, 55 (47%) reached rehabilitation readiness (RR), defined by a Western Neuro Sensory Stimulation Profile[6] score of at least 72, between 2 and 48 months after injury.

The RR and non-RR groups were not significantly different in terms of age, gender, or days from injury to first evaluation. Of the original sample, 37 (32%) progressed to RR in ≤ 6 months, 13 (11.2%) at 6–12 months, and 5 (4.3%) after 12 months. About 70% of patients who eventually became RR showed "slow, continuous progress," and 20% demonstrated an abrupt change in performance; 9% were inconsistent because of medical complications such as ventriculoperitoneal shunt malfunction, infection, and drug toxicities. The fact that all patients were privately insured raises questions of potential bias.

In summary, at 2–4 weeks after sustaining traumatic brain injury, approximately 50% of patients in vegetative state demonstrate evidence of neurologic (not necessarily functional) improvement in the first year.[189] Of those who show no neurologic improvement, many die in the first year.

Prediction of Outcome

A summary of factors that predict outcome in patients in vegetative state is found in Table 1. The few studies reporting outcome in anoxic coma indicate that prognosis can be estimated reliably within a few weeks of the hypoxic insult.[22,105,106,187,189]

Prediction of outcome after severe brain injury is both difficult and controversial.[13,25,183] Some have even suggested that patients destined for a good outcome do not pass through vegetative state.[91] It is quite important to determine whether a given study predicts mortality or morbidity.

Although Braakman[33] found that mortality can be predicted in the first 28 days after brain injury, the final severity of disability cannot. In general, consideration of multiple factors appears to increase the accuracy of prediction.[120,145]

It is somewhat discouraging that the most recent, and probably the most methodologically sound, study of outcome in vegetative state (by Levin and associates[103]) revealed no factors predictive of recovery. Factors considered include age, initial score on the Glasgow Coma Scale,[162] pupillary status, hypoxia, shock, pulmonary complications, initial findings with computed tomography (CT) of the brain, and intracranial diagnosis. Choi et al.[191] also identified no predictive factors for outcome at 3–6 months after injury in persons in vegetative state. These studies aside, older age seems to be a relatively consistent factor for predicting poor outcome.[17,34,189] Abnormal pupillary status at initial evaluation also has been cited as predictive.[13,32] Perhaps the best predictor is duration of unconsciousness; natural history studies clearly indicate a decreasing chance of significant recovery with time.[7,17,25,191] Despite their usefulness in the acute setting, neither initial GCS score[103,147] nor intracranial pathology[3,147] appears to be particularly predictive of chronic disability.

A few conflicting reports assess the prognostic value of neuroimaging studies, such as CT and MRI, specifically in persons in vegetative state. Neuroimaging in traumatic brain injury is discussed in detail in chapter 10. The Traumatic Coma Data Bank study[103] found no statistically significant difference in initial brain CT findings between patients in vegetative state at approximately 1 month after injury who did or did not progress over 3 years. More than 90% of both groups showed abnormalities on the initial CT scans. The study found a nonsignificant trend toward greater frequency of diffuse injury complicated by swelling or midline shift in the nonrecovery group. In addition, Narayan et al.[120] found CT imaging unhelpful in predicting outcome ("good" vs. "poor") after severe brain injury. CT prediction was markedly improved when clinical features were added. On the other hand, Van Dongen et al.[167] found that CT imaging could make relatively accurate predictions of mortality (death vs. survival) at 1 year. Once again, predictions were enhanced substantially when the clinical examination was added. The primary use for CT in the rehabilitation setting is the identification of surgically correctable processes, such as hydrocephalus.[158]

MRI is superior to CT in visualizing the brainstem and posterior fossa structures.[151,158] In addition to the technical difficulty of obtaining MRI scans in vegetative patients, no added benefit in prognostication of outcome has been documented. The same point can be made with physiologic imaging techniques such as single-photon emission computed tomography (SPECT) and positron emission tomography (PET) scanning.[151,158] Although the technology is useful in estimating cerebral blood flow in the acute setting,[1,164] much more research is necessary before such modalities can be recommended on a routine basis.[151]

A growing body of literature suggests that electrophysiologic (EP) testing, such as somatosensory evoked potentials (SSEP), brainstem auditory evoked potentials (BAEP), and visual evoked potentials (VEP), is helpful in predicting outcome after severe brain injury.[4,132,161,184] The objective nature of electrophysiologic testing provides an appealing mechanism to predict prognosis for patients in coma and vegetative state. SSEP provides information about the integrity of sensory pathways as well as about the severity of central nervous system damage.[132] In general, the greater the degree of abnormality on EP testing, the poorer the chances for significant functional recovery. Relatively normal responses indicate a relatively good prognosis for recovery.[161] BAEP and VEP may be better predictors of poor outcome, whereas SSEP can be helpful for prognosticating both good and poor outcomes.[4] One study found no significant benefit of EP testing over the standard neurologic examination.[108] A detailed discussion of this topic, including the technical aspects, is found in chapter 11. Other new modalities, such as cerebral blood flow studies,[90,151] have been reported as helpful in predicting outcome but are not universally available and require further investigation.

Implication for Rehabilitation Intervention

The delineation of periods for recovery is critical in determining the types and intensity of rehabilitation interventions. Although extenuating circumstances must always be considered (for example, prolonged, treatable medical complications), a breakoff at 6 months seems warranted.[189,191] By that point 93% of Braakman's patients had improved and 66.5% of Bricolo's were following commands. In Ansell's study, 67% of patients who became rehabilitation ready had done so by 6 months. Closer inspection reveals that most patients who progress beyond vegetative state will do so in the first 3 months.[189] Additional recovery from 6–12 months is not frequent, and

TABLE 2. Behaviorally Based Assessment Instruments for the Minimally Responsive Patient

Assessment Instrument	Test Sample Characteristics					Feasibility			
	n	M:F	Age (yr)	Time After Injury	Type of Injury	Target Population	Assessment Areas	Total No. Items	Administration Time
Western Neuro Sensory Stimulation Profile (Ansell & Keenan, 1989[6,7])	57	40:17	29 Range: 14–72	8 mo Range: 14–72	Closed	RL 2–5	Auditory and visual comprehension, tracking, object manipulation, tactile/olfactory arousal/attention	33	20–40 min
Coma Recovery Scale (Glacino et al., 1991[67])	28	15:13	32 Range: 16–63	2.7 mo Range: 1–9.5	Mixed: 19 TBI 3 Anoxia 2 Aneurysm 1 GSW	RL 2–5	Motor, visual, auditory, arousal/ attention, communication, oromotor	25	30 min
Sensory Stimulation Assessment Measure (Rader et al., 1989[128])	20	**	31 Range: 15–59	12.4 mo Range: 2–33	Mixed: 14 TBI 3 Anoxia 2 Aneurysm 1 GSW	RL 2–5	Visual, auditory, olfactory, tactile, gustatory	15	45–50 min
Coma/Near Coma Scale (Rappaport, 1992[130])	20	17:3	34.5 Range: 12–70	8.9 mo Range: 1–48	Mixed: 15 TBI 2 Stroke 1 Anoxia 1 Overdose 1 GSW	DRS Scores 21–29	Auditory, visual, threat, olfactory, tactile, pain, vocalization, command responsivity	11	15–20* min

* Estimated; **not available.
DRS = Disability Rating Scale, GSW = gunshot wound, M:F = male-to-female ratio, RL = Rancho level, RO = rank order coefficient.

(Columns continued on opposite page.)

recovery after a year is rare,[189] although it certainly has been reported.[8,119,138,160] Factors that predict group prognosis may not necessarily predict individual prognosis.[65] Maximal rehabilitation lengths of stay of 2–3 months seem reasonable.[85] Although at this point definitive guidelines are impossible, intensive rehabilitation efforts in minimally responsive patients are[144,184] (1) probably warranted up to 3 months after injury; (2) possibly warranted between 3 and 6 months after injury; and (3) questionable later than 6 months after injury in the absence of documentable and consistent neurologic improvement and behavioral response.[144,184,189]

Behaviorally Based Assessment Instruments

Among the most significant advances in research and care of minimally responsive patients has been the development of behaviorally based assessment instruments (BBAIs). Such scales generally expand on the concepts of the Glasgow Coma Scale.[162] BBAIs are considered to measure disability, albeit rudimentarily from a functional perspective.[56] Psychometric data are presented in Table 2, but published clinical applications of these scales are limited.[123] BBAIs are an important aspect of rehabilitation in the minimally responsive patient for various reasons:

1. BBAIs provide a structured approach by which neurologic and cognitive recovery can be monitored and documented. Scores also can be used to monitor the efficacy of pharmacologic, environmental, and behavioral interventions.

2. BBAIs can identify the patient's sensory, physical, and cognitive strengths, enabling the treatment team to maximize communication and consistency of responses. Weaknesses can be identified to focus the goals of further intervention.

TABLE 2. *(Columns continued)*

	Reliability				Validity			
IRR	**T-RT**	**Internal Consist-ency**	**RL**	**OCS**	**DRS**	**MSEP**	**Comments**
.94–.99 (except A/A and T/O at .64–.90)	**	Total = .95 A/A = .73 T/O = .59 (alpha)	.73 (RO p < .001)	**	**	**		Predictive validity: n = 50; 16/50 progressed to ≤ RL 5 with significantly lower scores in unimproved group in total score, auditory comprehension, visual tracking, and attention/arousal. Progressive decrease in variability of scores with time (RL 2 Æ RL 5)
.83 (kappa)	**	**	**	.90 (P; p < .01)	−.98	**		CRS scores showed a change of at least 1 point/week over 2 of 3 observational periods Mean change of 3.9 CRS points over 4 weeks % change of CRS was greater than DRS, GCS Outcome correlated best with change in CRS score rather than initial score Patients with score changes of ≤6 points over weeks tended to have poorer outcome
.89 (P; p < .01)	.93 (P; p < .01)	**	.68 (P; p < .01)	.70 (P; p < .01)	−.61 (P; p < .01)	**		Patients were mean of 12 months after injury and change may have been detected in a more acute sample SSAM did not show treatment effect in 19 patients undergoing sensory stimulation over 3 months
.98 (statistic not given)	**	.43–.65 (alpha)	**	**	.69 (P; p < .02)	.52 (RO; p < .05; n = 11)		CNC is expansion of the upper range of DRS (scores of 21–30) Correlations with MSEP is unique Initial CNC scores predicted "modest improvement" (those with scores ≤ 2 within 6–7 months of injury)

* Estimated; ** not available.
A/A arousal/attention, DRS = Disability Rating Scale, CNC = coma/near coma scale, CRS = coma recovery scale, GCS = Glasgow Coma Scale, IRR = interrater reliability, MSEP = multisensory evoked potentials, P = Pearson's correlation, RL = Rancho level, SSAM = sensory stimulation assessment measure, T/O = tactile/olfactory, T-RT = Test-retest reliability.

3. BBAIs provide a kind of shorthand for communication among the interdisciplinary team as well as a framework for team conferences.

4. Although current data are preliminary and based on small samples, BBAIs eventually may help to elucidate prognosis. Ansell[7] has already demonstrated the usefulness of one BBAI in tracking the natural history of recovery from severe brain injury.

5. Because BBAIs are standardized and relatively objective, information should be theoretically consistent among centers, thus facilitating multicenter research.

6. Finally, BBAI may serve as an early marker for changes in neuromedical status in minimally responsive patients as demonstrated by subtle decrements in cognitive performance.

All BBAIs are similar in that they represent ordinal scales; that is, they measure the direction but not necessarily the magnitude of change.[115] A brief description of four BBAIs is provided below, with the psychometric properties organized after Jette[94]: feasibility, reliability, and validity (see Table 2). Little is known about the precision of any BBAI.[123] Before using any assessment tool, interrater reliability should be determined among the team members involved in administration.[94]

The **Western Neuro Sensory Stimulation Profile (WNSSP)**[6] contains 33 items in 6 areas, yielding a score of 1–113. The score is based on responses to a variety of sensory stimulations and relies heavily on auditory and visual comprehension. Other areas include visual tracking, object manipulation, arousal/attention, and tactile/olfactory response. At admission, total scores, as well as scores on auditory comprehension, visual tracking and arousal/attention were higher in 16 minimally responsive patients at RL 2 and 3 who advanced to RL 5 than in 34 patients who did not advance. Despite overlap between the groups, these data suggest that the WNSSP has some predictive validity for recovery.

The **Sensory Stimulation Assessment Measure (SSAM)**[128] is an expansion of the three responses of the GCS (motor response, vocalization, and eye opening) to standardized sensory presentation. Patient responses to standardized visual, auditory, tactile, gustatory, and olfactory stimulations are rated from 1–6 in each of the three GCS areas, yielding a total score between 15–90. In a small study, Hall et al.[76] found that the SSAM detected differences in performance between phases of directed and nondirected sensory stimulation in 6 minimally responsive patients and was superior to the WNSSP in detecting daily fluctuations.

The **Coma Recovery Scale (CRS)**[67] theorizes hierarchical responses (from generalized to cognitively mediated) for 25 items in 6 areas: auditory, visual, motor, oromotor/verbal, communication, and arousal. For example, the visual score ranges from 0 (no response) to 6 (object recognition), and the auditory score ranges from 0 (no response) to 4 (replicable movement on command). The level of the highest response is scored for each of the 6 areas. Scores of 0–14 are considered "minimally responsive," whereas scores of 15–25 or higher indicate "emergent awareness." In their original study of 28 minimally responsive persons, Giacino et al.[67] found that changes in CRS scores showed stronger correlations with outcome [as measured by the Disability Rating Scale (DRS)] than initial, one-time scores. The change as a percentage of total score was greater for the CRS than for the GCS or DRS.[131]

Finally, the **Coma/Near Coma Scale (CNC)**[130] is an expansion of the upper range of the DRS, that is, "vegetative state" and "extreme vegetative state." Responses to stimulation for 8 items (outlined in Table 2) are scored, and patients are grouped into one of five categories from "no coma" to "extreme coma" (coma is not used in the strict sense as defined above). Changes in the CNC scores correlated with or predicted future changes in the DRS in a sample of 20 minimally responsive patients.[130]

Whyte has suggested that individualized assessments using a single-case experimental methodology also can be used in tracking progress of the minimally responsive patient.[174] Advantages to this approach include the ability to use virtually any modality available to a patient to document volitional behavior (without limitation to items in a standardized assessment instrument), the flexibility to choose more functional activities to track over time, and the cultivation of analytical thinking by team members. In addition, this technique allows control for spontaneous and reflexive responses. The inability to compare standardized data among centers and between patients is a significant limitation, however. The concomitant use of standardized and individualized approaches is quite feasible.

MEDICAL MANAGEMENT OF MINIMALLY RESPONSIVE PATIENTS

The medical management of minimally responsive patients requires close attention to maintenance issues, prevention of complications, treatment of acute events, and a high index of suspicion. Subtle alterations in cognition, vital signs, tone, and secretions may serve as the only clinical signs of an impending medical complication. Medical stability must be established, and current medications must be assessed critically before any arousal-specific intervention is attempted. The following discussion attempts to strike a balance between the theoretical and the practical, acknowledging that relevant research is sparse and interventions may be limited by available technology or expertise of staff. The overview presented in Table 3 may guide management but should not be applied rigidly.

Minimization of Medication

The minimally responsive patient may have numerous indications for specific medications (e.g., infections, seizures, increased tone). Many medications can affect the level of consciousness or quality of cognition. Early, critical analysis of all medications and constant vigilance in discontinuing all unnecessary drugs are essential. Medication can be assessed routinely at initial consultation, admission to the rehabilitation unit, or

TABLE 3.   Summary of Medical/Rehabilitation Interventions in the Minimally Responsive Patient*

Treatment Issue	Recommendations
Medication	Critically evaluate need for all medications Stop unnecessary medications Change "harmful" but necessary drugs to less offending alternatives
Neurologic deficit	Ensure adequate evaluation for reversible causes of coma Consider repeat neuroimaging studies to rule out hydrocephalus
Seizures	If present, avoid phenobarbital, ? avoid phenytoin Consider diagnosis of seizure in patients with rapid fluctuation in consciousness
Pulmonary disorders	If patient is on ventilator, attempt weaning when appropriate If patient has tracheostomy, begin capping when appropriate Prevent aspiration Maintain adequate pulmonary toilet Consider device to allow vocalization
Gastrointestinal disorders	Consider advantages of gastrostomy vs. jejunostomy tube Reflux precautions Sucralfate for ulcer prophylaxis/treatment Cisapride for gastroparesis, gastroesophageal reflux Maintain adequate nutrition
Autonomic functions	Hypertension—consider atenolol Fevers: medical evaluation to rule out fever of unknown origin; trial of bromocriptine in central fever Hypotension—gradually progress tolerance of upright position
Endocrine disorders	If clinically indicated, screen for syndrome of inappropriate antidiuretic hormone secretion, diabetes insipidus, anterior pituitary dysfunction
Oral hygiene	Initial daily oral hygiene Routine professional cleaning and care
Ophthalmologic care	Lubricate exposed cornea Evaluate for definite procedure or repair for eyelid closure
Skin	Initiate skin maintenance and healing program Consider specialized bed or seating systems, application of specialized surface treatment or protection
Incontinence	Male: condom catheter vs. adult diaper vs. intermittent catheterization Female: diaper (if no skin breakdown) vs. intermittent catheterization
Ethical concerns	Investigate existence of advance writings and establish legal consent for treatment
Social concerns	Family education, support referral to group or individual counseling

* These recommendations should serve only as a guide; actual care depends on many medical, social, and financial factors.

during weekly follow-up or prescription renewals. Two basic questions must be answered for each and every medication:

1. Is the medication essential? If so, is the dosage optimal?

2. Can another medication with fewer potential cognitive side effects or an alternative, nonpharmacologic program be substituted?

Methodologically sound, functional outcome studies of the effect of pharmacologic agents in minimally responsive patients are lacking. Classes of drugs theoretically to be avoided include catecholaminergic antagonists (noradrenergic and dopaminergic), anticholinergic agents, and gabaminergic agonists.[60,61,150,159] Some evidence, however, suggests that anticholinergic agents have theoretically beneficial effects in the acute stage of brain injury.[80]

Catecholamine receptor-blocking agents include the neuroleptics (major tranquilizers) and noradrenergic antihypertensives (e.g., methyldopa and beta- and alpha-blockers). Such drugs may impair motoric recovery after brain injury[159] and have been linked with deficits in attention, concentration, and memory.[71,157,185]

Feeney et al.[61] described decrements in task-specific recovery from unilateral ablation of the motor cortex in rats after a single dose of the neuroleptic haloperidol. Metoclopramide is chemically related to the phenothiazines and is frequently used in the management of gastroesophageal reflux (see below). H_2-receptor antagonists also have been associated with adverse CNS effects, including malaise, somnolence, and, in rare circumstances, reversible confusional states such as psychosis and hallucinations.[24,125] H_2 blockers should be used with additional caution in older patients with impaired renal function.[133,153]

Many medications have anticholinergic effects, including some tricyclic antidepressants (TCAs), which are reviewed thoroughly in chapter 23. In minimally responsive patients, use of TCAs is somewhat limited, because diagnosis of depression is difficult. Amitriptyline has been used in the treatment of agitation.[88,118] If treatment is necessary, agents with high anticholinergic properties should be avoided because of their cognitive side effects, including sedation and deleterious effect on memory.[185] Serotonin uptake inhibitors, a newer class of antidepressants, have a theoretical advantage because of their activating properties and lack of anticholinergic side effects. Recent research in motor recovery in brain-injured rats, however, suggests that the predominantly serotonergic agent trazodone, a nontricyclic antidepressant reported to be useful in stimulating arousal in minimally responsive patients,[39] also hinders recovery of locomotor performance.[29]

Gabaminergic agonists include the benzodiazepines as well as baclofen. Indications for their use include seizure management, regulation of sleep-wake cycles, and hypertonia. Seizure medication is discussed below and in chapter 13. Maintenance on a sedating medication such as diazepam should be avoided unless all other antiseizure medications have failed. Physical principles such as positioning and splinting should be attempted before the institution of a systemic medication for spasticity.[69] Motor point blocks and dantrolene sodium exert their effects at the level of the neuromuscular unit, thereby limiting sedation and cognitive side effects. Both diazepam and baclofen have central sedative effects, and their use should be limited to minimally responsive patients in whom demonstrable, functional difference in tone justifies the risk of cognitive side effects.

By definition, the patient in persistent vegetative state has sleep-wake cycles, but the cycles may be abnormal.[3] If regulation of the sleep-wake cycle is needed, environmental factors and sleep hygiene should be instituted before medications. The timing of procedures such as vital sign and enteral feeding/residual checks, medication administration, turning for pressure relief, and bathing may interrupt the circadian cycle. In practical terms, a 6–8 hour period should be established during which environmental stimuli are limited. In addition, one hour of early morning sunlight is thought to be helpful in establishing the wake part of the cycle.[46] If medication is necessary, short-acting hypnotics such as chloral hydrate are preferable to agents, such as flurazepam, that have a long half-life.[125] Zolpidem is a recently approved hypnotic agent that binds to benzodiazepine receptors in the brain. However, unlike the benzodiazepines, zolpidem does not alter the first two stages of the sleep cycle and thus, theoretically at least, enhances a more physiologic sleep pattern.[114]

Neurologic Issues

The anatomy and nomenclature of coma and "minimal responsiveness" are described above. Causes of coma include a variety or combination of factors arising from supratentorial lesions, subtentorial lesions, diffuse lesions, or metabolic disorders (Table 4). The clinical presentation of coma also varies, and coma may be seen with or without focal or lateralizing neurologic signs or alterations in cellular content of the cerebrospinal fluid (CSF).[137] If the cause of coma is uncertain, reversible causes must be entertained and ruled out. After traumatic injury, considerations include late-onset hygromas, hydrocephalus, infection, subclinical status epilepticus, and metabolic disorders.

Hydrocephalus refers to an enlarged ventricular system with an increase in the amount of cerebrospinal fluid. Obstructive hydrocephalus results from a blockage of the CSF pathways. Nonobstructive hydrocephalus results from either malabsorption of CSF or atrophy of brain substance, in which case it is termed hydrocephalus ex vacuo. Distinguishing between hydrocephalus and hydrocephalus ex vacuo can be difficult. The decision about whether to place a ventriculo-peritoneal shunt for drainage may be based on lack of continued recovery, decrement in the level of responsiveness, or improvement after performing the CSF tap test.[27] Cope1[3] found that 22% of sequentially CT-scanned patients required neurosurgical intervention to correct intracranial pathology, clinical improvement was noted in 7 of 9 patients.

The management of posttraumatic epilepsy is discussed at length in chapter 13; however, a few aspects are discussed below. Research results and subsequent recommendations for prophylaxis of posttraumatic seizures are mixed.[26,113,163] Some studies have found that the incidence of seizure correlates positively with the severity of injury and duration of unconsciousness,[36,75] whereas others have not.[50,182] Given that any seizure medication has side effects, no absolute threshold for prediction of late epilepsy and no specific recommendations for prophylaxis can be established.[93] Clinical practice varies enormously. Protocols in the United States range from universal prophylaxis to prophylaxis only after one or, at some institutions, two seizures. Sudden, erratic alterations in the patient's level of consciousness or vital signs may suggest seizure activity and should lead to further investigation, regardless of whether the patient has therepeutic antiseizure medication levels.

In patients selected for treatment, the rationale is to choose an efficacious drug with the fewest possible cognitive side effects. Although the most often used drug is carbamazepine, it is difficult to justify one agent over another. Some clinicians have suggested recently that valproic acid may be the best choice.[182] Multiple medications are required to control seizure activity in certain patients. Although monotherapy with felbamate has been shown to be efficacious in patients with uncontrolled partial seizures,[59] and a favorable side-effect profile (including few if any cognitive side effects) may be an added benefit in patients with TBI, the drug recently has been recalled due to hematologic toxicity.

Pulmonary Care

Adequate oxygenation, management of secretions, prevention of complications (including

TABLE 4. Approach to the Differential Diagnosis of Coma*

Normal brainstem reflexes, no lateralizing signs
1. Anatomic lesions of hemisphere found
   - Hydrocephalus
   - Bilateral subdural hematomas
   - Bilateral contusions, edema, or axonal shearing of hemispheres due to closed head trauma, subarachnoid hemorrhage
2. Bilateral hemispheral dysfunction without mass lesion (CT normal)
   - Drug-toxin ingestion (toxocologic analysis)
   - Endogenous metabolic encephalopathy (glucose, ammonia, calcium, osmolarity, PO_2, PCO_2, urea, sodium)
   - Shock, hypertensive encephalopathy
   - Meningitis (CSF analysis)
   - Nonherpetic viral encephalitis (CSF analysis)
   - Epilepsy (EEG)
   - Reye's syndrome (ammonia, increased intracranial pressure)
   - Fat embolism
   - Subarachnoid hemorrhage with normal CT (CSF analysis)
   - Acute disseminated encephalomyelitis (CSF analysis)
   - Acute hemorrhagic leukoencephalitis
   - Advanced Alzheimer's and Creutzfeldt-Jakob disease

Normal brainstem reflexes (with or without unilateral compressive third nerve palsy), lateralizing motor signs (CT abnormal)
1. Unilateral mass lesion found
   - Cerebral hemorrhage (basal ganglia, thalamus)
   - Large infarction with surrounding brain edema
   - Herpes virus encephalitis (temporal lobe lesion)
   - Subdural or epidural hematoma
   - Tumor with edema
   - Brain abscess with edema
   - Vasculitis with multiple infarctions
   - Metabolic encephalopathy superimposed on preexisting focal lesions (e.g., stroke)
   - Pituitary apoplexy
2. Asymmetric signs accompanied by diffuse hemispheral dysfunction
   - Metabolic encephalopathies with asymmetric signs (blood chemical determinations)
   - Isodense subdural hematoma
   - Thrombotic thrombocytopenic purpura (blood smear, platelet count)
   - Epilepsy with focal seizures or postictal state (EEG)

Multiple brainstem reflex abnormalities
1. Anatomic lesions in brainstem found
   - Pontine, midbrain hemorrhage
   - Cerebellar hemorrhage, tumor, abscess
   - Cerebellar infarction with brainstem compression
   - Mass in hemisphere causing advanced bilateral brainstem compression
   - Brainstem tumor or demyelination
   - Traumatic brainstem contusion-hemorrhage (clinical signs, auditory-evoked potentials)
2. Brainstem dysfunction without mass lesion
   - Basilar artery thrombosis causing brainstem stroke (clinical signs, angiogram)
   - Severe drug overdose (toxicologic analysis)
   - Brainstem encephalitis
   - Basilar artery migraine
   - Brain death

* These conditions should be at least considered for minimally responsive patients in whom the cause of decreased responsiveness is uncertain. (From Harrison's Textbook of Medicine, 12th ed., with permission.[46,137])

infection), and facilitation of speech are a few of the pulmonary issues pertinent to minimally responsive patients. The initial injury may involve compromise of the central respiratory drive, airway, chest wall, and lungs as well as loss of control or dysfunction of glottic structures protecting the trachea. Ensuing complications such as hypoxia, adult respiratory distress syndrome (ARDS), pulmonary emboli (fat or venous), and aspiration may add to morbidity.[21] Such factors place the brain-injured patient at increased risk for early and late pulmonary dysfunction that requires specific interventions and close monitoring.[170]

Airway Management

Potential complications associated with nasotracheal and orotracheal intubation include injury to the vocal cords, arytenoid, and mucosa. The incidence of tracheal stenosis is unclear. In one study[154] the incidence was documented at 9.1%, although the stenosis was of no clinical or functional significance. Early injury is promoted by agitation, posturing, motion of the tube due to inadequate fixation at the mouth, and tugging of the ventilation tubes.[56] Low-pressure cuffs have greatly reduced the incidence of serious tracheal stenosis, but the incidence of long-term laryngeal injury does not appear to have changed.[20,21] The length of time for which a patient may be maintained via translaryngeal intubation without increasing the risk of complications is not well defined.[81,99,110] Recommended times for conversion range from 7–14 days, depending on the clinical condition and stability of the patient and whether extubation is anticipated imminently.[81,110]

Indications for tracheostomy, aside from long-term mechanical ventilation, include relief of upper airway obstruction and, most commonly in the setting of brain injury, assistance with pulmonary toilet.[81] In addition to sparing further injury to the larynx, tracheostomy facilitates nursing care (especially airway suctioning), oral feeding, speech, and mobility.[41] Tracheostomy also facilitates transfer to a lower intensity of care (e.g., rehabilitation).

The cost and complications of tracheostomy are its primary limiting factors. Bleeding, pneumothorax, and damage to adjacent structures at the time of surgical placement are the immediate risks. With long-term use, tracheal injury and resultant stenosis occur at a low, but not yet definitively determined, rate.[20] Some investigations have reported an increased incidence of lower airway infections, typically with gram-negative bacilli, in patients with tracheostomy.[81]

Patients on mechanical ventilation or patients at risk for aspiration are usually managed with a silastic tube with a low-pressure, high-compliance cuff.[2] Cuff pressure should not exceed the capillary pressure of 20–30 mm H_2O. Tube size should be approximately 8–9 mm for men and 7–9 mm for women.[99] If tracheomalacia develops, a foam-cuffed tube may be used rather than progressively larger tubes or higher cuff pressures.[2] If aspiration is not a significant risk, an uncuffed nylon, silicone, or metal tube with removable inner cannula is used. Rigid silver tubes are reusable but may erode into the surrounding structures.

A relatively recent development is the tracheostomy button, which may be used in patients who are not at risk of aspiration of in need of ventilation. The "button" is a Teflon tube that may be inserted into the stoma and anchored against the anterior tracheal wall.[2] The tracheal lumen is unobstructed; this technique may facilitate speech and decrease irritation, thus lessening secretions. Inadvertent dislocation of the button is a disadvantage compared with standard tracheostomy units.

Speech can be facilitated by a fenestrated or "talking" tracheostomy. The tracheostomy tubes have an external lumen that forces compressed air through the vocal cords. Limitations include the high flow rates needed for adequate phonation[2] and the potential for growth of granulation tissue into the fenestration. The Passey-Muir valve, a one-way valve placed over the tracheostomy site, allows air to enter via the tracheostomy; exhalation through the oral cavity makes speech possible. Tolerance is limited by the inspiratory/expiratory effort of the patient.[48]

Recommendations for the care of tracheostomy tubes include daily cleaning of metal cannulas or replacement of synthetic inner cannulas.[2] Stomal cleaning should occur daily with replacement of pads and ties. The entire apparatus is replaced as often as weekly or as seldom as monthly.[99]

Although a few centers are capable of weaning mechanical ventilation,[21] tracheostomy discontinuation in minimally responsive patients is often left to the physiatrist. Rates of successful tracheal decannulation as high as 96% have been reported when weaning criteria include medical stability, minimal secretions, intact swallow, and tracheostomy capping of 24–48 consecutive hours.[36]

One approach to tracheostomy weaning begins with the use of progressively smaller, uncuffed tubes at 2–3 day intervals. Once an adult size of 4–5 mm is reached, plugging of the tube begins. Progression of plugged time and tolerance of plugging should be documented carefully. Once the patient can tolerate 24–48 hours of plugging, the tube may be removed and an occlusive dressing applied.[2,99] An alternate method is progressive plugging of the same-size tube, which is removed once plugging is tolerated for 24–48 hours. Close supervision of respiratory function with plugging and decannulation is imperative. Unfortunately, it may be difficult to determine clinically whether the tracheostomy facilitates clearance of secretions or acts as a foreign body that stimulates secretions. In patients who exhibit respiratory distress with plugging, consultation with an otolaryngologist for possible laryngoscopy is indicated.

Pulmonary Infection

The tracheostomy site is often colonized, because bacteria thrive in the warm, moist, nutrient-rich environment. Prophylactic antibiotics are not recommended for several reasons. In Goodpasture et al.'s study, prophylactic antibiotics led to earlier appearance of gram-negative bacilli.[72] In addition, chronic prophylaxis promotes development of resistant organisms that may prove extremely difficult to treat if a clinically significant infection develops.

Despite appropriate precautions and management, infection of the respiratory tract may occur and may be difficult to characterize. Frequently, a change in sputum color or alteration in vital signs or level of consciousness is the first indication of infection. Yellow or green sputum reflects the presence of numerous leukocytes in response to an offending organism.[170] Appropriate studies, such as sputum stain, sputum culture, radiographs, and blood work, may provide guidance in ferreting out the source of the infection.

Factors that predispose to oropharyngeal colonization with gram-negative organisms and pneumonia in minimally responsive patients include hospitalization, underlying disease, compromised host defenses, and recent antibiotic therapy.[170] Anaerobes in the oropharynx are the usual cause of aspiration pneumonia. Tuberculosis has recently become more prevalent in urban, indigent, immigrant, and immunocompromised patients. Diagnosis of infection with or reactivation of the tubercle bacillus may require special studies, such as the tuberculin skin test (PPD) and acid-fast staining of sputum.[170] Unexplainable fever, leukocytosis, or nasal discharge should alert the physician to include sinusitis in the differential diagnosis.[2]

Other Pulmonary Complications

Atelectasis may occur in patients with an impaired ability to mobilize respiratory secretions. Chest physiotherapy (CPT) may help to mobilize secretions from the lower respiratory tract and to prevent or reverse atelectasis. Because CPT is expensive and not without potential side effects, it should be reserved for patients with bronchorrhea and atelectasis, diagnoses in which a clear clinical benefit has been shown.[2]

The incidence of deep venous thrombosis (DVT) and pulmonary embolism (PE) in minimally responsive patients is not well documented. Kalisky et al.[96] found a 4% incidence of DVT in their review of a sample of severely brain-injured patients. A recent study suggests that routine screening for DVT at admission in the general brain-injured population[116] is not cost-effective.[116] The American Academy of Physical Medicine and Rehabilitation has formulated guidelines for patients undergoing stroke rehabilitation with altered mobility. The guidelines recommend prophylaxis with low-dose heparin, low-molecular-weight heparin, or external pneumatic compression for all patients with weakness. However, clinical evidence indicated conclusively that stroke-associated and brain injury-associated DVT should be treated in a similar manner.[31]

TABLE 5. Metabolic Changes after Brain Injury

- Increased urinary nitrogen excretion
- Alteration ion trace metal status with depressed serum zinc, increased urinary zinc excretion, and increased serum copper levels
- Increased acute-phase protein synthesis, including fibrinogen, alpha1-acid glycoprotein, serum c-reactive protein, and ceruloplasmin
- Decreased negative acute-phase protein synthesis, including albumin, retinol-binding protein, and thyroxine-binding prealbumin
- Fluid and electrolyte imbalance due, in some cases, to hypothalamus and pituitary gland dysfunction

From Hester DD: Nutrition Support: Diabetes Core Curriculum, 2nd ed. American Society for Parenteral and Enteral Nutrition, 1993, pp 229–241, with permission.

Gastrointestinal System

Management of the gastrointestinal tract is integrally related to the management of the pulmonary system. Nasogastric feeding tubes render the esophageal sphincters incompetent and may contribute to regurgitation or aspiration.[172] In addition, animal data indicate that acute and chronic brain injuries lower esophageal sphincter pressure, thus increasing the risk for relux.[169] Theoretically, placement of an ostomy tube that bypasses the esophagus reduces the risk of aspiration, because the tube is located distal to the pyloric sphincter.[135] In addition, prophylaxis against stress ulceration with histamine type-2 (H_2) blocking agents has been shown to increase gastric colonization with gram-negative bacilli in the critical care setting. Use of H_2 blockers is thought to facilitate retrograde bacterial colonization of the trachea, leading to an increased rate of pneumonia (35.7%) compared with sucralfate prophylaxis (10.3%).[54,57]

Providing adequate nutrition and avoiding complications of feeding are the primary gastrointestinal challenges in low-level patients. An understanding of the alterations in energy requirements after brain injury is essential. Some of these alterations are briefly reviewed below; the reader is referred to chapter 20 for additional information.

Enteral Nutrition

Robertson et al. reported that patients with GCS scores of 4–5 have the highest energy expenditure at an average of 26% above predicted.[134] Intermediate levels of nutrition were required in patients with a GCS > 8, and lower needs were found with GCS scores of 6–7. Energy expenditure with brain death or barbiturate coma averaged 14% below predicted. The characteristic metabolic changes that occur with brain injury are outlined in Table 5.

The goal of nutritional assessment is prevention of malnutrition. However, traditional parameters (e.g., albumin and transferrin) are not useful in studying efficacy of nutritional support during the first several weeks, because levels continue to decrease during the first 2 weeks after injury despite aggressive nutritional support.[82] Given the wide variability among minimally responsive patients, biweekly indirect calorimetry is recommended to determine energy requirements properly. Depending on the facility, this approach may or may not be practical. Alternatively, the Harris-Benedict equation may be used to estimate caloric requirements:

In men:
$$66 + (13.7 \times \text{weight in kg}) + (5 \times \text{height in cm}) - (6.8 \times \text{age})$$

In women:
$$655 + (9.6 \times \text{weight in kg}) + (1.85 \times \text{height in cm}) - (4.7 \times \text{age})$$

This basal energy expenditure is then multiplied by a factor of up to 1.75 for extremely stressed patients.[155] A subset of brain-injured patients requires caloric intake significantly higher than calculated. Sandel et al.[142] demonstrated that such patients are hypermetabolic; rather they are replacing muscle volume with very "caloric-dense" fat.

Enteral feedings are often not well tolerated in the acute phase. The cause of intolerance is probably multifactorial, including impaired gastric emptying, the effect of brain damage on the gastrointestinal system,[82,122,135] and medications that alter gastric emptying (e.g., bromocriptine, levodopa/carbidopa, narcotics). Intolerance of enteral feeding is significantly related to increased intracranial pressure and severity of injury.[82] Grahm et al.[73] demonstrated the benefits of early jejunal hyperalimentation in head-injured patients despite the absence of bowel sounds.

Benefits included increased caloric and nitrogen intake and improved nitrogen balance as well as reduction in the incidence of bacterial infections and length of stay in the intensive care unit. Technical availability and physician acceptance may explain in part the infrequency with which this feeding approach is used. Total parenteral nutrition (TPN) is an alternative route and may be given safely without causing serum hyperosmolality or affecting intracranial pressure. In summary, early feeding, by whatever route, improves survival and recovery.

Once an enteral route has been established, a general guide is to initiate isotonic feedings at 40 ml/hr and to increase the feedings by 10–20 mm every 8–12 hours until the target volume and caloric need are achieved. A dietitian may be helpful in establishing the dietary needs as well as in selecting the formula. Tube feeding should be held if the residual is greater than 2 times the hourly rate or greater than 100 ml. Fluid requirements vary, depending on the renal solute load, patient's weight, and additional water losses. Generally, 750–1000 ml/day of water are added to the nutritional supplements. Clinical monitoring of electrolytes or urine osmolality may be necessary to ensure adequate hydration. Bolus feedings are often used once tolerance of continuous drip infusions has been established. Feedings of less than 400 ml may be infused gradually over 20–40 minutes. The head of the bed should be elevated at least 30° during continuous feedings or kept elevated 1 hour after bolus feedings to help in preventing the risk of aspiration.

Advantages of bolus feeding include (1) stimulation of more physiologic feeding pattern; (2) greater mobility of the patient; and (3) administration of medication without reaction to the feeding supplement.[5] Disadvantages of bolus feeding include (1) added labor; (2) risk of delayed gastric emptying, which may increase the risk of aspiration pneumonia; and (3) more frequent association with bloating and diarrhea.[5]

Gastrostomy tubes have the advantage that bolus feedings may be used, whereas jejunostomy tubes theoretically have a lower risk of aspiration (although this is unclear[102]) and are not affected by disorders of gastric emptying. Prospective studies comparing the two types of tubes are needed to clarify optimal management.[49]

Other Gastrointestinal Issues

Gastroparesis refers to a delay in gastric emptying into the small bowel. The cause of gastroparesis after brain injury is unknown, but it is thought to be secondary to a brain-gut link.[135] Treatment is often required because of persistent symptoms of abdominal pain, nausea, and vomiting and intolerance of feedings. Metoclopramide has been the primary drug used to treat both gastroparesis and gastroesophageal reflux.[87] Concern over the antagonism of central dopamine receptors may limit its use.[24,61] Cisapride is a newer prokinetic agent structurally related to metoclopramide but devoid of extrapyramidal side effects and central antidopaminergic activity.[95] In clinical trials,[95] cisapride appears to be equivalent to metoclopramide in shortening gastric emptying time. Given the side-effect profiles and mechanism of action of each, cisapride appears to be preferable to metoclopramide for treatment of both gastroparesis and gastroesophageal reflux in minimally responsive patients. In addition, erythromycin may be used to facilitate gastric emptying, although its potential interaction with carbamazepine must be kept in mind.[181]

Stress ulceration in central nervous system injury has been reported in 26% of patients at admission to the Intensive Care Unit.[133] Using unknown selection criteria, Becker et al.[14] reported hematemesis in 75% and Hemoccult-positive stool in 25% of 16 patients in coma (length of coma: 28–133 days). Studies have shown negligible mortality from stress ulcers; the patient's underlying condition appears to be the major determinant of mortality.[57,177] Universal prophylaxis in the critical care setting has undoubtedly been the primary factor in reducing mortality from stress ulceration, but the best prophylactic agent is debated. Some consensus exists that antacids, H_2 blockers, and sucralfate protect against ulcers fairly equally.[28] Recent reports that patients receiving H_2-receptor blockers have higher rates of gram-negative pneumonia have led some authorities to recommend sucralfate.[54,57] No definitive studies address the appropriate long-term prophylaxis of stress ulcers in minimally responsive patients; thus, the relative risks of stopping a prophylactic agent at a certain point are difficult to ascertain. Endoscopically diagnosed ulcers should receive a standard 3–6-month course of treatment, depending on location of the ulcer and endoscopic reexamination. Recent evidence suggests that certain bacteria also may play a role in the pathogenesis of gastric ulcers; broad-spectrum antibiotics are used for treatment.[111]

Endocrine Dysfunction

Endocrine dysfunction, pathogenesis, and treatment are comprehensively discussed in chapter 21. Reported percentages of endocrine and hormonal abnormalities range from 4%, when diagnosis is based on overt clinical symptoms, to 20%, when a screening protocol is used.[89,96] In a recent review, Hansen and Cook[79] assert that most of the information about endocrine function in brain-injured patients is gleaned from case reports and that diagnosis of such abnormalities is often delayed, although signs and symptoms may be present for long periods.

The syndrome of inappropriate antidiuretic hormone (SIADH) secretion is estimated to occur in 30% of all neurosurgical patients; it is the most frequent endocrine complication in brain-injured patients in the acute care setting.[27,64] Treatment is initiated with fluid restriction and possibly demeclocycline. Disruption of the release of antidiuretic hormone is less frequent (1 in 200) and results in diabetes insipidus,[64] which is treated with intranasal or intramuscular desmovasopressin acetate (DDAVP). Repeated assessment of serum and urine sodium and osmolality is indicated for monitoring response to treatment, especially given recent evidence that in patients with TBI individual cognitive function varies widely with fluctuations of serum sodium.[9]

Menstrual irregularities are common after brain injury, although the cycle usually returns within the first several months. If the woman is of child-bearing age, a qualitative assessment of beta human chorionic gonadotropin should be performed, regardless of the sexual history. Low-dose combined oral contraceptive pills are useful in reestablishing the menstrual cycle, if clinically indicated.[27]

Miscellaneous Medical Problems

Autonomic disturbance secondary to damage in the upper brainstem or hypothalamus may lead to altered respiratory patterns, vasomotor instability, or difficulties in regulation of body temperature. In minimally responsive patients it may manifest as alterations in blood pressure, disturbances in cardiac rate or rhythm, and elevations of temperature. Autonomic dysfunction is difficult to diagnose, because it is a diagnosis of exclusion. Case reports that bromocriptine ameliorates autonomic dysfunction prove support for a clinical trial.[27,52] Propranolol and various other agents, such as dantrolene sodium and nonsteroidal anti-inflammatory drugs, have also shown some success.[27] Studies of chronic fever or long-term thermoregulatory deficits after brain injury have not been performed.[175]

Elevations of temperature in minimally responsive patients are most likely due to infection rather than autonomic dysfunction, especially in the presence of leukocytosis. Animal studies suggest that the preoptic anterior hypothalamus is the most important structure for regulation of internal temperature homeostasis. Response to many stimuli, including bacteria and their endotoxins, viruses, yeasts, spirochetes, immune reactions, hormonal substances, and drugs, may produce fever via endogenous pyrogens that engage neurons in the hypothalamus.[136] Thus, a search for the cause of fever may be quite complex. According to Bontke et al.,[26] pulmonary, urinary, and soft-tissue infections occur most frequently. Thus, these areas seem to be the appropriate starting points for investigating suspected infection. A less frequent cause—sinusitis in association with facial fractures or nasogastric feeding—is often elusive, unless sinus films are obtained.[2] In a general medical setting, other important causes include tuberculosis, drug fever, gastrointestinal organisms, bacterial infections in the bone (osteomyelitis) or abscesses (e.g., intracranial or intraperitoneal), neoplasm, and thrombophlebitis, with or without multiple pulmonary emboli. For a diagnosis of fever of unknown origin, elevations in temperature above 38.3° C (101° F) must be present for at least 2 weeks, with failure to produce an alternative diagnosis after 1 week of extensive study.[136] An infectious disease specialist may be helpful in the evaluation of fever of unknown origin.

Hypertension has been reported in 11–15% of head-injured patients with no history of elevated blood pressure.[96,100] In the acute stages of injury, hypertension may result from the release of catecholamines or increased intracranial pressure. Elevated blood pressure is accompanied by tachycardia and increased cardiac output. With this combination of signs, a beta-adrenergic blocking agent, such as atenolol,[176] is the preferred intervention; peripheral dilating drugs have been found to be ineffective.[62]

Other causes of hypertension should be considered, including autonomic dysreflexia from occult spinal cord injury, renal damage, adrenal hemorrhage, pheochromocytoma, or iatrogenic factors (e.g., major tranquilizers). Noxious stimuli also may produce elevations of blood pressures as part of the pain response. Potential sources include tracheostomy or gastrostomy tube sites (where application of a small amount of 2% viscous lidocaine is helpful), decubitus ulcers, unsatisfactory positioning or splinting, and occult fractures or injuries. Removal of noxious stimuli may alleviate the pain and forestall the need for systemic medication.

Hypotension in minimally responsive patients is most likely orthostatic and secondary to prolonged bed rest. Possible mechanisms include decreased plasma volume, lower skeletal muscle tone, and impairment of the baroreceptor reflexes.[2,48] Treatment consists of compression garments and gradual upright progression of the patient on a tilt table. Drugs such as ephedrine also may be of use in selected patients in whom more conservative treatment has failed. Profound hypotension may be associated with hypopituitarism that requires hormonal manipulation.[27]

Oral Care

Bruxism has been documented both in the general population and in brain-injured patients. The onset of bruxism has been correlated with return of sleep-wake cycles in a nontraumatically injured population.[127] Untreated, it may lead to a host of deleterious effects on ligaments and alveolar bone as well as undermine the stability and integrity of the immediately involved structures. Treatment consists of custom-fabricated biteguards to reduce dental destruction. Care should be taken that biteguards do not inadvertently occlude the airway in minimally responsive patients.

Oral hygiene has received little systematic attention in the brain-injured population.[186] Daily mouth and teeth care should be instituted as soon as possible. Routine cleaning and fluoride prophylaxis as well as restoration of carious areas should be initiated once the patient is stable.

Ophthalmologic Issues

Damage to the visual system after brain injury is relatively common and may result from direct trauma to the orbit and its structures, cranial nerve deficits, or visual pathway damage in the central nervous system. A recent review by Sadun and Liu provides a thorough analysis of posttraumatic visual disorders and treatments.[109,141] Protecting the cornea from exposure keratitis secondary to inadequate lubrication is of paramount importance, especially in patients with damage to cranial nerve VII.[19] An ophthalmologic lubricant should be used on a scheduled basis. Alternative management options and other rehabilitative issues have been discussed recently by Liu.[109]

Skin Care

The minimally responsive patient is at risk for loss of skin integrity secondary to the static forces of pressure and moisture as well as the active forces of shearing, friction, and abrasion. Prevention of decubitus ulcers includes proper nutrition, keeping the skin clean and dry, eliminating or minimizing pressure over susceptible areas, and prompt treatment of areas of breakdown.[15] Various options to decrease pressure and shearing have been developed for both mattresses and seating cushions, which must be selected with great care.

Incontinence

Management of incontinence is an ongoing issue in minimally responsive patients. Bowel programs should be established early in the course of rehabilitation by the use of softening and/or bulking agents as well as suppositories. This approach establishes an elimination schedule that aids in nursing care as well as in avoidance of constipation. Bladder management is optimal with an external collection device (condom catheter vs. diaper), which avoids the complications of indwelling catheters. An indwelling catheter may be necessary for healing of skin decubiti, but an intermittent catheterization program also may be appropriate. Repeated urinary tract infections should prompt urologic evaluation, including postvoid residuals and possibly cystometrographic studies or pharmacologic manipulation of bladder function.

AROUSAL-SPECIFIC INTERVENTIONS

Maximizing the medical status and minimizing the medication regimen is always the first, and probably most important, intervention for a minimally responsive patient. This first step is rooted in a basic knowledge of medication side effects and good medical care. Unfortunately, there is little protocol to provide guidance in treatment after this point. Few studies address the appropriate approach to arousal-specific interventions. The determination of "appropriate" ultimately falls on the attending physician, the institution, and, increasingly, third-party payors.[144] The actual and potential abuses of this rather subjective approach to treatment are underscored by the recent congressional investigation of the brain injury rehabilitation industry[42] and the new requirements for written ethical standards by the Commission for Accreditation of Rehabilitation Facilities.[40] Potential abuses aside, the generally young age of minimally responsive patients magnifies the ramifications of successful or unsuccessful interventions, in both human and financial terms. Arousal-specific interventions in minimally responsive patients can be classified in three broad groups:

nonpharmacologic (sensory stimulation), pharmacologic, and surgical.

Nonpharmacologic Interventions

Sensory stimulation has been defined as "the structured use of materials to stimulate the senses of the unresponsive patient."[58] Despite its wide availability,[121] the practice of sensory stimulation remains quite controversial.[58,147,183] The theoretical value of sensory stimulation lies in evidence that environmental deprivation deters optimal recovery from brain injury[107,117,180] and that structural changes in the central nervous system can be facilitated by environmental manipulation.[60,70,144,180] It is unclear whether such concepts, originally applied to developmental disorders, also apply to traumatic neurologic injury or whether passive stimulation is as effective as active participation in an enriched environment.[180]

Perhaps the most important role of the physiatrist in sensory stimulation is to establish the medical stability of the minimally responsive patient before initiating therapy and to discontinue therapy when medical status significantly changes.[58] The purpose of this discussion is not to provide a comprehensive review of the literature about the effectiveness of sensory stimulation in severely brain-injured patients. The reader is referred to recent reviews for further comments about efficacy.[58,183]

In brief, ample evidence suggests that sensory stimulation has a temporal effect on vital signs[58] and even electrophysiologic testing,[152] but no evidence indicates that it alters the natural history of the minimally responsive patient. Reports of efficacy differ substantially from striking[107] to moderate[117] to no[128] benefit. The relatively few published studies of efficacy are hampered most severely by small sample sizes,[76,117,179] lack of appropriate outcome measures,[178] lack of control groups,[128,179] mixed causes of injury,[128] lack of uniformity in definitions of responsiveness levels,[128] and poor definition of the stimulation procedures themselves.[179] However, several recently published studies are quite admirable, despite small sample sizes.[76,117,128] Because sensory stimulation poses little potential risk to patients, benefit and cost of treatment are the primary issues to be addressed.[144] Sensory stimulation should serve as only one component in the overall management of minimally responsive patients.[183]

For reasons outlined above, no gold standard guides selection of the type of sensory stimulation program. The distinction between directed (e.g., application of one of the assessment tools discussed above) and nondirected (e.g., a television or radio playing in the patient's room) seems logically appropriate.[76] Wood[179,180] uses the term "sensory regulation" for the controlled introduction of stimuli.

Nondirected programs imply the provision of sensory stimulation for purposes other than eliciting a specific response or simultaneous responses from multiple sensory modalities; they are essentially background noise.[180] Wood also includes such factors as skin care, range of motion, and bowel and bladder care. Directed programs imply sensory stimulation in a more therapeutic and observational context. A rehabilitation professional presents a stimulus designed to elicit a limited and predictable response in a single sensory modality (visual, auditory, tactile, olfactory, gustatory).[58,180] Directed sensory stimulation requires a method to qualitate, or preferably to quantitate, the patient's response.[144]

Nondirect sensory stimulation probably should not be considered in the context of therapy—and certainly not in the context of assessment. It is also inappropriate to provide nondirect sensory stimulation on a constant basis.[180] Because of the poor documentation of efficacy, directed sensory stimulation probably should be considered more in the context of assessment than therapy.

On the basis of the natural history of vegetative state, the length of treatment with sensory stimulation and intensive intervention in the setting of rehabilitation probably should not extend beyond 3 months after injury, in the absence of well-documented neurologic recovery.[32,34,103,144]

Pharmacologic Interventions

Pharmacologic interventions in minimally responsive patients are a new and exciting development. The metabolites of certain neurotransmitters (e.g., catecholamines) are known to be low after severe brain injury.[168] Conversely, levels of other neurotransmitters (e.g., acetylcholine and glutamate) may be elevated after acute brain injury and may exert a neurotoxic effect.[80] The first observations that recovery from brain injury could be facilitated pharmacologically were noted in the late 1970s and early 1980s.[53,59,140,168] The underlying principle is quite simple: if production of neurotransmitter substrates is impaired, replacement may either facilitate recovery or lessen the neurobehavioral sequelae of brain injury. Extensive animal studies provide a theoretical basis, especially the work of Fenney[60,61] and Goldstein and Davis.[70] Results from these and other research laboratories (detailed in chapter 4) indicate that pharmacologic manipulation can either facilitate[29,60,70] or hinder[24,25,60] recovery from brain injury in rats. The effect may be limited in more severe brain injury, however.[159] The studies also provide preliminary evidence that drugs best facilitate recovery when used in combination with "practice." Some have interpreted practice as the experimental equivalent of rehabilitation intervention.[29,60,61,70]

Almost no data document the frequency of pharmacologic intervention in minimally responsive patients, but the direct dopamine agonist bromocriptine (Parlodel) and the indirect agonist levodopa [in combination with carbidopa (Sinemet)] are the most commonly used agents. Amantadine (Symmetryl) may be used less often. Evidence suggests that norepinephrine and acetylcholine are more important for input processing and dopamine in response preparation.[173] However, Boyeson's recent animal data[30] suggest that norepinephrine may be more important than dopamine in facilitating motor recovery.

Among the pharmacologic interventions available for minimally responsive patients, dopamine agonists are probably the best known. Three expanded case series address dopaminergic agents in brain injury (Table 6).[53,101,168] The studies are variably limited by small sample sizes, lack of objective outcome measures, poor descriptions of sample characteristics, and inadequate descriptions of pharmacologic interventions (e.g., dosing, length of treatment).

TABLE 6. Pharmacologic Interventions for the Minimally Responsive Patient

Study	N	Etiology of Brain Injury	Methodology	Assessment
DiRocco, 1979[53]	15	Trauma—8 Surgery—6 Vascular—1	At least 7 days post injury No clinical/EEG improvement for 6 days prior to therapy Patients "generally vegetative" and medically stable	"Deep" coma—1 "Moderate coma"—3 "Obnubilation"—9 "Vigilant, but unconscious"—2
Van Woerkom, 1981[168]	38 patients 45 drug trials	All "post-traumatic": "majority" were traffic accidents	At least 4 weeks post-injury Most showed no improvement in "last weeks" GCS compared between 2 weeks before and 3 weeks after treatment 7 patients received 2 courses (separated by at least 5 weeks)	Glascow Coma Scale Glascow Outcome Scale
Lal, 1988[101]	11	Trauma—8 Anoxia—2 Gunshot wound—1 (1 patient withdrew due to side effects)	Plateaued for at least 1 month Original sample of 12; 1 patient withdrew ? Therapists blinded	

EEG = electroencephalogram, GCS = Glascow Coma Scale.   *(Columns continued on opposite page.)*

Nonetheless, aspects of each study seem to suggest a role for pharmacologic intervention. Lal et al.[53] reported that after initiation of Sinemet 3 patients at RL 2 progressed to RL 8, whereas patients at RL 3 progressed to RL 6 and 7. The patients progressed at 3.5, 3.7, 5.8, 9 and 19 months after injury, respectively. Spontaneous recovery is certainly possible within 6 months after injury but much less likely at the later times. Close examination of outcome descriptions suggests that levels of independence may not have been as high as the RL levels imply. In the best available study, Van Woerkom et al.[168] described 35/45 drug trials in which patients who were either stable or improving only slightly made substantial improvement after administration of L-dopa and/or physostigmine. All patients were treated at least 4 weeks after injury. DiRocco et al.[53] reported improvement in brain injury of mixed etiologies after initiation of L-dopa (up to 4 gm/day, with and without carbidopa). Despite a solid association between drug dose and clinical improvement, patients were treated so early after injury (7 days) that it is difficult not to attribute their improvement to spontaneous recovery. Haig and Ruess[78] reported that a patient at RL 2 improved substantially 6 months after injury. Vocalization was noted within a few days, and 3 months later the patient had progressed to RL 6 and could after introduction of Sinemet independently perform activities of daily living. Other case reports[24,44,140] suggest a beneficial effect of dopamine agonists in severe brain injury. Recent reports of the beneficial effect of bromocriptine in patients with nonfluent aphasia[10] strengthen the evidence for efficacy. Certainly, only a portion of the impairment in traumatic brain injury can be attributed to disturbances in neurotransmitter function. Van Woerkom suggested that replacement of neurotransmitters effectively treats "reversible functional disorders" but may have no effect on long-term neurologic outcome or structural damage unrelated to neurochemical processes.

Surgical Interventions

Several reports suggest a benefit from stimulators surgically placed in the mesencephalic reticular formation[98,166] or spinal dorsal column at the C2 level.[97] Tsubokawa[165] suggested that electrophysiologic studies can be used to select appropriate candidates for stimulator placement at 2 months or longer after injury. Researchers state that the stimulation needs to be continued for 6–8 months for adequate assessment of clinical response. Further delineation of complications and long-term side effects is advisable before

TABLE 6. *(Columns continued)*

Demographics	Drug(s) Used	Results/Comments
Not detailed	L-Dopa up to 4 grams/day (in majority) and L-Dopa plus carbidopa in rest	Outcome measures vague and confusing No side effects noted Short time post-injury makes natural recovery serious confounding variable Most patients improved; improvement related to dosing No statistical analysis offered
Mean age = 26 yr (range 7–54) 34 males, 4 females	L-Dopa with benzeracide (N = 23) Physostigmine (IV or IM) (N = 10)	No sedating medications given (except anti-seizures) 2 patients developed vomiting with L-dopa GCS scores higher for entire group after treatment (Wilcox rank test, p ≤ 0.05) Response better with higher GCS score and shorter time from injury
Age range 17–54 years 3–52 months post-injury "Most" on anti-seizure medication 8 inpatients/4 outpatients	Sinemet (starting dose 10/100 tid or 25/250 qid; no max given)	2 patients required long-term treatment All 7 subjects at ≤ 18 months post-injury improved, 4 patients at ≥ 18 months improved in cognition only 3 patients 3.5–5.8 months post-injury progressed from RL II → VIII (min. 3 months on Sinemet); 2 began at RL II → VII (9 and 19 months post-injury) Text indicates RL may have overestimated final functional status No toxic side effects noted; benefits seen at relatively low doses "Recent onset in severely involved patients seemed to make better gains"

GCS = Glasgow Coma Scale, RL = Rancho level.

undertaking this controversial and generally difficult surgical approach.

ETHICAL AND PSYCHOSOCIAL CONSIDERATIONS

The persistent vegetative state is defined and diagnostic criteria are set forth in a recent publication by the American Neurological Association.[3] "Persistent," which is defined as a period of at least 1 month, does not imply permanence or irreversibility, although the appropriateness of this definition continues to be debated. Etiology, duration, and the patient's age aid in prognosis. Persistent vegetative state after head trauma may require up to 6–12 months of observation before it is considered irreversible, the exact period is controversial. Advanced directives, family, physician, state law, or religious beliefs may determine the clinical management in persistent vegetative state of individual patients.

Diagnostic and prognostic criteria for minimally responsive patients have not been outlined clearly (see above). Given the current national debate over health care, allocation of resources to minimally responsive patients may prove to be a delicate balance between societal consensus and ability to pay for care. Outcome studies clearly indicate that long-term intervention and care have a lower success rate when functional improvement rather than survival is the paramount medical objective. Although studies of cost-effectiveness of management protocols and long-term care would clarify allocation of resources, to date no such studies exist. Therefore, as with patients in persistent vegetative state, postacute rehabilitative initiatives for minimally responsive patients depend primarily on family and physician involvement; soon they may depend largely on the funding source.

Societal duty and resource allocation involve a complex interplay of attitudes and beliefs, including quality of life, the patient's moral culpability and social role or contribution, and concepts of justice.[47] The process of obtaining a consensus on such issues should follow ethical guidelines so that rules of allocation can be applied to everyone, including those who formulate the rules. Families should not be required to bear the brunt or excessive burden of caring for the patient; as DeJong states, "One casualty should be enough."

By the time that a minimally responsive patient reaches the postacute care setting, a number of life-prolonging treatment decisions related to surgical interventions, ventilation, nutrition, and hydration already have been made. Authorization for continued treatment should be obtained from the patient's family, guardian, or conservator. Except in emergency situations, failure to do so may be considered battery—an unlawful and unpermitted touching of another person.[68] Inquiry should be made about an advance writing or other evidence of the patient's wishes, such as a living will, directive, or durable power of attorney for health care. When the patient's wishes are not documented, disagreement among family members about nonemergent treatment is best referred to the legal system for resolution. However, a recent study of ethics consultants documented a great variability in recommendations for life-prolonging treatment in persistent vegetative state, depending on family wishes, resource allocation, and personal preference.[63]

The decision of the family to treat the patient may come easily early in the postacute setting. Efforts to ensure that everything possible is done to help their loved one are common. Months later, if little or no recovery has occurred, decisions about ongoing treatment and placement become more difficult. Ultimately the family member(s) may be asked to make life-or-death decisions about such issues as ventilation, feeding, and treatment of infections.

In *Barber v. Superior Court*,[11] a court in California set forth the "proportionate treatment" test. Treatment is acceptable if a reasonable chance of benefit outweighs the burden of treatment. The Barber decision also stated that artificial administration of nutrition or hydration is tantamount to the use of a respirator and must be considered medical treatment. Another state court disagreed with this view of nutrition and hydration and in *Cruzan v. Harmon* ordered gastric feedings to be continued.[45]

Maintenance interventions, such as treatment of contracture that prevents range of motion, may not be covered by insurers, because they do not provide functional improvement; yet such interventions may have profound implications in the long-term care of minimally responsive patients.[85] Many health care facilities have ethics committees that may provide guidance to the physician and/or family. Ultimately, legal counsel and the courts may need to be involved if uncertainty persists at any treatment juncture.

The family's adjustment to the roles of decision maker and caregiver, added to the "loss" of the patient, is disruptive at best and devastating at worst. Rosin[139] describes a spectrum of six reaction stages in such families: grief and anxiety, guilt, denial, accommodation, disengagement, and rejection. These reactions are unlike those produced by death, because the mourning for a "partial death" is ongoing.[139] Stern et al.[156] postulate that families must choose either to give up hope for recovery or to continue to relate to the patient as a vital person. The choice may have consequences of either massive guilt for abandoning hope or profound resentment toward the patient for continuing to be alive yet unresponsive.[66]

Often such consequences create a mixture of emotionally charged feelings that may be vented as anger toward the professionals caring for the patient. This may be especially true when transfer to a lower level of care or long-term care facility is the issue. Professional support for the family is thus essential if such emotions are to be sorted out and processed. Quite often family members attempt to substantiate a level of consciousness and understanding on the part of the patient far above that which the team can document. Support groups for families are often helpful at either a facility or community level. Referrals for additional individual counseling may be necessary in certain situations. Before discharge or alternate placement of the patient, families should be provided with ongoing sources of long-term support.

ACKNOWLEDGMENTS. The authors thank M. Elizabeth Sandel, M.D., and John Whyte, M.D., Ph.D., for their review of the manuscript and Patty Williams for expert technical assistance.

REFERENCES

1. Abdel-Dayem H, Sadek SA, Kouris K, et al: Changes in cerebral perfusion after acute head injury: Comparison of CT with Tc-99m HM-PAO SPECT. Radiology 165:221–226, 1987.
2. Akers SM, Bartter TC, Pratter MR: Respiratory care. Phys Med Rehabil State Art Rev 4:527–542, 1990.
3. American Neurologic Association: Persistent vegetative state: Report of the American Neurologic Association Committee on Ethical Affairs. Ann Neurol 33:386–390, 1993.

4. Anderson DC, Bundlie S, Rockswold GL: Multimodality evoked potentials in closed head trauma. Arch Neurol 41:369–374, 1984.

5. Andrews K: Medical management. Phys Med Rehabil State Art Rev 4:495–515, 1990.

6. Ansell BJ, Keenan JE: The Western Neuro Sensory Stimulation Profile: A tool for assessing slow-to-recover head injured patients. Arch Phys Med Rehabil 70:104–108, 1989.

7. Ansell BJ: Slow-to-recover patients: Improvement to rehabilitation readiness. J Head Trauma Rehabil 8:88–98, 1993.

8. Arts WFM, van Dongen HR, van Hof-van Duin J, Lammens E: Unexpected improvement after prolonged post-traumatic vegetative state. J Neurol Neurosurgery Psychiatry 48:1300–1303, 1985.

9. Atchison JW, Wachendorf J, Haddock D, et al: Hyponatremia-associated cognitive impairment in traumatic brain injury. Brain Inj 7:347–352, 1993.

10. Bachman DL, Morgan A: The role of pharmacotherapy in the treatment of aphasia: Preliminary results. Aphasiology 2:255–228, 1988.

11. Barber v. Superior Court. 195 California, 484, 147 Cal. App. 3rd 1006 (1983).

12. Barlow P, Teasdale G: Prediction of outcome and the management of severe head injuries: The attitudes of neurosurgeons. Neurosurgery 19:989–991, 1986.

13. Bartokowski HM, Lovely MP: Prognosis in coma and the persistent vegetative state. J Head Trauma Rehabil 1:1–5, 1986.

14. Becker E, Sazbon L, Najensen T: Gastrointestinal hemorrhage in long-lasting traumatic coma. Scand J Rehabil Med 10:23–26, 1978.

15. Bergmann G, Thomas R: Nursing care. Phys Med Rehabil State Art Rev 4:517–526, 1990.

16. Berrol S: Considerations for the management of the persistent vegetative state. Arch Phys Med Rehabil 67:283–285, 1986.

17. Berrol S: Evolution and the persistent vegetative state. J Head Trauma Rehabil 1:7–13, 1986.

18. Berrol S: Persistent vegetative state. Phys Med Rehabil State Art Rev 4:559–567, 1990.

19. Berrol S: Cranial nerve dysfunction. Phys Med Rehabil State Art Rev 3:85–93, 1989.

20. Bishop MJ: Mechanisms of laryngotracheal injury following prolonged tracheal intubation. Chest 96:185–187, 1989.

21. Bishop MJ, Weymuller EA, Fink BR: Laryngeal effects of prolonged intubation. Anesth Analg 63:335–342, 1984.

22. Black PM: Predicting the outcome from hypoxic-ischemic coma: Medical and ethical implications [editorial]. JAMA 254:1215–1216, 1985.

23. Bleck TP, Smith MC: Diagnosing brain death and persistent vegetative state. J Crit Illness 4:60–65, 1989.

24. Bonfiglio RL, Costa JL, Bonfiglio RP: Awakenings II: Pharmacologic roles of metoclopramide and Sinemet in akinetic mutism [abstract]. Arch Phys Med Rehabil 72:817, 1991.

25. Bontke CF, Baize CM, Boake C: Coma management and sensory stimulation. Phys Med Rehabil Clin 3:259–272, 1992.

26. Bontke CF, Lehmkuhl LD, Englander J, et al: Medical complications and associated injuries of persons treated in the traumatic brain injury model systems programs. J Head Trauma Rehabil 8:34–46, 1993.

27. Bontke CF: Medical complications related to traumatic brain injury. Phys Med Rehabil State Art Rev 3:43–58, 1989.

28. Borrero E, Margolis IB, Bank S, et al: Antacid versus sucralfate in preventing acute gastrointestinal bleeding. Am J Surg 148:809–812, 1984.

29. Boyeson MG, Harmon RL: Effects of trazodone and desipramine on motor recovery in brain-injured rats. Am J Phys Med Rehabil 72:286–293, 1993.

30. Boyeson MG, Feeney DM: Intraventricular norepinephrine facilitates motor recovery following sensorimotor cortex injury. Pharmacol Biochem Behav 35:497–501, 1990.

31. Brandstater ME, Roth EJ, Siebens HC: Venous thromboembolism in stroke: Literature review and implications for clinical patients. Arch Phys Med Rehabil 73:379–391, 1992.

32. Braakman R, Jennett WB, Miderhoud JM: Prognosis of the posttraumatic vegetative state. Acta Neurochir 95:49–52, 1988.

33. Braakman R, Habbema JDF, Gelpke GJ: Prognosis and prediction of outcome in comatose head injured patients. Acta Neurochir 36 (Suppl):112–117, 1986.

34. Bricolo A, Turazzi S, Feriotti G: Prolonged posttraumatic unconsciousness. J Neurosurg 52:625–634, 1980.

35. Bricolo A: Prolonged posttraumatic coma. In Vinken PJ, Bruyn GW (eds): Handbook of Clinical Neurology. Amsterdam, North Holland, 1976, pp 699–755

36. Busch L, Duffy J: Tracheal decannulation of brain-injured patients [abstract]. Arch Phys Med Rehabil 70:A33, 19889.

37. Caveness WF, Meirowsky AM, Rish BL, et al: The nature of posttraumatic epilepsy. J Neurosurg 50:545–553, 1979.

38. Childs NL, Mercer WN, Childs HW: Accuracy of diagnosis of persistent vegetative state. Neurology 43:1465–1467, 1993.

39. Cohen P, Busch L: Use of trazodone in the traumatically brain injured [abstract]. Arch Phys Med Rehabil 70:A15, 1989.

40. Commission on the Accreditation of Rehabilitation Facilities: Standards Manual for Organizations Serving People with Disabilities, 1992, p 57.

41. Consensus Conference: Artificial airways in patients receiving mechanical ventilation. Chest 96:178–184, 1989.

42. Congressional Record. October 29, 1992. House Report 102-1059. Fraud and Abuse in the Head Injury Rehabilitation Industry. Committee on Governmental Operations. Washington, DC, United States Government Printing Office, 1992.

43. Cope DN, Date AS, Mar EY: Serial computerized tomographic evaluations in traumatic head injury. Arch Phys Med Rehabil 69:483–486, 1988.

44. Costa J, Rao N: Recovery in non-vascular lock-in syndrome following Sinemet [abstract]. Arch Phys Med Rehabil 69:770, 1988.

45. *Cruzan v. Harmon*. 760 S.W. 2nd 408 Mo. (1988).

46. Czeisler CA, Richardson GS, Martin JB: Disorders of sleep and circadian rhythm. In Wilson RA (ed): Harrison's Practice and Principles of Internal Medicine, 12th ed. New York, McGraw-Hill, 1991, pp 209–217.

47. DeJong G, Batavia AI: Societal duty and resource allocation for persons with severe traumatic brain injury. J Head Trauma Rehabil 4:1–12, 1989.

48. DeLisa JA, Gans BM (eds): Rehabilitation Medicine: Principles and Practice, 2nd ed. Philadelphia, J.B. Lippincott, 1993.

49. Demetrious AA: Current summaries on "Nutritional outcome and pneumonia in critical care patients randomized to gastric versus jejunal tube feedings." J Parenteral Enteral Nutr 17:191–192, 1989.

50. De Santis A, Sganzerla E, Spagnoli D, et al: Risk factors for late posttraumatic epilepsy. Acta Neurochir 55:64–67, 1992.

51. Deutsch PM: Life-care planning. Phys Med Rehabil State Art Rev 4:605–618, 1990.

52. Dieterich SC, O'Dell MW, Keebler PJ: Autonomic dysfunction in a pre-pubertal child: Successful treatment with bromocriptine [abstract]. Arch Phys Med Rehabil 74:1226, 1993.

53. DiRicco C, Maira G, Meglio M, Rossi GF: L-dopa treatment of comatose states due to cerebral lesions: Preliminary findings. J Neurosurg Sci 18:169–176, 1974.

54. Driks MR, Craven DE, Celli BR, et al: Nosocomial pneumonia in incubated patients given sucralfate as compared with antacids or histamine type 2 blockers. N Engl J Med 317:1376–1382, 1987.

55. Duckworth D: The need for a standard terminology and classification of disablement. In Granger CV, Gresham GE (eds): Functional Assessment in Rehabilitation Medicine. Baltimore, Williams & Wilkins, 1984, pp 1–13.

56. Dunham CM, LaMonica C: Prolonged tracheal intubation in trauma patients. J Trauma 24:120–124, 1984.

57. Eddleston JM, Vohra A, Scott P, et al: A comparison of the frequency of stress ulceration and secondary pneumonia in sucralfate- or ranitidine-treated intensive care patients. Crit Care Med 19:1491–1496, 1991.

58. Ellis DW, Rader MA: Structured sensory stimulation. Phys Med Rehabil State Art Rev 4:465–477, 1990.

59. Faught E, Sachdeo RC, Remler MP, et al: Felbamate monotherapy for partial-onset seizures. Neurology 43:688–692, 1993.

60. Feeney DM, Sutton RL: Pharmacotherapy for recovery of function after brain injury. Crit Rev Neurobiol 3:135–197, 1987.

61. Feeney DM, Gonzalez A, Law WA: Amphetamine, haloperidol, and experience interact to affect rates of recovery after motor cortex injury. Science 217:855–857, 1982.

62. Feibel JH, Baldwin CA, Joynt RJ: Catecholamine-associated refractory hypertension following acute intracerebral hemorrhage: Control with propranolol. Ann Neurol 9:340–343, 1981.

63. Fox E, Stocking C: Ethics consultant's recommendations for life-prolonging treatment of patients in a persistent vegetative state. JAMA 270:2578–2582, 1993.

64. Friedman W: Head injuries. CIBA Symp 35:24, 1983.

65. Friedman GD: Primer of Epidemiology, 3rd ed. New York, McGraw-Hill, 1987.

66. Frohman S: Family response to the coma-emerging patient. Phys Med Rehabil State Art Rev 4:593–603, 1990.

67. Giacino JT, Kezmarsky MA, DeLuca J, et al: Monitoring rate of recovery to predict outcome in minimally-responsive patients. Arch Phys Med Rehabil 72:897–901, 1991.

68. Gilfix M, Gilfix MG, Sinatra KS: Law and medicine: The persistent vegetative state. J Head Trauma Rehabil 1:63–71, 1986.

69. Glenn MB, Rosenthal M: Rehabilitation following severe traumatic brain injury. Semin Neurol 3:233–246, 1985.

70. Goldstein LB, Davis JN: Post-lesion practice and amphetamine-facilitated recovery of beam-walking in the rat. Restor Neurol Neurosci 1:311–314, 1990.

71. Goldstein LB, Matchar DB, Morgenlander JC, Davis JN: Drugs influence the recovery of function after stroke [abstract 85]. Presented at the 15th International Joint Conference on Stroke and Cerebral Circulation.

72. Goodpasture HC, Romig DA, Voth DW, et al: Prospective study of tracheobronchial bacterial flora in acutely brain-injured patients with and without antibiotic prophylaxis. J Neurosurg 47:228–235, 1977.

73. Grahm TW, Zadronzy DB, Harrington T: The benefits of early jejunal hyperalimentation in the head-injured patient. Neurosurgery 25:729–735, 1989.

74. Groswasser Z, Sazbon L: Outcome in 134 patients with prolonged posttraumatic unawareness. Part 2: Functional outcome of 72 patients recovering consciousness. J Neurosurg 72:81–84, 1990.

75. Guidice MA, Berchau RC: Posttraumatic epilepsy following head injury. Brain Injury 1:64–67, 1987.

76. Hall ME, MacDonald S, Young GC: The effectiveness of directed multisensory stimulation versus non-directed stimulation in comatose CHI patients: Pilot study of a single subject design. Brain Injury 6:435–445, 1992.

77. Hagen C, Malkmus D, Durham P: Levels of cognitive functioning. In Rehabilitation of the Head-Injured Adult: Comprehensive Physical Management. Downey, CA, Professional Staff Association of Rancho Los Amigos Hospital, 1979, pp 87–88.

78. Haig AJ, Ruess JM: Recovery from vegetative state of six months' duration associated with Sinemet (levodopa/carbidopa). Arch Phys Med Rehabil 71:1081–1083, 1990.

79. Hansen JR, Cook JS: Posttraumatic neuroendocrine disorders. Phys Med Rehabil State Art Rev 19993, pp 569–580.

80. Hayes RL, Povlishock JT, Singha B: Pathophysiology of mild head injury. Phys Med Rehabil State Art Rev 6:9–20, 1992.

81. Heffner, JE: Medical indications for tracheotomy. Chest 96:186–189, 1989.

82. Hester DD: Nutrition Support Dietetics Core Curriculum, 2nd ed. American Society for Parenteral and Enteral Nutrition, 1993, pp 229–241.

83. Higashi K, Sakata M, Hatano S, et al: Epidemiological studies on patients with a persistent vegetative state. J Neurol Neurosurg Psychiatry 40:876–885, 1977.

84. Higashi K, Hatano M, Abiko S, et al: Five-year follow-up study of patients with persistent vegetative state. J Neurol Neurosurg Psychiatry 44: 552–554, 1981.

85. Horn LJ: Systems of care for persons with traumatic brain injury. Phys Med Rehabil Clin 3:475–492, 1992.

86. Horn LJ, Glenn MB: Pharmacological interventions in neuroendocrine disorders following traumatic brain injury. Part II. J Head Trauma Rehabil 3:87–90, 1988.

87. Jackson MD, Davidoff G: Gastroparesis following traumatic brain injury and response to meclopramide therapy. Arch Phys Med Rehabil 70:553–555, 1989.

88. Jackson RD, Corrigan JD, Arnett JA: Amitriptyline for agitation in head injury. Arch Phys Med Rehabil 66:180–181, 1984.

89. Jacobs HE, Muir CA, Clince JD: Family reactions to persistent vegetative state. J Head Trauma Rehabil 1:55–62, 1986.

90. Jaggi JL, Obrist WD, Gennarelli TA, Langfitt TW: Relationship of early cerebral blood flow and metabolism to outcome in acute head injury. J Neurosurg 72:176–182, 1990.

91. Jennett B, Plum F: Persistent vegetative state after brain damage. Lancet 1:734–737, 1972.

92. Jennett B, Bond M: Assessment of outcome after severe brain damage: A practical scale. Lancet 1:480–484, 1975.

93. Jennett B: Epilepsy after Non-missile Head Injuries, 2nd ed. Chicago, William Heineman, 1975.

94. Jette AM: Concepts of health and methodologic issues in functional assessment. In Granger CV, Greshem GE (eds): Functional Assessment in Rehabilitation Medicine. Baltimore, Williams & Wilkins, 1984, pp 46–64.

95. Johnson AG (ed): Treatment of gastro-oesophageal reflux and gastic stasis: new perspectives with cisapride. In Proceedings of the 13th International Congress on Gastroenterology, Rome, 1988.

96. Kalisky Z, Morrison DP, Meyers CA, et al: Medical problems encountered during rehabilitation of patients with head injury. Arch Phys Med Rehabil 66:25–29, 1985.

97. Kanno T, Kamel Y, Yokoyama T, et al: Neurostimulation for patients in vegetative state. PACE 10:207–208, 1987.

98. Katayama Y, Tsubokawa T, Yamamoto T, et al: Characterization and modification of brain activity with deep brain stimulation in patients in a persistent vegetation state: Pain-related late positive component of cerebral evoked potentials. PACE 14:116–120, 1991.

99. Klingbeil GEG: Airway problems in patients with traumatic brain injury. Arch Phys Med Rehabil 69:493–495, 1988.

100. Labi MC, Horn LJ: Hypertension in traumatic brain injury. Brain Injury 4:365–370, 1990.

101. Lal S, Merbitz CP, Grip JC: Modification of function in head-injured patients with Sinemet. Brain Injury 2:225–233, 1988.

102. Lazarus BA, Murphy JB, Culpepper L: Aspiration pneumonia with long-term gastric versus jejunal feeding: A critical analysis of the literature. Arch Phys Med Rehabil 71:46–53, 1990.

103. Levin HS, Saydjari C, Eisenberg HM, et al: Vegetative state after closed-head injury: A Traumatic Coma Data Bank Report. Arch Neurol 48:580–585, 1991.

104. Levin HS, Williams D, Crofford MJ: Relationship of depth of brain lesions to consciousness and outcome after closed head injury. J Neurosurg 69:861–866, 1988.

105. Levy DE, Caronna JJ, Singer BH, et al: Predicting outcome from hypoxic-ischemic coma. JAMA 253: 1420–1426, 1985.

106. Levy DE, Bates D, Caronna JJ, et al: Prognosis in nontraumatic coma. Ann Intern Med 94:293–301, 1981.

107. LeWinn E, Dimancescu M: Environmental deprivation and enrichment in coma [letter]. Lancet 1:156–157, 1978.

108. Lindsay K, Pasaoglu A, Hirst D, et al: Somatosensory and auditory brain stem conduction after head injury: A comparison with clinical features in prediction of outcome. Neurosurgery 26:278–285, 1990.

109. Liu D: Posttraumatic visual disorders. Part II: Management and rehabilitation. Phys Med Rehabil State Art Rev 485–502, 1993.

110. Marsh HM, Gillespie DJ, Baumgartner AE: Timing of tracheostomy in the critically ill patient. Chest 96:190–194, 1989.

111. Marshall BJ: Campylobacter pylori: Its link to gastritis and peptic ulcer disease. Rev Infect Dis 12 (Suppl):S87–S93, 1990.

112. McLellan DR: The structural basis of coma and recovery. Phys Med Rehabil State Art Rev 4:389–407, 1990.

113. McQueen JK, Blackwood DHR, Harris P, et al: Low risk of late posttraumatic seizures following severe head injury: Implications for clinical trials of prophylaxis. J Neurosurg Psychiatry 46:899–904, 1983.

114. Medical Letter. Zolpidem for insomnia. 35:35–36, 1993.

115. Merbitz C, Morris J, Grip JC: Ordinal scales and the foundations of misinference. Arch Phys Med Rehabil 70:308–312, 1989.

116. Meythaler JM: Routine screening for deep venous thrombosis in brain injury patients [abstract]. Arch Phys Med Rehabil 74:1245, 1993.

117. Mitchell S, Bradley VA, Welch JL, Britton PG: Coma arousal procedure: A therapeutic intervention in the treatment of head injury. Brain Injury 4:273–279, 1990.

118. Mysiw WJ, Jackson RRD, Corrigan JD: Amitriptyline for posttraumatic agitation. Am J Phys Med Rehabil 67:29–33, 1988.

119. Najenson T, Sazbon L, Fiselzon, et al: Recovery of communication functions after prolonged traumatic coma. Scand J Rehabil Med 10:15–21, 1978.

120. Narayan RK, Greenberg RP, Miller JD, et al: Improved confidence of outcome prediction in severe head injury. J Neurosurg 54:751–762, 1981.

121. National Head Injury Foundation: Directory of Head Injury Rehabilitation Services. National Head Injury Foundation, Washington, DC, 1993.

122. Norton JA, Ott LG, McClain C, et al: Intolerance to enteral feedings in the brain-injured patient. J Neurosurg 68:62–66, 1988.

123. O'Dell MW: Coma assessment tools. Presented at the 54th Annual Meetings of the American Academy of Physical Medicine and Rehabilitation, San Francisco, 1992.

124. O'Neill B: Effectiveness of air bags [letter]. N Engl J Med 326:1091, 1992.

125. Physician's Desk Reference, 1991 ed. Medical Economics Company, Oradell, NJ, 1991.

126. Plum F, Posner JB: The Diagnosis of Stupor and Coma. Philadelphia, F.A. Davis, 1980.

127. Pretap-Chand R, Gourie-Devi M: Bruxism: Its significance in coma. Clin Neurosurg 87:113–117, 1985.

128. Rader MA, Alston JB, Ellis DW: Sensory stimulation of severely brain-injured patients. Brain Injury 3:141–147, 1989.

129. Ragnarsson KT, Thomas JP, Zasler ND: Model systems of care for individuals with traumatic brain injury. J Head Trauma Rehabil 8:1–11, 1993.

130. Rappaport M, Doughertey AM, Kelting DL: Evaluation of coma and vegetative states. Arch Phys Med Rehabil 73:628–634, 1992.

131. Rappaport M, Hall KM, Hopkins HK, et al: Disability rating scale for severe head trauma: Coma to community. Arch Phys Med Rehabil 63: 118–123, 1983.

132. Rappaport M: Brain evoked potentials in coma and the vegetative state. J Head Trauma Rehabil 1:15–29, 1986.

133. Reusser P, Gyr K, Scheidegger D, et al: Prospective endoscopic study of stress erosions and ulcers in critically ill neurosurgical patients: Current incidence and effect of acid-reducing prophylaxis. Crit Care Med 18:270, 1990.

134. Robertson CS, Clifton GL, Grossman RG: Oxygen utilization and cardiovascular function in head-injured patients. Neurosurgery 15:307–314, 1984.

135. Rombeau JL, Palac JC: Feeding by tube enterostomy. In Rombeau JL, Caudwell MD (eds): Clinical Nutrition: Enteral and Tube Feeding, 2nd ed. Philadelphia, W.B. Saunders, 1990, pp 230–249.

136. Root RK, Petersdorf RG: Chills and fever. In Wilson RA (ed): Harrison's Practice and Principles of Internal Medicine, 12th ed. New York, McGraw-Hill, pp 125–133.

137. Ropper AF: Coma and other disorders of consciousness. In Wilson RA (ed): Harrison's Practice and Principles of Internal Medicine, 12th ed. New York, McGraw-Hill, 1991, pp 193–200.

138. Rosenberg GA, Johnson SF, Brenner RP: Recovery of cognition after prolonged vegetative state. Ann Neurol 2:167–168, 1977.

139. Rosin AJ: Reactions of families of brain-injured patients who remain in a vegetative state. Scand J Rehabil Med 9:1–5, 1977.

140. Ross, ED, Stewart MD: Akinetic mutism from hypothalmic damage: Successful treatment with dopamine agonists. Neurology 31:1435–1439, 1981.

141. Sadun AA: Posttraumatic visual disorders. Part I: Injuries and mechanisms. Phys Med Rehabil State Art Rev 3:475–484, 1993.

142. Sandel ME, Norcross ED, Ross SE, et al: Protein metabolism after severe brain injury [abstract]. Arch Phys Med Rehabil 71:764, 1990.

143. Sandel ME, Ellis DW (eds): The Coma-Emerging Patient. Phys Med Rehabil State Art Rev Vol.4, 1990.

144. Sandel ME, Horn LJ, Bontke CF: Sensory stimulation: Accepted practice or expected practice? J Head Trauma Rehabil 7:115–120, 1993.

145. Sandel ME, Labi MLC: Outcome prediction: Clinical and research perspectives. Phys Med Rehabil State Art Rev 4:409–420, 1990.

146. Sandel ME, O'Dell MW: Persistent facial myoclonus as a poor prognostic indicator in severe brain injury. Arch Phys Med Rehabil 74:411–415, 1993.

147. Sazbon L, Groswasser Z: Outcome in 134 patients with prolonged posttraumatic unawareness. I: Parameters determining late recovery of consciousness. J Neurosurg 72:75–80, 1990.

148. Sazbon L, Costeff H, Groswasser Z: Epidemiological findings in traumatic post-comatose unawareness. Brain Injury 6:359–362, 1992.

149. Sazbon L: Prolonged coma. Prog Clin Neurosci 2:65–81, 1985.

150. Schallert T, Hernandez TD, Barth TM: Recovery of function after brain damage: Severe and chronic disruption by diazepam. Brain Res 379:104–111, 1986.

151. Seigal A, Alavi A: Brain imaging techniques. Phys Med Rehabil State Art Rev 4:433–446, 1990.

152. Sisson R: Effects of auditory stimuli on comatose patients with head injury. Heart Lung 19:373–378, 1990.

153. Slugg PH, Haug MT, Pippenger CE: Ranitidine pharmacokinetics and adverse central nervous system reactions. Arch Intern Med 152:2325–2329, 1992.

154. Satuffer JL, Olson DE, Petty TL: Complications and consequences of endotracheal intubation and tracheostomy. Am J Med 70:65–76, 1981.

155. Stein TP, Lazarus DD, Chatzidakis C: Human macronutrient requirements. In Rombeau JL, Caudwell MD (eds): Clinical Nutrition: Enteral and Tube Feeding. Philadelphia, W.B. Saunders, 1990, pp 54–72.

156. Stern JM, Sazbon L, Becker E, Costeff H: Severe behavioral disturbances in families of patients with prolonged coma. Brain Injury 2:229–262, 1988.

157. Streufert S, DePadova A, McGlynn T, et al: Impact of beta blockage on complex cognitive functioning. Am Heart J 116:311–315, 1988.

158. Stringer W, Balserio J, Fidler R: Advances in traumatic brain injury neuroimaging techniques. Neurorehabilitation 1:13–32, 1991.

159. Sutton RL, Weaver MS, Feeney DM: Drug-induced modifications of behavioral recovery following cortical trauma. J Head Trauma Rehabil 2:50–58, 1987.

160. Tanhehco J, Kaplan PE: Physical and rehabilitation of a patient after a 6-year coma. Arch Phys Med Rehabil 63:36–38, 1982.

161. Takashi T, Yamamoto T, Katayama Y: Prediction of outcome of prolonged coma caused by brain damage. Brain Injury 4:329–337, 1990.

162. Teasdale G, Jennett B: Assessment of coma and impaired consciousness. Lancet 2:81–83, 1974.

163. Temkin NR, Dikman SS, Wilneskey, et al: A randomized, double-blind study of phenytoin for the prevention of post-traumatic seizures. N Engl J Med 323:497–502, 1990.

164. Tenjin H, Ueda S, Mizukawa N, et al: Positron emission tomographic studies in cerebral hemodynamics in patients with cerebral contusion. Neurosurgery 26:971–979, 1990.

165. Tsubokawa T, Yamamoto T, Katayama Y: Prediction of outcome of prolonged coma caused by brain damage. Brain Injury 4:329–337, 1990.

166. Tsubokawa T, Yamamoto T, Katayama Y, et al: Deep-brain stimulation in a persistent vegetative state: Follow-up results and criteria for selection of candidates. Brain Injury 4:315–327, 1990.

167. Van Dongen KJ, Braakman R, Gelpke GJ: The prognostic value of computerized tomography in comatose head-injured patients. J Neurosurg 59:951–957, 1983.

168. Van Woerkom TCAM, Minderhoud JM, Gottschal T, Nicolai G: Neurotransmitters in the treatment of patients with severe head injuries. Eur Neurol 21:227–134, 1982.

169. Vane DW, Shiffler M, Grosfeld JL, et al: Reduced lower esophageal sphincter (LES) pressure after acute and chronic brain injury. J Pediatr Surg 17:960–973, 1982.

170. Weinberger SE: Principles of Pulmonary Medicine. Philadelphia, W.B. Saunders, 1992, pp 65–67.

171. Whitlock JA: Functional outcome of low-level traumatically brain-injured admitted to an acute rehabilitation programme. Brain Injury 6:447–459, 1992.

172. Whyte J, Glenn MB: The care and rehabilitation of the patient in a persistent vegetative state. J Head Trauma Rehabil 1:39–53, 1986.

173. Whyte J: Attention and arousal: Basic science aspects. Arch Phys Med Rehabil 73:940–949, 1992.

174. Whyte J: Individualized quantitative assessment of the minimally-responsive patient. Presented at the 54th Annual Meeting of the American academy of Physical Medicine and Rehabilitation, San Francisco, November, 1992.

175. Whyte J, Filion DT, Rose TR: Defective thermoregulation in a traumatic brain injury: A single subject evaluation. Am J Phys Med Rehabil 72:281–285, 1993.

176. Whyte J, Rosenthal M: Rehabilitation of the patients with traumatic brain injury. In DeLisa JA (ed): Rehabilitation Medicine: Principles and Practice, 2nd ed. Philadelphia, J.B. Lippincott, 1993, pp 825–860.

177. Wilcox CM, Spenney JG: Stress ulcer prophylaxis in medical patients: Who, what, and how much? Am J Gastroent 83:1199–1211, 1988.

178. Wilson SL, Powell GE, Elliott, Thwaites H: Sensory stimulation in prolonged coma: Four single case studies. Brain Injury 5:393–400, 1991.

179. Wood RL, Winkowski TB, Miller JL, et al: Evaluating sensory regulation as a method to improve awareness in patients with altered states of consciousness: A pilot study. Brain Injury 6:411–418, 1992.

180. Wood RL: Critical analysis of the concept of sensory stimulation for patients in vegetative states. Brain Injury 5:401–409, 1991.

181. Wroblewski BA, Singer WD, Whyte J: Carbamazepine-erythromycin interaction: Case studies and clinical significance. JAMA 255:1165–1167, 1986.

182. Yablon SA: Posttraumatic seizures. Arch Phys Med Rehabil 74:983–1001, 1993.

183. Zasler ND, Kreutzer JS, Taylor D: Coma stimulation and coma recovery: A critical review. Neurorehabilitation 1:33–40, 1991.

184. Zasler, ND, Taylor D, Decker M: Characteristics and outcome of coma following severe traumatic brain injury [abstract]. Arch Phys Med Rehabil 71:783, 1991.

185. Zasler ND: Advances in neuropharmacological rehabilitation for brain dysfunction. Brain Injury 6:1–14, 1992.

186. Zasler ND, Devany CW, Barman AL, et al: Oral hygiene following traumatic brain injury: A programme to promote dental health. Brain Injury 7:339–345, 1993.

187. American Congress of Rehabilitation Medicine: Recommendations for use of uniform nomenclature pertinent to patients with severe alterations in consciousness. Arch Phys Med Rehabil 76:205–209, 1995.

188. Multi-Society Task Force on PVS: Medical aspects of the persistent vegetative state (Part I). New Engl J Med 330:1499–1508, 1994.

189. Multi-Society Task Force on PVS: Medical aspects of the persistent vegetative state (Part II). New Engl J Med 330:1572–1579, 1994.

190. Giacino JT, Zasler ND: Outcome after severe traumatic brain injury: Coma, the vegetative state, and minimally responsive state. J Head Trauma Rehabil 10:40–56, 1995.

191. Choi SC, Barnes TY: Bullock R, et al: Temporal profile of outcomes in severe head injury. J Neurosurg 81:169–173, 1994.

NATHAN D. ZASLER M.D.

6

Neuromedical Diagnosis and Management of Postconcussive Disorders

We see what we look for. We look for what we know.

Goethe

Although rarely fatal, mild traumatic brain injury (MTBI) has a fairly high morbidity and accounts for approximately 80% of all hospitalizations for brain trauma.[158,159] Concussive brain injuries have been classified in many different ways, but there is no general agreement about nomenclature and categorization. Gennarelli divided concussive brain injuries into two variants: mild (no loss of consciousness) and classic (loss of consciousness). Although once deemed "benign" by many health care professionals, even mild concussive brain injuries may present with neuropsychological deficits of the same magnitude as classic concussive brain injuries.[170] Contrary to common belief, brain injury may result in significant pathology and impairment without loss of consciousness, particularly in children,[122] in whom death may result from subdural hematoma.

Many patients hospitalized after mild head and brain injury have transient somatic complaints that are a direct consequence of trauma not only to the brain but also to extraparenchymal structures, including the cranium, cranial adnexa, and cervical structures. Researchers historically have focused on the neuropsychological deficits and somatic complaints in this as yet poorly defined subset of symptomatic patients with whiplash and concussive cranial or brain injuries. Many so-called postconcussive symptoms in fact are related to extracerebral injury. Clearly, postconcussive disorders are real; because of their heterogeneity, however, it is wiser to avoid the catch-all term, postconcussive syndrome (PCS).

A large body of literature addresses the acute neuromedical presentation and management of patients with persistent postconcussional symptoms, but studies of postacute neuromedical and rehabilitative treatment are scarce. Also of note are the disparities across clinical disciplines regarding diagnosis, treatment, and prognosis for patients with MTBI and postconcussive disorder (PCD).[85,115,196] This chapter reviews the major acute and postacute neuromedical and rehabilitative issues in patients with MTBI.

ISSUES OF NOMENCLATURE

From both clinical and research perspectives, one of the major problems faced by rehabilitation professionals is inconsistent nomenclature. According to the Brain Injury Association (formerly National Head Injury Foundation) and the American Congress of Rehabilitation Medicine, the accepted term is **mild traumatic brain injury**. Modifiers such as subtle, minimal, and minor are to be discouraged. Practitioners must understand that the term "mild" describes only the initial insult relative to the degree of neurologic severity; there may be no correlation with the degree of short- or long-term impairment or functional disability. The term **head injury** should be reserved for cranial or cranial adnexal trauma. A particular patient, of course, may incur cerebral concussion (mild traumatic brain injury) as well as cranial, cranial adnexal, and/or cervical trauma.

Diagnostic terms such as whiplash injury have become outdated and should be replaced with more pathomechanically and physiologically correct terms such as **cervical acceleration/deceleration** (CAD) **injury**. The term postconcussive syndrome, as previously discussed, also should be avoided; although some symptoms (e.g., headache, dizziness, cognitive difficulties) occur with greater frequency, the variation among patients is great. Such terms as posttraumatic headache, posttraumatic visual dysfunction, and posttraumatic dizziness describe subjective symptoms, not medical diagnoses, and therefore should be avoided. Clinicians should seek instead to define the underlying pathophysiologic process responsible for the symptom; for example, headache may be due to migraine, referred myofascial dysfunction, and/or greater occipital neuralgia.

The Mild Traumatic Brain Injury Committee of the Head Injury Interdisciplinary Special Interest Group of the American Congress of Rehabilitation Medicine defines MTBI in clinical terms: traumatically induced physiologic disruption of brain function, as manifested by at least one of the following:

1. Any period of loss of consciousness;

2. Any loss of memory for events immediately before or after the accident;

3. Any alteration in mental state at the time of the accident;

4. Focal neurologic deficit that may or may not be transient but does not exceed (1) loss of consciousness of approximately 30 minutes or less; (2) an initial Glasgow Coma Scale score of 13–15 after 30 minutes; and (3) posttraumatic amnesia of no more 24 hours' duration.

Although this definition is not the end-all, it is a step in the right direction. Other recent attempts include sports concussion guidelines, which are based on a three-tier grading scale,[110] and the DSM-IV criteria for **postconcussional disorder**.[68] The multiple flaws in this definition, however, include the potential exclusion of less severely injured patients as well as overly strict or excessive criteria for symptom duration. The inclusion of posttraumatic seizures as a "defining" factor at any level in this categorization is misleading, because the incidence of seizures in patients with MTBI is analogous to the incidence of de novo seizures in the general population. Unfortunately, no attempt at definition has involved all of the various health care disciplines that diagnose and treat patients with MTBI (i.e., neurology, neurosurgery, physiatry, psychiatry, emergency medicine, and neuropsychology).

PATHOPHYSIOLOGY

One of the historical problems in studying MTBI has been the apparently silent nature of its pathophysiology. More recently, significant advances have been made in defining the acute events associated with MTBI in both animals and humans. Historically, the vast majority of the measures used to assess severity of traumatic brain injury have been too insensitive to document changes at either a microscopic or macroscopic level. Studies such as computed tomographic (CT) scans of the brain and standard electroencephalography (EEG) typically do not show abnormalities supportive of brain dysfunction and/or trauma.

Animal models have delineated the neuropathology and neurophysiology associated with mild brain injury.[98,99] The dilemma facing most clinicians is that the shear-strain changes commonly associated with mild brain injuries are beyond the resolution of most commonly used neurodiagnostic techniques; thus, "definitive" neurologic assessment and diagnosis of mild TBI are difficult, particularly in the postacute period. Strain has been theorized to be due to three main pathologic factors: (1) acceleration/deceleration of the head, (2) skull distortion with resultant pressure gradients, and (3) cervical spine stretching. Direct impact to the head or brain is not a hallmark of mild TBI (or TBI in general) and is by no means essential for brain injury. Instead, the magnitude, speed, and direction of the acceleration and deceleration forces on the skull and brain determine the extent of both transient and permanent axonal dysfunction. Many acute clinical findings can be explained by the centripetal nature of the strain and concomitant modulation of acceleration and deceleration forces by anatomic variations, including mass ratio of brain structures.

When strain occurs near the surface of the cortex, one anticipates problems with amnesia, short-term memory, and other higher level neuropsychological functions. Phenomena related to involvement of the lower brainstem include respiratory irregularities, apnea, vomiting, hypertension, and bradycardia. Upper pontine and mesencephalic phenomena include loss of consciousness, corneal and pupillary areflexia, and decerebration. Typically, phenomena related to the upper brainstem occur only with more significant force vectors. A small number of patients, particularly younger ones, also may suffer transient focal cortical neurologic deficits, including global amnesia and cortical blindness. Such transient deficits have been attributed to posttraumatic vascular hyperreactivity and may be equivalents of migraine.[112,116,298]

Studies examining the role of static and dynamic imaging modalities clearly indicate that MTBI may result in both focal and diffuse parenchymal insult. Of interest, some of the imaging abnormalities noted during the acute phase may be related to precontusional changes, which in turn may be related to alterations in permeability of the blood-brain barrier.[118] Axonal damage associated with diffuse shear injury has been observed by multiple researchers after experimentally induced traumatic brain injury.[219] The neocortical gray-white junction seems to be more prone to axonal shear injury in MTBI. Electron microscopy has revealed reactive swelling of the injured axon, which produces so-called retraction balls. As with brain injury in general, the neuropathologic continuum of diffuse axonal injury includes not only nerve fibers but also small blood vessels. Recent postmortem studies of patients with MTBI who died of other causes have shown multifocal axonal injury, consistent with fornix involvement, by immunostaining with an antibody to amyloid precursor protein (a marker of fast axonal transport).[32] One of the currently more active areas of research involves the role of delayed axonal injury in long-term neurologic impairment. Recent research in the neuropathologic correlates of memory dysfunction have demonstrated hippocampal involvement in animal models.[123] Other areas of research in the early pathophysiologic changes associated with MTBI include impact depolarization, alterations in neurotransmitter environment, changes in receptor binding, and altered immunoexpression of microglia and macrophages.[2,70] Additional research issues include the role of cytoskeletal proteins in maintaining neuronal integrity and function after MTBI as well as the potential role of neuroprotective agents and gene therapy in the early postacute period in minimizing residua associated with secondary brain injury.[70]

ACUTE NEUROMEDICAL ISSUES

Although most of the available literature suggests that the gross neurologic outcome from mild TBI is favorable, a few patients (5% or less) with normal or near-normal initial neurologic presentation may require neurosurgical intervention.[58,88,265] Although relatively rare, intracranial hematomas may occur after MTBI. The incidence of intracranial complications is significantly higher in patients with associated skull fractures.[58,254] In general, the presence of a linear skull fracture on standard skull films probably warrants additional neurodiagnostic assessment with CT scan. The presence of a skull fracture also increases the chance for neurosurgical intervention approximately by a factor of 20 and the chance of an intracranial hematoma approximately by a factor of 300. The phenomenon of a lucid interval after mild TBI and its relationship to intracranial hematomas as well as extraaxial collections (blood or cerebrospinal fluid between the brain and skull) also must be considered, particularly in patients with associated skull fractures.[9,195,254] Posttraumatic extraaxial collections without skull fractures are not uncommon in the pediatric population.[122] A Glasgow Coma Scale score of 13 or 14 in the emergency department, a focal elemental neurologic exam, and/or altered mental status may be associated with subsequent neurologic deterioration.[87] CT scans of the brain are standard practice for such patients because of their increased risk for intracranial pathology.

The use and potential overuse of skull radiographs remain controversial. Some clinicians advocate specific criteria for obtaining skull films, whereas others argue against such practices.[59,163,189,190] In 1987 Masters et al. published the classic recommendations for radiographic assessment of low-, moderate-, and high-risk groups.[190] A more recent study by Stein et al. advocates urgent cranial CT in any patient with a history of loss of consciousness. The authors noted that a near-normal or normal mental status exam in the emergency department did not rule out significant risk for intracranial injury as detected by CT scanning; Glasgow Coma Scale scores and the Reaction Level Scale scores were not helpful in making a differentiation between high- and low-risk groups.[266]

In a small group of patients, delayed traumatic intracerebral hemorrhage (DTICH) may cause deterioration 24–48 hours after injury, usually as a result of contrecoup contusions of the parietooccipital cortex that secondarily affect the frontotemporal lobes.[301] Patients with normal CT scans rarely have late neurologic deterioration requiring surgical intervention and generally may be observed at home.[265] On rare occasions, however, late deterioration occurs in patients with a normal CT scan.[226] Recent literature and clinical experience also suggest an acute role for magnetic resonance imaging (MRI) in this patient population.[197] In patients with mild TBI whose neurologic examination is inconsistent with CT findings, MRI has shown significant benefit in detecting axonal shear injury that may not be demonstrated on CT imaging.[267] Some authors advocate a separate classification system for patients with "complicated" MTBI (i.e., patients with parenchymal abnormalities on CT scan) because their neurobehavioral recovery profile is generally worse than that of patients with noncomplicated MTBI.[293]

The major issues in the acute setting after head and brain trauma include detection and removal of operative intracranial masses; treatment of depressed skull fractures, penetrating injuries, and elevated intracranial pressure; detection and management of cerebrospinal fluid leaks; and assessment of cranial adnexal structures and general musculoskeletal system for associated injuries. The Glasgow Coma Scale (GCS) score should be assessed as a simple yet sensitive neurologic screen, although it may be altered by concurrent alcohol or drug intoxication. The effect of alcohol on the neurologic examination is particularly significant when blood alcohol concentrations are greater than 0.20%.[142] Of interest, nicotine withdrawal in chronic heavy smokers may present neurobehaviorally with many parallels to the acute neurologic picture after mild-to-moderate brain injury.[21,209] An adequate history is particularly critical in the acute setting, including details about the accident (i.e., loss of consciousness, feeling dazed at time of accident, retrograde and/or anterograde amnesia, hemodynamic instability, prolonged extrication time) and recent or chronic use of alcohol, drugs, or tobacco (because of the potential for withdrawal syndromes). Use of passive restraint systems, including seatbelts and/or airbags, also should be noted.

Medical history, including present medications, prior loss of consciousness secondary to TBI, psychological or psychiatric history, and learning disability, should be documented when available. A thorough physical examination is critical in the acute period to assess focal neurologic deficits, both gross and subtle, and higher-level mental processes. Studies have shown that specifically designed cognitive screening tools may assist in identification of high-risk patients with PCD.[286] Particularly in children, the examiner must suspect abuse if the clinical presentation is consistent with such a scenario. Clinical situations that warrant hospitalization after mild TBI typically include alteration in mental status, GCS of 13 or 14, focal neurologic finding(s), skull fracture(s), abnormal CT, suspicion of abuse, clinical picture confounded by seizures, drugs, or alcohol, and/or lack of responsible supervision at home.[59]

Whether hospital admission or direct discharge from the emergency department results in better or worse outcomes in patients with MTBI remains controversial. Data from studies of the correlation between number and persistence of postconcussional symptoms and number of days in the hospital are inconsistent.[76,177] Logic dictates, however, that if stringent admission criteria were used, patients hospitalized for MTBI would have a greater incidence of long-term problems because of the more severe nature of their injury, which warranted admission in the first place.

POSTACUTE NEUROMEDICAL ISSUES

Practitioners dealing with patients with whiplash injuries, head trauma, and traumatic brain injury must realize that these are separate clinical phenomena and must be assessed and treated as such. It is not uncommon for one set of injuries to be properly diagnosed, whereas a complete set of other injuries is undiagnosed or misdiagnosed. A common scenario is the patient who is treated for headaches related to "brain injury" when in fact the headaches are myofascial in origin and associated with cervical acceleration/deceleration injury. The astute clinician assesses all potential causes (the so-called "3 Cs"— cerebral, cranial, and cervical) before developing an integrated, holistic treatment plan. The following sections discuss the diagnosis and treatment of various problems seen with cervical (whiplash) injuries, cranial and cranial adnexal trauma, and cerebral (brain) trauma.

Cervical Injuries

Injuries of the cervical spine are quite common, particularly after rear-end motor vehicle accidents.[216] Most patients recover from such injuries in a few weeks; however, others have longer-term sequelae due to a cornucopia of secondary complications. The

diagnostic and treatment challenges are relevant mainly to this group.

In the latter part of the 19th century, the so-called "railway spine" was the start of a controversial diagnosis that has received various responses from the medical community, particularly in relation to prognosis. Professional opinions about whiplash injury range from condemnation of an unscrupulous, litigious patient, presumed to be driven only by secondary gain, to belief in a true pathoanatomic basis with organic rather than primarily emotional symptoms.[184] A recent retrospective by Croft argues against the concept of "litigation neurosis" in cervical acceleration/deceleration trauma.[55] Acceleration/deceleration injuries of the cervical spine again received attention with the introduction of catapult-assisted take-off from aircraft carriers. A significant number of pilots had problems with persistent neck discomfort and pain; some even lost consciousness on take-off, resulting in crash landings. Further study noted that the major pathomechanics were those of a hyperextension neck injury produced by sudden acceleration.

Cervical whiplash injuries began to receive considerable attention in the late 1940s and early 1950s, when the full impact of the motor vehicle boom was noted. Since that time the debate about pathophysiology, incidence, prognosis, and treatment has been ongoing. According to current opinion, a significant number of patients (possibly 15–20%) have chronic disability due to soft-tissue neck injury not related to ongoing litigation. Recent well-controlled, prospective studies have refuted earlier perceptions about poor prognostic indicators for long-term recovery, such as cervical degenerative disk disease and reversal of the lordotic curve.[12,96] Earlier reports that women tended to have more chronic somatic symptoms and lower rates of return to work also have been refuted.[124]

Imaging recommendations for patients with cervical whiplash remain somewhat controversial, with no general agreement about what to get or when. The consensus seems to be that studies are of questionable usefulness. Depending on the issue at hand, plain radiography, CT, and MRI may have specific relative merits. The most common acute finding is straightening of the normal lordotic curve, which does not necessarily indicate a pathologic condition.[148,273] The primary purpose of acute radiographic assessment is to rule out correctable anatomic injuries. CT and MRI are generally used when the clinician has concerns about disk herniation or spinal cord insult. The correlation of clinical symptoms and imaging findings, even with MRI, remains at best debatable, with disparate results across studies.[217,243]

The most common acute symptoms of whiplash are neck pain, headache, and limitation in neck range of motion[10,124,216] Others include headache, visual disturbances, dizziness, cognitive dysfunction, weakness, and paresthesias.[279] A study by Sturzenegger et al. noted that several factors related to accident mechanics were associated with more severe symptoms: (1) an unprepared occupant; (2) a rear-end collision, with or without subsequent frontal impact; and (3) rotated or inclined head position at the moment of impact.[269]

Cerebral symptoms also may follow what seem like isolated whiplash injuries.[151] Two long-term studies involving cognitive disability and whiplash demonstrated that approximately 20–25% of patients were still symptomatic at 1 year after injury.[83,225] Ettlin et al. hypothesized that their findings in 21 patients with whiplash may be compatible with damage to basal, frontal and upper brainstem structures.

Whiplash injury typically involves a flexion-extension movement, but torsional components also may play a role. The essential cause of the acute injury is a postulated mechanical strain with or without contusion of ligaments and muscles supporting the cervical spine. Safety belts have been shown to increase the risk for cervical injury and, to a lesser extent, thoracic vertebral fractures.[275] Experimental studies have demonstrated significant potential tissue damage from whiplash injuries. MacNab used animal models to demonstrate lesions such as tears in the longus colli muscles and anterior longitudinal ligament, accompanied by retropharyngeal hematomas[185]; the more severe cases also involved tears extending into the spinal column, with detachment of a disk from the vertebral endplate. Such findings

have been confirmed by other investigators[208] in humans.

Probably one of the better studied pathomechanical events associated with vehicular accidents is cervical acceleration/deceleration injury secondary to rear-end impact. The head initially is displaced into extension as the shoulders are propelled anteriorly. After extension the inertia of the head is overcome, and it is accelerated forward, forcing the neck into flexion. Peak accelerations of 12 G have been noted during extension with relatively low rear-end impacts (20 miles/hour).[256] Because most cervical acceleration/deceleration injuries are not exclusively in the sagittal plane, the pathomechanics obviously become somewhat more complicated, with important implications for what part of the neck may be damaged by inclusion of rotational components. Structures that become more susceptible to injury with cervical rotational components include the zygapophyseal joint capsules, alar ligament complex, and intervertebral disks.[13] Forces that must be considered in analyzing cervical injury include extension, flexion, lateral flexion, and shear forces (usually horizontal). Cervical symptoms may be promulgated and maintained by injury to multiple structures within the neck, including intervertebral disks, muscles, ligaments, atlantoaxial complex, cervical vertebrae, zygapophyseal joints, and neurovascular structures.[279] Rare sequelae include cervical esophageal perforation.[262]

Chronic pain in association with CAD is most likely multifactorial. Causes may include myofascial dysfunction of the paracervical (anterior and posterior) and upper shoulder girdle musculature; injury to the C2–C3 zygapophyseal joint; greater and lesser occipital neuralgia; internal derangement of the temporomandibular joint; basilar artery migraine; and/or cervicothoracic somatic dysfunction.[272] Facial, neck, and shoulder dysesthesias may result from involvement of the upper cranial nerves and their superficial branches (greater auricular, superficial cervical nerve, and supraclavicular nerve) as well as the descending tract of cranial nerve V or its associated fibers.[5,7,9,10] Damage to the central trigeminal system in upper spinal cord segments and pontomedullary levels of the brainstem following soft-tissue injury of the cervical spine have been postulated on the basis of facial sensory changes in vibratory and temperature perception.[152] Some studies show a significant prevalence of chronic cervical zygapophyseal joint pain after CAD. Dwyer et al. mapped characteristic patterns of cervical zygapophyseal joint pain in normal volunteers, which may be useful for constructing pain charts.[75] The best treatment remains somewhat debatable.[14,15] Thorough assessment of cervical pain complaints relative to both pre- and postinjury history is critical if the clinician is to make a timely and appropriate diagnosis.[310]

Long-term follow-up studies (more than 2 years after injury) demonstrate that chronic disability due to soft-tissue neck injury alone is quite significant and not generally related to ongoing litigation or litigation resolution.[124,128,187] More recent, better controlled, prospective studies have refuted earlier perceptions about poor prognostic indicators for long-term recovery, such as reversal of the lordotic curve or presence of cervical spondylosis. Meenen et al. demonstrated no statistically significant relationship between preexisting cervical degenerative disease and exacerbation of the degenerative condition.[192] Prior positive relationships between female sex and chronic symptoms or rates of return to work also have been refuted.[124]

Various neurophysiologic phenomena have been theorized to be responsible for persistent symptoms after whiplash injury.[253] The second cervical nerve root is particularly susceptible to traction injury, because it is not protected by pedicles or facets. This fact, combined with the relatively high mobility of the atlantooccipital joint, leaves the posterior primary ramus of the C2 root highly vulnerable to trauma. Distally, the second cervical nerve becomes the greater occipital nerve (GON), which has a fairly significant cutaneous distribution over the scalp, neck, and face. Often posttraumatic attacks of hemicrania may be explained solely by a diagnosis of greater occipital neuralgia. Classically, left-sided GON involvement is more common in front-seat passengers, because the seat-belt shoulder restraint tends to restrict movement of the right shoulder girdle more than the left (the converse is true for

drivers). Frequently, this sequela is accompanied by ipsilateral retroorbital or periorbital eye pain related to the physiologic communication between the second cervical nerve and the ophthalmic branch of the trigeminal nerve at the medullary level.[249] Chronic greater occipital neuralgia may result from nerve entrapment, which is related to paracervical myodystonia involving the semispinalis capitis and/or traction stress from trapezius myodystonia as the GON penetrates the proximal tendinous insertion of the trapezius muscle.[281] So-called cervicogenic headache remains controversial; however, recent literature has reinforced its existence,[294] including the role of the C3 dorsal ramus in third occipital headache.[33]

Other potential causes of chronic pain and/or dysfunction after whiplash injury include nerve root irritation in the intervertebral foramina, foraminal encroachment, and vertebral artery compression. Posttraumatic vertebrobasilar insufficiency (VBI) may result from constriction or occlusion of the vertebral artery, most commonly at the second cervical level. The classic symptoms of VBI may accompany such occlusion, including diplopia, dizziness, drop attacks, dysmetria, and headache. Posttraumatic VBI secondary to vertebral artery compression has been demonstrated angiographically in symptomatic patients.[174] Rarely, the lower cranial nerves may be damaged by stretch injury, as in Collet-Sicard syndrome (involvement of cranial nerves 9–12).[117]

Cervicogenic vertigo or dizziness is a controversial condition that has been proposed to explain somatic complaints of nonvertiginous dizziness in the absence of true peripheral or central vestibular dysfunction after whiplash type injuries. Proposed mechanisms for cervicogenic dizziness include aberrations in the afferent input from positional proprioceptors in the cervical and lumbar regions,[126,228] overexcitation of the cervical sympathetic nerves,[127] compromise of vertebral artery blood flow,[239] and cervicolumbar hypertonicity.[127] Boquet et al. attempted to explain postconcussional vertigo by aberrations of cervical proprioceptive mechanisms through autonomic pathways etiologically related to ipsilateral cervical hypertonicity.[39] Most postconcussional patients in Boquet's study had positive triggerpoint findings and, on balance evaluation, posterolateral sway toward the hypertonic neck musculature. Ettlin et al. used comprehensive electronystagmography to evaluate 17 patients with whiplash injury and noted that over one-half had significant clinical abnormalities.[83] Kortschot's recent study of over 400 patients with PCD noted subjective complaints of vertigo and dizziness in 68%; 56% demonstrated central vestibular dysfunction.[154] The exact mechanism for cervicogenic vertigo remains unclear, although the available literature suggests that it is probably multifactorial.

Cervical hyperflexion and hyperextension injuries also may result in damage or irritation to posterior and anterior cervical sympathetics, respectively. Anterior cervical sympathetic dysfunction (ACSD), also called Bernard-Horner syndrome, is a well-recognized sequela of severe cervical hyperextension injury and typically presents with the triad of ipsilateral myosis, ptosis, and anhidrosis. Posterior cervical sympathetic dysfunction (PCSD), also known as Barre-Lieou syndrome, is a controversial clinical entity. Although rare as a posttraumatic phenomenon, PCSD is important clinically because it generally responds well to treatment regimens directed at decreasing cervical myodystonia and soft-tissue inflammation and increasing cervical spine mobility, both myoligamentous and osseous. Of interest, PCSD has been relatively lost in the historical medical literature.[16,175] It is theorized to result from irritation of the posterior cervical sympathetics, which consist of the vertebral nerve and the cervical sympathetic plexus and surround the vertebral artery and its branches. Alterations in sympathetic tone secondary to irritation cause transient ischemia to pontine and possibly occipital lobe structures. Alteration in cerebral blood flow secondary to cervical sympathetic stimulation has been demonstrated in animal models.[153] Although PCSD first was thought to be causally related only to degenerative changes in the lower cervical spine, it has been proposed that whiplash injuries may constitute another major etiologic factor.[97] Symptomatically, the major findings reported by patients with PCSD include vertigo, tinnitus, occipital headaches, blurry vision, and dysphonia.

Myofascial pain secondary to whiplash injury is an all too frequently overlooked cause of chronic pain and dysfunction after cervical hyperflexion/hyperextension injury. The anterior and/or posterior cervical musculature is usually involved. Of the anterior group, the muscle most commonly involved in whiplash injury is the sternocleidomastoid. The posterior cervical musculature occurs in four layers; from most superficial to deep, they include (1) trapezius, (2) splenius capitis and cervicis, (3) semispinalis capitis and cervicis, and (4) multifidi/rotatores.[281] Referred pain is one of the least understood clinical phenomena among physicians dealing with postconcussive injuries. Trapezius trigger points in the upper fibers may refer pain to the posterolateral neck, posterior ear, and temple, whereas lower fibers classically refer pain to the high cervical, suprascapular, and interscapular regions. Trigger points in the sternal portion of the sternocleidomastoid may refer pain to the vertex, occiput, cheek, eye, throat, and sternum, whereas trigger points in the clavicular portion of the sternocleidomastoid refer pain to the frontal and aural regions. Trigger points in the sternal branch of the sternocleidomastoid muscle also produce rather unusual symptoms related to autonomic phenomena; such symptoms typically involve the ipsilateral eye, nose, and, more rarely, ear. Trigger points in the clavicular branch of the sternocleidomastoid muscle may be associated with evidence of proprioceptive dysfunction, including postural dizziness, vertigo, syncope, and disequilibrium. Of interest, the relation of neck musculature to head and body orientation in space, although long recognized,[48] has been relatively ignored in whiplash patients with proprioceptive symptoms.

The splenius capitis refers pain to the vertex of the head, whereas the splenius cervicis refers pain to the eye (generally, retroorbital, sometimes with blurring of vision), angle of the neck, and diffusely into the cranium. Three main trigger points are associated with hyperflexion injuries of the cervical spine. The most common trigger point involves the multifidi or rotatores at the C4 or C5 level and produces referred pain into the suboccipital region and the upper shoulder girdle. The second common trigger point after cervical hyperflexion injury involves the semispinalis cervicis, with referred pain into the posterior occiput toward the vertex. Lastly, trigger points in the semispinalis capitis refer pain in a band-like fashion to the ipsilateral cranium, generally with maximal intensity in the frontotemporal area just above and behind the orbit. The scalene muscle group also may be injured by whiplash, particularly with severe lateral cervical displacement. Myofascial pain may be referred into the anterior chest and down the ipsilateral arm and hand as well as into the upper medial back. Often scalene referred pain may be mistaken for angina. Neurovascular entrapment secondary to compromise of the brachial plexus and subclavian vein also may occur, with symptoms of medial hand pain (ulnar distribution) and associated edema. Temporalis trigger points may be activated by local trauma as the person is tossed around in a struck vehicle or hit by an object on the side of the head. Referred pain may radiate to other areas of the temporalis muscle, upper dentition, and frontal eyebrow area as well as behind the orbit. An adequate knowledge of myofascial dysfunction is critical for appropriate management of patients with whiplash injuries. The seminal work by Travell and Simons remains the standard reference in this area of clinical diagnosis and treatment.[281]

Treatment for soft-tissue dysfunction secondary to whiplash must be individualized, given the heterogeneity of injuries. During the acute stage, the patient should be immobilized in a soft, contoured collar. Ice is generally recommended in the first 48–72 hours to minimize swelling; heat is used hereafter to decrease pain and to facilitate movement. Gradual mobilization should proceed after a few days, followed first by active mobilization and then by isometric strengthening exercises. Cervical traction may be helpful in subacute and chronic conditions, including Barre-Lieou syndrome. Medications, such as nonsteroidal antiinflammatory drugs and sometimes analgesics and muscle relaxants, may be necessary in both the acute and postacute period. Narcotic analgesics should be avoided. In patients with evidence of myofascial dysfunction, appropriate therapies directed to breaking up the pain cycle include spray-and-stretch techniques, trigger-point injections,[56,281] electrical stimulation, ultrasound, ischemic pressure, pulsed electromagnetic therapy (PEMT),[91] and acupuncture.[270] Once myofascial dysfunction is evident every attempt should be made to correct all biomechanical or environmental phenomena that may perpetuate the condition. In addition, some practitioners advocate prescription of phasic exercises for cervical rehabilitation, including rapid eye-head-neck-arm movements.[89] Recent literature suggests that manual therapy also may play a role in the treatment of the whiplash patient with cervicogenic headache,[143,287] although this approach remains somewhat controversial. Florian reviews the rationale or lack thereof for various therapies in the conservative management of neck pain.[90] Most recently, after reviewing the prevention, diagnosis, and management of whiplash injury, a task force in Canada concluded, to no great surprise, that "little rigorous information" was available; yet a specific patient care guideline was proposed.[263]

A relatively uncommon phenomenon after whiplash injury is basilar artery migraine (BAM), which seems to occur much more frequently in girls and young women.[138] BAM is commonly misdiagnosed by less sophisticated practitioners as malingering or conversional, when in fact it is a true organic sequela of whiplash trauma. BAM typically presents with intense vascular headache preceded by posterior circulation prodromata or aura accompanied by various symptoms, including visual impairment, ataxia, dysarthria, paresthesias, vertigo, drop attacks, and weakness.[25,268] The neurologic examination is usually normal if the patient is not having an attack. Recent studies have elucidated a neurotologic profile of this patient population, including abnormalities in clinical vestibular testing.[207] Electroencephalographic abnormalities have been reported in BAM,[139] as have cerebral SPECT abnormalities in the region of basilar vascular flow.[255] Typically, BAM is treated like other migrainous types of headache; however, anticonvulsants are occasionally an effective intervention.[108]

Temporomandibular joint disorders (TMJD) also may result from CAD injury; however, many clinicians overdiagnose this condition and do not adequately apportion symptoms to preexisting conditions, dental and otherwise. A recent study examining the biomechanics of TMJ injury during low-velocity extension-flexion injury revealed that the typical forces generated by rear-end collisions were inadequate to produce articular injury.[133] TMJD is marked symptomatically by pain in the muscles of mastication, range-of-motion restrictions, and muscle tenderness with or without joint crepitation and subluxation. Appropriate screening procedures for TMJ dysfunction are critical to clinical evaluation, including consideration of occult dental and facial fractures.[93] Internal joint derangement (intraarticular involvement) as a direct result of CAD injury is rare.[120, 223] Of interest, a large Australian study of somatic sequelae of traffic accidents noted that only 0.5% of whiplash patients presented with TMJD. The female-to-male ratio was 5:2.

The clinician must differentiate between intraarticular derangement secondary to trauma and sequelae of repeated microtrauma from hyperfunction (bruxism). Both may result in pathologic changes of the disk glenoid fossa, condylar head, and/or synovial linings of the TMJ. Myofascial dysfunction of the muscles of mastication (extraarticular involvement) with secondary TMJ involvement is much more common.[44]

Cranial Trauma

Damage to the cranium or cranial adenexal structures must be assessed in patients with so-called post-concussional symptoms. Many causes of prolonged somatic complaints after concussive injury are, on closer scrutiny, referable to damage to cranial structures, often without concomitant brain injury.

Skull fractures are relatively rare in MTBI (approximately 1 in 40 patients). Fractures may be closed or compound, depressed or nondepressed. Basilar skull fractures, as opposed to linear skull fractures of the cranial vault, may be clinically significant. If the dura mater is torn, the chance of a cerebrospinal fluid fistula is increased. A dural tear or basilar skull fracture increases the patient's risk of meningitis. Cerebrospinal fluid leaks through the nares (rhinorrhea) or ears (otorrhea) may be missed in the acute setting. Pneumocephalus, which may present as air within the subarachnoid space or cerebral ventricles, may be diagnosed by skull films or CT of the head. Operative management is indicated if air is noted within the brain parenchyma.[51] Approximately 4% of patients with mild head injury have an unsuspected temporal skull fracture.[46]

Hearing loss related to cranial adnexal sequelae of head trauma is not uncommon. Longitudinal fractures (about 80%) are more commonly associated with conductive hearing loss due either to ossicular chain disruption or to traumatic tympanic membrane tear and blood in the middle ear, although these fractures are not particularly common in PCD. Transverse temporal skull fractures (about 20%) may involve hearing loss, either mixed or profound sensorineural; hemotympanum; and dizziness; facial nerve injuries occur in about 50% of patients.[119,292] The conductive hearing loss associated with hemotympanum is typically temporary and resolves as the hematoma is resorbed. Progressive hearing loss after trauma should trigger further assessment for either perilymphatic fistula or endolymphatic hydrops.[179] Surgical correction of ossicular chain disruption may lead to restitution of hearing after separation of the incudostapedial joint, with or without dislocation of the body of the incus from the articulation with the malleus head (the most common type of ossicular dislocation in temporal skull fractures).

Complaints of dizziness after mild head trauma are extremely common. Appropriate clinical evaluation, including a clear delineation of the patient's symptoms, is critical. Neurodiagnostic evaluation of the dizzy patient may include audiologic testing, fistula test, electronystagmography, and posturography.[233] Labyrinthine concussion may result in transient auditory and vestibular symptoms without associated skull fracture. Sudden deafness after a blow to the cranium may be partially or completely reversible. Posttraumatic positional vertigo, so-called benign positional vertigo (BPV), is the most common of the neurootologic sequelae of closed head injury. Most patients demonstrate a paroxysmal positional nystagmus with rapid changes in position.[309] Posttraumatic BPV results from cupulolithiasis or dislodgement of calcium carbonate from the macula of the utriculus and attachment to the cupula of the posterior semicircular canal. Objective diagnosis can be made by bedside clinical examination; however, sensitivity is somewhat lacking because many patients may not have gross subjective symptoms that cue the clinician to look further. Often such patients have silent BPV and/or other vestibular disturbances despite grossly normal bedside examination.

Studies using electronystagmographic recordings (with caloric irrigation) suggest an inverse relationship between the occurrence of vestibular disorders and severity of associated neurologic injury as expressed by GCS. In addition, the frequency may be much higher than previously appreciated (> 50%).[205] A recent study found that dizziness associated with concussion was most commonly due to BPV, with an incidence of approximately 60%.[64] Electronystagmographic testing assists the clinician in differentiating central versus peripheral vestibular processes, as well as in delineating eye movement disorders, which occur on a central basis.[102] Ochs and Zasler speculated that silent BPV may contribute to the functional disequilibrium commonly experienced by patients with mild head injury. Of interest, many patients with BPV may awaken with morning headache, which some clinicians attribute to the patient's lying in the plane of the injured labyrinthine canal during the night and thereby inducing cocontraction of labyrinth-influenced neck musculature.[106] In general, the prognosis for posttraumatic BPV is quite good; symptoms resolve completely in most patients within 6 months and in the majority of the remainder within 2 years. As a general rule, vertigo after mild head or brain trauma is of peripheral origin in the postacute period rather than due to posttraumatic brainstem dysfunction.

Periodic exacerbations of BPV after symptoms have subsided are the exception rather than the rule. Vestibular suppressant medications may be used, but generally they should be considered only if symptoms are severe enough to compromise functional activities (e.g., frequent falls or significant nausea and/or vomiting). Research indicates that vestibular suppressants in fact may impede central nervous system adaptation to the aberrant vestibular input, thereby prolonging the symptomatic period of recovery. Patients with concomitant brain injury probably should avoid medications with significant sedative potential, such as benzodiazepines (e.g., diazepam), as well as anticholinergic medications (e.g., scopolamine). Both classes of drugs may have adverse effects on cognition, and anicholinergic agents also may cause visual disturbances. Newer agents, including flunarazine and phenytoin, have proved effective for the treatment of vertigo and may be reasonable alternatives in patients with head or brain injury.[49,206]

Vestibular exercises also may hasten neurologic and functional recovery via several proposed physiologic mechanisms, including central sensory substitution, rebalancing tonic activity, and physiologic habituation.[42,257,259] Behavioral interventions modeled after military aviation protocols to combat vertigo and nausea are useful.[260] The most recent literature recommends a three-pronged approach as part of an organized vestibular rehabilitation program: habituation exercises, postural control exercises, and general conditioning activities.[258] Surgery, a last resort for intractable BPV, is successful in the majority of cases (> 90%).[95]

The clinician should consider the possibility of posttraumatic endolymphatic hydrops (Meniere's syndrome), particularly in patients with an associated ipsilateral low-frequency hearing loss, tinnitus, and a sensation of fullness in the ear. Treatment of posttraumatic Meniere's disease may include vestibular suppressants if symptoms have significantly adverse effects on daily function. Head movements and rapid changes in head position should be avoided. In the remission phase, Meniere's disease may be treated with betahistine, a histamine derivative, and surgical procedures (both destructive and nondestructive).[41]

Posttraumatic perilymphatic fistula (PTPF) may result from rupture of the oval and, less commonly, the round window; the subsequent dehiscence between the inner ear and middle ear results in inappropriate stimulation of labyrinthine receptors. Symptoms of PTPF may include vertigo, fluctuating hearing loss (usually a late complication), tinnitus, chronic low-grade nausea, endolymphatic hydrops, cervical myodystonia, and persistent or exertional headache.[30] Patients with mild head trauma and PTPF often complain of nonspecific imbalance problems worsened by sudden turning and disequilibrium with perceptually complex external stimuli, such as patterns and wide-field motion (e.g., escalator rides, revolving doors, and crowds).[106] The sensation during ambulation has been described as "walking on pillows."[41] Such experiences tend to promote a mild agoraphobia. Some clinicians have speculated that symptoms of PTPF stimulate visual compensation for labyrinthine dysfunction. This compensatory mechanism subsequently causes disorientation in visually complex situations. Higher-level cognitive and language problems may result, presumably secondary to "attempted" sensory accommodation to aberrant afferent input as the result of PTPF rather than brain injury per se.[106] Although there is no definitive bedside clinical test for PTPF, application of pressure to the tympanic membrane with a pneumatic otoscope (Hennebert's fistula test) or application of pressure over the tragus may produce worsening of vertigo or nystagmus. Both tests are suggestive but not diagnostic for a perilymphatic fistula. Some investigators believe that caloric hypoexcitability or unexcitability associated with even partial conservation of cochlear function is a good indicator of PTPF.[168] Black, Lilly, and Nashner described the platform fistula test, which uses posturography for objective diagnosis.[29] The ability of posturographic testing to delineate perilymphatic fistulas has been questioned by this clinician as well as others[121]; however, further research is definitely indicated. There is no pathognomonic or characteristic electronystagmographic sign for PTPF.

Early treatment measures include bedrest, head elevation, and avoidance of straining.[41] The duration of bedrest is somewhat controversial, although most sophisticated clinicians advocate 5–10 days, given the functional and physiologic implications of prolonged immobilization. PTPFs usually heal spontaneously. Exploratory tympanotomy is necessary for definitive diagnosis of PTPF, but it is generally not recommended unless symptoms last longer than 1 month or

hearing loss is progressive. Chronic PTPF can be addressed surgically by patching the leaking oval or round window with temporal aponeurosis or stapeddectomy with interposition.[11] Recent studies examining different protein markers (e.g., beta$_2$ transferrin, apoproteins D and J) for more definitive identification of perilymphatic fluid during surgery show promising results.[276] Surgery generally is much more successful for control of vertigo than for restoration of hearing.[168]

Posttraumatic tinnitus is another common complaint that often eludes adequate diagnosis and treatment. Tinnitus has been reported in 30–70% of all head injuries.[231] Tinnitus is a symptom, not a disease entity; its etiology is still not well defined. Typically, posttraumatic tinnitus is due to an electrophysiologic derangement in the cochlea, cranial nerve VIII, or the central nervous system. Various grading systems may be used to track the natural history of tinnitus, response to treatment, and/or functional disability.[101] Appropriate audiologic battery testing is indicated in all patients with head injury and complaints of tinnitus. Hearing aids, cochlear implants, tinnitus maskers, and hearing instruments have been used to decrease subjective symptoms. No drug has been approved by the Food and Drug Administration for treatment of tinnitus, and current choices are at best controversial and poorly studied. Preliminary evidence suggests that oral tocainide may be effective.[79] Alprazolam has been advocated by one study,[147] but methodologic issues challenge its validity.[135] Electrical stimulation is also being explored as a potential treatment. Because tinnitus may be exacerbated by stress and anxiety, antidepressant medications, biofeedback, hypnosis, avoidance of stimulants (including caffeine), and proper sleep hygiene also have been recommended.[187]

Other common, yet frequently undiagnosed sequelae of cranial trauma are olfactory and gustatory deficits. Obrebowski et al. demonstrated that maxillofacial fractures were associated with a 16.7% incidence of anosmia, 23.2% incidence of hyposmia, and 0.9% incidence of asymmetric gustatory thresholds.[204] In patients without focal cortical contusion of central olfactory or gustatory centers in the anterior frontal and temporal lobes, one can assume that the cause is peripheral.[53] Dysfunction of cranial nerve I, which results in olfactory impairment, is quite common compared with other cranial nerve deficits in patients with mild cranial trauma. The incidence of olfactory dysfunction in patients with brain injury of all degrees of severity may be as high as 30–40%[52]; approximately one-third of patients suffer from total anosmia. Peripheral posttraumatic olfactory dysfunction may result from shearing injury to cranial nerve I at the cribriform plate as well as from mechanical injuries to the nose and nasal passages. Small contusions of the frontal and temporal central chemosensory centers also may contribute to olfactory dysfunction after even mild brain injury.[271]

Gustatory dysfunction is a much less common posttraumatic sequela than anosmia. Typically peripheral injury involves the cranial nerve VII, which is more prone to injury than cranial nerves IX and X (also involved in mediation of taste function).[53] Timely and appropriate rehabilitative interventions are important both for assuring safety and optimizing ADLs.[303]

Visual problems also may occur at a peripheral level unrelated to associated brain injury. Such deficits are not infrequently due to disorders of the vitreous element, both prefoveal and foveal; they are commonly associated with traction on the retina and subjective symptoms of floating spots (so-called "floaters").[57,60] Retinal injury, including detachment, tear and hemorrhage,[47,156] also may cause visual symptoms. In one study approximately 20% of patients with midfacial trauma were noted to have accommodative and/or convergence insufficiency.[3] A cursory assessment of the optic disk obviously misses the subtle lesions responsible for many posttraumatic visual symptoms. It is therefore important to refer patients with visual complaints to a skilled ophthalmologist or neuroophthalmologist.

Headache and neck pain are the most common physical complaints after concussion (mild brain injury) and are experienced early after injury by up to 70% of patients. Headache also occurs after more severe brain injury but for some reason, as yet unidentified, tends to be much less common. Postconcussive headaches may be quite persistent; however, they cannot be positively correlated with severity of injury.[297] Often injured persons seek medical care after concussion and/or cervical whiplash injury only to be diagnosed with posttraumatic headache (PTHA).

The majority of headache after mild brain injury is most likely benign, because it does not require surgical treatment. On occasion, however, complications may require surgical intervention, more often in patients with more severe brain injury. Specifically, persistent headache may result from subdural and epidural hematomas (blood collections between brain and skull), abscesses, and carotid cavernous fistulas (abnormal communication between venous and arterial blood flow). Such serious complications are ruled out through appropriate clinical examination and additional diagnostic tests.[212] The only definitive opinion about the utility of neuroimaging in the work-up of headache related to migraine; the investigators noted that in the absence of a recent change in headache pattern, seizures, or other focal neurologic findings, the routine use of neuroimaging was not warranted.[220]

There are multiple sources of head and neck pain, both inside and outside the head. Of interest, the brain itself is not a source of pain. The major structures inside the skull that produce pain are the thin coating over the brain at its base (dura), venous sinuses, blood vessels, and cranial nerves II, III, V, X, and XI. The major structures outside the skull that may produce posttraumatic pain include the skin, muscles, arteries, joint capsules, cavities within the head (e.g., sinuses, eyes, ears, nose, and oral cavity), cervical nerves I–III, and the thin layer of pain-sensitive tissue coating bones in the head and neck (periosteum). Headache typically results from six major physiologic phenomena: (1) displacement of intracranial structures, (2) inflammation, (3) ischemia and/or metabolic changes, (4) myodystonia, (5) meningeal irritation, and (6) increased intracranial pressure.

PTHA is not a diagnosis; it is a symptom. All too often, however, patients are diagnosed simply with PTHA, and the problem causing the pain is elaborated no further. Often PTHA is treated as vascular or migraine headache, when in fact the great majority are not due to migrainelike phenomena. It is therefore not surprising that patients often do not respond to prescribed treatment.

The clinician must keep the different mechanisms of PTHA in mind. In addition, the mechanism of injury responsible for the initial insult should be investigated. The clinician should inquire about history relevant to three main phenomena: (1) brain injury, (2) cranial or cranial/adnexal trauma, and (3) cervical acceleration/deceleration (CAD) insult (whiplash injury).

Major clues to the origin of the headache should come from the symptom profile and the preinjury history of headache. A patient with preinjury headache may develop a different type of headache or a worsening of the preinjury condition after trauma. The major questions relative to the symptom profile are expressed in the mnemonic **COLDER: C**haracter, **O**nset, **L**ocation, **D**uration, **E**xacerbation, and **R**elief. Other important descriptors include frequency, severity, associated symptoms, presence or absence of aura, degree of functional disability, and time of day that headaches develop. Such clues arm the clinician to conduct a clinical examination that allows a more specific conclusion about the origin of headache.

The major types of posttraumatic headaches are musculoskeletal headache, neuroma or neuralgic headache, sympathetic nerve dysfunction, and vascular (migraine) headache. Rare causes include seizure disorders, pneumocephalus, cluster, paroxysmal hemicrania,[283] and the potential surgical conditions mentioned above.

The most common cause of posttraumatic headache, and often one of the most overlooked, is referred musculoskeletal pain secondary to myofascial pain syndromes associated with cervical acceleration-deceleration insult. Temporomandibular joint dysfunction also should be considered (see below). Musculoskeletal headache that is cervicogenic typically presents with symptoms of pressure and tension, often with a caplike distribution. The headache tends to worsen with stooping, bending, or exertion and may be associated with other symptoms such as dizziness, sensitivity to light (photophobia), sensitivity to sound (phonophobia), and even imbalance. Clinicians must have a good understanding of relevant factors, including palpatory muscle examination, trigger vs. tender points, and pathognomonic clinical features such as "twitch response" and "jump sign." An understanding of referred pain patterns from trigger points—particularly for cervical muscles, which have a higher propensity for injury after whiplash—is critical (see cervical injury section).[306,310] Associated symptoms and factors that may perpetuate myofascial pain disorders also should be well understood.[131]

Cervical somatic (vertebral) dysfunction is often seen in association with cervical myofascial dysfunction. This condition is significantly underappreciated by the vast majority of clinicians. Subtle vertebral rotations, anterior as well as posterior, may cause pain, both local and referred to the head, through multiple mechanisms. Manual and/or manipulative therapy may be quite effective, either alone or in combination with other interventions, in resetting bony structures.[144] Manual therapy is helpful, when clinically indicated, for conservative short-term treatment and/or infrequent symptomatic treatment.[282] It is not recommended for long-term chronic treatment, because it does not address the underlying problem(s).

Temporomandibular joint dysfunction is a controversial consequence of whiplash injury. In this clinician's experience, posttraumatic headache sometimes results from injury to the muscles of mastication, which is much more common than injury to the joint itself. With significant muscle injury, however, the joint may become secondarily involved. TMJD is overdiagnosed as an explanation for PTHA. Another interesting and recently identified cause of PTHA, particularly presenting as temporal headache (as well as various other problems), is injury to the styloid process and/or its attachments (e.g., musculoligamentous structures).[295]

Large nerves in the scalp also may be injured, as a result of either direct trauma or entrapment from injured muscles in a state of "spasm" (more appropriately called myodystonia). The most common large nerves involved in headache pain are the greater and lesser occipital nerves; other candidates include the supra- and infraorbital nerves,[58,231] although any of the smaller nerves in the scalp may be affected. Headache generated by local contusion to the scalp with underlying scar formation in the nerves tends to be a shooting, stabbing pain. Particularly with greater occipital neuralgia, the classic finding is tenderness over the greater occipital nerve, with referred pain in the frontotemporal region and sometimes with associated pain around or behind the eye. The only way to make the diagnosis is to thoroughly palpate the soft tissue of the craniocervical junction; unfortunately, this aspect of the headache examination is often neglected.

Neuritic and neuralgic pain syndromes of the scalp and head may be managed by several methods, including local nerve blocks, treatment of associated muscle spasm, counterirritation techniques, topical medication (e.g., capsaicin) for pain mediated by small nerves in the scalp, cryoanalgesia, and, lastly and most aggressively, surgical intervention. As perineural edema subsides, many subacute neuralgias resolve. In the acute and subacute stage, mild diuretics, such as acetazolamide, may be beneficial in decreasing perineural edema and hastening recovery of transient nerve dysfunction. Diagnostic blocks with local anesthetics such as lidocaine may offer confirmation of clinically suspected neuralgic pain and cure at the same time.[56,289] Oral medications, such as tricyclic antidepressants, anticonvulsants, and nonsteroidal antiinflammatory drugs, also may be of benefit. Surgical intervention may be indicated for decompression when neuralgic pain is induced by local scar formation or neuroma formation.[78,253]

Certain nerve fibers in the neck (both anterior and posterior sections) also may be damaged by excessive flexion or extension of the neck, as in CAD insult. Anterior injury may produce various clinical conditions, including so-called dysautonomic cephalalgia. Whether the insult to anterior nerves is partial or total may affect medication choices (tricyclic antidepressants or beta blockers, respectively). Involvement of posterior cervical sympathetic dysfunction (Barre-Lieou syndrome) may produce symptoms of pain in the back of the head, tinnitus, blurry vision, and vertigo. Treatment is mainly directed at mobilization, control of inflammation, and pain management.

Migraine accounts for up to 20% of chronic posttraumatic headache. It is generally treated like nontraumatic migraine. The clinician should look at all factors that may influence headache, including so-called trigger factors (e.g., certain food groups as well as external and internal stressors). Treatment should be directed at minimizing the functional disability associated with the headache through interventions such as reduction of trigger factors and appropriate prescription of medication, which may be abortive, symptomatic, and/or prophylactic. McBeath and Nanda demonstrated the utility of dihydroergotamine and metoclopramide in postconcussive headache; of interest, relief of headache was accompanied by improvement in other symptoms, including memory and sleep problems and dizziness.[180] Birth control pills may exacerbate migraines in a small percentage of women, and this possibility should be considered in the overall holistic treatment of patients with posttraumatic migraine. Other interventions, such as relaxation training and biofeedback, may be included. Mixed headache syndromes (e.g., chronic daily headache with components of both tension myalgia headache and vascular headache) must be identified, particularly when they occur in conjunction with a treatable condition such as depression. It is also important for clinicians to be aware of other migrainelike headaches, including drug-induced headache, exertional headache, sexual headache, and rebound/withdrawal headache.

Atypical variants of posttraumatic migraine, such as basilar artery migraine, occur more frequently in young women, particularly after whiplash injury (see cervical spine section). The exact reason is still unclear. This type of vascular headache may be treated with atypical migraine medications, such as carbamazepine (Tegretol) or valproic acid (Depakote or Depakene), if it is unresponsive to more traditional approaches. Another atypical variant of migraine after trauma is transient cortical blindness, which is occasionally seen in children. Many rare causes of headache also should be considered in posttraumatic patients, including tension pneumocephalus, carotid cavernous fistulas, late extraaxial collections (e.g., subdural and epidural hematomas), subdural hygromas, paroxysmal hemicrania, and cluster headache. Neurodiagnostic tests such as CT or

MRI of the brain, plain radiographs, angiography or magnetic resonance angiography (MRA), and other vascular studies should be conducted as deemed appropriate by the treating clinician to rule out such disorders.

Multiple studies, some completed only in the past 3–5 years, demonstrate that ongoing litigation has little to no effect on the persistence of headache complaints. Studies have shown that patients continue to report significant symptoms even after litigation has ended.[211] Headache complaints seem to be more common in women for unexplained reasons.[143] A few patients develop intractable posttraumatic headache. In this practitioner's experience, most properly treated PTHA is not permanent or totally disabling over the long term.

By taking the appropriate time to acquire adequate pre- and postinjury histories, to conduct a careful clinical evaluation, and to order indicated diagnostic tests, the experienced clinician should be able to determine the underlying cause of PTHA. Once the appropriate diagnosis is made, treatment should be instituted in a holistic fashion with sensitivity to maximizing the benefit/risk ratio of particular interventions, prescribing treatment that encourages optimal compliance, and educating both patient and family about the condition, its treatment, and its prognosis.

Finally, vascular trauma may produce an array of sequelae, including aneurysms (both true and false), arterial dissection and/or occlusion, venous hemorrhage or thrombosis, and arteriovenous fistulas. Such conditions may occur extracranially or intracranially. In general, they are believed to be rare consequences of cranial, neck, or brain injury of any degree of severity; however, they have been reported even after mild injury.[92,149] The true incidence of vascular injury in patients with head or brain injury is difficult to assess accurately because of the inherent problems in diagnosing posttraumatic sequelae with such high rates of morbidity and mortality. Probably the best study to date[77] found only a 4.2% incidence of vascular injury in a large population of head-injured civilians. Nonetheless, because angiography is seldom done in the acute setting, particularly after mild cranial or brain trauma, the diagnosis of vascular injury depends mainly on bedside clinical examination. Vascular injury may manifest early, thereby hiding within the more generalized symptoms of trauma, or it may become evident only after a delay.[149] Thus, clinicians must have a good understanding of posttraumatic vascular syndromes to address them in a timely fashion, thereby minimizing morbidity and maximizing outcome.

Brain Trauma

Many practicing physicians believe that a patient with a normal CT and normal electroencephalogram is in fact normal. They should keep in mind, however, the old adage, "Absence of proof is not proof of absence." Historically, the lack of positive neurodiagnostic tests in patients with MTBI may have reflected a simple lack of sensitivity and/or specificity. Advances in basic neuroscience, acute care, neurodiagnostic evaluation, and rehabilitative care have provided evidence that patients with mild brain injuries may indeed suffer sequelae, albeit often subtle. Most patients, assuming the absence of complicating factors such as prior brain pathology (including prior brain injury), preinjury psychiatric or psychological problems, or history of learning disability or substance abuse, recover fairly expeditiously, without apparent long-term functional, neurologic, or neurobehavioral sequelae. The available literature suggests that a significant, albeit small, subset of patients with MTBI do not make full functional recovery. Patients with long-term impairments may show some resolution of symptoms over time, whereas others may have permanent impairments and permanent functional disabilities.[57,69,280]

Neurodiagnostic techniques have advanced at an astounding pace over the past decade. Such advances may open new frontiers for the evaluation of patients with mild brain injury (see Table 1).

Neurologic assessment alone is inadequate to ensure absence of intracranial pathology after MTBI. A recent study noted an 18.4% incidence of intracranial lesions in patients with MTBI and normal neurologic exams (5.5% required surgery).[266] Although other studies show similar findings, the most recent prospective studies suggest that the rate of

TABLE 1. Neurodiagnostic Testing for Specific Posttraumatic Sequelae

Posttraumatic Sequelae	Neurodiagnostic Procedure
Attentional deficits	Cognitive evoked potentials
Balance dysfunction	Posturographic assessment
Cerebral perfusion changes	Single-photon emission computerized tomography (SPECT)*
Cerebral metabolic changes	Positron emission tomography (PET)*
Electroencephalographic abnormalities	Sleep-deprived electroencephalography (EEG), 24-hour Holter EEG, video EEG, brain electrical activity mapping (BEAM),* magnetoencephalography (MEG)*
Erectile dysfunction	Nocturnal penile tumescence monitoring
Eye movement disorders	Electrooculography, rotary chair
Focal and/or diffuse brain dysfunction	Magnetic source imaging (MSI)
Neuralgic scalp pain, including cervical roots	Diagnostic/therapeutic local anesthetic block
Olfactory and gustatory dysfunction	Chemosensory evaluation for smell and taste
Perilymphatic fistula	Platform fistula test* on posturography, surgical exploration
Regional blood flow alterations	Transcranial color duplex/Doppler (TCD)
Sensorineural and conductive hearing loss	Audiologic evaluation, brainstem auditory evoked responses (BAERs), electrocochleography
Sleep disturbance	Polysomnography with median sleep latency test
Structural parenchymal changes	Magnetic resonance imaging
Vascular injury	Magnetic resonance angiography (MRA), angiography
Vestibular dysfunction	Electronystagmography with calorics, BAERs

* Questionable utility.
Modified from J Head Trauma Rehabil 8(3):20, 1993.

neurosurgical intervention in patients with MTBI is less than 1%.[40,146]

MRI studies of mild TBI are few and far between. Those that exist demonstrate somewhat discrepant results, which may be explained, at least in theory, by timing and technical aspects (e.g., strength of magnet, type of spin-echos, and thickness of cuts). Levin et al. performed one of the first good MRI studies of mild brain injury.[172] Although the small number of patients in each group precludes major generalizations, the results are noteworthy. The authors found a predominance of frontal and temporal abnormalities, which correlated with impairments demonstrated by neurobehavioral testing. In addition, and perhaps of greater significance, improvements in test scores coincided with resolution of MRI abnormalities. A more recent study assessed the utility of MRI in 134 patients with MTBI (GCS scores: 13–15) within 3 days of initial injury.[299] Cortical lesions were found in 25 patients, white matter lesions in 6, and basal ganglia lesions in 3. Cytowic used MRI to study nonhospitalized patients with acute mild brain injury and found results that differed from data published for hospitalized patients. The scans were largely normal, although some patients demonstrated so-called unidentified bright objects (UBOs).[57] UBOs, which are theorized to represent areas of demyelination or gliosis, are best visualized on T2-weighted spinecho. Of interest, they typically appear in white matter or at gray-white junctions and tend to occur in the periventricular region in the centrum semiovale rather than in the subependymal parenchyma. Such white matter changes are distinct from those seen with cerebrovascular disease associated with aging, which tend to be large, bilateral and symmetric, and located in the subependymal parenchyma (with a predilection for the frontal and occipital horns). Newer MRI techniques (such as spectroscopy, which at present remains a research tool) may assist in noninvasive demonstration of alterations in tissue metabolites and pH after mild brain injury.[267] Fluid attenuated inversion recovery (FLAIR) may prove a more sensitive technique for imaging T2-weighted sequences in patients with brain injury.[252]

Given the theorized low yield of static imaging by either CT or MRI in patients with MTBI, clinicians and researchers have begun to assess the utility of functional imaging for neurodiagnostic assessment.[267] At the present time, functional imaging remains more a research tool than an accepted means of clinical evaluation that has any bearing on treatment rendered. Aside from the potential to detect areas of hypoperfusion with single-photon emission computed tomography (SPECT) and areas of hypometabolism with positron emission tomography (PET), functional imaging may prove to be useful in the diagnosis and management of posttraumatic epilepsy, hypoxic-ischemic injury, and movement disorders as well in the quantification of neuroreceptors and monitoring of pharmacologic therapy.[5,137,267] SPECT may assist in delineation of unsuspected brain injury following head trauma[72] and in detection of sequelae of associated and/or suspected hypoxic-ischemic injury, even in the presence of normal CT and EEG findings.[250] Recent SPECT studies show significant promise as an adjuvant technique in assessing organic brain dysfunction in patients with PCD.[136,188] An interesting study using cerebral SPECT demonstrated a correlation between hyperemia and structurally normal (by CT and MRI) parenchymal tissue, lower morbidity and better outcomes. In addition, there was a higher incidence of this phenomenon in patients with MTBI than in patients with more severe brain injury.[238] Findings by Ruff indicate that patients with symptomatic mild brain injury and normal static imaging studies may have a predilection for PET abnormalities in the frontal and temporal lobes.[234] PET also demonstrated local cerebral glucose abnormalities in 3 cognitively impaired patients with mild brain injury (compared with 3 matched normal controls), none of whom had abnormalities on CT, MRI, or EEG.[134] Humayun et al. demonstrated significantly decreased glucose metabolism in medial and posterior temporal and posterior frontal parenchyma as well as in the left caudate. Increased metabolism was noted in the anterior temporal and frontal cortices.

Further research into functional imaging of patients with mild brain injury is obviously warranted, given the encouraging and fascinating findings to date.[27] Other strategies, including magnetic source imaging (MSI), may prove useful in evaluating brain function–structure relationships by combining neurophysiologic data from magnetoencephalography (MEG) with neuroanatomic data from MRI. Early studies have shown magnetic activity of abnormally low frequency in patients with TBI.[22]

EEG evaluation of postconcussive patients may demonstrate subtle abnormalities consistent with the diffuse dysfunction classically anticipated from the presumptive mechanism of injury, or, more rarely, it may show focal abnormalities, even in the presence of a nonfocal neurologic examination. The available literature shows no correlation between standard EEG findings and postconcussive symptoms,[140,245] particularly in the subacute and chronic periods after injury. Some studies have shown that if EEGs are performed immediately after concussion, abnormalities are much more common, although on serial testing they usually resolve quickly.[23] Low-voltage EEG and posterior theta rhythm, once considered to be pathognomonic for chronic mild brain injury,[54] are generally viewed at present as normal variants. Recent literature, however, has questioned our understanding of the pathogenesis and significance of abnormal nonepileptiform EEG rhythms.[242] From a clinical and medicolegal standpoint it is also difficult to establish a causal link between symptoms and an abnormal EEG. In other words, was the EEG abnormal before the injury as well?

The only study to examine pre- and postinjury EEGs found that 51% of patients had abnormal EEGs even before injury. Because preinjury EEGs were performed for neurologic or psychiatric reasons, however, the patients did not constitute a "normal" population.[178] Enomoto found that 42.5% of children had abnormal EEGs after mild brain injury.[81] The degree of abnormality seemed to be correlated with a positive history for loss of consciousness. The most frequent finding was occipital slow waves. The EEGs remained or became normal in 95% of cases.

More recent literature suggests a role for nonstandard EEG analysis of patients with

MTBI. Tebano used power spectral EEG analysis on the posterior lead of 18 patients with MTBI and compared the results with an age- and sex-matched control group.[274] He found a significant increase of the mean power of slow alpha, a reduction of fast alpha, with a shift of mean alpha frequency toward lower values, and a reduction of fast beta. Probably the best controlled study to date using power spectral analysis in MTBI was done by Thatcher.[277] Analysis yielded three classes of neurophysiologic variables: (1) increased coherence and decreased phase in frontal and frontal-temporal regions; (2) decreased power differences between anterior and posterior cortical regions; and (3) reduced alpha power in posterior cortical regions. Gross et al. presented preliminary data (with control populations) indicating four main functional differences in EEG categories: (1) more spike/sharp waves, (2) power differences in slow- and medium-frequency waves with eyes open and resting, (3) failure of slow- and medium-frequency waves to remain desynchronized while processing a continuous simple mental challenge and (4) lack of shift in power toward the frontal areas of the brain with mental activities.[107]

The role of newer electrographic diagnostic techniques using brain electrical activity mapping (BEAM) for diagnosis and management of the postconcussive patient remains controversial in general as well as in relation to TBI.[73,176,202] Several studies claim that BEAM demonstrates a higher level of sensitivity for electrographic and evoked potential abnormalities than conventional EEG, standard evoked responses, or static imaging.[130,290] General consensus dictates that BEAM information cannot be interpreted without concomitant assessment of a standard EEG recording. Some question the validity of many claims made by "evaluating clinicians" who perform quantitative EEG studies in the medicolegal setting. Criticism focuses on technical aspects of testing, interpretative issues, and lack of formal EEG training.[82] In 1994 a position paper reviewed the current state of quantitative EEG and addressed multiple questions about its utility.[74] Additional research is definitely needed to clarify the role of such technology in the clinical care of patients with postconcussive disorders.

Posturography has demonstrated utility in the assessment of balance disorders after brain injury. It has the potential to "diagnose" alterations in balance function due to sensory integration problems, motor disturbances, and vestibular dysfunction.[11,41] As noted above, the utility of posturographic assessment in the diagnosis of perilymphatic fistulas remains controversial, with the prevailing opinion on the negative side.

Electronystagmography (ENG) and electrooculography (EOG) can be useful in demonstrating posttraumatic deficits in eye movement function.[171] Cytowic et al. found that saccadic pursuits were the most common finding after mild brain injury.[57] Other investigators[205] have demonstrated significant eye movement disorders after brain injury, including aberrations in saccades, pursuit, and fixation as well as presence of square wave jerks. ENG and EOG obviously may serve as adjuvants to the standard neuroophthalmologic and ophthalmologic evaluation of the postconcussive patient by detecting subtle abnormalities that may not be apparent with bedside assessment. The exact neuropathologic correlates of eye movement disorders after mild brain injury have yet to be clarified; however, the major brain centers involved in normal eye movement have been elucidated.[171]

Autonomic nervous system evaluation (ANSE) has been suggested only recently as a neurodiagnostic modality in postconcussive patients. Lehrer demonstrated abnormal physiologic responsiveness in brain-injured adults during cognitive testing.[169] A more recent study demonstrating poor physiologic modulation of task performance after mild brain injury proposed a "physiological response battery," including frontal electromyography, electrodermal response, heart rate, finger pulse, finger temperature, and respiratory rate as well as a visual analog scale for measuring distress.[107] Further work is necessary to clarify the diagnostic utility of ANSE in postconcussive patients. The obvious implications for medical treatment relate to biofeedback training and potential pharmacologic interventions for patients with an aberrant ANSE.

Polysomnography also may prove useful in objectively quantifying and documenting alterations in sleep after concussive brain injury. Numerous investigators have shown alterations in rapid eye movement (REM) sleep,[230] decreased stage 1 sleep with a greater number of awakenings compared with controls,[222] and fragmented sleep with frequent awakenings and lack of dreaming.[57] Some investigators believe that although no finding in polysomnographic evaluation is pathognomonic, a complex of findings seem to be common, including maintenance insomnia, sleep architecture alterations with increased slow-wave sleep and decreased stage II and REM sleep, and failure of REM periods to increase and of sleep latency periods to decrease through the night.[107] Polysomnography also can demonstrate other conditions that may follow concussive brain injury, including sleep apnea, both central and peripheral; nocturnal myoclonus; restless leg syndrome; posttraumatic nocturnal seizures; and narcolepsy. In this author's opinion, polysomnography should be reserved for patients who are intractable to sleep hygiene education and/or pharmacologic intervention—unless there is strong clinical suspicion of a rare posttraumatic nocturnal disorder or medicolegal documentation is needed.

Several investigators have examined evoked potentials as a means of quantifying neural dysfunction and attempting to correlate abnormalities with postconcussive symptoms. Only a few studies examine the utility of multimodal evoked potentials (MEPs) in postconcussive patients. The literature indicates that auditory brainstem responses (ABRs) may be abnormal in 10–40% of patients after mild brain injury.[19,201,229,232,291] ABR results, however, have generally been inconsistent, and most studies demonstrate no statistically significant correlation of abnormal evoked potentials with postconcussive symptoms. The best study examining longitudinal evoked potentials in mild brain injury found a low incidence of abnormalities in patients tested by ABRs within the first 48 hours after injury. Of interest, there was no particular pattern on retesting 1 month later; in fact, some results were worse.[247] A recent study by Aleksanov et al.[4] noted that with 15 days after injury two-thirds of patients had decreased rates of conduction along the acoustic pathway of the brainstem, as assessed by short-latency evoked potentials.[4] Other studies have found no consistent correlation of ABRs with the prognosis of postconcussional symptoms.[244,246] Green et al. noted the potential utility of electronic brain imaging (EBI) in PCD.[103] A recent study examining multimodal evoked potential (MMEP) testing after acute injury (within 2 weeks) found no evidence to support the use of MMEPs in the documentation or prognosis of neurophysiologic deficits after mild brain injury.[291] One should carefully assess the literature related to MMEP for methodologic issues, such as the standards used for defining "abnormal" results and the timing of testing (the earlier the test, the more likely it is to be abnormal). Based on the available information, this author does not advocate general MMEP screening of postconcussive patients, particularly in the postacute period. This recommendation does not negate the appropriate use of select EP studies in patients with specific posttraumatic sequelae (e.g., dizziness, visual problems).

Cognitive evoked potentials (CEPs) and the P-300 wave have been studied to a limited extent in patients with mild brain injury. CEPs have been described in detail elsewhere for readers interested in the more technical aspects.[67] Normal amplitude and latency of the P-300 wave rely indirectly on the speed of information delivery, orientation, signal detection, stimulus evaluation time, and decision making.[221] CEPs are thought to be generated in response to attended, infrequent, task-relevant stimuli, thereby providing a neurophysiologic marker of disordered cognition. Several studies suggest that the P-300 response may be a marker for cerebral pathology; however, an abnormal P-300 is not pathognomonic for cerebral concussion, because it may be seen in dementing illnesses and aging.[71,214,221,227] Although further research is needed to clarify the exact role of CEPs after mild brain injury, the P-300 response may provide useful information about attentional processes, under both active and passive testing conditions, after concussive brain injury.

Professionals should have a clear understanding that neurodiagnostic procedures are not the penultimate tool to guide diagnosis and treatment. On the contrary, the information garnered from such tests should be used as an adjuvant to good clinical judgment, which ultimately dictates decisions about diagnosis and treatment.

Postconcussive neurologic deficits have been fairly well documented, although the literature is scattered through practically every discipline of medicine. Although grossly obvious neurologic sequelae of mild brain injury are rare, subtle but otherwise significant deficits occur with some frequency and should be assessed and treated appropriately.

Seizures are a relatively rare posttraumatic sequela of mild brain injury. The incidence of posttraumatic seizures is significantly higher in children than in adults; most cases occur in young children (i.e., less than 5 years of age) within the first 24 hours after injury. Most early pediatric seizures are not associated with an increased risk for future development of epilepsy.[59] Jennett's data indicate an incidence rate of 12% for late posttraumatic epilepsy (more than 1 seizure later than the first week after injury) in patients who experienced posttraumatic amnesia for less than 24 hours.[145] For the typical postconcussive patient with no risk factors (e.g., early seizures, subdural hematoma, focal cortical contusion, depressed skull fracture), the risk of late posttraumatic epilepsy is extremely low (less than 5%). In the first 1–2 years after injury, an occasional, patient may experience episodes that are suspicious for mild focal seizures but generally remit with time. More recent data suggest that the incidence is in fact much lower than Jennett previously calculated (closer to 1%).[62,296]

Cranial nerve deficits may occur after TBI of any degree of severity; however, dysfunction of cranial nerve I seems to be the most common problem after mild brain injury. Although there are no specific medical treatments for posttraumatic anosmia, numerous rehabilitative issues can and should be addressed, including compensatory strategies for activities of daily living, safety, and vocational and avocational pursuits.[303] Several chemosensory evaluation centers accept patients for objective verification of olfactory or gustatory dysfunction after MTBI (Table 2). Injury to the optic nerve is relatively rare in brain injury of any severity and especially rare after mild brain injury; however, it does occur, particularly with supraorbital and frontal impact, and should be evaluated in patients with visual complaints.[231,278] Oculomotor dysfunction secondary to third, fourth, or sixth nerve palsy may accompany MTBI.[156] Extraocular muscle paralysis secondary to cranial nerve injury typically shows good spontaneous recovery, particularly in patients with unilateral sixth nerve palsies and, to a lesser degree, unilateral fourth nerve palsies.[18] Surgical intervention should generally not be considered until 12 months after injury. Orthoptic intervention with Fresnel lenses[307] should be the early intervention of choice (as opposed to patching) for posttraumatic diplopia because it preserves binocular vision and thereby maintains more normal visual fields and depth

TABLE 2.   Chemosensory Clinics

Chemosensory Clinical Research Center
Monell Chemical Senses Center
3500 Market Street
Philadelphia, PA 19104-3308

Clinical Olfactory Research Center
SUNY Health Science Center at Syracuse
766 Irving Avenue
Syracuse, NY 13210

Connecticut Chemosensory Clinical Research Center
University of Connecticut Health Center
Farmington, CT 06032

MCV Taste and Smell Clinic
Virginia Commonwealth University
Medical College of Virginia Hospitals
Richmond, VA 23298-0551

Nasal Dysfunction Clinic
University of California, San Diego
Medical Center
225 Dickinson Street
San Diego, CA 92103

National Institute of Dental Research
National Institutes of Health
NIH Building 10, Room 1N-114
Bethesda, MD 20892

Rocky Mountain Taste and Smell Center
University of Colorado Health Science Center
4200 East Ninth Avenue
Denver, CO 80262

University of Cincinnati Taste and Smell Center
University of Cincinnati College of Medicine
231 Bethesda Avenue
Cincinnati, OH 45267-0528

University of Pennsylvania Smell and Taste Center
Hospital of University of Pennsylvania
3400 Spruce Street
Philadelphia, PA 19104-4283

perception. Botulinum injection into the antagonist of the paretic muscle also may be used in the interim period instead of surgery.[203] Less frequently, nuclear and supranuclear lesions may produce oculomotor disturbances. Divergence and convergence dysfunctions are not uncommon after mild brain injury.[236,213] Accommodative spasm, a rare clinical finding in this population, has been associated with psychiatric disorders, although some clinicians have claimed an association with organic brain dysfunction. Diplopia may occur after mild brain injury secondary to subtle cranial nerve palsies, breakdown of an underlying heterophoria, or extraocular muscle entrapment due to orbital fractures.

As noted above, cranial nerve VII is seldom injured centrally, but quite commonly damaged peripherally in association with temporal skull fractures; appropriate protection of the cornea is a must in such cases. Damage of cranial nerve VIII may result in sensorineural hearing loss (SNHL). A recent study found that 20% of patients with mild brain injury demonstrated conductive and sensorineural hearing loss; sensorineural loss affected mainly the high frequencies.[1] The prognosis for SNHL is universally poor. Progressive hearing loss in posttraumatic patients suggests either perilymphatic fistula or endolymphatic hydrops.[179] Dizziness after MTBI occurs rarely on a central basis and is generally peripheral in origin.[64] Cranial nerves V, IX, X, XI, and XII are seldom centrally injured in MTBI.

Postconcussive patients also may experience sensitivity to light and sound.[288] Clinicians commonly encounter such "vague" symptoms, which can be treated in a compensatory manner by prescription of transmittance absorptive lenses for photophobia (sensitivity to light)[278] and earplugs for phonophobia/sonophobia (sensitivity to sound).[57] Bohnen and colleagues performed one of the most methodologically sound studies of visual and acoustic hyperesthesia after MTBI. They found that as a group, patients were significantly less tolerant than controls to stimulus intensities of 71 dB and 500 lux.[35]

Sleep disturbance is seemingly quite common after concussive brain injury. Parsons and Ver Beek examined sleep-wake cycle disturbances in 75 postconcussive patients and found multiple alterations relative to pre-injury status, including: poorer sleep maintenance, more trouble getting back to sleep after awakening, longer periods of sleep and "wake-up" time on arising, fewer and less vivid dreams, and decreased sleep quality.[215] Kowatch recommended a treatment protocol that includes a thorough history, medication review, sleep hygiene measures, pharmacologic intervention, and, as necessary, polysomnographic evaluation, with a mean sleep latency test (MSLT) to assess objectively daytime somnolence.[157] Pharmacologic treatment may be necessary to normalize sleep-wake cycles as well as to improve daytime functional status. Studies have shown that normal sleep is mediated by two neurochemical systems: 5-hydroxytryptamine (5-HT) and norepinephrine/dopamine.[38] Sleep initiation problems are best treated with serotonergic agonists such as trazodone hydrochloride,[108] whereas sleep maintenance problems should be addressed with noradrenergic antidepressant medications such as nortriptyline.

Balance disorders and coordination problems are commonly seen in patients with MTBI. Most clinical experience indicates that incoordination is of a higher level and not necessarily apparent on bedside testing unless more sophisticated tests are used. Frontal lobe dysfunction may present with ipsilateral or bilateral impairment of motor integration on tasks such as fist-palm, fist-slap-chop, and the Mandrake test.[108] As noted earlier, posttraumatic inner ear problems may cause balance dysfunction and always should be considered, particularly in patients with dizziness; the clinician must keep in mind that vestibular dysfunction is sometimes "silent."[205] Sensory integration deficits may explain the majority of postconcussive balance problems; however, referral for balance assessment with posturographic evaluation and/or neurootologic examination should be considered as deemed appropriate.

Rare neurologic sequelae also have been reported in association with MTBI. Posttraumatic tremor may be delayed in onset and is typically of a mixed nature, demonstrating both postural and kinetic components.[24] Posttraumatic tremor has been treated with a number of pharmacologic agents, including clonazepam, propranolol, serotonergic agonists, and valproate.[306] Other types of movement disorder after mild brain injury include choreoathetosis[100] and dystonia.[65] Neuroendocrine dysfunction also has been reported in the form of diabetes insipidus.[36,300] Finally, cerebellar concussion, a rare clinical entity that typically is transient in nature and theoretically results from conjoint traumatic and ischemic events, has also been described.[94]

Neurobehavioral Dysfunction

Behavioral dysfunction is probably among the most challenging posttraumatic sequelae for clinicians, family, significant other(s), and patient on a day-to-day basis. Treatment should be multidimensional and include psychological, pharmacological, and patient/family training, counseling, and education. Differentiation between primary and secondary behavioral conditions is important to understanding implications for treatment as well as prognosis. Only recently has the issue of postconcussive disorder begun to be considered as a potential diagnostic category in the Diagnostic and Statistical Manual of Mental Disorders; however, it remains to some extent controversial.[4] The neuroscience community has begun no transdisciplinary effort to define MTBI behaviorally or otherwise.

An important diagnostic issue, unfortunately often missed by treating clinicians, is the distinction between PCD sequelae and posttraumatic stress disorder (PTSD). Despite the many parallels in their presentation, both treatment and prognosis involve significant differences. PTSD is a DSM-IV psychiatric diagnosis defined as an emotional reaction to a traumatic life event.[6] The severity of the condition is to a large extent dictated by pre- and postinjury psychological factors. PTSD symptoms include cognitive, affective, and somatic components,[183] much like postconcussive symptoms; however, the profile is different, as is the response to therapeutic intervention. Cognitive symptoms typically include attention and concentration problems, memory problems, and loss of the ability to sequence temporally. From an affective standpoint, the typical patient presents with an increased startle response, abulia, apathy, hypervigilance, and

generalized anxiety.[63] Sbordone recently noted that patients with MTBI who are amnestic for their injury "by definition" cannot develop PTSD.[241] Clearly, however, patients who lose consciousness and develop PTSD on the basis of recollections outside their amnestic timeframe or patients with no amnesia may indeed develop PTSD. Specific guidelines have been suggested for evaluating PTSD in a medicolegal context and for delineating potential malingers.[261]

Patients with PTSD tend to report persistent reliving of the event, including nightmares, avoidance of thoughts or feelings associated with the injury, and disturbed sleep.[108] On many occasions the differentiation between these two diagnostic entities is difficult, thereby stressing the importance of having a skilled psychiatrist as part of the treatment continuum. Treatment of PTSD and/or associated cognitive deficits is not analogous to brain injury related neurobehavioral sequelae. PTSD is best treated with psychotherapeutic intervention and adjuvant drugs such as tricyclic antidepressants, selective serotonergic reuptake inhibitors, valproic acid, and beta blockers, depending on the specific behavioral profile. A recent technique for PTSD treatment that has found both critics and advocates is eye movement desensitization reprocessing (EMDR).[285] Of interest, the incidence of PTSD has been found to be quite high in patients with chronic "posttraumatic headache."[50] This finding calls into question the true cause of the headache—physical trauma vs. secondary psychiatric response. Supporting a psychiatric element is recent research by Schreiber and Galai-Gat,[249] who noted that uncontrolled pain after physical injury may be at the core of PTSD. This theory further supports the general rehabilitation practice of early pain control in posttraumatic patients. Blanchard et al.[31] followed 98 victims of car accidents for development of PTSD symptoms. They found that among the patients who initially met the criteria for PTSD, avoidance and numbing symptoms declined significantly by 6-month follow-up, whereas most of the hyperarousal symptoms showed no significant decline.[31]

Pharmacologic intervention has been used for a multitude of posttraumatic sequelae

(Table 3), but no use has been more common than adjuvant therapy for behavioral management. As a general rule, pharmacotherapy should be used judiciously because of its potential for compromising cognitive function and retarding neural recovery. Responsible treatment demands a thorough understanding of neuropsychopharmacology. There is no doubt that certain agents may facilitate cognitive processes, whereas others may be inhibitory.[304] In addition, when used appropriately, drugs may serve as significant adjuvants to facilitate the rate of neural recovery. Anticonvulsants, such as carbamazepine and valproate, may be useful in addressing neurobehavioral sequelae such as severe emotional dyscontrol. Appropriate monitoring of drug levels, potential toxicities, and clinical response is critical.

Sleep disturbances, particularly disturbances of sleep initiation, may be treated with serotonergic agents such as trazodone; of interest, whether as a result of "good" sleep or the serotonergic agonism of the drug, patients commonly report improvements in daytime anxiety, irritability, and emotional lability.[108] Patients who are anxious and akathesic, with mild depressive symptoms, tend to do well with buspirone, a novel nonbenzodiazepine anxiolytic with antidepressant properties.[109] Prior research has shown that postconcussive patients are indeed at increased risk for depression.[8,240,245] Investigators have demonstrated that patients with PCD-related depression show a blunted prolactin response to buspirone, possibly suggesting a useful endocrine marker for postconcussive depression.[198] The investigators also hypothesized

TABLE 3. Pharmacologic Interventions for Common Posttraumatic Sequelae

Common Posttraumatic Sequelae	Pharmacologic Intervention
Anxiety	Serotonergic agonists: buspirone, sertraline, paroxetine, trazodone
Basilar artery migraine (BAM)	Antimigraine regimens psychotropic anticonvulsants
Cognitive dysfunction	Nootropes, catecholaminergic agonists, cholinergic agonists and/or precursors, neuropeptides,* vasoactive agents*
Depression	Tricyclic antidepressants (TCAs), selective serotonin reuptake inhibitors (SSRIs), venlafaxine, monoamine oxidase inhibitors (MAOIs), lithium carbonate, carbamazepine
Emotional lability and/or irritability	SSRIs, psychotropic anticonvulsants, TCAs, lithium carbonate, trazodone

Fatigue	Catecholaminergic agonists:
	    Methylphenidate
	    Amantadine
	    Dextroamphetamine
	Caffeine

Libidinal alteration:
    Decreased
    Increased
	Noradrenergic agonists, hormone replacement if low to borderline low
	SSRIs, trazodone, hormones—cyproterone or medroxyprogesterone acetate

Myofascial pain/dysfunction	NSAIDs, TCAs, SSRIs, mild muscle relaxants, capsaicin
Neuralgic and neuritic pain	Capsaicin, TCAs, SSRIs (?), carbamazepine and other antiepileptic drugs, NSAIDs, local anesthetic blockade
Posttraumatic stress disorder	Antidepressant medications, psychotropic anticonvulsants, propranolol, clonidine, MAOIs, lithium, benzodiazepines
Sleep initiation problems	Serotonergic agonists—trazodone, doxepin, amitriptyline
Sleep maintenance problems	Catecholaminergic agonists—nortriptyline
Tinnitus	Gingko biloba,* tocainide,* anti-migraine medications*

Vascular headache	Antimigraine regimens:
	    Symptomatic
	    Abortive
	    Prophylactic
	Atypical agents: valproic acid

* Questionable efficacy.
Modified from J Head Trauma Rehabil 8(3):21, 1993.

altered serotonergic function in postconcussive patients, which would provide further rationale for pharmacologic intervention to normalize the neurochemical environment.

At least in theory, one also would expect alterations in catecholaminergic function after mild brain injury. In practice, some of the neurobehavioral sequelae seem to correlate with a relative catecholaminergic deficiency based on their inherent nature and response to treatment with psychostimulants. Anergia and easy fatigability, abulia, inattention, and memory problems may respond to such drugs as methylphenidate or amantadine.

As a rule, personality changes tend to involve exacerbation of preexisting traits. This clinical picture may result to a large extent from damage to frontal and axial structures that are intimately involved with behavioral regulation. Several personality disorders may be amenable, at least to some degree, to treatment with psychopharmacologic agents.[284]

Sexual dysfunction also may be reported after mild brain injury.[155,161] Typically, postconcussive complaints center on reduced libido; however, problems with erectile function, orgasm, and vaginal lubrication also may be seen. First, the clinician must ensure that no significant posttraumatic affective component is presenting in part as sexual dysfunction. Secondly, appropriate neuroendocrine screens should be performed if primary or secondary hypothalmic-pituitary-gonadal dysfunction is suspected.[132] Male patients with complaints of erectile dysfunction may benefit from nocturnal penile tumescence (NPT) monitoring to assist in differentiation of organic and functional erectile disturbance.[302] Rehabilitative interventions for posttraumatic sexual dysfunction should always be discussed with the patient and significant other.[302,311]

Alcohol probably should be avoided in the acute and subacute recovery period for a multiplicity of reasons.[305] In addition, stimulants such as nicotine and caffeine may be relatively contraindicated in hypervigilant or irritable postconcussive patients. Conversely, natural stimulants such as caffeine may be used as psychopharmacologic agents in anergic, abulic, easily fatigable patients.[209]

Numerous other neuropsychiatric sequelae have been reported after mild brain injury, including mania,[264] depersonalization[105] and Capgras' syndrome.[26] Clearly, chronic pain issues, whether associated with posttraumatic headache or other conditions, must be factored into the analysis of postinjury behavior, along with cognitive complaints.[7,113,195] Clinicians should be aware that theoretically any DSM-IV condition may result from MTBI.[193] Familiarity with the neurobehavioral consequences of mild brain injury is critical if one is to offer appropriate intervention, both nonpharmacologic and pharmacologic.[108,210] Adequate neuropsychological and neuropsychiatric resources are essential in dealing with such posttraumatic deficits.

PEDIATRIC POSTCONCUSSIVE DISORDERS

The prevalence and long-term neuromedical and neuropsychological sequelae of MTBI and PCD have not been well studied in children. In general, studies suggest that in patients older than 2 years who are neurologically normal and without signs of depressed or basilar skull fracture, no CT scan is needed, even with an associated loss of consciousness.[66] One study proposed a possible link between occult brain injury, not necessarily leading to hospital admission, and various developmental disabilities in children, including hyperactivity, stuttering, mixed handedness, and aversion to mathematics.[251] A prospective study demonstrated that hospitalized adolescents with mild brain injury exhibited impairment mainly on measures of verbal learning, abstraction, and reasoning.[17] In their study of 53 children with MTBI and matched controls, Polissar et al. noted that a spectrum of neurobehavioral skills were affected weakly by MTBI.[218] A major controversy that continues to plague researchers as well as clinicians involved in forensic testimony is how, if at all, children with MTBI may exhibit "delayed expression" of deficits as a result of premature plateau of cognitive and personality maturity and physiologic developmental deficits.[212] Jaffe et al. reported that children with MTBI exhibited negligible deficits or change in performance during a 3-year follow-up study.[141] Further studies are obviously needed to clarify the long-term sequelae, if any, of MTBI in children.

TREATMENT ISSUES

Clearly, domain-specific therapy evaluations are needed to assess accurately the magnitude of subjective functional complaints. In addition, tried-and-true bedside clinical evaluation and appropriate neurodiagnostic testing are the foundation for the neuromedical and rehabilitative assessment that must precede specific recommendations for treatment.

Psychoemotional responses to injury must be acknowledged and managed, given their obvious contribution to symptoms in most patients. Appropriate psychological services to address such issues as symptom education, stress management, adjustment counseling, and psychotherapy are paramount.[150]

The following general recommendations can be made for assessment and treatment of patients with MTBI. Patients should be provided with compensatory strategies for executive function deficits by appropriate referrals to cognitive therapists (e.g., psychologists, occupational therapists, speech/language pathologists).

Adaptive strategies for higher-level activities of daily living should be pursued through occupational therapy. The patient's awareness of specific deficits should be emphasized, and "social rules" should be relearned to address higher-level linguistic deficits. An increase in awareness of functional performance should be stressed to facilitate implementation of individualized compensatory strategies.

As appropriate, cognitive remediation and retraining should be prescribed by the treating physician.[191] A neurologic physical therapist should treat higher-level balance deficits with vestibular habituation training and functional balance retraining as indicated. Referral for physical therapy may be appropriate for various sequelae of cranial trauma and CAD injury. Chiropractic and/or osteopathic referral may be appropriate if the treating clinician is not familiar with manual medicine diagnosis and treatment techniques, including high-impulse mobilization for posttraumatic cervical somatic dysfunction.[61] Of interest, although much evidence is of an empirical nature, craniosacral evaluation has demonstrated significant pathology in terms of low cranial rhythmic impulse and cranial strain patterns in patients with PCD.[104] Rehabilitative approaches to the patient with CAD injury are reviewed in Table 4.

A comprehensive neuropsychological evaluation should be performed to assess objective evidence of higher-level cognitive-behavioral, linguistic, and motor dysfunctions, which typically are not evident on bedside evaluation. Such evaluations also provide a basis for provision of compensatory strategies to both patient and family. Thorough physiatric and neuromedical assessment and treatment of sequelae related to MTBI vs. cranial adnexal trauma vs. CAD injury should be instituted as early as possible. The physician should prescribe pharmacologic agents in an appropriate manner to assist in facilitating neural, neuromusculoskeletal, and functional recovery (see Table 3). Clinicians should avoid drug prescriptions that may interfere with cognitive-behavioral recovery.[306,310] Appropriate instruction should be given about avoidance of alcohol early after injury. During the early recovery stages, patients should be encouraged to optimize diet, structure daily activities, and minimize controllable external stressors. Sleep hygiene education should be emphasized to optimize sleep efficiency and duration. Staged reentry into preinjury activities, including driving as well as vocational and avocational pursuits, is dictated by patient and family report as well as assessment findings.[310] Vocational rehabilitation is paramount for patients with more significant cognitive, behavioral, and/or physical disability. Patient and family education about MTBI and associated injuries, including basic pathophysiology, recovery course, and prognosis, should be an integral part of any comprehensive rehabilitation effort.[162] Supportive counseling services should be provided as indicated to deal with expected issues of emotional adjustment.

DETERMINATION OF ORGANICITY IN POSTCONCUSSIVE DISORDERS

Nonorganic contributions to the presenting condition, such as malingering, factitious disorders, somatoform disorders, and injury-related psychoemotional and psychiatric disorders (e.g,. PTSD, reactive depression) should be thoroughly explored.[234] Clinicians should

TABLE 4. Treatment Interventions for Cervical Acceleration/Deceleration Injury

Treatment Intervention	Description
Cervical passive mobilization techniques	Massage, muscle stretching, traction, manipulation, and passive joint mobilization
Cervicothoracic muscular stabilization techniques	Stabilization training: mobility, stability, flexibility, postural reeducation, exercise
Thermotherapy	Superficial heat, diathermy, cold (ice massage/ice packs), ultrasound, vapocoolant sprays
Intermittent cervical traction	30° neck flexion; 15–30 pounds with evidence of radiculopathy
Medications	NSAIDs, muscle relaxants. Avoid narcotic analgesics except for brief period during acute postinjury phase.
Trigger point injections	Sterile water, local anesthetic with or without steroids, dry needling
Bedrest	Early and only after severe injuries
Cervical zygapophyseal joint injections	Intraarticular local anesthetic or via blockade of the joint dorsal rami
Neural blockade	Occipital nerves and/or cervical epidural block
Correct any promulgating factors for myofascial pain	Postural issues, occlusal imbalance, leg length discrepancy, small hemipelvis, and short upper arms
Denervation and ablation procedures	Percutaneous denervation procedures, open neurectomy, and discectomy fusion
Manual medicine techniques	High velocity, low amplitude
Massage	Temporary benefit for pain relief
Exercise	Emphasize stretching and progressive increase in endurance
Transcutaneous electrical stimulation	For pain management
Education	Regarding disease process, prognosis and treatment goals
Cervical collars	Should not be prolonged and/or chronic. Need to wean.

be familiar with base-rate literature as it relates to postconcussive complaints.[166] Practitioners should not minimize or negate the validity of subjective complaints simply on the basis of incidence statistics. It is also important to compare the frequency, severity, and associated functional disability of the patient's postinjury subjective complaint with preinjury parameters. Solid evidence suggests that "naive subjects" are relatively good at endorsing symptoms on checklists for major depression and generalized anxiety disorder (96.9%) and PTSD (86%) as delineated in DSM-IIIR; 63.3% were able to identify 5 or more of 10 postconcussive symptoms.[167] Clearly, such data may lead clinicians away from the common practice of "patient checklists," which may generate examinee response bias.

Neuropsychological evaluation is a critical component in the evaluation of persons with MTBI, including determination of organicity. In addition, neuropsychological testing provides potentially critical medicolegal information that can be temporally followed to demonstrate initial and subsequent profiles

consistent with those seen after similar injuries. Examining neuropsychologists commonly make the following faux pas that may result in incorrect diagnoses in patients with presumptive MTBI:

1. Failure to consider preinjury intellectual functioning in relation to postinjury data. Educational and/or military records should be reviewed. Assessment must be made in relation to standardized scores; if they are not available, data should be corrected for the patient's age, education, and demographic characteristics (e.g., Heaton norms, Barona regression equation).

2. Failure to include unbiased collateral informants who can testify to pre- and/or postinjury status.

3. Adequate acknowledgement of preinjury medical and psychological history, including prior TBI.

4. Failure to consider factors potentially affecting test performance (e.g., psychoemotional issues, pain, vestibular symptoms).

5. Failure to use actuarial cut-off scores and norm-referenced actuarial methods to

support the diagnosis of organic brain dysfunction (e.g., T-scores, average impairment units, percentile ranks).

6. Failure to examine measures of validity, simulation, and/or dissimulation in the evaluation (e.g., validity measures on the Minnesota Multiphasic Personality Inventory, such as F-K score and subtle vs. obvious scores; malingering tests, such as forced-choice testing [e.g., Portland Digit Recognition], Rey 15-item memory test).

7. Failure to give adequate consideration to the initial degree of neurologic insult (as indicated by GCS score, duration of posttraumatic amnesia, and altered level of consciousness) or failure to correlate these parameters with severity and onset of symptoms and impairment.

8. Failure to analyze the pattern of change (if serial testing was performed) for consistency with anticipated recovery curves after central neurologic insult.

9. Failure to note the effects of medication—both positive and negative—on test performance.

10. Failure to assess the pattern of reported symptoms, their consistency with expected subjective reports after injuries of equal magnitude, correlation with neuropsychological test results, and temporal onset in relation to injury.

Clinicians evaluating litigating patients or, for that matter, patients with any type of potential secondary gain must be familiar with assessing nonorganic symptoms, both neurologic and musculoskeletal. Various procedures and clinical findings—such as Waddell's signs, Hoover's test, astasia-abasia, patchy or midline sensory loss, normal backwards gait with abnormal forward gait, and nonpronator drift—may increase the index of suspicion of a nonorganic condition.

In general, clinicians can best assess veracity by looking for telltale test-taking behaviors, analyzing performance in relation to test-item difficulty, evaluating test performance patterns, and becoming familiar with diagnostic procedures for the array of subjective complaints that may occur in patients with PCD.

Finally, familiarity with techniques for assessment of malingering may help in the evaluation of patient veracity and/or true organicity.[28,200] Clinicians, however, must keep in mind that there are only two ways to determine definitively that the patient is malingering: direct acknowledgment by the patient and direct or indirect observation by the clinician that the patient can do things that he or she denies the ability to do. Malingering tests are only tools that may increase the level of suspicion of nonorganicity, dissimulation, or symptom embellishment.

PROGNOSTICATION

Rehabilitationists must remain aware of how outcome and functional performance may be modified by a number of factors, including age, socioeconomic status, quality of family system, degree of anxiety and depression, symptom magnification, preinjury personality, pre- and postinjury psychiatric status, presence of litigation issues, potential for malingering, use (past or present) of drugs and alcohol, and chronic pain.

Prognoses must be made with specific impairments in mind. Each impairment typically has a different prognosis based on time to maximal medical improvement (MMI). Albeit rare, posttraumatic epilepsy has a different prognosis from other MTBI-related neurologic impairments, such as anosmia, tremor, and vascular headache.[84]

Functional prognosis must be considered separately from any and all neurologic prognoses. The presence of neurologic impairment after MTBI by no means rules out the possibility of full functional reentry into community, vocational, and avocational roles.[80] In general, negative prognostic factors for MTBI include older age, poor preinjury psychoemotional adjustment or intellectual status, and prior brain injury.[306] Fenton found that in a relatively small group of people with PCD (n = 45), chronic problems were more common in those who had more social difficulties before injury and in older women.[86] Multiple studies have examined the long-term outcome of MTBI relative to cognitive, behavioral, and vocational reentry. The conclusions of recent investigators about the risks for permanency of functional disability after MTBI are somewhat disparate.[37,173,184] In the author's opinion, no final neuromedical or functional prognoses should be made in patients with established MTBI until at least 18–24 months after injury, given the long-term nature of impairment in a small, albeit significant, number of patients.[34] The literature about cervical acceleration/deceleration injury suggests that approximately 60% of patients make a complete recovery, whereas approximately 8% are disabled to the point that they are unable to maintain employment.[12] Most patients reach a plateau by 1 year after injury.[96,183] The risk of disk rupture of sufficient magnitude to require surgical intervention has been estimated on the order of 0.5% of CAD injuries.[114] Duration of symptoms appears to be the most accurate prognostic factor, followed by symptom distribution; upper limb involvement is a particularly poor prognostic indicator.[12] The role of radiographic findings in prognostication remains controversial. Little evidence supports the claim that acute changes, other than in patients with preexisting cervical disease, are a poor prognostic indicator per se. Conversely, the absence of acute changes is not necessarily a harbinger of functional recovery.[12,237] The role of psychosocial stressors in recovery remains somewhat controversial.[224]

Litigation and psychological issues can definitely affect the course of recovery after MTBI, CAD injury, and cranial trauma. Many investigators have sought links between symptom persistence and ongoing litigation without success.[151,182] Kay noted that people in litigation are likely to report more symptoms, to have persistent symptoms, and not to return to work as quickly as people not involved in litigation.[151] Rutherford correctly points out that this observation may be related to negative effects of litigation or simply to the fact that people with more functional disability tend to be more likely to pursue litigation.[235] The process of litigation, at least from an experiential standpoint, tends to heighten and perpetuate symptoms in MTBI as well as associated injuries such as whiplash; whether this is a means of direct secondary gain or simply a result of the negative consequence of additional stress on an already over-stressed organism is unclear. Clinicians should realize that the incidence of gross malingering, a very different phenomenon, is probably low, although this issue has not been well studied in patients with either MTBI or CAD injury.[160]

MEDICOLEGAL CAVEATS

Medicolegal issues are quite common in postconcussive patients, in part because of the litigious nature of society and in part because of sincere efforts on the part of the injured person to get reasonable restitution. Although many of the conditions reviewed in this chapter are uncommon sequelae of brain or head injury, the medical and legal communities must keep in mind that they can and do occur. In addition, many of the more common and obvious posttraumatic sequelae often are misdiagnosed or remain undiagnosed by less sophisticated health care professionals. At the same time, the medical and legal systems must be aware that secondary gain, malingering, chronic pain, and pre- and postinjury psychological or psychiatric disorders may affect subjective symptoms. Furthermore, overly ambitious, albeit well-meaning, practitioners may overdiagnose the condition. Naivete aside, one must concede that some "injured" persons may indeed be coached by legal counsel about the "correct" postconcussional symptoms to maximize monetary settlement. Given the above pitfalls, the author recommends careful scrutiny for contributing factors, conscious and otherwise, as well as methodical neuromedical assessment before labeling any patient with a diagnosis that may affect negatively functional status and potential for community reintegration.

It is also important to understand the discrete differences between impairment and disability rating in both clinical and medicolegal contexts. All too often inexperienced clinicians confuse the two tasks and provide AMA impairment ratings when asked to do a disability evaluation. Several recent publications deal quite comprehensively with this topic.[125,312]

Multiple diagnostic tests may not be ordered for patients who do not have a medicolegal case—solely for the reason that the results would not alter patient management. When litigation is pursued, attempts to quantify and objectively document posttraumatic sequelae may be desired. As a rule, the earlier patients are sent for evaluation, the higher the yield in terms of abnormal results, regardless of the test. In general, clinical experience and available research data suggest that final neuromedical or functional prognoses should not be made until at least 18–24 months after injury unless *full* neurologic and functional recovery have already occurred.

CONCLUSIONS

It would be naive to think that chronic impairments due to mild brain injury do not result in emotional and psychological reactions on the part of the injured person as well as the family. Some of these reactions may be adaptive, whereas others may indeed be maladaptive—not to the fault of the patient per se but rather as a consequence of specific neuropathology and impairments. Physicians must remain sensitive to the neuropsychiatric, neuropsychological, and psychological aspects of mild brain injury to address such issues as they arise. Clinicians also must not minimize the importance of counseling[20] and education in patients with mild brain injury. One of the most critical components of education is prevention, particularly in view of the statistics on recurrent brain injury. An adequate continuum of clinical care for patients with mild brain injury should include resources for patients and families to deal with the above issues.[162]

Skilled physiatrists may play an integral part in this process, given their knowledge of functional assessment, rehabilitation medicine, neurology, musculoskeletal medicine, psychiatry, and internal medicine. Because of the complexity and variety of postconcussive neuromedical sequelae, an organized system of knowledgeable neuromedical follow-up is critical to ensure appropriate and timely intervention, rehabilitation, and, one hopes, staged reintegration into the community and workplace.

REFERENCES

1. Abd al-Hady MR, Shehata O, el-Mously M, Sallam FS: Audiological findings following head trauma. J Laryngol Otol 104(12)927–936, 1990.
2. Aihara N, Hall JJ, Pitts LH, Fukuda K, Noble LJ: Altered immunoexpression of microglia and macrophages after mild head injury. J Neurotrauma 12:53–63, 1995.
3. al-Qurainy IA: Convergence insufficiency and failure of accommodation following midfacial trauma. Br J Oral Maxillofac Surg. 33(2):71–75, 1995.
4. Aleksanov NS, Shchigolev IuS, Gizatullin ShKh: [Short-latency brain-stem auditory evoked potentials in patients with a brain concussion.] Zh Vopr Neirokhir Im N N Burdenko Apr-Jun:17–20, 1995.
5. American Academy of Neurology, Report of the Therapeutics and Technology Assessment Subcommittee: Assessment: Positron emission tomography. Neurology 41:163–167, 1991.
6. American Psychiatric Association: Diagnostic and Statistical Manual of Mental Disorders, 4th ed. Washington, DC, American Psychiatric Association, 1994, pp 704–706.
7. Anderson JM, Kaplan MS, Felsenthal G: Brain injury obscured by chronic pain: a preliminary report. Arch Phys Med Rehabil 71:703–708, 1990.
8. Atteberry-Bennett J, Barth JT, Loyd BH, Lawrence EC: The relationship between behavioral and cognitive deficits, demographics, and depression in patients with minor head injuries. Int J Clin Neuropsychol 8(3):114–117, 1986.
9. Bailey BN, Gudeman SK: Minor head injury. In Becker DP, Gudeman SK (eds): Textbook of Head Injury. Philadelphia, W.B. Saunders, 1990, pp 308–318.
10. Balla JI: Headache and cervical disorders: Report to the motor accidents board of Victoria on whiplash injuries. In Hopkins A (ed): Headache: Problems in Diagnosis and Management. London, Saunders, 1984, pp 256–269.
11. Baloh RW, Honrubia V: Clinical Neurophysiology of the Vestibular System, 2nd ed. Philadelphia, F.A. Davis, 1990.
12. Bannister G, Gargan M: Prognosis of whiplash injuries: A review of the literature. In Teasell RW, Shapiro AP (eds): Cervical Flexion-Extension/Whiplash Injuries. Philadelphia, Hanley & Belfus, 1993, pp 557–570.
13. Barnsley L, Lord S, Bogduk N: The pathophysiology of whiplash. In Teasell RW, Shapiro AP (eds): Flexion-Extension/Whiplash Injuries. Philadelphia, Hanley & Belfus, 1993, pp 329-353.
14. Barnsley L, Lord SM, Wallis BJ, Bogduk N: The prevalence of chronic cervical zygapophyseal joint pain after whiplash. Spine 20:20–25; 26 [discussion], 1995.
15. Barnsley L, Lord SM, Wallis BJ, Bogduk N: Lack of effect of intraarticular corticosteroids for chronic pain in the cervical zygapophyseal joints [see comments]. N Engl J Med. 330:1047–1050, 1994.
16. Barre JA: The posterior cervical sympathetic syndrome and its frequent cause: Cervical arthritis. Rev Neurol 33:1246, 1926.
17. Bassett SS, Slater EJ: Neuropsychological function in adolescents sustaining mild closed head injury. J Pediatr Psychol 15:225–236, 1990.
18. Beck RW: Ocular deviations after head injury. Am Orthop J 35:103–107, 1985.
19. Benna P, Bergamasco B, Bianco C, et al: Brainstem auditory evoked potentials in postconcussion syndrome. J Neurol Sci 3:281–287, 1982.

20. Bennett TL: Neuropsychological counseling of the adult with minor head injury. Cognit Rehabil Jan/Feb:10–16, 1987.
21. Benowitz NL: Pharmacologic aspects of cigarette smoking and nicotine addiction. N Engl J Med 319: 1318–1330, 1988.
22. Benzel EC, Lewine JD, Bucholz RD, Orrison WW Jr: Magnetic source imaging: A review of the Magnes system of biomagnetic technologies incorporated. Neurosurgery 33:252–259, 1993.
23. Bernad PG: Neurodiagnostic testing in patients with closed head injury. Clin Electroencephalogr 22(4):203-210, 1991.
24. Biary N, Cleeves L, Findley L, Koller W: Post-traumatic tremor. Neurology 39:103–106, 1989.
25. Bickerstaff ER: Basilar artery migraine. Lancet 1:15–17, 1961.
26. Bienenfeld D, Brott T: Capgras' syndrome following minor head trauma. J Clin Psychiatry 50: 68–69, 1989.
27. Bihan DL, Jezzard P, Haxby J, et al: Functional magnetic resonance imaging of the brain. Ann Intern Med 122:296–303, 1995.
28. Binder LM: Assessment of malingering after mild head trauma with the Portland Digit Recognition Test J Clin Exp Neuropsychol 15:170–182, 1993 [published erratum appears in J Clin Exp Neuropsychol 15:852, 1993].
29. Black FO, Lilly DJ, Nashner LM, et al: Quantitative diagnostic test for perilymph fistulas. Otolaryngol Head Neck Surg 96:125–134, 1987.
30. Black FO, Lilly DJ, Peterka RJ, et al: The dynamic posturographic pressure test for the presumptive diagnosis of perilymph fistulas. Neurol Clin 8:361–374, 1990.
31. Blanchard EB, Hickling EJ, Vollmer AJ, et al: Short-term follow-up of post-traumatic stress symptoms in motor vehicle accident victims. Behav Res Ther. 33:369–377, 1995.
32. Blumbergs PC, Scott G, Manavis J, et al: Staining of amyloid precursor protein to study axonal damage in mild head injury. Lancet 344:1055–1056, 1994.
33. Bogduk N, Marsland A: On the concept of third occipital headache. J Neurol Neurosurg Psychiatry 49:775–780, 1986.
34. Bohnen N, Jolles J, Twijnstra A: Neuropsychological deficits in patients with persistent symptoms six months after mild head injury. Neurosurgery 30:692–696, 1992.
35. Bohnen N, Twijnstra A, Kroeze J, Jolles J: A psychophysical method for assessing visual and acoustic hyperaesthesia in patients with mild head injury. Br J Psychiatry. 159:860–863, 1991.
36. Bohnen N, Twijnstra A, Jolles J: Water metabolism and postconcussional symptoms 5 weeks after mild head injury. Eur Neurol 33:77–79, 1993.
37. Bohnen N, Zutphen WV, Twijnstra A, et al: Late outcome of mild head injury: results from a controlled postal survey. Brain Inj 8:701–708, 1994.
38. Bonate PL: Serotonin receptor subtypes: Functional, physiological, and clinical correlates. Clin Neuropharmacol14:1–16, 1991.
39. Boquet J, Moore N, Boismare F, Monnier JC: Vertigo in post-concussional and migrainous patients: Implication of the autonomic nervous system. Agressologie 24:235–236, 1983.
40. Borczuk P: Predictors of intracranial injury in patients with mild head trauma. Ann Emerg Med 25:731–736, 1995.
41. Brandt T: Vertigo: Its Multisensory Syndromes. New York, Springer-Verlag, 1991.
42. Brandt T, Daroff RB: Physical therapy for benign paroxysmal positional vertigo. Arch Otolaryngol 106:484, 1980.
43. Briner W, House J, O'Leary M: Synthetic prostaglandin E1 misoprostol as a treatment for tinnitus. Arch Otolaryngol Head Neck Surg 119:652–654, 1993.
44. Brooke RI, LaPointe HJ: Temporomandibular joint disorders following whiplash. In Teasell RW, AP Shapiro (eds): Cervical Flexion-Extension/ Whiplash Injuries. Philadelphia, Hanley & Belfus. 1993, pp 443–454.
45. Brown SJ, Fann JR, Grant I: Postconcussional disorder: Time to acknowledge a common source of neurobehavioral morbidity. J Neuropsychiatry Clin Neurosci 6:15–22, 1994.
46. Browning GG, Swan IRC, Gatehouse S: Hearing loss in minor head injury. Arch Otolaryngol 108: 474–477, 1982.
47. Carter IR,. McCormick AQ: Whiplash shaking syndrome: Retinal hemorrhages and computerized axial tomography of the brain. Child Abuse Neglect 7:279–286, 1983.
48. Cohen LA: Body orientation and motor coordination in animals with impaired neck sensation. Fed Proc 18:28, 1959.
49. Chelen W, Kabrisky M, Hatsell C, et al: Use of phenytoin in the prevention of motion sickness. Aviat Space Environ Med Nov:1022–1025, 1990.
50. Chibnall JT, Duckro PN: Post-traumatic stress disorder in chronic post-traumatic headache patients. Headache 34:357–361, 1994.
51. Cooper PR: Skull fracture and traumatic cerebrospinal fistulas. In Cooper PR (ed): Head Injury. Baltimore, Williams & Wilkins, 1987, pp 89–107.
52. Costanzo RM, Zasler ND: Head trauma–sensorineural disorders: Diagnosis and management. In Getchell TV, Doty, RL, Bartoshuk LM, Snow JB (eds): Smell and Taste in Health and Disease. New York, Raven Press,1991, pp 711–730.
53. Costanzo RM, Zasler ND: Epidemiology and pathophysiology of olfactory and gustatory dysfunction in head trauma. J Head Trauma Rehabil 7:15–24, 1992.
54. Courjon J: Traumatic disorders. In Remond A (ed): Handbook of Electroencephalography and Clinical Neurophysiology, vol 15, pt 8. Amsterdam, Elsevier, 1972.
55. Croft AC: The case against "litigation neurosis" in mild brain injuries and cervical acceleration/deceleration trauma. J Neuromusculoskel Syst 1:149–155, 1993.
56. Cytowic R: Nerve Block for Common Pain. New York, Springer-Verlag, 1990.

57. Cytowic R, Stump DA, Larned DC: Closed head trauma: Somatic, ophthalmic, and cognitive impairments in nonhospitalized patients. In Whitaker HA (ed): Neuropsychological Studies of Nonfocal Brain Damage. New York, Springer-Verlag, 1988. pp 226–264.

58. Dacey RG, Alves WM, Rimel RW, et al: Neurosurgical complications after apparently minor head injury. Assessment of risk in a series of 610 patients. J Neurosurg 65:203–210, 1986.

59. Dacey RG, Dikmen SS: Mild head injury. In Cooper PR (ed): Head Injury. Baltimore, Williams & Wilkins, 1987, pp 125-140.

60. Daily L: Whiplash injury as one cause of the foveolar splinter and macular wisps. Arch Ophthalmol 97:360, 1979.

61. Dalby BJ: Chiropractic diagnosis and treatment of closed head trauma. J Manip Physiol Ther 16:392–400, 1993.

62. Dalmady-Israel C, Zasler ND: Post-traumatic seizures: a critical review. Brain Inj 7:263–273, 1993.

63. Davidoff DA, Kessler HR, Laibstain DF, Mark VH: Neurobehavioral sequela of minor head injury: a consideration of post-concussive syndrome versus post-traumatic stress disorder. Cognit Rehabil March/April:8–13, 1988.

64. Davies RA, Luxon LM: Dizziness following head injury: A neuro-otological study. J Neurol 242:222–30, 1995.

65. Davies E, Knox E, Donaldson I: The usefulness of nimodipine, an L-calcium channel antagonist, in the treatment of tinnitus. 28(3):125–192, 1994.

66. Davis RL, Mullen N, Makela M, et al: Cranial computed tomography scans in children after minimal head injury with loss of consciousness [see comments]. Ann Emerg Med 24:640–645, 1994.

67. Deacon-Eliott D, Campbell KB, Suffield JB, Prouix GB: Electrophysiological monitoring of closed head injury. III: Cognitive evoked potentials. Cognit Rehabil May/June:12–21, 1987.

68. Diagnostic and Statistical Manual of Mental Disorders, 4th ed. Post-concussional disorder. Washington, DC, American Psychiatric Association, 1994, pp 704– 706, 1994.

69. Dikmen S, Reitan RM, Temkin NR: Neuropsychological recovery in head injury. Arch Neurol 40:333–338, 1983.

70. Dixon CE, Taft WC, Hayes RL: Mechanisms of mild traumatic brain injury. J Head Trauma Rehabil 8(3)1–12, 1993.

71. Drake ME, John K: Long-latency auditory event-related potentials in the postconcussive syndrome. Clin Evoked Potentials 5:19–21, 1987.

72. Ducours JL, Roles C, Sangalli F, Guillet J: Craniofacial injuries and cerebral tomographic scintigraphy using N-isopropyl-iodo-amphetamine 123 I-AMP. Rev Stomato Chir Maxillofac 90(2): 89–94, 1989.

73. Duffy FH: Clinical value of topographic mapping and quantified neurophysiology. Arch Neurol 46:1133–1134, 1989.

74. Duffy FH, Hughes JR, Miranda F, Bernad P, Cook P: Status of quantitative EEG (QEEG) in clinical practice, 1994. Clin Electroencephalogr 25(4):6–22, 1994.

75. Dwyer A, Aprill C, Bogduk N: Cervical zygapophyseal joint pain patterns. I: A study in normal volunteers. Spine 15:453–457, 1990.

76. Edna T-H, Cappelen J: Late postconcussional symptoms in traumatic head injury. An analysis of frequency and risk factors. Acta Neurochir 86: 12–17, 1987.

77. El Gindi S, Salama M, Tawfik E, et al: A review of 2,000 patients with craniocerebral injuries with regard to intracranial haematomas and other vascular complications. Acta Neurochir 48:237–244, 1979.

78. Elkind AH: Headache and head trauma. Clin J Pain. 5:77–87,1989.

79. Emmett JR & Shea JJ: Treatment of tinnitus with tocainide hydrochloride. Otolaryngol Head Neck Surg 88:442–446, 1980.

80. Englander J, Hall K, Stimpson T, Chaffin S: Mild traumatic brain injury in an insured population: subjective complaints and return to employment. Brain Inj 6:161–166, 1992.

81. Enomoto T, Ono Y, Nose T, et al: Electroencephalography in minor head injury in children. Childs Nerv Syst 2(2):72–79, 1986.

82. Epstein CM: Computerized EEG in the courtroom. Neurology 44:1566–1569, 1994.

83. Ettlin TM, Kischka U, Reichmann S, et al: Cerebral symptoms after whiplash injury of the neck: A prospective clinical and neuropsychological study of whiplash injury. J Neurol Neurosurg Psychiatry 55:943–948, 1992.

84. Evans RW. Some observations on whiplash injuries. Neurol Clin 10:975–997 1992.

85. Evans RW, Evans RI, Sharp MJ: The physician survey on the post-concussion and whiplash syndromes. Headache 34(5):268–274, 1994.

86. Fenton G, McClelland R, Montgomery A, et al: The postconcussional syndrome: social antecedents and psychological sequelae. Br J Psychiatry 162:493–497, 1993.

87. Feurerman T, Wackym PA, Gade GF, Becker DP: Value of skull radiography, head computed tomographic scanning, and admission for observation in cases of minor head injury. Neurosurgery 22:449–453, 1988.

88. Fischer RP, Carlson J, Perry JF: Postconcussive hospital observation of alert patients in a primary trauma center. J Trauma 21:920–924, 1981.

89. Fitz-Ritson D: Phasic exercises for cervical rehabilitation after "whiplash" trauma. J Manip Physiol Ther 18:21–24, 1995.

90. Florian T: Conservative treatment for neck pain: Distinguishing useful from useless therapy. J Back Musculoskel Rehabil 1(3):55–66, 1991.

91. Foley-Nolan D, Moore, K, Codd M, et al: Low energy high frequency pulsed electromagnetic therapy for acute whiplash injuries. Scand J Rehabil Med 24:51–59, 1992.

92. Franges EZ: Assessment and management of carotid artery trauma associated with mild head injury. J Neurosci Nurs 18(5):272–274, 1986.

93. Friedman MH: Screening procedures for temporomandibular disorders. J Neuromuskel Syst 2:163–169, 1994.

94. Fumeya H, Hideshima H: Cerebellar concussion—three case reports. Neurol Med Chir (Tokyo). 34:612–615, 1994.

95. Gacek RR: Further observations on posterior ampullary nerve transection for positional vertigo. Ann Otol Rhinol Laryngol 87:300, 1978.

96. Gargan MF, Bannister GC: Long term prognosis of soft tissue injuries of the neck. J Bone Joint Surg 72B:901–903, 1990.

97. Gayral L, Toulouse F, Neuwirth E: Oto-neuro-ophthalmologic manifestations of cervical origin: Posterior cervical sympathetic syndrome of Barre-Lieou. N Y State J Med July:1920–1926, 1954.

98. Gennarelli TA, Adams JH, Graham DI: Acceleration induced head injury in the monkey. I: The model, its mechanical and psychological correlates. Acta Neuropathol 7(Suppl):23–25, 1981.

99. Gennarelli TA: Mechanisms and pathophysiology of cerebral concussion. J Head Trauma Rehabil 1(2):23–29, 1986.

100. George MS, Pickett JB, Kohli H, et al: paroxysmal dystonic reflex choreoathetosis after minor closed head injury [letter]. Lancet 336:1134–1135, 1990.

101. Goebel G, Hiller W: [The tinnitus questionnaire. A standard instrument for grading the degree of tinnitus. Results of a multicenter study with the tinnitus questionnaire.] HNO 42(3):166–172, 1994.

102. Goebel JA: Contemporary diagnostic update: Clinical utility of computerized oculomotor and posture testing. Am J Otol 13: 591-597, 1992.

103. Green J, Leon-Barth C, Dieter J, et al: Somatosensory evoked responses via electronic brain imaging (EBI). Clin Electroencephalogr 23(2):79–88, 1992.

104. Greenman PE, McPartland JM: Cranial findings and iatrogenesis from craniosacral manipulation in patients with traumatic brain syndrome. J American Osteop Assoc 95(3):182–188; 191–192, 1995.

105. Grigsby J, Kaye K: Incidence and correlates of depersonalization following head trauma. Brain Inj 7(6):507–512, 1993.

106. Grimm RJ, Hemenway WG, Lebray PR, Black FO: The perilymph fistula syndrome defined in mild head trauma. Acta Otolaryngol Suppl (Stockh) 464:1–40, 1989.

107. Gross H, Grove K, Tachiki K, et al: Multidimensional neurobehavioral indices of mild closed head/brain injury: convergent validations of softsigns. Presented at the National Head Injury Foundation, Annual Symposium. New Orleans, November 16, 1990.

108. Gualtieri T: Neuropsychiatry and Behavioral Pharmacology. New York, Springer-Verlag, 1991.

109. Gualtieri T: Buspirone: Neuropsychiatric effects. Update on pharmacology. J Head Inj Rehabil 6:90–92, 1991.

110. Guidelines for the management of concussion in sports. Sports Medicine Committee, Colorado Medical Society, May, 1990.

111. Haas DC, Lourie H: Trauma-triggered migraine: An explanation for common neurological attacks after mild head injury. Review of the literature. J Neurosurg 68(2):181–188, 1988.

112. Haas DC, Ross GS: Transient global amnesia triggered by mild head trauma. Brain 109:251–257, 1986.

113. Ham LP, Andrasik F, Packard RC, Bundrick CM: Psychopathology in individuals with post-traumatic headaches and other pain types. Cephalalgia 14(2):118–126 [discussion, 78], 1994.

114. Hamer AJ, Prasad R, Gargan MF, et al: Whiplash injury and cervical disc surgery. Presented at the British Cervical Spine Society Meeting, Bowness-on-Windermere, UK, Nov. 7, 1992.

115. Harrington DE, Malec J, Cicerone K, Katz HT: Current perceptions of rehabilitation professionals towards mild traumatic brain injury. Arch Phys Med Rehabil 74:579–575, 1993.

116. Harrison DW & Walls RM: Blindness following minor head trauma in children: A report of two cases with a review of the literature. J Emerg Med 8:21–24, 1990.

117. Hashimoto T, Watanabe O, Takase M, et al: Collet-Sicard syndrome after minor head trauma. Neurosurgery 23:367–370, 1988.

118. Hayes RL, Povlishock JT, Singha B: Pathophysiology of mild head injury. In Horn LJ, Zasler ND (eds): Rehabilitation of Post-Concussive Disorders. Philadelphia, Hanley & Belfus, 1992, pp 9–20.

119. Healy GB: Hearing loss and vertigo secondary to head injury. N Engl J Med 306:1029–1031, 1982.

120. Heise AP, Laskin DM, Gervin AS: Incidence of temporomandibular joint symptoms following whiplash injury. J Oral Maxillofac Surg 50:825–828, 1992.

121. Herdman S: Personal communication, 1991.

122. Hendrick EB, Harwood Hash DCF, Hudson AR: Head injuries in children: A survey of 4465 consecutive cases at the Hospital for Sick Children, Toronto, Canada. Clin Neurosurg 11:46–65, 1964.

123. Hicks RR, Smith DH, Lowenstein DH, et al: Mild experimental brain injury in the rat induces cognitive deficits associated with regional neuronal loss in the hippocampus. J Neurotrauma. 10:405–414, 1993.

124. Hildingsson C, Toolanen G: Outcome after soft-tissue injury of the cervical spine: A prospective study of 93 car-accident victims. Acta Orthop Scand 61:357–359, 1990.

125. Hinnant D, Tollison CD: Impairment and disability associated with mild head injury: Medical and legal aspects. Semin Neurol 14:84–89, 1994.

126. Hinoki M: Otoneurological observations on whiplash injuries to neck with special reference to the formation of equilibrial disorder. Clin Surg (Tokyo). 22:1683–1690, 1967.

127. Hinoki M: Vertigo due to whiplash injury: a neurootological approach. Acta Otolaryngol (Stockh) 419(Suppl):9–29, 1985.

128. Hodgson SP, Grundy M: Whiplash injuries: Their long-term prognosis and its relationship to compensation. Neuro-Orthopedics 7:88–91, 1989.

129. Holgers KM, Axelsson A, Pringle I: Ginkgo biloba extract for the treatment of tinnitus. Audiology 33(2):85–92.

130. Hooshmand W, Director K, Beckner E, et al: Topographic brain mapping in head injuries. J Clin Neurophysiol 4:233–234, 1987.

131. Horn L: Post-concussive headache: In Horn L, Zasler ND (eds): Rehabilitation of Post-Concussive Disorders. Philadelphia, Hanley & Belfus, 1992, pp 69–78.

132. Horn L, Zasler ND: Neuroanatomy and neurophysiology of sexual function. J Head Trauma Rehabil 5(2):14–24, 1990.

133. Howard RP, Hatsell CP, Guzman HM: Temporomandibular joint injury potential imposed by the low-velocity extension-flexion maneuver. J Oral Maxillofac Surg 53:256–262 [discussion, 263], 1995.

134. Humayun MS, Presty SK, Lafrance ND, et al: Local cerebral glucose abnormalities in mild closed head injured patients with cognitive impairments. Nucl Med Commun 10):335–344, 1989.

135. Huynh L, Fields S: Alprazolam for tinnitus. Ann Pharmacother 29:311–312, 1995.

136. Jacobs A, Put E, Ingels M, Bossuyt A: Prospective evaluation of technetium-99m-HMPAO SPECT in mild and moderate traumatic brain injury [see comments]. J Nucl Med 35:942–947, 1994.

137. Jacobson HG: Positron emission tomography—a new approach to brain chemistry. Council on Scientific Affairs, Report of the the Positron Emission Tomography Panel. JAMA. 260:2704–2710, 1991.

138. Jacome DE: Basilar artery migraine after uncomplicated whiplash injuries. Headache 26:515–516, 1986.

139. Jacome DE: EEG features in basilar artery migraine. Headache. 27:80–83, 1987.

140. Jacome DE & Risko M: EEG features in post-traumatic syndrome. Clin Electroencephalogr 15:214–220, 1984.

141. Jaffe KM, Polissar NL, Fay GC, Liao S: Recovery trends over three years following pediatric traumatic brain injury. Arch Phys Med Rehabil 76):17–26, 1995.

142. Jagger J, Fife D, Vernberg K, Jane JA: Effect of alcohol intoxication on the diagnosis and apparent severity of brain injury. Neurosurgery 15:303–306, 1984.

143. Jensen OK, Nielsen FF: The influence of sex and pre-traumatic headache on the incidence and severity of headache after head injury. Cephalalgia 10:285–293, 1990.

144. Jensen OK, Nielsen FF, & Vosmar L: An open study comparing manual therapy with the use of cold packs in the treatment of post-traumatic headache. Cephalalgia 10:241–250, 1990.

145. Jennett B: Epilepsy after Non-missile Head Injury. Chicago, Year Book, 1975.

146. Jeret JS, Mandell M, Anziska B, et al: Clinical predictors of abnormality disclosed by computed tomography after mild head trauma [see comments]. Neurosurg. 32:9–15 [discussion, 15–16], 1993.

147. Johnson RM, Brummett R, Schleuning A: Use of alprazolam for relief of tinnitus. Arch Otolaryngol Head Neck Surg 119:842–845, 1993.

148. Juhl JH, Miller SW, Roberts GW: Roentgenographic variations in the normal cervical spine. Radiology 78:591, 1962.

149. Kassell NF, Boarini DJ, Adams HP: Intracranial and cervical vascular injuries. In Cooper PR (ed): Head Injury, 2nd ed. Baltimore, Williams & Wilkins, 1987, pp 327–354.

150. Kay T: Neuropsychological diagnosis: disentangling the multiple determinants of functional disability after mild traumatic brain injury. In Horn L, Zasler ND (eds): Rehabilitation of Post-Concussive Disorders. Philadelphia, Hanley & Belfus, 1992, pp 109–127.

151. Kischka U, Ettlin TH, Heim S, Schmid G: Cerebral symptoms following whiplash injury. Eur Neurol 31:136–140, 1991.

152. Knibestol M, Hildingsson C, Toolanen G: Trigeminal sensory impairment after soft-tissue injury of the cervical spine: A quantitative evaluation of cutaneous thresholds for vibration and temperature. Acta Neurol Scand 82:271–276, 1990.

153. Kobayashi S, Waltz AG, Rhoton AL: Effects of stimulation of cervical sympathetic nerves on cortical blood flow and vascular reactivity. Neurology 21: 297–302, 1971.

154. Kortschot HW, Oosterveld WJ: [Otoneurologic disorders after cervical whiplash trauma.] Orthopadie 23:275–277, 1994.

155. Kosteljanetz M, Jensen TS, Norgard B, et al: Sexual and hypothalamic dysfunction in the post-concussional syndrome. Acta Neurol Scand 63: 169–180, 1981.

156. Kowal L: Opthalmic manifestations of head injury. Austr N Z J Ophthalmol 20:35–40, 1992.

157. Kowatch RA: Sleep and head injury. Psychiatr Med 7:37–41, 1989.

158. Kraus JF, Nourjah P: The epidemiology of mild, uncomplicated brain injury. J Trauma 28:1637–1643, 1988.

159. Kraus JF, McArthur DL, Silberman TA: Epidemiology of mild brain injury. Semin Neurol 14:1–7, 1994.

160. Kreutzer J, Marwitz J, Myers S. Neuropsychological issues in litigation following brain injury. Neuropsychology 4:249–259, 1991.

161. Kreutzer JS, Zasler ND: Psychosexual consequences of traumatic brain injury: Methodology and preliminary findings. Brain Inj 3:177–186, 1989.

162. Kreutzer, J.S., Zasler, N.D., Wehman P.H.: Neuromedical and psychosocial aspects of rehabilitation after traumatic brain injury. In Fletcher G, Jann B, Wolf S, Banja J (eds): Rehabilitation Medicine: State of the Art. Philadelphia, Lea & Febiger, 1992.

163. Lacey G, McCabe M, Constant O, et al: Testing a policy for skull radiography (and admission) following mild head injury. Br J Radiol 63:14–18, 1990.

164. Lee A, Mena IG, Miller B: Cerebral hypoxic injury detected by Tc-HMPAO SPECT. Clin Nucl Med 14:482–483, 1989.

165. Lee MS, Rinne JO, Ceballos-Baumann A, et al: Dystonia after head injury. 44:1374–1378, 1994.

166. Lees-Haley PR, Brown RS: Neuropsychological complaint base rates of 170 personal injury claimants. Arch Clin Neuropsychol 8:203–209, 1993.

167. Lees-Haley PR, Dunn JT: The ability of naive subjects to report symptoms of mild brain injury, post-traumatic stress disorder, major depression, and generalized anxiety disorder. J Clin Psychol 50: 252–256, 1994.

168. Legent F, Bordure P: [Post-traumatic perilymphatic fistulas.] Bull Acad Natl Med 178:35–44, 1994.

169. Lehrer PM, Groveman A, Randolph C, et al: Physiological response patterns to cognitive testing in adults with closed head injuries. Psychophysiology 26:668–675, 1989.

170. Leininger BE, Gramling SE, Farrell AD, et al: Neuropsychological deficits in symptomatic minor head injury patients after concussion and mild concussion. J Neurol Neurosurg Psychiatry 53: 293–296, 1990.

171. Leigh RJ, Zee DS: The Neurology of Eye Movements, 2nd ed. Philadelphia, F.A. Davis, 1991.

172. Levin HS, Amparo E, Eisenberg HM, et al: Magnetic resonance imaging and computerized tomography in relation to the neurobehavioral sequela of mild and moderate head injuries. J Neurosurg 66:706–713, 1987.

173. Levin HS, Mattis S, Ruff RM, et al: Neurobehavioral outcome following minor head injury: A three-center study. J Neurosurg 66:234–243, 1987.

174. Lewis RC, Coburn DF: Vertebral artery: Its role in upper cervical and head pain. Missouri Med 53: 1059–1063, 1956.

175. Lieou YC: Syndrome sympathetique cervical posterieur et arthrite cervicale chronique. These de Strasbourg, 1928.

176. Lopes da Silva FH: A critical review of clinical applications of topographic mapping of brain potentials. J Clin Neurophysiol 7: 535–551, 1990.

177. Lowden IMR, Briggs M, Cockin J: Post-concussional symptoms following minor head injury. Injury 20:193–194, 1989.

178. Lorenzoni E: Electroencephalographic studies before and after head injuries. Electroencephalogr Clin Neurophysiol 28:216, 1970.

179. Lyos AT, Marsh MA, Jenkins HA, Coker NJ: Progressive hearing loss after transverse temporal bone fracture. Arch Otolaryngol Head Neck Surg 121:795–799, 1995.

180. McBeath JG, Nanda A: Use of dihydroergotamine in patients with postconcussion syndrome. Headache 34(3):148–151, 1994.

181. McCaffrey RJ, Williams AD, Fisher JM, Laing LC: Forensic issues in mild head injury. J Head Trauma Rehabil 8(3):38–47, 1993.

182. McFarlane AC, Atchison M, Rafalowicz E, Papay P: Physical symptoms in post-traumatic stress disorder. J Psychosom Res 38:715–726, 1994.

183. McKinney LA: Early mobilization and outcome in acute sprains of the neck. BMJ 299:1006–1008, 1989.

184. Macciocchi SN, Reid DB, Barth JT: Disability following head injury. Curr Opin Neuro 6:773–777, 1993

185. MacNab I: Acceleration injuries of the cervical spine. J Bone Joint Surg. 46A:1797–1799, 1964.

186. MacNab J: The "whiplash syndrome". Orthop Clin North Am 2:389–403, 1971.

187. Marion MS, Cevette MJ: Tinnitus. Mayo Clin Proc 66:614–620, 1991.

188. Masdeu JC, Van Heertum RL, Kleiman A, et al: Early single-photon emission computed tomography in mild head trauma. A controlled study. J Neuroimaging 1994; 4(4):177–181.

189. Masters SJ: Evaluation of head trauma: efficacy of skull films. AJR 135:539–547, 1980.

190. Masters SJ, McClean PM, Arcarese JS, et al: Skull x-ray examinations after head trauma; recommendations by a multidisciplinary panel and validation study. N Engl J Med 316:84–91, 1987.

191. Mateer CA: Systems of care for post-concussive syndrome. In Horn LJ, Zasler ND (eds): Rehabilitation of Post-Concussive Disorders. Philadelphia, Hanley & Belfus, 1992, pp 143–160.

192. Meenen NM, Katzer A, Dihlmann SW, et al: [Whiplash injury of the cervical spine—on the role of pre-existing degenerative diseases.] Unfallchirurgie 20(3):138143 [discussion, 149], 1994.

193. Merskey H, Woodforde JM: Psychiatric sequelae of minor head injury. Brain 95:521–528, 1972.

194. Miller JD, Murray LS, Teasdale GM: Development of a traumatic intracranial hematoma after a "minor" head injury. Neurosurgery 27:669–673, 1990.

195. Miller L: Chronic pain complicating head injury recovery: Recommendations for clinicians. Cognit Rehabil Sept-Oct:12-19, 1990.

196. Mittenberg W, Burton DB: A survey of treatments for post-concussion syndrome. Brain Inj 8:429–437, 1994.

197. Mittl RL, Grossman RI, Hiehle JF, et al: Prevalence of MR evidence of diffuse axonal injury in patients with mild head injury and normal head CT findings. Am J Neuroradiol 15:1583–1589, 1994.

198. Mobayed M, Dinan TG: Buspirone/prolactin response to post head injury depression. J Affect Disord 19:237–241, 1990.

199. Newcombe F, Rabbitt P, Briggs M: Minor head injury: Pathophysiological or iatrogenic sequelae? J Neurol Neurosurg Psychiatry 57:709–716, 1994.

200. Nies KJ, Sweet JJ: Neuropsychological assessment and malingering: A critical review of past and present strategies. Arch Clin Neuropsychol 9:501–552, 1994.

201. Noseworthy JH, Miller J, Murray TJ, Regan D: Auditory brainstem responses in postconcussion syndrome. 38:275–278, 1981.

202. Nuwer MR: Uses and abuses of brain mapping. Arch Neurol 46:1134–1136, 1989.

203. Oates JA, Wood AJJ: Therapeutic uses of botulinum toxin. N Engl J Med 25:1186–1194, 1991.

204. Obrebowski A, Pruszewicz A, Baranczakowa Z, et al: [Early and delayed changes in olfactory and gustatory function following maxillofacial fractures]. Otolaryngol Pol 30:391–398, 1976.

205. Ochs AL, Zasler ND, Astruc J, O'Shanick GJ: Oculomotor dysfunction following traumatic brain injury. Presented at the Postgraduate Course on Rehabilitation of the Brain Injured Adult and Child, Williamsburg, VA, June 1991.

206. Olesen J: Calcium entry blockers in the treatment of vertigo. Ann N Y Acad Sci 522:690–697, 1988.

207. Olsson JE: Neurotologic findings in basilar migraine. Laryngoscope 101:141, 1991.

208. Ommaya AK: The neck: Classification, physiology and clinical outcome of injuries to the neck in motor vehicle accidents. In Aldeman B, Chapon A (eds): Biomechanics of Impact Trauma. Amsterdam, Elsevier; 1984.

209. O'Shanick GO, Zasler ND: Neuropsychopharmacologic approaches to traumatic brain injury. In Kreutzer J, Wehman P (eds): Community Integration Following Traumatic Brain Injury. Baltimore, Paul Brookes, 1989, pp 15–27.

210. O'Shanick G, Zasler ND: Neuro-psychopharmacological approaches to traumatic brain injury. In Kreutzer J, Wehman P (eds): Community Integration Following Traumatic Brain Injury. Baltimore, Paul Brookes, 1990.

211. Packard RC: Posttraumatic headache: Permanence and relationship to legal settlement. Headache 32:496–500, 1992.

212. Packard RC, Ham LP: Posttraumatic headache. J Neuropsychiatry 6:229–236, 1994.

213. Padula WV: A Behavioral Vision Approach for Persons with Physical Disabilities. Santa Ana, CA, Optometric Extension Program Foundation, 1988.

214. Papanicolaou AC, Levin HS, Eisenberg HM, et al: Evoked potential correlates of posttraumatic amnesia after closed head injury. Neurosurgery. 14:676–678,1984.

215. Parsons LC, Ver Beek D: Sleep-awake patterns following cerebral concussion. Nurs Res 31(5):260–264, 1982.

216. Pearce JMS: Whiplash injury: A reappraisal. J Neurol Neurosurg Psychiatry. 52:1329–1331, 1989.

217. Pettersson K, Hildingsson C, Toolanen G, et al: MRI and neurology in acute whiplash trauma. No correlation in prospective examination of 39 cases. Acta Orthop Scand 65:525–528, 1994.

218. Polissar NL, Fay GC, Jaffe KM, et al: Mild pediatric traumatic brain injury: Adjusting significance levels for multiple comparisons. Brain Inj 8:249–263, 1994.

219. Povlishock JT, Erb DE, Astruc J: Axonal response to traumatic brain injury: reactive axonal change, deafferentation and neuroplasticity. J Neurotrauma Suppl 1:S189–200.

220. Practice parameter: The utility of neuroimaging in the evaluation of headache in patients with normal neurologic examinations (summary statement). Report of the Quality Standards Subcommittee of the American Academy of Neurology. Neurology. 44:1353–1354, 1994.

221. Pratap-Chand R, Sinniah M, Salem FA: Cognitive evoked potential (P300): A metric for cerebral concussion. Act Neurol Scand 78:185–189, 1988.

222. Prigatano GP, Stahl ML, Orr WC, Zeiner HK: Sleep and dreaming disturbances in closed head injury patients. J Neurol Neurosurg Psychiatry 45:78–80, 1982.

223. Probert TC, Wiesenfeld D, Reade PC: Temporomandibular pain dysfunction disorder resulting from road traffic accidents—an Australian study. Int J Oral Maxillofac Surg 23(6 Pt 1):338–341, 1994.

224. Radanov BP, DiStefano G, Schnidrig A, Ballinari P. Role of psychosocial stress in recovery from common whiplash. Lancet 338:712–715, 1991.

225. Radanov BP, Sturzenegger M, DiStefano G, Schnidrig A: Relationship between early somatic, radiological, cognitive and psychosocial findings and outcome during a one-year follow-up in 117 patients suffering from common whiplash. Br J Rheumatol 33:442–448, 1994.

226. Ram Z, Hadani M, Spiegelman R, et al: Delayed nonhemorrhagic encephalopathy following mild head trauma. J Neurosurg 71:608–610, 1989.

227. Rappaport M, Clifford JO, Winterfield KM: P300 response under active and passive attentional states and uni- and bimodality stimulus presentation conditions. J Neuropsychiatry Clin Neurosci 2:399–407, 1990.

228. Reicke N: Der vertebrogene schwindel. Aetiologie und differntialdiagnose. Fortschr Med 96:1895–1902, 1978.

229. Rizzo PA, Pierelli F, Pozzessere G, et al: Subjective posttraumatic syndrome: a comparison of visual and brain stem auditory evoked responses. Neuropsychobiology 9:78–82, 1983.

230. Ron S, Algom D, Hary D, Cohen M: Time-related changes in the distribution of sleep stages in brain injured patients. Electroencephalogr Clin Neurophysiol 48:432–441, 1980.

231. Rouit RL, Murali R: Injuries of the cranial nerves. In Cooper PR (ed): Head Injury, 2nd ed. Baltimore, Williams & Wilkins, 1987, pp.141–158.

232. Rowe MJ, Carlson C: Brainstem auditory evoked potentials in postconcussion dizziness. Arch Neurol 37:679–683, 1980.

233. Rubin W: How do we use state of the art vestibular testing to diagnose and treat the dizzy patient? Neurol Clin 8:225–234, 1990.

234. Ruff R: Personal communication, 1991.

235. Rutherford WH: Postconcussion symptoms: Relationship to acute neurological indices, individual differences, and circumstances of injury. In Levin HS, Eisenberg HM, Bento AL (eds): Mild Head Injury. New York, Oxford University Press, 1989, pp 217–228.

236. Rutkowski PC, Burian HM: Divergence paralysis following head trauma. Am J Ophthalmol. 73:660–662, 1972.

237. Saal JA: Neck and back pain. Phys Med Rehabil State Art Rev 4, 1990.

238. Sakas DE, Bullock MR, Patterson J, et al: Focal cerebral hyperemia after focal head injury in humans: A benign phenomenon? J Neurosurg. 83:277–284, 1995.

239. Sandstrom J: Cervical syndrome with vestibular symptoms. Acta Otolaryngol (Stockh) 54:207–226, 1962.

240. Saran AS: Depression after minor closed head injury: role of dexamethasone suppression test and antidepressants. J Clin Psychiatr. 46:335–338, 1985.

241. Sbordone RJ, Liter JC: Mild traumatic brain injury does not produce post-traumatic stress disorder. Brain Inj 9:405–412, 1995.

242. Schaul N: Pathogenesis and significance of abnormal nonepileptiform rhythms in the EEG. J Clin Neurophysiol 7:229–248, 1990.

243. Schnarkowski P, Weidenmaier W, Heuck A, Reiser MF: [MR functional diagnosis of the cervical spine after strain injury.] Rofo Fortschr Geb Rontgenstr Neuen Bildgeb Verfahr 162:319–324, 1995.

244. Schoenhuber R, Gentilini M: Auditory brain stem responses in the prognosis of late postconcussional symptoms and neuropsychological dysfunction after minor head injury. Neurosurgery 19(4):532–534, 1986.

245. Schoenhuber R, Gentilini M: Anxiety and depression after mild head injury: A case control study. J Neurol Neurosurg Psychiatr. 51:722–724, 1988.

246. Schoenhuber R, Gentilini M, Orlando A: Prognostic value of auditory brain-stem responses for late postconcussion symptoms following minor head injury. J Neurosurg 68:742–744, 1988.

247. Schoenhuber R, Gentilini M, Scarano M, Bortolotti P: Longitudinal study of auditory brain-stem response in patients with minor head injuries. Arch Neurol 44:1181–1182, 1987.

248. Schreiber S, Galai-Gat T: Uncontrolled pain following physical injury as the core-trauma in post-traumatic stress disorder. Pain 54:107–110, 1993.

249. Schultz DR: Occipital neuralgia. J Am Osteop Assoc 76:335–343, 1977.

250. Reference deleted.

251. Segalowitz SJ: Mild head injury as a source of developmental disabilities. J Learn Disabil 24:551–559, 1991.

252. Segawa F, Kishibayashi J, Kamada K, et al: [FLAIR images of brain diseases.] No To Shinkei. 46:531–538, 1994.

253. Seletz E: Whiplash injuries: Neurophysiological basis for pain and methods used for rehabilitation. JAMA 168:1750–1755, 1958.

254. Servadei F, Ciucci G, Morichetti A, et al: Skull fracture as a factor of increased risk in minor head injuries. Surg Neurol 30:364–369, 1988.

255. Seto H, Shimizu M, Futatsuya R, et al: Basilar artery migraine. Reversible ischemia demonstrated by Tc-99m HMPAO brain SPECT. Clin Nucl Med 19:215–218, 1994.

256. Severy DM, Mathewson JH, Bechtol CO: Controlled automobile rear end collisions: An investigation of related engineering and medical phenomena. Can Serv Med J 11:727–759, 1955.

257. Shepard NT, Telian SA, Smith-Wheelock M: Habituation and balance retraining therapy: A retrospective review. Neurol Clin 8:459–475, 1990.

258. Shepard NT, Telian SA: Programmatic vestibular rehabilitation. Otolaryngol Head Neck Surg 112: 173–182, 1995.

259. Shumway-Cook A, Horak FB: Rehabilitation strategies for patients with vestibular deficits. Neurol Clin 8:441–457, 1990.

260. Shutty MS, Dawdy L, McMahon M, Buckelew SP: Behavioral treatment of dizziness secondary to benign positional vertigo following head trauma. Arch Phys Med Rehabil. 72:473–476, 1991.

261. Simon RI: Posttraumatic stress disorder in litigation: Guidelines for forensic assessment. Washington, DC, American Psychiatric Press, 1995.

262. Spenler CW, Benfield JR: Esophageal disruption from blunt and penetrating external trauma. Arch Surg 111:663–667, 1976.

263. Spitzer WO, Skovron ML, Salmi LR, et al: Scientific monograph of the Quebec Task Force on whiplash-associated disorders: redefining "whiplash" and its management. Spine 20(8 Suppl):1S–73S, 1995.

264. Starkstein SE, Mayberg HS, Berthier ML, et al: Mania after brain injury: neuroradiological and metabolic findings. Ann Neurol 27:652–659, 1990.

265. Stein SC, Ross SE: The value of computed tomographic scans in patients with low-risk head injuries. Neurosurgery 26:638–640, 1990.

266. Stein SC, Spettell C, Young G, Ross SE: Limitations of neurological assessment in mild head injury. Brain Inj 7:425–430, 1993.

267. Stringer W, Balseiro J, Fidler R: Advances in traumatic brain injury neuroimaging techniques. NeuroRehabilitation 1(3)11–30.

268. Sturzenegger MH, Meienberg O: Basilar artery migraine: A follow-up study of 82 cases. Headache 25:408–415, 1985.

269. Sturzenegger MH, DiStefano G, Radanov BP, Schnidrig A: Presenting symptoms and signs after whiplash injury: the influence of accident mechanisms. Neurology. 44:688–693, 1994.

270. Su HC, Su RK: Treatment of whiplash injuries with acupuncture. Clin J Pain. 4:233–247, 1988.

271. Takahashi T, Kobayashi Y, Okamoto S, et al: [MRI of traumatic anosmia.] No Shinkei Geka. 23:207–211, 1995.

272. Teasell RW, Shapiro AP (eds): Cervical flexion-extension/whiplash injuries. Spine State Art Rev 7:329–578, 1993.

273. Teasell RW, Shapiro AP, Mailis A: Medical management of whiplash injuries: An overview. Spine State Art Rev 7:481–499, 1993.

274. Tebano MT, Cameroni M, Gallozzi G, et al: EEG spectral analysis after minor head injury in man. Electroencephalogr Clin Neurophysiol 70(2):185–189, 1988.

275. Teifke A, Degreif J, Geist M, et al: [The safety belt: effects on injury patterns of automobile passengers.] Rofo Fortschr Geb Rontgenstr Neuen Bildgeb Verfahr 159:278–283, 1993.

276. Thalmann I, Kohut RI, Comegys TH, et al: Protein profile of human perilymph: In search of markers for the diagnosis of perilymph fistula and other inner ear disease. Otolaryngol Head Neck Surg 111:273–280, 1994.

277. Thatcher RW, Walker RA, Gerson I, Geisler FH: EEG discriminant analyses of mild head trauma. Electorencephalogr Clin Neurophysiol 73(2):94–106, 1989.

278. Tierney DW: Visual dysfunction in closed head injury. J Am Optometr Assoc 59:614–622, 1988.

279. Tollison CD, Satterthwaite (eds.): Painful Cervical Trauma: Diagnosis and Rehabilitative Treatment of Neuromusculoskeletal Injuries. Baltimore, Williams & Wilkins. 1992.

280. Tom-harald E: Disability 3–5 years after minor head injury. J Oslo City Hosp 37:41–48, 1987.

281. Travell JG, Simons DG: Myofascial Pain and Dysfunction: The Trigger Point Manual. Baltimore, Williams & Wilkins, 1983.

282. Turk Z, Ratkolb O: Mobilization of the cervical spine in chronic headaches. Manual Med 3:15–17, 1987.

283. Turkewitz LJ, Wirth O, Dawson GA, Casaly JS: Cluster headache following head injury: a case report and review of the literature. Headache 32: 504–506, 1992.

284. Tyrer P, Seivewright N: Pharmacological treatment of personality disorders. Clin Neuropharmacol 11:493–499, 1988.

285. Vaughan K, Armstrong MS, Gold R, et al: A trial of eye movement desensitization compared to image habituation training and applied muscle relaxation in post-traumatic stress disorder. J Behav Ther Exp Psychiatry 25(4):283–291, 1994.

286. Veltman RH, VanDongen S, Jones S, et al: Cognitive screening in mild brain injury. J Neurosci Nurs 25(6):367–371, 1993.

287. Vernon H (ed.): Upper Cervical Syndrome: Chiropractic Diagnosis and Treatment. Baltimore, Williams & Wilkins, 1988.

288. Waddell PA, Gronwall DMA: Sensitivity to light and sound following minor head injury. Acta Neurol Scand 69(5):270–276, 1984.

289. Waldman SD: The role of neural blockade in the evaluation and treatment of common headache and facial pain syndromes. Headache Q Curr Treat Res 2(4):286–291, 1991.

290. Walker SH, Patton ES: Brain Electrical Activity Mapping (BEAM) in the Evaluation of Traumatic Brain Injury. Nicolet Instrument Corporation, 1988.

291. Werner RA, Vanderzant CW: Multimodality evoked potential testing in acute mild closed head injury. 72:31–34, 1991.

292. Williams GH, Giordano AM: Temporal bone trauma. In Becker DP, Gudeman SK (eds): Textbook of Head Injury. Philadelphia, W.B. Saunders, 1990, pp 367–377.

293. Williams DH, Levin HS,Eisenberg HM: Mild head injury classification. Neurosurgery 27: 422–428, 1990.

294. Wilson PR: Chronic neck pain and cervicogenic headache. Clin J Pain. 7:5–11, 1991.

295. Wong E, Lee G, Mason DT: Temporal headaches and associated symptoms relating to the styloid process and its attachments. Ann Acad Med Singapore 24:124–128, 1995.

296. Yablon SA: Posttraumatic seizures. Arch Phys Med Rehabil 74:983–1001, 1993.

297. Yamaguchi M: Incidence of headache and severity of head injury. Headache 32:427–431, 1992.

298. Yamamoto LG, Bart RD: Transient blindness following mild head trauma: Criteria for a benign outcome. Clin Pediatr 27:479–483, 1988.

299. Yokota H, Kurokawa A, Otsuka T, et al: Significance of magnetic resonance imaging in acute head injury. J Trauma 31(3):351–357, 1991.

300. Yoshida J, Shiroozu A, Zaitsu A, et al: Diabetes insipidus after trauma of two extremes in severity. Yonsei Med J 31:71–73, 1990.

301. Young HA, Gleave RW, Schmidek HH, Gregory S: Delayed traumatic intracerebral hematoma: Report of 15 cases operatively treated. Neurosurgery 14: 22–25, 1984.

302. Zasler ND, Horn L: Rehabilitative management of sexual dysfunction. J Head Trauma Rehabil 5(2): 14–24, 1990.

303. Zasler ND, McNeny MR, Heywood PG: Rehabilitative management. J Head Trauma Rehabili 7(1):66–75, 1992.

304. Zasler ND: Pharmacologic aspects of cognitive function following traumatic brain injury. In Kreutzer JS (ed): Cognitive Rehabilitation: A Functional Approach. Baltimore, Paul H. Brookes, 1991, pp 87–93.

305. Zasler ND: Update on pharmacology. Neuromedical aspects of alcohol use following traumatic brain injury. J Head Trauma Rehabil 6(4):78–80, 1991.

306. Zasler ND: Advances in neuropharmacological rehabilitation for brain dysfunction. Brain Inj 6(1): 1–14, 1992.

307. Zasler ND, McClintic N: Functional orthoptic evaluation after traumatic brain injury. Presented at the Post-graduate Course on Rehabilitation of the Brain Injured Adult and Child, Williamsburg, VA. June 1991.

308. Zasler ND, McNeny R, Heywood P: Rehabilitative management of olfactory and gustatory dysfunction following brain injury. J Head Trauma Rehabil 7(1):66–75, 1992.

309. Zasler ND, Ochs A: Oculovestibular dysfunction in symptomatic mild traumatic brain injury. Arch Phys Med Rehab. 73:963, 1992.

310. Zasler ND: Mild traumatic brain injury medical assessment and intervention. J Head Trauma Rehabil 8(3):13–29, 1993.

311. Zasler ND: Sexual function in traumatic brain injury. In Silver JM, Yudofsky SC, Hales RE (eds): Psychiatric Aspects of Traumatic Brain Injury. Washington, DC, American Psychiatric Press, 1994.

312. Zasler ND: Impairment and disability evaluation in post-concussive disorders. In Rizzo M, Tranel D (eds): Head Injury and Post-Concussive Syndrome. New York, Churchill Livingstone, 1995.

7

Pediatric Brain Injury Rehabilitation

EPIDEMIOLOGY

Mortality from traumatic brain injury (TBI) in young people aged 0–19 years has been estimated by Kraus to be approximately 7,000 deaths for 1985 or about 29% of all deaths from injury in children and adolescents.[60] Extrapolating from his 1981 survey of brain injury in San Diego County residents[59] and from data in the National Head and Spinal Cord Injury Survey, he estimates a brain injury rate of 219.4/100,000/per year, with the incidence being 2.1 times higher for males than for females. The estimates are compatible with previous data from Minnesota[2] and Maryland.[73] Both the Minnesota and San Diego County data show an abrupt peak in incidence between 15 and 19 years (see figure on p. 10).

Kraus again extrapolated his data to estimate that this incidence represents over 550,000 bed days/year. He also projected that each year 29,000 young people aged 0–19 years have a disability due to brain injury, with estimated disability rates of 10%, 90%, and 100% for mild, moderate, and severe brain injuries, respectively.

DiScala and colleagues[28] reviewed the data from the National Pediatric Trauma Registry from 1985 to 1988 and found that of 4,870 cases younger than 20 years, 44.8% sustained a traumatic brain injury. Of the head-injured population, over 50% also sustained extracranial injury. The combination of head injury and extracranial injury was associated with higher mortality and morbidity, a fact that has been confirmed in other studies.[75,111,122]

In an analysis of all brain injuries in children and adolescents in San Diego County during 1981, Kraus found that the majority of injuries resulted from falls and motor vehicle accidents (Table 1). Two-thirds of the injuries in infants less than 1 year of age were due to falls, but of these, only 8% were serious. Among preschool children, 51% of brain injuries were caused by falls, of which 6% were serious. Conversely, 22-55% of motor vehicle accidents were associated with serious injuries in all age groups. Assault was associated with a higher incidence of severity than in the younger age groups (0–4 years) in the older groups. Both Kraus and Discala et al. showed that a nearly linear increase in the incidence of motor vehicle accidents was paralleled by a nearly linear decrease in the incidence of falls with increasing age during the first two decades of

TABLE 1. Brain Injuries by Major External Cause and Percentage Seriously Injured by Age, San Diego County, California, 1981*

Age Group, y	No. of Cases	External Cause, %											
		Motor Vehicle		Falls		Assault		Sports/ Recreation		All Others		Total	
		All Brain Injury	Serious Brain Injury	All Brain Injury	Serious Brain Injury	All Brain Injury	Serious Brain Injury	All Brain Injury	Serious Brain Injury	All Brain Injury	Serious Brain Injury	All Brain Injury	Serious Brain Injury
1	54	7	50	69	8	17	56	2	100	6	67	100	24
1–4	185	22	23	51	6	5	90	16	3	6	45	100	16
5–9	229	31	31	31	4	1	0	32	7	5	18	100	14
10–14	241	24	22	18	9	5	25	43	7	10	4	100	12
15–19	525	55	31	9	10	17	28	10	4	10	19	100	25
All ages	1234	37	29	24	7	10	34	21	6	8	20	100	18

* Percent seriously injured includes those patients with moderate, severe, or fatal brain injuries.
From Kraus JF, et al: Brain Injuries among infants, children, adolescents and adults. Am J Dis Child 144: 687, 1990, with permission.

life. Chorba and associates,[21] however, reported that the involvement of children under the age of 5 years in fatal and nonfatal motor vehicle accidents has increased in recent years, despite the use of restraints.

A recent National Crime Survey[128] found that 67 of 1,000 teenagers experienced violent crimes each year compared with 26 of 1,000 adults. In a study based in Massachusetts, Guyer et al.[41] found that 1 of 132 children/year were victims of an intentional injury requiring medical attention. Baker et al.[6] found that

the most marked increases in homicide rates during the past three decades were among children and adolescents. In 1986, 1,100 children are estimated to have died as a result of abuse or neglect, most of whom were under 2 years of age.[19] According to the same source, children in the United States are over 10 times more likely to be victims of homicide than European children (Fig. 1), and deaths and hospitalizations due to injury represent only a small portion of actual incidents.

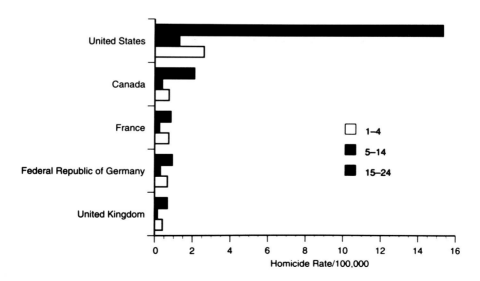

FIGURE 1. Homicide rate in individuals 24 years and under in Europe and North America. (From Children's Safety Network: A Data Book of Child and Adolescent Injury. Washington, DC, National Center for Education in Maternal and Child Health, 1991.)

PREDISPOSING FACTORS

Of the many studies that have attempted to identify risk factors for pediatric injury, most have relied on retrospective methodology or lacked controls. However, several studies have used epidemiologic methods[2,37,88,98] or prospective designs.[11,27] Bijur et al. found that 5-year-old boys with high aggression scores were 2.4 times more likely than other children to have significant injury between the ages of 5 and 10 years.[11] Aggressive behavior was increased with such variables as low socioeconomic conditions, frequent moves, and working mothers who were distressed and unhappy; once such variables were controlled, aggression and overactivity as measured on the Rutter Child Behavior Questionnaire were still associated with increased risk for injury. However, as this study and others have pointed out, the majority of injuries occur in children who are not considered at high risk.

A prospective cohort study of preschool children by Davidson et al.[27] confirmed the previous association of injury rate with gender (males were at a 1.52 increased rate of injury compared with females) as well as with specific behavior problems, including difficulty with discipline, encopresis (in boys only), and fearfulness. However, overactivity and decreased concentration were not associated with an increased rate of injury. Of interest, difficulty with discipline was associated with an increased risk of injury only in the children of mothers with intermediate and high neuroticism scores.

Pless et al.[88] undertook an epidemiologic analysis of traffic injuries in children aged 7–16 years and found that two child-related factors (fidgety and "abnormal" behavior) and three family-related risk factors account for only a small percentage of childhood injuries, suggesting that the most appropriate preventive approach is community-wide environmental passive interventions.

OUTCOMES AND ASSESSMENT

It is generally believed that children and young people have better outcomes after traumatic brain injury than adults. However, evaluation of outcome in children is limited by the tools used for initial assessment,

whether or not the care was delivered by personnel with pediatric expertise, and by methods used for assessment of function.

Because of the limited applicability of the Glasgow Coma Scale (GCS)[112] to very young children, two variations have been suggested: the Children's Coma Scale (CCS)[42,90] and the Pediatric Coma Scale (PCS).[92] The CCS is commonly used in many centers around the United States and is appropriate for children under the age of 36 months. More recently the Pediatric Coma Scale was prospectively evaluated for use in children from 9–72 months of age and found to be reliable.[107] The PCS relies heavily on brainstem reflexes because of the unreliability of judging consciousness in children under the age of six years (Table 2). Furthermore, norms were established for each age group between birth and 5 years; in evaluating the overall prognostic value of the PCS, the group found that children whose coma scores were below the norm for age tended to have poorer outcomes.

Evaluation of post-traumatic amnesia also has proved to be challenging. Because questions on the Galveston Orientation and Amnesia Test (GOAT) are inappropriate for children, an orientation test specifically for children has been developed: the Children's Orientation and Amnesia Test (COAT). The COAT is reliable for children between the ages of 4 and 15 years.[32] The Galveston group found that verbal and nonverbal memory were more impaired at 6 and 12 months after injury in patients with posttraumatic amnesia (PTA) of more than 3 week's duration; they also found that PTA was correlated more strongly with outcome than the GCS score. One retrospective observational study[69] found no significant difference in outcome among children with a GCS score of 3–5 versus children with a score greater than 6. This finding suggests that PTA is a more accurate method of judging severity in very young children as well as in older children and adults. Although the COAT is useful in the age range established by its authors, a method for evaluating PTA in children under the age of 4 years has not been established.

Similarly, standard outcome scales such as the Functional Independence Measure (FIM) or the Barthels are inappropriate for

TABLE 2. Comparison of Glasgow Coma Scale, Children's Coma Scale, and Pediatric Coma Scale

Glasgow Coma Scale (Teasdale)	Children's Coma Scale (Raimondi)	Children's Coma Scale (Hahn)	Pediatric Coma Scale
Eye Opening	**Eyes**	**Eye Opening**	**Eyes Open**
4 Spontaneous	4 Pursuit	4 Spontaneous	4 Spontaneous
3 Reaction to speech	3 Extraocular muscle intact, pupils reactive	3 Reaction to speech	3 To speech
2 Reaction to pain		2 Reaction to pain	2 To pain
1 No response	2 Fixed pupils or EOM impaired	1 No response	1 None
Verbal	1 Fixed pupils or EOM paralyzed	**Verbal**	**Best verbal response**
5 Oriented		5 Smiles, oriented to sound, follows objects, interacts	5 Orientated
4 Confused/disordered	**Verbal**	*Crying* *Interacts*	4 Words
3 Inappropriate words	3 Cries	4 Consolable Inappropriate	3 Vocal sounds
2 Incomprehensible sounds	2 Spontaneous respiration	3 Inconsistently Moaning consolable	2 Cries
1 No response	1 Apneic	2 Inconsolable Irritable, restless	1 None
Motor	**Motor**		**Best motor response**
6 Spontaneous (obeys verbal commands)	4 Flexes and extends	1 No response	5 Obeys commands
5 Localizes pain	3 Withdrawal from painful stimuli	**Motor**	4 Localizes to pain
4 Withdraws in response to pain	2 Hypertonic	6 Spontaneous (obeys verbal command	3 Flexion to pain
3 Abnormal flexion to pain (decorticate posture)	1 Flaccid	5 Localizes pain	2 Extension to pain
2 Abnormal extension response to pain (decerebrate posture)		4 Withdraws to pain	1 None
1 No response		3 Decorticate response to pain	**Age norms**
		2 Decerebrate response to pain	0–6 months = 9
		1 No response	6–12 months = 11
			12–24 months = 12
			2–5 years = 13
			>5 years = 14

EOM = extraocular movement.

many pediatric age groups. Because of the normal developmental processes, the baseline for measurement shifts constantly. The WeeFIM has some use for evaluating functional independence in children under the age of 6 years, and the FIM can be used in older age groups. The Pediatric Evaluation of Disability Inventory (PEDI) has been developed by the group at Tufts[36] and has the advantage of scores that are expressed as a percentage of the expected age-appropriate performance rather than absolute numbers, thus permitting longitudinal tracking. However, it is somewhat complicated to use and to score. Other common assessment tools standardized for the pediatric age group include the Bruinicks-Oseretsky Test of Motor Proficiency, the Peabody Individual Achievement Test, the Beery Test of Visual Motor Integration, the Battelle Developmental Inventory and the Bayley Scales of Infant Development (Table 3).

The Wechsler Intelligence Tests have been used extensively in the evaluation of outcome in pediatric brain trauma. Klonoff et al.[57] conducted a 5-year follow-up study of brain-injured children and found persistent deficits in neuropsychologic functioning and academic achievement. Chadwick and Rutter[18] found that the performance IQ was more affected than the verbal IQ in children with TBI, but believed that neuropsychologic testing in addition to the Wechsler Intelligence Scale for Children-Revised (WISC-R) was not necessary. However, Berger-Gross and Shackelford[9] found that the WISC-R was not sensitive enough to identify many deficits and disagreed with the conclusion that additional neuropsychological testing in children with TBI was noncontributory. Several other groups have noted that speeded testing is a more sensitive measure of deficit, as is the assessment of academic performance.[42,68,97,131] Levin believed that the Selective Reminding Test was especially sensitive to TBI.[67]

Children with less severe trauma may not be as obviously impaired, but the Seattle group provided evidence for true cognitive sequelae in children with mild TBI in a prospective study of mildly, moderate, and

TABLE 3. *Standardized Assessment Tools for Children and Adolescents*

Test	Age Range	Used For
Conners Rating Forms	School Age	Identifying behavioral problems
Child Behavior Checklist	4–16 years	Assessing social competence and behavior
Bayley Scales of Infant Development	2–30 months	Measuring mental and motor development in infants
Stanford-Binet Intelligence Scale	2 years through adulthood	Measuring verbal and nonverbal intelligence
Wechsler Scales	5–6 years (WPPSI), 6–16 years (WISC-R)	Assessing intelligence and identifying strengths and weaknesses
McCarthy Scales of Children's Abilities	2.5–8.5 years	Assessing intelligence in young children
Kaufman Assessment Battery for Children	2.5–12.5 years	Assessing intelligence and achievement
Wide Range Achievement Test (WRAT)	5–<12 years (level 1), 12 years to adult	Assessing academic achievement
Peabody Individual Achievement Test (PIAT)	Kindergarten through high school	Assessing academic achievement
Bender Visual Motor Gestalt Test	5–11 yr 11 mo (Koppitz)	Assessing development and visuomotor skills
Beery Test of Visual Motor Integration (VMI)	2–15 years	Assessing visual memory, perception, and motor maturation
Halstead-Reitan Test Battery	5–18 (Reitan-Indiana), 9–14 (Halstead)	Assessing abilities of children with brain injuries
Luria Nebraska Neuropsychological Battery	8–12 years	Assessing abilities of children with brain injuries
Vineland Scales	Birth to adulthood	Assessing social competence
Bruinicks-Oseretsky Scales of Motor Development	4.5–14.5 years	Quantitating fine and gross motor scales by age
Wide Range Assessment of Memory and Learning	5–17 years	Assessing memory

severely brain-injured children and controls. Among the mildly injured children (defined as initial GCS greater than 13), a small but significant difference was found in speeded motor tasks and long-term verbal memory tasks compared with matched controls 1 year after injury.[51] Such findings are similar to Gulbrandsen's study, which compared performance of complex neuropsychological tasks at 4–8 months after injury with noninjured controls.[40] Levin and Eisenberg also noted storage and retrieval difficulties in mildly brain-injured children on short-term follow-up.[68] However, at 3-year follow-up, testing of the mildly injured students by the Seattle group demonstrated subtle deficits without functional significance.[34]

Vargha-Khadem's group observed that language deficits secondary to TBI appear to be more profound when injury occurs before the age of 5 years,[118] and in her 10–15-year follow-up Thomsen found that people who are severely injured at a younger age (15–21 years) are at higher risk of late behavioral and emotional sequelae than older patients.[115] Basso and Scarpa noted a clear difference in aphasia patterns and recovery that was related to age of injury,[7] yet Klonoff's prospective study of 231 children between the ages of 2.7 and 15.9 years of age found no difference in outcome between older and younger groups.[57] Because Klonoff's study included no separate analysis of degrees of severity, some interplay of variables between etiology and age of injury may have been overlooked. Kriel and Krach found that children younger than 6 years of age appeared to have poorer outcomes than older children.[62] Although the younger age group included children who had suffered abuse and, hence, the possibility of cumulative injury, the data still suggest poorer outcomes for younger children, regardless of etiology.

Because of the variability in etiology of injury, developmental stage at the time of injury, and assessment tools, it is difficult to make prognostic statements about TBI in individual children even when referring to the best-designed studies. One trend, however, is clear: the worst outcomes occur when multiple trauma is present. In a prospective study of 369 pediatric patients Walker et al.[122] found a mortality rate of 12%; in the remaining 88% outcome ranged from good to moderately disabled when serious TBI was not accompanied by multitrauma. However, in the presence of multitrauma, the mortality rate rose to 33%, only 66% made a good-to-moderate recovery, and 1% were vegetative. Splaingard et al.[111] found that by 2 years after trauma, 45% of children with serious TBI who required gastrostomies and tracheostomies had achieved functional independence and were cared for at home. They also found that all children achieving even partial independence by 6 months after injury could be cared for at home within 2 years.

Boyer and Edwards[13] did a retrospective review of 220 consecutive patients with TBI between the ages of 6 and 21 years admitted to a pediatric rehabilitation hospital in New Jersey. Patients were accepted at any level of consciousness. At the time of admission 55% of the children were at a Rancho Los Amigos (RLA) level of I–III. At 1 year, only 17% were still at a RLA level of less than IV. Of all patients, 71% were able to return home, 10% went to a nursing home, and the others were placed in institutions. Although 79% achieved independent mobility (46% of these without assistive devices), at 1 year after injury only 8% were enrolled in regular education, 39% were enrolled in special education, and 17% in cognitive remediation, whereas 25% were unable to participate in any type of educational program. Some improvement was noted up to 3 years after injury, at which time 14% of children were able to attend regular classes. In contrast to Ward's data,[123] the authors found no obvious shift in Glasgow Outcome Scale (GOS) categories between years 1 and 3 after injury. Of interest, the number of patients achieving RLS level VIII increased from 40% at 1 year to 61% at 2 years and to 67% at 3 years, without an accompanying shift in GOS category. This discrepancy no doubt reflects the relative insensitivity of the GOS as an outcome measure.

In a similar study in Holland, Ruijs[97] looked at 70 patients with closed head injury aged 4–18 years. Sixty-three patients were discharged home; 4 were sent to a rehabilitation center, where 2 still remained at the time of the study; 2 went to nursing homes; and 1 was sent to a psychiatric crisis center. The patients and their families were interviewed 2–4 years after the injury. In all of the children with coma of more than 1 week's duration and in 29% with coma of less than 1 week's duration, personality change was noted, including uninhibited behavior, inhibited behavior, a combination of both, and, in 3 patients, changes that could not be classified. Of the 38 children with coma of less than 15 minute's duration, 21% experienced "school problems," 21% had difficulty in concentrating, and 16% experienced memory impairment. Of the 66 school-aged children, 47% were able to continue their education, 23% had to repeat a grade, 5% continued their education at a lower level, and 12% required individual education. The researchers found that coma of 1 week's duration was the outside limit for which regular education could be continued and that significant school problems were present in 59% of children and adolescents with coma duration between 15 minutes and 1 week.

Costeff et al.[25] reviewed 31 consecutive children who suffered severe TBI (defined as coma for at least 7 days) and were admitted to the Loewenstein Hospital for rehabilitation. All patients were followed for 5 years or more, and age at injury ranged from 3–15 years. Twenty-four (80%) had significant disability, and 7 had seizure disorders. Ataxia and hemiballismus were more common in this age group than in adults, and 13 of the 30 survivors had significant behavioral and social problems. Although the mortality rate of children with TBI was lower than that of adults with TBI from the same region, as was the incidence of persistent vegetative state, the overall severity of disability was judged by the authors to be similar in both groups.

Kriel and Krach[61] recently reviewed 37 children with TBI aged 0.15–18.9 years, with coma of 3 months' duration or longer. Outcomes were rated with the Modified Glasgow Outcome Scale. Seventy-five percent eventually regained consciousness, although by 5 years 50% of children who remained in a persistent vegetative state had died.

The crucial issues in evaluation of outcome in children appear to be longevity of follow-up and definition of outcome. Short-term studies looking at motoric or cognitive outcome or longer-term studies using such insensitive measures as the GOS or standard achievement tests have led to the widespread belief, particularly among personnel involved in the care of adults, that outcome is significantly better in children than in older individuals.

It is becoming increasingly clear, however, that children often grow into their deficits.[45,55,68] Because of the inability to measure many temporal and frontal lobe functions in young children, clinicians and educators may consider them to be free of deficits. However, ongoing long-term studies reveal the academic and social difficulties that such young people often experience. In their long-term, case-control study of mild, moderately, and severely head-injured youth, the Seattle group found that at 3 years after injury moderately and severely injured children did significantly worse on 40 of 53 variables than controls, even though some performance was still within the range of normal.[35] Higher-order cognitive skills were more profoundly affected, and deficits were reflected in progressively poorer performance in academic testing of reading, writing, and arithmetic. Furthermore, outcome variables were associated with severity of injury, as demonstrated in the earlier 1-year follow-up data. Although for over two decades a direct relationship between severity and outcome has been noted in children as well as in adults,[14,51,52,67,68,97,130] the Seattle group also found that as a group the most severely injured children also showed the most recovery.

Klonoff[56] recently published a 23-year outcome study of his 1967 study group. Of the original 231 subjects (only 10% of whom suffered moderate-to-severe TBI), 175 were located and 159 agreed to participate in a follow-up interview. Klonoff's group found that 31% of the sample reported subjective sequelae, which also were related to severity of injury. Difficulties with learning and memory, depressed mood, and anxiety disorders were reported most commonly. Furthermore 15.1%

reported recurrent head injuries, and 8.8% had lost consciousness. Although this study suffers from lack of case controls and external verification of self-reports it is compatible with other long-term studies[57,97,115] as well as more recent short-term studies.[34,51,52]

A retrospective review of 200 schizophrenics found an increase in the history of head trauma during childhood with loss of consciousness or confusion lasting more than 1 hour; compared to similar numbers of patients with bipolar disease or major depression as well as surgical controls, the difference was significant.[130] In the majority of cases, the head injury had occurred before the age of 5 years.

Abstract thinking skills and executive functions begin to develop during early adolescence; thus behavioral and academic difficulties may begin to emerge in children with preadolescent TBI who have performed satisfactorily during their primary school years. As their peers move onto higher cognitive tasks, they lag behind. The above studies of Klonoff and the Seattle group support the concern that such youngsters are at risk for serious behavior and academic difficulties over the long term. Research into how to provide the most effective and appropriate rehabilitation services is urgently needed.

The immediate outcome of TBI in adolescents sometimes may be difficult to assess with purely subjective criteria, because adolescent behavior is typically disinhibited, oppositional, and labile. For most adult neuropsychological tests, norms have been developed for subjects as young as 16 years, but below age 16 other measures must be used. Although an adolescent version of the Minnesota Multiphasic Personality Inventory (MMPI) has been developed, mental health professionals whose practices are confined primarily to adults may not have the adolescent version and may attempt to substitute the adult MMPI. The adolescent norms must be used for testing this age group, or the results may be invalid.

The reliability of cerebral imaging studies in predicting outcome has been disappointing overall. The prognostic value of the computed tomographic (CT) scan generally has been poor,[67,95] although Levin found that a left temporal mass effect was associated with residual impairment of verbal memory, and Kriel and colleagues[63] as well as Costeff[25] found that CT evidence of cerebral edema in the acute phase was associated with a poorer outcome. Positron emission tomography (PET) shows some promise.[114]

Michaud et al.[75] found that the GCS 75 hours after injury as well as Injury Severity Scale (ISS), pupillary responses, and oxygenation in the emergency department were predictive of outcome; as mentioned above, Walker also found that extracranial injury was associated with poorer prognosis than intracranial injury alone.[122] Wagstyl et al. found that abnormal plantar and pupillary light reflexes in the emergency department predicted death or severe disability (using the GOS) with 99% certainty in the cases that they reviewed.[121] Although persistently increased intracranial pressure is treated aggressively in children, it appears to be mediated by autonomic responses in many instances and does not carry as grave a prognosis in children as in adults with TBI.[108]

In summary, the effect of various factors on outcome has been evaluated over the years. Because of differing study designs and assessment techniques, various researchers have drawn conflicting conclusions. It seems safe to conclude that children and adolescents have a lower mortality rate than adults and on short-term follow-up appear to have less morbidity. Severity as measured by initial GCS scores, by ISS scores, or by evaluation of PTA has a direct relationship to morbidity, particularly in the domains of intelligence and adaptive problem solving, memory, academic performance, motor performance, and psychomotor problem solving.[9,18,51,57] In addition, motor disability tends to be less severe in children than in adults.[13,14] However, language deficits acquired during the preschool years are worse than later acquired aphasias,[118] and difficulties in behavior and academic performance, particularly in the nonverbal domains, are prevalent, even in the less severely injured youth.[57] One group found that an intact family was predictive of better outcome in preschool-age patients.[117] This variable did not emerge in studies of older children, but premorbid behavior difficulties were associated with poorer outcomes and may have reflected family instability.

SENSORY DEFICITS

Visual disturbances due to TBI are common in both children and adults. However, the acute management differs in the very young. Because a preschooler with ocular dysmotility has a great capacity to suppress permanently the vision in the weaker eye, immediate consultation with a pediatric ophthalmologist is vital when ophthalmoplegia occurs. Careful visual assessment and alternating patching, as appropriate, may prevent a permanent loss of vision due to suppression. If a preschool child requires patching, the patch usually must be taped in place because of noncompliance with removable patches; thus the corneas must be monitored carefully.

In an outstanding review of oculomotor abnormalities due to TBI, Baker and Epstein[5] describe the types of visual disturbances that can be encountered in both adults and children. Neither incidence nor outcome is addressed, but the descriptions of injuries, including orbital fractures, cranial neuropathies, brainstem syndromes, and disturbances of saccades and pursuit due to cerebral lesions are compatible with clinical observations in children and youth. As with adults, any optic nerve trauma must be evaluated immediately for potential decompression.

Retinal hemorrhages in preschoolers with traumatic brain injury are considered pathognomonic for nonaccidental trauma and are believed to be due to rotational forces, which are typically of low velocity.[29,44]

Transient cortical blindness after pediatric TBI has been described by Griffith[38] as lasting no longer than two days. However, prolonged transient blindness has been reported in preschool children and is certainly familiar to most pediatric clinicians. The author has observed transient cortical blindness in a preschool child that lasted up to 30 days and was followed by nearly complete recovery of vision. However, cortical blindness lasting more than several days generally carries a grave prognosis for children of school-age and older.

Because children often have difficulty describing accommodation defects and diplopia or even visual field cuts, assessment generally must be observational in nature. Each state has a Department of the Visually Handicapped, which usually can supply a pediatric functional vision assessment by a trained specialist. This assessment supplements the diagnostic and prescriptive services of a pediatric opthalmologist. Such services may be administered through the local department of education or, in some instances, the health department. Inpatient pediatric rehabilitation programs can apply to the state vision services for a specialist to be assigned to evaluate pediatric patients on a regular basis, to make recommendations to the rehabilitation team, and to make referrals on discharge for local services, if they are needed.

The best management of accommodation defects is usually reassurance that the difficulty is temporary and will resolve without need for intervention. Diplopia in school-age and adolescent patients can be managed with patching. Because teenagers usually reject eye-patches, a pair of inexpensive glasses or sunglasses can be adapted to allow for alternate patching; often the sunglass lens can be popped in or out, depending on the side that is to be occluded. In patients with prolonged or severe diplopia, prisms can be attached to the lens of standard glasses and then changed as ocular motility improves. In youth, ocular dismotility of central origin may improve for up to 12 months after trauma, and most opthalmologists prefer to use conservative management for this period of time before suggesting surgical intervention.

Hearing loss is also common in pediatric TBI. Longitudinal fractures of the temporal bone—the most common basilar skull fractures—are associated with conductive hearing loss.[99] The traumatic conductive triad consisting of hearing loss, bloody otorrhea, and unconsciousness is well-known to clinician. Transverse fractures of the temporal bone are associated more often with sensory hearing loss. Fracture of the labyrinthine capsule should be suspected when tinnitus, vertigo and a sense of fullness in the ears are associated with fluctuating hearing loss. Low scores in speech discrimination with vertigo and little or no hearing loss may mean that a fistula is present. Simple concussion has been associated with hearing loss, most frequently at 4,000–6,000 Hz. Because of the difficulty that very young children have in describing symptoms, a high index of suspicion must be maintained. Furthermore, accurate testing requires an audiologist with extensive experience in both pediatrics and in traumatic hearing loss; audiologists with little pediatric experience may consider very young children untestable and those with little TBI experience may not test beyond 4,000 Hz.

In a retrospective review of 62 consecutive patients with TBI admitted to a pediatric inpatient rehabilitation unit, each of whom received standardized audiologic evaluation, 16% were found to have a conductive hearing loss, 13% a sensorineural hearing loss, and 16% a central auditory processing problem.[24] This study is compatible with the findings of a study by Vartianen and colleagues.[119] Although, according to Miltenberger et al. a peripheral hearing loss may confound a central auditory processing (CAP) disorder,[77] only two of the children in the first study were found to have a combined sensorineural hearing loss and CAP disorder; in both cases the two deficits were clearly separate entities.[24] Thus, if the audiologist is aware of the potential confusion, the deficiencies can be identified clearly.[55] Review of the literature suggests that all children with moderate-to-severe traumatic brain injuries should have a thorough audiologic evaluation consisting of standard and/or adaptive audiometry, impedance audiometry, and, when suspicion for CAP is high, the Screening Test for Auditory Processing (SCAN) for patients between the ages of 3 and 10 or the Willeford Test Battery and Staggered Spondaic Word List for patients with a cognitive age over 10 years. Furthermore, when behavioral or academic problems are noted after minor traumatic brain injury, a thorough audiologic evaluation should be considered.

The importance of identification of sensory deficits in pediatric patients cannot be overemphasized. In the case of ophthalmologic problems, patching, glasses, or preferential classroom seating may help to alleviate the difficulty. When audiologic deficits are present, hearing aids, an FM transmitter, or preferential classroom seating may be indicated. Academic performance is affected adversely by sensory deficits, most of which can be easily addressed by proper evaluations, follow-up, and a thoughtful rehabilitation plan.

NUTRITIONAL AND ENDOCRINE DISORDERS

The nutritional needs of infants, children, and adolescents have been well-described throughout the pediatric literature. In the United States virtually all hospitals serving children employ registered pediatric dieticians. It is inappropriate to calculate fluid requirements, caloric needs, and minimum daily requirements on the basis of adult data. In particular, tube feedings specific for infants and children must be used in patients below 6 years of age. Serious fluid and electrolyte disturbances may result when pediatricians or pediatric dieticians are not consulted about appropriate intravenous fluids or enteral feedings.

Proper nutrition must be ensured, not only to maintain the child during the period of recovery, but also to allow growth. The weight of the brain of a 24-month-old child is 75% that of an adult; by age 6 years, the brain has reached 90% of its adult weight. The majority of the brain is myelinated by the second year of life, but myelination continues throughout the second decade of life. Somatic growth is most rapid during the first 2 years of life and again during puberty. Failure to provide adequate nutrition during these crucial growth periods can lead to unnecessary complications, including growth failure, skin breakdown, and anemia.

One method for calculating caloric needs uses an age versus weight method (for example, newborn, 50 cal/kg/24hr; 1 week–6 months, 65–70 cal/kg/24hr; 6–12 months, 50–60 cal/kg/24hr).[45] This method yields the standard basal caloric expenditure (SBC). Actual expenditure is then calculated by taking into account temperature, activity level, stress, and other factors. Spasticity and flaccidity profoundly affect nutritional requirements in children, and need for growth must always be taken into account.

Oral intake often becomes an issue with a pediatric or adolescent patient. Because so much of the maternal-child interaction centers around feeding, children quickly discover food refusal as a powerful means of control. Such behavior is often exaggerated during severe illness or injury and may become particularly acute in the rehabilitation unit. It is important to deemphasize the aspect of oral intake while protecting the child's nutrition. Often well-meaning staff facilitate food-refusal by silently or even overtly communicating their anxiety; for this reason, all staff, including aides, housekeepers, and volunteers, as well as other clinical personnel, must be enlisted in a consistent approach to food refusal. If the child already has a nasogastric or gastric tube in place, food refusals may be approached in a more relaxed manner. In the child without enteric access, consistent food refusal for more than a few days that does not respond to a behavioral approach should be managed with nonpunitive institution of tube feedings.

Pediatric and adolescent patients must be weighed at least weekly and preferably twice weekly. Frequent, appealing snacks must be offered in addition to meals and usually can be incorporated into pleasant activities, such as social-skills groups, cooking groups, outings, and playtime. Toddlers should receive small portions with particular emphasis on finger foods, when appropriate. A toddler may be easily discouraged by the sight of an adult-sized meal on a large plate. On the other hand, adolescents often request and require double portions as well as free access to milk and other fluids.

Superior mesenteric artery syndrome (also known as cast syndrome) may occur in asthenic children in body jackets or body casts. It has also been observed in brain-injured children[87] and should be suspected when a thin child who spends the majority of time in the recumbent position develops further weight loss and an ileus. It is managed as in adults: avoidance of the supine position, removal of abdominal compression garments or molded jackets, if possible, and refeeding, usually jejunal.

Although rare, hypopituitarism with impaired growth,[76] cachexia, and hypogonadism[85] has been reported in children after traumatic brain injury, as has precocious puberty.[12,110] Linear growth and weight should be followed carefully in all children during both inpatient and outpatient courses. Growth points must be plotted on a growth chart, and any deviation must be investigated.

Syndrome of inappropriate secretion of antidiuretic hormone (SIADH) and diabetes insipidus may occur during the intensive care phase of treatment but rarely occur first during the rehabilitative phase. However, Anmuth et al. reported a case of chronic SIADH in a 14-year-old boy with TBI, who responded to treatment with demeclocycline until intake of fluid could be restricted.[3]

MISCELLANEOUS MEDICAL COMPLICATIONS

Heterotopic ossification (HO) occurs in children and adolescents but not as frequently as in adults. Hurvitz et al. (1992) reviewed 90 brain-injured patients under the age of 19 years who had been comatose for more than 24 hours.[48] They found the incidence of HO to be 14% and identified risk factors as age greater than 11 years, and longer length of coma; in addition, HO was associated with poorer overall outcome. However, only 3 of 13 patients with HO had residual impairments secondary to HO. In a prospective study at DuPont of 82 youths (60 with TBI), aged 4 months to 21 years, bone scans uncovered 16 sites of HO, only 6 of which were identified before the scans.[109] In 3 of the patients, all of whom were older than 13 years of age, progress was impeded by HO. A previous study reported by the same center found evidence of HO in 25 of 111 patients, only 3 of whom had significant impairment related to the HO.[22] All of these studies have comparable results, suggesting that HO rarely results in functional impairment in younger children. The use of etidronate in children and adolescents has been reported to result in osteoporosis and should be avoided.[20,106] In preadolescent patients, treatment with medication is probably not necessary, and in adolescents anti-inflammatory agents are probably the most appropriate choice. In all cases, gentle but persistent range-of-motion exercises are imperative.

The prospective study of Sobus also looked at the incidence of undetected musculoskeletal trauma in pediatric rehabilitation patients.[109] Of 60 children with TBI, a total of 25 previously unnoticed fracture sites were identified by bone scan in 16 patients and 19 were found to have newly detected sites of soft-tissue trauma.

An occasional complication of childhood skull fractures is the so-called growing fracture. Scarfo et al. hypothesized that this phenomenon results from the interaction of three basic conditions: head injury with a large gaping fracture, corresponding dural tear, and occurrence during infancy, the period of most rapid brain growth.[103] Intracranial pressure vectors are thus altered, and the ventricular system begins to deform. A significant cranial defect may require surgical correction. Although pediatric skull fractures do not require longitudinal follow-up in the majority of patients, the convergence of the above factors or the presence of a persistent palpable cranial defect over a known skull fracture should clue the physician to follow up with skull films or a CT of the head with bony windows. An excellent review of the subject has been published by Arseni and Ciurea.[4]

Although rare, traumatic intracranial aneurysms occur more frequently in children than in adults. In a review of the literature, Buckingham concluded that aneurysms secondary to penetrating trauma occur more often in teenagers.[16] Aneurysms due to nonpenetrating trauma are more common at the base of the skull or in the periphery, and peripheral traumatic aneurysms are more common in younger patients.[16] Delayed acute intracranial hemorrhage was the most common presenting symptom. Others included epistaxis, progressive cranial nerve palsy, or a growing fracture.

Delayed neurologic deterioration in apparently mildly brain-injured children was investigated retrospectively by Snoek. Of 967 patients aged 2 months to 17 years, 42 experienced deterioration after a "lucid" or symptom-free interval; of these, only 1 had an intracranial hematoma, and 3 died. Various causes appeared to play a role, but the author concluded that the autonomic flow to the juvenile brain is different and may result in a delayed manifestation of increased intracranial pressure.

MANAGEMENT OF TRACHEOSTOMY

Management of tracheostomy in children and adolescents differs from that in adults. Fenestrated tracheostomy tubes are inadvisable, because granulation tissue forms much more rapidly in youthful patients than in adults and may grow into the fenestrations within 1 week, making removal difficult and dangerous. Furthermore, subglottic stenosis secondary to tracheal granulation is more frequent in children than in adults. A recent study from DuPont Institute found that 30% of pediatric patients with TBI tracheostomies had tracheal granuloma, whereas 13% had tracheal stenosis.[22] An overall 90% complication rate in pediatric patients with TBI who arrived at the rehabilitation unit with tracheostomies suggests that such patients should be decannulated with caution. The authors suggest the following protocol for decannulation of children with prolonged intubation: (1) oxygenation and ventilation must be adequate; (2) mechanisms for management of secretions must be intact; (3) medical complications must be treated; (4) nutritional status must be satisfactory; (5) risks of aspiration and poor airway protection must be assessed; and (6) radiography and selective bronchoscopy should be performed.

Gradual reduction of the size of the tracheostomy tube without the above protocol may be successful in older children, but the practitioner must be aware that sizes of the external diameters of the Shiley and Portex tubes differ. In a child's airway, a slight increase in the external diameter of a tracheostomy tube may cause partial airway obstruction; thus changes in types of tubes must be done carefully.

MANAGEMENT OF SPASTICITY

Spasticity in prepubertal children often may be managed with positioning and splinting alone because of the child's smaller size and relative weakness. In a larger child who is not forcefully posturing, serial casting may be successful both in the intensive care unit and throughout the rehabilitative phase. Bivalved fiberglass casts usually are managed by the nursing staff, except in patients with extreme posturing problems. In such patients bivalved casts may be used if the nursing staff pays meticulous attention to proper application, performs frequent skin checks, and adheres to the splinting schedule established by the physiatrist or therapy staff.

Excessive posturing may be controlled with Tranxene or Dantrium (Table 4). However, posturing often reflects agitation rather than spasticity and should be managed as much as possible by controlling pain and reducing environmental stimuli or by attempting to identify and treat previously undetected musculoskeletal trauma.

In the intensive care unit, complications due to fisting frequently may be reduced by inserting rolled terry washcloths into the fisted hand; this approach generally is better tolerated than the use of cones, at least initially. As the patient's course progresses, dorsal splints with thumb abduction may be more useful than palmar resting splints, which may further stimulate the palmar grasp reflex.

In the intensive care unit, maintenance of hip and knee flexion with sandbags and pillows is generally more successful than footboards or positioning splints in breaking up trunk and lower-extremity extensor posturing. If such measures, in combination with ankle splints, do not control the extension and if side-lying is impractical, then positioning casts may be warranted. However, they must be applied carefully by an individual skilled in casting and must be changed every 3–5 days to prevent skin breakdown. Usually such casts cannot be successfully bivalved because of the extreme force of posturing.

During the rehabilitation phase, a combination of side-lying, hammocks, hip and knee flexion, and splinting usually controls spasticity. When necessary, medications may be used. Dantrolene sodium (Dantrium) may be useful, although its sedating properties may be undesirable. However, sedation is usually less marked in younger children than in adults. In the past, oral baclofen has been used for the long-term management of cerebral spasticity, although it has not proved to be clinically effective at the normally recommended dose. Sometimes it is useful in combination with Dantrium. Valium can be used for spasticity but may be associated with increased agitation in children who are emerging from coma.

Baclofen pumps have some application in older children and adults for treatment of spinal and supraspinal spasticity.[100] The adult pump is the size of a hockey puck; a smaller pediatric pump has been developed

TABLE 4. Commonly Used Medications and Doses

Name	Dosage	Side Effects	Monitoring
Acetaminophen	10–15 mg/kg/dose q4h Max 5 doses/24 h	Hepatotoxicity from overdose; contraindicated in G6PD deficiency	Liver enzymes, if multiple hepatotoxic medications
Baclofen (Lioresal)	1–4 yr: 2.5–5 mg BID–TID 5–12 yr: 2.5 mg–10 mg TID	Drowsiness, constipation, nausea, muscle weakness, hallucination with abrupt withdrawal	Renal function; EEG if patient has known seizure disorder
Carbamazepine (Tegretol)	Initial 10 mg/kg/24 hr, increase in increments to to 20 mg/kg/24 hr Max 100 mg dose BID	Drowsiness, dizziness, diplopia, urinary retention, Stevens-Johnson, hepatotoxicity	CBC, liver enzymes, drug levels
Chlorazepate dipotassium (Tranxene)	1–3 yr: $\frac{1}{2}$ of a 3.75 mg tab BID–TID 4–9 yr: 3.75 mg BID–TID 9–12 yr: 7.5 mg BID–TID	CNS depression	Liver enzymes
Clonidine (Catapres)	5–12 yr: 0.05 mg BID, increasing in increments of 0.05 mg/day to a max of 0.2 mg/day	Drowsiness, which resolves in a few days; hypotension (rare); hypertension with abrupt withdrawal	Blood pressure
Codeine	0.5–1.0 mg/kg/dose q4–6hr IM or PO Max 30–60 mg/dose	Constipation, cramping, respiratory depression, CNS depression	Respiratory status
Dantrolene (Dantrium)	0.5 mg/kg/dose BID; gradually increase to max of 3 mg/kg QID Max 100 mg QID	Drowsiness, weakness, malaise diarrhea	Liver function studies
Diazepam (Valium) — As sedative:	0.12–0.8 mg/kg/24 hr q6–8 hr PO; Max 0.6 mg/kg within an 8-hr period	Hypotension, respiratory depression, do not use in neonates, give no faster than 2 mg/min undiluted	Respiratory status
Status epilepticus:	0.2–0.5 mg/kg/dose IV q15–20 min; <5 yr total 5 mg, >5 yr total 10 mg		
Docusate (Colace)	<3 yr: 10–40 mg/24 hr 3–6 yr: 20–60 mg/24 hr 6–12 hr: 40–120 mg/24 hr >12 yr: 50–240 mg/24 hr	Diarrhea Liquid form extremely bitter	Stool consistency; hydration
Imipramine (Tofranil)	0.5 mg/kg/q hs PO; increase by 0.5 mg/kg Max PO dose 1.5 mg/kg	Drowsiness, dry mouth, constipation, dizziness	BP, CBC; ECG if doses >1 mg/kg are to be used. Drug levels at high doses
Lithium	15–60 mg/kg/day BID-TID PO	Goiter, nephrogenic diabetes insipidus, sedation; seizures or death at levels >2.5 mEq/L	Thyroid functions, electrolytes, hydration, drug levels (0.6–1.2 mEq/L
Lorazepam (Ativan)	Status epilepticus: 0.05 mg/kg dose IV or PR up to max of 4 mg/dose. May repeat in 15–20 min × 1	Respiratory depression, sedation, dizziness, ataxia	Respiratory status
Methylphenidate (Ritalin)	0.25 mg/kg/dose PO with breakfast and lunch; may double weekly until 1–2 mg/kg/24 hr Max 60 mg/24 hr	Insomnia, weight loss, rash, nausea, anorexia, hallucinations, tics	Weight, sleep pattern
Phenytoin (Dilantin)	4–7 mg/kg/24 hr BID IV or PO Max 300 mg/24 hr	Dermatitis, ataxia, hepatotoxicity, nystagmus, SLE and Stevens-Johnson syndromes, blood dyscrasias	CBC, liver enzymes, drug levels (10–20 mg/L)
Ranitidine (Zantac)	2–4 mg/kg/24 hr PO BID	Headache, malaise, insomnia, sedation, arthralgia, hepatotoxicity	Liver enzymes
Trazodone (Desyrel)	25–150 mg q hs PO; not approved for children <13 yr	Nausea/vomiting	Liver enzymes

Max = maximum, BID = twice daily, TID = three times daily, QID = four times daily, PO = orally, IM = intramuscularly, IV = intravenously, CNS = central nervous system, EEG = electroencephalogram, BP = blood pressure, CBC= complete blood count, ECG = electrocardiogram, PR = rectally, SLE = systemic lupus erythematosus.

that is satisfactory for older children but still too large for very young children.

Selective dorsal rhizotomy has become a popular modality for the control of persistent cerebral spasticity. Long-term follow-up of patients originally operated on by pioneers of the technique has yielded no evidence of serious complications due to partial laminectomies in young children.[10] However, the surgery is extensive and requires intensive postoperative therapy. Furthermore, strength does not reach premorbid levels until at least 6 months after surgery. Selective dorsal rhizotomy has produced satisfactory control of severe spasticity in many patients and should be considered a reasonable option for treatment of static severe spasticity that lasts more than 2 years and does not respond to other modalities. Its efficacy, however, remains controversial. In an editorial published in 1990, Landau and Hunt conclude that as yet there is no convincing evidence of efficacy and that long-term complications are as yet unknown.[64] One gait laboratory study concluded that spasticity and gait dynamics were positively affected by the procedure but that basic patterns of muscle activation were not.[17] Various centers report differing results from selective dorsal rhizotomy, some of which appear to be related to surgical technique, some to the presurgical screening process, and some to postsurgical rehabilitation. In this author's experience, function certainly can be improved in selected patients. However, the physicians and the family must have realistic goals for the surgery (for example, improved positioning) and not expect a miraculous result.

Nerve and motor point blocks may be used successfully in children but usually require general anesthesia. Because the effects generally do not last for more than 6 months, it is debatable whether such methods are cost-effective when general anesthesia must be used. Recent work on the use of Botox in children with spastic diplegia is promising. The procedure can be performed successfully in the office without use of anesthesia, and electromyographic monitoring has shown fairly successful results.[58] The use of the topical anesthetic EMLA (lidocaine 2.5% and prilocaine 2.5%) has further reduced the painfulness of the procedure. The fact that the paralysis induced by Botox is nondestructive and reversible makes it an appealing modality. As with the more standard neurolytic procedures, the effects last for about 3–6 months in most patients.

Muscle lengthening procedures produce a longer-lasting effect. However, because of growth, such procedures may have to be repeated several times during childhood and adolescence. Each lengthening procedure results in some weakening of muscle and so must be undertaken with serious consideration of stage of development and overall rehabilitation plan.

Spasticity may result in contractures during periods of rapid growth, particularly during adolescence. For this reason, it is advisable to monitor outpatients every 3 months during growth spurts, and to consider more aggressive splinting, casting, and stretching during these periods. If the purpose and temporary nature of the intervention are explained to the child and family, compliance is often excellent and surgery can sometimes be avoided.

Tone-reducing ankle-foot orthoses have become popular in many centers. These orthoses have a footplate with a longitudinal arch as well as two transverse arches and extend over the dorsum of the foot. Similar casts can be fabricated. Several groups have found them to be useful in reducing lower-extremity spasticity and in improving gait.[15,46,49,102] The braces have the disadvantage of being more difficult to apply and need to be replaced more frequently than standard AFOs. However, if the family is informed of such inconveniences, they can be used quite successfully and are generally well-tolerated by the child if they are properly fabricated.

Biofeedback to control spasticity has been evaluated by Nash and colleagues.[79] They taught two 5-year-olds and 1 eight-year-old with spastic diplegia to use biofeedback for spasticity control. Although the technique was successful, and although carry-over to muscles other than the trained muscle was observed, long-term follow-up was not done. This technique may hold promise.

Soft thumb-abduction splints may successfully reduce increased hand tone and allow better function. They are inexpensive, unobtrusive, and generally well-liked by patients.

Splinting and bracing often are rejected by adolescents, particularly during the school day. Rather than becoming involved in a power struggle, it may be more productive for the health care provider to allow the adolescent to go to school without braces, if such a decision is not medically contraindicated, and to wear splints in the evening or at night and during the summer vacation.

SEIZURES

In a 1986 review of the literature, Kennedy and Freeman concluded that early posttraumatic seizures were more common in children than in adults, that late seizures were more common in adults, and that prophylaxis had not been demonstrated to prevent the development of late seizures.[54]

In an evaluation of early seizures in children, Hahn et al. reviewed a series of children with TBI under the age of 17 years who were admitted to Children's Memorial Hospital from 1980–1986.[43] Excluded from the sample were children with fluid and electrolyte imbalances, hypoxic or ischemic brain injury, or a premorbid history of seizures. Of the 937 children 87 experienced early seizures; 3 experienced seizures between 24 hours and 7 days after admission; and only 2 developed seizures after 7 days. Development of early seizures was associated with a GCS score of 8 or less, diffuse cerebral edema, acute subdural hematoma, and open, depressed skull fractures with damage to the parenchyma. Both children who developed seizures after 1 week had depressed skull fractures. Based on their observations and a review of the literature, the authors advocated seizure prophylaxis for children with factors associated with a higher incidence of seizures, but no specific duration of prophylaxis was recommended.

The long-term prophylactic use of antiepileptic drugs in children should not be undertaken lightly, particularly in view of the 1990 study of Farwell et al., which investigated the use of prophylactic phenobarbital for febrile convulsions and its effect on intelligence.[33] In this large-scale prospective study, some children with febrile convulsions were treated with prophylactic phenobarbital, and others were not. The prophylactic use of antiepileptic drugs did not decrease the incidence of epilepsy, but was found to have a small but significant negative effect on IQ.

In a 1991 review of the neurobehavioral effects of phenytoin, valproate, and carbamazepine in adult patients with TBI, Massagli found no definite proof of the desirability of one agent over another and recommended a study of the behavioral and cognitive effects of antiepileptic drugs in patients with TBI.[94] In general, all of the drugs evaluated in this review produced negative cognitive effects, particularly at higher levels.

Mitchell et al. reported a blinded study of antiepileptic drugs in 111 epileptic children aged 5–13 years, in which the children were evaluated for simple and complex reaction times, attention, and impulsivity; in addition, blood levels of the drugs were drawn.[78] Although higher levels of most of the agents were associated with more impulsive errors on complex reaction times, the authors found an improvement in complex reaction time in 54 children treated with higher levels of carbamazepine monotherapy. Minimal dose-related effects were noted with phenobarbital.

Clonazepam is commonly used in pediatrics in the management of difficult-to-control seizures. However, its common side effect of increased oral and bronchial secretions makes it an undesirable drug in patients with poor cough, oropharyngeal weakness, or oromotor apraxia.

Based on current knowledge of the possible negative effects of phenobarbital on cognition in the developing brain and on the frequency of idiosyncratic agitation in children treated with phenobarbital (over 50% in one series),[1] most intensive care units now use phenytoin rather than phenobarbital for acute prophylaxis; thus, when the patient arrives in the rehabilitation unit, he or she is often taking enteral phenytoin and tube feedings. If the receiving physician feels uncomfortable weaning the patient from phenytoin, plasma levels must be assessed immediately, because tube feedings interfere with absorption.[8] Furthermore, after approximately 3 weeks of treatment, all phenytoin receptor sites are occupied and plasma concentration may increase suddenly to toxic levels. Dilantin stays in suspension poorly, and if it is administered in the suspension form, doses may vary considerably, particularly if the drug is not vigorously resuspended by shaking before administration. For these reasons, if Dilantin is to be continued, levels must be monitored carefully until oral feedings and pharmacologic equilibrium are established.

A 1986 study of the effects of nonfebrile seizures on intellectual functioning in children demonstrated no evidence of intellectual deterioration over time, regardless of the anticonvulsant therapy. On the basis of the available literature, it appears that ongoing prophylaxis of early posttraumatic seizures is probably not indicated; if seizures are present, however, phenytoin is satisfactory in most patients and has the advantage of less frequent dosing as well as less cost. No solid evidence in the literature supports a change to carbamazepine, despite the theoretical advantages.

Agitation

Children and adolescents emerging from coma move through the Rancho levels in a similar fashion to adults. However, the agitated phase is often not as prolonged as in adults. When faced with severe agitation that lasts for more than 24 hours, the clinician should determine what factors are involved and attempt to manipulate them rather than resort immediately to pharmacologic management.

Overstimulation by well-meaning staff, parents, and friends often contributes to the agitation. Many families believe that by talking loudly and turning on lights, television, and radios they can help to "bring the child around." Some families resist suggestions to decrease visitors and stimuli, and in many acute medical settings, children with TBI are placed in multibed rooms with higher staff ratios to facilitate closer observation. As with adults, restraints often increase agitation and should be used as little as possible. Heavy sedation may prolong recovery, as indicated in the adult literature, and thus should be avoided.

It may be necessary for the rehabilitation team to set up an "agitation protocol" for children with TBI in the acute medical unit, consisting of a single room with no television or telephones, limited visitors, and visual monitors. When a family member or team member is in the room, restraints may be discontinued. If the child does not attempt to remove tubes, a single restraint consisting of a sheet folded around the waist and pelvis and fastened to the bed frame is often sufficient. Although some units have rooms with mattresses on the floor, patients are still at risk of falling against a wall when they stand. In the rehabilitation unit, patients should receive the initial therapies in their room until the agitation has nearly subsided. If a family member can spend the night with the child, nighttime restraints often may be avoided. If no tubes or intravenous lines that can be dislodged are present, a veil bed may be used to contain the patient.

Occult fractures (see previous discussion), broken teeth, and headaches are frequent causes of pain and hence of agitation that may be easily overlooked. Careful examination, particularly of the oral cavity, and aggressive pain management often reduce agitation. Administration of acetaminophen with codeine (Table 4) every 4 hours while the patient is awake frequently reduces the amount of agitation and usually avoids oversedation. However, stool softeners and a moderately aggressive bowel program should be implemented to avoid impaction.

Constipation and urinary tract infections also may exacerbate agitation and must be treated if present. Colace elixir is quite bitter and usually unacceptable to children who are able to take medications by mouth. However, it is useful when medications are administered by gastric or jejunal tubes. Milk of magnesia is a highly satisfactory stool softener and is well-accepted by younger children, but most older children prefer and can be managed with Colace tablets.

If no source of pain or other cause of agitation is identified and if agitation increases in the evening or results in poor sleep at night, a trial of a low-dose antidepressant in the evening may be considered. Imipramine has been used in children for many years, and dosage guidelines are readily available (Table 4). Many young children below the age of 5 years respond to a single 5-mg dose at bedtime with improved sleep patterns. School-age children may be started at 10 mg, at bedtime. Dosages may be increased as needed. Adolescents aged 13 years or older tolerate trazadone well and often respond to an evening dose as low as 25 mg, although 50 mg is generally a good starting dose.

When prescribing tricyclic antidepressants, the clinician must keep in mind that they can be associated with cardiac rhythm changes in both children and adults[123] and that they lower the seizure threshold.[50] However, at the lower doses described above, such side effects are rare. Once the sleep cycle is normalized and agitation has resolved, it is usually desirable to attempt to discontinue the nighttime antidepressants during the rehabilitation program.

If agitation does not resolve, clonidine may be used. Clonidine has been used successfully in attention deficit disorder in children with high aggression levels[123] and is rarely associated with side effects other than initial drowsiness or hypotension. Blood pressure should be monitored and a single dose withheld if it is low. Although clonidine is not officially approved for use in patients under the age of 12 years, it has been successfully prescribed by pediatricians for certain types of attention deficit disorder-hyperactivity disorder with components of agitation for several years. The initial dose of 0.05 mg orally twice daily in a school-aged child may be increased in 0.05 mg daily increments to a maximum of 0.2 mg/day. There is little experience with clonidine in preschool children.

Clonidine may be dosed orally or transdermally. The transdermal patch is convenient, but doses are difficult to titrate, and the full activity of the drug is not observed for at least 24 hours. However, in cases of severely agitated and aggressive patients, transdermal delivery may be quite useful, minimizing the amount of medication that has to be administered orally or by gastric tube.

Propranolol (Inderal) also has been helpful in reducing agitation, particularly in preschool children. However, its sedative and hypotensive effects may outweigh its benefits. Inderal is most useful for decreasing agitation in the acute phases of injury to the central nervous system, especially in the intensive care unit, because it can be administered intravenously. The usual pediatric dose is 2–4 mg/day orally, divided in 2–4 equal doses. Treatment should be discontinued gradually.

Movement Disorders

Roig[96] has reported the successful management of nonhereditary chorea with carbamazepine. However, first-line agents continue to be haloperidol, chlorpromazine, reserpine, and phenobarbital. Successful pharmacologic management of post-TBI tremor in children has not been reported, although Inderal may be tried.

PHARMACOLOGIC MANAGEMENT OF BEHAVIORAL ISSUES

Inattention, Impulsivity, and Disinhibition

The pediatric rehabilitation team often can successfully enlist the patient's family in carrying out a behavioral program for the brain-injured child. However, such a program may need to be supplemented with medication.

A child with a significantly decreased attention span needs to be thoroughly evaluated to determine the cause. Visual or auditory distractibility often is not responsive to medical management and must be addressed environmentally. However, children who meet the criteria for attention deficit disorder with or without hyperactivity may respond well to medication, particularly if they have a premorbid history of the disorder. Methylphenidate is a good initial choice, particularly because the results are immediate. Children are quite susceptible to placebo effect, as are the adults surrounding them. For this reason, cognitive tasks should be targeted and a baseline established. If possible the medication should be given in a blinded fashion and data collected in an ABAB protocol (i.e., two trials on medication [A] interspersed with two trials off [B] medication) to determine whether any positive effects are the result of recovery or of medication. In low dosages, methylphenidate raises the seizure threshold, but in high doses it is believed to lower seizure threshold. Side effects of methylphenidate include depressed appetite and insomnia, which usually subside after treatment has continued for 2 weeks. Growth retardation also has been reported at high doses over prolonged periods.[123]

Werry found improvements in hyperactive children with both imipramine and methylphenidate.[124] The structural relationship between imipramine and carbamazepine may explain some of the positive performance effect reported with carbamazepine in epileptic patients (see related information under seizures).

If methylphenidate does not improve concentration and attention, a trial of imipramine or trazodone may be warranted. Evaluation of the effects is more difficult, because maximal benefit is not seen for 1–2 weeks. When used in a single evening dose, the tricyclic antidepressants may improve the quality of sleep in posttraumatic patients and thus improve daytime concentration ability, in addition to the benefits observed in noninjured patients with attention deficit-hyperactivity disorder. Collection of baseline data and vacations from medication are important tools in evaluating effectiveness.

Gualtieri evaluated amantidine in a group of patients that included three children aged 5, 14, and 16 years, all with symptoms of severe disinhibition.[39] All three children demonstrated a good response with minimal side effects. Amantidine has been used successfully in the treatment of viral infections in children; the same doses may be used in the management of disinhibition.

Outbursts and Mania

Episodic dyscontrol is managed in both children and adults by a structured behavioral approach, with clear consequences for out-of-control behavior, and medication if needed. If episodes of rage are not associated with mania, carbamazepine is usually the drug of choice. If manic episodes are present, lithium may be preferable, although carbamazepine alone has been used successfully in the treatment of bipolar disease in adolescents.[65] Children are said to tolerate lithium well,[91] but long-term effects are unknown, and higher doses may be required in children than in adults. The therapeutic margin of lithium is narrow, the half-life is long, and dehydration may lead quickly to increased blood levels. In addition, affective disorders in children are difficult to diagnose; thus, before lithium is considered, it is advisable to consult a pediatric psychiatrist with experience in treating children with traumatic brain injuries.

The combination of lithium and carbamazepine is potentially toxic,[84] and levels must be monitored closely if the drugs are used concurrently.

Some clinicians are concerned that even the act of prescribing medication for childhood behavioral problems may carry the message that the child is inadequate and needs drugs to control his or her behavior. In response to this concern, Whalen and Henker recommend the attributional approach, which compares the situation to that of a child who needs glasses or crutches but who is getting stronger and beginning to take control of his or her behavior.

Prevention

Various programs aimed at preventing TBI in children, most of which are educational, have been established throughout the country. Many of these programs, however, have been created at great expense without evaluating either the target audience or the results.

Some investigators have indeed looked at target populations in an attempt to establish meaningful prevention programs. An important study from Harborview in Seattle evaluated the parental expectations of traffic skills of children and found that parents overestimated such skills in younger age groups (5–6 years-old).[30] This finding was consistent across all socioeconomic levels. However, parental expectations were appropriate in the older age groups. Salvatore evaluated the ability of school-aged children to estimate the velocity of oncoming cars and found that boys underestimated and girls overestimated the speed of oncoming traffic across all age groups.[101]

Jordan et al. evaluated the efficacy of educational interventions with adolescent mothers and found that the incidence of injury to their children was successfully reduced.[53] Ozanne-Smith found an 80% rate of compliance with helmet use and decreased incidence of injury in Victoria, Australia, after helmet legislation was passed.[81] In a 1989 study of traffic injuries in children, Pless et al. were unable to identify strong predictors

TABLE 5. Intervention Sites and Topics for Childhood Injury Prevention Programming

Interven-tion Site	Prenatal	Birth	1–4 Years	5–9 Years	10–14 Years	15–19 Years
Prenatal care	Parenting skills training Parent seat belts Infant safety seats Education Home safety training	Parenting skills training Parent seat belts Infant safety seat loans				
Hospitals	Infant safety seat loans	Infant safety seat loans	Gates	Bike helmets	Bike helmets	Bike helmets
Women, infants, and children parenting classes		Infant, toddler safety seats	Infant, toddler safety seats Pedestrian safety Home safety			
Primary health care settings		Infant, toddler safety seats	Infant, toddler safety seats Pedestrian safety Home safety	Seat belts Pedestrian safety Bicycle safety Helmets	Farm machinery Recreational safety Bicycle safety, helmets Alcohol counselling	Farm machinery Recreational safety Bicycle safety, helmets Alcohol counselling
Homes			Home, toy safety Motor vehicle safety products	Home, toy safety Motor vehicle safety products	Motor vehicle safety	
Schools				Safe playgrounds, sports Pedestrian skills Bike skills Bike helmets After school programs	Safe playgrounds, sports Farm machinery Child labor legisla-tion enforcement Bike helmets After school programs	Violence reduction Education Farm machinery Child labor legisla-tion enforcement
Day care centers			Playground safety			
Worksites	Infant safety seats	Infant safety seats	Toys, home safety		Child labor legisla-lation enforcement Training for adoles-cent employees	Child labor legisla-tion enforcement Training for adoles-cent employees
Social serv-ices, youth services	Family support	Family support	Family support	Family support	Suicide crisis centers Out-of-home care	
Local law enforcement		Safety seat laws	Safety seat laws	Seat belt laws Helmet laws Handgun storage/control	Seat belt laws Helmet laws Alcohol sales/con-sumption laws Handgun storage/control	Seat belt laws Helmet laws Alcohol sales/con-sumption laws Handgun storage/control
Code enforcement		Tap water regu-lators, building codes, smoke detectors, pool fences, gates	Tap water regu-lators, building codes, smoke detectors, pool fences, gates	Tap water regu-lators, building codes, smoke detectors, pool fences, gates	Tap water regu-lators, building codes, smoke detectors	
State and federal government			Reduce television violence	Reduce television violence	Reduce television violence	Reduce television violence Drivers license at 18 Handgun control
Local community				Bike trails, side-walks Helmet legislation Off-street play areas Organized sports	Bike trails, side-walks Helmet legislation Off-street play areas Organized sports	Bike trails, side-walks Helmet legislation Server and point-of-sale interventions
Media		Infant safety seats	Toddler seats Safe play areas	Seat belts Reduce televised violence Bike helmets	Seat belts Reduce televised violence Bike helmets	Seat belts Reduce televised violence Bike helmets Occupational safety Drinking/driving

From Children's Safety Network: A Data Book of Child and Adolescent Injury. Washington, DC, National Center for Education in Maternal and Child Health, 1991.

for traffic injuries in children and concluded that an environmental approach to prevention would be most effective.[81] Several studies comparing educational with legislative approaches found that educational approaches have short-term effects, whereas legislative approaches are particularly effective in the long term.[26,86,93,104] Legislation mandating the use of helmets, seatbelts, and athletic safety measures has a major role, as well as environmental manipulations, such as bicycle and pedestrian paths, overpasses at busy intersections, and safe playgrounds. As Widome stated, "Injury prevention is as much a community and public responsibility as it is an individual one."[129] Society pays for each individual who is injured, and societal responsibility for prevention as well as provision of services must be recognized. Prevention, however, must be multifaceted and constantly reevaluated (Table 5).[19]

Educational Issues

Like return to previous employment for the brain-injured adult, return to an academic environment may present seemingly insurmountable challenges for the child or adolescent. Because of the propensity of TBI to affect vision and hearing, new learning, memory, concentration, impulse control, and organizational skills, previously achievable academic tasks, and even the classroom environment, may become particularly taxing. In addition to the academic expectations from the student, peer interaction is a vital part of the school environment, and children or adolescents with TBI frequently find themselves socially isolated from peer groups. Because the child may have little physical evidence of the injury, social and academic expectations may be unrealistic, and the child may become frustrated and depressed. Occasionally a parent refuses to allow information about the child's deficits to be communicated to the school because he or she believes that the child is "completely recovered." Parental denial has been identified up to 10 years after injury[115] and may present a significant barrier to recovery.

By law (PL 94-142) all school children with disabilities must be provided an appropriate educational program in the least restrictive environment possible. All disabled students have an individual education plan (IEP), that must, by federal law, undergo review at a minimum of every 2 years. School districts receive federal funds for compliance with this mandate. However, the law leaves room for a great deal of individual interpretation.

Unless the school has expertise in TBI, the child may be assigned to a learning disabled or severely emotionally disturbed placement. Although such placements may be appropriate in some cases, the continued, sometimes remarkable, recovery during the first 2 years after TBI in children requires frequent, sometimes bimonthly, program evaluation, and the presence of both emotional and cognitive difficulties requires a multifaceted approach. Furthermore, the law has recently recognized "brain injury" as a separate category of impairment. Legal recognition, however, does not mean that the school is required to set up a separate program for brain-injured students; in many cases, because of shortage of funds and staff, existing resources must be adapted to the brain-injured student. For the student with severe motor impairment but fairly good cognitive skills, it is reasonable to expect the school to provide assistance for activities of daily living, mobility, and motoric academic tasks, such as note-taking. Generally such students can learn to use computers effectively for word-processing and to interface with augmentative communication, if needed. In such cases, the school should be urged strongly to provide access to an appropriate computer at school and for homework.

School therapy services must be "educationally related" but this requirement leaves room for a fair amount of interpretation. Some schools provide occupational therapy, physical therapy, and speech services at least weekly, whereas others provide strictly academically related speech and occupational services. The rehabilitation professional has the responsibility to communicate the need for therapy services and their relationship to the child's academic achievement as well as potential for improvement. It is also important for the rehabilitation team to communicate with the school in a positive and supportive fashion and to avoid unrealistic expectations, such as requesting all rehabilitative services to be provided by the school system.

In an excellent review of educational issues in TBI, Telzrow identifies several deterrents to successful academic reentry,[113] including conflict between the treatment center and the educational agency. Such conflict most often occurs when the school is approached in an aggressive fashion without an understanding of legal mandates and policies. In addition, the treatment center must recognize that the school requires several weeks to prepare for the student. Thus it is wise for the rehabilitation team to contact the school as soon as they become aware of the student and to plan jointly for reentry. Reentry often is facilitated when qualifying evaluations required by the school are administered by the treating team.

Telzrow also cites the lack of TBI-specific programs as a deterrent to successful reentry. The child with TBI often performs at a nearly age-appropriate level on achievement batteries, which refer to previously learned material. Yet the cognitive skills for further academic advancement frequently are impaired. Thus students sometimes may not be identified by achievement screenings as having special needs, or the initial academic placement may be too high. Aspects of existing programs for learning disabled, severely emotionally disturbed, and sensory or orthopedically impaired students may need to be pulled together to address successfully the needs of the student with TBI.

The prolonged summer vacation may cause the student with TBI to lose headway in academic achievement. If an extended school year cannot be arranged for children and adolescents who appear to need it, the treatment center may need to provide supplemental cognitive therapy services.

Telzrow also identifies ten aspects of educational services that enhance the program of most children with TBI: controlled environment (such as a self-contained or modified classroom) with gradual reintegration into the general classroom; low pupil-to-teacher ratio; repetition and multimodality presentation; emphasis on process; behavioral programming; integration of rehabilitative therapies; simulations for generalization of skills to real life; cuing and shadowing (in adult vocational programs); readjustment counseling; and home-school liaison. In the author's experience, most of the above services are required for successful academic progress, particularly with the moderately to severely involved student.

It is not unusual for school-aged patients to return to school successfully with little intervention but to develop significant academic and social problems in the preadolescent years. Thus, the students must be followed longitudinally, and the school must be made aware of the possibility of difficulty once the academic and organizational demands are accelerated.

Preschoolers with traumatic brain injuries are entitled by law (PL99-457) to specialized services until the third birthday. Early intervention services may be administered locally through the school districts or health department and provided by various agencies including hospitals, home-health agencies, county health departments, and schools. However, each program must serve young children "at risk" and establish an Individual Family Service Plan (IFSP) for each client. Although the rehabilitation team may include an early education specialist, an occupational therapist, a physical therapist, and a speech pathologist, the primary therapist who delivers most of the care may be assigned from any of those disciplines. Some early intervention services are not free or may be billed to the insurer; thus, before a referral is made, the rehabilitation professional should instruct the family to inquire about cost and procedures. Some insurance plans offer limited benefits for outpatient therapy, and it is vital for the treatment team to try to utilize such benefits in the most cost-effective manner. Sometimes an early intervention program meets the insurer's criteria, but decisions must be made by the rehabilitation professionals and family in a knowledgeable fashion.

A recent study indicated that physical therapy isolated from an integrated system was not useful in improving performance in infants with cerebral palsy.[82] Several insurers have used this study as a basis for denial of therapy services to infants and preschool children. Although the study demonstrated the importance of integrated programming, it has been widely interpreted as proving the ineffectiveness of therapy. Rehabilitation professionals must be aware of this and similar studies and prepared to refute the third-party denials with evidence of the child's progress and the efficacy of specific therapeutic interventions.

The student with TBI who is planning to attend college must be made aware of the services available on many campuses for disabled students. National guides to colleges and universities with services for learning disabled students and students with physical impairments are available from Academic Press.[70,71]

ISSUES INVOLVED IN DEFINING CHRONIC CONDITIONS

At the heart of advocating for services for brain-injured children and adolescents is the definition of chronic disabling conditions. Perrin et al. have provided an excellent discussion of assessment of chronic health conditions in children.[89] They suggest that the child's condition be described by a multi-faceted approach that includes duration, age of onset, limitation of age-appropriate activities, visibility, mobility, cognition, emotional and social factors, sensory functioning, and communication among other aspects. They recommend that a condition be considered chronic if it lasts more than 3 months and that it be described in terms of its impact on the child. Children with traumatic brain injuries can be fairly evaluated with this approach and thus receive services and/or compensation commensurate with their needs.

Chronic disabling conditions in children produce profound family issues. Several authors have described both acute and chronic family reactions, including denial,[115] inability to identify needs or locate support systems,[72,120] sibling distress,[80,120] and the belief that identified needs are not met by the rehabilitation professionals involved in the child's care. The rehabilitation team must actively assist each family with learning how to identify personal and family needs, and how to seek and accept support from friends and extended family. The team also must empower family members to speak confidently when their concerns are not given due consideration by medical and education professionals.

PEDIATRIC REFERRALS TO REHABILITATION SERVICES

Although the last decade has seen an increase in the number of pediatric rehabilitation programs in the United States, most clinicians still find that the number of referrals is quite small in comparison with the expected number of traumatic brain injuries in their geographic area. Wesson and colleagues evaluated persistent disabilities in children 6 months after injury and found that of brain-injured children with an Abbreviated Injury Score of 4 or higher and only one injury or with a score of 2 or higher and more than two injuries, 55% continued to manifest inabilities to perform age-appropriate activities.[126] Although they did not assess cognitive or behavioral deficits, the authors recommended that children receive more rehabilitation services.

Similarly, a survey of 4,870 children with TBI admitted to hospitals participating in the National Pediatric Trauma Registry found that 16.2% had 1–3 impairments at discharge; of these, only 2.9% were discharged to rehabilitation or extended care facilities. Of the 5.9% with four or more impairments, only 42% were discharged to rehabilitation or extended care facilities.[28] The reasons for nonreferral to rehabilitation services were not clear, but the fact that 58% of severely impaired children were not referred is of concern.

Hence, pediatric rehabilitation specialists must strive to make services accessible and cost-effective and to gather additional outcome data that prove the effectiveness of rehabilitation services for children and adolescents.

REFERENCES

1. Abu-Arafeh IA, Wallace SJ: Unwanted effects of antiepileptic drugs. Dev Med Child Neurol 30:115–121, 1988.
2. Annegers JF, Grabow JD, Kurland LT, Laws ER: The incidence, causes and secular trends of head trauma in Olmsted County, Minnesota, 1935–1974. Neurology 30:912–919,1980.
3. Anmuth CJ, Ross BW, Alexander MA, et al: Chronic syndrome of inappropriate secretion of antidiuretic hormone in a pediatric patient after traumatic brain injury. Arch Phys Med Rehabil 74: 1219–1221, 1993.

4. Arseni C, Ciurea AV: Clinicotherapeutic aspects in the growing skull fracture: A review of the literature. Childs Brain 8:161–172, 1981.

5. Baker RS, Epstein AD: Ocular motor abnormalities from head trauma. Surv Opthalmol 35:245–267, 1991.

6. Baker S, O'Neill B, Ginsburg MJ, LiG: The Injury Fact Book. New York, Oxford University Press, 1992, p 5.

7. Basso A, Scarpa TM: Traumatic aphasia in children and adults: A comparison of clinical features and evolution. Cortex 26:501–514, 1990.

8. Bauer LA: Interference of oral phenytoin absorption by continuous nasogastric feedings. Neurology 32:570–572, 1982.

9. Berger-Gross P, Shackelford M: Closed-head injury in children: Neuropsychological and scholastic outcomes. Percept Mot Skills 61:254, 1985.

10. Berman B, Vaughan CL, Peacock WJ: The effect of rhizotomy on movement in patients with cerebral palsy. Am J Occup Ther 44:511–516, 1990.

11. Bijur P, Golding J, Haslum M, Kurzon M: Behavioral predictors of injury in school-age children. Am J Dis Child 142:1307–1312, 1988.

12. Blendonohy PM, Phillip PA: Precocious puberty in children after traumatic brain injury. Brain Inj 5:63–68, 1991.

13. Boyer MC, Edwards P: Outcome one to three years after severe traumatic brain injury. Br J Acc Surg 22:315–320, 1991.

14. Brink JL, Garrett AL, et al: Recovery of motor and intellectual function in children sustaining severe head injuries. Dev Med Child Neurol 12:565–571, 1970.

15. Bronkjorst AJ, Lamb GA: An orthosis to aid in reduction of lower limb spasticity. Orthot Prosthet 41:23–28, 1987.

16. Buckingham MJ, Crone KR Ball WS, et al: Traumatic intracranial aneurysms in childhood: Two cases and a review of the literature. Neurosurgery 22:398–408, 1988.

17. Cahan LD, Adams JM, Perry J, Beeler LM: Instrumented gait analysis after selective dorsal rhizotomy. Dev Med Child Neurol 32:1037–1043, 1990.

18. Chadwick O, Rutter M, Shaffer D, Shrout PE: A prospective study of children with head injuries. IV:Specific cognitive deficits. J Clin Neuropsych 3:101–120, 1981.

19. Children's Safety Network: A Data Book of Child and Adolescent Injury. Washington, DC, National Center for Education in Maternal and Child Health, 1991, p 5.

20. Chiodo AE, Nelson V: Rickets associated with etidronate use in a pediatric head injured patient. Arch Phys Med Rehabil 68:539–542, 1987.

21. Chorba TL, Klein TM: Increases in crash involvement and fatalities among motor vehicle occupants younger than five years old. Pediatrics 91:897–901, 1993.

22. Citta-Pietrolungo TJ, Alexander MA, Cook SP, Padman R: Complications of tracheostomy and decannulation in pediatric and young patients with traumatic brain injury. Arch Phys Med Rehabil 74:905–909, 1993.

23. Citta-Pietrolungo TJ, Alexander MA, Steg NL: Early detection of heterotopic ossification in young patients with traumatic brain injury. Arch Phys Med Rehabil 73:258–252, 1992.

24. Cockrell JL, Gregory SA: Audiological deficits in brain-injured children and adolescents. Brain Inj 6:261–266, 1992.

25. Costeff H, Grosswasser Z, Goldstein R: Long-term follow-up review of 31 children with severe closed head trauma. J Neurosurg 73:684–687, 1990.

26. Cote TR, Sacks JJ, Lambert-Huber DA, et al: bicycle helmet use among Maryland children: Effect of legislation and education. Pediatrics 89:1216–1220, 1992.

27. Davidson LL, Hughes SJ, O'Connor PA: Preschool behavior problems and subsequent risk of injury. Pediatrics 82:644–651, 1988.

28. DiScala C, Osberg JS, Gans BM, et al: Children with traumatic head injury: Morbidity and post-acute treatment. Arch Phys Med Rehabil 72:662–666, 1991.

29. Duhaime AC, Alario AJ, Lewander WJ, et al: Head injury in very young children: Mechanisms, injury types and ophthalmologic findings in 100 hospitalized patients younger than 2 year of age. Pediatrics 90:179–185, 1992.

30. Dunne RG, Asher KN, Rivara FP: Behavior and parental expectations of child pedestrians. Pediatrics 89:486–490, 1992.

31. Ellenberg JH, Hirtz DG, Nelson KB: Do seizures in children cause intellectual deterioration? N Engl J Med 314:1085–1088, 1986.

32. Ewing-Cobbs L, Levin HS, Fletcher JM, et al: The Children's Orientation and Amnesia Test: Relationship to severity of acute head injury and to recovery of memory. Neurosurgery 27:683–691, 1990.

33. Farwell JR, Lee YJ, Hirtz DG, et al: Phenobarbital for febrile seizures: Effects of intelligence and on seizure recurrence. N Engl J Med 332:364–369, 1990.

34. Fay GC, Jaffe KM, Polissar NL, et al: Mild pediatric traumatic brain injury: A cohort study. Arch Phys Med Rehabil 74:895–901, 1993.

35. Fay GC, Jaffe KM, Polissar NL, et al: Outcome of pediatric traumatic brain injury at three years: A cohort study. Arch Phys Med Rehabil 75:733–741, 1994.

36. Feldman AB, Haley SM, Coryell J: Concurrent and construct validity of the Pediatric Evaluation of Disability Inventory. Phys Ther 70:602–610, 1990.

37. Goldstein FC, Levin HS: Epidemiology of pediatric closed head injury: Incidence, clinical characteristics and risk factors. J Learn Disabil 20:518–525, 1987.

38. Griffith , Dodge PR: Transient blindness following head injury in children. N Engl J Med 278:648–651, 1968.

39. Gualtieri T, Chandler M, Coons RB, Brown LT: Amantidine: A new clinical profile for traumatic brain injury. Clin Neuropharmacol 12:258–270, 1989.

40. Gulbrandsen GB: Neuropsychological sequelae of light head injuries in older children six months after trauma. J Clin Neuropsychol 6:257–268, 1984.

41. Guyer B, Lescohier I, et al: Intentional injuries among children and adolescents in Massachusetts. N Engl J Med 321:1548–1589, 1989.

42. Hahn YS, Chyung, C, Barthel MJ, et al: Head injuries in children under 36 months of age. Childs Nerv Syst 4:34–39, 1988.

43. Hahn YS, Fuchs S, Flannery AM, et al: Factors influencing posttraumatic seizures in children. Neurosurgery 22:864–867, 1988.

44. Harcourt B, Hopkins D: Ophthalmic manifestations of the battered baby syndrome. BMJ 3:398–401, 1971.

45. Harriet Lane Handbook, 13th ed. St Louis, Mosby, 1991.

46. Hinderer KA, Harris SR, Purdy AH, et al: Effects of 'tone-reducing' vs. standard plaster-casts on gait improvement of children with cerebral palsy. Dev Med Child Neurol 30:370–377, 1988.

47. Holmes GL: Prolonged cortical blindness after closed head trauma. South Med J 71:612–613, 1978.

48. Hurvitz EA, Mandac BR, Davidoff G, et al: Risk factors for heterotopic ossification in children and adolescents with severe traumatic brain injury. Arch Phys Med Rehabil 73:459–462, 1992.

49. Hylton NM: Postural and functional impact of dynamic AFO's and FO's in a pediatric population. J Prosthet Orthot 2:40–53, 1989.

50. Jabbari B, Bryan GE, Marsh EE, Gundersen C: Incidence of seizures with tricyclic and tetracyclic antidepressants. Arch Neurol 42:480–481, 1985.

51. Jaffe KM, Fay GC, Polissar NL, et al: Severity of pediatric traumatic brain injury and neurobehavioral recovery at one year—a cohort study. Arch Phys Med Rehabil 74:587–595, 1993.

52. Jaffe KM, Fay GC, Nayak LP, et al: Severity of pediatric traumatic brain injury and early neurobehavioral outcome: A cohort study. Arch Phys Med Rehabil 73:540–547, 1992.

53. Jordan EA, Duggan AK, Hardy JB: Injuries in children of adolescent mothers: Home safety education associated with decreased injury risk. Pediatrics 91:481–487, 1993.

54. Kennedy CR, Freeman JM: Posttraumatic seizures and posttraumatic epilepsy in children. J Head Trauma Rehabil 1:66–73, 1986.

55. Keith RW, Novak KK: Relationships between tests of central auditory function and receptive language. Semin Hear 5:243–249, 1983.

56. Klonoff H, Clark C, Klonoff PS: Long-term outcome of head injuries: A 23 year follow-up study of children with head injuries. J Neurol Neurosurg Psychiatry 56:410–415, 1993.

57. Klonoff H, Low MD, Clark C: Head injuries in children: A prospective five-year follow-up. J Neurol Neurosurg Psychiatry 40:1211–1219, 1977.

58. Koman LA, Mooney JF, Smith BP et al: Management of cerebral palsy with botulinum A toxin: Preliminary investigation. J Pediatr Orthop 13:489–495, 1993.

59. Kraus JF, Fife D, Conroy C: Pediatric brain injuries: The nature, clinical course, and early outcomes in a defined United States population. Pediatrics 79:501–507, 1987.

60. Kraus JF, Rock A, Hemyari P: Brain injuries among infants, children, adolescents and young adults. Am J Dis Child 144:684–691, 1990.

61. Kriel RL, Krach LE, Jones-Saete C: Outcomes of children with prolonged unconsciousness and vegetative states after acquired brain injuries. Presented at the 47th Annual Meeting of the American Academy for Cerebral Palsy and Developmental Medicine, Nashville, 1993.

62. Kriel RL, Krach LE, Panser LA: Closed head injury: Comparison of children younger and older than 6 years of age. Pediatr Neurol 5:296–300, 1989.

63. Kriel RL, Krach LE, Sheehan M: Pediatric closed head injury: Outcome prolonged unconsciousness. Arch Phys Med Rehabil 69:678–681, 1988.

64. Landau WM, Hunt CC: Dorsal rhizotomy, a treatment of unproven efficacy. J Child Neurol 5:174–178, 1990.

65. Lapierre YD, Raval KJ: Pharmacotherapy of affective disorders in children and adolescents. Psychiatr Clin North Am 12:951–961, 1989.

66. Lehr E: Psychological Management of Traumatic Brain Injuries in Children and Adolescents. Chicago, Rehabilitation Institute of Chicago, 1990, p 227.

67. Levin HS, Eisenberg HM: Neuropsychological impairment after closed head injury in children and adolescents. J Pediatr Psychol 4:289–401, 1979.

68. Levin HS, Eisenberg HM: Neuropsychological outcome of closed head injury in children and adolescents. Childs Brain 5:281–292, 1979.

69. Lieh-Lai MW, Theodorou AA, Sarnaik AP, et al: Limitations of the Glasgow Coma Scale in predicting outcome in children with traumatic brain injury. J Pediatr 120:195–199, 1992.

70. Liscio, MA: A Guide to Colleges for Learning Disabled Students. Orlando, FL, Academic Press, 1986.

71. Liscio, MA: A Guide to Colleges for Mobility Impaired Students. Orlando, FL, Academic Press, 1986.

72. Marks M, Sliwinski M, Gordon WA: An examination of the needs of families with a brain-injured child. Neurorehabilitation 3:1–12, 1993.

73. Marganitt B, MacKenzie EJ, Deshpande JK, et al: Hospitalization for traumatic injuries among children in Maryland: Trends in incidence and severity: 1979–1988. Pediatrics 89:608–613, 1992.

74. Massagli TL: Neurobehavioral effects of phenytoin, carbamazepine and valproic acid: Implications for use in traumatic brain injury. Arch Phys Med Rehabil 72:219–226, 1991.

75. Michaud LJ, Rivara FP, Grady MS, Reay DT: Predictors of survival and severity of disability after severe brain injury in children. Neurosurgery 31:254–264, 1992.

76. Miller WL, Kaplan SL, Grumbach MM: Child abuse as a cause of post-traumatic hypopituitarism. N Engl J Med 302:724–728, 1980.

77. Miltenberger G, Dawson G, Raica A: Central auditory testing with peripheral hearing loss. Arch Otolaryngol 104:11–15, 1978.

78. Mitchell WG, Yi Zhou MS, Chavez JM, Guzman BL: Effects of antiepileptic drugs on reaction time, attention and impulsivity in children. Pediatrics 91:101–105, 1993.

79. Nash J, Neilson PD, O'Dwyer NJ: Reducing spasticity to control muscle contracture of children with cerebral palsy. Dev Med Child Neurol 31:471–480, 1989.

80. Orsillo SM, McCaffrey RJ, Fisher JM: Siblings of head injured individuals: A population at risk. J Head Trauma Rehabil 8:102–115, 1993.

81. Ozanne-Smith J, Sherry K: Bicycle related injuries: Head injuries since legislation. Hazard 6:1–8, 1990.

82. Palmer FB, Shapiro B, Wachtel RC, et al: The effects of physical therapy on cerebral palsy: A controlled trial in infants with spastic diplegia. N Engl J Med 318:803–808, 1988.

83. Parmalee DX, O'Shanick GS: Neuropsychiatric interventions with head injured children and adolescents. Brain Inj 1:41–47, 1987.

84. Parmalee DX, O'Shanick G: Carbamazepine-lithium toxicity in brain-damaged adolescents. Brain Inj 2:305–308, 1988.

85. Paxson CL Jr, Brown DR: Post-traumatic anterior hypopituitarism. Pediatrics 59:948–950, 1976.

86. Pendergrast RA, Ashworth CS, DuRant RH, Litaker M: Correlates of children's bicycle helmet use and short-term failure of school level interventions. Pediatrics 90:354–358, 1992.

87. Philip PA: Superior mesenteric artery syndrome in a child with brain injury. Am J Phys Med Rehabil 70:280–282, 1991.

88. Pless IB, Peckham CS, Power C: Predicting traffic injuries in childhood: A cohort analysis. J Pediatr 115:932–938, 1989.

89. Perrin EC, Newacheck P, Pless IB, et al: Issues involved in the definition and classification of chronic health conditions. Pediatrics 91:787–793, 1993.

90. Raimondi A, Hirschauer J: Head injury in the infant and toddler: Coma severity and outcome scale. Childs Brain 11:12–35, 1984.

91. Rancurello, M: Antidepressants in children: Indications, benefits and limitations. Am J Psychother 40:377–392, 1986.

92. Reilly PL, Simpson DA, Sprod R, Thomas L: Assessing the conscious level in infants and young children: A pediatric version of the Glasgow Coma Scale. Childs Nerv Syst 4:30–33, 1988.

93. Rivara FP: Child pedestrian injuries in the United States: Current status of the problem, potential interventions, and future research needs. Am J Dis Child 144:692–696, 1990.

94. Rivara FP, Booth CL, Bergman AB, et al: Prevention of pedestrian injuries to children: Effectiveness of a school training program. Pediatrics 88:770–775, 1991.

95. Rivara F, Tanaguchi D, Parish RA, et al: Poor prediction of positive computed tomographic scans by clinical criteria in symptomatic pediatric head trauma. Pediatrics 80:579–584, 1987.

96. Roig M, Monserrat L, Gallart A: Carbamezepine: An alternative drug for the treatment of nonhereditary chorea. Pediatrics 82:492–495, 1988.

97. Ruijs MBM, Keyser A, Gabreels FJM: Long-term sequelae of brain damage from closed head injury in children and adolescents. Clin Neurol Neurosurg 92:323–328, 1990.

98. Rutter M: Psychological sequelae of brain damage in children. Am J Psychiatry 138:1535–1544, 1981.

99. Sakai CS, Mateer C: Otological and audiological sequelae of closed head injury. Semin Hear 5:157–173, 1984.

100. Saltuari L, Kronenberg M, Marosi MJ, et al: Long-term intrathecal baclofen treatment in supraspinal spasticity. Acta Neurol (Napoli) 14:195–207, 1992.

101. Salvatore S: The ability of elementary and secondary school children to sense oncoming car velocity. J Safety Res 6:118–125, 1974.

102. Sankey RJ, Anderson DM, Young JA: Characteristics of ankle-foot orthoses for management of the spastic lower limb. Dev Med Child Neurol 31:466–470, 1989.

103. Scarfo GB, Mariottini A, Tomaccini D, et al: Growing skull fractures: Progressive evolution of brain damage and effectiveness of surgical treatment. Childs Nerv Syst 5:163–167, 1989.

104. Scheidt PC, Wilson MH, Stern MS: Bicycle helmet law for children: A case study of activism in injury control. Pediatrics 89:1248–1250, 1992.

105. Shaul PW, Towbin RB, Chernausek SD: Precocious puberty following severe head trauma. Am J Dis Child 139:467–469, 1985.

106. Silverman SL, Hurvitz EA, Nelson VS, et al: Rachitic syndrome after disodium etidronate therapy in an adolescent. Arch Phys Med Rehabil 75:118–120, 1994.

107. Simpson DA, Cockington RA, Hanieh A, et al: Head injuries in infants and young children: The value of the Pediatric Coma Scale. Review of the literature and report on a study. Childs Nerv Syst 7:183–190, 1991.

108. Snoek JW, Minderhoud JM, Wilmink JT: Delayed deterioration following mild head injury in children. Childs Brain 107:15–36, 1984.

109. Sobus KML, Alexander MA, Harcke HT: Undetected musculoskeletal trauma in children with traumatic brain injury or spinal cord injury. Arch Phys Med Rehabil 74:902–904, 1993.

110. Sockalosky JJ, Kriel RL, Krach LE, et al: Precocious puberty after traumatic brain injury. J Pediatr 110:373–377, 1987.

111. Splaingard ML, Gaebler D, Havens P, Kalichman M: Brain injury: Functional outcome in children with tracheostomies and gastrostomies. Arch Phys Med Rehabil 70:318–321, 1989.

112. Teasdale G, Jennett B: Assessment of coma and impaired consciousness. A practical scale. Lancet 2:81–84, 1974.

113. Telzrow, CF: Management of academic and educational problems in head injury. J Learn Disabil 20:536–545, 1987.

114. Tenjin H, Ueda S, Mizukawa N, et al: Positron emission tomographic studies on cerebral hemodynamics in patients with cerebral contusion. Neurosurgery 26:971–979, 1990.

115. Thomsen IV: Late outcome of very severe blunt head trauma. A 10–15 year second follow-up. J Neurol Neurosurg Psychiatry 46:870–875, 1984.

116. Thomsen IV: Do young patients have worse outcomes after severe blunt head trauma? Brain Inj 3:157–162, 1989.

117. Tompkins CA, Holland AL, Radcliff G, et al: Predicting cognitive recovery from closed head injury in children and adolescents. Brain Cogn 13:86–97, 1990.

118. Vargha-Khadem F, O'Gorman AM, Watters GV: Aphasia and handedness in relation to hemispheric side, age at injury and severity of cerebral lesion during childhood. Brain 108:677–696, 1985.

119. Vartianen E, Karjolainen S, Karja J: Auditory disorders following head injuries in children. Acta Otolaryngol (Stockholm) 99:529–536, 1985.

120. Waaland PK, Raines SR: Families coping with childhood neurological disability: Assessment and therapy. Neurorehabilitation 1:19–27, 1991.

121. Wagstyl J, Stucliffe AJ, Alpar EK: Early prediction of outcome following head injury in children. J Pediatr Surg 22:127–129, 1987.

122. Walker ML, Storrs BB, Mayer T: Factors affecting outcome in the pediatric patient with multiple trauma. Childs Brain 11:387–397, 1984.

123 Ward JD, Alberico AM: Pediatric head injuries. Brain Inj 1:21–25, 1987.

124. Water BGH: Psychopharmacology of the psychiatric disorders of childhood and adolescence. Med J Aust 152:32–39, 1990.

125. Werry JS, Aman M, Diamond E. Imipramine and methylphenidate in hyperactive children. J Clin Psychol Psychiatry 21:27–35, 1980.

126. Wesson DE, Williams JI, Spence LJ, et al: Functional outcome in pediatric trauma. J Trauma 29:589–592, 1989.

127. Whalen CK, Henker B: Social impact of stimulant treatment for hyperactive children. J Learn Disabil 24:231–240, 1991.

128. Whitaker C, Bastian L: Teenage Victims: A National Crime Survey Report. Pub. no. NCJ-129129. Washington, DC, US Department of Justice, Bureau of Justice Statistics, 1991.

129. Widome MD: On the relevance of poor judgement. Pediatrics 84:724–726, 1989.

130. Wilcox JA, Nasrallah HA: Childhood head trauma and psychosis. Psychol Res 21:303–306, 1987.

131. Winogron HW, Knights RM, Bawden HN: Neuropsychological deficits following head injury in children. J Clin Neuropsychol 6:269–286, 1984.

MARK V. JOHNSTON   Ph.D.

KARYL HALL   Ed.D.

GEORGE CARNEVALE   Ph.D.

CORWIN BOAKE   Ph.D.

8

Functional Assessment and Outcome Evaluation in Traumatic Brain Injury Rehabilitation

The assessment of patient function after rehabilitation for traumatic brain injury (TBI) is essential to prognosis, treatment planning, and evaluation of treatment effectiveness. Outcome assessment is fundamental to the justification of rehabilitative interventions for patients with TBI. Functional assessment in TBI rehabilitation, however, currently faces a series of problems.

The functional sequelae of TBI are highly complex. All areas of life may be affected by TBI, resulting in innumerable cognitive, social, behavioral, emotional, or physical problems; thus, the set of relevant domains is large. The complexity of relevant outcomes, combined with the limited resources for research, has led to the use of functional assessment tools developed for other fields, especially physical rehabilitation and mental health. Although such procedures are relevant and necessary, many professionals have misgivings about their use in TBI. Such measures sometimes have items or features that can be misleading when applied to TBI. The last decade or so has seen the publication of various functional measures specific to TBI and partial validation of a few, but there are still major gaps. In addition, severity of

symptoms greatly influences the choice of appropriate measures. In sum, the current state of the art leads both researchers and clinical managers to question how they should assess the function and progress of patients with TBI.

Many still claim that rehabilitation is so complex, holistic, and ideographic that it is impossible to measure or even express its specific effect. Given the complexity of TBI rehabilitation, these claims deserve a sympathetic hearing. But we cannot accept these claims, as they amount to a denial that rehabilitation can possibly document robust effects across patients. If rehabilitation is to justify its expense, it must demonstrate that it routinely engenders sustained improvements in the everyday lives of persons served.

There is no single best way to assess patients with TBI, but the number of logical options with empirical support is limited. This chapter lays the groundwork for progress in functional assessment of patients with TBI, reviews the best-developed measures, and lists other options deserving consideration, with an emphasis on better-developed, standardized measures. The degree of valid standardization, however, is still limited, and

197

programs need to strike a balance between individualized and standardized assessment.

Criteria for choice of outcome measures include sensitivity to improvement and logical relation to treatment interventions. Sensitivity to the life problems experienced by persons with TBI is a paramount criterion. This chapter emphasizes measures of function at the level of disability, that is, defined activities or performances. Because outcome measures are not clinically interpretable without adjustment for severity, both neuromedical and neuropsychological measures of impairment are reviewed. The type of brain injury and knowledge of brain-behavior relationships are important in interpretation of patient function; the literature on this topic is too extensive to review here.

Indices of handicap in the community are probably most relevant to the continued success and growth (or contraction) of TBI rehabilitation over the long term. In some parts of the United States (e.g., California), managed care organizations have cut back on referrals to programs that specialize in rehabilitation of patients with TBI. The prosperity and perhaps even the existence of such programs rest on public justification and evidence of their efficacy and cost-effectiveness.

STANDARDIZED FUNCTIONAL ASSESSMENT

Programs need to justify their interventions in terms of outcomes not only to the patient but also to payers, regulators, referral sources, managed care organizations, and families.[71] As managed care organizations mature, they demand objective evidence that programs deliver effective, high-quality services and produce the outcomes they project for patients.[34,71] The emerging paradigm includes treatment guidelines and practice parameters,[30] which involve standardization of assessment and treatment strategies, demonstrated effectiveness or efficacy, and reduced variation in medical interventions. Theories of rehabilitative interventions increasingly are questioned unless supported by evidence.

There is evidence that clinical professionals frequently do not agree on what constitutes severity in TBI.[169] Such disagreement reflects the relative youth of TBI rehabilitation and the complexity of approaches to functional assessment, but it also speaks to the need for standardization. Standardized measures and terminology[107] facilitate communication within the rehabilitation team as well as with case managers, families, and other professionals; they also enhance respect for the field.

The Individual vs. the Group. Standardized measures give a useful framework for clinical assessment, a point of departure for more individualized assessment and interventions. Because virtually all current functional assessment involves significant error, it is unjustified to project on the basis of a single measure that a patient's outcome will be the same as the group average. Standards in medical rehabilitation state that multiple measures and sources of information are necessary for planning of treatment and projection of outcome.[96] Formal functional assessment gives a few points of reference, but clinical judgment and experience must fill in the gaps to address the individual patient.

Formal measures remain most useful in research, outcome evaluation, program evaluation, and quality improvement in moderate-sized groups of patients. They are technically of limited validity when applied to individuals. The prescriptive validity of functional measures—their logical connection to optimized treatment strategies—is also wanting. These lacunae can be ameliorated by the next generation of researchers, but a complete solution is nowhere in sight.

Uses of Functional Assessment

Functional scales in rehabilitation have multiple uses, but are not used in quite the same way, for instance, as serum tests, which may give a simple positive or negative indication of pathology and even imply treatment. Clinical logic in rehabilitation differs from that in acute medical care. Specific uses of functional measures in rehabilitation include:

- Evaluation of rehabilitation potential for an individual patient.
- Understanding of patients' deficits, strengths, and needs in initial clinical evaluation, including both formal inferences and informal clues to how and where progress may be made.

• Tracking progress and response to treatment to obtain objective evidence of whether meaningful progress has been made[146] toward priority treatment objectives (see below).

• Decisions about readiness for discharge to home or other level of care—a major use of formal functional assessment that has not been exploited fully.

• Demonstration of the quality, effectiveness, and outcomes of a rehabilitation program to case managers, professional audiences, and the public.

• Systematic monitoring of quality in rehabilitation.[95,97]

Most outcome measures have been developed for overall program evaluation or for research purposes. Their applicability to planning of interventions for individual patients, however, leaves something to be desired. Scales usually need greater sensitivity and highly specific content to inform treatment decisions. Attempts have been made to develop systems involving both general outcomes based on handicap level and measures of specific functional objectives that give direction to rehabilitative planning for individual patients[66,67,69]; such systems, however, have not been well validated or widely adopted.

CONCEPTUAL BASIS FOR ASSESSMENT

The Wood-World Health Organization's (WHO) taxonomy of impairment, disability, and handicap[180] provides a framework for understanding of outcomes. For applications to clinical rehabilitation, however, the taxonomy should be extended or refined.

The three WHO levels reflect the biologic, personal, and societal levels of analysis. An **impairment** is an abnormality in an organ system. A **disability** is a limitation of the ability to perform a needed activity. Disability includes assessments of performances in basic activities of daily living (ADLs), such as mobility and self-care; instrumental ADLs (IADLs), such as household chores, community mobility, and shopping; and cognitively-loaded activities, such as financial management, daily scheduling, and communication with others. A **handicap** is a disadvantage arising from an inability to perform a normal role in the actual environment. Handicap reflects the person-in-environment, not the person alone. Community integration, independent living as a whole, performance of social roles, and vocational status are examples of handicap. The term **social disadvantage** is a valuable near-synonym for handicap.[124] For example, a person with TBI may have memory deficits (impairment) that lead to an inability to manage finances (disability) and ultimately to the need to live with another person who provides supervision (handicap).

Uses of the Levels

Understanding the three WHO levels is important, for interventions that positively affect one level may not affect another. A common problem in TBI rehabilitation is that, despite a measurable or statistically significant reduction of impairment, disability in a practical sense may not change.[174] With comatose patients, numerous impairments may be remedied without alteration of long-term disability or consciousness. On the other hand, rehabilitation may lead to alterations in disability and handicap without significant change in neurological status.[33,174] For instance, studies have demonstrated improvement in practical communicative tasks with no change in aphasia scores.[77] Patients with TBI commonly learn to use memory aids (e.g., a written schedule) without change in tests of memory impairment.

Clinically, assessment of the role demands likely to be faced after discharge is necessary to understand the patient and helpful in prioritizing interventions. Haffey[66–68] described methods by which team conferences project rehabilitation outcomes on the basis of living arrangement and primary productive activity after discharge. Interventions are then prioritized in terms of whether they are likely to reduce the primary barriers to such outcomes. Adjusting interventions to address those needs that are most essential to independent living, for instance, is much more cost-effective than simply working on the most abnormal of current impairments or functional limitations.

In sum, impairments must be measured to understand and prescribe appropriate medical and therapeutic interventions. Measures of impairment indicate whether the outcome is due to neurophysiologic recovery or to environmental changes or compensatory adaptation. Measures of clinical disability or functional limitations can indicate whether the improvements in function are likely to be meaningful to the patient. Real-world measures of disability indicate whether patients in fact use skills they were trained in. Measures of handicap indicate whether multifaceted interventions cumulate to outcomes valued by most persons in society.

Critique and Extension

The WHO taxonomy was developed for broad epidemiologic studies, and certain extensions are valuable to advance understanding of clinical effectiveness.

The term disability is used in two senses. First, it is used to express the results of performance testing in a clinical or at least well-defined situation. In this chapter the term **clinical disability** denotes such tests, which assess ability in the person. The term **functional limitation** also is used to denote specific clinical disabilities. Secondly, the term disability is used to denote activity deficits in the patient's actual, uncontrolled environment (e.g., in a follow-up interview). **In situ** or **real-world disability** is close to being a measure of handicap but is much narrower than the WHO definition of handicap.

For medical applications, an additional level must be added: **pathologic processes**, or abnormalities at the cellular or molecular level. Diseases are based on pathologic processes.

Handicap

Handicap or social disadvantage is the ultimate outcome in that it is based on social norms[180] and thus directly reflects social values. But it also is the most problematic level from a practical clinical perspective. Hospital rehabilitation programs treat primarily at the level of impairment and disability. In acute rehabilitation settings, it may be difficult to project the long-term level of handicap. A major product of rehabilitation is reduced dependence in basic activities, and this is measured at the level of clinical and real-world disability (actual dependence in basic activities at follow-up). Broader handicap is routinely assessed in only one respect: whether the patient is placed in a nursing home or with family in the community.

Certain limitations of handicap measures need to be kept in mind. Some dimensions of handicap may be highly affected by factors other than brain injury or even general health. Occupation and economic handicap, for instance, depend on prior employment status, age, sex, wealth, family support, rates of unemployment in the community, or societal tolerance for unusual behavior.[21,22,173] Rehabilitative interventions can modify some social and environmental factors, but many such factors are beyond the control of health-related programs. Exogenous social and environmental factors need to be measured or at least considered in interpreting the level of handicap.

Handicap is also problematic because it is so broad. Broad roles such as physical independence or occupation involve many skills. Therapists must work on selected skills, in the hope that they will lead to a greater improvement in the patient's status. Moreover, normal role expectations are unclear in our individualistic, multicultural society. The person's personal goals and values may differ from the norm.

The current WHO concept of handicap encompasses the notions of broad normative roles, personal disadvantage, and person–environment interaction. These elements need to be assessed more specifically to help a person with TBI. For example, one often needs to know a person's particular functional limitations or skills to assist in the return to independent living or work. One may need to know whether the family can accept and care for the newly impaired person, whether the house is wheelchair-accessible, or whether the employer is willing to make allowances. Factors in the social and physical environment need to be distinguished from factors in the person.

Rehabilitation programs have been shown repeatedly to reduce handicap, even in persons chronically disabled by TBI years after injury.[33] An increased focus on long-term level of handicap is a constructive response to increasing pressures to demonstrate the value and cost-effectiveness of TBI rehabilitation programs.[71,75]

Criteria for Choice of Measures

There is broad agreement among practitioners of medical rehabilitation that functional assessment needs to be improved and standardized. Assessment systems must demonstrate both greater validity (from which to make a larger number of useful inferences or projections) and greater reliability. The consensus on this issue led to publication of *Measurement Standards for Interdisciplinary Medical Rehabilitation* in 1992.[96] Practical criteria for selection and interpretation of measures in TBI can be derived from these standards.

Validity, the ultimate criterion for judging a scale, hinges on the uses to which the scale is put. The validity of a scale initially must be judged by understanding its content (**content validity** or sensibility[50]). Empirical proof of the validity of key inferences is typically needed. In particular, a valuable scale should predict some event in the future: **predictive validity** is a key indicator of the value of a functional scale. **Construct validity** is the highest form of validity. In brief, it means that a measure behaves as expected, according to theory, and is free from key confounding factors. Validity needs to be explained in terms of a sensible construct. In sum, validity is always validity *for* a delimited construct, purpose, and type of problem; it is not a global yes-no attribute.

All measures involve some probability of error. Published information about the degree of **reliability** and potential biases of the scale is essential to professional interpretation. Information about the number of dimensions in a scale (e.g., homogeneity measures, factor analysis, Rasch analysis) indicates whether it measures one or several dimensions and when it is meaningful to add dimensions together for a summary score.

As a rule of thumb, measures need to be sensitive to patient change during rehabilitation. Most existing functional scales have **ceiling** and **floor** limitations; that is, they are not sensitive to improvement among patients whose function is relatively high or very low, respectively. Basic ADL measures, such as the Functional Independence Measure (FIM), for instance, are insensitive to progress of high-level patients, who need speed, endurance, and planning abilities to function in the community.[114] Very low functioning patients may have technical nursing problems, the resolution of which is not included in ADL scales. The danger is obvious: one may infer that the patient is not improving or not responding to treatment, when in fact the assessment is insensitive at the patient's level of function.

A professional scale requires a manual that includes such information as instructions for use and data about validity and reliability. Users of scales have obligations. They should read the manual and follow the instructions to ensure valid results. Proper use of some scales requires training.

These standards differ from the *AMA Guide to the Evaluation of Permanent Impairment*.[3] The AMA system may have content validity for certain diagnoses, in the sense that a panel of physician experts agrees that the content is adequate or as good as possible, but its adequacy for brain injury is questionable. No scientific studies establish the predictive validity of the system for its common use in establishing the inability of persons with brain injury to work or their needs for long-term assistance. Data about the reliability of recommended measures are not reported in the publication. The system harkens back to an era when it was hoped that disability could be predicted entirely by evaluation of simple physical impairments. Many studies over recent decades have demonstrated that this assumption is false. Human performance, after all, depends on individual strengths as well as weaknesses, and return to work depends on how job demands interact with personal abilities and disabilities as well as on environmental modifications and the supportiveness of the employer.

Effective Treatment and Related Measures

The overarching question is not only measurement of outcomes but also inference of effective treatment. Effective treatment is inferred from a pattern of input (including severity and type of brain damage and baseline functioning), process (types of treatment), and outcomes over time. Both technical impairment and broader quality-of-life measures are needed to infer effective treatment.

The validity of a **long-term treatment objective** depends on two key characteristics: (1) the objective must be interpretable in terms of socially valued activities in the person's likely real life; and (2) it must be at least logically sensitive to the effects of current rehabilitative interventions.[66,67,95] Ideally, a measure of a treatment objective is validated in a controlled trial, but improvement in the measure should have at least some correlation with intensity of relevant treatment(s). Specific treatment objectives in rehabilitation are often, but not always, at the level of clinical disability or functional limitation. Measures of handicap may be necessary to demonstrate the social value of interventions, and impairment level measures are needed to infer causation and to select an intervention strategy.

FUNCTIONAL OUTCOME MEASURES BY LEVEL OF SEVERITY

What constitutes severity in TBI? Cost-effective case management and rehabilitation planning is all but inconceivable without assessment of severity. Understanding of severity is also essential to choose a measure that can gauge patient progress and avoid misinterpretation due to ceiling and floor problems. Sensitive assessment of a particular patient's key problem in active medical rehabilitation may require a measure more commonly used at another level of care.

The following sections begin with indices of global severity and proceed to measures appropriate to active rehabilitation, ending with measures of function in the community.

Assessments of Global Status

Assessment of overall severity of injury or disability is the essential starting point for functional assessment of patients with TBI. Three measures of overall status are prominent: the Glasgow Outcome Scale, the Rancho Los Amigos Level of Cognitive Function Scale, and the Disability Rating Scale.

The *Glasgow Outcome Scale* (GOS) is a simple, ordinal rating of global outcome. The GOS originally had 4 points and was later refined to have 5 points: death, vegetative state, severe disability, moderate disability, and good recovery. Clinicians can assign a GOS rating in less than 5 minutes. GOS ratings correlate strongly with measures of severity of TBI, such as the Glasgow Coma Scale (GCS), shortly after injury.[86,88] In recent decades, numerous other predictive relationships have been established in international neurosurgical outcome studies.[87]

GOS ratings correlate strongly with tests of motor speed or coordination. Grooved pegboard scores, for instance, predict 80% of variation of GOS scores.[29] GOS ratings have significant but weaker correlations with neuropsychological performances, such as Controlled Oral Word Association (verbal fluency), Trailmaking Part B (processing speed and attention), and Rey-Osterreith Complex Figure Delayed Recall (memory).[29]

As a rather simplistic characterization of overall patient level, the GOS has limited sensitivity. Several works, for instance, have noted the limited sensitivity of the GOS levels of moderate disability and good recovery.[43] Most severely injured patients with "good recovery" exhibit persisting neuropsychological deficits.[35]

A further problem is that GOS ratings must be made on a partly subjective basis. For example, a criterion for the category of good recovery is that the patient is employable[88]; the clinician is required to predict the employability of patients who are not working. Although early reports claimed that the GOS had adequate inter-rater reliability, a recent study found that general practitioners tended to make overoptimistic GOS assessments compared with psychologists. Any rating of patient outcomes in simple, global terms will no doubt at times be ambiguous.

GOS ratings tend to plateau at 6 months.[88] Thus the GOS is insensitive to the gains shown by patients after rehabilitation. For example, most clients in postacute rehabilitation programs fall in the categories of "moderate disability" and "good recovery," and their GOS ratings infrequently change with improvement. Although useful for comparison of results with previous research, the

GOS is not a good choice as a measure of long-term outcome for rehabilitation patients.

The Rancho Los Amigos Level of Cognitive Function Scale (Rancho or LCFS) was designed to describe the typical stages of neurobehavioral recovery following severe TBI during inpatient rehabilitation.[70] The Rancho is an 8-level ordinal scale in which each level corresponds to a stage of recovery. For example, level III corresponds to "early recovery" patients who intermittently follow commands and level IV to agitated patients in posttraumatic amnesia. The Rancho is widely used for evaluation of patients with TBI in North American inpatient rehabilitation units because of its simplicity, close correspondence with clinical features, and integration with treatment protocols in most therapies.

After many years, data have demonstrated at least limited validity and reliability for the Rancho LCFS. Rancho scores at admission to rehabilitation correlate significantly with 24-hour GCS scores, length of coma, and duration of posttraumatic amnesia.[74] Their correlation at admission with the Disability Rating Scale (DRS) is 0.72; with motor subscales of the Functional Independence Measure (FIM), 0.48; and with the FIM cognitive subscale, 0.66.[74] The Rancho has been shown to correlate moderately with more specific, objective measures of cognitive function (e.g., the Brief Test of Head Injury[83] [BTHI] and DRS[62]). Patients at Rancho LCFS level III at admission to rehabilitation (displaying localized responses to stimuli) are substantially more likely to improve than those admitted at level II (general responsiveness).[162] The Rancho has been used in a number of studies to characterize patient groups. The LCFS is modestly related to vocational outcomes (but not as well as the Functional Assessment Inventory [FAI] or even the GOS[123]).

The Rancho has been used to define in part the criteria for admission to rehabilitation. Levels III (localized response) and IV (agitated, confused) have been stated as minimal admission levels. A traditional criterion for admission to active, practice-based rehabilitation is the ability to follow commands. This criterion is appropriately broadened to include responses that demonstrate specific discrimination of the nature of the stimulus; for example, use of the arm to push away a noxious stimulus as opposed to a localized withdrawal reflex. Research to develop empirically based criteria for cost-effective admission and discharge is sorely needed.

Although the Rancho scale has acceptable reliability when used as an initial description of cognitive level,[62] limitations to its reliability become apparent when one attempts to apply it precisely. A minority of patients skip a stage of recovery (e.g., confused-agitated) or meet the requirements of two stages simultaneously (e.g., mute patients who can communicate through other channels). As an assessment of neurobehavioral functioning in higher-level patients, the Rancho does not assess communicative or behavioral deficits that are important for many patients. Scales based on more specific behaviors rather than multifaceted "levels" are more reliable and objective.

The Rancho LCFS was not designed as an outcome measure, and its use has far outstripped its original role. The Rancho cannot serve as a primary assessment of cognitive function or as a measure of outcome. The Rancho remains useful as an initial description or summary of patients' neurobehavioral functioning during inpatient rehabilitation and orients the team to likely treatment issues.

Rappaport's *Disability Rating Scale* (DRS) is probably the best-validated method for assessment of general functioning and recovery after TBI. Many studies have reported good reliability and validity coefficients for the DRS.[48,55,62,72,74,127,133–135,149] The DRS is a sum of ratings over different scales of disability and impairment. The DRS is fairly easy to use and can be completed in under 5 minutes if the clinician is familiar with the patient. It can be scored by direct observation of the patient, interview, or telephone. An advantage of the DRS is its ability to track a patient from coma to community reintegration.[55,72,127] The DRS is more reliable than the Rancho LCFS.[62] The DRS has been shown to be sensitive to change in medical rehabilitation programs[72,74] and in postacute programs designed to decrease disabilities or restore work roles.[32,55,126,133] It is more sensitive to change than either the GOS or Rancho.[72,74] The DRS is one of the best predictors of length of stay in inpatient rehabilitation units.[108]

A major disadvantage of the DRS is its relatively insensitivity to mild and moderate TBI, because it was designed for severe TBI. For patients with an FIM score above 25, the FIM may have greater sensitivity to change in rehabilitation than the DRS.[23] Despite its name, items in the DRS address impairment and handicap as well as disability. At levels of intermediate severity the DRS requires assessment of cognitive capacity for self-care rather than observation of dependence in self-care activities. This assessment requires familiarity with the patient and subjective judgments by the clinician, the basis of which is unclear. The DRS also requires subjectivity in rating patients' employability and capacity for independent living. An additional disadvantage is that patients can receive the same DRS rating for different reasons; thus DRS ratings do not imply directly what interventions may be appropriate.

Logically, the DRS should be useful, in conjunction with more detailed measures, to bracket a range of function for admission and discharge in inpatient rehabilitation programs. Patients should be out of coma and vegetative state to respond to active learning and practice-based rehabilitation. This implies a DRS score of no more than 21 at admission. By comparison, the TBI Model Systems have not usually admitted minimally responsive patients to rehabilitation; they have reported an average DRS of 12 at admission.[108] The level at which a patient is discharged depends on family support and resources for needed assistance and supervision. The TBI Model Systems report an average DRS of 6 at discharge, with a range of 5–7, depending on initial severity.[108]

The DRS has been recommended for assessment of outcome in neurosurgical trials.[28] The authors recommend the DRS as a basic component in clinical TBI data systems to characterize caseload severity and to establish rough caseload comparability across different rehabilitation programs.

Multidimensional Assessments

The multidimensionality of function after TBI is a problem with all global status ratings. A patient with TBI may be severely disabled in one functional dimension (e.g., activities requiring intact declarative memory) but normal in others (e.g., physical ADLs). The above global ratings are useful to establish rough comparability of patient samples and to assess global severity. Global ratings, however, are not sufficiently sensitive for clinical management or planning rehabilitation treatment. Measures that reflect more specific disabilities are currently the appropriate standard for assessment of function after TBI. A multidimensional profile of patient function is needed in rehabilitation.

The *Portland Adaptability Inventory* (PAI) consists of 24 outcome items that the clinician rates on a 4-point scale.[113,117] The items are summed to yield a total score that may range from 0 (best outcome) to 72 (worst outcome). PAI items were specifically designed to sample problems that are typically encountered in long-term TBI survivors, particularly problems with behavior and social isolation. Items represent domains termed Temperament and Emotionality, Activities and Social Behavior, and Physical Capabilities. Studies of outcomes of postacute programs have shown significant improvement in PAI scores.[117] Based on its design and content, the PAI appears to have substantial promise as an outcome measure for TBI programs. Endorsement for routine use requires evidence of the PAI's reliability, internal structure, and validity.

Measures of independence in basic self-care ADLs and mobility have been designed primarily for general rehabilitation populations but are applicable to TBI patients with similar problems. Patients with brain injury enter medical rehabilitation hospitals with disabilities in basic self-care and mobility skills, and therapy aims to reduce these dependencies. General rehabilitation disability measures, such as the FIM[65] and Program Evaluation Conference System (PECS),[146] are clearly sensitive to improvement in inpatients with TBI. A significant minority of patients with TBI in residential community integration programs have dependencies in such ADLs.[92,93] In sum, improved independence in basic ADLs remains the most widely accepted means of marking patient progress in inpatient rehabilitation programs.

The Functional Independence Measure (FIM) is currently the most widely used measure of disability; it is used to assess significant patient improvement in hundreds of comprehensive medical rehabilitation programs nationwide. The FIM requires therapists, nurses, physicians, or other clinicians to assess the degree of assistance needed on a 7-point scale in 18 items. The FIM can be completed in 30 minutes or less by clinicians who know the patient. The FIM is a general disability scale, designed to be applicable across a wide range of physical and neurologic impairments. Norms for typical improvement are available.[65] Inter-rater agreement among trained personnel appears to be relatively good.[76] Rasch analysis has shown that the 13 ADL items can be meaningfully aggregated and transformed to an interval-level measure of motor or physical disability; similarly, the 5 communication, cognition, and psychosocial items comprise a rougher measure of cognitive function.[114] The same analysis, however, reveals ceiling and floor insensitivities and possible misfit problems; for example, with bowel and bladder function. FIM motor scores at admission have been found to be the best predictors of length of stay for nearly all impairment groups.[181] The FIM clearly predicts burden of care in patients with multiple sclerosis[63] or stroke.[64] The FIM has been used to assess TBI outcomes[42] and is more sensitive for assessing functional change during inpatient rehabilitation than the DRS.[18]

The FIM was designed originally as a minimal data set; it was not designed for TBI. Studies to date support the validity, reliability, and sensitivity of the FIM as a measure of disabilities commonly treated in inpatient rehabilitation. The physical ADL items in the FIM may be adequate, but its cognitive, behavioral, and community-related items seem inadequate for patients with TBI. Few clinical professionals in TBI rehabilitation accept the FIM as an adequate measure of cognitive and psychosocial function. The FIM needs to be augmented for patients with TBI.

The Functional Assessment Measure (FAM), which is used in the Traumatic Brain Injury Model Systems project, adds 12 items to the FIM. The combined scale (FIM-FAM) is designed for greater sensitivity to the problems of brain-injured patients.[73,74] Many FAM items relate to community functioning (e.g., car transfers, employability, community mobility). FAM items rated at admission correlate with severity of injury in a pattern similar to the FIM.[74] FAM items involving "attention" and other abstract concepts may have poorer inter-rater reliability than FIM items involving directly observable behaviors.[73]

The *Program Evaluation Conference System* (PECS) is a well-developed, multidimensional system designed to be used both in clinical team conferences and for program evaluation.[79,119,146] With 79 items, the PECS is much longer than the FIM, but it also provides substantially greater information about patient function. The PECS has items not found in the FIM relating to assessment of instrumental ADLs and community skills, cognition, and nursing and family needs. The PECS assesses five primary dimensions of function: motoric competence, cognitive competence, applied self-care, communication, and various physical impairments.[147] The 21 items related to cognitive competence have been refined to produce an interval-level measure.[148] The PECS discriminates level of care (inpatient hospital or nursing home, vs. day program) in a mixed stroke-TBI population.[80] Accuracy of prediction ranged between 73% and 100%. Applied self-care (rehabilitation nursing) and motoric competence (physical mobility and ADLs) were the primary discriminating factors, although cognitive competence contributed somewhat. The PECS correlates modestly with the Brief Symptom Inventory and with CT scan lesions.[119] Total PECS and PECS cognition scores also predict return to work or school.[133] Clinicians probably need to consider factors not assessed in the PECS (e.g., extremes of substance abuse, family support or its lack, financial need) to predict return to work by individual patients.

The *Sickness Impact Profile* (SIP) is well-developed and has been widely used to assess general health outcomes.[119,153] The SIP is a 136-item questionnaire that assesses physical ADL outcomes—including ambulation, mobility, and body care—but goes far beyond. Psychosocial outcomes include social interaction, alertness, and emotional behavior. Other independent subscales include sleep and rest, eating, work, home management, and recreational pastimes. The breadth of assessed domains is exemplary and useful in patients with TBI. The SIP has been used in several studies of TBI.

The *Glasgow Assessment Schedule* (GAS) has 40 items dealing with 6 domains: personality change, subjective complaints, occupational function, cognitive functioning, physical examination, and ADLs.[116] Inter-rater agreement is adequate, and the GAS has been shown to correlate with the GOS, but no report of its use has been published since its initial publication in the mid-1980s.

Other multidimensional disability assessments relevant to TBI include the *European Head Injury Evaluation*,[165] the *Comprehensive Assessment Inventory for Rehabilitation* (CAIR),[66,67] and others.[119,152]

Instruments from the Rand Medical Outcomes Study have attained great popularity for assessment of the outcomes of medical care in the United States. Short-form questionnaires (e.g., the SF-36) have items relevant to TBI but lack assessment of cognitive problems and in all probability are inadequate for assessment of TBI outcomes[156]; long-form instruments have more relevant items, but no data about their validity in TBI are available.

Summary

General rehabilitation measures aimed at ADLs have limitations when used in TBI, but the degree of limitation is a controversial topic for current research. The FIM, for instance, appears to be insensitive to supervision needs[46]; this shortcoming is likely to be a significant problem in patients with TBI. Few professionals in TBI rehabilitation believe that measures of independence in ADLs, developed largely for physically disabled geriatric populations, are adequate for their patients. ADLs depend primarily on physical abilities and make relatively limited cognitive demands, drawing as they do on overlearned habits. Independence only in at-home activities is necessary but profoundly insufficient as a measure of outcome in patients with TBI. Psychosocial and cognitive dysfunctions, which may be manifested most clearly in social and occupational roles, are

for most patients the most disabling consequences of TBI.[140]

COGNITIVE IMPAIRMENTS AND DISABILITIES

Assessing Cognitive Impairments

Impairments of cognition and behavioral changes are seen in virtually all survivors of TBI and are the major causes of their disability. As the best-developed method of assessing cognitive and behavioral deficits in brain-injured persons, neuropsychological testing plays a major role in rehabilitation. This section discusses uses of neuropsychological tests, both for evaluation of outcome and for clinical work, and briefly describes the more widely used tests.

In general, neuropsychological tests are developed with the goal of either measuring a specific cognitive function or detecting the presence of brain dysfunction. They can be viewed as ways to extend the neurologic examination for more accurate evaluation of deficits in higher brain functions. Like other parts of the neurologic examination, most neuropsychological tests are designed to focus on a limited subset of neurologic functions and to minimize demands on other neurologic functions. Neuropsychological tests are usually quite different from everyday tasks, which may involve too many cognitive functions to be useful diagnostically. To eliminate extraneous effects on performance, neuropsychological testing is done in a quiet, nondistracting setting such as an office. Neuropsychological tests are sufficiently narrow or specific that they are usually interpreted as indicators of brain functioning (i.e., functional impairments). They do not directly assess broader goal-oriented activities (i.e., disabilities). Because they are performance tests, however, test scores do not reflect single areas of brain function.

If neuropsychological tests are good measures of brain functions, should they be used to measure the outcome of rehabilitation? Neuropsychological tests are useful as measures of outcome for certain specific purposes but not as measures of the general outcome of rehabilitation. An important specific use of neuropsychological tests is to measure the outcome of treatments (e.g., medications or neurosurgery) that are expected to diminish brain impairment or pathology. Recommended neuropsychological tests for neurosurgical trials[28] are summarized in Table 1. Several studies have used neuropsychological tests to measure the outcome of cognitive retraining, which may attempt to target specific cognitive functions such as attention and memory.[150]

Measuring outcomes with neuropsychological tests helps to determine how much recovery of brain functioning has occurred but not how the patient's life has been affected. Measures of brain functions are not equivalent to measures of independent living, successful return to work or school, or other real-world outcomes. In short, neuropsychological tests are measures of impairment rather than of disability or handicap.

In addition, neuropsychological tests may be insensitive to the impact of the many therapeutic techniques designed to teach compensatory strategies that allow the patient to perform an activity by using preserved abilities and circumventing deficits. Such techniques are expected to reduce the level of disability and handicap without reducing the patient's deficits. For example, written memory aids such as a notebook or calendar are intended to compensate for memory deficits rather than improve the brain's ability to store or retrieve information. Neuropsychological tests are not expected to show changes in cognitive functioning that result from compensatory therapy, although the therapy may improve aspects of the patient's life. Studies of improvement in TBI survivors many years after the injury, when neurologic function is asymptotic, have reported substantial reductions of disability and especially handicap.[33,92,93,140] It is inappropriate to use neuropsychological testing as the only measure of rehabilitation outcomes because test results do not reflect the success or failure of treatment.

The main role of neuropsychological assessment in rehabilitation is to aid in understanding the patient's difficulties and in planning the appropriate therapy. The reasons for a patient's difficulties in performing an everyday activity may not be clear, yet the proper rehabilitation strategy depends on

TABLE 1. Recommended Outcome Measures for Neurosurgical Trials

Measure	Domain, Severity, Comment
Glasgow Coma Scale (GCS)	Depth of coma
Galveston Orientation and Amnesia Test (GOAT)	Posttraumatic amnesia/orientation Moderate and severe Indicates capability for more extensive neuropsychological testing
Digit Symbol Substitution	Attention Moderate and severe
Paced Auditory Serial Addition Test (PSAT)	Attention Moderate
Rey Complex Figure	Memory Moderate and severe
Selective Reminding	Memory Moderate and severe
Controlled Oral Word Association	Language Moderate and severe
Trail Making B	Mental processing, concentration, and response speed Moderate and severe
Wisconsin Card Sort	Mental processing Moderate only
Grooved Peg Board	Motor function Moderate and severe
Neurobehavioral Rating Scale (NBRS)	Behavior and psychopathology Moderate and severe
Glasgow Outcome Scale (GOS)	Global functional outcome over all functional levels Needed because of extensive experience with it
Disability Rating Scale (DRS)	Global cognitive and functional outcome More sensitive than GOS

From Clifton GL, Hayes RL, Levin HS, et al: Outcome measures for clinical trials involving traumatically brain-injured patients: Report of a conference. Neurosurgery 31:975–978, 1992, with permission.

such an understanding. For example, one person may have difficulty on the job because deficits in memory cause him or her to forget to complete assignments. Another person may have difficulty because of slowed motor or cognitive processing. The deficits responsible for poor job performance may have existed even before the injury, as in persons with learning disabilities or attention-deficit disorder. Understanding of the basis for the difficulty is essential in modifying job-related duties or placing the person in a different position. Neuropsychological assessment is concerned with the patient's strengths as well as weaknesses; both types of findings are essential for both diagnosis and treatment.[39,131,159]

In summary, neuropsychological assessment is useful in identifying the deficits responsible for the patient's difficulty with certain activities, in establishing which goals may be realistic or unrealistic at that time, and in designing interventions to improve function and independence. In addition, when neuropsychological assessment is repeated at later times in recovery, the results can be compared in order to monitor the rate and extent of cognitive recovery (or decline).

In principle, neuropsychological measures can be used to adjust or interpret outcomes in terms of the severity of cognitive impairment. Such adjustment is critical, because disability and handicap outcomes are usually uninterpretable without considering the severity of impairment. Outcomes themselves, however, are best assessed in terms of improvements in clearly important aspects of everyday life.

Assessment Strategy. Neuropsychological evaluation should include not only testing but also a detailed clinical interview, review of pertinent records, and interview with collateral informants about the patient's everyday functioning and emotional-behavioral problems. The patient's history, goals, family, and interpersonal adjustment need to be assessed to form a holistic understanding.[39,131] The clinical use of neuropsychological and other tests involves an understanding of brain-behavior relations. The enormous variety of neurologic conditions mandates flexibility in the approach to assessment. Thus there are no simple rules for conducting a "proper" assessment. Several works present caring and technically astute strategies for neuropsychological assessment.[39,112,131,160]

Although flexibility in assessment is needed, standardization also has advantages. Many neuropsychologists use a core battery approach in which they give the same set of tests to all patients in a diagnostic group, supplemented with tests chosen for each patient. In addition, the use of neuropsychological assessment in research studies generally requires that patients receive the same battery of tests and questionnaires.

One such research battery is used in the *Traumatic Brain Injury Model Systems*, a multicenter study of outcome after TBI.[40,105] The summary of tests below is based on the Model Systems assessment battery.

Perceptual Impairments. The patient's ability to sense and perceive stimuli in different modalities is routinely tested, particularly in the visual modality. Visual assessment generally includes testing of the visual fields, lateral visual inattention, and performance on more complex visual perceptual tasks such as copying designs with blocks. Assessment of basic sensory functions is critical, because sensory deficits may cause poor performance on tests of higher cognitive functions that rely on accurate perception of the test stimuli. Examples of perceptual tests commonly used in neuropsychological assessment are the Facial Recognition Test, Judgment of Line Orientation, Line Bisection, and cancellation tests.[53,112]

Memory and Learning. Impairment of memory is experienced by most patients following TBI.[39,105,159] Memory testing focuses on the ability to learn and recall new, unfamiliar information (i.e., recent memory) as opposed to the ability to recall old, familiar information (i.e., remote memory). Memory tests usually require the patient to recall information that was presented earlier in the evaluation, such as stories, word lists, and geometric diagrams. The subject may be asked to recall the information immediately after presentation or after a delay, usually of about 30 minutes. *The Wechsler Memory Scale–Revised* (WMS–R), perhaps the most frequently used test of memory impairments, is well standardized and has clearly established norms.[53,112] The WMS–R has subscales for verbal, visual, delayed, and general memory. Floor effects may make it insensitive to the varied memory function of patients with severe memory impairments. Other commonly used memory tests are the *Buschke Selective Reminding Test*[78] and the *Rey-Osterreith Complex Figure*.[28]

Attention and Concentration. Attention and concentration are also commonly impaired after brain injury. Attention refers to awareness of incoming stimuli and ability to process one stimulus while screening out others. Because virtually all tasks involve attention, attentional deficits lower performance on most neuropsychological tests. One type of test, such as the Digit Span and Visual Memory Span subtests of the WMS–R,[53,112] asks the patient to repeat stimulus sequences immediately after they are presented. Another type of attentional test asks the patient to perform a simple task as many times as possible within a set time limit. Such tests assess processing speed as well as attention; the *Trailmaking Test* and *Symbol Digit Modalities Test* are examples.[53,112] Brain-injured patients may perform markedly better in distraction-free environments.[39,105,150,159]

Executive Functions. The executive functions refer to the patient's ability to plan, initiate, follow through, and monitor the success of activities.[112] Such functions depend on the prefrontal areas of the frontal lobes. In everyday life, problems in executive functions may be manifested most clearly as difficulty in coping with unfamiliar problems. Tests of executive functions, such as the *Wisconsin Card Sorting Test*, examine the ability to develop strategies for solving unfamiliar problems. Many neuropsychologists believe that executive functions are not well assessed by available tests and include observations of the patient's test behavior and personality to improve assessment of executive functions.

General Intelligence. Traditional intelligence tests are often used in neuropsychological assessment. The standard intelligence tests in the United States are the *Wechsler Adult Intelligence Scale– Revised* (WAIS–R) and the *Wechsler Intelligence Scale for Children–III* (WISC–III).[53,112] Both are good predictors of academic performance, which is important in youthful survivors of TBI who need to return to school. However, measured intelligence may be well preserved after TBI despite debilitating problems with executive functions or memory.

Brief Tests of Cognitive Function. Table 2 lists five potentially useful but brief assessments of cognitive function that can be completed in 20-30 minutes or less. Data specific to TBI are available for the first three. These tests are sometimes called screening tests, because they are used to screen for significant impairments that deserve more detailed evaluation. Screening tests are designed to be used preliminary to—not as a substitute for—comprehensive neuropsychological evaluation. Brief assessments do not have the reliability needed to distinguish clearly among levels and types of brain deficits in individual patients. Given the massive human and economic costs of TBI,[90,108,118] a full neuropsychological evaluation is surely justifiable at some point in the course of recovery from moderate or severe TBI.

Assessment of Cognitive Disability

Cognitive disability refers to the impact of cognitive impairments on daily activities. Measures of cognitive disability (1) reflect activities valued by the person and (2) are sensitive to cognitive impairment. This topic is currently controversial and changing. To the most logical of readers, the term cognitive disability will seem paradoxical, because decreased cognition is preeminently an impairment. To others, thinking is obviously a basic activity in human life that manages all daily behaviors. Many significant cognitive impairments do not manifest themselves clearly as disabilities in basic ADLs or other activities that are highly dependent on motor function or long-term memory, relatively simple, or overlearned. But other life problems and patterns of disruption of everyday activities are more sensitive to cognitive impairments.

Assessment Approaches. Assessment based on disability in daily life has a long history in rehabilitation. Numerous attempts have been made to assess neurobehavioral function broadly and with a content that fairly directly reflects activities in daily life.[85] Such assessments differ from traditional tests by using problem situations that typically occur in daily life. Patients' responses to such realistic problems are observed and difficulties in action are rated.

Occupational therapists, for instance, frequently infer the patient's strengths and weaknesses by observation of problems in

TABLE 2. Brief Measures of Cognitive Function

Scale Name	Comments on Content, Validity, and Reliability
Neurobehavioral Cognitive Status Examination (NBSE)[101]	Assesses intellectual functioning in 5 areas, along with attention and orientation. Fair validity; no reliability data.
Barry Rehabilitation Inpatient Screening of Cognition (BRISC)[10]	Designed to assess broad range of below-normal functioning in 8 areas. Good reliability (except digits backward). Some validity data in TBI.
Brief Test of Head Injury (BTHI)[83]	Emphasis on expressive linguistic communication, with some receptive/gestural items. Assesses general cognitive ability, correlating fairly highly (0.75) with Rancho LCFS scores.
Strub and Black Mental Status Examination[155]	One of the more comprehensive of the brief screens. Few reliability or validity data provided.
Mini-Mental Status Examination (MMSE)	Very well known. Simple. Identifies demented patients. Shortest of the screens. Too brief to be used alone after TBI.

instrumental daily living activities. The approach is dynamic, as the therapist alters the situation to discover what facilitates and what interferes with a patient's performance.[163]

The *Comprehensive Assessment Inventory for Rehabilitation* (CAIR) involves a similar logic but is a more formal assessment. The CAIR was specifically designed for TBI rehabilitation. It contains many items that require therapists (1) to observe the person's daily behavior and (2) to assess patterns of errors and the impact of numerous specific factors that hinder performance.[66,67] For example, therapists are asked to rate the type of sensory and perceptual problems manifested in the patient's daily activities, the type and severity of attentional errors, and memory/learning problems manifested in daily activities in the facility and in the community.

The *Cognitive Behavior Rating Scale* (CBRS) asks an observer familiar with the patient to rate ability or the degree to which certain items describe the person in actual life.[177] Although designed to assess dementia, several dimensions are relevant to TBI rehabilitation.

Another strategy is to assess patient performance in life activities that depend highly on cognitive functions. Such activities may include organizing and carrying out a daily schedule, financial management, chores necessary to maintain a household, shopping and purchasing needed items, driving an automobile, community mobility, and safety behavior. Instrumental ADL and community activity scales, such as the CAIR,[66,67] contain such items. Although such activities are broader and less standardized than

neuropsychological tests, their content is more directly relevant to daily life. This direct relevance is advantageous for predicting the patient's required level of supervision and for planning skills to be taught in rehabilitation. Assessment of abilities used in daily life is central to outcome evaluation in rehabilitation.

General Ratings. Many of the attempts to assess cognitive disability with rating scales completed by clinicians are parts of multidimensional disability assessments.

The FIM goes beyond its progenitor, the Barthel Index, in ratings of comprehension, expressive communication, social interaction, problem solving, and memory. Such items, which comprise a measure of cognitive function that is psychometrically separate from motor ADL items, have adequate but not high unidimensionality.[114] The FIM indicates whether a patient is completely aphasic or demented, but its adequacy in TBI is widely questioned. Evidence for the predictive validity of FIM cognitive items is a matter of current research. A recent study found substantial inconsistencies among ratings of communication by nurses and speech-language pathologists.[1]

As noted previously, *Functional Assessment Measure* (FAM)[74] ratings may be somewhat unreliable, but the FAM may be more sensitive than the FIM to functional changes during the postacute period.[74]

The PECS contains ratings of cognitive competence (e.g., short-term memory), applied self-care, and communication that are especially relevant to TBI.[79,146–148,153] In one study of patients with TBI, the PECS total score and cognitive subscores predicted return to work or school better than the DRS or Rancho, with 84% accuracy.[133] None of these indices were designed to measure employment, however, and additional measures are needed to predict return to work accurately.

There are many general ratings of cognitive disability,[152,153] all of which rely to a greater or lesser degree on professional judgment and somewhat uncontrolled patient responses. The advantages are simplicity and breadth. The disadvantages are loss of reliability and objectivity.

Measures Sampling More Realistic Behaviors. An alternative approach to assessment is to test the patient with situations that simulate real-world problems. This approach is used in the *Rivermead Behavioral Memory Test* (RBMT), which consists of simulated everyday memory tasks, such as remembering where a personal belonging was hidden in the testing room earlier in the session. The RBMT has adequate reliability and has been shown to correlate well with therapists' ratings of memory problems.[179] In one study, RBMT scores were highly predictive of amnesic patients' ability to live independently.[178] Other attempts also use everyday memory tasks, such as memory for names and faces and self-report of memory abilities.[115]

More work is needed to develop the ecological or real-world validity of cognitive assessment procedures. In principle, this goal can be accomplished either by developing assessment procedures that resemble real-world activities or by research that establishes stronger correlations between neuropsychological tests and desired real-world outcomes. Assessments based on testing the person in meaningful activities currently give the most exact results.

Communicative Impairment and Disability

Communication is closely entwined with cognitive functioning, and many neuropsychological tests include communication as a cognitive activity. Nonetheless, communication and language are so important that they deserve specific assessment. The limitations of neuropsychological testing also apply to technical tests of communicative function, most of which are measures of impairment. Both are valuable for understanding the basis for the patient's problems but may be related only indirectly to daily life activities valued by the patient and by society.

Communicative Impairments. Tests of aphasia are useful in the assessment of language dysfunction due to brain injury, although they were developed primarily for patients with aphasia secondary to stroke. Such tests may underestimate substantially the communicative success of aphasic adults in natural settings but overestimate the communicative performance of patients with TBI.[77] The *Boston Diagnostic Aphasia Examination* (BDAE), for example, is a comprehensive, lengthy assessment of "components of language" with 34 subtests.[61] Other measures of linguistic impairment include the *Multilingual Aphasia Examination* (MAE), the *Token Test*, the *Porch Index of Communicative Ability*, the *Western Aphasia Battery*, *Word Fluency*, and the *Reitan-Indiana Aphasia Screening Test Scoring System*.[72,112] Clinicians no longer need to make up their own routine, brief batteries. The *Brief Test of Head Injury* (BTHI), for instance, is suitable for bedside use in acute settings. Information about its internal scaling characteristics and concurrent validity is available.[83]

Well-developed measures of dysarthria and the resulting disability—decreased intelligibility—are also available.[77,112] The *Assessment of Intelligibility of Dysarthric Speech* summarizes communicative function by the "communication efficiency ratio." Reliability is good, and normative data are available.[182]

Auditory perception tests include the *Wepman Auditory Discrimination Test*, the *Seashore Rhythm Test*, and the *Speech-Sounds Perception Test*.[53,112]

Like other tests of cognitive impairment, tests of communicative impairment are useful to understand patients' communicative problems and recovery. However, a number of pragmatic features of communication, such as initiation of spontaneous communication and use of gestures, may not be well assessed. Most critically, measures of communicative impairment may lack sensitivity to compensatory or learning-based improvements in real-life communicative activities that result from rehabilitative therapy. In fact, inappropriate use of communicative impairment measures to evaluate speech-language therapy has led to false conclusions that rehabilitative interventions are ineffective.[9,77,144]

Communicative Disability.   Assessments of communicative disability are not as numerous or well-developed as measures of communicative impairment. Development and validation of such measures are much needed.

Developed in 1969 before the WHO framework, Sarno's *Functional Communication Profile* (FCP) contains many items that measure whole communicative tasks (disability) and a few narrower items that measure functional impairments.[77,112,141,143,144] Overall the FCP is broad enough to be considered as a measure of communicative disability. The FCP is based on a rating of verbal and written comprehension and expression in aphasic adults. Reliability is only fair, but it predicts functional communication.

Many scales attempt to assess communicative disability using broad ratings of expressive and receptive communication. Examples include the FIM/FAM[73,74,114] and PECs.[79,147]

The *Communicative Abilities in Daily Living* (CADL) uses structured conversation and role playing (e.g., doctor's visit).[9,77,112] The use of simulated activities makes the CADL a more specific—and more laborious—measure of communicative disability than global ratings.

Haffey and Johnston's Comprehensive Assessment Inventory for Rehabilitation (CAIR) involves a rating of the success of communicative tasks in real settings.[66,67] It provides a number of examples of ecologically valid outcomes based on the frequency of problems in different real-world communicative situations, such as talking to friends over the phone, expressing basic daily needs, and buying an item in a store. Such items are promising as measures of communicative outcomes.[26]

Neurobehavioral Syndromes and Maladaptive Behaviors

Works by Bond,[21] Brooks,[24,25] and others[140] have established that emotional and behavioral changes are the most stressful consequences of TBI for relatives of survivors. Despite evidence that behavioral problems are critical factors in outcome after TBI, relatively few measures have been designed specifically to assess them. However, evidence of validity and reliability is now available for several scales relevant to behavioral and emotional problems.

Bond's Social Scale (BSS)[21,22] was an early and simple attempt to rate significant social outcomes after TBI. It requires a 3–5 point rating of 6 items—work, leisure pursuits, family cohesion, legal offenses, sexual problems, and alcohol abuse. Such topics are clearly practical and important to both the patient and society. Statistically significant agreement has been shown between the patient with TBI and other informants.[44] The BSS correlates significantly with the Katz Adjustment Scale and many other outcome measures (except time off work since injury).[44] Any simple scale, of course, must omit some important behaviors.

Levin's *Neurobehavioral Rating Scale* (NBRS), derived from the Brief Psychiatric Rating Scale, is a clinical rating scale designed to measure common behavioral and psychiatric symptoms after TBI.[111] Its 27 items assess cognitive and emotional disturbances, sometimes in terms of complex syndromes. Inter-rater reliability is satisfactory, but training is required to use the NBRS reliably. Data support its definite, if limited or moderate, validity in brain injury. Factor analysis revealed three principal components in the NBRS: cognitive/energy, self-appraisal, and somatic/anxiety. The NBRS has been used primarily to track neurobehavioral recovery after TBI but also may be useful as a measure of behavioral change in response to neurosurgical and psychopharmacological interventions.[28]

Several studies have used the *Katz Adjustment Scale*, especially the Relatives Form (KAS-R), to measure behavioral changes after TBI.[84] The KAS assesses adjustment from the perspectives of both patient and family. Behavioral problems assessed by the KAS-R include belligerence, apathy, social irresponsibility and judgment, emotional sensitivity, paranoid ideation, psychotic anxiety, bizarreness, depression, antisocial behavior, and suicidal inclinations. The KAS has satisfactory interrater reliability and concurrent validity. Normative data are available for non-TBI groups. The KAS-R is fairly lengthy, but its breadth may be valuable.

The *Patient Assessment of Own Functioning*[27] is a 47-item self-report by patients of their awareness and perception of disability. Little information about reliability or objective validity is available. The *Patient Competency Rating Scale* is a 30-item, 5-point rating of behavioral competencies.[52] Forms are available for use by the patient and staff or others, and some reliability data are available. The results of both scales may be useful clinically when compared with more objective criteria.

Measures of personality, depression, and other behavioral problems from mental health appear to be logically relevant to TBI. Few of these measures, however, have been validated in this population.

The *Minnesota Multiphasic Personality Inventory* (MMPI) has been widely used for decades to assess psychopathology in clinical settings and has been used in TBI. The MMPI is long (566 items) and requires training to interpret. Patients with closed head injury respond to a number of MMPI items in a pathologic direction. Two groups (factors) of abnormal MMPI responses have been identified: cognitive/sensory-motor and emotional/somatic.[2] Because a number of items on the MMPI describe physical and cognitive sequelae of brain injury, artifactual elevations may be produced on certain subscales.[57] Other mental health instruments also assess complaints (e.g., fatigue, poor memory, confusion) that may result from brain injury rather than from psychiatric disorder.

Other scales used to assess psychosocial and behavioral problems after TBI include the *Social Adjustment Scale* (SAS)[26] and the *Psychosocial Rating Scale* (PRS).[55] Wallace reviews 11 functional scales in mental health, most with social behavior components.[168]

Frequency and Severity of Actual Maladaptive Behaviors. Frequency counts of specific behaviors may be more objective than general ratings or self-reports. Behavior observations also entail problems of reliability, observer error, and attitudinal bias.

Haffey and Johnston present an approach using actual counts of various behavioral symptoms of emotional distress (e.g., anxiety, depressive behavior) and social behavior problems (e.g., aggressive, disruptive behavior, polydrug abuse).[66,67] The disruptiveness of social behaviors can be clearly graded in terms of real-world consequences (e.g., did it interrupt others' activities? did it result in expulsion from the room or facility?). This approach makes it possible to compare behavioral outcomes across patients and provides a vocabulary of behavioral treatment goals. A major problem, shared with other assessments of social behavior outcomes, is how to aggregate counts of specific behavioral problems into more general dimensions. The approach is close to the level of handicap in that frequency of actual events rather than abilities is assessed, but it is much narrower than most measures of handicap. Disruptive events reveal both actual behaviors and social responses. The circumstances that elicit the maladaptive behavior are important to understand, but little research has focused on the validity and reliability of methods for assessing the eliciting circumstances.

As in the wider population, alcohol and drug abuse are frequent problems among patients with brain injury. Many questionnaires ask about current and preinjury drug abuse. The *Michigan Alcoholism Screening Test* (MAST) asks 25 face-valid questions about drinking behavior; a short form is available.[146] Current alcohol and drug abuse is under-reported but remains a significant issue.

Most scales conceive of adequate functioning in terms of typical or "normal" behavior or optimal mental states. But it is also possible to conceive of adequate functioning as behaviors that do not have a particularly adverse impact on self or others. Bond's Social Scale and the Haffey-Johnston CAIR are among the few attempts to develop assessments based on such an approach. Pressure to increase cost-effectiveness will escalate the need for practical approaches to assessment of neurobehavioral outcomes.

Awareness of Deficits. Persons who suffer a major, permanent injury need to understand their new selves. This concept overlaps with adjustment to disability, but emphasizes the understanding of new limitations and preserved strengths. Unawareness or denial of impairments is a common behavioral problem after TBI and has been cited as a critical predictor of success in vocational rehabilitation programs.[132]

One major approach in measuring awareness of deficit is to evaluate the agreement between reports by the patient and family members about behavioral problems and difficulties in various activities. The *Patient Competency Rating Scale* (PCRS)[52] is perhaps the best-known scale used to elicit such reports. The PCRS has been used to predict vocational outcome after a 6-month outpatient treatment program.[52]

A second approach is to obtain the patient's self-report of errors in everyday life that are due to memory, perception, communication, or some other specific cognitive function. The *Everyday Memory Questionnaire* is an example.[167] The *Patient Assessment of Own Functioning* (PAF), a 47-item self-report instrument, elicits subjective ratings of everyday functioning in memory, communication, and other functions.[27] Haffey and Johnston[66,67] present one rating scale for adjustment to disability. Prigatano and Schacter describe the full complexity of self-awareness after brain injury.[132] The relation of scales of awareness of deficit to more objective measures of outcome is currently undocumented or poorly documented. Although the validity of these scales is limited, they may be clinically useful approaches to understanding patient progress.

Independent Living, Household, and Community Skills

Persuasive evidence indicates that training in practical household, community, and occupational skills is an effective strategy for reintegrating patients with TBI into the community.[32,33,55,92,93] Measures of these skills are highly valuable in assessing outcomes for postacute programs, higher-level patients, and long-term follow-up studies. Standardized assessment is valuable for prioritizing needed skills.

Independent living and household skills include such activities as cooking and kitchen management, scheduling of daily activities,

cleaning, fixing and other chores, financial management, and shopping. Fine motor coordination, endurance, strength, and/or more complex cognitive abilities are required for activities reviewed below. IADLs are more difficult to measure than ADLs.[148,151]

Community mobility is often a problem. Speed and endurance in ambulation, negotiation of environmental obstacles, safety, and the ability to plan and execute an itinerary are required for independent community mobility. Use of public transportation and driving are major issues.

The PECS has items related to social issues, vocational and educational activity, recreation driving, home management, and other skills.[79,119,146] As mentioned elsewhere, a number of studies have established the real but limited predictive validity of the PECS in patients with TBI; thus it is a leading candidate for use in TBI rehabilitation.

The CAIR was developed for TBI and has items related to such skills as household management, community mobility, and financial management.[66,67] Unfortunately, the CAIR has not received the necessary validation and testing to be applied with confidence.

The "home integration" items of the *Community Integration Questionnaire* (CIQ) are essentially an index of simple home activities or IADLs. Because the CIQ asks about actual performance rather than ability, it is discussed more fully under handicap.

The *Life Skills Profile*[139] (LSP) has 39 items assessing constructs relevant to function and adaptation in the community. Although the LSP was developed for schizophrenia, the assessed skills are relevant to TBI.

Pfeffer's *Functional Activities Questionnaire* (FAQ) deserves consideration in TBI, because it assesses skills such as managing financial affairs, reading, remembering appointments, shopping alone, recreational or hobby skills, and travel out of the neighborhood.[119,129] The FAQ, which has 10 items and is completed by a relative or close friend, is designed for study of normal aging and mild senile dementia. Research and experience are needed before it can applied with confidence to patients with TBI.

Most of the other IADL scales were designed for use in gerontology and also include ADL items. Examples include the *Multilevel*

Assessment Instrument,[106] the *Older Americans Resources and Services* (OARS) questionnaire, adaptive tasks in the *Rapid Disability Rating Scale* (RDRS-2), and others.[119,121]

Assessment of health or productive social and recreational abilities remains poorly developed. The scales above have items dealing with social and recreational activities.

Prevocational Skills

Rehabilitation programs frequently target the development of prevocational skills. The intermediate outcomes of such programs may be assessed in terms of employability. Ben-Yishay and others have shown that employability ratings based on observation of performance in simulated work situations can have high predictive validity in samples of brain-injured persons.[11] His *Employability Rating Scale* provides 10 options for rating productive activities. The FAM and CAIR also have ratings of employability for paid or unpaid occupations. The DRS has an employability rating and predicts return to work.[32,126]

Several more specific scales have been moderately successful in predicting employment of patients with TBI. The *Functional Assessment Inventory* (FAI),[38,123] predicts return to work. The FAI assesses abilities and disabilities in a fairly comprehensive (multidimensional) but simple (practical) way.[38] It has good content and concurrent validity,[123] although prescriptive utility is less clear. PECS scores also correlate with return to work in patients with TBI, although the PECS was designed primarily for inpatient assessment.[79,133]

Neuropsychological tests of higher cognitive function predict employment significantly but inconsistently.[140] A key issue is what additional measures are necessary to increase accuracy of prediction. Another issue is how to identify person-job interactions where neuropsychological tests predict strongly and to distinguish them from situations where they do not predict strongly. The number of variables involved in vocational evaluation is large, but uniform evaluation and goal-setting procedures are still feasible. Transferrable skills need to be assessed. One needs to progress rapidly from basic evaluation to situational or community-based assessment.[54] Works on general vocational

outcome analysis[15] and employment evaluation in patients with TBI[54,170] discuss vocational issues in more detail.

Mild Brain Injury

Assessment of mild brain injury is primarily beyond the scope of this chapter but is so common that it deserves mention. To identify the specific impact of mild brain injury may be difficult or impossible, but current functional limitations certainly can be assessed. Cognitive screens and ratings of independence in ADLs are usually insensitive in patients with mild brain injury. Likely or at least attributed real-life losses or handicaps (e.g., days off from work due to headaches, unemployment due to repeated loss of concentration and low productivity) can be documented. The *Subjective Complaint Checklist* of symptoms may be useful.[49] A key problem is inaccuracy of assessment of preinjury function or preexisting deficits. The *Psychosocial History Checklist*[75] allows some assessment of prior function.

HANDICAP AND COMMUNITY INTEGRATION

This section briefly reviews tools for the assessment of household and community skills and broader handicap-level outcomes for persons with TBI. Preceding sections described instruments which have items or subscales useful for the assessment of function in the community. Many individuals continue to have marked cognitive, communicative, and neurobehavioral problems that can be assessed by tools described in preceding sections (e.g., assessment of frequency and severity of maladaptive social behavior[21,22,66,67]). A minority of persons with TBI in the community remain so highly dependent on others for basic skills that inpatient disability measures are relevant.[92,93] Inpatient rehabilitation measures, however, are insensitive to real improvements among higher-level patients (ceiling problems).[114] They typically assess independence only in household mobility and self-care ADLs, whereas life involves a great deal more. Assessment of TBI outcomes requires measures of broader real-life outcomes, including independent living skills, productive roles, and level of handicap in other psychosocial areas.

Independent living, household, social, community, and vocational skills interrelate. For instance, a person trained to do a job also may need training in how to commute. Vocational skills do not diminish handicap if the person is in fact unemployed. Even money can be hollow without someone to love and share. One must assess the degree to which the system as a whole works in practice. General handicap measures are needed.

Multidimensional Indices of Handicap and Community Integration

Some aspects of handicap are easily assessed. A few instruments have been developed recently, although data about their reliability and validity remain limited.

The *Community Integration Questionnaire* (CIQ)[175,176] was developed specifically for the assessment of patients with TBI. Using factor analysis, three dimensions were identified from a larger number of items: home, social, and vocational integration (the home and vocational scales assess independence and productivity).

The CIQ distinguishes between persons with disability due to TBI and nondisabled controls and among at least three levels of disability within the TBI population. It is designed to measure integration in a way relevant to TBI, but, like other handicap-level measures, it is not designed to discriminate TBI from other impairments. The CIQ is simple and easy to complete. The 15 items can be completed in 10–15 minutes by brain-injured patients or family members by telephone or personal interview. The CIQ shows satisfactory reliability. Answers by the person with brain injury correlate highly with those of family members. If the patient with TBI is able to communicate, a personal interview is recommended.[6] To differentiate the effect of TBI and rehabilitation from preinjury factors, retrospective preinjury activities need to be assessed. The CIQ comprises an excellent but minimal set for assessment of community outcomes.

The *Craig Handicap Assessment and Recording Technique* (CHART) was developed

to assess handicap after spinal cord injury.[172] Psychometric properties, reliability, and validity have been demonstrated. The CHART is currently being expanded to include activities that often are limited by cognitive problems. A number of the items in the CHART, however, are problematic in patients with TBI, and its use with TBI is currently experimental.

Many other scales assess one or more aspects of community integration. Scales developed to assess actual quality of life, productive activities, psychosocial adjustment, and instrumental ADLs after discharge may be relevant. The WHO-Wood taxonomy itself has not been subjected to direct empirical test in patients with TBI or most other disability groups. The taxonomy posits "orientation" to the environment as a dimension of handicap, but the dimension is unclear. Other important dimensions of handicap are also difficult to measure exactly, including the role of an "independent person," social integration, and needed recreational activities. Long-term social outcomes are a complex and perhaps even heterogeneous domain.[44]

Employment and Productive Activities

Humans need a productive or socially valued occupation—paid employment and/or unpaid contributions to family, friends, or the community. Absence of a rewarding occupation, despite independence in basic ADLs, is a depressingly frequent problem after TBI. Lost work is the largest social cost produced by TBI, albeit an indirect one.[34,90]

Employment is simple to measure—so simple that it is often measured inadequately and inaccurately. Return to work can be meaningfully measured by simple counts, but such counts may not take into account changes in hours of work, rate of pay, or stability of employment. To assess employment, it is important to assess hours of work or at least whether the work is full- or part-time. Earnings per hour more frequently decline than improve[92,93]; thus decline in earnings must be assessed to characterize fully the impact of injury. Long-term stability of employment is a key issue; employment level at 90 days is a more questionable measure of vocational outcomes in patients with TBI than in physically disabled groups. Employment before the injury (and before admission for chronic clients living in the community before admission) also needs to be assessed.

The monthly employment ratio is based on the number of months a person has been employed and the number of months a person has been available for employment during the past year.[171] Full- or part-time workers are considered employed. Months spent in full-time attendance at school or in an institution are considered not available for employment.

Although paid work is the main productive activity valued in American society, it is not the only option, and for many persons it may be not be appropriate, expected, or feasible. Contribution to family and household, parenting, and volunteer work can be appropriate and productive occupations for some individuals. There is no well-validated, precise way of assessing the broader dimension—occupation or productive activity—across whole TBI populations, although attempts have been made. Ordinal scales of productive activities have been proposed.[41] Many scales rate such alternative productive activities. Cope and colleagues gave credit for recreational and volunteer time in addition to paid employment.[32] There are also a number of employability scales, but employability is a disability rating. Handicap is assessed by whether the person in fact has the desired or normatively expected productive occupation.

Independent Living

Living arrangement provides a rough estimate of level of dependence and cost to society. The fact that an individual lives at home with family may reflect the dedication of the family, cultural influences, or economic resources, rather than independence. Nevertheless, discharge to private residence is considered a good outcome and transfer to a chronic care facility a poor outcome. Simple descriptions of living arrangement can be ordinated to characterize independent living.[41] Placement immediately after discharge is meaningful, but follow-up over time is necessary to assess independence accurately.

Levels of assisted care or required supervision are direct methods of determining level of independence. The CHART, for instance, directly asks for hours of assistance per day.[172] Difficulties in current methods of obtaining such information include the uncertainties of supervision versus direct care needs, paid versus unpaid assistance, effects of insurance payment for attendant care, variations in skill level of assistance, and discrepancies between needed and received care. Despite uncertainties, global independence remains central to assessment of rehabilitation outcome.

In summary, handicap is a complex of activities in the person's actual environment. It is essential to measure handicap in the community, which is the bottom line for measurement of rehabilitation outcomes and has great implications for long-term cost-effectiveness.

OTHER ENDPOINT OUTCOMES

Costs and Economic Outcomes. To payors, costs are the ultimate outcome, and outcome assessment can no longer ignore costs to society. Charges or actual expenditures are only the starting point for assessment of costs, but are problematic. The medical care industry is hardly a classic free competitive market. Many facilities maintain high cost-to-charge ratios, and charges for the same service vary substantially, depending on legal subsidies and contractual arrangements. Charges for rehabilitation hospital care for persons with brain injury average $51,416 in Model Systems, and prior acute hospital care averages $66,368.[108] Such averages provide a benchmark, but costs for individual patients vary enormously above and below them. Treatment and rehabilitation of more severe injuries involve higher costs. At minimum a measure of general severity (e.g., the DRS[32,108]) is needed to assess appropriateness of rehabilitation costs.

Rehospitalization and nursing home costs have been estimated at $4.49 billion dollars annually in the United States.[118] Losses due to mortality and morbidity—work loss and disability—are much higher ($20.6 and $12.7 billion, respectively). Other estimates have put the cost of lost work alone at $25.9–$34.4 billion annually in 1980 dollars.[90] Costs of lost work by family members and of unpaid supervision are probably substantial but have not been fully estimated.[75] All estimates agree that lost work is the largest cost associated with TBI.[34,90] Payors are clearly responsible for survival and cannot easily renounce their responsibility for basic ADL needs, which are linked to survival, but they are frequently not responsible for costs of long-term care and supervision and lost productivity. The restriction of treatment objectives to the bare-bones basics implies an effort to shift costs of TBI-related dependency, behavioral problems, and unemployment from insurers to Medicaid, welfare, society at large, and, above all, to the family and patient. Justification of rehabilitation needs to be based on reduced long-term costs and improved productivity for all parties, including the patient, family, payor, and society as a whole.

Payors ought to consider not only costs but also cost-effectiveness. Cost-effectiveness in rehabilitation is a complex matter, and the few works on the topics provide merely an orientation.[8,90,108] One fruitful method of investigating cost-effectiveness in rehabilitation is consideration of cost per unit of functional gain.[89,90,155] The idea is that the relation of effort to result indicates cost-effectiveness. Normative data based on hundreds of American inpatient rehabilitation hospitals are available for cost/gain relationships using FIM scores.[65] Cost-effective TBI rehabilitation programs should show a statistical correlation between effort and result, and programs can be identified that are not cost-effective by this criterion.[90,93,155] There are numerous potential pitfalls in analyses using gain per day or gain per dollar, which are simplistic surrogates for full cost-effectiveness analyses. Early admission of survivors of serious TBI to specialized rehabilitation programs has repeatedly been associated with reduced costs and greater cost/gain relationships.[31,90,108]

Stress.   Although life satisfaction and stress are not stable phenomena, they suffuse the human interaction between professionals, clients, and families. Clinical rehabilitation staff need to understand the values, goals, and sources of life satisfaction and stress for the person with injury and significant others.

Extreme levels of stress and related problems have been documented repeatedly among family members of persons with TBI and often are much higher than with physically disabling injuries.[17,104] Various subjective burden questions have been used to assess family stress after TBI,[104] including a number of useful single-item questions (e.g., the Bradburn or delighted-terrible scale).[119] More elaborate instruments include the *Katz Adjustment Scale*, the *Leeds Anxiety and Depression Scales*, the *Social Adjustment Schedule*, the *Dyatic Adjustment Scale*, the *Personal Assessment of Intimacy in Relationship*, the *Family Crisis Oriented Personal Evaluation Scales*, the *Hassles Scale*, the *Ways of Coping Inventory*, and the *Symptom Checklist 90* (SCL-90).[104]

Life Satisfaction.   Life satisfaction is a crucial but difficult-to-measure outcome that has been infrequently studied in TBI rehabilitation. Measures of life satisfaction include the *Life Satisfaction Index-A* (LSIA), the *Quality of Life Scale*, and the *Personal Well-Being Scale* (PWB).[56,119] Measures of life satisfaction are subjective and rather unstable and may depend on factors irrelevant to the quality of rehabilitative care (e.g., prior wealth).[56] Likely life satisfaction is a key ethical and practical issue in regard to life-saving measures for the most severely injured patients, but its implications extend much further. Life satisfaction and other means of engaging the subjective values, beliefs, and feelings of the person with TBI are critical issues regardless of the difficulties in measuring them.

SUMMARY AND CONCLUSIONS

Neither brain dysfunction nor its impact on life is simple. Multiple domains of function need to be assessed, depending on the severity and type of brain injury and the functional and life problems facing the patient. Many instruments have been developed in the last decade or so to assess function in patients with TBI. Use of novel, completely non-standardized, locally developed measures is no longer needed or justifiable for most domains in TBI rehabilitation. No gold standard of measures, however, is evident, because the predictive and construct validity of existing tools remains insufficiently developed to meet measurement standards for medical rehabilitation.[96] Further work will help to identify the best scales for different applications.

Assessment of Severity. Global case severity needs to be routinely assessed in rehabilitation with standardized measures. Valid, practical measures of general severity of TBI are available, including the GCS, duration of posttraumatic amnesia (preferably assessed by GOAT scores), the DRS, and multidimensional measures of disability commonly used in rehabilitation hospitals, such as the FIM and the PECS. The DRS is currently the best validated method of assessing global case severity.

Multidimensional Assessment. The authors recommend assessment of function in multidimensional terms. Physical sequelae need to be distinguished from the primary outcomes of TBI, which are usually cognitive and neurobehavioral. Although functional independence remains the bread and butter of inpatient TBI rehabilitation, vocational skills and productive activities are keys to long-term success as judged by the person and by society.

The amount of research done to predict level and type of care, supervision needs, and optimal admission in patients with TBI has been grossly inadequate, given the enormous practical and theoretical importance of such criteria. Projection of current care needs is the basis of level-of-care assessment, but this approach is unsatisfactory when the question is whether the patient has the potential to live more independently after astute rehabilitative interventions. Similarly, likelihood of return to work can be estimated only roughly at present, and much more research is needed to improve the ability to forecast likelihood of success in alternative types of work.

Particularly critical is the need to develop and establish measures for assessment of cognitive disabilities, that is, practical measures demonstrated to be highly sensitive to the impact of cognitive impairments on socially valued activities in daily life. Clarifying the life activities most likely to be disrupted after different types of TBI is a

first step. Likely activities include instrumental ADLs, community activities, behavioral or psychosocial disorders, adjustment to disability, and planning and problem-solving activities. Without compelling objective data that prove their essential role in improving outcomes valued by the patient and society, funders will save money by ignoring psychosocial and behavioral outcomes.

Neuropsychological and neurophysiologic measures are needed to understand the patient's problems. In conjunction with other information, they are needed to plan rehabilitative interventions. Although such technical tests predict outcomes to a certain degree,[140] they give only a partial picture of outcome.

Handicap and Disability. Measures of performances—of disability and handicap—are interpretable in terms of daily life and remain the basis for outcome and progress assessment in rehabilitation. Both neuropsychological tests and broader assessments of disability help to clarify the functional strengths and deficits of the patient as well as therapeutic goals and objectives, and provide essential information for decisions about level of care and discharge or placement.

Handicap or social disadvantage is currently the best level for measurement of general outcome goals for comprehensive rehabilitation programs.[95] It is currently quite feasible to describe the outcomes of TBI rehabilitation in terms of independence in basic self-care ADLs and mobility, household and community IADLs, return to work, and other productive roles.[92,93,95] Although current measures of handicap are limited, they have proved to be sensitive to change associated with participation in intensive TBI rehabilitation programs.[33,92]

Assessment of handicap is also important clinically, because it can help to prioritize treatment interventions toward life issues most valued by society and the patient.[66–68] Reduction of handicap, however, is a long-term, global goal, and clinical rehabilitation also needs more concrete, proximal objectives.

Treatment Objectives. Clinical rehabilitation needs proximal as well as ultimate measures of outcome. The further development and validation of measures of long-term treatment objectives are critical needs in rehabilitation practice and outcomes research.[66,67] Treatment objectives should be linked to a treatment protocol based on validated theory. The theory need not be elaborate and may be based, for example, on more obvious features of learning theory, exercise physiology, or well-established medical interventions. Ideally, validation of measures of long-term treatment objectives requires controlled studies. But even in the absence of ideal experimental evidence, astute clinicians have some knowledge of effective rehabilitative interventions and know roughly where to look for an effect.

Examples. Treatment objectives are typically neither as global as measures of handicap nor as specific as most measures of impairment. Treatment objectives may be described in terms of what the patient will be able to do at discharge, that is, in fairly familiar functional terms.[66,67,95] Several systems for measurement of life skills (specific disabilities or functional limitations) are promising as measures of treatment objectives. The Haffey-Johnston CAIR,[66,67] for example, includes indices of independence in self-care ADLs and mobility as well as higher-level skills. Also included are household IADLs and community skills, such as financial management, parenting skills, driving, cooking, shopping, and financial management. Merely staying outside a nursing home is not enough.

Treatment objectives in communication can be expressed in functional terms. An item such as "client will communicate needs in purchasing groceries in market 95% of the time" is directly interpretable in terms of real-life needs and is probably responsive to practice-based interventions. Communicative objectives include expressive, receptive, oral, and written communication with feasible augmentative devices, as demonstrated by problems in real settings and tasks.[66,67]

Some treatment objectives may be described in terms of a mix of impairments and independent management skills; obvious examples are bowel and bladder problems. Health-related self-management includes both reliable self-regulation and specific medications. Musculoskeletal and body-movement impairments include general weakness, problems with coordination, balance, or endurance and other concerns. To be valid treatment objectives in the present sense, they may be assessed not in terms of impairment but in terms of the degree to which they restrict the patient's independence.[66,67] Similarly, cognitive impairments may be assessed not in terms of neuropsychological severity but in terms of impact on daily activities.[66,67] Ratings of specific cognitive disability and more ecologically valid cognitive measures may serve as valid treatment objectives.

Counts of the frequency and disruptiveness of maladaptive social and emotional behaviors are eminently suitable treatment objectives.[66,67] Ratings of well-established psychological syndromes may be outcome measures for combinations of pharmacologic and psychotherapeutic interventions. The danger, however, lies in use of ratings of less established psychological syndromes as treatment objectives, because their reality and value may be questionable. Awareness of the need to compensate and adjustment to limitations and prosocial behavior are important treatment objectives, although only general ratings of these domains are currently available. Tests of work or academic skills or ratings of employability or even leisure skills also may serve as treatment objectives.

Reductions in impairment sometimes may be used as long-term treatment objectives, with certain caveats. For example, for patients in the months following severe TBI, treatment objectives may include prevention of extreme weight loss, decubitus ulcers, and spasticity; control of hydrocephalus; and mobilization.[66,67] There are, however, dangers to uncritical acceptance of all current medical-nursing goals as validated treatment objectives. Severely injured patients have many impairments, alteration of which may have little effect on practical long-term outcomes, (e.g., range of motion in permanently comatose patients). An impairment measure must have a strong relationship to long-term disability or handicap to serve as a proxy for functional treatment objectives. A number of medical-nursing impairments may meet this criterion,[66,67,95] but work is needed to sort out stronger from weaker candidates.

Critique. One difficulty with treatment objectives is that comprehensive rehabilitation involves so many interventions that documenting the outcomes of each is excessively burdensome. One solution is to monitor progress only toward treatment objectives that are most critical to stable independent living or productive activity outcomes.[66–68] Such monitoring would be less burdensome than current documentation of therapy in micro (15-minute) units.

The relationship between treatment objectives and broader outcomes is also an issue. Documented treatment objectives deal with only part of patient function and part of the comprehensive rehabilitation program. Wider handicap outcomes still need to be assessed to determine whether the program as a whole makes a substantial difference in the person's life. Programs that claim to restore prevocational skills, for instance, need to measure not only job skills but also whether the client actually gets a job. Programs that improve independence need to assess the degree of supervision that the person receives and needs after discharge. Handicap-level outcomes are valuable for prioritizing treatment objectives.[67,68] Treatment objectives are necessary to link global outcomes to what the team is doing.

The Individual vs. the Group. Current standardized measures of outcome are most valid and useful at the group or program level. These measures can determine whether appropriate patients are admitted, whether severity-adjusted outcomes are as good as other rehabilitation programs, and whether length of stay is normatively justified; they also demonstrate the value of rehabilitation.[97] Comparisons of persons are implicit in the attempt to discern patterns of effective treatment.

Clinicians should choose outstanding measures and become familiar with them. These measures will provide structure to clinical assessment and planning, but they should not become more than a theme that inspires variations. Clinicians must adjust goals and interventions to the needs of individual patients.

ACKNOWLEDGMENTS. The authors thank Samuel C. Shiflett, Ph.D., for assistance with summarizing scales; Miriam Maney, M.A., for assistance with general outcome measures; John DeLuca, Ph.D., for criticisms which strengthened the work; and Margaret Crater, M.A., for editorial assistance. Preparation of this work was supported by grants H133B30041 from the National Institute for Disability and Rehabilitation Research, 108 from the Henry Kessler Foundation, and H128A00022 from the Rehabilitation Services Administration.

REFERENCES

1. Adamovich BLB: Pitfalls in functional assessment: A comparison of FIM ratings by speech-language pathologists and nurses. NeuroRehabilitation 2(4):42–51, 1992.
2. Alfano DP, Paniak CE, Finlayson HJ: The MMPI and close injury: A neurocorrective approach. Neuropsychiatry Neuropsychol Behav Neurol 6(2):111–116, 1993.
3. American Medical Association: Guide to the Evaluation of Permanent Impairment, 3rd ed (revised). Milwaukee, WI, American Medical Association, 1990.
4. Anastasi A: Psychological Testing, 6th ed. New York, Collier, 1988.
5. Anderson SI, Housley AM, Jones PA, et al: Glasgow Outcome Scale: An inter-rater reliability study. Brain Inj 7:309–317, 1993.
6. Antonal RF, Livneh, Antonak C: A review of research on psychosocial adjustment to impairment in persons with traumatic brain injury. J Head Trauma Rehabil 8(4):87–100, 1993.
7. Ansell BJ, Keenan JE: The Western Neuro-sensory Stimulation Profile: A tool for assessing slow-to-recover head-injured patients. Arch Phys Med Rehabil 70:104–108, 1989.
8. Ashley MJ, Persedel CS, Krych DK: Changes in reimbursement climate: Relationship among outcome, cost, and payor type in the postacute rehabilitation environment. J Head Trauma Rehabil 8(4):30–47, 1993.
9. Aten J, Caligiuri Â, Holland A: The efficacy of functional communicative therapy for chronic aphasic patients. J Speech Hearing Disorders 47:93–96, 1982.
10. Barry P, Clark DE, Yaguda M, et al: Rehabilitation inpatient screening of early cognitive recovery. Arch Phys Med Rehabil 70:902–906, 1989.
11. Ben-Yishay Y: Relationship between employability and vocational outcome after intensive holistic cognitive rehabilitation. J Head Trauma Rehabil 2(1):35–48, 1987.
12. Blackersby LVF, Baungarten A: A model treatment program for the head-injured substance abuser: Preliminary findings. J Head Trauma Rehabil 5(3):47–59, 1990.
13. Bohannon RW, Smith MB: Interrater reliability of a modified Ashworth scale of muscle spasticity. Phys Ther 67:206–207, 1987.

14. Bohannon RW, Warren ME, Cogman KA: Motor variables correlated with the hand-to-mouth maneuver in stroke patients. Arch Phys Med Rehabil 72:682–684, 1991.

15. Bolton B: Outcome analysis in vocational rehabilitation. In Fuhrer M: Rehabilitation Outcomes: Analysis and Measurement. Baltimore, P. Brooks, 1987, pp 57–70.

16. Born JD: The Glasgow-Liège Scale: Prognostic value and evolution of motor response and brain stem reflexes after severe head injury. Acta Neurochir (Wien) 91:1–11, 1988.

17. Brooks DN: The head-injured family. J Clin Exp Neuropsychol 13:155–188, 1991.

18. Bowers DN, Kofroth LK: Comparisons of Disability Rating Scale and Functional Independence Measures during recovery from traumatic brain injury. Arch Phys Med Rehabil 70:855–892, 1985.

19. Bowler RM, Thaler CD, Becker CE: California Neuropsychological Screening Battery (CNS/B I & II). J Clin Psychol 42:946–955, 1986.

20. Born JD, Albert A, Hans P, Bonnal J: Relative prognostic value of best motor response and brain stem reflexes in patients with severe had injury. Neurosurgery 16:595–601, 1985.

21. Bond MR: Assessment of the psychosocial outcome after severe brain injury. In Porter R, Fitzsimmons DW (eds): Outcome of Severe Damage to the Central Nervous System. CIBA Foundation Symposium 34, Amsterdam, Elsevier, 1975.

22. Bond MR: Assessment of the psychosocial outcome after severe head injury. Acta Neurochir (Wien) 34:57–70, 1976.

23. Bowers DN, Kofroth LK: Comparisons of Disability Rating Scale and Functional Independence Measures during recovery from traumatic brain injury. Arch Phys Med Rehabil 70:A58, 1989.

24. Brooks DN, Aughton ME: Cognitive recovery during the first year after severe brain injury. Int Rehabil Med 1:160–165, 1979.

25. Brooks N, Campsie L, Symington C, et al: The effects of severe brain injury on patient and relative within seven years of injury. J Head Trauma Rehabil 2(3):1–13, 1987.

26. Burton LA, Volpe B: Social Adjustment Scale assessments in traumatic brain injury. J Rehabil 59(4):34–37, 1993.

27. Chelune G, Heaton R, Lehman R: Neuropsychological and personality correlates of patients complaints of disability. In Goldstein G (ed): Advances in Clinical Psychology, vol. 3. New York, Plenum, 1986.

28. Clifton GL, Hayes RL, Levin HS, et al: Outcome measures for clinical trials involving traumatically brain-injured patients: Report of a conference. Neurosurgery 31:975–978 , 1992.

29. Clifton GL, Kreutzer JS, Choi SC, et al: Relationships between Glasgow Outcome Scale and neuropsychological measures after brain injury. Neurosurgery 33:34–38, 1993.

30. Committee to Advise the Public Health Service on Clinical Practice Guidelines, Field MJ, Lohr KN (eds): Clinical Practice Guidelines. Washington, DC, National Academy Press, 1990.

31. Cope DN, Hall K: Head injury rehabilitation: Benefit of early intervention. Arch Phys Med Rehabil 63:433–437, 1982.

32. Cope DN, Cole JR, Hall KM, Barkan H: Brain injury: Analysis of outcome in a post-acute rehabilitation system. Part 1: General Analysis. Brain Inj 5:111–125, 1991.

33. Cope DN: Effectiveness of traumatic brain injury: A review. Brain Inj 1994 (in press).

34. Cope DN, O'Lear J: A clinical and economic perspective on head injury rehabilitation. J Head Trauma Rehabil 8(4):1–14, 1993.

35. Conzen M, Ebel H, Swart E, et al: Long-term neuropsychological outcome after severe head injury with good recovery. Brain Inj 6:45–52, 1992.

36. Corrigan JD: Development of a scale for assessment of agitation following traumatic brain injury. J Clin Exp Neuropsychol 11:261_277, 1989.

37. Crosby L, Parsons LC: Clinical neurologic assessment tool: Development and testing of an instrument to index neurologic status. Heart Lung 18: 121–129, 1989.

38. Crew NM, Athelstan GT: Functional assessment in vocational rehabilitation: A systematic approach to diagnosis and goal setting. Arch Phys Med Rehabil 62(70:299–305, 1981.

39. Cripe LI: Neuropsychological and psychosocial assessment of the brain-injured person: Clinical concepts and guidelines. Special Issue: Traumatic brain injury rehabilitation. Rehabil Psychol 34(2): 93–100.

40. Dahmer ER, Shilling MA, Hamilton BB, et al: A model systems database for traumatic brain injury. J Head Trauma Rehabil 8(2):12–25, 1993.

41. DeJong G, Hughes J: Independent living: Methodology for measuring long-term outcomes. Arch Phys Med Rehabil 63:68–73, 1982.

42. DiScalas C, Grant CC, Brooke MM, Gans BM: Functional outcome in children with traumatic brain injury: Agreement between clinical judgement and the Functional Independence Measure. Am J Phys Med Rehabil 71:145–148, 1992.

43. Ditunno JF: Functional assessment measures in CNS trauma. J Neurotrauma (Suppl 1):S301–S305, 1992.

44. Dodwell D: The heterogeneity of social outcome following head injury. J Neurol Neurosurg Psychiatry 51:833–838, 1988.

45. Diller L, Ben-Yishay Y: Analyzing rehabilitation outcomes of persons with head injury. In Fuhrer MJ (ed): Rehabilitation Outcomes: Analysis and Measurement. Baltimore, Brooks, 1987, pp 209– 220.

46. Disler PB, Ropy CW, Smith BP: Predicting hours of care needed. Arch Phys Med Rehabil 74:139–143, 1993.

47. Eisenberg HM, Weiner RL: Input variables: How information from the acute injury can be used to characterize groups of patients for studies of outcomes. In Levin HS, Grafman J, Eisenberg HM (eds): Neurobehavioral Recovery from Head Injury. New York, Oxford, 1987, pp 13–29.

48. Eliason MR, Topp BW: Predictive validity of Rappaport's Disability Rating Scale in subjects with acute brain dysfunction. Phys Ther 64:1357–1360, 1984.

49. Englander J, Hall KM, Simpson T, Chaffin S: Mild traumatic brain injury in an insured population: Subjective complaints and return to employment. Brain Inj 6(2):161–166, 1992.

50. Feinstein AR: Clinimetrics. New Haven, Yale University Press, 1987.

51. Folstein MF, Folstein SE, McHugh PR: Minimental state: A practical method for grading the cognitive state of patients for the clinician. J Pyschiatr Res 12:189–198, 1975.

52. Fordyce DS, Roueche JR: Changes in perspectives of disability among patients, staff and relatives during rehabilitation of brain injury. Rehabil Psychol 31:217–229, 1986.

53. Franzen MD: Reliability and Validity in Neuropsychological Assessment. New York, Plenum, 1989.

54. Fraser RT: Vocational evaluation. J Head Trauma Rehabil 6(3):46–58, 1991.

55. Fryer J, Haffey W: Cognitive rehabilitation and community readaptation: Outcomes from two program models. J Head Trauma Rehabil 2:51–63, 1987.

56. Fuhrer MJ: Subjective well-being of persons with physical disabilities: Implications for medical rehabilitation outcomes and models of disablement. Am J Phys Med Rehabil (in press).

57. Gass CS: MMPI-2 interpretation and closed head injury: A correction factor. Psychol Assess 3:27–31, 1991.

58. Gensemer IB, Smith JL, Walker JC, et al: Psychological consequences of blunt head trauma and relation to other indices of severity of injury. Ann Emerg Med 18:9–12, 1989.

59. Giacino JT, Kezmarski M, DeLuca J, Cicerone KD: Monitoring rate of recovery to predict outcome in minimally-responsive patients. Arch Phys Med Rehabil (in press).

60. Giannota SL, Weiner JM, Karnaze D: Prognosis and outcome in severe head injury. In Cooper PR (ed): Head Injury, 2nd ed. Baltimore, Williams & Wilkins, 1987, pp 464–487.

61. Goodglass H, Kaplan E: Boston Diagnostic Aphasia Examination. Philadelphia, Lea & Febiger, 1972.

62. Gouvier WD, Blanton PD, LaPorte KK, Nepomeceno C: Reliability and validity of the Disability Rating Scale and the Levels of Cognitive Functioning Scale in monitoring recovery from severe head injury. Arch Phys Med Rehabil 68:94–97, 1987.

63. Granger CV, Cotter AC, Hamilton BB, et al: Functional assessment scales: A study of persons with multiple sclerosis. Arch Phys Med Rehabil 71: 870–875, 1990.

64. Granger CV, Cotter AC, Hamilton BB, Fiedler RC: Functional assessment scales: A study of persons after stroke. Arch Phys Med Rehabil 74:133–138, 1993.

65. Granger CV, Hamilton BH: The Uniform Data System for Medical Rehabilitation report of first admissions for 1991. Am J Phys Med Rehabil 72: 33–38, 1993.

66. Haffey WJ, Johnston MY: An information system to assess the effectiveness of brain injury rehabilitation. In Wood R, Eames P (eds): Models of Brain Injury Rehabilitation. London, Chapman Hall, 1989.

67. Haffey WJ, Johnston MV: A functional assessment system for real world rehabilitation outcomes. In Tupper D, Cicerone K (eds): The Neurophysiology of Everyday Life. Boston, Martinus Nijhoff, 1990.

68. Haffey WJ, Lewis FD: Programming for occupational outcomes following traumatic brain injury. Rehabil Psychol 34(2):142–158, 1989.

69. Haffey W, Lewis F: Rehabilitation outcomes following traumatic brain injury. Phys Med Rehabil State Art Rev 3:293–318, 1989.

70. Hagan C: Language cognitive disorganization following closed head injury: A conceptualization. In Trexler LE (ed): Cognitive Rehabilitation: Conceptualization and Intervention. New York, Plenum, 1982, pp 131–151.

71. Hagen C: Managed care: It may be an opportunity. NeuroRehabilitation 4:58–61, 1994.

72. Hall K, Cope DN, Rappaport M: Glasgow Outcome Scale and Disability Rating Scale: Comparative usefulness in following recovery in traumatic head injury. Arch Phys Med Rehabil 66:35–37, 1985.

73. Hall KM: Overview of functional assessment scales in brain injury rehabilitation. NeuroRehabilitation 2:98–113, 1992.

74. Hall KM, Hamilton BB, Gordon WA, Zasler ND: Characteristics and comparisons of functional assessment indices: Disability Rating Scale, Functional Independence Measure, and Functional Assessment Measure. J Head Trauma Rehabil 8(2):60–74, 1993.

75. Hall KM, Karzmark P, Stevens M, et al: Family stressors in traumatic brain injury: A two-year follow-up. Arch Phys Med Rehabil 1994 (in press).

76. Hamilton BB, Laughlin JA, Granger CV, Kayton RM: Interrater agreement of the seven-level Functional Independence Measure (FIM). Arch Phys Med Rehabil 72:790, 1992.

77. Hartley LL: Assessment of functional communication. In Tupper DE, Cicerone KD (eds): The Neuropsychology of Everyday Life: Assessment and Basic Competencies. Boston, Kluwer Academic, 1990, pp 125–166.

78. Hannay HJ, Levin HS: Selective reminding test: An examination of equivalence of four forms. J Clin Exp Neuropsychol 7:251–263, 1985.

79. Harvey RF, Jellinek HM: Patient profiles: Utilization in functional performance assessment. Arch Phys Med Rehabil 64(6):268–271, 1983.

80. Harvey RF, Silverstein B, Venzon MA, et al: Applying psychometric criteria to functional assessment in medical rehabilitation: III. Construct validity and predicting level of care. Arch Phys Med Rehabil 73:887–892, 1992.

81. Heinemann AW, Linacre JM, Wright BD, et al: Relationships between impairment and physical disability as measured by the Functional Independence Measure. Arch Phys Med Rehabil 75: 133–143, 1994.

82. Heinemann AW, Linacre JM, Hamilton BB: Prediction of rehabilitation outcomes with disability measures. Arch Phys Med Rehabil 75:123–143.

83. Helm-Estabrooks N, Hotz G: Brief Test of Head Injury: Normed Edition Manual. Chicago, Riverside, 1991.

84. Jackson HF, Hopewell CA, Glass CA, et al: The Katz Adjustment Scale: Modification for use with victims of traumatic brain injury and spinal surgery. Brain Inj 6(2):109–127, 1992.

85. Jacobs HE: The Los Angeles head injury survey: Project rationale and design implications. J Head Trauma Rehabil 2:37–50, 1987.

86. Jennett B, Teasdale G, Braakman R, et al: Prediction of outcomes in individual patients after severe head injury. Lancet 1:1031–1035, 1976.

87. Jennett B, Teasdale G, Murray G, Murray L: Head injury. In Evans RW, Baskin DS, Yatsu FM (eds): Prognosis of Neurological Disorders. New York, Oxford University Press, 1992.

88. Jennett B, Teasdale G: Management of Head Injuries. Philadelphia, F.A. Davis, 1981.

89. Johnston MV: Cost-benefit methodologies in rehabilitation. In Fuhrer M (ed): Rehabilitation Outcomes: Analysis and Measurement. Baltimore, Brooks, 1987.

90. Johnston MV: The economics of brain injury. In Miner ME, Wagner K (eds): Neurotrauma, No. 3. Boston, Butterworth, 1989.

91. Johnston MV, Cervelli L: Systematic care for persons with head injury. In Bach-y-Rita P (ed): Traumatic Brain Injury. New York, Demos, 1989, pp 203–219.

92. Johnston MV, Lewis FD: The outcomes of community re-entry programs for brain injury survivors. Part 1: Independent living and productive activities. Brain Inj 5(2):141–154, 1991.

93. Johnston MV: The outcomes of community re-entry programs for brain injury survivors. Part 2: Further investigations. Brain Inj 5(2):155– 168.

94. Johnston MV, Findley TW, DeLuca J, Katz RT: Research in physical medicine and rehabilitation. XII: Measurement tools with application to brain injury. Am J Phys Med Rehabil 70(1):40– 56, 1991.

95. Johnston MJ, Wilkerson DL: Program evaluation and quality improvement systems in brain injury rehabilitation. J Head Trauma Rehabil 7(4):68–82, 1992.

96. Johnston MV, Keith RA, Hinderer S: Measurement Standards for Interdisciplinary Medical Rehabilitation. Arch Phys Med Rehabil 73(Suppl):S6–S23, 1992.

97. Johnston MV, Wilkerson DL, Maney M: Evaluation of the quality and outcomes of medical rehabilitation programs. In DeLisa J, et al (eds): Rehabilitation Medicine: Principles and Practice. Philadelphia, J.B. Lippincott, 1993.

98. Johnstone AJ, Lohlun JC, Miller JD, et al: A comparison of the Glasgow Coma Scale and the Swedish Reaction Level Scale. Brain Inj 7:501–506, 1993.

99. Karoly P (ed): Measurement Strategies in Health Psychology. New York, Wiley, 1985.

100. Katz RT, Rovai GP, Brait C, Rymer WZ: Objective quantification of spastic hypertonia: Correlation with clinical findings. Arch Phys Med Rehabil 73:339–347, 1992.

101. Kiernan RJ, Mulller J, Langston JW, Van Dyke C: The neurobehavioral cognitive status examination: A brief but differentiated approach to cognitive assessment. Ann Intern Med 197:481–485, 1987.

102. Keenan JE: Assessment tools for severely head-injured adults. Cognit Rehabil 7(2):24–26, 1989.

103. Kreutzer JS, Leninger B, Doherty K, Waaland P: General Health and History Questionnaire: Richmond, VA, Rehabilitation Research and Training Center on Severe Traumatic Brain Injury, Medical College of Virginia, 1987.

104. Kreutzer JS, Marwitz JH, Kepler K: Traumatic brain injury: Family response and outcome. Arch Phys Med Rehabil 73:771–778, 1992.

105. Kreutzer JS, Gordon WA, Rosenthal M, Marwitz J: Neuropsychological characteristics of patients with brain injury: Preliminary findings from a multicenter investigation. J Head Trauma Rehabil 8(2):47–59, 1993.

106. Lawton MP, Moss M, Fulcomer M, Kleban MH: A research and service oriented multilevel assessment instrument. J Gerontol 37:91, 1982.

107. Lehmkuhl LD: Brain Injury Glossary. Houston, HDI Publishers, 1993.

108. Lehmkuhl LD, Hall KM, Mann N, Gordon WA: Factors that influence costs and length of stay of persons with traumatic brain injury in acute care and inpatient rehabilitation. J Head Trauma Rehabil 8(2):88–100, 1993.

109. Levin HS, O'Donnell VM, Grossman RG: The Galveston Orientation and Amnesia Test: A practiced scale to assess cognition after head injury. J Nerv Ment Dis 167:675–684, 1979.

110. Levin HS, Grafman J, Eisenberg HM: Neurobehavioral Recovery from Head Injury. New York, Oxford University Press, 1987.

111. Levin HS, et al: The neurobehavioral rating scale: Assessment of the behavioral sequelae of head injury by the clinician. J Neurol Neurosurg Psychiatry 50:183–193, 1987.

112. Lezak MD: Neuropsychological Assessment, 2nd ed. New York, Oxford University Press, 1983.

113. Leak MD: Relationship between personality disorders, social disturbances, and physical disability following traumatic brain injury. J Head Trauma Rehabil 2:57–69, 12987.

114. Linacre JM, Heinemann AW, Wright BD, et al: The structure and stability of the Functional Independence Measure. Arch Phys Med Rehabil 2:57–69, 1987.

115. Little MM, Williams JM, Long CJ: Clinical memory tests and everyday memory. Arch Clin Neuropsychol 1:323–333, 1986.

116. Livingston MG, Livingston HM: The Glasgow Assessment Schedule: Clinical and research assessment of head injury outcome. Int Rehabil Med 7(4):145–149, 1985.

117. Malec JF, Smnigelski JS, DePompolo RW, Thompson JM: Outcome evaluation and prediction in a comprehensive, integrated post-acute outpatient brain injury rehabilitation programme. Brain Inj 7:15–29, 193.

118. Max W, MacKenzie EJ, Rice DP: Head injuries: Cost and consequences. J Head Trauma Rehabil 6(2):76–91, 1991.

119. McDowell I, Newell C: Measuring Health: A Guide to Rating Scales and Questionnaires. New York, Oxford University Press, 1987.

120. McLean A, Dikmen SS, Temkin NR: Psychosocial recovery after head injury. Arch Phys Med Rehabil 74:1041–1046, 1993.

121. Meyers AM: The clinical Swiss army knife: Empirical evidence of the validity of IADL functional status measures. Med Care 30(Suppl): MS96–MS111, 1992.

122. Miller L: Neuropsychology, personality, and substance abuse: Implications for head injury rehabilitation. Cognit Rehabil 7(5):26–31.

123. Mysiw WJ, Corrigan JD, Hunt M, et al: Vocational evaluation of traumatic brain injury patients using the Functional Assessment Inventory. Brain Inj 3(1):27–34, 1989.

124. National Institutes of Health, National Institute of Child Health and Human Development (U.S. Department of Health and Human Services, Public Health Service): Research Plan for the National Center for Medical Rehabilitation Research. NIH Publ. No. 93-3509.Rockville, MD, National Institutes of Health, 1993,

125. National Head Injury Foundation: Professional Council Substance Abuse Task Force White Paper. Southborough, National Head Injury Foundation, 1988.

126. Novack TA, Bennett G, Bergquist TF: Disability Rating Scale scores during recovery from head injury. Poster presentation, AAPM&R/ACRM Conference, Seattle, 1988.

127. Novack TA, Berquist TF, Bennett G, Gouvier WD: Primary caregiver distress following severe head injury. J Head Trauma Rehabil 2:69–77, 1992.

128. Oddy M, Coughlan T, Tyerman A, Jenkins D: Social adjustment after closed head injury: A further follow-up seven years after injury. J Neurol Neurosurg Psychiatry 48:564–568, 1985.

129. Pfeffer RI, Kurosaki TT, Chance JM, et al: Use of the Mental Function Index in older adults: Reliability, validity, and measurement of change over time. Am J Epidemiol 120:922–935, 1984.

130. Porkorny AD, Miller BA, Kaplan HB: The brief MAST: A shortened version of the Michigan Alcoholism Screening Test. Am J Psychiatry 129: 342–345, 1972.

131. Prigatano GP, Klonoff PS: Psychotherapy and neuropsychological assessment after brain injury. J Head Trauma Rehabil 3:45–56, 1968.

132. Prigatano GP: Disturbances of self-awareness of deficit after traumatic brain injury. In Prigatano GP, Schachter DL (eds): Awareness of Deficit after Brain Injury: Clinical and Theoretical Issues. New York, Oxford University Press, 1991, pp 111–126.

133. Rao N, Kilgore KM: Predicting return to work in traumatic brain injury using assessment scales. Arch Phys Med Rehabil 73:911–916, 1992.

134. Rappaport M, Hall KM, Hopkins HK, et al: Disability Rating Scale for severe head trauma: Coma to community. Arch Phys Med Rehabil 51:118–123, 1970.

135. Rappaport M, Herrero-Backe C, Rappaport ML, Winterfield KM: Head injury outcome up to ten years later. Arch Phys Med Rehabil 70:885–892, 1989.

136. Rappaport M, Dougherty AM, Keltring DL: Evaluation of coma and vegetative states. Arch Phys Med Rehabil 73:628–634, 1992.

137. Rinel R, Giordani B, Barth J, Jave J: Moderate head injury: Completing the clinical spectrum of brain trauma. Neurosurgery 11:344–351, 1982.

138. Rocca B, Martin C, Vivland K, et al: Comparison of four severity scores in patients with head trauma. J Trauma 29:299–305, 1989.

139. Rosen A, Hadzi-Pavlovic D, Parker G: The life skills profile: A measure assessing function and disability in schizophrenia. Schizophr Bull 15:325–337, 1989.

140. Rosenthal M, Millis S: Relating neuropsychological indicators to psychosocial outcome after traumatic brain injury. NeuroRehabilitation 2(4):1–8, 1992.

141. Sarno MT: The Functional Communication Profile: Manual of Directions. New York, New York University Medical Center, Institute of Rehabilitation Medicine, 1969.

142. Sarno MT, Levita E: Some observations on the nature of recovery in global aphasia. Brain Lang 13:1–12, 1981.

143. Sarno MT (ed): Acquired Aphasia. New York, Academic Press, 1981.

144. Sarno MT: Functional measurement in verbal impairment secondary to brain damage. In Granger CV, Gresham G (eds): Functional Assessment in Rehabilitation Medicine. Baltimore, Williams & Wilkins, 1984, pp 210–222.

145. Reference deleted.

146. Selzer ML: The Michigan Alcoholism Screening Test: The quest for a new diagnostic instrument. Am J Psychiatry 127:1653_1658, 1971.

147. Silverstein B, Kilgore KM, Fisher WP, et al: Applying psychometric criteria to functional assessment in medical rehabilitation. I: Exploring unidimensionality. Arch Phys Med Rehabil 72: 631–637, 1991.

148. Silverstein B, Fisher KM, Kilgore KM, et al: Applying psychometric criteria to functional assessment in medical rehabilitation. III: Defining interval measures. Arch Phys Med Rehabil 73:507–518, 1992.

149. Smith RM, Fields FR, et al: Functional scale of recovery from severe head trauma. Clin Neuropsychol 1:48–50, 1979.

150. Sohlberg MM, Mateer C: Effectiveness of an attention training program. J Clin Exp Neuropsychol 9:117–130, 1987.

151. Spector WD, Katz S, Murphy JB, et al: The hierarchical relationship between activities of daily living and instrumental activities of daily living. J Chronic Dis 40:481, 1987.

152. Spector WD: Functional disability scales. In Spilker B (ed): Quality of Life Assessments in Clinical Trials. New York, Raven, 1990, pp 115–129.

153. Spilker B (ed): Quality of Life Assessments in Clinical Trials. New York, Raven, 1990.

154. Spittler JF, Langenstein H, Calabrese P: Die quantifizierung krankhafter bewusstseinsstörungen: Gütekritierien, Zwecke, handlichkeit. [Quantifying pathological disorders of consciousness. Reliability, aims, feasibility.] Anasthesiol Intensivmed Notfallmed Schmerzther 28(4):213– 221, 1993.

155. Spivack G, Spettell CM, Ellis DW, Ross SE: Effects of intensity of treatment and length of stay on rehabilitation outcomes. Brain Inj 6:419–434, 1992.

156. Stewart AL, Ware JE Jr (eds): Measuring Functioning and Well-being. Durham, NC, Duke University Press, 1992.

157. Strub RL, Black FW: The Mental Status Examination in Neurology, 3rd ed. Philadelphia, F.A. Davis, 1993.

158. Stuss DT, Benson DF: The Frontal Lobes. New York, Raven Press, 1986.

159. Stuss DT, Buckle L: Traumatic brain injury: Neuropsychological deficits and evaluation at different stages of recovery and in different pathologic subtypes. J Head Trauma Rehabil 7(2):40–49, 1992.

160. Tankle RS: Application of neuropsychological test results to interdisciplinary cognitive rehabilitation with head-injured adults. J Head Trauma Rehabil 3:24–32, 1988.

161. Teasdale G, Knill-Jones R, Van der Sande J: Observer variability in assessing impaired consciousness and coma. J Neurol Neurosurg Psychiatry 41:603–610, 1978.

162. Timmons M, Gasquoine L, Scibak JW: Functional changes with rehabilitation of very severe traumatic brain injury survivors. J Head Trauma Rehabil 2(3):64–73, 1987.

163. Toglia JT: Approaches to cognitive assessment of the brain-injured adult: Traditional methods and dynamic investigation. Occup Ther Pract 1:36–57, 1989.

164. Tupper D, Cicerone KM (eds): The Neuropsychology of Everyday Life. Boston, Kluwer Academic, 1990.

165. Truelle JL, Brooks DN, Zomeran AD, et al: A European head injury evaluation chart. Scand J Rehabil Med Suppl 26:115–125, 1992.

166. Udin-Aronow H: Rehabilitation effectiveness with severe brain injury: Translating research into policy. J Head Trauma Rehabil 2:224–236, 1987.

167. Wade DT: Measurement in Neurological Rehabilitation. New York, Oxford University Press, 1992.

168. Wallace CJ: Functional assessment in rehabilitation. Schizophr Bull 12:604–630, 1986.

169. Wanlass RL, Reutter SL, Kline AE: Communication among rehabilitation staff: "Mild," "moderate," or "severe" deficits? Arch Phys Med Rehabil 73:477–481, 1992.

170. Wehman P, Kreutzer JS (eds): Vocational Rehabilitation for Persons with Traumatic Brain Injury. Rockville, MD, Aspen, 1990.

171. Wehman P, Kreutzer J, West M, et al: Employment outcomes of persons following traumatic brain injury: Pre-injury, post-injury, and supported employment. Brain Inj 3:397–412, 1989.

172. Whiteneck G, et al: Quantifying handicap: A new measure of long-term rehabilitation outcomes. Arch Phys Med Rehabil 73:519–526, 1992.

173. Whiteneck GG: Outcome evaluation and spinal cord injury. NeuroRehabilitation 2(4):31–41, 1992.

174. Whyte J: Towards a methodology for rehabilitation research. Am J Phys Med Rehabil (in press).

175. Willer B, Rosenthal M, Kreutzer JS, et al: Assessment of community integration following traumatic brain injury. J Head Trauma Rehabil 8(2):75–87, 1993.

176. Willer B, Ottenbacher KJ, Coad ML: The community integration questionnaire: A comparative examination. Am J Phys Med Rehabil 1994 (in press).

177. Williams JM, Klein K, Little M, Haban G: Family observations of everyday cognitive impairment in dementia. Arch Clin Neuropsychol 1:103–109, 1986.

178. Wilson BA: Long-term prognosis of patients with severe memory disorders. Neuropsychol Rehabil 1:117–134, 1991.

179. Wilson B, Cockburn J, Baddeley A: Assessment of everyday memory functioning following severe brain injury. In Miner ME, Wagner K (eds): Neurotrauma, No. 3. Boston, Buttersworth, 1989, pp 83–89.

180. World Health Organization: International Classification of Impairments, Disabilities, and Handicaps. Geneva, World Health Organization, 1980.

181. Wright BC, Linacre JM: Rasch Analysis BIGSTEPS version 2.26. Chicago, MESA Psychometric Laboratory, University of Chicago, 1992.

182. Yorkston K, Beukelman D: Assessment of Intelligibility of Dysarthric Speech. Tigard, OR, C.C. Publications, 1981.

183. Zung B, Charalampous K: Item analysis of the Michigan Alcoholism Screening Test. J Study Alcohol 40:502–504, 1979.

LOUIS E. PENROD M.D.

9
Medicolegal Aspects
of Traumatic Brain Injury

Traumatic brain injury almost certainly alters an individual's function within society, at least transiently, and thus results in critical interactions between medical management and the individual's legal status. The exact legal precedents and procedures to be followed are not clear in many cases; both theory and case law are rapidly evolving from a limited state of development. A new decision in case law could alter drastically the standards of practice, even in jurisdictions outside the one in which the case was heard. Therefore, this chapter focuses more on the current status of theory to give the practitioner a basis for action, especially when theory may be the only guideline. The practitioner must seek legal advice about local application of theory. First, however, the practitioner should perform an analysis of the case to permit efficient management of difficult medicolegal problems.

The most critical question is a determination of the individual's ability to act autonomously in a competent manner. This general topic is pivotal in determining whether an individual can participate in treatment decisions that range from taking the next dose of medication to continuance of life-prolonging technology. The reasons that an individual

may or may not be capable of decision making range from an obvious medical condition (e.g., coma) to subtle legal questions (e.g., do statements made socially by the individual bear enough weight to withdraw life-prolonging measures). The first part of the chapter explores the basic concepts of autonomy and mental competency and suggests how these concepts may be integrated into physiatric practice. This discussion should provide the practitioner with a basis for action when confronted with difficult questions about competency, guardianship, consent to treatment, and proxy decision making.

Another important medicolegal aspect is how the physiatrist interacts with the legal system. Medical training usually does not address this issue well, if at all. The discrepancies between basic fundamentals of scientific and legal thought are a serious pitfall that may compromise the practitioner's integrity or credibility. An additional complication is the fact that the applicable case law governing expert witness testimony continues to evolve. Health care reform also will affect the physician's role in the legal arena. The second part of the chapter explores the differences between legal and scientific thought and the development of case law and regulations governing expert witness testimony. Such background provides the basis for the formal set of "Guidelines for Expert Witness Testimony" adopted by the American Academy of Physical Medicine and Rehabilitation. The second part of the chapter concludes with practical information intended to guide the practitioner.

TRAUMATIC BRAIN INJURY AND INDIVIDUAL RIGHTS

Medical Ethics Framework

The key question for the practitioner confronted with a new case of traumatic brain injury is the proper relationship of the physician to the patient. In formulating the initial rehabilitation plan, the practitioner must decide whether the patient can participate in decisions pertaining to case management. The many facets of this question revolve around the central issue of whether or not the patient is autonomous. The extent to which this issue is addressed explicitly may vary greatly as a function of the practitioner as well as the specifics of the case. In some cases, the proper course of action may not be clear even to a well-informed and proficient practitioner. Whatever action is chosen should be based on principles as clear as those that govern the selection of a particular pharmacologic agent. Such ethical principles provide a framework for thought and action. The subject of autonomy as a basic principle of medical ethics has a central role in this analysis. In general, the framework of medical ethics presented in this chapter follows that defined by Beauchamp and Childress in *Principles of Biomedical Ethics*.[6] This standard text of biomedical ethics provides much of the basis for currently accepted thought about autonomy, competency, and proxy decision making. Furthermore, Beauchamp and Childress provide practical advice for resolving conflicts between the basic principles of medical ethics in particular cases.

In general, the development of ethical theory has followed one of two basic assumptions. The oldest tradition in Western thought is known as deontology, which attributes intrinsic values to persons or actions. Such intrinsic values rather than the potential outcome(s) are the basis of making ethical decisions. In contrast to deontology, the consequentialist theories are more concerned with outcome than with intrinsic values at the foundation of the decision. Consequentialist thought is best known in the form of utilitarianism, which seeks to maximize the utility that results from a decision. The intrinsic value of a person or principle is weighed against the outcome and may be sacrificed to maximize overall utility. Often utilitarianism is summarized by the statement that the end justifies the means, but this summary is an oversimplification. Utilitarianism does not deny the existence of intrinsic values; instead, it attempts to provide an explicit framework for balancing these values against outcome. From the consequentialist viewpoint, deontology fails because it does not explicitly address the balances of intrinsic values against outcome, and may lead to unethical outcomes because a basic principle was upheld as supreme. Both deontology and utilitarianism exist as a spectrum of thought with considerable overlap.

Beauchamp and Childress developed a system that is consistent with both major theories and can be applied in a practical fashion. All decisions are based on the four basic principles of **respect for autonomy, nonmaleficence, beneficence,** and **justice**. Each of these principles is held to be binding in a prima facie manner; that is, the decision maker must meet each of these principles. However, in cases involving a conflict between two or more principles, the decision may violate one of the principles to ensure the best outcome. The strength of the system lies in the process to be followed when a principle is violated; the decision maker is forced to address explicitly and minimize the violation while maximizing the outcome. This system also acknowledges that ethical theory and decision making may not be consistent with policy (regulations or laws). Again, the system of counterbalancing basic principles against outcome may help to manage such difficulties. Furthermore, a wide range of ethical problems can be readily analyzed in terms of basic principles, including use of life-support technology, proxy decision making, competency, and justification of research on persons who cannot consent to participate.

The principle of respect for autonomy is an outgrowth of the Western tradition of placing value on the right to self-determination. Central to this principle is the concept that individuals have the ability to act autonomously. Autonomous action requires that the individual acts "(1) intentionally, (2) with understanding, and (3) without controlling influences that determine the action."[6] Any action may vary in the extent to which it is strictly autonomous. An individual may choose to follow a legal or religious tradition rather than some unique course. If the individual understands what the decision entails in a substantial fashion, the decision can be autonomous even if it may appear to have been externally dictated. An individual may also decide to act autonomously with less than perfect understanding. When a contract is signed without reading the fine print, understanding is imperfect. If the individual knows that this is the case, the decision may remain autonomous. This distinction is extremely important in informed consent. Practitioners often struggle with what information is necessary to obtain informed consent. The recent trend toward greater disclosure of information demands a reasonable attempt to impart understanding to the patient. Informed consent does not require total understanding, which would be impossible; patients cannot be expected to grasp completely concepts that the professional with extensive training and experience understands imperfectly. The patient, however, has a right to information to the extent that he or she deems necessary. In some cases the educational process may be legitimately terminated when the patient indicates, "You are the doctor; do what you think is best," whereas other cases may require extensive explanations. The crucial criterion for meeting informed consent is an assurance that the patient has the information that he or she believes is essential to make an autonomous decision. Respect for autonomy obligates the practitioner to create an environment that maximizes the possibility of autonomous action. Once this autonomous decision has been made, the practitioner is then obliged to honor the decision. In the framework of ethics advanced by Beauchamp and Childress, respect for autonomy generally takes precedence over the other three principles. But, as it is only a prima facie principle, in special situations this principle may be violated.[6]

Nonmaleficence is often viewed in the context of the ubiquitous medical maxim, primum non nocere ("first of all, do no harm"). Avoiding harm to the patient is easy to understand when unproved or harmful therapeutic methods are involved. On the other hand, in decisions to withdraw life-supporting technologies, the extent to which the individual may be harmed is not always clear. Beauchamp and Childress discuss the principle of nonmaleficence extensively in the context of withdrawing support, determining quality of life, and proxy decision making (see individual discussions below).

The principle of beneficence obliges the practitioner to act in a manner that advances the interests of patients. This principle is at the core of medical care. Avoiding harm alone, without providing beneficial therapies, is not considered adequate medical practice. Beneficence requires a careful weighing of the potential benefit against the potential risk in deciding to what extent beneficence is an obligation. Providing emergency medical care is usually considered an obligation, even when it may entail some risk or inconvenience to the provider. On the other hand, providing extensive nonemergency care without compensation or at substantial personal risk is not obligatory. Paternalism arises as a complication of beneficence, usually in conflict with respect for autonomy. The physician may feel obliged to pursue a course "for the good of the patient" that involves withholding information. In current practice, this decision would be extremely hard to defend, given the importance placed on autonomy. However, if autonomy is in serious question, as during suicidal depression, paternalistic action may be justified.

The principle of justice requires that all individuals be treated equally to the extent that they are equal. This principle becomes important in medical rehabilitation practice in two aspects. First, all individuals have the right to a reasonable minimum of health care, despite their socially disadvantaged status or limited capacity in some important function. Cases in which this is not possible (e.g., rationing) require a means to ensure equitable distribution of risk and benefit. The second aspect of the principle of justice is the ability to participate in research. To the extent that individuals with TBI cannot autonomously agree to participate, they should be carefully protected. It may be acceptable to select a comatose patient as a research subject, providing the risk is limited and the research is expected to benefit others. When risk becomes substantial, justice demands reasonable certainty that the research will provide direct benefit to the patient.

It is not always possible to meet all of the obligations demanded by the four basic principles. This situation is handled by recognition that the four principles are binding only in a prima facie manner. Infringement may be ethical if the following conditions are met: (1) a realistic possibility of achievement; (2) infringement is judged to be necessary; (3) the necessary infringement is the least infringement possible; and (4) the practitioner seeks to minimize the effects of the infringement.[6] The strength of this system lies in thorough and systematic resolution of conflict. When confronted by a difficult situation, the practitioner may apply the four basic principles, seeking to minimize infringement when it cannot be avoided. By proceeding in an explicit manner, the practitioner has acted ethically even if certain aspects of the action seem ethically unclear.

Competency

Competency is probably the most critical issue in the medicolegal status of the patient with TBI. The term competency is commonly used clinically to indicate the patient's ability to make reasonable decisions. Strictly speaking, the determination of competency is a legal rather than a medical process. Medical judgment determines that the individual appears to have the capacity to make decisions. Proceeding from this medical determination to a subsequent legal determination is not routinely necessary. The need for legal clarification varies with the particulars of the case, both medically and socially. In all cases the practitioner is obliged to determine the extent of the patient's capacity to decide and to project how this capacity is expected to evolve in the context of eventual societal demands. To this extent the clinician determines competency for practical purposes in many if not most cases. At either extreme, competence and incompetence are clinically obvious. The continuum between coma and return to employment presents an unclear and often fluctuating picture of competence. This section explores the general aspects of competency as well as modifications for specific cases; discusses how to proceed from clinical data to legal determinations; and points out limitations to this process.

In American society, individuals are assumed to be generally competent. This assumption allows the individual to make a wide range of decisions independently—from making selections on a dinner menu to planning a mountain-climbing expedition. Society allows this freedom because individuals are expected to be able to assess risk independently and to act rationally. When it appears that an individual is not competent, a legal determination is required to infringe on the individual's rights. Legal determination can be directed at either general competence or a focal area of specific competence. General competence entails the global ability to act on decisions in all aspects of the person's life. Limitations of specific competence may meet the individual's needs more exactly, especially in patients with TBI. The patient may be competent to live independently but not to manage financial affairs. The exact process or guidelines used in a specific jurisdiction vary greatly. Governing statutes are usually vague and allow the judge great latitude in determining what is required for determination of competence in a particular case.

Many methods have been proposed to establish clinically whether or not an individual is competent. The "sliding scale" approach, in which the nature of the decision and its possible outcome determine the rigor of the criteria for competence, has received much attention.[15] This approach is used implicitly in many cases of decision making by or for a patient with questionable competency, although the subjectivity of interpreting the patient's wishes and the risks associated with specific outcomes make it problematic.

Appelbaum and Gutheil[3] proposed standards of competency to guide clinical investigations for both general and specific cases.

Although they are concerned specifically with mental illness, their system appears to be applicable to TBI. Establishing general competence involves clinical investigation to ensure that the individual has (1) an awareness of the situation; (2) a factual understanding of the issues; (3) an appreciation of the likely consequences of any decision; (4) the ability to rationally manipulate information; (5) an ability to function in one's own environment; and (6) an ability to meet the imposed demands. Data about most of these criteria are readily available to the rehabilitation team.

The task remaining to the physician is a compilation of the facts of the particular case. Typically the team is aware of the need to meet the particular environmental and social needs of the patient. For the purpose of a legal determination with serious consequences, it may be necessary to observe individual performance over time in the relevant environment. Evaluations of functional performance, which are familiar to rehabilitation teams, may be of more relevance to competency than more formalized testing.[38] Use of specific mental status tests to predict the capacity for self-care has been questioned.[50] The commonly used Folstein Mini-Mental Status Examination is sensitive to both age and educational level and thus may give either falsely elevated or falsely depressed scores compared with an individual's daily functional performance.[12] Evidence also suggests that a multidisciplinary competency panel often rates as competent individuals whom formalized tests rate as impaired.[43] By virtue of training and experience the rehabilitation team should be able to provide the interpretation of the "cold facts" necessary to determine whether an individual is competent.

For an individual with TBI, the question may focus more on specific than general competence. The individual may be restricted in specific ways but capable of autonomy in a more general manner. For example, informed consent to a risky medical procedure or management of finances may be curtailed, although the individual may be permitted to live independently otherwise. Appelbaum and Gutheil propose that specific competence requires (1) communication of a choice; (2) factual understanding of the issues; (3)

appreciation of the situation and its consequences; and (4) rational manipulation of information. On a superficial level, these criteria appear to parallel those for general competence, but they are qualitatively distinct in that they are applied focally and with somewhat less rigor. For example, the communication of a choice may entail only that a choice has been made and communicated. Yet the choice must have a degree of stability to ensure that it can be implemented. This is often a problem in patients recovering from TBI, whose mental status may fluctuate. The ability to manipulate information rationally also requires interpretation. The cognitive process must involve a reasonable analysis of the situation and its possible consequences, but the end result (or decision) is not required to be "rational" by the standards of the evaluator.

On a practical basis clinicians frequently make decisions about competence and manage the case on the basis of that determination. In the postinjury period the physician, in agreement with the family, typically makes substantial decisions on behalf of the patient. Considering that many therapeutic interventions (e.g., surgery, psychoactive or anticoagulant drugs) may be associated with serious and permanent risks, this practice raises difficult ethical and legal questions. Strictly speaking, the potential for abuse of the individual's rights is significant. On the other hand, in almost all cases this process appears to work well in protecting the individual's interests by promoting recovery. Submitting all cases to legal review would produce extensive delays in provision of care with little benefit in protection of the individual. This informal system of assessing competence has been supported by the President's Commission on Ethical Problems in Medicine and Biomedical and Behavioral Research.[39] The system of biomedical ethics outlined above should assist the practitioner in developing a justified approach to such problems. The principle of respect for autonomy demands that the practitioner make every reasonable attempt to establish autonomy on the part of the patient. However, if the patient is not capable of autonomy, the other principles will guide an ethical course of action. Deciding for the patient infringes on autonomy. Ensuring that the decision minimizes harm (nonmaleficence), maximizes potential benefits (beneficence), and does not subject the patient to unreasonable risks in light of potential benefit (justice) follows Beauchamp and Childress's procedure for resolving conflicts in meeting the obligations of the basic principles.

Proceeding from informal assessment to legal determination of competence should be an extension of the functioning of a well-run rehabilitation team. Critical to the process is a systematic evaluation and documentation of the patient's behavior. The patient's level of participation and interaction is a basis for therapeutic decisions such as use of medications for restlessness and agitation. As detailed elsewhere in this book, the use of such medications should entail objective measures to ensure that the desired effect is achieved. Such data also may be used to demonstrate impaired or fluctuating mental status in a legal determination. High-quality neuropsychological assessments are particularly valuable in guiding decisions about competence. A psychosocial evaluation of the family dynamics also may be a determining factor in how an individual case is handled. In the patient who has an intact family structure with a reasonably intelligent and caring spouse and who is expected to recover substantially, only informal mechanisms of decision making are needed. If, however, the patient is a young single adult with adversarial divorced parents and the prospect of significant residual impairment, a legal determination becomes essential. The formal decision allows the rehabilitation team to function effectively, because decision making on behalf of the individual is legally clarified. The team attempts to explain to the family the issues of proxy decision making from both a practical and legal viewpoint. The family then uses its judgment about how to proceed. Formal documentation of the family-team discussion should be included in the chart. In extreme cases, the team may choose to exercise the right to petition directly for a competency determination. This step should be taken with the assistance of the hospital's legal staff and possibly also a formal ethics committee.

The clinician must be aware of and seek to minimize the limitations of competency determinations. Probably the most significant is an inappropriate finding of incompetence. Despite the recent emphasis on specific rather than global incompetence, it is not clear that the courts are applying the concept of limited incompetence. It is easier to judge the individual to be generally incompetent than to expend the time and effort to delineate specific areas of competence and incompetence. For patients with TBI, this outcome may be particularly problematic, because some abilities may remain intact, whereas others may be devastated. The rehabilitation team must provide clearly understood information about specific abilities and impairments to the legal professionals trying the question of competence. On the other hand, the existence of specific deficits in a generally intact individual may be missed by superficial assessment. Again, carefully collected performance data from various settings can minimize the problem.

Many jurisdictions do not require that the individual assessed for competence be informed of the proceedings. Although this approach seems to be contrary to the spirit of rehabilitation, it has occurred within the mental health setting, where the desire to restore the patient to a high level of function is as honest as in rehabilitation. Certainly, the comatose individual has no capacity to understand the importance of a competency determination. On the other hand, the patient with limited capacity during recovery from TBI has an unclear ability to understand such issues. The team should err on the side of attempting to impart understanding to the patient.

Another pitfall in determination of probable competence is the influence of congruence between the stated wishes of the patient and the treating clinician(s). If the recommendations of the team are followed by the patient or family, the question of competence is easy to ignore. On the other hand, if disagreement over how to proceed arises, issues of competence are more likely to be raised. Finally, a determination of incompetence in patients with TBI may have long-reaching implications as recovery proceeds. Reversal of the decision varies from one jurisdiction to another. Routine follow-up should specifically address the area(s) of incompetence and determine whether the initial decision should be reversed.

Guardianship

The concept of guardianship, which dates from the founding of the Roman Empire, was intended initially to protect individual property rather than the individual herself or himself. As the concept developed through history, guardianship was extended from cases of physical incapacity, mental retardation, or minor status to include other cases such as mental illness. Recently the concept evolved to include protection of the individual as well as the individual's property, and the guardian was granted the authority to decide issues such as consent to treatment and living conditions as well as disposition of finances. As stated above, the most recent change has been the consideration of specific incompetence, which restricts the powers of a guardian to narrower bounds. In addition, the consequences to the ward of a particular action or decision by the guardian may be considered in delimiting the guardian's authority. For example, in some cases the ward retains the power to make a will but not to handle daily finances or to enter into contracts. Because the will has little impact on the deceased ward, it is scrutinized less closely than a contract that may lead to financial ruin of the living ward.[3]

The implications of a determination of incompetency vary with the particulars of the case. For an individual in a persistent vegetative state who is otherwise medically stable, the judgment of incompetence has little impact on autonomy or self-esteem. On the other hand, for an individual in the process of recovery or with a significant degree of independent function, the finding of incompetence has a wide range of effects. The necessity of deferring to the decisions of the guardian may undermine the level of independence that has been achieved. Alternatively, if the ward is relieved of the task of managing finances, which may entail significant risk of failure, the ward is free to concentrate on tasks and decisions that can be successfully managed. With the appointment of a guardian, the rehabilitation team has a clearly delineated mechanism for reaching decisions on behalf of the patient. Furthermore, the guardian's formal charge with decision-making authority entails the responsibility of ensuring that all decisions are in the best interest of the ward. Particularly in the case of financial matters, the court typically establishes a formal reporting mechanism to ensure that the guardian is adequately discharging his or her responsibilities. If someone believes otherwise, the court may be petitioned to review the situation and to hold the guardian accountable for any unacceptable actions.

Characteristics of the ideal guardian, as suggested by Appelbaum and Gutheil,[3] include availability, competence, empathic intuition, freedom from conflict of interest, willingness to serve, and availability of adequate remuneration and protection from liability. Such characteristics are intended to ensure that the interests of the ward are likely to be protected. In the setting of mental health, the ward often has limited family and financial resources. For this reason, Appelbaum and Gutheil argue forcefully for a system of professional guardians to serve the best interests of their wards. Although the situation for patients with TBI is likely to be different from that of persons with chronic mental illness, most of the above criteria also have validity in TBI.

Availability is important, because at times clinical decisions must be made rapidly, without regard to holidays, weekends, or vacations. Competence may seem self-evident, but the effort must be made to educate the guardian about relevant issues so that decisions are well founded. Empathic intuition refers to the guardian's ability to make decisions that reflect the likely wishes of the incompetent individual. This ability implies that the concept of substituted judgment is followed. The nature of substituted judgment and its limitations are addressed in more detail below.

Freedom from conflict of interest is a particularly difficult criterion. On one hand, although a guardian chosen from the family is more likely to reflect the values of the incompetent individual, decisions reached by the family member are unlikely to be free from conflict of interest. Another problem related to conflict of interest is the struggle between the desire to choose a relatively easy management strategy, such as institutionalization, rather than to deal with the need to reach decisions on behalf of the ward repeatedly or frequently. This problem is ameliorated by the criterion of willingness to serve as a guardian.

The criterion of adequate remuneration and protection from liability is related more to the system of care in which the guardian serves rather than to the guardian per se. This issue is probably not as important in TBI as in mental health, but the truth of this assertion has not been tested. According to Appelbaum and Gutheil, remuneration and protection from liability strongly affect the characteristics of the relationship, and adequacy of both is essential to ensuring that the job of guardianship is taken seriously, with the best interest of the ward in mind. Because individuals with TBI are probably more likely to have intact social supports than those with chronic mental illness, this criterion may not need to be so rigorous, at least in the early postinjury period. On the other hand, in severely incapacitated individuals with a limited support system, it assumes more importance.

Consent to Treatment and Substituted Decision Making

Whether the situation is governed by formal guardianship, previous legal documents such as a durable power of attorney for health care decisions, or an informal arrangement between the family and the rehabilitation team, significant decisions must be made on behalf of the incapacitated individual. Even when the situation has been formalized, the potential for ethical conflict should be kept in mind. This potential conflict arises from the possible discrepancy between what the individual may have decided and the decisions reached on his or her behalf.

At the root of any substituted or proxy decision for an individual who was previously competent must be the principle of respect for autonomy, as outlined in the system of Beauchamp and Childress.[6] The individual has the right to choose what is done to her or his body in the course of receiving health care. This right is paramount, even when the individual's decision is not the decision reached by the caregiver, as long as the decision can be shown to be autonomous. When an individual no longer can be construed as autonomous, a method of proxy decision making is necessary. Because any proxy decision violates the principle of respect for autonomy, this violation must be minimized to the extent possible. The

approach to this problem has evolved through several mechanisms throughout history.

The earliest concept of substituted decision making was that of parens patriae. This concept is based on the belief that some ultimate authority, usually the government, has the power to protect persons under its jurisdiction, as a parent protects a child. This concept fell out of favor because of the obvious conflict between the interests of the state and the interests of the individual. Supplanting the parens patriae concept was an attempt to make judgments in the best interest of the individual. The proxy decision maker attempts to maximize the benefit to the incapacitated person. The unacceptable drawback to this system is the recognition that in fact a proxy is unlikely to understand the best interest of the other person. Especially in the case of a family member, the desires of the decision maker are likely to influence the analysis of what the best decision may be. To overcome this limitation, the concept of substituted judgment was adopted. The proxy decision maker attempts to decide as the incapacitated individual would decide if able. This concept implies that the decision maker has an understanding of the values and beliefs of the person for whom the decision is made. Furthermore, the decision must be made without regard for the interests or values of the proxy. As detailed below, this system has limitations at least as significant as its predecessors.

For a balanced approach, the reader is referred to the method of resolving ethical conflict developed by Beauchamp and Childress.[6] Because the decision maker must violate autonomy and exercise a certain degree of paternalism, the action must be tempered by explicit attention to the principles of nonmaleficence and beneficence. All decisions must minimize potential harm and at the same time attempt to maximize benefit. At first glance, this approach may seem to be a return to the concept of best interest. However, Beauchamp and Childress have proposed a method that combines best interest judgments with substituted judgments, in accordance with the particulars of the case, rather than insists on either approach exclusively. Theirs is a more active analysis within the overall system of medical ethics. Proxy decision making is an exceedingly complex issue for which no rigid approach holds up to careful scrutiny in all situations. This section attempts to provide a framework for action by reviewing pertinent case law, medical ethics literature, and legislative history.

An emergency situation is probably the easiest problem for the clinician to resolve. A true emergency allows no time to seek input from proxy decision makers, either explicitly or implicitly. In patients with TBI, this scenario occurs more often in the acute care phase. On the other hand, rehabilitation may involve situations, such as status epilepticus or elopement from treatment, in which action must be taken immediately. The law allows the clinician to take action without fear of retribution as long as the action is within the guidelines of currently accepted practice. It is assumed that the incapacitated individual has given implied consent.

The decision to withdraw or withhold life support for individuals in a persistent vegetative state is probably the most difficult issue that can arise in proxy decision making. To date, only one professional medical society has published a position paper: the Council on Scientific Affairs and Council on Ethical and Judicial Affairs of the American Medical Association.[11] The paper was reviewed in a report from the Council on Ethical and Judicial Affairs in 1992.[10] Both documents support current ethical thought in holding that it is acceptable either to withdraw or to withhold life support if the patient is in a persistent vegetative state. Also supported is the opinion that artificially supplied nutrition and hydration are medical treatments that can be withdrawn. The physician who objects to such actions is not required to participate, but he or she is expected to transfer the care of the patient to another physician who will follow through with the decision to withdraw support. The first document highlights the variability of the legal situation among states and suggests the involvement of an ethics committee to help to sort through the issues.

A number of important cases have contributed to the development of current legal thought about proxy decision making. Most of these cases are reviewed in the article by Miles and August discussed below.[36] Within the context of brain injury, the most significant cases have involved cessation of life support for individuals in a persistent vegetative state. The two most publicized cases centered on Karen Ann Quinlan and Nancy Cruzan.

Karen Ann Quinlan became vegetative after an apparent drug overdose. Her father, who had been appointed as guardian, eventually sought to have the respirator disconnected. This request was approved by the New Jersey Supreme Court based on the argument that if she were able to express an opinion, she would not want to be kept on life support in her current condition. Of interest, the suit was brought over the objections of her physicians, who believed that withdrawing the respirator would be unethical. Two other factors of this case deserve mention. In the course of the proceedings, the father expressed the opinion that to withdraw nutrition would not be acceptable. In addition, when the respirator was disconnected, Quinlan was able to sustain respiration and did not die immediately as expected.[28]

Nancy Cruzan was vegetative as the result of a TBI sustained in a motor vehicle accident. Her father, who also had been appointed guardian, sought to discontinue artificial nutrition and hydration. The argument that she would not have wanted to be artificially sustained was rejected by the Missouri Supreme Court. The Missouri court held that the state had a parens patriae obligation to protect its citizens unless the individual had indicated otherwise in a "clear and convincing" statement. Because Cruzan had left no written instructions to discontinue life support if she became vegetative, the state insisted that artificial nutrition and hydration be maintained. The case received a large amount of attention, with many special interest groups providing "friend of the court" briefs in an attempt to sway the decision. The United States Supreme Court eventually upheld the Cruzan decision, on the basis that each state had the right to decide the necessary criteria to reach a decision to terminate life support.[13]

The Cruzan decision has aroused much controversy. The State of Missouri has adopted a "clear and convincing" standard by requiring an indication from the individual that she or he would not want to be maintained on artificial life support in "hopeless" situations. Furthermore, in written support of this decision, the state has taken the position that an individual by definition cannot make an informed refusal of treatment in advance. This position effectively blocks able-bodied, mentally competent individuals from successfully requesting withdrawal of artificial nutrition and hydration if they should become persistently vegetative. The severity of this standard has been decried, but some authors believe that the U.S. Supreme Court expects additional cases to delineate further the range of acceptable procedure, with eventual adoption of a less rigorous standard.[42]

Several important points can be drawn from the two cases. First, decisions involving such a momentous outcome as expected death may expand to involve many persons and groups that have no relationship to any of the original parties. A means of anticipating and dealing with this potential is important. Explicit formal discussion of the particulars of a case is the first step. However, when a team member is at odds with the group as a whole, she or he may choose to involve outside parties rather than face opposition alone. Secondly, although ethical thought has evolved to the position that withdrawal of a life-sustaining intervention is equivalent to not beginning the intervention and that all interventions are equivalent (whether ventilators or feeding tubes), this view is not necessarily supported by the population at large, special interest groups, or the legal system. Existing legal decisions, strictly speaking, apply only within the jurisdiction in which they were reached. Typically a court takes decisions from other jurisdictions into consideration but is under no obligation to do so. Thus, following a precedent from another jurisdiction is not necessarily safe. Finally, once the decision has been made and the action carried out, the outcome may be much different from what was anticipated, as in the Quinlan case.[31] For this reason, the existence of a formal mechanism for ongoing discussion and guidance, such as an ethics committee, is essential.[22]

The selection of a proxy decision maker may occur without the appointment of a guardian. The following qualifications have been suggested by Beauchamp and Childress: (1) ability to make reasoned judgments (competence), (2) adequate knowledge and information, (3) emotional stability, and (4) a commitment to the incompetent patient's interests that is free of conflicts of interest and free of controlling influence by others who may not seek the patient's best interest.[6] These criteria are similar to those proposed by Appelbaum and Gutheil for the ideal guardian. Of note, Beauchamp and Childress do not expect the proxy to be impartial. Instead, the proxy must actively work to secure the best interests of the incompetent individual and resist all influences that may conflict with this best interest, such as the emotional or financial interests of family members.

Two issues related to substituted decision making are disturbing: (1) uncertainty about its conceptual validity and (2) evidence of a substantial gender bias in applying the concept. For the concept to have validity, the proxy must have sufficient information on which to base a decision. Few individuals have detailed their views with enough precision and thoroughness to cover all eventualities. Even if prior discussions and/or written instructions exist, a certain amount of interpretation or extrapolation probably will be necessary for application to the immediate situation. In addition, most relevant discussions take place with a spouse, close family member, or friend, none of whom is likely to be free of conflict of interest in recalling and applying the information. Furthermore, certain deeply held values or beliefs may have been too personal to share. As a result, the proxy makes decisions consistent with his or her values rather than the values of the incompetent individual. Several studies have found a frequent and significant discrepancy between the choices of the proxy and what the individual would choose.[16,44,51] An additional problem is the assumption that the values or opinions of an able-bodied and cognitively intact individual have relevance after physical and cognitive compromise.[40] Judgments on the value of a particular state of existence may be relevant only after that state has been experienced. Therefore, previously expressed wishes may be no longer valid. The proxy may then fall back to a best-interest judgment, but, because the proxy cannot experience the altered state of the incompetent person, the validity of any judgment can be legitimately questioned.

The evidence of significant gender bias in applying substituted judgment is also disturbing. This topic was explored by Miles and August in a review of appellate-level decisions about "the right to die."[36] The review analyzes the legal thought involved in 22 decisions concerning 8 men and 14 women in a total of 14 states. Evidence of the incompetent person's previously expressed opinion ranged from none to extensive discussions with close family members over a period of years and formal advance directive documents. The authors found an apparently systematic difference in how the cases were resolved, depending on the sex of the incompetent individual. Any opinion expressed by the man, no matter in what context, was held to be the result of careful analysis and thus was likely to be honored in constructing a substituted decision. On the other hand, the prior opinions of women typically were held to be an emotional response and were ignored in drafting the decision. This bias occurred even with an advance directive or designation of durable power of attorney for health care decisions. In effect, the court decisions valued the autonomy of the men but disregarded the autonomy of the women. Of note, the Cruzan decision was cited by Miles and August as an example of gender bias. The Missouri State Supreme Court ordered continuation of life support over her family's objections and a construction of her views about life support.

Given the limitations of proxy decision making and the sometime capricious, always expensive results of legal cases, as well as the delays involved, several attempts have been made to clarify the legislative background so that most decisions can be made without resorting to litigation. The Patient Self-Determination Act of 1990 is the only federal legislation that addresses the need for written advance directives. This law has had a major impact to the extent that all individuals admitted to the hospital are now presented with information about advance directives and encouraged to draw up their own. However, little evidence indicates that the legislation has affected the frequency with which individuals actually complete this process.[30] Moreover, some evidence suggests that treating physicians are often unaware of the existence or intent of an advance directive completed by the patients under their care.[49] The patient would have to be alert and mentally competent to accomplish this task. It is almost certain that the Patient Self-Determination Act will have no impact on clarifying the decision-making process for patients with TBI.

The problem also has been addressed through legislation that provides for the statutory appointment of a surrogate decision maker when an advance directive does not exist. The guidelines adopted vary greatly by state. To date, only a minority of states have addressed the issue, despite evidence that the majority of the population favors an approach that prevents sustaining life through artificial means.[17,20]

The Health Care Surrogate Act of Illinois, signed into law in 1991, is an example of a statutory means of appointing a surrogate without resorting to a court proceeding. The act applies to individuals who have not executed a living will or a durable power of attorney for health care or whose clinical condition is not covered by advance directives. The initial step required by law is a determination that the individual meets one of three "qualifying conditions":

1. A "terminal condition," defined as irreversible illness and imminent death. However, the meaning of "imminent" is not clarified.

2. A state of "permanent unconsciousness" in which "initiating or continuing life-sustaining treatment, in light of the patient's medical condition, provides only minimal medical benefit." This condition is clearly applicable to individuals in a persistent vegetative state.

3. An "incurable or irreversible" condition that will "ultimately" cause death, even with life-sustaining treatment. The condition must cause "severe pain or otherwise impose an inhumane burden on the patient." It is unclear what injuries or diseases may fall under this category; apparently physicians were meant to have some discretion in dealing with situations such as severe neurologic damage due to hypoxia that does not strictly meet the criteria for persistent vegetative state.

An interesting aspect of the Illinois law is that the attending physician, along with a second physician, has the responsibility of determining whether one of the three qualifying conditions is met. If so, the physician then must determine through "reasonable inquiry" whether a surrogate decision maker is available. The following order of priority is specified: legal guardian; spouse; adult son or daughter; parent; adult brother or sister; adult grandchild; close friend; and guardian of the person's estate. Only when all of these possibilities have been exhausted is it necessary to resort to court action. Of note, the standing given to a close friend is unusual in such legislation. The surrogate is expected to make a decision, in consultation with the physician, on the basis of what the individual would have wanted under the circumstances. If no prior indication has been made, then a best-interest course of action is taken. If objections to a chosen course of action are raised, it is still possible to initiate formal guardianship proceedings. Health care providers acting in accordance with a surrogate's decision are protected from liability. A quirk of the law is that decisions are limited to withdrawing life support; the surrogate does not have the authority to make other, less significant, health care decisions.[45]

In the state of New York, a Task Force on Life and the Law was appointed by Governor Cuomo in 1985 to address various issues related to the provision or withholding of care. The 1992 report, entitled *When Others Must Choose: Deciding for Patients Without Capacity*, recommends various methods of reaching proxy decisions for patients who cannot decide for themselves and who have not appointed a surrogate decision maker.[47] The recommendations of the Task Force are similar to the provisions of the Illinois law, although the proxy is empowered with the ability to make all decisions. If no surrogate is identified, the treating physician is given broad decision-making powers; requirements for review by peers or an ethics board depend on the nature of the decisions. Although the final form of any legislation is uncertain, previous recommendations of the Task Force about life-sustaining treatment and do-not-resuscitate orders were adopted with little modification.[37]

The Rehabilitation Team and Ethical Conflict

For practical purposes, the problem becomes how to translate theory into action when decisions about patient management must be made. Banja advocates transforming the TBI team into a functioning ethics committee,[5] arguing that the team is used to dealing with difficult decisions and also has the most expertise in analyzing relevant issues. In the present author's opinion, this proposal involves two major problems:

1. The TBI team is unlikely to possess sufficient background in ethics to deal with all potential problems. Through an educational effort, of course, this shortcoming may be overcome. On the other hand, focusing the education of the team on the rapidly evolving aspects of TBI care is of much greater importance to the welfare of the patient.

2. Unavoidable conflicts of interest occur when the team responsible for patient management attempts to function as an ethics committee. Although the ethical issues of team function and patient management are legitimate topics for the team to tackle, emotional attachment to the patient develops even within the bounds of professional conduct and raises doubt that serious life-and-death decisions can be made with sufficient detachment.

It would be a more acceptable alternative to involve an institutional ethics committee that has neither limitation. This team should be familiar with the concepts of biomedical ethics so that their approach to patient management is ethically as well as scientifically acceptable. Beauchamp and Childress's approach is a workable and understandable framework for taking action in an ethically acceptable manner.

This recommendation presupposes that an institutional Ethics Committee exists. For most large hospitals, this is the case. The committee usually consists of members with a variety of backgrounds, including an attorney and a member from the lay community as well as health care providers of several descriptions (physicians, nurses, therapists, and/or social workers). This broad representation is intended to provide the opportunity for the discussion of various viewpoints. For freestanding rehabilitation programs and nursing homes, such a committee may not exist, and this deficiency should be addressed in some fashion. For example, if the suggestions of the New York Task Force (see above) are enacted, a functioning bioethics review committee is essential. Smaller institutions may cooperate in supporting a common committee.

In any case, the clinician leading the rehabilitation team needs to possess a strong working knowledge of ethical analysis. Even among individuals drawn from ethics committees, divergence of opinion may be considerable. One study surveyed such individuals on the proper action to be taken in a number of scenarios.[19] The results, in general, found little agreement on how each situation should be handled. This study, however, depended on individual answers from the respondents. Perhaps in open discussion the divergence of opinion would be useful for a full exploration of the topic before a consensus is reached. In any case, the recommendations of an ethics committee are only recommendations; they are not a legal judgment. This underlines the importance of ethical understanding on the part of the clinician.

ETHICS OF PROVIDING AN EXPERT OPINION

Expert Witness Testimony and Peer Review

The increasing importance of expert witness testimony over the last decade reflects the increasing frequency of litigation. The probability that a practitioner will serve as an expert witness is high. This section discusses several factors, both technical and ethical, that provide a basis for testifying in an ethical and professional manner. Peer review is discussed as an extension of the concepts developed for expert witness testimony.

The problems inherent in the role of the expert witness are addressed succinctly by Brent in an article appropriately entitled, "The Irresponsible Expert Witness: A Failure of Biomedical Graduate Education And Professional Accountability."[12] Brent acknowledges the many factors that the medical profession cannot affect directly, such as the litigation-prone public, the current status of the judicial process, and the control of legislatures and congress by the legal profession. However, he notes several factors that the medical profession can address to improve its performance in the legal area:

1. The "deteriorating image of the physician in the public's mind, making him more likely to be sued;

2. Improper communication with the patient by physicians, nurses, residents, and students;

3. Failure to eliminate incompetent physicians from the practice of medicine; and

4. Inappropriate testimony by expert witnesses."

Brent deals specifically with the fourth factor, pointing to two major problems that contribute to inappropriate expert witness testimony. The first is a "lack of veracity and objectivity," which is complicated by substantial fees. In addition, the ego gratification of being called an "expert" leads some witnesses to lose their objectivity. However, the factor that Brent believes to be most important is the expert's unawareness of his or her proper role in the courtroom. Because of such poor understanding the expert functions as a partisan in the litigation, rather than as a scholar. Brent attributes this lack of understanding to a failure of graduate medical education.

This section attempts to delineate the proper role of an expert witness. As Black pointed out, the legal system must look to expert witnesses to answer

> questions that lie beyond the understanding and knowledge of non-scientists, but at the same time judges without scientific training must determine whether those answers are reliable enough to warrant their use at trial. This need to evaluate expertise while simultaneously depending on it, creates a fundamental tension that permeates and shapes the way in which courts decide the admissibility of scientific evidence.[17]

This dichotomy may be understood more clearly by comparing the different views of causation within the scientific and legal communities. Newtonian physics portrays causation in a quantitative manner: mechanical contacts or collisions between particulate objects follow the physical laws defined by mathematics. By the late nineteenth century, this concept, known as corpuscularianism, was combined with positivism or the belief that scientific knowledge expanded unceasingly. This philosophy emphasizes deductive reasoning and mechanistic interpretations based on a causal chain. Since development of quantum mechanics in the early twentieth century, however, science has depended on inductive reasoning and probabilistic techniques. Although scientists continue to use causal language, they depend primarily on understanding of probabilistic reasoning and statistical analysis to determine causation.[18]

On the other hand, the legal system tends to assume the existence of a clearly delineated causal chain. The procedures in the courtroom attempt to identify what is called a "but for" cause: the event but for which another event would not have occurred. The "but for" cause is not self-evident in every case. For this reason, judges use the notion of proximate cause: the one cause picked from many that can be addressed to enforce specific policy goals of the judicial system. The proximate cause, however, is provided within the context of a causal chain analysis. The proximate cause was rationalized further by Calabresi,[9a] who introduced the concept of the "cheapest cost-avoider."[9a] This approach is a search through the causal chain to determine at what point the cheapest intervention could have prevented the eventual outcome. Quite often proponents of this approach conveniently find that the cheapest cost-avoider is an individual or institution with sufficient means to pay the cost of damages. Thus, the municipality that does not notice the missing stop sign is often responsible for the accident rather than the driver who acted in an inappropriate manner.[26] This approach to truth closely resembles corpuscularianism. When the legal emphasis on deductive causal chain reasoning confronts the scientific emphasis on probabilistic reasoning, a significant amount of confusion necessarily results.[18]

A review of the history of expert witness testimony helps to provide a basis for outlining the ideal role of an expert witness. As Black notes, the general acceptance test for introduction of scientific or medical evidence was established by *Frye v the United States* in 1923.[7] This decision involved a murder case in which the conviction was appealed on the basis that the defendant had passed the systolic blood pressure deception test, a precursor of the polygraph lie detector. The introduction of the blood pressure test into the trial was denied with the following explanation:

Just when a scientific principle or discovery crosses the line between the experimental and demonstrable stages is difficult to define. Somewhere in this twilight zone, the evidential force of the principle must be recognized and while courts will go a long way in admitting expert testimony deduced from a well-recognized scientific principle or discovery, the thing from which the deduction is made must be sufficiently established to have gained general acceptance in the particular field in which it belongs.

Thus, the validity of the reasoning used by an expert witness was not accorded the same importance as the starting principles. This position was eventually superseded by Rule 702 of the *Federal Rules of Evidence*, which addresses the admissibility of expert testimony:

If scientific, technical, or other specialized knowledge will assist the trier of fact to understand the evidence or to determine a fact in issue, a witness qualified as an expert by knowledge, skill, experience, training, or education may testify thereto in the form of an opinion or otherwise.

Therefore, the "expert" needs only to possess "some special knowledge" that would be useful to the litigation. This "special knowledge" is not defined.

The adoption of the *Federal Rules of Evidence* did not clarify the approach to expert witness testimony in a practical sense. Many courts continued to apply the *Frye* rule, with strict adherence to the position that any knowledge or principle must have reached general acceptance. This conservative view led to many judgments that resulted in injustice because a new, and eventually validated, technique was not accepted into evidence. The most celebrated of such cases involved the judgment that the actor Charlie Chaplin must pay support for a child who, according to blood testing, could not be his.[26]

On the other hand, use of too lenient a screen involves the danger that any "expert" promoting unique and unfounded theories may sway judgments, opening the legal arena to decisions with no thread of scientific merit. This danger has been of particular concern in cases of toxic tort litigation. Many instances of such outcomes are detailed by Huber,[26] although he focuses on the litigation arising out of purported birth defects secondary to use of the drug Bendectin for morning sickness. Despite extensive epidemiologic evidence to the contrary, various claims seeking damages for birth defects were brought against Merrill Dow Pharmaceuticals. Most of the cases were dismissed as having no validity. However, in its review of *Daubert v Merrill Dow Pharmaceuticals* in 1993 the United States Supreme Court handed down a landmark decision. The case involved alleged damages brought by two sets of parents on behalf of their respective children, who were born with limb deformities. Their cases rested on the testimony of an expert who claimed that a novel epidemiologic technique showed that the limb deformities may have been caused by the drug. Both a federal trial court and an appeals court refused to hear the case through strict application of the *Frye* rule. The legal question involved whether the *Federal Rules of Evidence* had superseded the guidelines of *Frye* or incorporated their intent.

The Supreme Court returned the case to the lower court, with the instructions that Federal Rule 702 had indeed replaced the guidelines of *Frye*. The court also offered further clarification of when evidence is admissible through expert witness testimony, insisting that the expert's opinion must have "a reliable basis in the knowledge and experience of his discipline." This criterion forces the judge to decide the validity of any testimony to be admitted into evidence. The Supreme Court suggested that the following factors be used in reaching the decision:

1. Is the theory or technique testable, and has it been tested?
2. Has it been subjected to peer review and publication?
3. In the case of a particular scientific technique, what is the known or potential rate of error?
4. What (if any) are the standards that control the technique's operation?
5. To what extent is the theory or technique accepted in the scientific community?

None of the five factors was held to be either a necessary or a sufficient condition in determining the admissibility of testimony. However, whereas the stringent standards of the *Frye* rule were relaxed, the court seemed to affirm that knowledge or techniques are admissible only if they are based on application of the scientific method and subject to further scientific review.

The case received considerable attention; at least 20 friend-of-the-court briefs were submitted.[12] The outcome has been positively received at least in the scientific and medical community.[23,24] However, the ultimate effect of the decision is still not clear. Judges will be placed more frequently in a position of weighing evidence that they do not have the background to understand, with the inherent tension described by Black.[7] Courts may seek their own experts rather than rely on those brought by parties to the suit. This method has been used successfully in other countries, but a previous attempt in the United States was viewed by some as a failure.[27] Until the situation is clarified further, the author recommends adherence to the guidelines for testimony as adopted by professional societies (see below).

Usually more than one expert witness testifies in a given case. Often, their testimony is to some extent in conflict. This further complicates the proceedings, because the judge must sort between various viewpoints that he or she does not understand individually. The decision is often made in a manner that seems capricious to the scientific or medical community. The courts rely on licensure or board certification as evidence of expert status. This interpretation of "expert" is clearly different from that within the profession and to some extent has led to comparison of qualifications in the game of "your expert witness versus mine." Alternatively, the court may give preferential weight to the testimony of the treating physician, who may rely on anecdotal evidence rather than a true understanding of the problem.

It is easy to have a smug attitude when comparing standards within the scientific and legal systems. However, another aspect of expert witness testimony gives cause for reflection. Rule 703 of the *Federal Rules of Evidence* addresses hearsay, which typically is strictly forbidden within the judicial system. However, in the case of the expert witness, hearsay may be admitted into the proceedings.[19] Medical professionals do not appreciate the fact that much of the information on which they base life-and-death decisions would be considered hearsay by the legal profession and, therefore, totally unreliable. Examples would include reports of nurses or therapists about the patient's physiologic or psychological behavior. In cases of rehabilitation, the expert witness should keep in mind that he or she may be reporting information obtained by a therapist rather than directly by the witness. The reliability of this source of information may be critical to the outcome of the case.

Another unusual situation occurs when the treating physician functions as an expert witness and is placed in the position of being a "fact witness" as well as an expert witness.[2] A fact witness provides information about what actually occurred in a given situation. As both the treating physician and an expert witness, the physician has an incredible amount of power to influence the outcome of the case. It is easy to blur the lines between reporting what happened and providing a medical interpretation.

The medical profession cannot single-handedly bring order to the chaos inherent in legal decision-making. However, delineation of proper conduct for an expert witness and education of the members of the profession may greatly improve the situation. The expert witness has been invited to participate because he or she possesses abilities essential to making a decision in as fair a manner as possible. The expert witness must attempt to educate the judge, jury, and lawyers on both sides of the issue to the best of his or her ability. The testimony should be as clear, sincere, and dispassionate as possible. The expert witness should keep in mind at all times that he or she represents the medical profession and the body of knowledge at its core. The bounds of what is and is not within that core knowledge should be respected at all times.

Guidelines for Expert Witness Testimony, which was prepared for the American Academy of Physical Medicine and Rehabilitation (AAPM&R) and addresses the above issues, is based on the *Principles of Medical Ethics* published by the American Medical Association (AMA) as well as the guidelines of other specialty societies. The AMA's *Principles of Medical Ethics* and *Guidelines for Expert Witness Testimony* are contained in the current

Opinions of the Council on Ethical and Judicial Affairs of the American Medical Association.[14] The AMA's *Principles* are part of the orientation packet received by new members (Appendix A). The specific instance of medical testimony is addressed in section 9.07 of the current *Opinions*:

> As a citizen and as a professional with special training and experience, the physician has an ethical obligation to assist in the administration of justice. If a patient who has a legal claim requests his physician's assistance, the physician should furnish medical evidence with the patient's consent in order to secure the patient's legal rights.
>
> The medical witness must not become an advocate or a partisan in the legal proceeding. The medical witness should be adequately prepared and should testify honestly and truthfully. The attorney for the party who calls a physician as a witness should be informed of all favorable and unfavorable information developed by the physician's evaluation of the case. It is unethical for a physician to accept compensation that is contingent upon the outcome of litigation.

Guidelines for expert witness testimony also have been adopted by the disciplines of pediatrics,[25] neurosurgery,[41] and orthopedics as well as by the American College of Surgeons.[46] In addition, the subject has received extensive debate in the psychiatric literature, particularly in regard to forensic psychiatry. Guidelines for other specialty societies, however, were not identified by a review of the literature. The guidelines adopted by the AAPM&R were modeled primarily after the *Guidelines for Pediatrics*. One of the most important aspects of the *Principles of Medical Ethics* of the AMA as well as guidelines for expert witness testimony prepared by other specialty societies is their clearly understood language. The AAPM&R guidelines, as adopted by the Board of Governors in 1992, attempt to maintain clarity while addressing the range of issues anticipated for the expert witness who is a physiatrist (Appendix B).

Various mechanisms may be used for enforcement of guidelines. As noted by Rovit and Hauber, professional associations retain the ability to enforce an ethical code among their members, provided that the code does not interfere with basic constitutional rights, such as due process.[41] The American Association of

Neurological Surgeons (AANS) has established a mechanism that ensures due process without significant infringement on individual neurosurgeons. A repository of expert witness testimony has been established. The testimony is submitted—strictly on a voluntary basis—by parties to litigation for whom neurosurgeons have served as expert witnesses. Records contain the case name, name of the expert witness, and other key words useful for cross-indexing. In response to qualified requests, the previous activity of an expert witness can be extracted from the repository. Rovit and Hauber suggest that the repository should be used to discredit "itinerant testifiers." Specific issues that they suggest for exposition are a clear delineation of the expertise of the testifier, the nature and scope of relevant past activities, as well as previously expressed opinions under oath.

The mechanism for enforcement within the AAPM&R has not yet been decided. It is clear, however, that without a central repository of information, we can have no reliable methods of policing our members.

To some extent peer review is related to expert witness testimony. Although no extensive guidelines have been adopted, the current *Opinions of the Council of Ethical and Judicial Affairs of the American Medical Association* addresses peer review in section 9.10:

> Medical society ethics committees, hospital credentials and utilization committees, and other forms of peer review have been long-established by organized medicine to scrutinize physicians' professional conduct. At least to some extent, each of these types of peer review can be said to impinge upon the absolute professional freedom of physicians. They are, nonetheless, recognized and accepted. They are necessary. They balance the physician's right to exercise his medical judgment freely with his obligation to do so wisely and temperately.[25]

Within the *Principles of Medical Ethics*, points 2, 3 and 7 are referenced as specifically applicable to peer review, but they are useful only in general terms. In the AAPM&R's *Guidelines*, guidelines 3–5 can be used to define the relationship between the peer reviewer and the reviewee. The reviewer should understand that the practice of medicine remains a mixture of art and science; thus there is often more than one legitimate

approach to a clinical problem. The approach taken by the reviewee, although not the same as that of the reviewer, may still be within the bounds of acceptable practice and should not be censured. In addition, variations in practice do not necessarily relate to variations in outcome. Substandard practice should not be condoned in any form, be it poor documentation or outright negligence. However, the reviewer should give the reviewee the benefit of the doubt whenever appropriate.

Concern that an individual physician or medical society may incur risk of countersuit in peer review or in enforcing standards of behavior has been an impediment to effective implementation. In certain cases, individuals have been sued for participation in peer review activities.[32] A recent opinion of the Federal Trade Commission (FTC) appears to put this concern to rest by establishing the right of professional societies to conduct peer review and to sanction their members. The decision dealt specifically with setting of fees, but the FTC ruling should hold for any peer review activities.[48]

Two recent developments may change substantially the future of expert witness testimony. The first is the case of *Philip Knight v Richard Cordry*.[29] Knight, a pediatric surgeon, was sued after the death of a 2-year old boy whom he had treated. After 27 months of legal maneuvering, the case against Knight was dismissed. Knight then sued the plaintiff's attorney, Richard Cordry, claiming that the original lawsuit was unnecessary. The jury eventually awarded Knight $150,000 for damages. Part of Knight's defense was built on an inaccurate and inadequate reading of the facts by an expert witness. This example should deter the so-called expert witness who is willing to testify to any position for a fee—the proverbial "hired gun."

The second development was a proposal by former President Bush to replace litigation with mediation and arbitration.[32] Refusal by the plaintiff to participate in mediation or arbitration, followed by loss of the suit in litigation, would make the plaintiff liable for the defendant's legal costs. With the transition to the Clinton administration, the shape of tort reform is unclear, but certainly it will be a central issue in the battle over health care reform. If a mediation process is adopted, it will be the responsibility of the medical profession to provide testimony and decision-making capability. If this responsibility is not embraced enthusiastically, the results of mediation are likely to be as capricious as the results of litigation have proved to be.

The Mechanics of Testimony

Most physicians find their interactions with the legal system to be confusing or frustrating, partly because of lack of familiarity with the mechanics of the legal process. This section provides rudimentary information about basic issues such as responding to a summons, depositions, requests for independent medical examinations, and setting of fees for legal work.

The receipt of a summons may be shocking or distressful for a physician. The situation is best handled by finding out the details of the issue in question. Approaching the problem with the same methodical manner used in medical management allows time to find the best solution. The summons may demand the physician's appearance at a hearing with little notice, but most courts accommodate the other demands of the physician's schedule and often allow considerable leeway for negotiation in responding to the summons. Another mechanism, such as a deposition, may be used in lieu of a personal appearance. Before taking action, the physician should seek legal counsel or assistance from an individual more familiar with the legal system.

The deposition is the legal proceeding most frequently encountered by a physician. Depositions usually occur during the phase of the legal process known as discovery, which is often the key phase of the litigation. Both sides of the dispute are involved in fact-finding and testing of their position in the case. The testimony of the expert witness(es) may be critical in reaching a settlement or forcing the case to trial.[21] The deposition itself is a formal legal proceeding in that the deposed physician is under oath and a court reporter records the statements of all involved. Attorneys for both sides are present to cross-examine the deposed. Occasionally the proceeding is recorded on videotape, but this procedure is not typical. During the deposition, the above guidelines for testimony should be kept in mind. One needs to proceed as calmly and dispassionately as possible. Especially when testifying as an expert witness rather than a fact witness, the physician must avoid becoming a partisan to the suit and should not respond to a question if its intent is unclear. The witness has the right to ask for clarification as well as to clarify his or her own statements if deemed necessary. If the witness has difficulty with confusion or other factors, it is permissible to ask for a recess to regain self-composure.

The physician should enter the proceeding adequately prepared. Preparation should include a review of the details of the case as well as any pertinent background from medical literature. An experienced attorney usually ensures that a retained witness is prepared before allowing testimony. The physician should request a predeposition meeting if he or she is uncomfortable about the situation or has questions about the case. The witness should ensure that all pertinent information is available before testimony. Because all information and materials presented to the expert are discoverable, the retaining attorney may try to limit the information available to the expert. Any supporting information should be available during the deposition. It is wise to review this source of information with the attorney before the deposition.

Prior writings or testimony by the witness may be questioned during the testimony. Discrepancies in opinions rendered by the witness are particularly discrediting and may be grounds for a perjury charge.[33] As outlined in the above discussion of codes of conduct for witnesses, the testimony must not be biased by the position of the retaining side.[1,14,25,41,46] Both positive and negative opinions should be presented. It is acceptable to discuss adverse opinions or findings with the retaining attorney before the deposition.

Finally, two critical points must be kept in mind. First, although the witness is deposed under oath, neither attorney is under oath. The attorneys are not required to tell "the truth, the whole truth, and nothing but the truth." Their only job is to win for their client. Secondly, any testimony presented in a deposition may be reviewed in court. A false deposition is subject to the same penalties for perjury as false testimony given in court. Because most cases are settled out of court, a physician's interaction with the proceedings typically ends with the deposition. Because of its critical role in settling the case, the deposition should be approached with the same seriousness as a court appearance, although usually it is not as stressful. At the conclusion of the deposition, the witness is usually given an opportunity to review the transcript for accuracy. The necessity of review depends on the nature of the case, but in many cases this right is waived.

The de bene esse deposition is another alternative to courtroom testimony in which the proceeding is recorded on videotape for presentation in court. This mechanism, which is used most commonly when the expert cannot easily appear in court, has two drawbacks: (1) it is static to the extent that further questions are not possible, and (2) the nonverbal communication of the expert is sometimes obscured. As technology evolves, additional methods have been experimented with to permit testimony without the physical presence of an expert. Two-way closed circuit video has received the most attention.[35] Whether such efforts will become more commonplace is uncertain.

A courtroom appearance places the expert witness in an unfamiliar setting that in some respects is theatrical. Before this appearance, the witness should thoroughly review all information pertinent to the case. In particular, the depositions of other expert witnesses should be analyzed. A good attorney prepares the witness by reviewing the testimony to be presented. In some cases, the attorney may cross-examine the expert with much greater intensity than an opponent would use so that the witness is prepared to respond with professional deportment to whatever may arise in court. During the trial, the expert should be highly conscious of the image that he or she presents. A calm, professional manner is essential. The expert should be prepared to use language that neither loses the jury in technical jargon nor gives the impression of condescension. Because the jury knows that the expert has been retained by one side in the suit, they are naturally skeptical of the testimony. An educational, professional, dispassionate but interesting presentation is essential in establishing credibility.[21]

When asked to perform an independent medical examination for the purpose of future legal testimony, extensive and explicit communication with the requesting party is essential. A "typical work-up" is probably not sufficient to answer the questions that will be asked. By reviewing the goals of the examination, the expert is not as likely to be faced with unforeseen questions while under oath. As an extension of this approach, data from objective testing are often helpful in supporting an opinion. For clinical management, the subjective or semiquantitative findings of a clinical examination are usually sufficient. However, under oath one may be asked to place a numerical value on such diagnostic qualifiers as "moderate" or "two-plus." The more quantitative data that can be collected, the more supportable the opinion. However, the expert needs to be cognizant of the limitations of any test and should be prepared to explain such concepts as "false-negative."

When retained by one of the parties to a suit, the physician must maintain a clear line of communication with the representing attorney. This necessity is reflected in the guidelines for expert testimony discussed above. Most lawyers welcome the chance to explore issues in depth with the expert, and close communication dispels some of the tension that is natural in such interactions. All findings relevant to the outcome of the case, both positive and negative, should be shared explicitly, including the strengths and weaknesses of the opposing position. Of particular interest is the expert's prior testimony, as discussed above in relationship to the enforcement mechanism adopted by the American Academy of Neurological Surgeons.[41] It is easy to discredit an expert who makes a living by testifying to a variety of opinions, depending on the particulars of the case.

Above all, the expert should remember that he or she is testifying as a representative of the medical profession rather than as a partisan. As discussed above, the Supreme Court decision in *Daubert* may alter radically the involvement of expert witnesses.[23,24] Certainly, if the expert witness is retained by the court, the likelihood of change is high. Despite the admonition for the expert witness to present impartial testimony, the current system fosters the impression that the expert is influenced on some level by the retaining party.

Finally, the subject of fees deserves attention. As the guidelines for testimony clearly state, a fee that is contingent on the outcome of the case is not ethical. Otherwise the expert has little guidance in setting a fee for legal work. An informal survey by the author found that physicians use various mechanisms. Most physicians based the fee in part on what they would charge for an equivalent amount of clinical time. Often "hassle factor" was added to the typical fee for clinical work. No respondent reported an instance in which a fee was disputed, although the fee, how it is arrived at, and how it is distributed are legitimate questions that may be explored as part of the testimony. In the author's university-based independent practice group, this issue is handled explicitly. The group determined that work for present or former patients was different from work for persons with whom no clinical relationship exists. For this reason, a differential fee structure that addresses preparation time was adopted. When a member of the group is contacted about a case, the fee structure is discussed and presented in writing. Payment of the fee for a deposition is required before the deposition is scheduled. This plan was adopted to prevent the experience that other groups at the university had encountered. Frequently depositions had been canceled at the last minute, leaving gaps in the schedule that could have been used for other activities. The requirement of advance payment has virtually eliminated this problem. Obviously, this approach is in part a function of the location and type of the author's practice. Other practitioners should use a similar approach to the extent that it can be implemented prospectively and explicitly. The handling of issues such as preparation time, telephone calls, written reports, and billing may legitimately vary from one situation to the next. Careful consideration and preparation in each case help the expert to deal smoothly with the issue of fee. To avoid consuming great amounts of time with little or no reward, careful records of preparation time must be kept. The attorney may accept an aggregate time or make a legitimate request for more detailed records.

CONCLUSION

This chapter serves as a primer for a wide range of medicolegal topics related to the care of individuals with traumatic brain injury. Some issues, such as competency and consent to treatment, apply to almost all cases. On the other hand, expert witness testimony may be a small part of a physician's practice. No single chapter (or book, in fact) can elucidate fully the complexity of medicolegal issues. Although certain underlying concepts and precedents are operative throughout American society, their application varies greatly. Even federal law may be interpreted differently in different jurisdictions. The information in this chapter therefore serves only as a starting point. The practitioner must be aware that the local situation may be somewhat different. Local ethics committees, hospital and personal legal services, and the experience of other physicians are valuable resources. It would be foolish to rely only on the information presented in this chapter in dealing with weighty medicolegal issues.

APPENDIX A

American Medical Association
*Principles of Medical Ethics**

  I. A physician shall be dedicated to providing competent medical service with compassion and respect for human dignity.
 II. A physician shall deal honestly with patients and colleagues and strive to expose those physicians deficient in character or competence, or who engage in fraud or deception.
III. A physician shall respect the law and also recognize a responsibility to seek changes in those requirements which are contrary to the best interests of the patient.
 IV. A physician shall respect the rights of patients, of colleagues, and of other health professionals and shall safeguard patient confidences within the constraints of the law.
  V. A physician shall continue to study, apply and advance scientific knowledge, make relevant information available to patients, colleagues and the public, obtain consultation, and use the talents of other health professionals when indicated.
 VI. A physician shall, in the provision of appropriate patient care except in emergencies,

be free to choose who to serve, with whom to associate, and the environment in which to provide medical services.

VII. A physician shall recognize a responsibility to participate in activities contributing to an improved community.

*Adopted in 1980.

APPENDIX B

White Paper on Expert Witness Testimony

Ethical Issues Subcommittee, American Academy of Physical Medicine and Rehabilitation*

After review of the general Principles of Medical Ethics of the American Medical Association and guidelines for expert witness testimony published by several other specialty societies, the Ethical Issues Subcommittee recommends the adoption of the following guidelines. These guidelines are based primarily on those adopted by the American Academy of Pediatrics with several modifications. Central to these guidelines is the concept that the expert witness functions in education of the court as a whole. It is not the function of the expert witness to be representing either of the parties involved, even though the expert witness may have been contracted primarily by one party.

1. The physician should have current experience and ongoing knowledge about the areas of clinical medicine in which he or she is testifying and familiarity with practices during the time and place of the episode being considered as well as the circumstances surrounding the occurrence. The physician should refuse to offer opinions on subjects which are beyond his/her area of expertise. The bounds of the expert's field of expertise should be clearly stated in testimony.

2. The physician's review of medical facts should be thorough, fair, and impartial and should not exclude any relevant information to create a view favoring either the plaintiff or the defendant. The ultimate test for accuracy and impartiality is a willingness to prepare testimony that could be presented unchanged for use by either the plaintiff or defendant.

3. The physician's testimony should reflect an evaluation of performance in light of generally accepted standards, neither condemning performance that clearly falls within generally accepted practice standards nor endorsing or condoning performance that clearly falls outside accepted practice standards. The physician should identify as such opinions which are

personal and not necessarily held by other physicians. When equally acceptable approaches to a clinical problem exist, these should be detailed impartially in the testimony.

4. The physician should make a distinction between medical malpractice and medical maloccurrence when analyzing any case. The practice of medicine remains a mixture of art and science; the scientific component is a dynamic and changing one based to a large extent on concepts of probability rather than absolute certainty.

5. The physician should make every effort to assess the relationship of the alleged substandard practice to the patient's outcome, because deviation from a practice standard is not always causally related to a less-than-ideal outcome.

6. The physician should be willing to submit transcripts of depositions and/or courtroom testimony for peer review.

7. The physician expert should cooperate with any reasonable efforts undertaken by the courts or by plaintiffs' or defendants' carriers and attorneys to provide a better understanding of the expert witness issue.

8. It is unethical for a physician to accept compensation that is contingent upon the outcome of litigation.

*Presented in October, 1991.

REFERENCES

1. Advisory statement. AAOS Bull 40:5, 1992.
2. Alt HA: The treating physician as an expert witness. Tex Med 83:74–76, 1987.
3. Appelbaum PS, Gutheil TG: Clinical Handbook of Psychiatry and the Law, 2nd ed. Baltimore, Williams & Wilkins, 1991.
4. Banja J: Ethical aspects of treatment for coma and the persistent vegetative state in the coma-emerging patient. Phys Med Rehabil State Art Rev 4:581–585.
5. Banja JD: Patient rights, ethics committees, and the 1992 Joint Commission standards: Implication for traumatic brain injury programs. J Trauma Rehabil 7(4):46–56, 1992.
6. Beauchamp TL, Childress JF: Principles of Biomedical Ethics. New York, Oxford University Press, 1989.
7. Black B: Evolving legal standards for the admissibility of scientific evidence. Science 239:1508–1512, 1988.
8. Brennan TA: Untangling causation issues in law and medicine: Hazardous substance litigation. Ann Intern Med 107:741–747, 1987.
9. Brent RL: The irresponsible expert witness: A failure of biomedical graduate education and professional accountability. Pediatrics 70:754–762, 1982.
9a. Calabresi G: The Cost of Accidents: A Legal and Economic Analysis. New Haven, CT, Yale University Press, 1970.

10. Council on Ethical and Judicial Affairs, American Medical Association: Decisions near the end of life, Council report. JAMA 267:2229–2233, 1992.

11. Council on Scientific Affairs and Council on Ethical and Judicial Affairs: Persistent vegetative state and the decision to withdraw or withhold life support. JAMA 263:426–430, 1990.

12. Crum RM, Anthony JC, Bassett SS, Folstein MF: Population-based norms for the mini-mental state examination by age and educational level. JAMA 269:2386–2391, 1993.

13. Cruzan by Cruzan v Director, Missouri Dept. of Health, et al, 110 S.Ct. 2841

14. Current Opinions of the Council on Ethical and Judicial Affairs of the American Medical Association. Chicago, American Medical Association, 1986.

15. Drane JF: The many faces of competency. Hastings Cent Rep, 15(2) April 1985.

16. Emanuel EJ, Emanuel LL: Proxy decision making for incompetent patients: An ethical and empirical analysis. JAMA 267:2067–2071, 1992.

17. Emanuel LL, Barry MJ, Stoeckle JD, et al: Advance directives for medical care-a case for greater use. N Engl J Med 324:889–895, 1991.

18. Firestone MH: Exception to the exception: Expert medical testimony and behavioral hearsay under federal rule 703. J Leg Med 3:117–135, 1982.

19. Fox E, Stocking C: Ethics consultants' recommendations for life-prolonging treatment of patients in a persistent vegetative state. JAMA 270:2578–2582, 1993.

20. Gamble ER, McDonald PJ, Lichstein, PR: Knowledge, attitudes, and behavior of elderly persons regarding living wills. Arch Intern Med 151:277–280, 1991.

21. Gianna DJ: A primer for the expert witness preparation for deposition and the courtroom. J Disabil 3:111–119, 1993.

22. Gilfix M, Gilfix MG, Sinatra KS: Law and medicine: The persistent vegetative state. J Head Trauma Rehabil 1:63–71, 1986.

23. Gold JA, Zaremski MJ, Lev ER, Shefrin DH: Daubert v Merrell Dow: The Supreme Court tackles scientific evidence in the courtroom. JAMA 270:2964–2967, 1993.

24. Greene S: Supreme court ruling receives warm welcome. Nature 364:94, 1993.

25. Guidelines for expert witness testimony. Pediatrics 83:312–313, 1989.

26. Huber PW: Galileo's Revenge: Junk Science in the Courtroom. New York, NY, Basic Books, 1991.

27. Imwinkelried EJ: The court appointment of expert witnesses in the United States: A failed experiment. Law Med 8:601–609, 1989.

28. In the Matter of Quinlan, 355 A.2d 647.

29. Kansas doctor wins suit against plaintiff lawyer. Am Med Assoc News 35(8):8, 1992.

30. LaPuma J, Orentlicher D, Moss RJ; Advance directives on admission: Clinical implications and analysis of the patient self-determination act of 1990. JAMA 266:402–205, 1991.

31. Lee DK, Swinburne AJ, Fedullo AJ, Wahl GW: Withdrawing care: Experience in a medical intensive care unit. JAMA 271:1358–1361, 1994.

32. McCormick B: Alternatives to courtroom key to Bush reform plan. Am Med Assoc News 35(8):27, 1992.

33. McCormick B: Perjury charges stem from medical expert's testimony. Am Med News, March 16, 1992, p 7.

34. Medical News and Perspectives: What constitutes an expert witness? JAMA 269:2057, 1993.

35. Miller RD: The presentation of expert testimony via live audio-visual communication. Bull Am Acad Psychiatry Law 19:5–20, 1991.

36. Miles SH, August A: Courts, gender and "the right to die". Law Med Health Care 18:86–95, 1990.

37. Moreno JD: Who's to choose? Surrogate decision-making in New York State. Hastings Cent Rep 23(1):5–11, 1993.

38. Nolan BS: Functional evaluation of the elderly in guardianship proceedings. Law Med Health Care 12(5):211–218, 1984.

39. President's Commission for the Study of Ethical Problems in Medicine and Biomedical and Behavioral Research: Making Health Care Decisions: the Ethical and Legal Implications of Informed Consent in the Patient-Practitioner Relationship, vol 1. Washington, DC, United States Government Printing Office, 1982.

40. Robertson JA: Second thoughts on living wills. Hastings Cent Rep 21(6):6–9, 1991.

41. Rovit RL, Hauber C: The expert witness: Some observations and a response from neurosurgeons. Bull Am Coll Sur 74:(7):10–16, 1989.

42. Rouse F: Advance directives: Where are we heading after Cruzan? Law Med Health Care 18:353–359, 1990.

43. Rutman D, Silberfeld M: A preliminary report on the discrepancy between clinical and test evaluations of competence. Can J Psychol 37:634–639, 1992.

44. Seckler AB, Meier DE, Mulvihill M, Cammer Paris BE: Substituted judgment: How accurate are proxy predictions? Ann Intern Med 115:92–98, 1991.

45. Sounding Board: Beyond advance directives— health care surrogate laws. N Engl J Med 327:1165–1169, 1992.

46. Statement on the Physician Expert Witness. Professional Liability Committee, American College of Surgeons. Bull Am Coll Surg 74(8):6–7, 1989.

47. The New York State Task Force on Life and the Law: When Others Must Choose: Deciding for Patients Without Capacity. New York. New York State Task Force on Life and the Law, 1992.

48. United States of America Federal Trade Commission, Office of the Secretary: Letter to Johnson and Peterson Re: The Power of Medical Societies to Regulate Members, Washington, DC, Feb. 14, 1994.

49. Virmani J, Schneiderman LJ, Kaplan RM: Relationship of advance directives to physician-patient communication, (AHCPR grant HSO6912). Arch Intern Med 154:909–913.

50. Winograd CH: Mental status tests and the capacity for self-care. J Am Geriatr Soc 32:49–55, 1984.

51. Zweibel NR, Cassel CK: Treatment choices at the end of life: A comparison of decisions by older patients and their physician-selected proxies. Gerontologist 29:615–621, 1989.

PART TWO
Assessment and Management of Specific Posttraumatic Stress Disorders

10

Neuroimaging in Traumatic Brain Injury

Neuroimaging has become vital in the care of survivors of traumatic brain injury. Most patients suffering traumatic brain injury are evaluated, at some time, with one of many types of neuroimaging. Rehabilitation professionals should be familiar with various neuroimaging modalities, which can be used to predict outcome, to assess affected brain regions, to determine risk for various complications, and to depict focality of damage. This chapter describes basic concepts behind each of the neuroimaging techniques, focusing on its specific usefulness in the rehabilitation setting. It is clearly beyond the scope of this chapter to cover the broad range of possible neuroradiologic abnormalities; instead, the discussion focuses on the abnormalities that are most germane to the rehabilitation professional caring for patients with traumatic brain injury.

COMPUTED TOMOGRAPHY

Computed tomography (CT) was developed in the 1970s. The initial CT scanner was installed in the United Kingdom in 1971. Today there are thousands of CT scanners throughout the world; almost every hospital in the United States that cares for survivors

of traumatic brain injury has access to CT imaging. Modern CT scanners are a vast improvement over earlier models.

Image Generation

Unlike conventional radiographs, CT imaging involves a process by which the x-ray beam passes through the brain at many vectors, as uniformly as possible. A portion of the radiation is absorbed by the structures of the brain; the portion that is not absorbed is detected by electronic scanners. Thus, the amount of radiation detected by the scanners reflects the density of the imaged structures,[1] which are moved through the CT scanner in a symmetric and smooth fashion to keep the beams focused on one point. Computerized manipulation allows axial and reconstructed images. One can now obtain a CT scan of the brain in 5–10 minutes.

A key point in the interpretation of CT imaging is the notation of relative densities. Bone tends to appear white on CT imaging, whereas air appears black. This difference is a product of the amount of radiation that reaches the electronic detectors. Variations in tissue intensity depend on the amount of radiation that each tissue absorbs. Thus bone, which is quite a dense structure, absorbs much of the radiation. The fact that little radiation reaches the detectors produces a white appearance on CT scan; conversely, air permits much of the radiation to pass onto the detectors and thus appears as dark or black. Therefore, tissues that are scanned with CT produce images between the whiteness of bone and the blackness of air because of their density.[2] The ability to compare and contrast fine gradations of tissue density makes CT imaging so valuable. Relative densities tend to occur in the following order, from most dense to least dense: bone, acute blood, postacute blood, edema, brain, cerebrospinal fluid, fat, air.[3] Fast CT speeds effectively limit motion artifact. Scan speeds of less than 5 seconds are routine for most modern scanners, and rapid scanning of about 2 seconds decreases the need for sedation of patients.[4] For head and brain imaging, 10-mm sections are routinely used, whereas so-called thin sections (5-mm) are used to assess occult bone fracture. CT images can be reformatted for multiplanar or 3-dimensional views.

The rehabilitation specialist evaluating CT imaging of the brain should avoid the temptation to turn immediately to obvious structural abnormalities. A methodical approach helps to prevent overlooking of subtle abnormalities. Evaluation should include familiarity with various anatomic structures in the normal state. Our protocol tends to evaluate in a structured fashion (Table 1).

Extraaxial Lesions

Extraaxial lesions arise outside the brain itself. Often they arise from the dura or nearby structures. Extraaxial processes include subdural or epidural hematomas and dermoid or arachnoid cysts. Classically extraaxial lesions expand to displace the brain to the innermost table of bone. Extraaxial hematomas may well be associated with

TABLE 1. Computed Tomography Assessment

Bone	Presence of shift
Cisterns	Extraaxial lesions
Ventricles	Intraaxial lesions

occult skull fracture, and care must be taken to observe for such fractures. Extensive displacement of the brain by extraaxial lesions may cause shift of midline brain structures and herniation syndromes. Acute extraaxial hemorrhage (< 1 week old) has a high attenuation coefficient and is accordingly high in density on CT scan. Subacute blood continues to decrease in attenuation and thus becomes darker. Because chronic hematomas have a further decrease in attenuation, the resultant image is relatively isodense compared with brain tissue.

Epidural Hematoma

Epidural hematomas often result from arterial trauma, usually to the meningeal arteries. Meningeal arteries ascend between the dura and the bone. Fractures occur in up to 91% of patients with epidural hematomas.[5] Epidural hematomas that are venous in origin are generally due to coagulation disorder and occasionally to torsional trauma. Epidural hematomas from a venous source are more likely to occur in the posterior fossa, whereas epidural hematomas from an arterial source usually occur in the temporoparietal region of the brain.[5] Typically epidural hematomas assume a biconvex or almost egg-shaped appearance because the dura is separated from the brain and fluid collects in the newly created space. Epidural hematomas appear to have a high recurrence rate. Some authors believe that epidural hematomas involve a lower risk of posttraumatic epilepsy than other intracranial lesions (Fig. 1).

Subdural Hematoma

Subdural hematomas are located under the dural space adjacent to the brain; hence their name. Because of their proximity to the surface of the brain, subdural hematomas tend to assume a crescent shape, following the course of the brain tissue below them. Subdural hematomas rarely assume a convex shape, which makes them more difficult to distinguish from epidural hematomas. The convex shape is associated with extremely brisk hemorrhage or confounding artifact. Unlike their epidural counterparts, subdural hematomas are rarely associated with underlying fracture. Density changes tend to reflect a somewhat shorter time span than

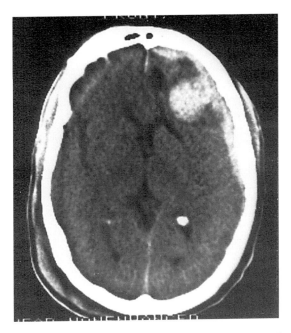

FIGURE 1. CT image of classic egg-shaped epidural hematoma. Of note, a subdural hematoma is also present.

that of epidural hematomas. Acute subdural blood has a high attenuation factor, which gradually diminishes to an isodense status over 14–21 days.[6] Subsequent bleeding into a more chronic hematoma is not uncommon, and the more acute and higher attenuation blood may produce a layering effect. Differentiation from hygromas is often difficult, and mixed attenuation lesions are common in the chronic stages. Because blood is an irritant, lesions in which blood is the major causative factor tend to produce further gyri retraction. Acute mixed-density lesions tend to carry a worse prognosis and a higher incidence of herniation syndromes because of their tendency for rapid expansion (Figs. 2–4).

Intraaxial Lesions

Subarachnoid Hemorrhage

Subarachnoid hemorrhage (SAH) is an area of increasing interest to specialists in traumatic brain injury. SAH appears to be a major cause of posttraumatic vasospasm. Vasospasm may cause secondary injury to tissues.[7] SAH may result from trauma, aneurysm, arteriovenous malformation, coagulopathy or,

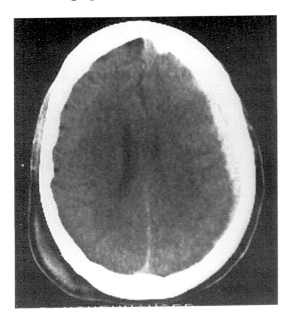

FIGURE 2. Curvilinear density of a high-intensity (bright) represents subdural hematoma.

rarely, infarct. SAH appears as a high-density lesion located in the cerebrospinal fluid spaces. As blood is cleared, the density of the

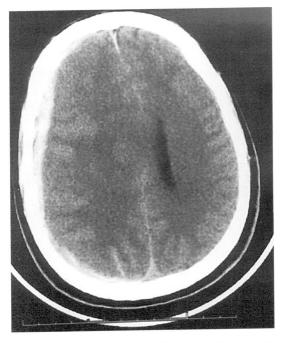

FIGURE 3. Curvilinear density of an acute nature (subdural hematoma) causes shift of midline brain structures and obliteration of adjacent ventricle.

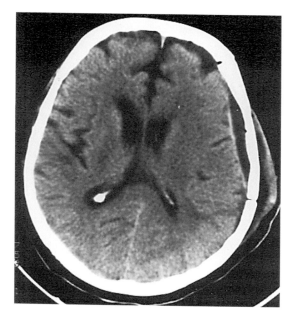

FIGURE 4. Isodense lesion of a curvilinear nature. The dark image reflects that it is more chronic in nature.

lesion consequently diminishes. Of note, CT imaging is more sensitive than MRI in detecting acute SAH (Fig. 5). Because SAH and

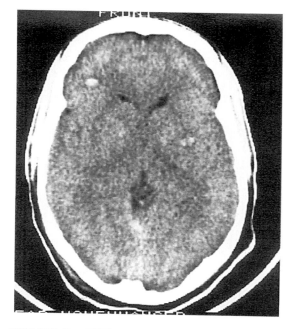

FIGURE 5. Diffuse subarachnoid hemorrhage that follows the path of the gyri, especially in the posterior aspect. Also seen are multiple small punctate intracerebral hemorrhages.

resulting vasospasm have a significant effect on outcome, early identification and management of consequent vasospasm are paramount.[8] SAH may produce vasospasm as late as 2–3 weeks after the initial event, although the typical time period is within the first week. Arteriography, transcranial Doppler, and single-photon emission computed tomography are useful in assessing the patient for vasospasm.[9,10]

Intraparenchymal and Intraventricular Hemorrhage

As a primary event, intraventricular hemorrhage may result from hypertensive hemorrhage, trauma, arteriovenous malformation, or tumor. Acute intraventricular hemorrhage is visualized as a high-density lesion on CT imaging. Of note, as hemoglobin breaks down over time, a more isodense lesion is appreciated.[11] In the acute stages of hemorrhage, CT imaging is clearly more accurate than MRI.[12]

Contusion

A contusion results from blunt trauma to the surface of the brain, usually the temporal, parietal, and frontal regions. Contusions may be at the site of the lesion (coup) or at a site almost opposite to the side of the lesion (contrecoup). Contusions are often superficial but may blossom into a larger lesion within several days of the injury (Fig. 6). CT may be relatively insensitive to small focal contusions, and minimal hemorrhages may be sequestered by their proximity to the bone table. MRI is nearly twice as sensitive as CT in detecting contusions.[13,14]

Intraparenchymal Hematoma

Intraparenchymal hemorrhage from trauma may result in a wide variety of lesions. Clearly both superficial and deep intraparenchymal hematomas are common. Severe intraparenchymal lesions close to the ventricular system may well rupture into the ventricles. Significant intraparenchymal hematomas may cause mass effect and result in significant ventricular compromise and/or herniation. Most common posttraumatic intraparenchymal hematomas involve the temporal and frontal lobes because of the bony encasement (Fig. 7).

Diffuse Axonal Injury

Diffuse axonal injury (DAI) is a shear phenomenon that results in disturbance in cellular structures after a traumatic brain injury.[15,16] While the clinical situation may be quite severe, the CT findings may be limited. It is not uncommon, however, to see small punctuate hemorrhages, white matter lesions, and corpus callosal hemorrhages (see Fig. 8). Small hemorrhages adjacent to the third ventricle are also seen in DAI. Of note, the CT findings in DAI may be without abnormality, especially in those cases where no punctate hemorrhage is noted.[17]

Hydrocephalus

Cerebrospinal fluid (CSF) is a clear ultrafiltrate of the plasma that supports the brain and spinal cord structures. Approximately 150 ml of CSF is present within the dura and spine. Hydrocephalus results from an accumulation of CSF within the cranium. Hydrocephalus most commonly results from an inability to absorb CSF at the rate at which it is produced. Deficits may be due to blockage of CSF absorption by the arachnoid villi or to disturbance of CSF flow into the venous system. Ventriculomegaly may represent merely an ex vacuo phenomenon rather than true clinical hydrocephalus. Depending on the assessment tool, the incidence of posttraumatic ventricular dilation has been reported as high as 72%.[19] Fortunately, the incidence of clinical hydrocephalus is much lower (1–7%).

Posttraumatic hydrocephalus is usually associated with symptoms such as lethargy, behavioral disturbance, ataxia, and incontinence. Noncommunicating and communicating varieties of hydrocephalus are possible in patients with traumatic brain injury. In the noncommunicating variety, abstraction prevents CSF from entering the subarachnoid space. Imaging evaluation should note the point of obstruction. The temporal horns are a sensitive indicator of hydrocephalus and may be the first sign on imaging. Communicating hydrocephalus, which is characterized by a free system between the ventricular and subarachnoid space, usually is due to disturbance in the flow of CSF from the basilar cisterns or to a deficit in reabsorption from the arachnoid villi. Patterns of hydrocephalus

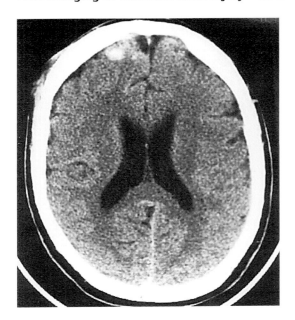

FIGURE 6. Bilateral frontal contusions, more distinctly seen on the right.

may be relatively similar for both types; however, in communicating hydrocephalus the third ventricle may be less distended and the amount of interstitial edema decreased.[20]

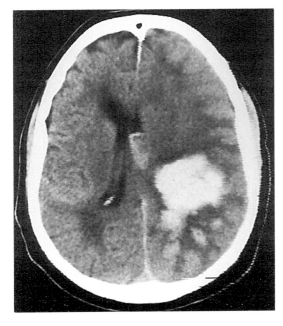

FIGURE 7. A rather spectacular and large acute left intracerebral hematoma with penetration into the ventricles. Midline shift is also observed.

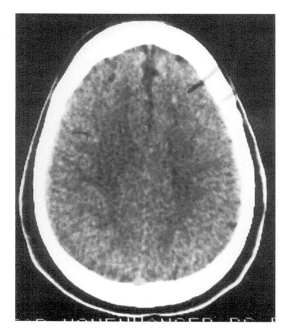

FIGURE 8. Punctate hemorrhages are noted by the black line on the left. This scan is representative of diffuse axonal injury.

The distinction between ex vacuo phenomenon and true hydrocephalus remains difficult with CT imaging; however, the pattern of

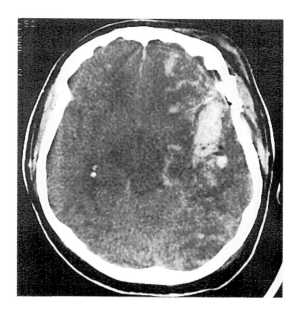

FIGURE 9. A large left intracerebral hematoma and diffuse subarachnoid hemorrhage. Virtual obliteration of the cisterns is noted, along with herniation.

ventricular enlargement may be different. Ex vacuo phenomenon tends to spare the temporal horns, which, although larger than normal, may be small compared with the lateral ventricles. Frontal horn angle in ex vacuo phenomenon is often greater than 95°, whereas in communicating or noncommunicating hydrocephalus the standard angle of the frontal horns is often less than 95°.[21,22]

Fractures

Posttraumatic fractures are common, especially in direct assault injuries. Fractures of the skull may lead to numerous complications, such as CSF leak, epidural hematoma, or pneumocephalus. Careful evaluation of the bone-window images on initial CT imaging, especially in patients with clinical evidence of a basilar or middle fossa fracture, is crucial. CT imaging is usually the most helpful neuroimaging technique in identifying occult bone lesions, especially lesions of the temporal bone and orbital wall.

Herniation Syndromes

Herniation syndromes result from displacement of the brain parenchyma by an expanding mass lesion and involve serious clinical consequences.

Uncal Herniation

The uncus is the most medial portion of the temporal lobe and abuts the suprasellar cistern. A traumatic lesion located ipsilateral to the uncus may expand sufficiently to compress the suprasellar cistern with resultant herniation (Fig. 9).

Subfalcine Herniation

Subfalcine herniation occurs when an expanding mass pushes the ipsilateral cerebral cortex under the falx. Obstructive hydrocephalus often results if the herniation has closed off the contralateral foramen of Monro. In subfalcine herniation the corpus callosum and often the ventricle ipsilateral to the side of the lesion shift into the opposite side of the cranium.

Transtentorial Herniation

If a mass of sufficient size occupies a space in the fixed margins of the cranium, herniation results. If continued expansion occurs in uncal herniation, the brain is pushed caudally through the tentorium. Of note, the brainstem is shifted to the side opposite the lesion with enlargement of the ambient cistern and concomitant compression of the suprasellar and interpedunclar cisterns. Effacement of the quadrigeminal plate cistern may follow.[23] Clinical concerns of a rather grave nature involve brainstem compression and posterior cerebral artery perfusion.

Edema

Various forms of edema may be seen on neuroimaging; all forms, however, appear as a low-attenuation region on CT. Hypoxic or cytotoxic edema may occur from ischemic injury or as a primary posttraumatic event. In the second instance, edema occurs as a diffuse phenomenon involving the entire cortical region but generally sparing posterior fossa structures. Often the signal of the white matter has greater density than that of the gray matter. Vasogenic edema, which in general is considered white matter, results from at least a partial disruption in the blood-brain barrier. Hallmark evidence is swelling of white matter with sparing of gray matter. Ischemic edema may be an important secondary complication in traumatic brain injury (Fig. 10). Difficulty with the cellular pump mechanism results in accumulation of intracellular fluids. Edema accrues in both the gray and white matter, and a sectional pattern may occur in association with infarction. Periventricular edema may result from hydrocephalus or extensive intraventricular hemorrhage.[23a] Pressure causes tearing of the ventricular lining with resultant accumulation of fluid adjacent to the frontal and lateral horns.[24] These high signal-intensity changes are best demonstrated on T2-weighted magnetic resonance imaging.

Penetrating Injuries

The most common cause of penetrating injury is gunshot wounds. One can usually identify the missile fragments, bone elements, and hemorrhage associated with the tract of the injury. CT imaging is the study of choice for imaging penetrating injuries, because metal-

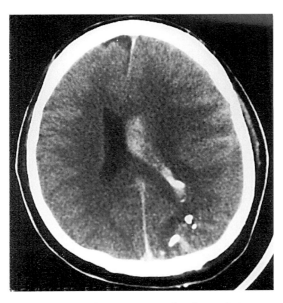

FIGURE 10. Fragments and a large intraventricular hemorrhage with resultant diffuse edema.

lic artifact and image dissolution are greater concerns with MRI. Pneumocephalus, subarachnoid hemorrhage, and diffuse cerebral edema are commonly noted with missile injuries.[25] Even without scan imaging, streak artifacts from the metallic fragments may severely compromise detail, especially along the lines of the bullet tract[26] (Figs. 11 and 12). Other objects also may penetrate the cranial cavity and cause extensive damage.[27]

Classification Systems

The classification of posttraumatic CT findings is controversial. The system used by the Traumatic Coma Data Bank (TCDB) involves assessment for cisternal compression, midline shift, operative lesion, and presence or absence of 25 ml of blood. The TCDB has used this system to predict mortality.[18] The value of other classification systems that assess lesion side, size, and location has yet to be established (Table 2).

Contrast vs. Noncontrast Imaging

Noncontrast imaging appears to be more valuable than contrast imaging for acute evaluation and assessment of either intraaxial or extraaxial lesions. Contrast is most

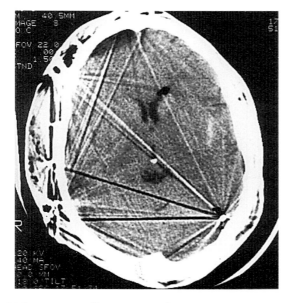

FIGURE 11. Scatter secondary to multiple missile fragments of a metallic nature.

useful for differentiating tumor or infectious mass from a posttraumatic lesion. Although this distinction is usually made on a clinical basis, neuroimaging may be needed. Because the blood-brain barrier is a relatively sturdy

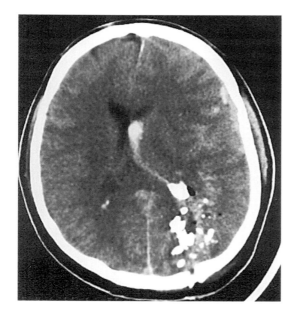

FIGURE 12. Multiple intracerebral hematomas and retained metallic fragments. Intraventricular hemorrhage and subarachnoid hemorrhage are also noted.

entity under normal conditions, iodine-labeled substances have been designed to emphasize regions with a deficit. Under normal conditions iodine-labeled substances respect the blood-brain barrier and do not show enhancement, whereas uptake of contrast into the parenchyma reveals a disturbance in the blood-brain barrier. Patterns of enhancement may give significant clues to the specific diagnosis; however, they should be reviewed with an experienced radiologist, because subtle changes may affect categorization of the lesion.

Special Scan Techniques

Dynamic Imaging

Rapid-sequence scanning (acquisition of images as fast as 30 seconds) followed by intravenous contrast allows evaluation of selected regions of interest with flow imaging. This method of assessing vascular abnormalities has had limited application. Newer techniques, such as spiral CT or double-contrast CT imaging, may allow vascular imaging that is equal or superior to magnetic resonance angiography.

TABLE 2. Classification System of the Traumatic Coma Data Bank

Category	Definition
Diffuse injury I (visible pathology)	No visible intracranial pathology on CT
Diffuse injury II	Cisterns are present with midline shift of 0–5 mm and/or lesion densities; no high- or mixed-density lesion > 25 ml; may include bone fragments and foreign bodies
Diffuse injury III (swelling)	Cisterns compressed or absent with midline shift of 0–5 mm; no high- or mixed-density lesion > 25 ml
Diffuse injury IV (shift) Evacuated mass lesion Nonevacuated mass lesion	Midline shift > 5 mm; no high- or mixed-density lesion > 25 ml, any lesion surgically evacuated; high- or mixed density lesion > 25 ml, not surgically evacuated

Xenon Inhalation Scan Imaging

Inhalation of stable xenon with dynamic CT imaging allows assessment and quantification of regional blood flow. Because xenon crosses the blood-brain barrier, it provides a stable method of assessing cerebral perfusion. Care must be taken, however, because xenon concentrations of 50% or greater act as an anesthetic agent. This technique has become a valuable research tool, but it is not widely available clinically.

Air or Contrast Cisternography

Contrast cisternography may be performed to assess flow abnormalities. It is usually recommended that scanning immediately follow intrathecal injection of contrast. One may position the contrast toward the region of interest by using the tilt table. Shunts may be investigated by small injection followed by both immediate and delayed scanning. This method helps to detect shunt stenosis or obstruction. Air or carbon dioxide contrast CT scanning is useful in assessing patients for a rare lesion at the cerebropontine angle. This procedure involves the intrathecal instillation of a small bolus of air or carbon dioxide to provide a contrast medium. Most commonly this procedure is used to investigate possible tumor location and has minimal application in posttraumatic patients.

Summary

Computed tomography is clearly the most widely available neuroimaging technique and in the acute setting remains the most useful. Its ability to detect acute hemorrhage and to delineate regions of compression or herniation syndromes is excellent. Rapid acquisition of images reduces not only scanner time but also motion artifact and need for sedation. Its inability to provide functional and detailed information about the posterior fossa and white matter leaves room for other modalities.

MAGNETIC RESONANCE IMAGING

Magnetic resonance imaging (MRI) has multiple advantages over CT because it often provides a more sensitive indicator of brain abnormalities. At present the uses and practical applications of MRI are exploding. Although CT remains a superior modality for assessing acute hemorrhage, calcification, and fracture, MRI is superior in virtually all other areas. MRI provides superior identification of posterior fossa structures, delayed hemorrhage, and subtle cortical abnormalities as well as a contrastlike image without the obligation to use contrast.[28]

Principles of Scanning

It is beyond the scope of this chapter to discuss in detail all of the physical principles involved in MRI scanning, but a basic understanding is necessary. Whereas CT resolution depends on variation in attenuation secondary to density differences, MRI depends on the relative presence of hydrogen—in particular, mobile hydrogen. Hydrogen generates the largest MRI signal of all typical nuclear components in the body. Via a powerful external magnetic field, individual particles align themselves either in parallel to the field or against the field. Application of radiofrequency forces can change against the parallel component to a parallel component. In reality, the situation is not so simple; individual components form a cone around the axis of the external magnetic field with a magnetic moment occurring in the direction of the external magnetic field. Precession frequency (all components together), called the Larmor frequency, is a function of the specific nuclei and the strength of the magnetic field. All excitation radiofrequency pulses are applied at the Larmor frequency and in the direction perpendicular to the axis of the external field. The excessive energy from the radiofrequency pulse tips this group of precise nuclei into another plane (the x-y plane). Once a radiofrequency pulse is turned off, the excessive energy decreases dramatically and the precise nuclei begin to return to their original alignment.[29] This process induces an alternating current that is detectable. The phase of decreased excitation or relaxation is important,[30] because at this point the precision group causes recovery of the magnetic field along the z axis and loss of the magnetic field along the x-y axis. Loss of magnetic field along the x-y plane is due to T2

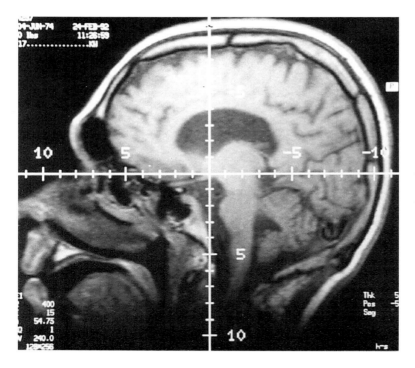

FIGURE 13. Coronal section with a T1 relaxation time. Cerebrospinal fluid is dark, whereas fat is bright.

or transverse relaxation and recovery along the z axis to T1 or longitudinal relaxation.[31] Thus, the image becomes a function of how the precise nuclei are allowed to relax once they have been tipped into another plane.

Signal Issues and Definitions

Because relaxation times play an important role in determining the image, a brief discussion of specifics is in order. T1 is the time required for magnetization in the z axis to reach 63% of its original value. In practice, water and other liquids have long T1s, whereas more compact structures have shorter T1s. T2 is a product of the rate of loss of magnetization in the x-y plane. Specifically, T2 is the time required for the reduction of magnetization in the x-y plane to 37% of its original value. Because tissues vary in relaxation times, they produce a variation in signal intensity. In general, tissues with long relaxation times appear with low signal on T1 and high signal on T2 imaging. In contrast, tissues with short relaxation times appear with high signal on T1 and low signal on T2. Thus, cerebrospinal fluid, which is a liquid component, has a long relaxation time and appears with low signal on T1 and high

signal on T2 imaging. MRI signals are stronger from tissues than from bone,[32] because bone has a relatively low population of mobile hydrogen and is nearly devoid of MRI signals. Paramagnetic substances also have an effect on the signal generation. Examples of paramagnetic substances include iron (as it occurs in methemoglobin and gadolinium).[33] The effects of paramagnetic substances include T1 hyperintensity and T2 hypointensity when observed in sufficient concentrations (Fig. 13).

Artifacts and Precautions

Patient motion is the most common form of artifactual disturbance. Moving objects tend to result in ghost images. Although certain sequencing modalities make artifacts less apparent, as little movement as possible is warranted for optimal image production. Pulsating blood and cerebrospinal fluid may cause ghost images and signal void. Metallic artifacts, produced by ferromagnetic and other metallic substances,[34] cause major distortions that are easily recognized. MRI must be used with caution in patients with metallic fragments, pacemakers, ferromagnetic aneurysmal clips, neurostimulators, and metallic cranial or facial plates. The magnetic field is so extremely strong that pens and scissors may be dangerous in the magnetic field room. Magnetic field-induced current may heat tissues adjacent to any wire or metallic structure. One should question each MRI site about its policy in evaluating patients with indwelling metallic substances.

Extraaxial Lesions

MRI scanning of the acutely injured patient with suspected intra- or extraaxial lesions is difficult because of the time involved. MRI is most useful for evaluation of parenchymal and extraaxial lesions several days to 1 week after injury. Oxyhemoglobin in the early period after injury does not carry the intensity of MRI signal as well as more oxidized hemoglobin products. Chronic subdural hematomas show characteristics of deoxyhemoglobin and methemoglobin. Subdural hygroma appears crescent in shape but may appear more continuous with the adjacent subarachnoid space and thus produce "normal flowing" interdigitation on scanning.[35] MRI of acute epidural hematomas is usually as accurate as CT; however, as previously noted, acute intervention and timing issues make early MRI scanning more difficult. Some care must be taken in the analysis of both epidural and subdural hematomas with MRI, because identifying portions adjacent to the inner table of bone may be difficult.

Intraaxial Lesions

Contusions and Parenchymal Hemorrhage

Cortical contusions tend to occur with the greatest frequency in the frontal regions. Classically cortical contusions spare the white matter and involve only superficial cortical structures. Such contusions typically occur along the frontal inferior aspect of lateral regions and similarly in association with the temporal lobe. Contusions frequently occur with diffuse axonal injury, and at least one-half contain some hemorrhagic component. MRI reflects lesion size and edema effect more accurately than CT scanning. Of note, MRI is far more accurate for evaluation

of contusions without a hemorrhagic component. As stated previously, MRI more accurately identifies lesions within the posterior fossa and thus plays a superior role in localizing cerebellar or brainstem contusions.[36] Large intraparenchymal lesions are best evidenced acutely by CT. MRI and magnetic resonance angiography may be helpful in differentiating other occult causes of intraparenchymal hemorrhage, such as vascular lesion or tumor. In addition, the extent of associated edema with a subacute hemorrhage is best evaluated with MRI.[37]

Diffuse Axonal Injury

Diffuse axonal injury (DAI) results from stress and shearing forces and is the most typical lesion of traumatic brain injury. Typical sites include the frontal and temporal regions, corpus callosum, internal capsule, and brainstem.[38] Often DAI is associated with other lesions of either extraaxial or contusional origin. MRI is clearly superior to CT in demonstrating these subtle lesions, about 20% of which are associated with a hemorrhagic component.[39] Hemorrhagic DAI lesions most typically affect the white matter regions and internal capsule. Most DAI lesions are not associated with hemorrhage, but they are rarely singular and tend to occur in a more diffuse fashion along the axis of the axons.[40] Often seen are regions of enhancement termed unidentified bright objects (UBOs). UBOs are thought to be focal regions of demyelination or gliosis.

Subarachnoid Hemorrhage

Subarachnoid hemorrhage often results from the tearing of small subarachnoid vessels. Posttraumatic subarachnoid hemorrhage rarely shows the same amount of blood in the cisterns as a typical postaneurysmal hemorrhage. In some posttraumatic cases further work-up is obligatory, and the presence of an aneurysm on magnetic resonance angiography or conventional angiography leads to the "chicken-or-egg" dilemma. Of note, subarachnoid hemorrhage has an interdigitating appearance on MRI and, to a lesser extent, on CT.[41] The importance of subarachnoid hemorrhage and its possible implications in secondary injury are identified above in the discussion of CT.

Intraventricular Hemorrhage and Subcortical Lesions

The reported incidence of intraventricular hemorrhage and subcortical lesions in post-traumatic states varies. Massive hemorrhage into the ventricles may require ventriculostomy or other drainage; hydrocephalus is a possible complication. MRI is superior to CT in identifying associated contusions or parenchymal hemorrhage and far more specific for identifying and localizing subcortical and brainstem lesions. MRI is also clearly superior in identifying midbrain and pontine lesions, specifically lesions of the nonhemorrhagic variety.[42]

Hydrocephalus

The differences between communicating and noncommunicating hydrocephalus are discussed in the section about CT. Noncommunicating hydrocephalus is associated with frontal and temporal horn dilatation as well as periventricular edema. Periventricular edema is most apparent on T1-weighted imaging, which best contrasts the hypointense cerebrospinal fluid with the edema surrounding the ventricle. The edematous fluid contains an increased amount of myelinlike proteins that produce a more intense image on T1 imaging. Posterior fossa causes of obstruction, such as rare posttraumatic cysts, are more easily located with MRI imaging.[43] Although cerebrospinal fluid produces a flow-void signal and pulsatile flow may be seen, its role in diagnostic MRI is not clear. Of note is the newer application of MRI specifically to assess the flow of cerebrospinal fluid, which also depends on flow-void and pulsatile phenomena.[44] Some argue that the presence of sulci on MRI is a key differentiating factor between ex vacuo and true hydrocephalus.

Ventricular Shunting

In true hydrocephalus a shunt is placed usually into the lateral ventricles. Both CT and MRI can be used to assess the placement of such a shunt. Shunts, however, are not without complications, including malfunction, ventriculitis, subdural hematomas, and an isolated fourth ventricle.

Magnetic Resonance Angiography

A great deal of energy is currently directed at refinement of the techniques for magnetic resonance angiography. A three-dimensional image is obtained with the gradient echo technique. This image is produced by synchronizing flow effect images in the vasculature. Although magnetic resonance angiography remains a promising and exciting technique, some authorities believe that it may be replaced by more advanced CT techniques. From a clinician's point of view magnetic resonance angiography is valuable in investigating occult causes of posttraumatic subarachnoid hemorrhage, vasospasm, sagittal sinus pathology, or carotid cavernous fistula.

Magnetic Source Imaging and Magnetoencephalography

Magnetoencephalography is an exciting new technique that allows almost real-time images of brain activity. Current flow within dendrites generates a magnetic field that is detected within the superconducting circuitry. This technique is not widely available; it requires a shielded room and a sophisticated superconductivity detector. Lewine and others have investigated the use of magnetoencephalograpy in minor head trauma. Its potential for evaluating occult cognitive and motoric deficits, as well as the success of pharmacologic programs, is enormous.

Summary

MRI offers detailed assessment that is virtually unsurpassed. New and exciting schemes have created opportunities to evaluate cerebrospinal fluid and vascular flow. MRI appears to be a superior modality in the postacute period and offers better visualization of posterior fossa and white matter shear lesions.

ANGIOGRAPHY

The role of angiography in posttraumatic patients clearly focuses on ruling out occult causes of hemorrhage. Angiography may also show value in assessing posttraumatic patients for vasospasm, fistulas, and arterial dissection. Newer low-osmolarity contrast media have made angiography safer. The advent of digital subtraction angiography (DSA) allows rapid manipulation of multiple images with subtraction of osseous structures from the examination. The reader is referred to one of several angiography atlases for a full discussion.

Carotid Angiography

Carotid angiography is now generally performed by percutaneous femoral catheterization, which allows selective examination of the internal or external carotid artery. Once contrast is introduced, it is standard to obtain rapid-sequence images at about 1 second so that arterial capillary and venous phases can be evaluated. Vasospasm may be a life-threatening complication and lead to increased neurologic deficit and other comorbidities. Detailed evaluation for vasospasm with angiography or other techniques and aggressive treatment are advocated.

Vertebral Angiography

Direct needle puncture is now superseded by catheter techniques. Usually the left vertebral artery is easier to catheterize than the right vertebral artery. If the subclavian artery can be catheterized, an indirect vertebral angiogram may be performed.

Digital Subtraction Angiography

One of the advantages of digital subtraction angiography (DSA) is that relatively adequate studies can be obtained with limited arterial concentrations of contrast. Venous injections are also possible, but resolution is not as good. Movement in uncooperative patients may blur findings, and superimposition of vessels is an issue in the lateral view.[45] Intraarterial DSA allows selective study and decreased dosage of contrast bolus.

Dural Sinus Studies

During normal angiographic studies (specifically carotid angiography), the region of the superior sagittal sinus can be seen, but detail is often obscured. DSA provides more accurate imaging of the sinuses, the importance of which includes imaging of potential sagittal sinus thrombosis.

FUNCTIONAL IMAGING

Functional neuroimaging is an exciting new area. Such methods allow measurement of metabolic activity or its relative correlate, cerebral blood flow. Although static neuroimaging (MRI, CT) provides valuable information about anatomic structures, it provides little information about dynamic functional cerebral activity. A dynamic image can be constructed with nuclear isotopes labeled to a ligand. Both positron emission tomography and single-photon emission tomography have potential for assessment of occult pathology, inconsistent findings, seizure disorders, perfusion disorders, and movement disorders, as well as prognostication. Care should be taken in the evaluation and clinical correlation of each scan. Accurate evaluation requires experience, and a critical review of the interpretation and resolution of the scanning equipment is warranted. Other techniques of functional imaging include nuclear ventriculography and transcranial Doppler ultrasound.

Positron Emission Tomography

Positron emission tomography (PET) allows evaluation of dynamic metabolic activity within the brain. It continues to serve as the gold standard by which other metabolic and perfusion parameters are measured. In its original application with use of isotopes, PET simply measures metabolic activity for glucose. With use of 18-fluorodeoxyglucose or oxygen inhalation, PET is able to show a change in metabolic activity. Classic experiments began with showing that increasing visual stimulus led to increased uptake in the occipital region. Two important concepts in functional imaging are contrast and spatial resolution. Contrast refers to the intensity of an image, the ability to measure accurately the concentration of positron-emitting tracer within the subject that is scanned. This feature also allows quantification of intensity. Spatial resolution refers to the ability to represent various subdivisions of the subject that is scanned.

Contrast Issues

Imaging resolution and clarity vary greatly with choice of radionucleotide. Currently under development are various ligands linked to dopamine, opiate, and mixed (dopaminergic and serotonergic) receptors. Potential distortions and limitations of spatial and contrast resolution are inherent to each radioligand.

Process

The region of the brain in which positron-emitting radionucleotide decays is determined by the radionucleotide's biologic properties. Decay results in the production of positrons that are annihilated by collision with an electron. Detectors note variations in arrival time and record differences. Resolution is limited by two major factors: (1) positrons must travel to the point of inhalation, and (2) some of the positrons are absorbed or deflected as they pass through tissue. The size, shape, and quality of the detection scanners are clearly crucial. Current systems use multiple scanning detectors that move, in general, along the scanner axis; thus planar image resolution is superior to axial resolution. Various modifications of scanner geometry can change the resolution effect. Most PET scanners are unable to identify small structures accurately. Specific resolution numbers are important in evaluating a particular scanner. The partial volume effect explains some of the resolution deficits; the effect of items below detection threshold is averaged with adjacent tissues. Of note, objects approaching a cylindrical shape are somewhat more sensitively detected in most scanning systems.

Analysis

Qualitative visual inspection requires experience and care. To date there is no agreement on the best method for quantitative analysis of data. Regions of interest that either can be drawn or conform to predetermined geometrically structured areas are analyzed in a more quantitative fashion. Computer programs can be designed to assess pixel transition across a range of image intensities and regional subdivisions, thus producing a more quantitative measure. Various anatomic imaging techniques have been correlated with PET via computer enhancement to produce anatomic parallels to regions of interest. Care must be taken with any type of interpretation, and critical review is necessary. Of major concern is the over- or under-interpretation of scans when medicolegal issues are involved.

Clinical Uses

PET has become a useful clinical and research tool. It remains the benchmark for functional imaging. It has been used for the assessment of epilepsy (posttraumatic), depression, detection of occult deficits, and medication effects.[46] Focal hypometabolism is common in patients with interictal epilepsy. Many PET studies have been carried out in patients with known complex partial epilepsy and reveal focal areas of hypometabolism corresponding to predicted epileptogenic areas. In patients with temporal lobe epilepsy, which causes temporal hypometabolism, ipsilateral frontal hypometabolism also has been reported. This may be due in part to undetected frontal complex partial epileptiform activity or to unexplained loop mechanisms. Local increases in oxygen fraction may indicate epileptiform activity more reliably than local decreases in either cerebral blood flow or metabolic activity. Several specific neurotransmitters can be used to study local alterations in one receptor system.[47] Ictal studies reveal regions of hyper- or hypometabolism.

PET also is useful in determining the extent of hypoxic ischemic injury. Global decreases in metabolic activity and bilateral hypometabolic activity appear to carry a relatively poor prognosis.[48] In anecdotal reports, patients who are slow to recover from hypoxic ischemic injury maintain reasonable metabolic activity on PET and subsequently recover to a "reasonable" functional status. PET studies also have been useful in detecting and assessing lesions not accounted for by conventional anatomic imaging. Several studies have demonstrated the superiority of functional imaging in assessing patients for pathology.[49] As noted previously, care must be taken not to over-interpret scans; however,

PET appears to provide a greater scope of functional involvement, and early studies show that functional imaging is somewhat superior for predicting deficits. Few, if any, studies have assessed long-term outcome with PET; functional outcome predictors are discussed in more detail at the end of the chapter.

Functional imaging has been helpful in assessment of depression and evaluation of treatment. PET techniques also have been useful in detecting unrecognized depression in correlation with clinical symptoms. No strong studies detail the usefulness of PET in evaluating various medications or predicting depression in patients with traumatic brain injury.[50] The future of PET in predicting which patients with traumatic brain injury may experience movement disorders is quite good. PET also may be helpful in differentiating prior injury from occult neoplastic pathology.[51]

Disadvantages

The disadvantages of functional imaging, specifically PET, must be taken into account. PET requires a rather long and arduous processing time in most scanners, thus making it difficult to use in uncooperative patients with traumatic brain injury. Because PET systems tend to be exquisitely sensitive to motion, a cooperative patient is essential. PET equipment is quite costly, scanning costs are relatively high, and maintenance is an ongoing issue; thus PET studies are relatively expensive for the patient. Long scanning time also makes PET difficult to use in the acute or periacute period. As discussed above, partial volume effect limits resolution; in irregularly shaped or thin regions, such as the lateral frontal cortex, metabolic rates may be underestimated.[52] Such technical hazards make quantitative analysis more desirable for assessing the results of clinical trials. In addition, medications and alcohol may result in a general depression of activity and skew results if they are not taken into account. The effect of normal aging on both metabolic and perfusion functional imaging is controversial; lack of standardization makes interpretation of results difficult. Finally, PET imaging requires the use of an on-site cyclotron.

Summary

PET appears to be a useful tool; its ability to assess metabolic activity is unsurpassed. At present, PET may be a useful research and clinical tool. We do not use PET for all patients but rather advocate its use when standard anatomic imaging does not explain clinical concerns. Careful analysis of the equipment, the context of the interpretation, and the experience of the staff is warranted. Among its greatest promise in the future is the potential of PET to study receptor ligands and to map specific deficits. The ability to assess the effectiveness of pharmacotherapy is a significant part of its future.

Single-Photon Emission Computed Tomography

Single-photon emission computed tomography (SPECT) is a method of assessing perfusion and attempts to correlate perfusion with metabolic activity. Care must be taken because perfusion is not necessarily linked to metabolic activity in all cases. SPECT is much less expensive than PET and does not require the presence of a cyclotron. Like PET, SPECT is superior to more standard anatomic imaging in the detection of lesions.[53]

Process

During SPECT a radioligand is injected into the patient before scanning, and images are constructed via computer enhancement after radiodetection. General principles of photon emission and annihilation are similar to those discussed in the outline of PET imaging. Partial volume effects remain; geometric alignment of the scanners, number of scanning cameras, and color capability play major roles in image construction. Scanners dedicated to brain injury are certainly preferable. Multiple-headed scanners produce increased resolution of the subject. It is important to know the resolution of the particular scanner that one uses. Color vs. monochromic imaging has created a considerable controversy. Color produces more vivid prints that are easier to interpret. However, it is best to assess SPECT scans on the original screens. Original screen evaluation prevents loss of detail; thus monochromic images appear relatively equal in sensitivity. The multiple gradations of color prints involve the potential for oversensitivity and abusive interpretation (Fig. 14).

Isotopes

The isotopes in most common use are HM-PAO (Ceretec) and 123-I para iodoamphetamine (IAMP). At present, only HM-PAO is available for commercial use in the United States. Both agents are useful for perfusion scanning because of their rapid achievement of peak concentrations in the cerebral tissues: 70–90% extraction on the first pass.[54] IAMP is still a popular agent outside the United States. It provides a unique look at both immediate and delayed or "refill" perfusion. IAMP, an amphetamine-like agent, also has presynaptic and postsynaptic receptor site binding properties, which may provide another means of evaluation. IAMP has special value in evaluating perinumbral ischemic regions and in assessing patients for posttraumatic vasospasm because of its reperfusion effects. HM-PAO is almost a pure blood perfusion agent. It has the unique property of sticking to cerebral tissues and thus provides an image that represents the time at which the patient was injected.[55] This feature is advantageous in evaluating patients who are uncooperative, agitated, or experiencing seizures. Radiopharmaceuticals that can image the dopaminergic system (specifically d2 and d1 receptor antagonists) are under development. Opiate receptors have been studied with the mu-receptor

binding agent, carfentanil.[56] Such newer agents have enormous potential for assessing specific pathway deficits and documenting the efficacy of pharmacotherapy.[57]

Analysis

Like PET, SPECT can be analyzed by experienced visual observation or evaluation of regions of interest. Evaluation can be done with computer quantification of pixel counts or reporting of percent change, with the cerebellum as the baseline. Fortunately, normal scans should be relatively homogeneous throughout cortical regions. The rater's experience appears to be the most important factor in interpretation of SPECT scans.

Clinical Uses

SPECT appears to have similar uses to PET; however, its lower cost and quicker imaging time and the convenience of its radiopharmaceutical make it somewhat more user-friendly. SPECT can be used to detect seizures and to evaluate behavioral changes, depression, vasospasm, headaches, and pharmacologic efficacy. On rare occasions SPECT helps to evaluate posttraumatic occult arterial dissections, revealing perfusion abnormalities. When SPECT is used to assess patients for seizures, one must remember that interictal activity may not produce perfusion changes, although some metabolic deficits may be noted (thus the superiority of PET over SPECT in rare cases). HM-PAO allows assessment of behavioral disturbance and captures the disturbance as a moment in time.

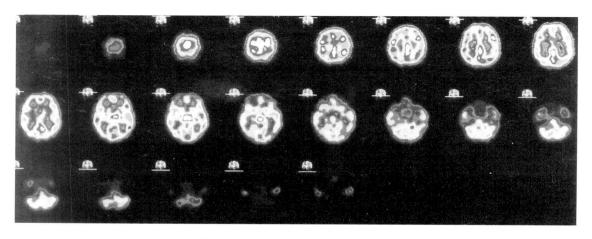

FIGURE 14. SPECT image with frontal region hypoperfusion.

Both SPECT and PET have been shown to detect lesions not seen in static imaging. Patients with persistent deficits on cognitive assessment may show regions of hypoperfusion, predominantly in the frontal and temporal regions. Frontal hypoperfusion produces persistent complaints of behavioral problems and problem-solving deficits. Further studies are clearly warranted to determine the role of functional imaging in the assessment of mild injury.[58,59]

Summary

SPECT provides a relatively quick and somewhat less expensive method for the assessment of function. Problems include limited resolution, correlation with metabolic activity, and cost. Variations in equipment and skill of interpreters leads to significant discrepancies and potential abuses.

Nuclear Ventriculography

Nuclear ventriculography (NV) is a method for diagnosing hydrocephalus and assessing shunt patency. Radiopharmaceuticals are injected intrathecally, and images are obtained at 2 hours and over the next 48 hours, as appropriate. In normal subjects, early scans show high uptake over the basal cisterns and sylvian fissures, whereas later scans show gradual transport activity over the vertex as activity in the basilar regions fall. Little activity is noted, and lack of cerebral activity at 2 hours may indicate obstruction within the thecal space. In hydrocephalus, activity in the ventricles persists well beyond 24 hours, whereas little activity is noted over the hemispheres, indicating a lack of free flow of cerebrospinal fluid.[60] This pattern tends to occur in communicating hydrocephalus, whereas noncommunicating hydrocephalus tends to show obstruction in the region of the basal cisterns. NV may be used to evaluate shunt patency. When injected into a patent shunt, a radiopharmaceutical should be delivered rapidly into the circulation. If the shunt is obstructed, the radiopharmaceutical accumulates in the reservoir of the shunt. NV may be enhanced for assessment of rhinorrhoea and fistula formation.

Transcranial Doppler Ultrasound

Since its development in the early 1980s, transcranial Doppler ultrasound has improved remarkably its ability to measure cerebral blood flow in a noninvasive manner. Accurate and reproducible evaluations of blood flow velocity and vascular diameter are easily accomplished.[61] Transcranial Doppler ultrasound has become an increasingly important method for the detection of vasospasm in patients with subarachnoid hemorrhage. Newer applications include assessment of cerebral blood volume.[62]

FUNCTIONAL OUTCOME PREDICTION: STATIC AND FUNCTIONAL IMAGING

Static anatomic imaging (CT and MRI) has been most valuable in assessing patients with traumatic brain injury for acute lesion phenomena and in determining the need for intervention. Much of the literature has focused on acute mortality outcomes and/or measures determined by the Glasgow Outcome Scale. Early studies determined that patients with cisternal compression have a worse prognosis.[63] As expected, large focal lesions have a higher incidence of motor loss, and patients with herniation syndromes have a higher mortality rate.[64,65] Most studies focus on the ability to predict survival or vegetive status.

CT imaging has distinct limitations, and a single CT scan may be less predictive than clinical examination.[66] Thatcher did not find a strong link between CT and Disability Rating Scale status.[67] Van Dongen noted that bilateral cisternal compression and lesions of the brain parenchyma are the best prognostic factors in comatose patients.[68] Reider-Grosswasser noted that late CT findings of an abnormal third ventricle ratio correspond with cognitive and behavioral disturbance.[69] A small study at our institution indicated that the worst CT image within 72 hours has little predictive capability for functional outcome in in-patient rehabilitation.[70]

MRI may be a more appropriate method to assess severity of diffuse axonal injury, yet few studies look at long-term outcomes. MRI has also been found superior for assessing more chronic lesions, contusions, and posterior fossa lesions.[71] Levin reviewed the MRI findings of patients with mild or moderate injury. The predominance of frontal and temporal lesions correlated with neuropsychologic testing, and deficits appeared to improve with visual resolution of the lesion on MRI scan.[72] Lesion site, as imaged by MRI, appears to be related to neuropsychological deficit.[73] Few definitive studies examine the role of MRI in predicting functional outcome, either at admission to rehabilitation or at community integration. Static imaging appears to be a good predictor of acute survival and helps to determine which patients may experience further deficits, but more detailed evaluation and studies are clearly needed to increase the prognostic capabilities of static examinations.

Functional imaging has been evaluated in even fewer studies, but it shows great promise because it images relatively true activity. Magnetoencephalography and magnetic source imaging are new venues for predicting functional and cognitive performance.[74,75] An initial study in Kuwait demonstrated that SPECT was superior in determining lesion size and in identifying patients with poor outcomes (death or vegetative state).[76] Patients who remain in lower-level states have been noted to have profound and significant decrease in metabolism, as assessed by PET imaging. Continued study of the role of promising modalities in determining functional prognosis is warranted.

REFERENCES

1. Ossman CB: Basic radiological principles of computed tomography. In Gonzales CF, Grossman CB, Masdeu JC (eds): Head and Spine Imaging. New York, John Wiley & Sons, 1985, pp 43–47.
2. Chuang SH, Fitz CR: Computed tomography of head trauma. In Gonzalez CF, Grossman CB, Masdeu JC (eds): Head and Spine Imaging. New York, John Wiley & Sons, 1985, p 525.
3. New PFJ, Aronow S: Attenuation measurements of whole blood and blood fractions in computed tomography. Radiology 121:635–640, 1976.
4. Norman D, Axel L, Berninger W, et al: Dynamic computed tomography of the brain: Techniques, data analysis and applications. AJR 136:759–770, 1981.
5. Zimmerman RA, Bilaniuak LT: Computed tomographic staging of traumatic epidural bleeding. Radiology 144:809–812, 1982.
6. Reed D, Robertson W, Graeb D, et al: Acute subdural hematomas. Atypical CT findings. AJNR 7:417–421, 1986.
7. Levy M, Rezei A, Masri L, Litofsky S, et al: The significance of subarachnoid hemorrhage after penetrating craniocerebral injury: Correlations with angiography and outcome in a civilian population. Neurosurgery 32:532–540, 1993.
8. Eisenberg H, Gary H, Aldrich E, et al: Initial CT findings in 753 patients with severe head injury. J Neurosurg 73:688–698, 1990.
9. Grolimund P, Weber M, Seiler R, et al: Time course of cerebral vasospasm after severe head injury. Lancet 2:1173, 1988.
10. Suwanela C, Suwanela N: Intracranial arterial narrowing and spasm in acute head injury. J Neurosurg 36:314–323, 1972.
11. Cusamano F, Bertolino GT, Pichezzi P, et al: Computed tomography in severe head trauma. Acta Neurol 7:1114–1120, 1985.
12. French B, Dublin A: The value of computerized tomography in the management of 1000 consecutive head injuries. Surg Neurol 7:171–183, 1983.
13. Bradley W: Pathophysiologic correlates of signal alteration. In Brandt-Zawadzkim, Norman D (eds): Magnetic Resonance Imaging of the Central Nervous System. New York, Raven Press, 1987.
14. Zimmerman R, Bilanick L, Hackney D, et al: Head injury: Early results of comparing CT and high field MR. AJNR 7:757–761, 1986.
15. Zimmerman R, Bilaniuk L, Gennerelli T: Computed tomography of shearing injuries of the cerebral white matter. Radiology 127:393–396, 1978.
16. Gennerelli T, Thiabult L, Adams J, Graham J: Diffuse axonal injury and traumatic coma in the primate. Ann Neurol 12:546–574, 1986.
17. Sasiadek M, Marciniak R, Bem Z: CT appearance of shearing injuries of the brain. Bildgebung 58(3):148–149, 1991.
18. Marshall L, Marshall S, Klauber M, et al: A new classification system of head injury based on computerized tomography. J Neurosurg 75:S14–S20, 1991.
19. Grossman CB: Hydrocephalus and atrophic and degenerative disorders. In Magnetic Resonance Imaging and Computed Tomography of the Head and Spine. Baltimore, Williams & Wilkins, 1990.
20. Benson D, Le May M, Patten D: Diagnosis of normal pressure hydrocephalus. N Engl J Med 283:609–615, 1970.
21. Gonzalez C, Reyes P: Hydrocephalus, atrophic and degenerative disorders. In Gonzalez C, Grossman C, Masdeu J (eds): Head and Spine Imaging. New York, John Wiley & Sons, 1985, pp 435–450.
22. Grossman CB: Cranial and intracranial trauma. In Magnetic Resonance Imaging and Computed Tomography of the Head and Spine. Baltimore, Williams & Wilkins, 1990.
23. Steinhoff H, Lange S: Principles of contrast enhancement in computerized tomography. In Lanksch W, Kazner E (eds): Cranial Computerized Tomography. Berlin, Springer-Verlag, 1976, pp 60–88.

23a. Mirivis SE, Wolf AL, Numaguchi Y, et al: Posttraumatic cerebral infarction diagnosed by CT: Prevalence, origin, and outcome. AJR 154: 1293–1298, 1990.

24. Katyama Y, Tsubokawa T, Miyazaki S, et al: Oedema fluid formation within contused brain tissue as a cause of medically uncontrollable elevation of intracranial pressure: The role of surgical therapy. Acta Neurochir Suppl (Wein) 51:308–310, 1990.

25. Levi L, Borovich B, Guilburd J, et al: Wartime neurosurgical experience in Lebanon: Craniocerebral injuries. Isr J Med Sci 26:555–558, 1990.

26. Kane N, Jamjoom A, Temiory M: Penetrating orbitocranial injury. Injury 22:326–327, 1991.

27. Shaffery ME, Polin RS, Phillips C, et al: Classification of civilian craniocerebral gunshot wounds. A multivariate analysis predictive of mortality. Neurotrauma 9(Suppl):S279–S285, 1992.

28. Orrison WW, Gentry L, Stimac GD: Comparison of cranial CT and MR in closed head injury evaluation. AJR 15:351–356, 1994.

29. Carlson J, Arakawa M, Kaufman L, et al: Depth focused radiofrequency coils from MR imaging. Radiology 165:251–255, 1987.

30. Jacobsen HG: Fundamentals of magnetic resonance imaging. JAMA 258:3417–3423, 1987.

31. Balter S: An introduction to the physics of magnetic resonance imaging. Radiographics 7:371–383, 1987.

32. Wehrli F, Mac Fall J, Newton T: Parameters determining the appearance of NMR images. GE Publications, 1984.

33. Drayer B, Burger P, Darwin R: Magnetic resonance imaging of brain iron. AJNR 7:373–380, 1986.

34. Pusey E, Lufkin R, Brown R, et al; Magnetic resonance imaging artifacts: Mechanism and clinical significance. Radiographics 6:891–911, 1986.

35. Lusine J, Levy E: MRI documentation of hemorrhage into post-traumatic subdural hygromas. Mt Sinai J Med 60:161–162, 1993.

36. Salcman M, Pevsner P: Value of MRI in head injury. Comparison with CT. Neurochirurgie 38:329–332, 1992.

37. Derosier C, Brinquin L, Bonsignour J, et al: MRI and cranial trauma in the acute phase. J Neuroradiol 18:309–319, 1991.

38. Adams A, Mitchell G, Graham D, et al: Diffuse brain damage of immediate impact type: Its relationship to primary brain stem damage in head injury. Brain 100:489–502, 1977.

39. Sasiadek M, Marcinicak R, Bem Z: CT appearance of shearing injuries of the brain. Bildgebung 58(3):148–149, 1991.

40. Levi L, Guilburd J, Lemberger A, et al: Diffuse axonal injury analysis of 100 patients with radiologic signs. Neurosurgery 27:429–432, 1990.

41. Levy ML, Rezae A, Masri L, et al: The significance of subarachnoid hemorrhage after penetrating craniocerebral injury: Correlations with angiography and outcome in a civilian population. Neurosurgery 32(4):532–540, 1993.

42. Sklar E, Quencer R, Bowen B, et al: Magnetic resonance applications in cerebral injury. Radiol Clin North Am 30:353–366, 1992.

43. El Gammal T, Allen M, Brooks B, et al: Evaluation of hydrocephalus. AJNR 8:591–597, 1987.

44. Bradley W: Pathophysiologic correlates of signal alterations. In Brant-Zawadzki M, Norman D (eds): Magnetic Resonance Imaging of Nervous System. New York, Raven Press, 1987, pp 23–42.

45. Sutton D: Interventional radiology. In A Textbook of Radiology and Imaging. New York, Churchill Livingstone, 1993, pp 1445–1498.

46. Theodore W, Fishbein D, Larson S: Neuroimaging in refractory partial seizures: Comparison of PET, CT, and MRI. Neurology 36:750–759, 1986.

47. Frost J, Mayberg H, Doglass K, et al: Alterations in cerebral mu-opiate receptors in temporal lobe epilepsy and following ECT. J Cereb Blood Flow Metab 7(Suppl):421, 1987.

48. Levy D, Sitidis J, Rottenberg: Differences in cerebral blood flow and glucose utilization in vegetive versus locked in patients. Ann Neurol 122:673–682, 1987.

49. Alavi A: Functional and anatomic studies of head injury. J Neuropsych 1(Suppl):S45–S50, 1989.

50. Ichise M, Chung D, Wang P, et al: Technetium-99m-HMPAO SPECT, CT and MRI in the evaluation of patients with chronic traumatic brain injury: A correlation with neuropsychological performance. J Nucl Med 35:217–226, 1994.

51. Moseley I, Sutton D, Kendall B, et al: Intracranial lesions. In A Textbook of Radiology and Imaging. New York, Churchill Livingstone, 1993, pp 1499–1574.

52. Engel J: The use of PET scanning in epilepsy. Ann Neurol 15(Suppl):S180–S191, 1984.

53. Prayer L, Wimberger D, Oder W, et al: Cranial MR imaging and cerebral 99mtc HM-PAO-SPECT in patients with subacute or chronic severe closed head injury and normal CT examinations. Acta Radiol 4:593–599, 1993.

54. Kuhl D, Barrio J, Huang S, et al: Quantifying local cerebral blood flow by N-isopropyl(123-I) iodoamphetamine (IMP) tomography. J Nucl Med 23:196–203, 1982.

55. Ell P, Hocknell J, Costa D, et al: A new regional cerebral blood flow agent with 99mTc-labelled compound. Lancet 2:50–51, 1985.

56. Frost J, Mayberg H, Fisher R, et al: Relationship of opiate receptor binding and temporal lobe epilepsy using C-11 carfentanil. J Nucl Med 27:1027, 1986.

57. Kojima A, Tsuji A, Takaki Y, et al: Correction of scattered photons in Tc-99m imaging by means of a photopeak dual-energy window acquisition. Ann Nucl Med 6(3):153–158, 1992.

58. Gray B, Ichise M, Chung D, et al: Technetium-99M-HMPAO SPECT in the evaluation of patients with a remote history of traumatic brain injury: A comparison with x-ray computed tomography. J Nucl Med 33(1):52–58, 1992.

59. Newton M, Greenwood R, Britton K, et al: A study comparing SPECT with CT and MRI after closed head injury. J Neurol Neurosurg Psychiatry 55:92–94, 1992.

60. Davies E: Radionuclide scanning. In Davies E (ed): A Textbook of Radiology and Imaging. New York, Churchill Livingstone, 1993, pp 1572–1574.

61. Newell D, Aaslid R: Transcranial Doppler: Clinical and experimental uses. Cerebrovasc Brain Metab Rev 4:122–143, 1992.

62. Chan K, Dearden N, Miller J: The significance of posttraumatic increase in cerebral blood flow velocity: A transcranial Doppler ultrasound study. Neurosurgery 30:697–700, 1992.

63. Toutant S, Klauber M, Marshall L, et al; Absent or compressed basal cisterns on first CT scan: Ominous predictors of outcome in severe head injury. J Neurosurg 61:691–694, 1984.

64. Sweet R, Miller J, Lipper M, et al: Significance of bilateral abnormalities on CT scan in patients with severe head injury. Neurosurgery 3:16–21, 1978.

65. Murphy A, Teasdale G, Matheson M, et al: Relationship between CT indices of brain swelling and intracranial pressure after head injury. In Ishii S, Nagai H, Brock M (eds): Intracranial Pressure. Berlin, Springer-Verlag, 1983, pp 562–566.

66. Naryan R, Greenburg R, Miller J, et al: Improved confidence of outcome prediction in severe head injury: A comparative analysis of the clinical examination, multimodality evoked potentials, CT scanning, and intracranial pressure. J Neurosurg 54:751–762, 1981.

67. Thatcher R, Cantor D, McAlaster, et al: Comprehensive predictions of outcome in closed head-injured patients. Ann N Y Acad Sci 82–101, 1991.

68. Van Dongen K, Braakman R, Gelpke G: The prognostic value of computerized tomography in comatose head-injured patients. J Neurosurg 59:951–957, 1983.

69. Reider-Grosswasser I, Cohen M, et al: Late CT findings in brain trauma: Relationship to cognitive and behavioral sequelae and to vocational outcome. AJR 160:147–152, 1993.

70. Zafonte R, Atty E, Dade R, et al: Neuroimaging classification in TBI: Predictors of functional status. Arch Phys Med Rehabil 74:1279, 1993.

71. Gentry L, Godersky J, Thompson B, et al: Prospective comparative study of intermediate field MR and CT in the evaluation of closed head trauma. AJR 150:673–682, 1988.

72. Levin H, Williams D, Crofford M, et al: Relationship of depth of brain lesions to consciousness and outcome after closed head injury. J Neurosurg 69:861–866, 1988.

73. Wilson J, Wiedman K, Hadley D, et al: Early and late magnetic resonance imaging and neuropsychological outcome after head injury. J Neurol Neurosurg Psychiatry 51:391–396, 1988.

74. Schwartz B, Gallen C, Aung M, et al: Magnetoencephalographic detection of focal slowing associated with head trauma [abstract]. Biomag 93, Vienna 48–49, 1993.

75. Lewine JD: Magnetoencephalography and magnetic source imaging. In Orrison W, Lewine J, Sanders J, Hartshore M (eds): Functional Brain Imaging. St. Louis, Mosby, 1994, pp 82–102.

76. Abdel-Dayem H, Sade K, Kouris K: Changes in cerebral perfusion after acute head injury: Comparison of CT with tc-99HMPAO SPECT. Radiology 165:221–226, 1987.

11

Electrophysiologic Assessment

This chapter focuses on evoked potential (EP) findings in traumatic brain injury (TBI). The EP technique can help to evaluate the extent and severity of brain and other central nervous system (CNS) or sensory impairments. It can also help in predicting outcome among patients with brain injury.

WHAT ARE EVOKED POTENTIALS?

Evoked potentials (EPs) as used in this chapter refer to electrophysiologic and neuropsychologic central nervous system responses to either external stimulation of one or more sensory modalities or to internally generated brain responses associated with the processing of information precognitively or cognitively. EPs can be obtained upon stimulation of various senses, such as sight, hearing, smell, taste, and balance. In addition they can be obtained by stimulating receptors for touch, pain, heat, and vibration. They are also obtained upon requiring individuals to carry out various cognitive tasks such as counting, recognizing, or detecting differences between stimuli and even recognizing the absence of a sensory stimulus.

Many variables affect the physical characteristics of EP patterns, including patient variables such as age, sex, and physical, neurologic, and psychological status as well as medication and other drug substances (e.g., alcohol, marijuana, cocaine). In addition, both voluntary and involuntary muscle activity and various physiologic activities such as heart rate and eye movements can affect EP patterns. Equipment characteristics such as type of electrode, electrode locations, and equipment recording parameters (e.g., gain, sensitivity, and bandpass settings) can affect EPs. Signal characteristics, including stimulus intensity and duration, stimulus modality, temporal sequencing, stimulus probability, and external electrical interference, also affect EP patterns. Damage to the CNS, whatever the cause (traumatic injury, anoxia, infection, congenital abnormalities, tumors, hydrocephalus, drug use or drug abuse), can also affect the configuration of EP patterns.

EP pattern characteristics that may be affected are the latencies of various peaks, conduction times between peaks, peak amplitudes, pattern configurations, pattern symmetry, and pattern replicability upon repeat stimulation.

When working with long-latency EP patterns (up to 500 msec or greater after stimulus onset), variability is relatively high from run to run. Consequently, relatively small effects, such as those of drugs, are not readily detectable. When working with persons with severe head injury, drug effects do not constitute a major problem for interpretation in most patients, because one is searching for changes in brain function much greater than the relatively subtle effects associated with medications commonly used for pain, tranquilization, sleep, spasticity, and epileptiform activity. These and other chemical substances (such as alcohol and a number of illegal drugs), however, can be important when examining short-latency (< 30 msec) EP responses. Relatively large changes and nonsubtle effects on long-latency cortical evoked responses in patients with severe brain injury are associated with damage or death of large numbers of neurons, destruction of white matter, intracranial pressure associated with hematomas, hydrocephalus and displaced brain tissue, or effects associated with major toxic, inflammatory, edematous, or infectious processes.

The overall gestalt of EP patterns, including left-right assymmetry and anterior-posterior voltage differences, yields useful information about the location, extent, and severity of brain dysfunction, particularly in patients with severely traumatized brain injury.

HOW ARE EVOKED POTENTIALS OBTAINED?

The theory behind EPs stems from signal-averaging considerations, a technique that has been used for some time in the physical sciences. When a signal is quite small, such as a few millionths of a volt produced by the brain when it is stimulated, it cannot be detected readily, particularly when it is buried in the larger thousandth of a volt produced by ongoing background electroencephalographic activity. A signal-averaging technique, however, allows extraction of the smaller signal. By presenting a signal repeatedly and measuring the brain's electrical activity each time for a short, fixed duration after onset of the signal (e.g., a brief

auditory tone, a brief flash of light, or a brief tactile stimulation of the skin), it is possible to acquire and obtain an average of the brain's response to repeated stimulation. In the course of this signal-averaging procedure, the background electrical activity of the brain behaves approximately like random noise. In other words, for every positive-going electrical potential there is also, in general, a negative-going electrical potential; therefore, signals tend to cancel each other. The evoked pattern of brain electrical potentials based on the averaging of repeated stimulus presentations that yield consistent electrophysiologic brain responses, however, will become increasingly robust and emerge from the background brain activity, which becomes less prominent because of the canceling process just described. In this context the lily emerges from the mud. One can then begin to study and analyze the configuration of EP patterns under different conditions for different subjects.

General Methodologic Considerations

Position. A patient may be tested sitting up, lying down, or in any position. The main consideration is to have the patient as relaxed as possible. This minimizes muscle artifact and the relatively large muscle-generated voltages that mask and distort the smaller voltages emanating from the brain.

Sedation. At times it is necessary to introduce sedation by using small amounts of medication such as chloral hydrate (500–1000 mg), diphenhydramine hydrochloride (25 or 50 mg), or diazepam (5, 10, or 20 mg) about 30 minutes before testing. As mentioned above, such medications do not seriously interfere with pattern interpretations, particularly interpretations of long-latency cortical responses, in patients with severe brain damage. Long-latency cortical EP patterns, though suppressed, are even readable in pentobarbital coma.[115,137]

Limitations. Skull topography after head injury sometimes makes it difficult to place electrodes in accordance with the 10-20 system[80]—a system that specifies placement of scalp recording electrodes (Fig. 1). Patient inability to cooperate in the testing, much muscle and movement artifact, and the pulling off of electrodes also make it difficult at times to test patients with TBI. Because of such difficulties it is often necessary to use the smallest number of scalp and other electrodes that is consistent with obtaining useful and readable EP patterns. From a practical point of view testing should be completed in a reasonable time—the "reasonableness" being related to the physical and mental status of the patient. The technician should have special training in obtaining long-latency evoked potentials in addition to training in obtaining short-and intermediate-latency responses. The technician must be patient and understanding with a high frustration tolerance. The interpreting physician also needs special orientation and training before attempting to read, interpret, and integrate the meaning of multimodality late cortical EP responses. The management of a rehabilitation facility must understand enough about the evoked potential procedure to be willing to support the cost of equipment and maintenance as well as the required personnel and ongoing educational expenses. Another important limitation is reflected in the need for additional short-, intermediate-, and long-term follow-up studies to establish firmly the reliability and validity of EP patterns in predicting outcome among patients who have experienced severe brain trauma.

Differences in methods used by various investigators also constitute an important limitation. Analyses of short-latency EP responses that reflect sensory afferent data do not yield the same information as attempts to analyze long-latency data that reflect corticocortical connections and higher level cognitive activities. Even the definition of "long latency" varies. Ahmed's[3] long latency is 40 msec and Yamada's[189] is 113 msec; whereas Pfurtscheller et al.'s[127] extends to 200 msec, Keren et al.'s[86] to 250 msec, and Greenberg et al.'s[64] and Rappaport et al.'s[134] to 500 msec. Other values fall between, and longer values are also used.

Differences in the sensitivity of tools and techniques used to evaluate the clinical condition of patients who have sustained traumatic brain injury also affect findings. For

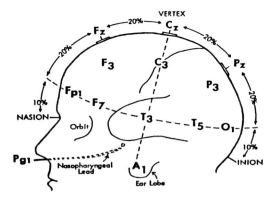

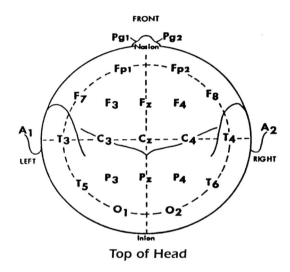

FIGURE 1. International (10-20) scalp recording electrode placements. (By permission of Ellen R. Grass, Grass Instruments Co.)

example, Keren et al.[86] indicate that the long-latency somatosensory EP (SEP) response was not particularly helpful in predicting outcome in patients with prolonged postcomatose unawareness after traumatic brain injury. On the other hand, Pfurtscheller et al.,[127] Greenberg et al.,[64] and Rappaport et al.[134] found significant relationships between long-latency evoked potential patterns and clinical outcome. Both Pfurtscheller et al. and Rappaport et al. noted that long-latency SEPs are more sensitive to outcome in patients with severe disabilities, whereas short-latency SEPs may be more sensitive in some patients with relatively mild disabilities associated with brain trauma.

The method of measurement of the degree of abnormality of long-latency EP patterns also affects findings. For example, Greenberg et al.[64] and Rappaport et al.[135] used a fairly systematic method of rating abnormality for which interrater reliability can be established. Keren et al.[86] did not. Outcome measurement scales are also differentially sensitive, as reported by Rappaport et al.[135] For example, the Disability Rating Scale (1982) is more highly correlated with clinical condition than the Glasgow Coma and Outcome Scales,[67,135,171] particularly when tracking patients with severe traumatic brain injury over extended periods. More informative comparisons of EP findings in patients with TBI require the establishment of accepted standards for short-, intermediate-, and long-latency EP testing, evaluation of EP abnormalities, and evaluation of patients' clinical condition at the time of testing and follow-up.

Stimuli

Auditory. To obtain auditory nerve and brainstem responses, brief (100-μsec) clicks are presented at a rate of 10 per second at a loudness of about 80 db until the responses to 2000 clicks have been averaged. Rate of presentation can be varied up to about 25 clicks per second without major changes in peak latencies or central conduction times. When multiple sclerosis is suspected, an auditory "stress" test can be performed in which 70 or more clicks per second are presented to determine whether there is a breakdown in the transmission of auditory information. Higher stimulation rates result in an increase in peak latencies in normal subjects. Intensity affects peak latencies. As the signal intensity is increased, latency decreases, particularly for peak V, which occurs usually less than 6 msec after stimulus onset at 80 db. The peak V response is thought to originate in the midbrain (mesencephalon) in the area of the inferior colliculus. Normal variations in brainstem responses have been reported by Chiappa et al.[24]

As described in greater detail below, the relationship between stimulus intensity and peak latency can be used to detect not only the approximate hearing threshold but also different types of hearing impairments, such as impairments in bone conduction or sensorineural hearing loss. Tones can be used instead of clicks in certain situations (described below) but not to obtain auditory nerve and brainstem responses. The length of time needed to present tones overshadows and obscures auditory nerve and brainstem responses, which require very brief inputs for best results.

Visual. As discussed in more detail below, visual stimuli may be presented to one eye at a time as either quickly changing or shifting checkerboard patterns (pattern reversal [PR]) on a televisionlike monitor or as brief (e.g., 10-msec) flashes of light that can be presented either on a monitor or by using special goggles. Either an eyepatch or independently controllable goggles are used to obscure the eye not being tested. In PR testing, check size, field size, light intensity, contrast, and pupil dilation can influence the EP configuration. Usually 100–200 stimuli are presented to each eye, and the evoked brain responses are averaged.

Pattern reversal EPs can be used to evaluate acuity of vision and detection of field defects (for example, those associated with tumor pressure on the optic chiasm), retinal responsivity, disease processes such as optic neuritis, multiple sclerosis, and neuropathy associated with diabetes mellitus or other neuropathologic conditions. Flash EPs provide less specific information. They can indicate whether there is peripheral responsivity to light stimulation, transmission of light information through the optic pathways to the cortex, and the degree of abnormality of cortical responses. Flash EPs do not provide information about visual acuity.

Somatosensory. Somatosensory evoked potential (SEP) stimuli, which are discussed in more detail below, usually consist of briefly presented electrical square wave pulses (usually 200–400 μsec) via stimulating electrodes applied to various parts of the body such as the wrist, ankle, or knee. Stimuli usually are presented at an intensity of about 2 milliamperes (ma) above motor threshold (at which a reflex motor response is observed in the tested limb). Sensation threshold (at which an individual reports awareness of stimulation) is noted before the motor threshold is reached. Stimulation is nonnoxious and well tolerated unless one deliberately seeks information in response to pain by increasing the intensity of the stimulus. Depending on the somatosensory response to be evaluated, the number of repeat stimulations that are averaged usually ranges between 100 and 500.

Prior to stimulation the skin must be prepared. Cleansing removes surface debris, and electrode jelly is used to facilitate the transmission of each brief pulse. Stimulating electrodes are then secured with tape to ensure good contact with the skin. A number of suitable stimulating electrodes are available commercially. Caution must be used to make sure that the gels at the positive and negative electrodes do not make contact. The positive electrode should be distal. Caution also must be exercised in placing electrodes to ensure that current is not transmitted across the cardiac region. Proper electrical grounding must be used. During testing the patient must be isolated from the current source. Modern equipment is designed to take into account these safeguards. Needle stimulating electrodes placed subcutaneously may be used, when appropriate, instead of surface stimulating electrodes.

Somatosensory EPs provide information not only about sensory and motor thresholds but also about transmission times from the periphery (e.g., the upper or lower extremities, face, spinal areas, and other areas of interest) to and through the spinal cord to subcortical and cortical areas of the brain. Latency and amplitude findings can be compared with known normative data to determine the location and degree of impairment as well as left-right side difference.

Pain. A number of SEP-type studies have been undertaken to examine the relationship between EP patterns and pain.[10,20,22,70,79,109,166,167] Although various pain-inducing stimuli have been used, electrical short-duration stimulus pulses of different intensities appear to be the most common. Electrical stimuli have been applied to tooth pulp, fingertips, and various dermatomal sites on the upper and lower extremities. EP patterns in response to

pain have been elicited by laser stimuli.[17,94] Pain responses also have been induced in olfactory studies by stimulating the trigeminal nerve with carbon dioxide (CO_2). Pain responses have been the basis for evaluating analgesic substances such as pentazocine, aspirin, and ibuprofen.[76,89] Becker, Yingling, and Fein[10] suggested that in studying responses to painful stimuli three components must be distinguished: pain stimuli per se, stimulus intensity below the pain threshold, and the cognitive component reflected in the P300 response. Peak latency and topographic overlap in these components cause difficulties of interpretation. Nonetheless, Becker et al.[10] reported that the pain and intensity components associated with somatosensory stimulation are larger at Cz than Pz and occur within the window 260–360 msec, whereas the P300 component is larger at Pz than Cz and occurs later, at about 400 msec. Kunde and Treede[94] found that the mean peak latency for pain from a heat laser stimulus was longer than the latency for electrically induced pain (176 msec vs. 110 msec, respectively). At these latencies, which are not in the window identified by Becker et al., maximal responses were found in the parietotemporal-temporal region contralateral to the side of stimulation. Again, the topographic location is different from that described by Becker et al.,[10] according to whom responses may have been generated in the secondary somatosensory cortex.

Kakigi et al.[84] reported a large positive component at P320 when obtaining pain-related somatosensory EPs upon stimulation with a CO_2 laser. They indicated, however, that pain-specific cognition may have been involved. This theory appears likely in light of findings by other investigators mentioned above. Bromm et al.[17] reported that laser heat stimulation applied to hairy skin is able "to objectify disturbances in the pain and temperature senses." The investigators noted no alteration in SEPs obtained by conventional electrical nerve stimulation. Although they state that cutaneous heat stimuli "did not correspond to the severity of the subjectively reported sensory deficit," it may be possible to develop this technique further for use in evaluating the sensory status of persons with brain injury. Rosenfeld et al.[152] reported that the P300 amplitude decreases and latencies increase as pain is increased. Wright et al.[188] reported that SEP amplitudes correlated with changes in the perception of pain. Lekic et al.[97] related pain to tooth pulp evoked potentials and found shorter latencies in patients suffering from trigeminal neuralgia and higher amplitudes on the affected side. Patients with thalamic lesions and decreased touch and vibration sensibility are reported to show relatively large effects on SEP patterns obtained upon stimulation of the median and tibial nerves.[74]

In most pain studies, subjects are alert and can indicate the degree of their discomfort. Indication of discomfort may be a problem in some patients with brain injury, particularly those with severe brain injury. Ethical considerations are also involved in dealing with painful stimuli. At present we appear limited in observing clinical responses to short-duration discomforting stimuli administered in the course of neurologic examination or specified in various disability rating scales.[136,146] In light of peak latency overlap, it appears impractical to distinguish a pain response from a typical SEP response in patients with severe head injury who cannot reliably report their subjective experience. The trigeminal pain response in olfactory assessment is a possibility but seems to require so many controls (see olfactory section below) that it may not offer a practical approach, except possibly in cooperative individuals with mild head injury. Only future research will determine whether, ultimately, we can extract useful information about specific responsivity to pain by EP testing of persons with brain injury.

N18.   The N18 peak is obtained by SEP testing of the median nerve at the wrist. It is useful in determining the approximate level of damage in the subcortical portion of the CNS. Its exact origin is controversial. Urasaki et al.[176] found a decreased or absent N18 amplitude "in patients with midbrain pontine lesions but not in those with thalamic or putaminal lesions." In another study[177] Urasaki et al. found that upon stimulation of the posterior tibial nerve and median nerve changes in P30 and N33 (peaks generated by stimulation of the lower extremity) correlated with

those of P14 and N18 (peaks generated by stimulation of the upper extremity). They concluded that scalp P30 and P14 originate from activity near dorsal column nuclei, whereas N33 and N18 originate from the brainstem below the thalamus. In still another study,[178] Urasaki et al. implanted depth electrodes in epileptic patients and suggested that N18a and N18b originate in "the upper pons to midbrain region which projects to the rostral subcortical white matter of the frontal lobe." Based on their study of median nerve responses in normal subjects and in patients with high cervical, brainstem, and thalamic lesions, Sonoo et al.[161] concluded that it is "most probable the main part of N18 corresponds to the ventro-rostral negative pole of the dipolar potential generated at the cuneate nucleus." Although the exact origin of N18 is still uncertain, these conclusions represent progress in our knowledge. At one time it was thought that N18 was associated primarily with thalamic or thalamocortical activity.

Other Modality Stimulation.   Smell, taste, and equilibrium functions also can be tested. At this time they are quite limited in helping to evaluate persons with traumatic brain injury.

Smell.   Evoked potential responses can be elicited by stimulating the olfactory modality by various techniques.[38] Increasing olfactory deficits correlate with increasing severity of brain injury—with deficits reported in 20–30% of patients with brain injury. Epidemiologic data are presented by Constanzo and Zasler.[31] Hummel and Kobal[77] showed differences in the topographic representation of EP responses to olfactory substances such as vanillin and acetaldehyde compared with trigeminal substances such as ammonia and sulfur dioxide. Parietocentral sites appear to be involved for olfactory substances, whereas the vertex area appears to be involved for trigeminal substances.[77] It is difficult, however, to determine the exact source of olfactory stimulation because of the frequent overlap of stimulation of olfactory and somatosensory systems. Contamination of less than rigidly controlled olfactory studies by thermal, mechanical, and other extraneous stimuli, such as those that cause pain (see above) makes interpretation difficult. Habituation is another problem that must be considered in olfactory testing.

Nevertheless, Hummel and Kobal[77] offer the opinion that further investigations of the topographic distribution of cortical SEPs may help to evaluate olfactory disturbances. They demonstrated that olfactory evoked potentials (OEP) are sensitive to the concentration of odorous substances and that this sensitivity is reflected in the amplitude ratio N1/P2. With increased concentration there is also a decrease in the latencies of peaks N1 (at about 485 msec) and P2 (at about 650 msec). No latency differences were found among the four odorants tested. They found that all of 30 patients who suffered frontobasal craniocerebral trauma had a complete loss of smell and could not respond to vanillin or hydrogen sulfide. There was, however, a response to CO_2, mediated, as mentioned above, by the trigeminal nerve.[90] Because of this differentiation the investigators concluded that OEPs "constitute a specific tool suitable for investigating the olfactory system."

Auffermann, Gerul and Mathe[8] reported objective diagnosis of olfaction by using a combination of contingent negative variation of (CNV; discussed below) and OEP. Their approach requires a relatively wide window of about 2.6 seconds. They report that anosmia can be determined by both CNV and OEP, although CNV shows less variability. Parosmia "is accessible by CNV only." Hyposmia can also be detected when the odor is just above the threshold, but the CNV amplitude "tends to be large whereas OEP amplitudes may be undetectable." Because of the relative difficulty of OEP testing, which requires instructing subjects to breathe in a special way (velopharyngeal closure to avoid respiratory flow of air inside the nasal cavity) and to attend carefully to the stimuli, routine olfactory testing of patients with severe brain injury appears to involve practical difficulties. Hummel and Kobal[77] conclude that "the diagnosis of patients suffering from olfactory disturbances . . . remains a problem despite . . . methodological advances."

Taste.   The incidence of gustatory impairment after brain injury is much lower than the incidence of olfactory impairment. Constanzo and Zasler[31] report the incidence to be less than 0.5%. Doty[38] described various nonevoked response techniques for evaluating regional responses on the tongue to different gustatory stimuli. Plattig[129] discussed gustatory evoked potentials and electrogustometry techniques, reporting differential gustatory evoked potentials (GEPs) with different substances such as sodium chloride, tartaric acid, sucrose, and quinine hydrogen chloride. GEPs are also sensitive to different concentrations. Response times vary widely. For sweet stimuli, the response time is 1540 msec; for bitter, 1530 msec; for salty, 370 msec; and for sour, 410 msec. The GEP response can be influenced by the galvanic skin response. Fewer stimulations, however, appear to be needed than, for example, with auditory brainstem evoked potentials (24 vs. 2000 repetitions, respectively). In gustatory testing as well as in olfactory and vestibular EP testing (discussed below) the technical problems pose a barrier to routine testing of patients with brain injury, mild or severe. Requirements in terms of apparatus, time, sustained attention, and controls to prevent contamination from olfactory, tactile, temperature, and other concomitant stimuli are among the factors that have to be considered. A special laboratory environment geared to this type of testing is needed.

Vestibular Function.   Parker[122] described a number of nonevoked potential methods for evaluating vestibular function, including electronystagmorgraphy, oculomotor screening, positional testing, caloric stimulation, rotational testing, and dynamic posturography. Few articles address evoked potential responses to vestibular stimulation. Short-latency vestibular evoked responses to acceleration stimuli have been recorded in 10 normal as well as 3 deaf individuals with impaired vestibular function. Elidan et al.[46] report that short-latency peaks were measured at 3.5, 6.0, and 8.4 msec, whereas middle-latency peaks occurred at 8.8, 18.8, and 26.8 msec. The subjects with vestibular impairment did not show clear and consistent middle-latency responses. One study of a cat reported that the major site of initiation of the short-latency vestibular response associated with angular acceleration is the crista ampullaris of the lateral semicircular canal.[99]

A search of the literature reveals little information about tests of vestibular function in persons with head injury. The nature of the test (sudden acceleration and deceleration) may be helpful in cooperative patients with mild head injury. In all likelihood this type of vestibular function test would not be suitable for many patients with severe head injury. Furthermore, the yield does not appear promising if the results of Durrant and Furman[43] are replicated and remain valid. They found no difference in long-latency rotational evoked potentials (LLREP) between normal subjects and patients with bilateral vestibular loss. They concluded that LLREPs elicited by using a conventional rotary chair were not of vestibular origin but probably reflected somatosensory components. They cite differences between their findings and reports of vestibular responses but provide no satisfactory explanation except to postulate an association with differences in techniques.[15,72] Such findings and considerations suggest that the time is not yet at hand when vestibular evoked potential testing can be used routinely or profitably in the evaluation of patients with brain injury, mild or severe.

Contingent Negative Variation. Contingent negative variation (CNV) is a slowly developing negative potential in the brain discovered by Walter.[180] It is associated with expectancy, attention, and decision making. To elicit this response, a warning signal must be followed by a delay of up to several seconds, which, in turn, is followed by a stimulus input requiring an "imperative" response. Brain electrical activity that demonstrates CNV is usually recorded from a minimum of three scalp electrodes, FZ, CZ and PZ. The CNV begins about 400 msec after the warning stimulus. Chiappa[25] suggests at least two components: a frontally located negative response that may be related to an orienting response and a later centrally located negativity that may be related to a premotor potential. In general, the CNV phenomena has not had much clinical utility. Auffermann et al.[8] reported its use, as mentioned above, in evaluating olfaction. A recent study by Rockstroh et al.,[149] however, may point the way to using the CNV for evaluation of brain injury.

Auditory click probe stimuli were presented with different delays after the onset of a warning stimulus. Subjects were instructed to press a button as quickly as possible after a probe stimulus was presented. Reaction time was measured. The investigators found that reaction times were faster late during the anticipatory interval and the probe evoked potentials were enhanced. It was proposed that slow cortical potentials indicate the timing of excitability in cortical neuronal networks. If this is true, one would expect to find delayed and diminished excitability in the cortical neuronal networks of selected brain-damaged patients, including longer reaction times, longer times of onset of EP patterns, with the degree of delay and diminishment related to the severity of brain impairment. Further research is needed. Drake[40] offers the opinion that the CNV "may be generated in the frontal lobes" and is attenuated in patients with complex parietal seizures.

Cognitive Responses. Evoked potential responses in relation to neuropsychologic activity are discussed below in conjunction with active and passive P300 responses.

Recording Electrodes

Recording electrodes may be made of gold, silver-silver, or other metals. It is beyond the scope of this chapter to go into technical detail about the effect of metals on electrode performance, impedance levels, and attachment site preparations. One should follow the recommendations of the manufacturer of the evoked potential signal-averaging equipment.

Placement of scalp recording electrodes for evoked potential testing may vary, depending on purpose. The number of electrodes also varies. One can place 20–28 electrodes at one time, using either an electrocap or the more tedious hand placement technique. In some studies 128 electrodes have been placed, and 256 have been suggested to obtain exquisite detail about specific brain topographic sensory and motor functioning.[54] The use of relatively few recording electrodes, however, is satisfactory for the evaluation of patients with TBI unless the investigator is interested in special research projects.

A basic configuration found to be useful in evaluating patients with severe head injury calls for the placement of four scalp recording electrodes, each with a cephalic or non-cephalic reference electrode and a common ground, which may be on the center forehead, shoulder, tip of the nose, or elsewhere. Designations for electrode scalp placement generally conform to the ten-twenty system[80] (see Fig. 1). One configuration used to evaluate peripheral sensory and CNS impairment in patients with TBI calls for recording electrodes at C3' (central sensory area over the left hemisphere, 2 cm posterior to C3), C4' (central sensory area over the right hemisphere, 2 cm posterior to C4), 01 (left occipital area), and 02 (right occipital area). An Erb's point electrode helps to detect a brachial plexus response during testing of the median nerve. An electrode at C3 or C7 (over the third or seventh cervical vetebral process below the occiput) is helpful, particularly when one wants to ensure that somatosensory information is transmitted through the spinal cord upon stimulation of the upper and lower extremities. Linked ear lobes (or mastoids) are used often as a cephalic reference. Frequently an electrode at Fpz (midforehead) is used as ground. Electrodes to detect eye movement, heart activity, and other physiologic artifacts are commonly used. Other electrode placements are possible.[4,25,27,65,86,162]

Evoked Potential Tests for Traumatic Brain Injury

Testing procedures to obtain EP patterns in patients with severe traumatic brain injury in long-term rehabilitation vary widely. In addition, no internationally accepted protocol for evaluation of brain function in patients with severe brain injury encompasses short-, intermediate-, and long-latency brain evoked potential responses. Thus it is simpler to describe one approach, with the recognition that many modifications are possible. Eleven multisensory EP patterns are obtained, scored, and interpreted using a test protocol summarized below and discussed in further detail in a later section. Each of the eleven EP patterns is obtained two times at each testing session to determine the degree of replicability of each pattern. EP recordings described below are obtained upon independent stimulation of the left and right sides (except, of course, the P300 response).

Sample Protocol for the Multisensory-Evoked Potential Tests in Patients with Traumatic Brain Injury

1. Brainstem auditory evoked potential (BAEP)
   Left and right auditory nerve and brainstem short-latency (0–10 msec) evoked potentials using C3' and C4' (ipsilateral and contralateral) far-field scalp recordings.
2. Cortical auditory evoked potential (CAEP)
   Left and right long latency (0–500 msec) cortical auditory evoked potentials using C3' and C4' (ipsilateral and contralateral) near-field scalp recordings; at times an intermediate latency (0–60 msec) response is obtained.
3. Visual evoked potential (VEP)
   Left and right visual long latency (0–500 msec) flash evoked potentials using C3', C4', 01, and 02 (ipsilateral and contralateral) near-field scalp recordings.
4. Somatosensory evoked potential (SEP)
   • SEP intermediate latency (I)
   Left and right intermediate-latency (0–60 msec) somatosensory evoked potentials based on stimulation of the median nerve using C3' and C4' (ipsilateral and contralateral) scalp recordings.
   • SEP long latency (L)
   Left and right long-latency (0–500 msec) somatosensory evoked potentials based on stimulation of the median nerve using C3' and C4' (ipsilateral and contralateral) scalp recordings.
   • P300 and PP300 responses
   Long latency (750 msec) event-related potentials (ERP) obtained in response to the presentation of brief infrequent stimuli (20% occurrence) inserted randomly into a sequence of brief frequent stimuli (80% occurrence). Unimodality (auditory-auditory tones of different frequencies) and/or bimodality (visual flash-auditory tone) stimulus conditions may be presented. The montage involves scalp recording electrodes at Fz, Pz, C3', and C4'.

For subjects who can cooperate by counting the infrequently occurring stimuli, a P300 response is obtained. For subjects who cannot count because of severe brain injury, a passive P300 (PP300) can be obtained, provided the brain injury is not extreme.

When an evaluation of peripheral conduction time in the upper extremity is needed, the brachial plexus response can be used. This response provides information about conduction time between the wrist and the brachial plexus in the region of the axilla before the somatosensory signal enters the spinal cord. A surface recording electrode is placed at Erb's point (at the shoulder posterior to the clavicle and medial to the acromioclavicular junction) and referenced to the ipsilateral mastoid or ear lobe. Often this response can also be detected by scalp electrodes.

When the lower extremities must be tested to evaluate the transmission of peripheral somatosensory information from the ankle, knee, perianal, or other areas to and through the spinal cord, surface recording electrodes can be placed at various points along the spine as well as at Cz (or Cz', 2 cm posterior to Cz), the midline (vertex) of the scalp. Stimulating surface electrodes are placed typically in the region of the posterior tibial nerve at the ankle posterior to the medial malleolus; near the sural nerve at the ankle posterior to the lateral malleolus; or near the peroneal nerve posterolateral to the knee.

Short-latency BAEPs and intermediate-latency SEPs are referred to as far-field responses because the scalp recording electrodes are relatively far from the brainstem or other subcortical areas where signals are generated. In contrast, in near-field responses electrodes pick up nearby underlying cortical responses, such as long-latency cortical auditory EPs (CAEPs), long-latency visual evoked potentials (VEPs), and long-latency somatosensory evoked potentials (SEPs). Most investigators prefer to obtain the responses in visual testing by using a pattern reversal technique, which provides more useful information than a flash technique. In the pattern reversal technique a number of small black and white squares subtending an angle of about 20' appear on a television-like monitor. The black and white squares reverse about 2 times a second (usually 1.1 or 1.8 times per second to avoid a harmonic frequency associated with the 60-Hz current used to power equipment).

Unfortunately, most patients with severe traumatic brain injury are unable to cooperate sufficiently and to fixate steadily on the monitor. Consequently, flash stimulation is used. Under this condition eyes can be open or closed. When the eyes are closed, the eyelids are transparent to light. In fact, somewhat better patterns can be obtained with closed eyes, because less artifact may be associated with eye movements or visual distractions. VEP pattern abnormalities and clinical disability in patients with severe traumatic brain injury have been discussed by Rappaport et al.[141]

Specific descriptions of the various auditory, visual, and somatosensory evoked potential testing techniques applications are found in a number of sources,[25,91,162] and additional information is provided later in this chapter. All of the aforementioned sensory tests are primarily electro- or neurophysiologic responses of relatively short latency and do not generally reflect neuropsychologic or cognitive activity that may be initiated between 150 and 250 msec after stimulus onset, with a particularly prominent response at about 300 msec.

Precognitive or early cognitive testing is obtained, as mentioned above, by using the P300 paradigm.[124,125,128,154,162,169] In this technique two different stimuli are presented, one with a low probability and one with a high probability. Subjects are usually asked to count the number of low-probability stimuli, which in some cases may be random absence of stimuli. Under either condition one can identify event-related potentials (ERP) in which a major positive-going peak occurs approximately 300 msec after stimulus onset.

A passive P300 (PP300) response also has been found; that is, a P300 response can be detected without requiring the subject to count and keep track of the number of stimuli presented.[28,130,139,143,145,148,168] This technique has potential usefulness for the neuropsychological as well as the neurophysiologic evaluation of severely brain-injured patients, as discussed in greater detail in the section about assessment of cognitive functioning.

APPLICATIONS OF EVOKED POTENTIAL TESTING

Although the primary focus of this chapter is to discuss the application of EP testing in evaluating patients with severe traumatic brain injury, brief mention is made of various other clinical applications of the same EP techniques that may contribute important information in evaluating persons with brain injury. As described in greater detail below, SEP testing can help to determine whether patients with TBI also have spinal cord injury, particularly when they cannot cooperate adequately in the physical examination.

EP testing complements evaluation of structural changes after head injury by providing information on functional changes. Radiographs, computerized tomography (CT), magnetic resonance imaging (MRI), and related techniques are excellent in displaying anatomical relationships and abnormalities, but they usually do not provide information about neurophysiologic function. For example, an MRI scan of the brain shortly after death does not necessarily indicate that one is looking at a cadaver. EPs, however, provide information about neurophysiologic activity and degree of electrophysiologic impairment. A combined anatomic and functional evaluation may provide the most useful information for assessing types of impairments in patients with TBI. Newer MRI and other techniques discussed elsewhere in this text are beginning to provide functional as well as structural information.[29,53,96]

EPs can help to identify a variety of neurologic disorders, many of which may precede head injury. Examples include deafness or impaired hearing, multiple sclerosis, optic neuritis, acoustic neuroma, scotoma, dementia, stroke, hydrocephalus, and various neurologic lesions associated with different diseases.[25,162] EPs have been used to assess the effects of pain and various analgesics. Other clinical applications of EP testing are described elsewhere.[138]

USES OF EVOKED POTENTIALS IN TRAUMATIC BRAIN INJURY

Evaluation of Sensory Function

Auditory, visual, and somatosensory EPs represent the sensory modalities most frequently evaluated in patients with head injury. As mentioned above, however, it is possible in selected cases to assess olfactory, gustatory, and vestibular modalities and responses to painful stimuli as well as impairment in urinary, bowel, and sexual function and response to vibratory stimulation. Methods for carrying out the latter assessments are provided in various texts and articles.[1,9,19,25,43,66,77,162] In this section only auditory, visual, and somatosensory EP tests are discussed.

Auditory. Far-field short-latency recordings of brainstem auditory evoked potentials (BAEPs) provide information not only about the response of the auditory nerve to auditory stimulation but also about central conduction times between different relay points in the brainstem (medulla, pons) and beyond (mesencephalon, thalamocortical radiations, and cortex). In a patient with head injury, unless one is aware of premorbid hearing impairment, BAEPs provide useful information about left-right side hearing problems associated with traumatic injury. Rehabilitation staff can use this information when approaching the patient and when carrying out rehabilitation interactions.

In addition, BAEPs can be used to monitor changes in peripheral hearing ability. Figure 2 shows an idealized auditory nerve and brainstem response pattern prepared by Grass Instruments in 1979. The BAEP pattern can be used to determine hearing threshold but with some limitations.[25,158] It also can be used to determine whether hearing loss is associated with poor bone conduction or a sensorineural problem.[158,162] Figure 3 shows short-latency auditory EP responses. Curve C depicts the results in a patient with a bone conduction problem. Note the delay in the peak V latency at all levels of stimulus intensity. Pattern S-N shows the results in a patient with sensorineural hearing loss. Note that the peak V latency is delayed until the signal intensity becomes relatively high, at which point the latency decreases to close to the normal range (n). It is as if a person who is hard of hearing says that he cannot hear what you are saying in a normal voice, but when you shout loudly, he says, "Stop yelling at me." At that point, of course, enough residual hearing fibers have been recruited that the hard-of-hearing person finally can make out what is said. Information about bone conduction and sensorineural hearing problems can be useful in a rehabilitation context.

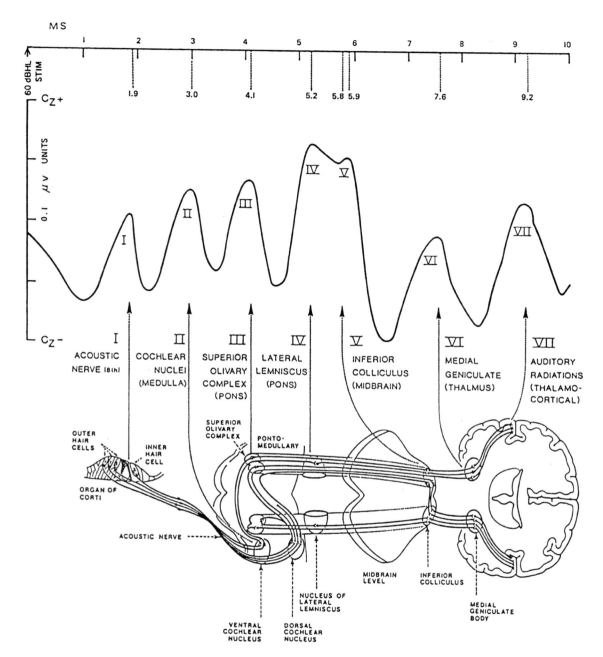

FIGURE 2. Auditory nerve and brainstem short-latency auditory evoked potential (BAEP) pattern with proposed functional-anatomic correlations. Diagram of normal latencies for vertex-positive brainstem auditory potentials; waves I through VII evoked by clicks at 60 dbHL (60 db above normal hearing threshold) at a rate of 10 per second. Lesions at different levels of auditory pathway tend to produce response abnormalities beginning with indicated components, although this does not specify the precise generators of the response; the relative contributions of synaptic and axonal activity to the response are as yet unknown. Intermediate latency (5.8 msec) between wave I and waves IV and V is mean peak latency of fused wave IV/V, when present. Cz+, Cz− = vertex positivity, represented by an upward pen deflection, and vertex negativity, represented by a downward pen deflection. (By permssion of Ellen R. Grass, Grass Instruments Co.)

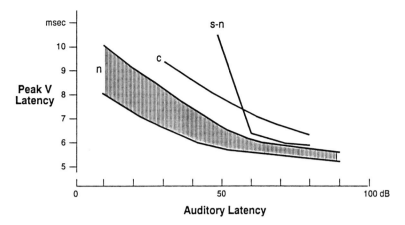

FIGURE 3. Relationship between the latency of wave V and the intensity of the auditory stimulus. Shadowed band labeled n shows the normal range. Curve c shows response configuration with conductive hearing loss. Curve s-n shows response configuration with sensorineural hearing loss. (Modified from Spehlman R: The abnormal BAEP. In Spehlman R (ed): Evoked Potential Primer: Visual, Auditory, and Somatosensory Evoked Potentials in Clinical Diagnosis. Boston, Butterworth, 1985, p. 234.)

Near-field long-latency cortical auditory evoked potentials (CAEPs) provide information about how the cortex responds to auditory input once the BAEP test has demonstrated that the peripheral auditory system is intact, functions adequately, and transmits auditory information to the cortex. The degree of abnormality of the cortical response contributes to understanding about relatively high-level impairment in responding to auditory information. As indicated below, when this information is added to similar information obtained by testing the visual and somatosensory modalities, the emerging picture reflects the extent and severity of cortical damage. The CAEP obtained in response to click stimulation does not provide information about specific higher level deficits in processing auditory information. In general, the CAEP response is less highly correlated than long-latency SEP patterns with disability and outcome. Nevertheless, in a multimodal EP testing procedure, the CAEP response increases the correlation with both clinical disability and outcome. Figure 4 shows typical long-latency CAEP patterns reflecting two successive runs obtained from a 47-year-old normal woman. Auditory EP testing contributes additional information to patient evaluation and prediction of outcome when the P300 response to tones is examined, as discussed in

the section on cognitive event-related potentials (ERPs).

Visual. Long-latency visual evoked responses in a patient with TBI provide information

Normal CAEP — F47

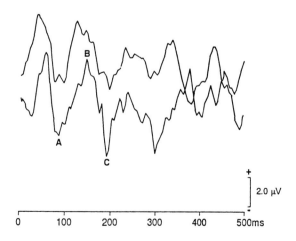

FIGURE 4. Long-latency cortical auditory evoked potential (CAEP) pattern obtained from a normal 47-year-old woman presented with click stimuli at 80 db. Two successive runs. Average of 100 presentations. Clicks presented every 1.1 seconds. Major consistent peaks are A, negative peak about 90 msec after stimulus onset and B, positive peak at about 150 msec; negative peak C at about 200 msec. Latencies and configurations variable.

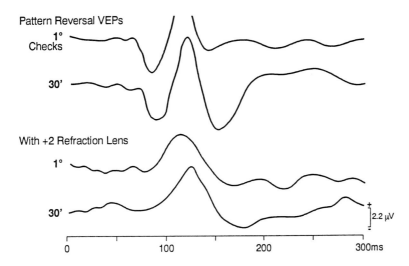

FIGURE 5. Visual evoked potential (VEP) in response to a reversing (1.88 times per second) black and white checkerboard pattern presented to one eye. Two check sizes (1° and 30'); 120 averages per run. Upper two runs based on normal vision without glasses. Bottom two runs based on blurred vision induced by a +2 refraction lens. Note also slightly longer peak latency for the smaller check size. Patterns smoothed.

about peripheral and CNS responsivity to visual stimulation as well as left-right side differences. Retinal responsivity in each eye can be evaluated as well as impairments in the transmission of visual information through the optic nerve, optic chiasm, and geniculocalcarine tract to the visual cortex and surrounding visual association areas in the occipital regions of the brain.[25,91] Prechiasmal, chiasmal, and postchiasmal damage can sometimes be identified.[25,69] Information can be obtained to identify conditions such as homonymous hemianopsia, optic neuritis, multiple sclerosis, and various other disease entities.[25,162]

In patients with TBI who cannot respond to a Snellen chart or other tests of acuity, it is even possible to carry out refraction tests to fit them with appropriate lenses. This test is performed by placing different lenses before each eye while exposing the patient to repeated stimulation of reversing checkerboard patterns until the VEP that shows the sharpest and most robust amplitude is found. Figure 5 shows a VEP pattern in a 46-year-old women in response to pattern reversal stimuli as well as the effects on the VEP pattern of a two plus diopter lens that impaired vision. This test, in which a subject must watch reversing black and white squares on a monitor, can be given only to patients who can fixate on a point in the center of a monitor for about 60 seconds. Figure 6 shows pattern reversal VEP results in a patient with scotoma in the right eye; the normal left eye is shown for comparison. Zihl and Schmid[192] found that pattern reversal stimuli were helpful in evaluating blurring in brain-damaged patients.

The pattern-reversal VEP test cannot be given to patients with TBI who cannot cooperate. For such patients a flash VEP test is

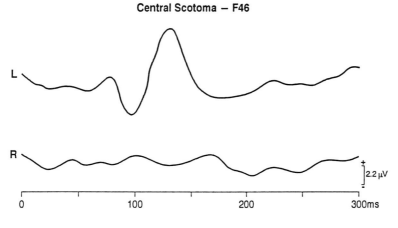

FIGURE 6. Visual evoked potential (VEP) response to pattern-reversal stimuli presented to a 46-year-old woman with a normal left eye and a right eye with a scotoma.

used. Figure 7 shows a severely brain-injured patient with distinct left-right side differences in response to flash stimulation. As mentioned above, this test provides limited information; however, it can indicate whether there is a response to light stimulation presented independently to the left and right eyes. Caution must be used in interpreting responses to flash stimuli. A flash VEP pattern may be seen in the presence of cortical blindness.[51,71] This pattern may be related to the phenomenon of blind sight or unconscious vision.[157,183] From recordings over the sensory areas of the left and right hemispheres (at C3' and C4') and over the left and right occipital areas (01 and 02), flash VEPs can yield information about the degree of abnormality of cortical responses in these regions and, at times, allow identification of left-right side differences. Occipital responses, in general, are more robust than central cortical responses except in the presence of marked occipital damage. In addition, flash VEP patterns can provide information about differences in the ipsilateral and contralateral transmission of visual stimuli. This information not only provides data about cortical responsivity in these regions but also helps to identify problems in the regions of the optic chiasm (where optic fibers converge that carry information from both the nasal and temporal fields) and the geniculocalcarine tract.[25,162] Among patients in coma it has been reported that as delta activity in the EEG decreases, VEP patterns return toward normal.[13] Alter et al.[5] reported that by using both flash and auditory stimuli it is possible to "discriminate between globally good and poor outcomes following severe head injury."

Interpretations of VEPs can be confusing, unless one is aware of the effects of different electrode placements (montages) as well as differences in VEP patterns associated with pattern reversal (PR)[95] and flash stimuli. Figure 8 shows VEP configurations in response to pattern reversal and flash stimuli with different scalp recording montages.

Somatosensory
This section discusses both intermediate (I)-latency (0–60 msec) and long (L)-latency (0–500 msec) cortical somatosensory evoked

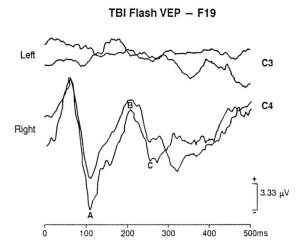

TBI Flash VEP – F19

FIGURE 7. Visual evoked potential (VEP) responses to flash stimuli presented independently to the left and right eyes in a 19-year-old woman with traumatic brain injury. Averages based on 100 brief (10-msec) flashes. Two successive runs for each eye. Note distinct left-right side differences. Patterns were obtained despite patient's inability to cooperate during her physical examination because of the severity of brain injury.

responses. SEP testing has multiple uses in the rehabilitation context. Like CAEP and VEP patterns, it can help to assess the extent and severity of brain injury, because somatosensory information is transmitted to parts of the cortex and subcortex that are different from areas that respond primarily to auditory and visual stimulation. In addition, SEP testing provides information about the integrity of the spinal cord. In patients who are unable to cooperate in the physical examination there is often a question about whether abnormal muscle observations are due to upper motor neuron problems, spinal cord damage, or both. SEP patterns help to differentiate the nature of the problem. If, for example, the posterior tibial nerve is stimulated at the ankle, the SEP pattern can show by recordings at L1–L3 (lower lumbar area) whether peripheral transmission of nervous information from the leg to the cord is impaired. Similarly, if a recording electrode is placed over the cervical region at C3 or C7 at the back of the neck, it is possible to detect impairment in transmission from the lower lumbar part of the cord to the cervical region. A scalp electrode, usually

Normal VEP – F47

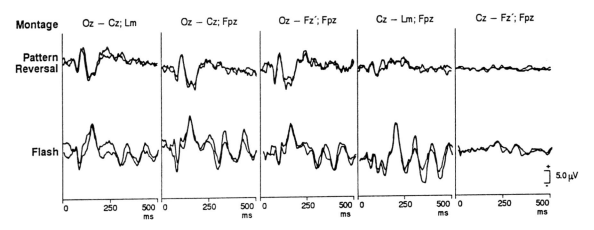

FIGURE 8. Normal pattern reversal (PR) and flash (F) visual evoked potentials (VEP) using different scalp recording electrode arrangements (montages) showing active-reference electrode pairs (Oz-Cz) and ground electrode (LM, where LM refers to linked mastoids). Note three differences. In the PR patterns the positive peak at about 100 msec after stimulus onset (P100) is more consistent and robust; for the flash pattern a P100 is also present but appears relatively diminished only because of the adjacent robust positive-going peak at 150 msec. Also, for the PR pattern note the negative-positive-negative complex between 135 and 170 msec, whereas for the F pattern note the single prominent positive-going peak at 150 msec. Note also the diminishment or absence of robust repetitive positive peaks ("ringing") after about 240 msec for the PR pattern. See text for further explanation. Subject: 47-year-old normal woman wearing lens correcting vision to 20/20.

placed midline at Cz' (2 cm posterior to Cz), provides information about impairment at the cortical level in this and surrounding areas.

Further information can be obtained if the median nerve is tested by placing stimulating electrodes at the midline anterior portion of the wrist, with the positive electrode at a distal site. Scalp recording electrodes placed at C3' or C4' provide information about impairments in contralateral and ipsilateral cortical responses. In addition, it is possible to determine whether peripheral transmission is impaired by measuring conduction time from the wrist to an EP peak that reflects activity in the area of the brachial plexus (approximately 9 msec in a normal individual). This electrical activity occurs just before the signal enters the cord. Thereafter, a peak sometimes is identified at approximately 11–12 msec, which reflects neural activity in the area of synapses in dorsal column nuclei portion of the spinal cord. This peak sometimes cannot be seen clearly because it merges into the next positive peak. The next

peak, frequently bimodal and occurring at 13–14 msec after stimulus onset, is believed to reflect activity in the cervicomedullary junction near the dorsal column.

The N18 response discussed above is now thought to be a prethalamic response originating between the upper pons and midbrain. By measuring conduction time between the cord and prethalamic response, it is possible to detect CNS damage in this area, which usually manifests as a delay in transmission. Responses around 21–24 msec after stimulus onset are thought to come from the thalamic and thalamocortical areas. Later responses reflect activity in the primary somatosensory cortex. A nonspecific major positive-going peak occurs at about 45 msec. Delays and distortions in these and later peaks occur with CNS damage in affected areas. SEP patterns, according to one study, may ultimately be able to provide information about midline brain damage affecting interhemispheric communication.[147] The foregoing peaks are obtained from subcortical and early cortical responses during intermediate-latency recordings (up to 60 msec after stimulus onset). Figure 9 shows recordings from both the contralateral cortex (C3) and the ipsilateral Erb's point upon stimulation of the right median nerve.

Long-latency recordings (up to 500 msec after stimulus onset) provide additional information about the general impairment in cortical responsivity to somatosensory stimulation. Typical arrays of contralateral and ipsilateral peak latencies and amplitudes in normal subjects to about 240 msec after stimulus onset have been reported[147] (Fig. 10). As explained below, the level of abnormality of EP patterns can be rated with evoked potential abnormality (EPA) scores, similar to EPA scores given to BAEP, CAEP, and VEP patterns.[134,135] EPA scores given to such multisensory EP patterns provide information about the extent and severity of brain damage and are correlated significantly with dysfunctional behavior and cognitive impairments as well as clinical outcome up to 2 years after injury.[135,136] Such findings hold up in replication studies.[6,116]

Facco et al.[47] also found that median nerve SEP patterns were significantly related to outcome. Specifically, they discussed improved outcome prediction by combined parietal N20 and frontal N30 analysis and reported that assessment may be improved by using motor evoked potentials in addition to SEPs. Synek and Trubuhovich[170] presented a number of cases to illustrate the usefulness of intermediate-latency SEP patterns in patients in coma early after injury. Ahmed[2] reported that SEP data for 60 comatose patients with head trauma, hypoxia, and cerebrovascular disease provided useful quantitative information about the functional state of the cerebral cortex. Several authors have found that by tracking changes in SEP (and other modality EP) patterns it is possible to distinguish between patients who will and will not show meaningful progress.[86] Figure 11 shows multimodality EPs for a 33-year-old woman who was in an extreme vegetative state when first tested after head injury in an auto accident. The initial auditory, visual, and somatosensory EP patterns as well as changes in these patterns over a 7-month period are shown, along with Disability Rating (DR) scores (discussed below), which show improvement

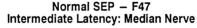

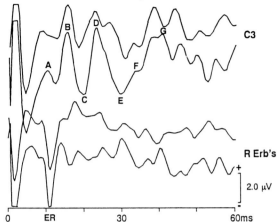

FIGURE 9. Intermediate-latency somatosensory evoked potential patterns obtained upon stimulation of the right median nerve of a normal 47-year-old woman. At the top are two successive recordings obtained from the contralateral hemisphere (C3') based on averaging 100 stimulations of 400-μsec duration presented at a rate of 5.3 stimulations per second at 2 ma above twitch threshold with the contralateral mastoid as reference. A = activity associated with activity in the area of the brachial plexus before the signal enters the spinal cord. The sharp downward peak at about the same latency in the lower two recordings is a more robust reflection of this activity recorded from the Erb's point electrode (ER) at the shoulder medial to the acromioclavicular junction posterior to the clavicle. B = activity in the vicinity of the thalamus (preceding activity at the synaptic connections within the dorsal column of the spinal cord is obscured in the upward going portion of this peak). C is thought to be associated with activity in the area of the thalamocortical radiations. D is probably associated with early activity in the primary somatosensory cortex. E, F, and G are nonspecific later cortical activity. The G response (P45) is usually robust but may be markedly diminished and show poor replicability in traumatic brain injury.

in clinical condition (i.e., DR scores decrease over time). Improvement in brain responsivity reflected in EPA scores preceded clinical evidence of recovery. This pattern has been seen a number of times in our laboratory and has been reported also by Greenberg et al.[64] and Newlon et al.[116] Its theoretical basis is discussed below. Correlations also have been shown between SEP patterns and sensory

Normal Cortical SEP — F27
Long Latency: Median Nerve

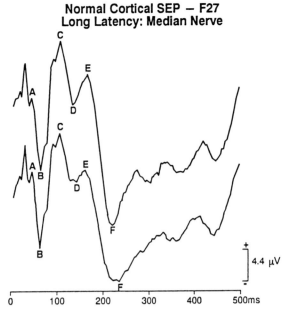

FIGURE 10. Long-latency somatosensory evoked potential patterns obtained from the contralateral scalp electrode, C3, upon stimulation of the right median nerve of a normal 27-year-old woman. Repeat runs, each based on averaging 100 stimulations of 400-μsec duration presented at a rate of 1.1 stimulations per second at 2 ma above twitch threshold. Letters A–F represent nonspecific cortical responses; latencies, amplitudes, and standard deviations are reported in Rappaport M, Hemmmerle AV, Rappaport ML: Intermediate and long latency SEPs in relation to clinical disability in traumatic brain injury patients. Clin Electroencephalogr 21(4):188–191, 1990.

disturbances in stroke patients as well as overall outcome.[23,182] The value of serial multimodality evoked potential testing is discussed briefly below.

Cognitive. Inroads have been made in neuropsychological evaluation via brain evoked potential testing. Although perhaps at a relatively primitive level, cognitive brain activity beyond early sensory neurophysiologic responses can be detected with evoked potential testing and reflects higher level CNS functioning as well as impairments in such functioning. This advance holds promise for improving our ability to assess and evaluate the extent and severity of brain dysfunction as well as the accuracy of prediction of outcome in patients with TBI and other

brain damage. It also can increase our understanding of neurophysiologic activity in various cognitive processes such as short-term memory.

At this time the main evoked potential approach to neuropsychological assessment is the use of the P300 technique.[128,132,162] This technique can be used with patients who cannot cooperate in testing, including those with severe brain injury.[39,130,139,145,148,168] In such cases, because the response is obtained while the patient is passive and cannot respond to instructions to count relatively infrequent stimuli, the evoked potential pattern is referred to as a passive P300 (PP300) event-related response. Variables that influence the latencies and amplitudes of this response include age, task difficulty, habituation to repeated stimuli, changes in probability of the stimuli,[42] sequence of stimuli, interstimulus interval, distraction stimuli, and disease processes.[25,37,128,132,143,162]

Of particular interest and in need of follow-up research, especially with respect to brain injuries, are relationships between the P300 response and measurements of deficits in information processing,[27] attention,[28,113] intelligence,[124,125] cognitive decline associated with injury and aging,[185] posttraumatic amnesia,[120] and isolated areas of CNS injuries.[92,93,119,186] Other relevant relationships need to be investigated further, such as exposure to toxic substances,[111,181] presence of seizures,[114] and the effects of various diseases such as multiple sclerosis,[75] human immunodeficient virus infection,[108] and nontraumatic coma.[61]

Another reason to anticipate that P300 and PP300 ERPs will shed light on cognitive brain dysfunction in patients with TBI is evidence that abnormal and aberrant thought patterns in schizophrenia and dementia are associated with both abnormal anatomic and abnormal ERP and EEG patterns.[7,55,62,81,104,106,107,123,126,172]

It has been proposed that P300 as well as PP300 responses reflect both cortical and subcortical activity.[93,148,190] The PP300 appears to be part of a reflex-like orienting response to a novel stimulus before the stimulus is processed at a higher cortical level where conscious awareness and stimulus analysis occur. This preconscious and

EP Changes Over Time in a Head Injury Patient — F33

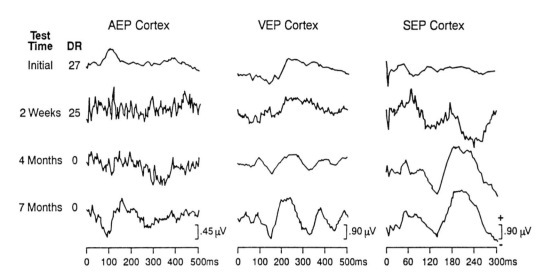

FIGURE 11. Evoked potential changes over time in a 33-year-old woman with traumatic brain injury. Changes in the late cortical auditory, visual (flash), and somatosensory (median nerve) responses are shown at 2 weeks and 4 and 7 months after the motor vehicle accident. Changes in disability ratings (DR scores—see text) are also shown. Positive changes in long-latency (cortical) EP patterns precede positive changes in clinical condition. BAEP and intermediate-latency SEP patterns were essentially nonpredictive of outcome.

conscious neurocognitive activity (which also occurs in species lower than humans) is embedded in the positive-going peak(s) that occurs approximately 300 msec after a relatively rare signal is presented randomly and intermittently in the course of presenting a different but relatively frequent signal.[59,128,162]

The P300 response is enhanced by focused attention when, for example, a subject is required to count stimuli.[143] It is degraded or obliterated when a subject is distracted or must attend to a different task.[128,143] It is speculated that this CNS response has evolutionary and survival value. A sudden unexpected event—be it sound, light, or movement—causes attention to be focused on it. (Examine your attention when a traffic light suddenly turns red.) Then evaluation helps to determine whether the event is associated with potential danger. In the lower animal kingdom, alerting to the snap of a twig may help to avoid being eaten. In civilization, alerting to the sudden squeal of brakes may help to avoid harm associated with such signal events. Experimentation in our laboratory

has shown that the usual P300 paradigm is not needed to elicit a P300 type of response. Mere presentation of an infrequent, randomly presented stimulus without the presence of a frequently presented stimulus can also produce a P300 response. It is believed that a sudden, unexpected stimulus such as a gunshot can produce a robust P300 without a frequently occurring contrasting stimulus.

The P300 and PP300 responses have been reported to be sensitive to different tasks and different clinical conditions. For example, the P300 response has been shown to be delayed and/or diminished in head injury, dementia, Alzheimer's disease, and other neurologic abnormalities, whether caused by trauma, infection, circulatory problems, or congenital conditions.[25,148,162] Prolonged P300 responses have been reported in severe traumatic brain injury,[148] Parkinson's disease,[60] Huntington's disease,[151] metabolic encephalopathies,[58] chronic renal failure,[30] Down syndrome,[163] alcoholism,[11] and schizophrenia.[48,126] It has also been used to investigate prosopangnosia,[159] anosognosia,[105] blind sight,[157] visual neglect

PP300 Comparison

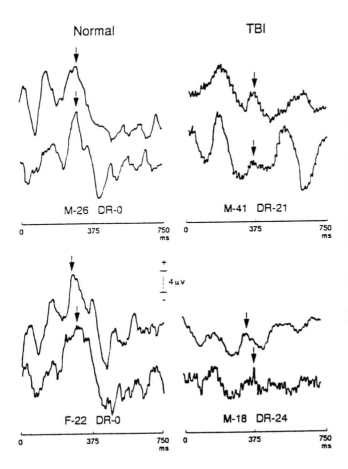

FIGURE 12. Passive P300 (PP300) event-related potential (ERPs) responses (arrows) in two normal subjects and two patients with TBI. The patients with TBI have increased latencies, decreased amplitudes, and increased variability of responses. The 41-year-old man (M-41) had a disability rating (DR) score of 21 (extremely severe disability); see text and Figure 19. The 18-year-old man (M-18) had a DR score of 24 (vegetative state). (From Rappaport M, Clifford JO: Comparison of passive P300 brain evoked potentials in normal and severely traumatically brain injured subjects. J Head Trauma Rehabil 9:94–104, 1994, with permission.)

following unilateral parietal lobe lesion,[98] and inattention following prefrontal lesion.[87,88] In addition, it has been used to evaluate closed head injury.[155] Clark et al.[27] used event-related potentials to measure deficits in information processing after moderate-to-severe closed head injury. They found a correlation between P2/N2 amplitudes and time since injury, which suggests that this parameter "offers the prospect of a sensitive, non-behavioral measure of recovery in cognitive processing."

At this stage the sensitivity of the P300 or PP300 technique to make subtle differentiations among different degrees of brain trauma is not great. The technique yields sufficient information, however, to differentiate normal subjects from patients with severe traumatic brain injury, particularly those who have a poor prognosis.[145,148] Figure 12 presents examples of PP300 patterns in two

normal subjects and two traumatically brain-injured patients with severe cognitive disabilities. Attempts have been made to increase the sensitivity of the PP300 technique by using stimuli from two rather than one modality. The working hypothesis is that the more severe the brain injury, the less likely a patient under the PP300 condition will respond to a rare signal if the two signals are from the same modality. The patient who shows a PP300 response when the rare and frequent signals are from different modalities (e.g., auditory and visual), however, is likely to show a better prognosis than the patient who shows no response to unimodal or bimodal stimulus presentation. Initial findings support this hypothesis.[143] Figure 13 shows clear evidence of differences in peak latencies and amplitudes in the PP300 response between normal subjects and patients with TBI.[120,148] In addition, a patient who suffered

FIGURE 13. Mean latencies in milliseconds and amplitudes in microvolts for the passive P300 peak as well as the preceding and following negative peaks in normal subjects and patients with TBI. (From Rappaport M, Clifford JO: Comparison of passive P300 brain evoked potentials in normal and severely traumatically brain injured subjects. J Head Trauma Rehabil 9:94–104, 1994, with permission.)

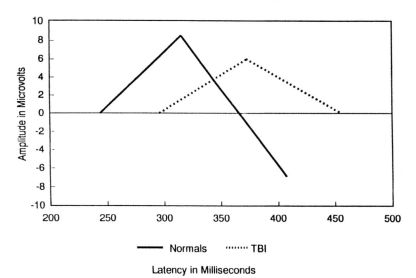

severe TBI and died within 1 month of testing showed virtually no PP300 response (Fig. 14). Similar results were found in a patient who had been in an extreme vegetative state with no signs of improvement for over 3 years.[139]

Serial Evoked Potentials

Serial studies of multimodality evoked potentials in patients with severe brain injury help to identify whether patients are likely or not likely to make progress. The case cited above (see Fig. 11) is one example. Cases reported by Greenberg et al.[64,65] provide other examples and also indicate how sensory EPs allow predictions of residual sensory deficits that in a number of instances are more accurate than clinical predictions. Underlying neurologic repair must precede recovery of neuropsychological function and the ability to relearn old skills or to learn new skills. Serial EPs can provide information about neurologic repair, which is reflected in normalization of EP patterns over time. The absence of such change does not augur well for patients with severe brain injury. Positive changes, although encouraging, are not completely predictive of ultimate outcome. Further research is obviously needed to understand better the relationship between various improvements in EP configurations over time and degree of clinical change likely to be found in patients with severe brain injury.

EVOKED POTENTIAL EVALUATION OF PATIENTS WITH TRAUMATIC BRAIN INJURY

Acute vs. Long-term Traumatic Brain Injury

Although EP testing close to the time of an acute TBI has been done,[64,65,115,116,184] a number

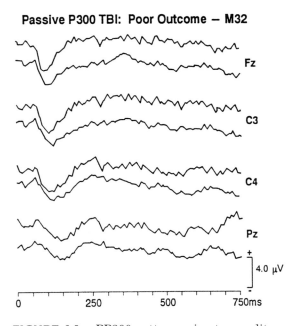

FIGURE 14. PP300 pattern using two auditory stimuli (a frequent 3000 Hz and an infrequent 1000 Hz) in a patient with TBI who died within 1 month after testing.

of practical and logistic considerations tend to diminish its use in this context. In acute situations the primary mission is to remove quickly threats to life and potential brain impairment. Breathing must be maintained, bleeding must be stopped, and developing physiologic crises—such as those associated with expanding subdural hematomas, pressure from skull fractures, and hydrocephalus—must be detected and controlled. After a patient is stabilized, further evaluation can be undertaken, including evaluation by brain evoked potential testing. If the clinical condition of the patient is sufficiently understood after medical stabilization, EP testing may not contribute enough additional useful information to be required. Also, shortly after brain trauma, developing edema and the effects of fresh trauma may yield false-positive EP findings that are not immediately helpful. Patients have to be monitored over time with repeat testings to obtain a true picture of residual neurophysiologic deficits. At least 2–4 weeks may be needed in severe brain injury cases before EP results, particularly long-latency cortical responses, have reasonable clinical and prognostic reliability and validity.[14] Furthermore, because of the time required for multisensory EP testing in an acute setting with many people bustling around the patient until stabilization has been achieved, it is frequently impractical and logistically impossible to do such testing without markedly interfering with the critical work of others. In addition, the acute use of medications may distort EP findings. EP testing, in general, does not constitute a life-preserving procedure. It is better used after the acute phase is over to monitor long-term slow changes in brain function associated with clinical changes and to help in assessing the need for ongoing intensive rehabilitation efforts.

Mild vs. Severe Brain Injury

In cases of mild head injury such as post-concussive syndrome, short-latency evoked potentials have "failed to show definite differences" compared with normal subjects, according to Drake.[41] Yet Montgomery et al.[110] reported that short-latency auditory EPs were abnormal in 13 of 26 patients immediately after head injury. Four patients had abnormal patterns for 6 months. Brown et al.[18] refer to other electrophysiologic irregularities. After reviewing the literature about relationships between evoked potentials and neural dysfunction, Zasler reported that "ABR [auditory brainstem responses] results have generally been inconsistent and most studies demonstrate no statistically significant correlation of abnormal evoked potentials with post-concussive symptoms."[191] Similar conclusions are drawn by other investigators.[184] In general, short-latency responses show mixed findings and cannot be depended on to show consistent abnormalities in patients with minor brain injury.

This is not surprising in light of findings reported by Rappaport et al. in a series of studies involving patients with severe brain injury far beyond a postconcussive condition.[137,142,144] Short-latency ABRs as well as short- and intermediate-latency SEPs obtained upon median nerve stimulation showed relatively little change in abnormalities with increasing severity of cortical brain damage. Because of the relative lack of correspondence between short- and intermediate-latency EPs and clinical disability, these EPs have not been consistently useful in evaluating patients with either mild or severe brain injury. Increased severity of brain damage, however, was associated with increased abnormalities in long-latency (cortical) evoked responses (Figs.15 and 16).

As discussed below, in patients with severe head injury higher correlations are found between long-latency multimodality evoked potentials and both clinical condition at time of testing and outcome several years after injury. It is possible that ABRs and other short- and intermediate-latency EP responses are not closely related to degree of brain injury and clinical disability because the structures responsible for generating these responses are buried deep in the brain and, in many instances, are relatively protected from the effects of head trauma. This interpretation is supported by analyses of parts of the brain most likely to be injured during head trauma—such as the frontal lobes, the temporal and occipital poles, the temporo-parietal and relevant contre-coup areas, and

BAEP & CAEP Abnormality Comparisons

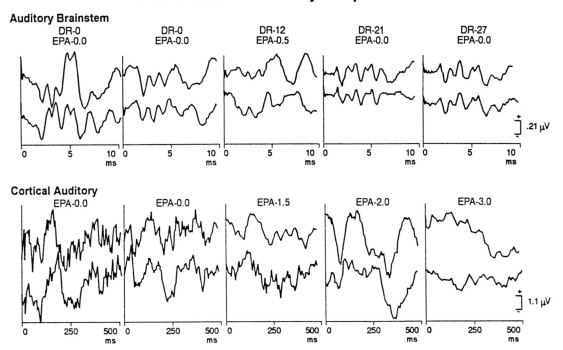

FIGURE 15. Comparison of short-latency (BAEP) and long-latency (CAEP) auditory evoked potential abnormality (EPA) scores in relation to the clinical disability rating (DR) scores. Note the relative absence of EPA change with DR change in the top row where BAEP patterns are presented. In contrast, in the bottom row of CAEP patterns, the systematic changes in EPA scores with increasing DR scores reflect increasing clinical disability. See text for further explanation. (From Rappaport M, Hemmerle AV, Rappaport ML: Intermediate and long latency SEPs in relation to clinical disability in traumatic brain injury patients. Clin Electroencephalogr 22(4):201, 1991, with permission.)

the white matter—when the forces of injury generate shearing responses.

In mild head injury most long-latency cortical responses also yield little useful information and, in general, cannot be distinguished from normal responses. Exceptions include P300 and CNV responses.[41,103] CNV responses in such cases have been reported to be persistently attenuated or asymmetric with frontal lobe involvement.[41] In one well-defined case, a patient who sustained a skull fracture and subsequently developed depression and change in behavior initially showed no P300 response as well as quantitative EEG (QEEG) abnormalities. Within 2 weeks after successful treatment with carbamazapine and clonazepam, both QEEG and P300 patterns had normalized.[103] Abnormal P300 responses were also observed in another instance of early mild-to-moderate brain trauma cited and illustrated below. Finally,

multisensory evoked potential testing has been found useful in evaluating the extent and severity of brain dysfunction and in predicting clinical outcome in persons with severe TBI.[34,49,64,65,100,116,127,133,135,137,156]

Although a number of reports in addition to those cited above have demonstrated some utility of EP testing in the acute stage shortly after brain trauma,[6,65,85] this section is devoted primarily to EP testing in evaluating surviving patients with severe head injury who have been stabilized medically and can be or have been placed in a long-term rehabilitation facility. As indicated above, emphasis is placed on examining long-latency cortical EP responses. Damage to the cortex, as opposed to damage to the brainstem, deserves close examination, because it is primarily responsible for abnormal psychological and behavioral manifestations after severe brain injury.

SEP(I) & SEP(L) Abnormality Comparisons

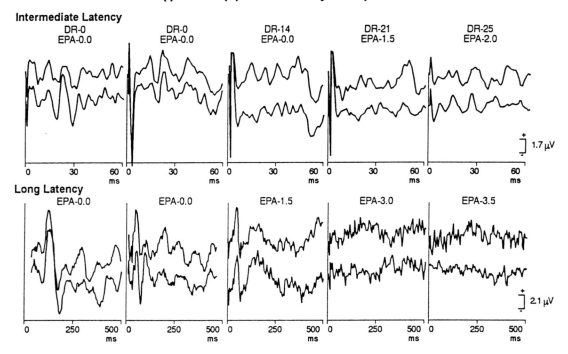

FIGURE 16. Comparison of intermediate (I)- and long-latency (L) SEP evoked potential abnormality (EPA) scores in relation to the clinical disability rating (DR) scores. Note the relatively minor EPA changes in the intermediate-latency patterns with increasing clinical disability reflected in the DR scores (higher DR scores are associated with greater disability). In contrast, note in the bottom row of SEP patterns the clear increasing degradation of long-latency SEP patterns with increasing clinical disability as reflected in the DR scores. See text for further explanation. (From Rappaport M, Hemmerle AV, Rappaport ML: Intermediate and long-latency SEPs in relation to clinical disability in traumatic brain injury patients. Clin Electroencephalogr 21(4):190, 1990, with permission.)

Relation between Evoked Potential Abnormality and Clinical Condition

The approach described in this section calls for testing of three sensory modalities—auditory, visual, and somatosensory—and of cognition, as reflected in the P300 response. For the auditory and somatosensory modalities short- and intermediate-latency responses are obtained in addition to long-latency cortical responses. These five EP tests done on the left and right sides of the body plus the P300 response yield a total of 11 EP patterns (enumerated above) that can be analyzed and interpreted. Analyses are based on ratings of the degree of abnormality of the evoked potential patterns. The patterns provide information about subcortical and cortical responsivity to the presented stimuli. They

also provide information about left-right side differences. The degree of abnormality and its location are correlated not only with degree of sensory recovery but also with overall clinical condition and outcome.[64,65,135] The highest correlation occurs when all long-latency cortical responses (AEP, VEP, SEP) are examined in relation to condition at time of testing and outcome up to 2 years after injury.[135] Evoked potential abnormalities are correlated significantly with clinical condition and outcome as measured by the Disability Rating Scale[136] and its 1987 revision. When the Glasgow Coma Scale is used, the correlations are lower.[67,135,171] Rehabilitation outcome can also be predicted using the DR scale by itself.[50] Greenberg et al.[64] demonstrated that evoked potential patterns predicted sensory deficits much better than clinical judgment (Table 1). One study that

TABLE 1. Forecasts of Focal Deficits 3–30 Months after Head Trauma

Somatosensory Evoked Potential			Visual Evoked Potential			Auditory Evoked Potential		
Hemiparesis	I–II	III–IV	Visual Dysfunction	I–II	II–IV	Auditory Dysfunction	I–II	III–IV
Resolved	6	0	Vis. Dys.	1	9	Deaf	1	5
Permanent	0	9	No Vis. Dys.	20	3	Not Deaf	24	3
n = 15	p < .001		n = 33	p < .001		n = 33	p < .001	
Correct clinical prediction*								
	40% (6/15)			30% (3/10)			17% (1/6)	
Correct EP prediction*								
	100% (15/15)			90% (9/10)			83% (5/6)	

* Note better prediction of outcome in terms of focal deficits using EP results in contrast to clinical impressions.
Modified from Greenberg RP, Moyer DJ, Becker DP, et al: Evaluation of brain function in severe head trauma with multimodality evoked potentials. J Neurosurg 47:150–162, 1977.

followed patients with TBI for up to 10 years after injury found no significant relationship between early EP testing and long-term outcome beyond about 2 years.[140]

A study by Rappaport et al.[135] demonstrated that each sensory EP pattern was correlated significantly with the clinical condition of a patient with severe head injury placed in a long-term rehabilitation facility. The lowest correlation involved BAEP patterns alone (r = 0.35, p < 0.01, n = 88); the highest single modality correlation was with long-latency cortical SEP (median nerve) patterns (r = 0.55, p < 0.01, n = 41). The highest overall correlation occurred when the EPA scores of all three modalities were used in the analysis (r = 0.78, p < 0.01, n = 39).[135] In general, as mentioned above, short-latency auditory and intermediate-latency somatosensory responses are not nearly as closely related to clinical condition or outcome as are the late cortical responses.[142,144] Figure 15 compares short- and long-latency (cortical) SEP patterns as well as disability rating (DR) and evoked potential abnormality (EPA) scores for subjects with no traumatic brain injury and patients with intermediate and severe traumatic brain injuries. Figure 16 makes a similar comparison for relatively short- and long-latency (cortical) SEP patterns. Both examples indicate relatively little change in the short-latency auditory or the intermediate-latency SEP patterns (median nerve) with increasing severity of clinical disability as reflected in DR scores. On the other hand, marked degradation in the long-latency cortical EP

patterns (both auditory and somatosensory) is associated with increasing disability (i.e., increasing DR scores). This difference has been noted a number of times. Such findings, as mentioned previously, may be due to the fact that the structures involved in short- and intermediate-latency EPs are buried relatively deeply within the brain or brainstem and are, therefore, relatively protected in most instances of brain trauma. One study involving anoxia associated with drowning found that adding BAEP EPA scores *decreased* the significance of the correlation between EPA and clinical outcome.[137] For the above reasons and observations, it is believed that the significance of relationships between outcome in long-term survivors of severe brain injury and evoked potential patterns depends primarily on the degree of abnormality of cortical rather than subcortical auditory or somatosensory EP responses. In the acute state shortly after injury, however, short-latency EP patterns do have predictive value,[6,65,85] although, as mentioned above, results are not consistent.[191] For the patient placed in a long-term rehabilitation facility, the long-latency cortical responses are more valuable in predicting outcome.

Readers interested in knowing more about how to rate the degree of abnormality of evoked potential patterns should review the articles by Greenberg et al.,[65] Rappaport et al.,[134] Pfefferbaum et al.,[126] Newlon et al.,[116] and Firsching and Frowein.[49] EPA scores are usually based on a number of criteria, such as the following:

- Presence or absence of major EP peaks usually seen in persons without brain dysfunction
- Degree of deviance of major peaks from expected latencies
- Degree of deviance of major peaks from expected amplitudes
- Degree of overall pattern abnormality (i.e., "noisiness"; irregularity of size and shape of pattern envelope; diffuseness and abnormality of peak configurations)
- Degree of pattern dissimilarity for recordings obtained simultaneously over the left and right hemispheres
- Replicability of pattern upon repeat testing

With training, correlation among blind raters is in the upper 0.80s. More sophisticated approaches to finding EP features to predict outcome have been used. Alter, John, and Ransohoff[5] have shown that a combination of several automatically extracted quantitative features of evoked potentials can discriminate between globally good and poor outcomes following severe head injury. Peak-to-peak variance appears to be a single EP feature with predictive value. Figure 17 provides three examples of auditory EP patterns associated with five major levels of evoked potential abnormality (EPA). Figure 18 provides similar examples for long-latency VEP patterns and for intermediate- and long-latency median nerve SEP patterns.

Auditory Evoked Potentials

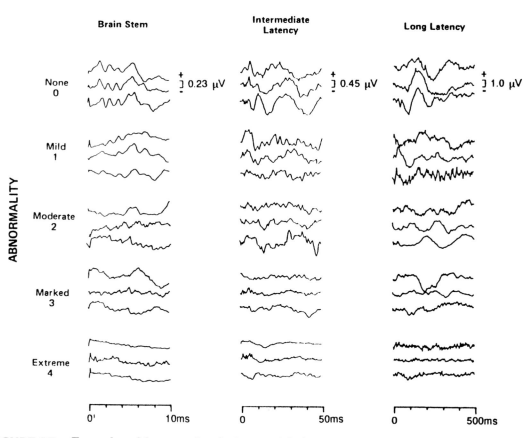

FIGURE 17. Examples of degrees of evoked potential abnormality (EPA) for short-latency (BAEP), intermediate-latency, and long-latency (CAEP) auditory evoked potential patterns. Three examples for each major level of EP abnormality: none (0); mild (1); moderate (2); marked (3); and extreme (4). (Modified from Rappaport et al: Evoked potentials and head injury 1. Rating of evoked potential abnormality. Clin Electroencephalogr 12(4):163, 1981, with permission.)

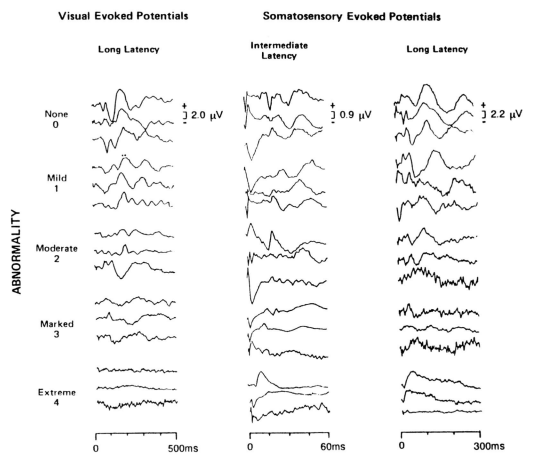

FIGURE 18. Examples of degrees of evoked potential abnormality (EPA) for long-latency visual evoked potentials and intermediate- and long-latency somatosensory evoked potentials (median nerve). Three examples for each major level of EP abnormality: none (0); mild (1); moderate (2); marked (3); and extreme (4). (Modified from Rappaport, M, Hall KM, Hopkins HK, et al. Evoked potentials and head injury 1. Rating of evoked potential abnormality. Clin Electroencephalogr 12(4):163, 1981, with permission.)

The correlation of EPA scores with a patient's clinical condition, as mentioned above, can be based on a number of rating scales, including the Glasgow Outcome Scale,[82] the Disability Rating (DR) Scale,[136] the Coma/Near-Coma (CNC) Scale,[146] and various other functional assessment scales such as those cited by Hall.[68] The DR scale is more sensitive than the Glasgow scale in assessing the clinical condition and outcome in patients who have suffered severe brain injury.[45,50,63,67,135,136] Whereas the DR score can be used to follow patients for their entire posttrauma career, acute hospital and rehabilitation settings as well as after discharge, the CNC scale was designed primarily to monitor small changes in the clinical condition of very low-level patients within a hospital or rehabilitation facility. Such patients have a DR score of at least 21 (essentially they have an extremely severe disability or are in a vegetative or extreme vegetative state). Figure 19 shows the 1987 revision of the DR scale.[136] Instructions on its use are found on the back of the scale (Fig. 20). The relation between DR scores and level of disability is shown in the lower right of Figure 19. Figure 21 shows the CNC scale, whereas Figure 22 (taken from the back of the CNC form) shows the relation between CNC scores and levels of near-coma and coma. The CNC scale is more sensitive than the DR scale;

DISABILITY RATING (DR) SCALE●

Name _____ Sex _____ Birthdate _____ Brain Injury Date _____

Cause of Injury: _____ MVA/MCA* _____ Head Trauma** _____ Infection _____ Stroke _____ Anoxia

_____ Developmental (Congenital) _____ Degenerative _____ Metabolic _____ Drowning

_____ Other (Specify) _____

*MVA = Motor Vehicle Accident; MCA = Motorcycle Accident. *Circle one.*

**Gun shot, blunt instrument, blow to head, fall, etc.

DATE OF RATING

CATEGORY	ITEM ▲									
Arousability	Eye Opening[1]									
Awareness and	Communication Ability[2]†									
Responsivity●●	Motor Response[3]									
Cognitive Ability for	Feeding[4]									
Self Care	Toileting[4]									
Activities	Grooming[4]									
Dependence on Others●●●	Level of Functioning[5]									
Psychosocial Adaptability	"Employability"[6]									
COMMENTS:	**Total**									

[1]Eye Opening

0 Spontaneous
1 To Speech
2 To Pain
3 None

[2]Communication Ability†
Either Verbal; Writing or Letter Board;
or Sign (viz. eye blink, head nod, etc.)

0 Oriented
1 Confused
2 Inappropriate
3 Incomprehensible
4 None

[3]Best Motor Resp.

0 Obeying
1 Localizing
2 Withdrawing
3 Flexing
4 Extending
5 None

[4]Cognitive Ability for Feeding,
Toileting, Grooming (Does patient
know how and when? Ignore motor disability.)

0 Complete
1 Partial
2 Minimal
3 None

†In presence of tracheostomy (place T next to score); for voice or speech dysfunction (place D next to score if there is dysarthria, dysphonia, voice paralysis, aphasia, apraxia, etc.)

[5]Level of Functioning
(Consider both physical &
cognitive disability)

0 Completely independent
1 Independent in special environment
2 Mildly dependent — (a)
3 Moderately dependent — (b)
4 Markedly dependent — (c)
5 Totally dependent — (d)

[6]"Employability"
(As a full time worker,
homemaker or student)

0 Not restricted
1 Selected jobs, competitive
2 Sheltered workshop,
   non-competitive
3 Not employable

Disability Categories	
Total DR Score	**Level of Disability**
0	None
1	Mild
2-3	Partial
4-6	Moderate
7-11	Moderately severe
12-16	Severe
17-21	Extremely severe
22-24	Vegetative state
25-29	Extreme vegetative state
30	Death

a **needs limited assistance (non-resident helper)**
b **needs moderate assistance (person in home)**
c **needs assistance with all major activities at all times**
d **24-hour nursing care required**

● Rappaport et al. Disability Rating Scale for Severe Head Trauma Patients: Coma To Community. Arch Phys Med Rehab. 63:118-123, 1982
●● Modified from Teasdale, Jennett, Lancet 2:81-83, 1974
●●● Modified from Scranton et al. Arch Phys Med Rehab. 51:1-21, 1970

▲ See over for item definitions
Revised 8/87

FIGURE 19. Revised Disability Rating (DR) Scale. (Modified from Rappaport M, Hall KM, Hopkins HK, et al. Disability rating scale for severe head trauma: Coma to community. Arch Phys Med Rehabil 63:119, 1982, with permission.)

ITEM DEFINITIONS

Eye opening

0— SPONTANEOUS: eyes open with sleep/wake rhythms indicating active arousal mechanisms; does not assume awareness.

1— TO SPEECH AND/OR SENSORY STIMULATION: a response to any verbal approach, whether spoken or shouted, not necessarily the command to open the eyes. Also, response to touch, mild pressure.

2— TO PAIN: tested by a painful stimulus.[1]

3— NONE: no eye opening even to painful stimulation.

Best communication ability (If patient cannot use voice because of tracheostomy or is aphasic or dysarthric or has vocal cord paralysis or voice dysfunction then estimate patient's best response and enter note under comments.)

0— ORIENTED: implies awareness of self and the environment. Patient able to tell you a) who he is; b) where he is; c) why he is there; d) year; e) season; f) month; g) day; h) time of day.

1— CONFUSED: attention can be held and patient responds to questions but responses are delayed and/or indicate varying degrees of disorientation and confusion.

2— INAPPROPRIATE: intelligible articulation but speech is used only in an exclamatory or random way (such as shouting and swearing); no sustained communication exchange is possible.

3— INCOMPREHENSIBLE: moaning, groaning or sounds without recognizable words; no consistent communication signs.

4— NONE: no sounds or communications signs from patient.

Best motor response

0— OBEYING: obeying command to move finger on best side. If no response or not suitable try another command such as "move lips," "blink eyes," etc. Do not include grasp or other reflex responses.

1— LOCALIZING: a painful stimulus[1] at more than one site causes a limb to move (even slightly) in an attempt to remove it. It is a deliberate motor act to move away from or remove the source of noxious stimulation. If there is doubt as to whether withdrawal or localization has occurred after 3 or 4 painful stimulations, rate as localization.

2— WITHDRAWING: any generalized movement away from a noxious stimulus that is more than a simple reflex response.

3— FLEXING: painful stimulation results in either flexion at the elbow, rapid withdrawal with abduction of the shoulder or a slow withdrawal with adduction of the shoulder. If there is confusion between flexing and withdrawing, then use pin prick on hands, then face.

4— EXTENDING: painful stimulation results in extension of the limb.

5— NONE: no response can be elicited. Usually associated with hypotonia. Exclude spinal transection as an explanation of lack of response; be satisfied that an adequate stimulus has been applied.

Cognitive ability for feeding, toileting and grooming.

Rate each of the three functions separately. For each function answer the question, does the patient show *awareness of how and when* to perform each specified activity. *Ignore motor disabilities* that interfere with carrying out a function. (This is rated under Level of Functioning described below.) Rate best response for toileting based on bowel and bladder behavior. Grooming refers to bathing, washing, brushing of teeth, shaving, combing or brushing of hair and dressing.

0— COMPLETE: *continuously shows awareness that he knows how* to feed, toilet or groom self and can convey unambiguous information that he *knows when* this activity should occur.

1— PARTIAL: *intermittently shows awareness that he knows how* to feed, toilet or groom self and/or can intermittently convey reasonably clearly information that he *knows when* the activity should occur.

2— MINIMAL: shows *questionable* or *infrequent awareness that he knows in a primitive way how* to feed, toilet or groom self and/or shows infrequently by certain signs, sounds or activities that he is *vaguely aware when* the activity should occur.

3— NONE: *shows virtually no awareness at any time* that he knows how to feed, toilet or groom self and *cannot convey information by signs, sounds, or activity that he knows when* the activity should occur.

Level of functioning

0— COMPLETELY INDEPENDENT: able to live as he wishes, requiring no restriction due to physical, mental, emotional or social problems.

1— INDEPENDENT IN SPECIAL ENVIRONMENT: capable of functioning independently when needed requirements are met (mechanical aids).

2— MILDLY DEPENDENT: able to care for most of own needs but requires limited assistance due to physical, cognitive and/or emotional problems (e.g., needs non-resident helper).

3— MODERATELY DEPENDENT: able to care for self partially but needs another person at all times.

4— MARKEDLY DEPENDENT: needs help with all major activities and the assistance of another person at all times.

5— TOTALLY DEPENDENT: not able to assist in own care and requires 24-hour nursing care.

"Employability"

The psychosocial adaptability or "employability" item takes into account overall cognitive and physical ability to be an employee, homemaker or student. This determination should take into account considerations such as the following:

1. able to understand, remember and follow instructions; 2. can plan and carry out tasks at least at the level of an office clerk or in simple routine, repetitive industrial situations or can do school assignments; 3. ability to remain oriented, relevant and appropriate in work and other psychosocial situations; 4. ability to get to and from work or shopping centers using private or public transportation effectively; 5. ability to deal with number concepts; 6. ability to make purchases and handle simple money exchange problems; 7. ability to keep track of time schedules and appointments.

0— NOT RESTRICTED: can compete in the open market for a relatively wide range of jobs commensurate with existing skills; or can initiate, plan, execute and assume responsibilities associated with homemaking; or can understand and carry out most age relevant school assignments.

1— SELECTED JOBS, COMPETITIVE: can compete in a limited job market for a relatively narrow range of jobs because of limitations of the type described above and/or because of some physical limitations; or can initiate, plan, execute and assume many but not all responsibilities associated with homemaking; or can understand and carry out many but not all school assignments.

2— SHELTERED WORKSHOP, NON-COMPETITIVE: cannot compete successfully in job market because of limitations described above and/or because of moderate or severe physical limitations; or cannot without major assistance initiate, plan, execute and assume responsibilities for homemaking; or cannot understand and carry out even relatively simple school assignments without assistance.

3— NOT EMPLOYABLE: completely unemployable because of extreme psychosocial limitations of the type described above; or completely unable to initiate, plan, execute and assume any responsibilities associated with homemaking; or cannot understand or carry out any school assignments.

Instructions: Place date of rating at top of column. Place appropriate rating next to each of the eight items listed. Add eight ratings to obtain total DR score.

---

[1]*Standard painful stimulus is the application of pressure across index fingernail of best side with wood of a pencil; for quadriplegics pinch nose tip and rate as 0, 1, 2 or 5.*

FIGURE 20. Instructions for use of the Disability Rating (DR) Scale.

RAPPAPORT COMA/NEAR-COMA SCALE

(For patients with a Disability Rating (DR) score ≥21, i.e., Vegetative State)[1]

(Complete form twice a day for 3 days then weekly for 3 weeks; every two weeks thereafter if DR score ≥21. If DR <21 follow monthly with DR scores.)[†]

NAME _____ SEX ___ BIRTHDATE _____ TYPE OF INJURY: MVA___ STROKE___ DR___

DATE OF INJURY/ILLNESS _____ DATE OF ADMISSION _____ HEAD INJURY___ ANOXIA___ DATE___

FACILITY _____ RATER _____ OTHER (describe) _____ TIME___

Parameter	Stim No.	Stimulus	No. of Trials	Response Measure	Score Options	Score Criteria
AUDITORY*	1	Bell ringing 5 sec. at 10 sec. intervals	3*	Eye opening, or orientation toward sound	0 / 2 / 4	≥3X / 1 or 2X / No response
COMMAND RESPONSIVITY with priming**	2	Request patient to open or close eyes, mouth, or move finger, hand or leg	3	Response to command	0 / 2 / 4	Responds to command 2 or 3X / Tentative or inconsistent IX / No response
VISUAL with priming** Must be able to open eyes; if not, score 4 for each stimulus situation (items 3, 4, 5) and check here ___ ***	3	Light flashes (1/sec. X5) in front; slightly left, right, and up and down each trial	5	Fixation or avoidance	0 / 2 / 4	Sustained fixation or avoidance 3X / Partial fixation 1 or 2X / None
	4	Tell patient "Look at me"; move face 20" away) from side to side	5	Fixation & tracking	0 / 2 / 4	Sustained tracking (at least 3X) / Partial tracking 1 or 2X / No tracking
THREAT	5	Quickly move hand forward to within 1-3" of eyes	3	Eye blink	0 / 2 / 4	3 blinks / 1 or 2 blinks / No blinks
OLFACTORY (block tracheostomy 3-5 seconds if present)	6	Ammonia capsule/bottle 1" under nose for about 2 seconds	3	Withdrawal (w/d) or other response linked to stimulus	0 / 2 / 4	Responds 2 or 3X quickly (≤3 sec.) / Slowed/partial w/d; grimacing IX / No w/d or grimacing
TACTILE	7	Shoulder tap - Tap shoulder briskly 3X without speaking to patient; each side	3*	Head or eye orientation or shoulder movement to tap	0 / 2 / 4	Orients toward tap 2 or 3X / Partially orients IX / No orienting or response
	8	Nasal swab (each nostril; entrance only - do not penetrate deeply)	3*	Withdrawal or eye blink or mouth twitch	0 / 2 / 4	Clear, quick (w/in 2 sec.) 2 or 3X / Delayed or partial response IX / No response
PAIN (Allow up to 10 sec. for response) If spinal cord injury check here ___ & go to stimulus 10	9	Firm pinch finger tip; pressure of wood of pencil across nail; each side	3*	See Score Criteria	0 / 2 / 4	Withdrawal 2 or 3X / Gen. agitan./non-specific movmnt IX / No response
	10	Robust ear pinch/pull X3; each side	3*	Withdrawal or other response linked to stimulus	0 / 2 / 4	Responds 2 or 3X / Gen. agitan./non-specific movmnt IX / No response
VOCALIZATION** (assuming no tracheostomy) If trach. present do not score but check here ___	11	None. (Score best response)	-	See Score Criteria	0 / 2 / 4	Spontaneous words / Non-verbal vocaliz. (moan, groan) / No sounds

Total CNC Score (add scores)	A
Number of items scored	B
Average CNC Score (A + B)	C
Coma/Near-Coma Level (0-4)[†]	D

COMMENTS: (Include important changes in physical condition such as infection, pneumonia, hydrocephalus, seizures, further trauma, etc.)

[1] Rappaport et al. Disability Rating Scale for Severe Head Trauma Patients: Coma to Community. Arch Phys Med Rehabil. 63:118-123, 1982 (Revised Form 1987)

[†] See back for TRAINING NOTE and COMA/NEAR-COMA LEVELS.

*If possible use brain stem auditory evoked response (BAER) test at 80 db nHL to establish ability to hear in at least one ear.

**Whether or not patient appears receptive to speech, speak encouragingly and supportively for about 30 sec. to help establish awareness that another person is present and advise patient you will be asking him/her to make a simple response. Then request the patient to try to make the same response with brief priming before 2nd, 3rd and subsequent trials.

***Make sure patient is not sleeping. Check with nursing staff on eye opening ability and arousability.

*Each side up to 3X if needed.

*Consult with nursing staff on arousability; do not judge solely on performance during testing. If patient is sleeping, repeat the assessment later.

Revised 8/90

FIGURE 21. The Coma/Near-Coma (CNC) Scale. (From Rappaport M, Dougherty AM, Kelting DL: Evaluation of coma and vegetative states. Arch Phys Med Rehabil 73:630, 1992, with permission.)

COMA/NEAR-COMA CATEGORIES

Level	Range	Level of Awareness/Responsivity
0	0.00 - 0.89	**NO COMA**; consistently and readily responsive to at least 3 sensory stimulation tests● plus consistent responsivity to simple commands.
1	0.90 - 2.00	**NEAR COMA**; consistently responsive to stimulation presented to 2 sensory modalities and/or inconsistently or partially responsive to simple commands.
2	2.01 - 2.89	**MODERATE COMA**; inconsistently responsive to stimulation presented to 2 or 3 sensory modalities but not responsive to simple commands. May vocalize (in absence of tracheostomy) with moans, groans & grunts but no recognizable words.
3	2.90 - 3.29	**MARKED COMA**; inconsistently responsive to stimulation presented to one sensory modality and not responsive to simple commands. No vocalization.
4	3.50 - 4.00	**EXTREME COMA**; no responsivity to any sensory stimulation tests; no response to simple commands. No vocalization.

●Sensory stimulation tests are items 1, 2, 3, 4, 5, 6, 7, 8, 9, 10

TRAINING NOTE TO NEW RATERS:

While one person does the testing, 2, 3 or more observers rate each item <u>independently</u> (without discussion). Afterwards discuss ratings. If rating is changed, leave initial rating but place changed rating in parenthesis next to it. Repeat this process on 5 to 10 patients or until raters train themselves to place patients at least in the same category range. Thereafter single ratings can be used but, for purposes of reliability, a minimum of two independent ratings per patient is encouraged. Ratings should be done at about the same time each day if possible. Under "Comments" record special information that may have had an extraordinary effect on the ratings on a given day -- such as: Patient was severely ill with pneumonia; patient was vomiting; patient had known increase in intracranial pressure (viz., hydrocephalus), patient fell out of bed; etc.

ADDITIONAL COMMENTS:

FIGURE 22.   Coma/Near-Coma (CNC) Scale categories and training note.

low-level patients improve on the CNC scale, whereas they remain relatively fixed on the DR scale[146] (Fig. 23). The CNC scale has been found useful in identifying low-level patients who can benefit from ongoing active rehabilitation therapy when otherwise they might be moved prematurely to lower levels of care. The CNC scale correlates significantly with evoked potential abnormalities[146] (Fig. 24).

Figures 25 and 26 show EP patterns from patients in a long-term rehabilitation setting with good and poor outcomes, respectively, and include EPA scores for each of ten EP tests. Each figure shows the sex and age of the patient; the initial disability rating (DRi) at time of EP testing; the disability outcome rating (DRo); the elapsed time in months between

DRi and DRo (ET); and the elapsed time between date of injury and EP testing (ETep). The higher the DR score, the greater the disability. The figures show two successive runs yielding BAEP, CAEP, and VEP (flash) EP patterns recorded from the ipsilateral scalp (at C3' or C4') and SEP (I) and SEP (L) patterns recorded from the contralateral scalp (at C3' or C4'). Evoked potential abnormality (EPA) scores are shown for each pattern (the higher the EPA scores, the greater the abnormality). Prognosis depends on these numbers. The lowest (best) EPA scores are associated with the BAEP and SEP(I) short-latency patterns, but these EP patterns are *least* helpful in predicting outcome in long-term survivors of TBI. The long-latency patterns of CAEP,

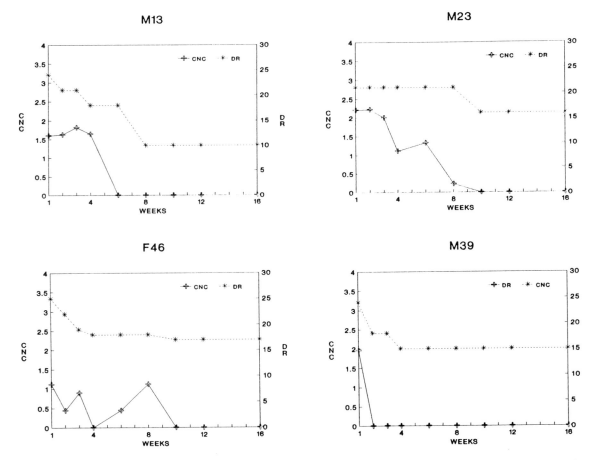

FIGURE 23.   Comparison of sensitivity of Disability Rating (DR) and Coma/Near-Coma scores for evaluating very low-level (essentially vegetative state) patients with TBI. Note that the improvement in CNC scores (movement to lower CNC scores) is not shown as dramatically in the DR scores. M = male; F = female. Number is age in years. See text for further explanation. (From Rappaport M, Dougherty AM, Kelting DL: Evaluation of coma and vegetative states. Arch Phys Med Rehabil 73:631, 1992, with permission.)

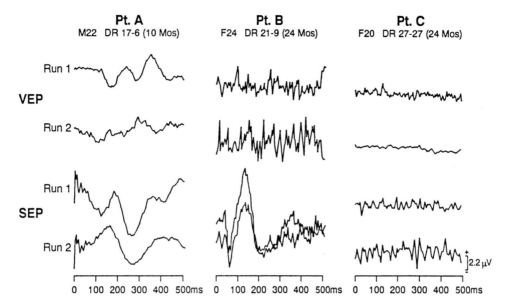

FIGURE 24. Examples of relationships between initial visual and somatosensory (median nerve) evoked potential patterns and clinical change in level of disability as reflected in the DR scores. Subject A, a male 22 years old, who showed distinct but irregular long-latency VEP and SEP patterns, went from a DR 17 (extremely severe disability) to a DR 6 (moderate disability) after 10 months of active rehabilitation. Similar results are shown for patient B. For patient C, however, a female 20 years old, the VEP and SEP patterns were extremely abnormal, and this patient showed no change in her level of disability DR 27 (extreme vegetative state) over a 24-month period despite active rehabilitation efforts. See text for further information. (Modified from Rappaport M: Evoked potentials and head injury in a rehabilitation setting. In Neurotrauma: Treatment, Monitoring, and Rehabilitation Issues. Stoneham, MA, Butterworth, 1985, p 191.)

VEP, and SEP(L) are better predictors of outcome. The individuals presented in Figures 24 and 25 were injured in separate automobile accidents. The elapsed time between DRi and DRo in the patient with good outcome was 13 months; elapsed time since injury until EP testing was 5 months. For the patient with poor outcome, the numbers were 60 and 8 months, respectively.

Note the array of the cortical EPA profile scores [CAEP, VEP, and SEP(L)] in the patient who showed improvement (22-year-old man). There are no markedly-to-extremely or extremely abnormal EPA scores (3.5 or 4.0, respectively). There is only one markedly abnormal (3.0) score—the CAEP in the left hemisphere. Otherwise, the worst scores are moderately-to-markedly abnormal (2.5), occurring in the left hemisphere in response to visual flash stimulation and in the right hemisphere in response to auditory stimulation. Most of the remaining EPA scores range between mildly-to-moderately abnormal (i.e.,

1.0, 1.5, and 2.0). The right hemisphere shows a somewhat better response to flash stimulation than the left hemisphere.

On the basis of all recorded patterns, the following interpretations can be made. BAEP EPA scores indicate that the patient can process auditory information adequately at the periphery (auditory nerve and brainstem responses appear less than mildly abnormal, with EPA scores of only 0.5), although clinically the patient has a disability rating of 21 (extremely severe on the DR scale). Despite evidence of widespread impairment in cortical responsivity to sensory stimulation presented to the auditory, visual, and somatosensory modalities, impairment is primarily in the moderately-to-markedly abnormal range (EPAs of 2 or 2.5) or less with no markedly-to-extremely abnormal patterns (EPA scores of 3.5 or 4.0). The TBI report at initial EP testing concluded that "This array of cortical responsivity suggests there can be further . . . improvement in the patient's

TBI EP Test Protocol Results: Improvement Shown — M22
DRi 21, DRo 3, ET 13 Mos, ETep 5 Mos

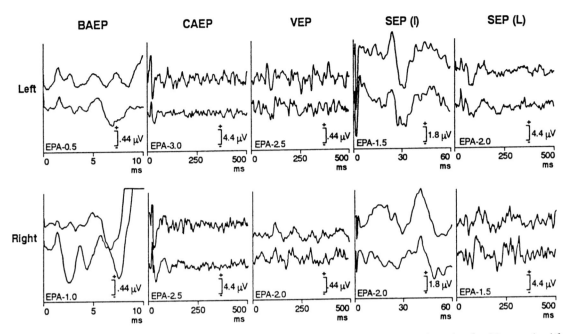

FIGURE 25. Ten patterns from a typical TBI EP test protocol showing a patient (male, 22 years) with a relatively good outcome. The initial disability (DRi) score was 21 (extremely severe disability); the elapsed time (ET) was 13 months until the outcome disability rating (DRo) of 3 (partial disability) was recorded. The elapsed time between admission to a rehabilitation facility and initial EP testing (ETep) was 5 months. Left and right BAEP, CAEP, VEP, intermediate-latency SEP (median nerve), and long-latency SEP patterns are shown (two runs each). In the left lower corner of each pattern is the evoked potential abnormality (EPA) score (the higher the number, the greater the abnormality). Note the lower EPA scores for this good outcome patient than for the patient with poor outcome shown in Figure 26. See text for further information.

clinical condition with ongoing intensive rehabilitation therapy." When the patient was evaluated 13 months later, his DR score was 3 (partial disability)—a considerable improvement over his DR score of 21 (extremely severely disability) at initial EP testing.

Now note in Figure 26 the array of EPA patterns for the patient who showed no improvement (m, 31 yrs). BAEP EPA scores show moderate impairment (EPA = 2.0) on the left and moderate-to-marked impairment (EPA = 2.5) on the right. Although not normal, these responses are still compatible with ability to process auditory information at the auditory nerve and brainstem level. Similarly, the SEP (I) patterns are slightly better than the late cortical SEP (L) patterns. Nevertheless, the SEP (I) patterns are markedly abnormal (EPA = 3.0) when the left and right median nerves are stimulated. EPA scores are worse

than those of the patient with good outcome. When the late cortical responses are examined upon stimulation of the auditory, visual, and somatosensory modalities, their EPA patterns are markedly-to-extremely (3.5) or extremely (4.0) abnormal. Such high degrees of abnormalities, particularly when they occur in more than one sensory modality, usually have a grave outcome. The TBI EP report provided after initial testing concluded that "This array of patterns indicates a very poor prognosis with relatively little responsivity to be expected from ongoing intensive rehabilitation activities." When the patient was evaluated 60 months later, his disability rating was still DR 28 (extreme vegetative state)—the same as at EP testing 5 years earlier.

In general, experience has shown that when EPA scores are 3.0 (markedly abnormal), 3.5 (markedly-to-extremely abnormal),

TBI EP Test Protocol Results: No Improvement Shown — M31
DRi 28, DRo 28, ET 60 Mos, ETep 8 Mos

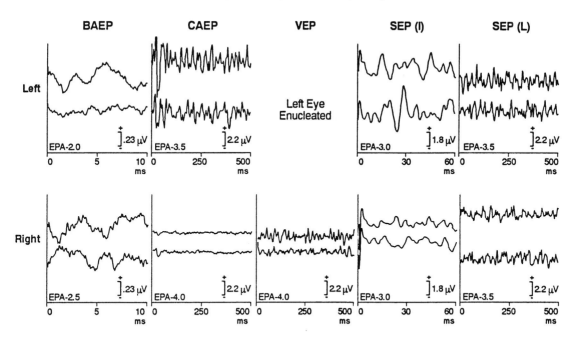

FIGURE 26.   Nine patterns from a typical TBI EP test protocol showing a patient (male, 31 years) with poor outcome. The initial disability (DRi) score was 28 (extreme vegetative state); the elapsed time (ET) was 60 months until the outcome disability rating (DRo) of 28 was recorded. Essentially no change in the patient's clinical condition occurred despite rehabilitation efforts. Elapsed time between admission to a rehabilitation facility and initial EP testing was 8 months. In the left lower corner of each pattern is the evoked potential abnormality (EPA) score (the higher the number the greater the abnormality). Note the higher EPA scores for the patient with poor outcome than for the patient with good outcome shown in Figure 25. See text for further information.

or 4.0 (extremely abnormal), the prognosis for meaningful clinical improvement is poor, particularly if long-latency cortical SEP patterns are involved and if two or more long-latency cortical EP patterns have an EPA score greater than 3.0. Poor clinical improvement refers to a change in the DR score only within a single category (see Fig. 19) or, if a patient is at the lowest disability level within a category, improvement only to the upper levels of the next lower category. This pattern has been found not only among patients with TBI but also among young victims in drowning incidents.[137]

The sensitivity of EPA scores extends to patients in prolonged coma or near-coma as defined by the Coma/Near-Coma scale.[146] EPA scores in this group of patients, who generally have a poor prognosis, can predict which patients will show modest improvement with

ongoing intensive rehabilitation efforts.[146] This distinction can be important in identifying patients for whom it is justified to request authorization for further intensive rehabilitation before considering a premature move to lower levels of care, where meaningful rehabilitation may be absent or minimal and progress is likely to be aborted. In this context multisensory EP testing and interpretation can be helpful in promoting cost-effective care.

The PP300 ERP neuropsychological test is currently being evaluated to determine whether it improves further our ability to identify patients with TBI who are most likely to make meaningful progress with ongoing intensive rehabilitation efforts. The above examples show that in selected cases the test has utility in evaluating the effects on the brain of mild head injury. It has also been demonstrated that the PP300 in brain-injured patients is quantitatively significantly different in terms of peak latencies and amplitudes from similar patterns in normal subjects. Furthermore, the absence of a PP300 response in patients with extreme brain injury is associated with a very poor outcome and failure to emerge from coma—and perhaps with imminent death. What has not been demonstrated yet is a significant correlation between the degree of abnormality of P300 or PP300 responses and outcome for patients with head injuries who fall into the mild, moderate, marked, and severe ranges of brain injury. A recent research communication by Martin Ford (1995), however, demonstrates that P300 deficits can be identified in individuals with only mild head injury. Further research is obviously needed. Suggestions that may improve the sensitivity of the event-related potential response in assessing degree of brain impairment and in predicting clinical outcome are presented in the concluding research section below.

Evoked Potentials Complement Electroencephalography and Other Brain Assessment Procedures

The development of EP technology has permitted identification of neurophysiologic abnormalities not obtainable through EEG testing. Cannon and Drake[21] demonstrated significantly longer central conduction times between BAEP peaks I–V and III–V in brain-injured patients with rage attacks and self-injurious behavior than in controls. EEG patterns showed no specific identifying features. Hutchinson et al.[78] found that SEP patterns were better than EEG in predicting outcome of severe head injury when patients were examined within 3 days of injury and followed for 6 months. In studying patients with alpha-coma, Ganji et al.[52] reported that auditory and somatosensory EP patterns were helpful in localizing areas of lesion in the brain in the absence of specific EEG information and evidence of a mass lesion on CT scan. Tsao et al.[174] reported that SEP patterns were helpful in predicting recovery in a child in a persistent vegetative state who exhibited a "generalized delta activity

of variable amplitude and questionable pattern changes on stimulation."

The P300 response and quantitative electro-encephalotopography (QEEG). Because EEG and QEEG are described and discussed in other chapters, comments here are limited to the utility of QEEG findings in evaluating the P300 responses. Although this technique holds promise, a number of inherent difficulties must be recognized, particularly in patients with severe head injury. QEEG involves placement of many scalp recording electrodes, usually 20–28. Placement of so many electrodes may be quite difficult in patients with severe head injury, not only because of absent or uneven scalp contours but also because irritability, voluntary and involuntary muscle activity generating voltages that obscure EP patterns, and general uncooperativeness of patients with TBI are compounded by the length of time it takes to place electrodes. Even with a relatively cooperative patient and a skilled technician, it may take 30–45 minutes or more before testing can begin and then a number of hours before multimodality and P300 testing is completed. Nevertheless, at least in cooperative patients with relatively minor head injury, it is possible to extract information about brain function that is not as readily available by either regular EEG or more limited EP testing.

Before presenting an example of EP brain mapping, several caveats are in order. It has been said the QEEG technique sometimes may not provide information that is already available in the raw EEG.[25,118] This may be true to a certain extent. It is comparable to saying that if one looks hard enough at a plain radiograph, one probably can see things that are much clearer in an MRI scan. In addition, the use of color in topographic brain displays can be misleading. The colors are selected arbitrarily by the programmer and the borders between colors do not represent distinct and sudden changes in brain function. Color borders reflect instead an artifact not only of programming but of mathematical interpolation of likely changes in voltages between adjacent recording electrodes. These same artifacts can also distort QEEG EP patterns. Nevertheless, useful information can be extracted that may not be seen as readily in other brain evaluation methods.[175]

Figure 27 shows significant differences (z-score differences color coded) in QEEG (quantitative electroencephalography) patterns between a 52-year-old male engineer complaining of increasing problems with both short- and long-term memory associated with earlier head trauma and averaged QEEG patterns obtained from normal subjects matched for age and sex. Note in Figure 28 the distinct topographic voltage configuration differences in two P300 patterns—the one on the left shows the response of a normal subject, and the one on the right shows the abnormal P300 response of the 52-year-old male engineer who demonstrated abnormal QEEG patterns (Fig. 27). The normal subject shows symmetric voltages with maximum voltages appearing in the vertex region, whereas patient voltages are asymmetric and diminished, with an overall configuration that appears quite irregular. Figure 29 shows the actual ERP P300 patterns recorded from eight scalp electrodes (C3, C4, Cz, Pz, P3, P4, F3, F4). The ERP patterns for all 8 recording sites are comparable for the normal subject. For the patient, however, some patterns are diminished, diffuse, asymmetrical, and irregular, particularly in the central and left parietal areas. Because the patient was beginning to think that his problems were psychological in light of previous negative EEG, CT, and MRI findings, it was reassuring to learn that a physical problem was present, although cause and treatment could not be specified at the time of evaluation of the QEEG results. Presenile dementia was suspected.

In patients with dementia and Alzheimer's disease, ERP patterns have been found to be different from those in normal individuals.[57,131,132] P300 test results have shown that latencies are longer and amplitudes generally are smaller. St. Clair[165] found that 70% of 15 patients with dementia of Alzheimer's type had latency and amplitude abnormalities with no false positives. Similar findings have been reported by other investigators,[128] including findings in investigation of P300 responses in severely brain injured patients.[148]

Several studies in the literature discuss relationships between EP and QEEG results.

Wirsen et al.[186] evaluated 18 patients with frontal trauma using EEG, QEEG, and auditory P300 EPs. They reported that "some regional abnormalities were more easily detected by topographic mapping" when there was significant reduction in P300 amplitude in the frontal areas compared with posterior areas. Jordan et al.[83] reported the application of standard EEG and both EP and QEEG testing in the evaluation of early dementia. They found that both EEG and EP studies helped to differentiate various cases of dementia. They also found that QEEG studies helped to differentiate dementia from depression. Verma et al.[179] found that evoked potentials obtained during a QEEG analysis at N1 (negative peak at about 100 msec after stimulus onset), P2 (positive peak at about 190 msec), and N2 (negative peak at about 260 msec) were correlated differentially with cognitive functions. They reported that N1 and P2 are correlated with mental speed and N2 with short-term memory. Such findings obviously suggest the need for research with brain-injured patients.

EPs in relation to other brain assessment methods. As mentioned earlier, MRI and CT scans provide primarily anatomic or structural information but relatively little information about neurophysiologic functioning (although, as indicated in other chapters, this is changing). By providing information about neurophysiologic functioning, EP testing is complementary to structural evaluation techniques. One study that evaluated 100 patients with TBI observed that relatively often neurophysiologic and neuropsychological impairments in patients with severe head injury showed no outstanding neuroanatomic changes on CT scans.[14] Multimodality EP patterns, however, were consistently quite abnormal. Markland et al.[102] demonstrated the correlation between BAEP patterns and MRI scans and their utility in identifying the presence of unilateral brainstem lesions. Papanicolaou et al.[121] demonstrated localization of auditory EP response sources using magnetoencephalography and MRI scans. Correspondence between MRI and visual evoked potential changes was found in patients with a definite (but not probable) diagnosis of multiple sclerosis.[112]

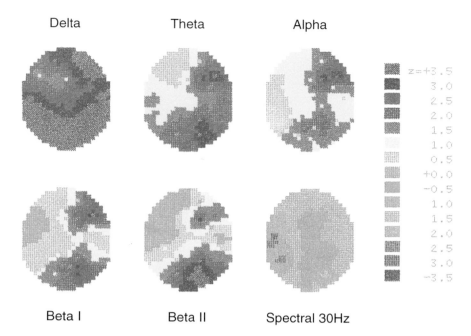

Delta   Theta   Alpha

Beta I   Beta II   Spectral 30Hz

FIGURE 27. Topographic quantitative EEG (QEEG) brain map of a 52-year-old male complaining of increasing problems with both short- and long-term memory compared with similar data from normal subjects. Previous routine EEG and both MRI and SPECT scans were negative. Pink/magenta colors in the right frontal and right central parietal regions identify areas of brain electrical activity that are three standard deviations away from the EEG activity demonstrated by normal subjects matched for age and sex. Presenile dementia is suspected. See also P300 response in Figures 28 and 29.

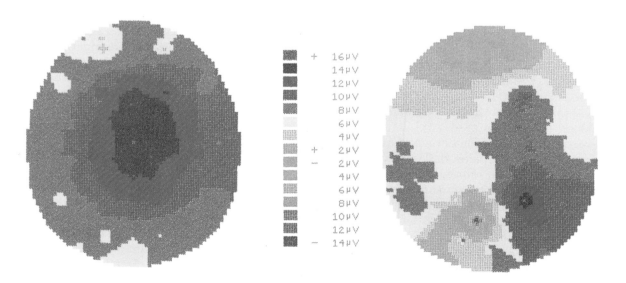

FIGURE 28. Comparison of P300 brain responses in a 32-year-old normal female (left) and a 52-year-old male (right) complaining of short- and long-term memory problems associated with previous head trauma. Note symmetric and generally higher voltages in the normal subject compared with the patient. Same patient as in Figure 27.

P300 ERP

Normal — F32   Abnormal — M52

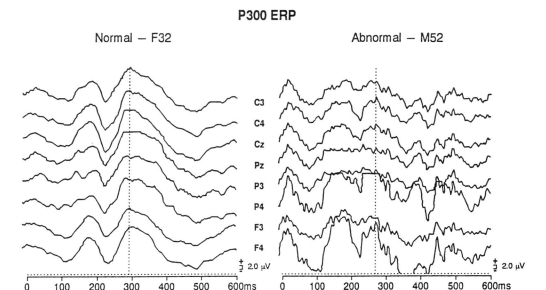

FIGURE 29. P300 evoked response potential (ERP) patterns from a 32-year-old normal female and 52-year-old male complaining of increasing problems with both short- and long-term memory. (QEEG topographic brain maps shown in Figure 28.) Note the absence of robust and congruent patterns affecting the central (Pz) and right side (P4) of the parietal area in contrast to the left and right patterns recorded in the frontal (F3 and F4) and central areas (C3 and C4).

Positron emission tomography (PET) and single-photon emission computer tomography (SPECT), specialized techniques in which radioactive material is injected into the patient so that areas of differential metabolism in the brain can be studied, have been shown to be related to EP findings. Cusumano et al.[33] reported that SEP results, particularly the parietal P25 component, "showed a superior prognostic power" in predicting outcome at 1 year in 68 severely head-injured, comatose patients. SPECT results, which showed severely reduced uptake of the injected material, were associated with reduced amplitudes of SEP components. SPECT scans also have been shown to be related to behavioral dysfunctions.[173] In a group of brain-disordered schizophrenics, PET scan results showed a decreased anteroposterior metabolic gradient.[35] Passive P300 responses demonstrated that the anteroposterior scalp gradient found in normal subjects was absent in patients with severe TBI.[148] Regional cerebral blood flow (rCBF) has also been correlated with EP, PET, SPECT, and EEG as well as neuropsychologic findings.[44,73,150] In addition, the psychiatric literature has shown meaningful associations between SPECT findings and unusual thought and cognitive processing, many of which are frequently exhibited by patients with TBI who consistently show abnormal EP patterns. Obsessive-compulsive disorders, schizophrenia, and depression are current examples.[101,104,117,153] Because of their high incidence in the general population (approximately 15%, mostly affective disorders) and a probably higher incidence among severely brain-injured patients, who generally have a poorer premorbid mental history, such psychiatric disorders and their EP correlates should be kept in mind.[16,103,106]

SPECT scans can be useful in distinguishing primary organic neurologic disease, such as cerebrovascular disease, dementia, and epilepsy, from primary psychopathology.[36] It is also helpful in evaluating disturbances in perfusion and metabolism,[187] which may be associated with impaired CNS function and abnormal EP patterns.

With the above correlations in mind, further research may allow use of the relatively inexpensive EP technique to extract useful information that improves both understanding of the extent and severity of brain injury and prediction of the need for extensive and intensive rehabilitation.

FUTURE DIRECTIONS

Brain evoked potential testing, whether done simply or with the aid of computerized sophistication that allows brain mapping, has much to recommend it. It is innocuous, noninvasive, and relatively inexpensive compared with other current procedures that provide information about the status of the brain. EP testing correlates significantly with the extent and severity of brain injury and is predictive of clinical outcome in stabilized long-term rehabilitation patients with severe brain injury, although further work in this area is needed. It is also correlated with other tests of brain status and function, such as routine EEG, MEG (magnetoencephalography), rCBF, CT, MRI, SPECT, and PET scans. It complements anatomic studies by providing insight into the neurophysiologic and neuropsychological functioning of normal and injured brains.

EP testing is useful in helping to assess patients with traumatic brain injury, particularly those who are so severely injured that they are unable to cooperate adequately in physical and mental examinations. Multimodality evoked potential testing in traumatic brain injury and its current utility and limitations have been described above. The question naturally arises, where do we go from here? Research should be pursued in several directions to improve the ability of EP testing to provide increasingly sophisticated and useful information on behalf of patients with injured brains.

Integrated anatomic-functional research. The literature to date indicates a growing body of information about anatomic-functional interactions. Much more work needs to be undertaken, particularly efforts to define as precisely as possible intracranial topography and origins of evoked responses, especially the source(s) of the P300 response.[56,160] The three-dimensional EP plots reported by Clifford and Williston[28] are of great interest, and work of this type should be pursued further. From information gleaned from the literature so far, it appears quite possible to study simultaneous and near-simultaneous

left-right brain responsivity in normal subjects and patients with TBI presented with a variety of challenging stimulus situations. Researchers should follow up early findings that EP testing can be used to assess midline brain impairment, particularly impairment that impacts interhemispheric communication.[147] These studies should be undertaken concurrently with MRI, SPECT, PET, MEG, and other brain function evaluation techniques whenever feasible, including concurrent neuropsychological assessment.

There is a pressing need to gather more data about the relationship between long-latency EP patterns and outcome (short-, intermediate-, and long-term) in relation to the severity of brain injury in surviving patients. Only a few studies have been undertaken so far, and the validity of outcome prediction needs to be examined more closely with additional studies.

Another avenue of research that should be pursued is cognitive functioning in the normal and injured brain. In light of modern technology, there is every reason to believe that it should be possible to evaluate a number of neuropsychological processes with the evoked potential technique. This can become an increasingly important area of investigation in light of the limitations of neurologic assessment in mild head injury.[164] The EP paradigm reported by Clark et al., in which deficits in information processing following moderate-to-severe closed head injury were demonstrated using event-related potentials, is suggestive of one direction in which future research can be undertaken.[27] Other relatively recent findings showing relationships between ERPs and tests of intellectual functioning as well as ERPs and semantic expectancy lend further support to the expectation that ultimately the ERP technique can be used to assess the effects of "minor" head injury on brain function.[32,124]

The EP technique can and should be used to study brains challenged under different conditions. Psychophysical perceptions as well as cognitive discriminations can be challenged. For example, a patient may be requested to say yes or no to whether a tachistoscopically presented comparison is the same or different or whether what has been presented is correct or incorrect. The tachistoscopic presentation provides a time-definite onset of a stimulus that is needed for EP testing. A psychophysical test may consist of judging whether the lengths of two lines are the same or different; whether two geometric patterns or two simultaneous tones or two colors or shades of gray are the same or different. Moving to a higher cognitive level, subjects could be asked if two faces, two words, two numbers (of different lengths), or the answers to two simple mathematical problems (additions, subtractions, multiplications, or divisions) are the same or different. Observing and comparing EP patterns obtained under a placebo (i.e., a tachistoscopic flash without content) condition and under a brain challenge task condition may prove rewarding in understanding brain responsivity in normal subjects and patients with TBI. It may also help to improve our ability to judge which patients with TBI are likely to derive the greatest benefit from intensive rehabilitation and provide a marker of progress or lack of progress over time. Therefore, it can help to determine when limited intensive rehabilitation resources should be conserved and when a patient with severe traumatic brain injury should be moved to a lower level of care.

Many other avenues of investigation will emerge as one pursues the research directions suggested above. To paraphrase Goethe, the larger grows the circle of our knowledge, the larger is the circumference of ignorance upon which it touches and, therefore, the larger the number of questions that can be pursued productively.

REFERENCES

1. Abbruzzese G, Abbruzzese M, Favale E, et al: The effect of hand muscle vibration on the somatosensory evoked potential in man: An interaction between lemniscal and spino-cerebellar inputs? J Neurol Neurosurg Psychiatry 43:433– 437, 1980.
2. Ahmed I: Use of somatosensory evoked responses in the prediction of outcome of coma. Clin Electroencephalogr 19(2):78–86, 1988.
3. Ahmed I: Can somatosensory evoked potentials predict outcome from coma? Clin Electroencephalogr 23(3):126–131. 1992.
4. Alster J, Pratt H, Feinsod M: Density spectral array, evoked potentials, and temperature rhythms in the valuation and prognosis of the comatose patient. Brain Inj 7(3):191–208, 1993.
5. Alter I, John ER, Ransohoff J: Computer analysis of cortical evoked potentials following severe head injury. Brain Injury 4(1):19–26, 1990.
6. Anderson DC, Bundlie S, Rockswold GL: Multimodality evoked potentials in closed head trauma. Arch Neurol 41:369–374, 1984.
7. Andreasen NC (ed): Brain Imaging: Applications in Psychiatry. Washington, DC, American Psychiatric Press, 1989.
8. Auffermann H, Gerull G, Mathe F, Mrowinski D: Olfactory evoked potentials and contingent negative variation simultaneously recorded for diagnosis of smell disorders. Ann Otol Rhinol Laryngol 102 (1 Pt 1):6–10, 1993.
9. Badr G, Carlsson CA, Gall M, et al: Cortical evoked potentials following stimulation of the urinary bladder in man. Clin Neurophysiol 54:494–498, 1982.
10. Becker DE, Yingling CD, Fein G: Identification of pain, intensity and P300 components in the pain evoked potential. Electroencephalogr Clin Neurophysiol 88:290–301, 1993.
11. Begleiter H, Porjesz B, Bihari B, et al: Event-related brain potentials in boys at risk for alcoholism. Science 225:1493–1496, 1984.
12. Begleiter H, Porjesz B, Wang W: A neurophysiologic correlate of visual short-term memory in humans. Electroencephalogr Clin Neurophysiology 87:46–53, 1993.
13. Bergamasco B, Bergamini L, Mombelli AM, Mutani R: Longitudinal study of visual evoked potentials in subjects in post-traumatic coma. Schweiz Arch Neurol Neurochir Psychiatr 97:1–10, 1966.
14. Berrol S, Rappaport M, Cervelli L, et al: Severe head trauma: A comprehensive medical approach (collaborative). Head Injury Rehabilitation Project. Final Report to the National Institute for Handicapped Research from the Institute for Medical Research at Santa Clara Valley Medical Center, San Jose, November 1982, p VIII–65.
15. Bohmer A, Henn V Lehmann D: Vestibular evoked potentials in the awake rhesus monkey. Adv Otorhinolaryngol 30:54–57, 1983.
16. Boutros NN, Zouridakis G, Overall J: Replication and extension of P50 findings in schizophrenia. Clin Electroencephalogr 22(1):40–45, 1991.
17. Bromm B, Frieling A, Lankers J: Laser-evoked brain potentials in patients with dissociated loss of pain and temperature sensibility. Electroencephalogr Clin Neurophysiol 80:284–291, 1991.
18. Brown SJ, Fann JR, Grant I: Postconcussional disorder: Time to acknowledge a common source of neurobehavioral morbidity. Neuropsychiatry Clin 6:15–22, 1994.
19. Buchner H, Höpfner U, Biniek R, et al: High frequency vibration induced gating of subcortical and cortical median nerve somatosensory potentials: Different effects on the cervical N13 and on the P13 and P14 far-field SEP components. Electromyogr Clin Neurophysiol 32:311–316, 1992.
20. Buchsbaum MS: Quantification of analgesic effects by evoked potentials. In Bromm B (ed): Pain Measurement in Man: Neurophysiological Correlates of Pain. Amsterdam, Elsevier, 1984, pp 291–300.
21. Cannon PA, Drake ME: EEG and brainstem auditory evoked potentials in brain-injured patients with rage attacks and self-injurious behavior. Clin Electroencephalogr 17(4):169–172, 1986.
22. Chatrian GE, Canfield RC, Knauss TA, Lettich E: Cerebral responses to electrical tooth pulp stimulation in man. Neurology 25:745–757, 1975.

23. Chester SC, McLaren CE: Somatosensory evoked response and recovery from stroke. Arch Phys Med Rehabil 70:520–525, 1989.

24. Chiappa KH, Gladstone KJ, Young RR: Brainstem auditory evoked responses: Studies of waveform variations in 50 normal human subjects. Arch Neurol 36:81–87, 1979.

25. Chiappa KH, (ed): Evoked Potentials in Clinical Medicine, 2nd ed. New York, Raven Press, 1990.

26. Ciganek L: The EEG response (evoked potential) to light stimulus in man. Electroencephalogr Clin Neurophysiol 13:165–172, 1961.

27. Clark CR, O'Hanlon AP, Wright MJ, et al: Event-related potential measurement of deficits in information processing following moderate to severe closed head injury. Brain Inj 6:509–520, 1992.

28. Clifford JO, Williston JS: The effects of attention and context on the spatial and magnitude components of the early responses of the event-related potential elicited by a rare stimulus. Int J Psychophysiol 14:209–226, 1993.

29. Cohen MS, Rosen BR, Brady TJ: Ultrafast MRI permits expanded clinical role. Magn Reson 26 Winter, 1992.

30. Cohen SN, Syndulko K, Rever B, et al: Visual evoked potentials and long latency event-related potentials in chronic renal failure. Neurology 33:1219–1222, 1983.

31. Constanzo RM, Zasler ND: Epidemiology and pathophysiology of olfactory and gustatory dysfunction in head trauma. J Head Trauma Rehabil 7(1):15–24, 1992.

32. Curran T, Tucker DM, Kutas M, Posner M: Topography of the N400: Brain electrical activity reflecting semantic expectancy. Electroencephalogr Clin Neurophysiol 88:188–209, 1993.

33. Cusumano S, Paolin A, Di Paola F, et al: Assessing brain function in post-traumatic coma by means of bit-mapped SEPs BAEPs, CT, SPET and clinical scores. Prognostic implications. Electroencephalogr Clin Neurophysiology 84:499–514, 1992.

34. Dauch WA: Prediction of secondary deterioration in comatose neurosurgical patients by serial recording of multimodality evoked potentials. Acta Neurochir (Wien) 111(3–4):84–91, 1991.

35. DeLisi LE, Buchsbaum MS, Holcomb HH, et al: Clinical correlates of decreased anteroposterior metabolic gradients in positron emission tomography (PET) of schizophrenic patients. Am J Psychiatry 142:78–81, 1985.

36. Devous MD: Comparison of SPECT applications in neurology and psychiatry. J Clin Psychiatry 53 (Suppl 11):13–19, 1992.

37. Donchin E, Tueting P, Ritter W, et al: On the independence of the CNV and the P300 components of the human averaged evoked potential. Electroencephalogr Clin Neurophysiol 38:449–461, 1975.

38. Doty RL: Diagnostic tests and assessment. J Head Trauma Rehabil 7:47–65, 1992.

39. Drake ME, Phillips BB, Pakalnis A: Passive long-latency event-related potentials in mental retardation. Electromyogr Clin Neurophysiol 32:637–640, 1992.

40. Drake ME: EEG and event-related potentials in epilepsy. Clin Electroencephalogr 24(1):51–52, 1993.

41. Drake ME: Value and limitations of evoked potentials in head injury. Clin Electroencephalogr 25(1):46–47, 1994.

42. Duncan-Johnson CC, Donchin E: On quantifying surprise: The variation of event-related potentials with subjective probability. Psychophysiology 14:456–467, 1977.

43. Durrant JD, Furman JMR: Long latency rotational evoked potentials in subjects with and without bilateral vestibular loss. Electroencephalogr Clin Neurophysiol 71:251–256, 1988.

44. Eberling JL, Reed BR, Baker MG, Jagust WJ: Cognitive correlates of regional cerebral blood flow in Alzheimer's disease. Arch Neurol 50:761–766, 1993.

45. Eliason MR, Topp BW: Predictive validity of Rappaport's disability rating scale in subjects with acute brain dysfunction. Phys Ther 64:1357–1360, 1984.

46. Elidan J, Leibner E, Freeman S, et al: Short and middle latency vestibular evoked responses to acceleration in man. Electroencephalogr Clin Neurophysiol 80:140–145, 1991.

47. Facco E, Munari M, Donà B, et al: Spatial mapping of SEP in comatose patients: improved outcome prediction by combined parietal N20 and frontal N30 analysis. Brain Topogr 3:447–455, 1991.

48. Finley WW, Faux SF, Hutcheson J, et al: Long-latency event-related potentials in the evaluation of cognitive function in children. Neurology 35:323–327, 1985.

49. Firsching R, Frowein RA: Multimodality evoked potentials and early prognosis in comatose patients. Neurosurg Rev 13(2)141–146, 1990.

50. Fleming JM, Thy B, Maas F: Prognosis of rehabilitation outcome in head injury using disability rating scale. Arch Phys Med Rehabil 75:156–163, 1994.

51. Frank Y, Torres F: Visual evoked potentials in the evaluation of "cortical blindness" in children. Ann Neurol 6:126–129, 1978.

52. Ganji S, Peters F, Frazier E: Alpha-coma: Clinical and evoked potential studies. Clin Electroencephalogr 18(3):103–113, 1987.

53. Gevins A, Le J, Brickett P, et al: Seeing through the skull: Advanced EEGs use MRIs to accurately measure cortical activity from the scalp. Brain Topogr 4(2):125–131, 1991.

54. Gevins A: High resolution EEG. Brain Topogr 5:321–325, 1993.

55. Giesser BS, Schroeder MM, LaRocca NG, et al: Endogenous event-related potentials as indices of dementia in multiple sclerosis patients. Electroencephalogr Clin Neurophysiol 82:320–329, 1992.

56. Goldman-Rakic PS: Topography of cognition: Parallel distributed networks in primate association cortex. Annu Rev Neurosci 11:137–156, 1988.

57. Goodin DS, Squires KC, Starr A: Long latency event-related components of the auditory evoked potential in dementia. Brain 101:635–648, 1978.

58. Goodin DS, Starr A, Chippendale T, et al: Sequential changes in the P3 component of the auditory evoked potential in confusional states and dementing illnesses. Neurology 33:1215–1218, 1983.

59. Goodin DS, Aminoff MJ, Mantle MM: Subclasses of event-related potentials: Response-locked and stimulus-locked components. Ann Neurol 20:603–609, 1986.

60. Goodin DS, Aminoff MJ: Electrophysiological differences between demented and nondemented patients with Parkinson's disease. Ann Neurol 20: 603–609, 1986.

61. Gott PS, Rabinowicz AL, DeGiorgio CM: P300 auditory event-related potentials in nontraumatic coma. Arch Neurol 48:1267–1290, 1992.

62. Gottlieb D, Wertman E, Bentin S: Passive listening and task related P300 measurement for the evaluation of dementia and pseudodementia. Clin Electroencephalogr 22(2):102–107, 1991.

63. Govier WD, Blanton PD, LaPorte KK, Nepomuceno C: Reliability and validity of the disability rating scale and the levels of cognitive functioning scale in monitoring recovery from severe head injury. Arch Phys Med Rehabil 68:94–97, 1987.

64. Greenberg RP, Mayer DJ, Becker DP, et al: Evaluation of brain function in severe human head trauma with multimodality evoked potentials. J Neurosurg 47:150–162, 1977.

65. Greenberg RP, Newlong PG, Hyatt MS, et al: Prognostic implications of early multimodality evoked potentials in severely head-injured patients. J Neurosurg 55:227–236, 1981.

66. Haldeman S, Bradley WE, Bhatia NN, et al: Pudendal evoked responses. Arch Neurol 39:280–283, 1982.

67. Hall KM, Cope DN, Rappaport M: Glasgow outcome scale and disability rating scale: Comparative usefulness in following recovery in traumatic head injury. Arch Phys Med Rehabil 66:35–37, 1985.

68. Hall KM: Overview of functional assessment scales in brain injury rehabilitation. Neuro Rehabil 2(4):98–113, 1992.

69. Halliday AM, Halliday E, Kriss A, et al: The pattern-evoked potential in compression of the anterior visual pathways. Brain 99:357–374, 1976.

70. Harkins SW, Chapman CR: Cerebral evoked potentials to noxious dental stimulation: Relationship to subjective pain report. Psychophysiology 15:248–2 52, 1978.

71. Hess CW, Meienberg O, Ludin HP: Visual evoked potentials in acute occipital blindness. J Neurol 227:193–200, 1982.

72. Hofferberth B: Evoked potentials to rotary stimulation. Acta Otolaryngol 406(Suppl):134–136, 1984.

73. Holman BL, Devous MD: Functional brain SPECT: The emergency of a powerful clinical method. J Nucl Med 33(10):1888–1904, 1992.

74. Holmgren H, Leijon G, Boivie J, et al: Central post-stroke pain—somatosensory evoked potentials in relation to location of the lesion and sensory signs. Pain 40:43–52, 1990.

75 Honig LS, Ramsay E, Sheremata WA: Event-related potential P300 in multiple sclerosis. Relation to magnetic resonance imaging and cognitive impairment. Arch Neurol 49:44–50, 1992.

76. Hummel T, Huber H, Pauli E, Kobal G: Differences in analgesic effects of ibuprofen (acid) and ibuprofen lysinate in using an experimental evoked potential pain model. Nauym-Schmidberg Arch Pharmacol (Suppl:R104):341, 1990.

77. Hummel T, Kobal G: Differences in human evoked potentials related to olfactory or trigeminal chemosensory activation. Electroencephalogr Clin Neurophysiol 84:84–89, 1992.

78. Hutchinson DO, Frith RW, Shaw NA, et al: A comparison between electroencephalography and somatosensory evoked potentials for outcome prediction following severe head injury. Electroencephalogr Clin Neurophysiol 78:228–233, 1991.

79. Jacobson RC, Chapman CR, Gerlach R: Stimulus intensity and inter-stimulus interval effects on pain-related cerebral potentials. Electroenceph Clin Neurophysiol 62:352–363, 1985.

80. Jasper HH: The ten–twenty electrode system of the international federation. Electroencephalogr Clin Neurophysiol 10:371–375, 1958.

81. Javitt DC: Neurological approaches to analyzing brain dysfunction in schizophrenia. Psychiatr Ann 23(3):144–150, 1993.

82. Jennett B, Snoek J, Bond MR, et al: Disability after severe head injury: Observations on use of Glasgow Outcome Scale. J Neurol Neurosurg Psychiatry 44:258–293, 1981.

83. Jordan SE, Nowacki R, Nuwer M: Computerized electroencephalography in the evaluation of early dementia. Brain Topogr 1(4):271–282, 1989.

84. Kakigi R, Shibasaki H, Ikeda A: Pain-related somatosensory evoked potentials following CO_2-laser stimulation in man. Electroencephalogr Clin Neurophysiol 74:139–146, 1989.

85. Karnaze DS, Marshall LF, McCarthy CS, et al: Localizing and prognostic value of auditory evoked responses in coma after closed head injury. Neurology 32:299–302, 1982.

86. Keren O, Groswasser Z, Sazbon L, et al: Somatosensory evoked potentials in prolonged postcomatose unawareness state following traumatic brain injury. Brain Inj 5:233–240, 1991.

87. Knight RT: Decreased response to novel stimuli after prefrontal lesions in man. Electroencephalogr Clin Neurophysiol 59:9–20, 1984.

88. Knight RT, Scabini D, Woods DL, Clayworth C: Contributions of the temporal-parietal junction to the human auditory P3. Brain Res 13:109–116, 1989.

89. Kobal G, Hummel C, Nurnberg B, Brune K: Effects of pentazocine and acetylsalicylic acid on pain-rating, pain-related evoked potentials and vigilance in relationship to pharmacokinetics parameters. Agents Action 29:342–359, 1990.

90. Kobal G, Hummel T: Olfactory evoked potentials in humans. In Getchell TV, Doty RL, Bartoshuk LM, Snow JB Jr (eds): Smell and Taste in Health and Disease. New York, Raven Press, 1991, pp 255–275.

91. Kooi KA, Marshall RE: Visual Evoked Potentials in the Central Disorders of the Visual System. Philadelphia, Harper & Row, 1979.

92. Kropotov JD, Etlinger SC, Ponomarev VA, et al: Event-related neuronal responses in the human strio-pallido-thalamic system. I. Sensory and motor functions. Electroencephalogr Clin Neurophysiol 84:373–385, 1992.

93. Kropotov JD, Etlinger SC, Ponomarev VA, et al: Event-related neuronal responses in the human strio-pallido-thalamic system. II. Cognitive functions. Electroencephalogr Clin Neurophysiol 84:386–393, 1992.

94. Kunde V, Treede R-D: Topography of middle-latency somatosensory evoked potentials following painful laser stimuli and non-painful electrical stimuli. Electroencephalogr Clin Neurophysiol 88:280–289, 1993.

95. Kurita-Tashima S, Tobimatsu S, Nakayama-Hiromatsu N, Kato M: Effect of check size on the pattern reversal visual evoked potential. Electroencephalogr Clin Neurophysiol 88:280–289, 1993.

96. Kwong KK, et al: Dynamic magnetic resonance imaging of human brain activity during primary sensory stimulation. Natl Acad Sci 89:5675, 1992.

97. Lekic D, Cenic D: pain and tooth pulp evoked potentials. Clin Electroencephalogr 23(1):37–46, 1992.

98. Lhermittte F, Turell E, LeBrigand D, et al: Unilateral visual neglect and wave P300. Arch Neurol 42:567–573, 1985.

99. Li G, Elidan J, Sohmer H: The contribution of the lateral semicircular canal to the short latency vestibular evoked potentials in cat. Electroencephalogr Clin Neurophysiol 88:225–228, 1993.

100. Lindsay KW, Carlin J, Kennedy I, et al: Evoked potentials in severe head injury: Analysis and relation to outcome. J Neurol Neurosurg Psychiatry 44:796–802, 1981.

101. Machlin SR, Harris GJ, Pearlson GD, et al: Elevated medial-frontal cerebral blood flow in obsessive-compulsive patients: A SPECT study. Am J Psychiatry 148:1240–1242, 1991.

102. Markland ON, Farlow MR, Stevens JC, et al: Brainstem auditory evoked potential abnormalities with unilateral brain-stem lesions demonstrated by magnetic resonance imaging. Arch Neurol 46:295–299, 1989.

103. Mas F, Prichep LS, Alper K: Treatment resistant depression in a case of minor head injury: An electrophysiological hypothesis. Clin Electroencephalogr 24:118–122, 1993.

104. Mauer K, Dierks T, Strik WK, Frolich L: P3 topography in psychiatry and psychopharmacology. Brain Topogr 3:79–84, 1990.

105. Mauguiere F, Brechard S, Pernier J, et al: Anosognosia with hemiplegia: Auditory evoked potential studies. In Courjon J, Mauguiere F, Revol M (eds): Clinical Applications of Evoked Potentials in Neurology. New York, Raven Press, 1982, pp 271–278.

106. McCarley RW, Shenton ME, O'Donnell BF, et al: Auditory P300 abnormalities and left posterior superior temporal gyrus volume reduction in schizophrenia. Arch Gen Psychiatry 50:190–197, 1993.

107. McConaghy N, Stanley VC, Michie PT, et al: P300 indexes thought disorder in schizophrenics, but allusive thinking in normal subjects. J Nerv Mental Dis 181(3):176–182.

108. Messenheimer JA, Robertson KR, Wilkins JW, et al: Event-related potentials in human immunodeficiency virus infection. Arch Neurol 49:396–400, 1992.

109. Miltner W, Johnson R, Braun C, Larbig W: Somatosensory event-related potentials to painful and nonpainful stimuli: Effects of attention. Pain 38:303–312, 1989.

110. Montgomery EE, Fenton RJ, McClellan RJ, et al: The psychobiology of minor head injury. Psychol Med 21:375–385, 1991.

111. Morrow LA, Steinhauer SR, Hodgson MJ: Delay in P300 latency in patients with organic solvent exposure. Arch Neurol 49:315–320, 1992.

112. Müller FAJ, Hänny PE, Wichmann W, et al: Cerebrospinal fluid immunoglobulins and multiple sclerosis. Arch neurol 46:367–371, 1989.

113. Naatanen R: The role of attention in auditory information processing as revealed by event-related potentials and other brain measures of cognitive function. Behav Brain Sci 13:201–288, 1990.

114. Nelson CA, Collins PF, Torres F: P300 brain activity in seizure patients preceding temporal lobectomy. Arch Neurol 48:141–147, 1991.

115. Newlon PG, Greenberg RP, Enas RP, et al: Effects of therapeutic pentobarbital coma on multimodality evoked potentials recorded from severely head injured patients. Neurosurgery 12: 613–621, 1983.

116. Newlon PG, Greenberg RP, Gudeman SK: Evoked potentials in the management of severely head-injured patients. In Becker DP, Gudeman SK (eds): Textbook of Head Injury. Philadelphia, W.B. Saunders, 1989, pp 278–307.

117. Nordahl TE, Benkelfat C, Semple WE, et al: Cerebral glucose metabolic rates in obsessive compulsive disorder. Neuropsychopharmacology 2:23–28, 1989.

118. Nuwer MR: Uses and abuses of brain mapping. Arch Neurol 46:1134–1136, 1989.

119. Onofrj M, Curatola L, Malatesta G, et al: Delayed P3 event-related potentials (ERPs) in thalamic hemorrhage. Electroencephalogr Clin Neurophysiol 83:52–61, 1992.

120. Papanicolaou AC, Levin HS, Eisenberg HM, et al: Evoked potential correlates of posttraumatic amnesia after closed head injury. Neurosurgery 14:676–678, 1984.

121. Papanicolaou AC, Baumann S, Rogers RL, et al: Localization of auditory response sources using magnetoencephalography and magnetic resonance imaging. Arch Neurol 47:33–37, 1990.

122. Parker SW: Vestibular evaluation—electronystagmography, rotational testing, and posturography. Clin Electroencephalogr 24(4):151–159, 1993.

123. Pechura CM, Martin JB (eds): Mapping The Brain and Its Functions. Integrating Enabling Technologies Into Neuroscience Research. Washington, DC, National Academy Press, 1991.

124. Pelosi L, Holly M, Slade T, et al: Wave form variations in auditory event-related potentials evoked by a memory-scanning task and their relationship with tests of intellectual function. Electroencephalogr Clin Neurophysiol 84:344–352, 1992.

125. Pelosi L, Holly M, Slade T, et al: Event-related potential (ERP) correlates of performance of intelligence tests. Electroencephalogr Clin Neurophysiology 84: 515–520, 1992.

126. Pfefferbaum A, Wenegrat BG, Ford JM, et al: Clinical application of the P3 component of event-related potentials. II. Dementia, depression and schizophrenia. Electroencephalogr Clin Neurophysiol 59:104–124, 1984.

127. Pfurtscheller G, Schwartz G, Gravenstein N: Clinical relevance of long-latency SEPs and VEPs during coma and emergence from coma. Electroencephalogr Clin Neurophysiol 62:888–98, 1985.

128. Picton TW, Hillyard SA: Endogenous event-related potentials. In Picton TW (ed): Human Event-Related Potentials. Handbook of Electroencephalography and Clinical Neuophysiology, rev ser vol. 3. New York, Elsevier 1988, pp 361–426.

129. Plattig K-H: Gustatory evoked brain potentials in humans. In Getchell et al (eds): Smell and Taste in Health and Disease. New York, Raven Press, 1991, pp 277–286.

130. Polich J: P300 from a passive auditory paradigm. Electroencephalogr Clin Neurophysiol 74:312–320, 1989.

131. Polich J: P300 in the evaluation of aging and dementia. In Brunia M, Mulder G, Verbaten MN (eds): Event-Related Brain Potential Research. Amsterdam, Elsevier, 1991.

132. Polich J: P300 in clinical applications: Meaning, method, and measurement. In Niedermeyer E, da Silva FL (eds): Basic Principles, Clinical Applications, and Related Fields, 3rd ed. Baltimore, William & Wilkins, 1993, pp 1005–1018.

133. Rappaport M, Hall K, Hopkins K, et al: Evoked brain potentials and disability in brain-damaged patients. Arch Phys Med Rehabil 58:333–338, 1977.

134. Rappaport M, Hall KM, Hopkins HK, et al: Evoked potentials and head injury: 1. Rating of evoked potential abnormality. Clin Electroencephalogr 12(4):154–166, 1981.

135. Rappaport M, Hopkins HK, Hall KM, et al: Evoked potentials and head injury: 2. Clinical applications. Clin Electroencephalogr 12(4):167–176, 1981.

136. Rappaport M, Hall KM, Hopkins K, Belleza, et al: Disability rating scale for severe head trauma: Coma to community. Arch Phys Med Rehabil 63: 118–123, 1982.

137. Rappaport M, Maloney JR, Ortega H, et al: Survival in young children after drowning: brain evoked potentials as outcome predictors. Clin Electroencephalogr 16(4) 183–191, 1985.

138. Rappaport M: Evoked potentials. In Hall RCW, Beresford TP (eds): Handbook of Psychiatric Diagnostic Procedures, vol. II. Spectrum, 1985.

139. Rappaport M: Brain evoked potentials in coma and the vegetative state. J Head Trauma Rehabil 1:15–29, 1986.

140. Rappaport M, Herrero-Backe C, Rappaport ML, et al: Head injury outcome: Up to ten years later. Arch Phys Med Rehabil 70:885–892, 1989.

141. Rappaport M, Herrero-Backe C, Winterfield KW, et al: Visual evoked potential pattern abnormalities and disability in severe traumatic brain injury patients. Head Trauma Rehabil 4(2):45–52, 1989.

142. Rappaport M, Hemmerle AV, Rappaport ML: Intermediate and long latency SEPs in relation to clinical disability in traumatic brain injury patients. Clin Electroencephalogr 21(4):188–191, 1990.

143. Rappaport M, Clifford JO, Winterfield KM: P300 response under active and passive attentional states and uni- and bimodality stimulus presentation conditions. J Neuropsychiatry Clin Neurosci 2:399–407, 1990.

144. Rappaport M, Hemmerle AV, Rappaport ML: Short and long latency auditory evoked potentials in traumatic brain injury patients. Clin Electroencephalogr 22(4):199–292, 1991.

145. Rappaport M, McCandless KL, Pond W, et al: Passive P300 response in brain injury patients. J Neuropsychiatry Clin Neurosci 3:180–185, 1991.

146. Rappaport M, Dougherty A, Kelting DL: Evaluation of coma and vegetative states. Arch Phys Med Rehabil 73:628–634, 1992.

147. Rappaport M, Leonard J, Portillo SR: Somatosensory evoked potential peak latencies and amplitudes in contralateral and ipsilateral hemispheres in normal and severely traumatized brain-injured subjects. Brain Inj 7:3–13, 1993.

148. Rappaport M, Clifford JO: Comparison of passive P300 brain evoked potentials in normal and severely traumatically brain injured patients. J Head Trauma Rehabil 9:94–104, 1994.

149. Rockstroh B, Müller, Wagner M, et al: "Probing" the nature of the CNV. Electroencephalogr Clin Neurophysiol 87:235–241, 1993.

150. Roper SN, Mena I, King WA, et al: An analysis of cerebral blood flow in acute closed-head injury using technetium-99m-HMPAO SPECT and computed tomography. J Nucl Med 32(9):1684–1687, 1991.

151. Rosenberg C, Nudleman K, Starr A: Cognitive evoked potentials (P300) in early Huntington's disease. Arch Neurol 42:984–987, 1985.

152. Rosenfeld JP, Johnson MM, Koo J: Ongoing ischemic pain as a workload indexed by P3 amplitude and latency in real-versus feigned-pain conditions. Psychophysiology 30:253–260, 1993.

153. Rubin RT, Villaneuva-Meyer J, Ananth J, et al: Regional xenon 133 cerebral blood flow and cerebral technetium 99m HMPAO uptake in unmedicated patients with obsessive-compulsive disorder and matched normal control subjects: Determination by high resolution single-photon emission computed tomography. Arch Gen Psychiatry 49:695–702, 1992.

154. Ruchkin DS, Sutton S, Tueting P: Emitted and evoked P300 potentials and variation in stimulus probability. Psychophysiology 12:591–595, 1975.

155. Rugg MD, Cowan CP, Nagy ME, et al: Event related potentials from closed head injury patients in an auditory "oddball" task: Evidence of dysfunction in stimulus categorization. J Neurol Neurosurg Psychiatry 51:691–698, 1988.

156. Seales DM, Rossiter VS, Weinstein ME: Brain stem evoked responses in patients comatose as a result of blunt head trauma. J Trauma 19:347–353, 1979.

157. Shefrin SL, Goodin DG, Aminoff MJ: Visual evoked potentials in the investigation of "blindsight." Neurology 38:104–109, 1988.

158. Silman S, Silverman CA: Brainstem auditory-evoked potentials. In Auditory Diagnosis: Principles and Applications. New York, Academic Press, 1991, pp 266–274.

159. Small M: Visual evoked potentials in a patient with prosopagnosia. Electroencephalogr Clin Neurophysiol 71:10–16, 1988.

160. Smith ME, Halgren E, Sokolik M, et al: The intracranial topography of the P3 event-related potential elicited during auditory oddball. Electroencephalogr Clin Neurophysiol 76:235–248, 1990.

161. Sonoo M, Genba K, Zai W, et al: Origin of the widespread N18 in median nerve SEP. Electroencephalogr Clin Neurophysiol 84:418–425, 1992.

162. Sphelmann R: Evoked Potential Primer: Visual, Auditory, and Somatosensory Evoked Potentials in Clinical Diagnosis. Boston, Butterworth, 1985.

163. Squires NK, Galbraith GC, Aine CJ: Event related potential assessment of sensory and cognitive deficits in the mentally retarded. In Lehmann D, Callaway E (eds): Human Evoked Potentials: Applications and Problems. New York, Plenum Press, 1979, pp 397–413.

164. Stein SC, Spettell C, Young G, Ross SE: Limitations of neurological assessment in mild head injury. Brain Inj 7:425–430, 1993.

165. St. Clair D, Blackwood D, Muir W: P300 abnormality in schizophrenic subtypes. J Psychiatry Res 23:49–55, 1989.

166. Stowell H: Cerebral slow waves related to the perception of pain in man. Brain Res Bull 2:23–30, 1977.

167. Stowell H: Event related brain potentials and human pain: A first objective overview. Int J Psychophysiol 1:137–151, 1984.

168. Surwillo WW, Iyer V: Passively produced P3 components of the averaged event-related potential in aging and in Alzheimer's type dementia. Neuropsychiatry Neuropsychol Behav Neurol 1:177–189, 1989.

169. Sutton S, Braren M, Zubin J, John ER: Evoked potential correlates of stimulus uncertainty. Science 150:1187–1188, 1965.

170. Synek VM, Trubuhovich RV: Important abnormalities in recordings of somatosensory evoked potentials in coma. Clin Electroencephalogr 22(22):118–126, 1991.

171. Teasdale G, Jennett B: Assessment of coma and impaired consciousness. Lancet ii:81–84, 1974.

172. Thatcher RW, Cantor DS, McAlaster R, et al: Comprehensive predictions of outcome in closed head-injured patients. The development of prognostic equations. Ann NY Acad Sci 620:82–101, 1991.

173. Trzepacz PT, Hertweck M, Starratt C, et al: The relationship of SPECT scans to behavioral dysfunction in neuropsychiatric patients. Psychosomatics 33(1):62–71, 1992.

174. Tsao CY, Ellingson RJ, Wright FS: Recovery of cognition from persistent vegetative state in a child with normal somatosensory evoked potentials. Clin Electroencephalogr 22(3):141–143, 1991.

175. Turgay A, Gordon E, Vigdor M: Comparison of conventional electroencephalography (EEG) and quantitative EEG/dynamic brain Integr Psychiatry 8(2):121–127, 1992.

176. Urasaki E, Wada S, Kadoya C, et al: Amplitude abnormalities in the scalp far-field N18 of SSEPs to median nerve stimulation inpatients with midbrain-pontine lesion. Electroencephalogr Clin Neurophysiol 84:232–242, 1992.

177. Urasaki E, Tokimura T, Yasukouchi H, et al: P30 and N33 of posterior tibial nerve SSEPs are analogous to P14 and N18 of median nerve SSEPs. Electroencephalogr Clin Neurophysiol 88:525–529, 1993a.

178. Urasaki E, Uematsu S, Lesser RP: Short latency somatosensory evoked potentials recorded around the human upper brain-stem. Electroencephalogr Clin Neurophysiol 88:92–104, 1993b.

179. Verma NP, Nichols CD, Greiffenstein MF, et al: Waves earlier than P3 are more informative in putative subcortical dementias: A study with mapping and neuropsychological techniques. Brain Topogr 1(3):183–191, 1989.

180. Walter WG: Slow potential waves in the human brain associated with expectancy, attention and decision. Archiv Psychiatrie Zeitschrift f.d. ges. Neurologie 206:309–322, 1964.

181. Wasch HH, Estrin WJ, Yip P, et al: Prolongation of the P-300 latency associated with hydrogen sulfide exposure. Arch Neurol 46:902–904, 1989.

182. Watanabe Y, Shikano M, Ohba M, et al: Correlation between somatosensory evoked potentials and sensory disturbance in stroke patients. Clin Electroencephalogr 20(3):156–161, 1989.

183. Weiskrantz L: Unconscious vision. Sciences Sept/Oct:23–28, 1992.

184. Werner RA, Vanderzant CW: Multimodality evoked potential testing in acute mild closed head injury. Arch Phys Med Rehabil 72:31–34, 1991.

185. Williamson PC, Merskey H, Morrison S, et al: Quantitative electroencephalographic correlates of cognitive decline in normal elderly subjects. Arch Neurol 47:1185–1188, 1990.

186. Wirsén A, Stenberg G, Rosén, et al: Quantified EEG and cortical evoked responses in patients with chronic traumatic frontal lesions. Electroencephalogr Clin Neurophysiol 82:127–138, 1992.

187. Woods SW: Regional cerebral blood flow imaging with SPECT in psychiatric disease: Focus on schizophrenia, anxiety disorders, and substance abuse. J Clin Psychiatry 53 Suppl II:20–25.

188. Wright A, Davies I, Riddell JG: Intra-articular ultrasonic stimulation and intracutaneous electrical stimulation: Evoked potential and visual analogue scale data. Pain 52(2):143–155, 1993.

189. Yamada T, Shivapour E, Wilkinson T, Kimura J: Short- and long-latency somatosensory evoked potentials in multiple sclerosis. Arch Neurol 39:88–94, 1982.

190. Yingling CD, Hosobuchi Y: A subcortical correlate of P300 in man. Electroencephalogr Clin Neurophysiol 59:72–76, 1984.

191. Zasler ND: Neuromedical diagnosis and management of post-concussive disorders. Phys Med Rehabil State Art Rev 6:33–67, 1992.

192. Zihl J, Schmid C: Use of visually evoked responses in evaluation of visual blurring in brain-damaged patients. Electroencephalogr Clin Neurophysiol 74:394–398, 1989.

JAMES T. McDEAVITT M.D.

12

Electroencephalographic Technologies in Traumatic Brain Injury

The past three decades have witnessed impressive growth in relatively noninvasive techniques to probe the central nervous system. Computed tomography (CT) and magnetic residence imaging (MRI) provide anatomic information, whereas single proton emission computed tomography (SPECT) and positron emission tomography (PET) provide information about relative cerebral blood flow and metabolism, respectively. Electroencephalography (EEG) remains the only commonly available direct measure of cerebral neurophysiology and provides useful information about cerebral function. However, most physicians in rehabilitation settings rarely use EEGs except in the diagnosis of epilepsy.

This chapter reviews basic technical and neurophysiologic aspects of both conventional EEG and the growing array of automated and computerized quantitative electroencephalographic (QEEG) technologies. Also discussed are potential prognostic and diagnostic uses specific to traumatic brain injury.

CONVENTIONAL ELECTROENCEPHALOGRAPHY

Hans Berger (1873–1941) is generally considered to be the discoverer of the human EEG,[56] recording electrical activity directly from the cerebral cortex in 1924. The significance of this event was not acknowledged by the mainstream medical community for more than a decade; once established, however, the field grew rapidly until the 1970s when the introduction of CT slowed its growth and limited some of its applications.[43]

The typical EEG recording apparatus consists of several components.[42] Scalp electrodes are placed with particular care to minimize impedance. Although potentials recorded directly from the cerebral cortex are fairly large (500–1500 mv), by the time the signal passes through the meninges, cerebrospinal fluid, dura, and skull, it is substantially attenuated and measures only 10–100 mv at the surface.[57] The signal therefore passes through a series of amplifiers to boost the weak scalp potential and through filters to minimize unwanted signal artifact. Finally, the signal is recorded on paper, usually by an electromechanical device that displaces a pen by a distance proportional to the amount of current passing through the device.

The EEG recording is usually obtained simultaneously from multiple electrodes. Electrodes are arranged in a standardized array

317

TABLE 1. **Summary of Major Electroencephalographic Rhythms**

Rhythm	Frequency	Origin	Significance
Delta	0.1–4 Hz*	Various	Deep sleep (stages 3–4)
Theta	4–7.5 Hz	Hippocampus	Increased in some forms of arousal
Alpha	8–13 Hz	Unknown	Relaxed wakefulness
Beta	13–40 Hz	Brainstem/thalamus	Attentive states
Sleep spindle	7–14 Hz (in bursts)	Thalamus	Light sleep (stage 2)

* Some sources classify delta activity as waves with frequencies of 1–4 Hz and anything slower as "slow waves." (Adapted from Sklar B, Hanley J, Simmons WW: A computer analysis of EEG spectral signatures from normal and dyslexic children. IEEE Trans Biomed Eng 20:20–26, 1973, with permission.)

referred to as a montage. Many electrode montages have been used in the past for both clinical and research purposes. The majority of studies performed today use the international 10–20 system, in which anatomic landmarks of the skull are identified and electrodes are placed at intervals of 10% or 20% of the distance between landmarks. Thus the montage is standardized for relative distance and can be used on heads of all sizes, even those of premature infants.[66]

The EEG recording consists of several lines that on first glance may appear to be oscillating randomly. However, careful inspection and experience allow identification of families of rhythms that are similar in shape, duration, and frequency. EEG rhythm patterns have been recently discussed at length by Steriade[75] and are reviewed briefly here.

Beta rhythms have the fastest frequency (13–40 Hz) of all normal rhythms. Beta activity increases in attentive states. For example, occipital beta activity increases in dogs during periods of intense visual attention. Generation of beta waves requires intact neuronal connection between the brainstem reticular activating system, thalamus, and cerebral cortex. Transection of the brainstem at the mesopontine junction eliminates beta waves and produces coma.

Alpha rhythms, which are relatively fast at 8–13 Hz, also are normal and typically are seen in states of relaxed wakefulness, as when the eyes are closed in a quiet room. Stimulation, especially visual stimulation, and increased mental effort eliminate alpha waves from the recording, a normal phenomenon known as alpha suppression or blocking.[57]

Theta and delta rhythms comprise the majority of the slower frequency rhythms, oscillating at 4.0–7.5 Hz and 0.1–4.0 Hz, respectively. Theta rhythms may originate in the hippocampus. Delta rhythms probably originate from various sources and are normally seen in the deeper stages (3 and 4) of sleep.

A final rhythm pattern deserves mention, because it is a central character in the discussion of EEG changes in head injury. Spindle oscillations or sleep spindles, which occur during normal stage 2 sleep, consist of 1–2 second bursts of 7–14 Hz waves. They are believed to originate in the thalamus. The various EEG rhythms are summarized in Table 1.

Conventional Electroencephalography in Traumatic Coma

One of the earliest studies of EEG changes after traumatic brain injury, performed in 1941, examined injuries sustained in war.[87] Of the 74 patients, 31 were classified as exhibiting abnormal EEG findings. The study demonstrated two weaknesses in design that were to plague EEG research into brain injury for four decades: (1) the author had difficulty in classifying the wide range of nonspecific findings,[69] and (2) the study population was heterogenous, including patients with mild concussions as well as patients in deep coma.

During the next several years, the sophistication of the EEG literature related to coma increased in three general areas: (1) identification of specific EEG findings that confer either a favorable or unfavorable prognosis, (2) improvement in coma classification, and (3) improvement in the systematic classification of EEG findings.

Specific Prognostic Indicators

At the time of the earliest studies of coma, diffuse delta activity was believed to be the predominant finding in most comatose states. Variations in electroencephalographic patterns that appeared to have some value in predicting ultimate prognosis were gradually identified. As previously discussed, in normal stages of sleep bursts of 7–14 Hz activity known as sleep spindles are frequently seen. Chatrian[15] first reported a case series of 11 comatose patients with favorable outcomes who displayed normal sleep spindles on EEG. A subsequent retrospective review examined the records of 184 patients, of whom only 19 were comatose as a result of trauma. Patients whose EEG recording included normal-appearing sleep potentials had a better prognosis. Later studies[11] confirmed the favorable prognostic value of normal sleep spindles, which are present in the majority of comatose patients acutely but frequently disappear or are replaced by atypical potentials after 48 hours. The persistence of normal sleep potentials beyond 48 hours appears to confer a favorable functional prognosis.[69]

Additional factors suggest an unfavorable prognosis. Comatose patients whose EEGs display predominant activity that is morphologically similar to alpha waves (alpha coma) tend to have a worse prognosis for survival.[86] The finding of alpha coma is less ominous if the electroencephalographic changes resolve within 24 hours.[35] Similarly, coma with predominant theta activity on EEG (theta coma) proved to be uniformly fatal in about a dozen reported cases.[76,77] There are no reports of survival in patients with theta coma.

These early prognostic studies certainly added to the understanding of electroencephalographic changes after traumatic coma. However, they are of little use in a rehabilitation setting, because they generally predict survival rather than function.

Improvement in Coma Classifications

EEG research into brain injury has been hampered by imprecise classification of injury severity. An early study[72] of comatose patients included a "light coma" group, defined as patients in whom "arousal and cooperation [are] at times possible; more often there is confusion, disorientation and sometimes restlessness." Such imprecision in the definition of coma produced confusing and contradictory results in early coma studies.

This confusion was eased in the late 1960s by increased sophistication in the classification of coma. Plum and Posner[64] described a classification system, contemporaneously with Gerstenbrand and Lücking,[27] based on the concept of rostral-caudal progression. The concept holds that an unrelieved supratentorial mass lesion results in an orderly progression of diencephalic, midbrain, pontine, and medullary failure, which can be tracked clinically by examining the patient's respiratory pattern, pupillary responses, ocular reflexes, and motor responses. The two classification systems are summarized in Table 2.

TABLE 2. Stages of Coma: Rostral-Caudal Progression

Coma Stage		Clinical Findings			
Plum and Posner[64]	Gerstenbrand and Lücking[27]	Respiratory Pattern	Pupillary Response	Oculocephalic/ Oculovestibular Reflexes	Motor Response
Early diencephalic	MBS1/MBS2	Normal, possible Cheyne-Stokes	Small/reactive	Normal	Hypertonic
Late diencephalic	MBS3	Cheyne-Stokes	Small/reactive	Normal	Decorticate
Midbrain/upper pons	MBS4	Central hyper-ventilation	Slightly dilated/ unreactive	May be impaired	Decerebrate
Lower pontine/ upper medullary	BBS1	Rapid and shallow	Unreactive	Absent	Flaccid
Medullary	BBS2	Irregular in rate and depth	Unreactive	Absent	Flaccid

MBS = midbrain syndrome, BBS = midbrain bulbar syndrome.

Investigators soon incorporated the more sophisticated strategies of coma classification into studies to define more precisely patterns of EEG findings in head injury, and certain clear relationships between the degree of rostral-caudal progression and EEG findings have emerged. Rumpl[68] studied 80 comatose patients, classified by Gerstenbrand and Lücking's criteria. As subjects progressed from diencephalic to midbrain, pontine, and medullary involvement, EEG activity changed in favor of predominantly slower rhythms (i.e., delta rhythms), and the signals became more homogeneous. Although the study was not designed to evaluate EEG as a prognostic tool, Rumpl observed that the absence of normal-appearing sleep spindles seemed to confer an unfavorable prognosis for survival.

Of note, Gerstenbrand and Lücking's classification system, based on stages of midbrain syndrome (MBS) and midbrain bulbar syndrome (BBS), was a strong prognostic tool. Only 3 of 19 patients classified as MBS-1 died or remained vegetative, compared with 12 of 31 patients classified as MBS-2. Essentially all patients (70 of 71) with more caudal involvement (MBS-3 through BBS-2) died or remained vegetative. Such data must be interpreted with caution, because prognosis was not the intended focus of the study and the length of follow-up of the vegetative patients was not specified.

The work discussed thus far is limited in that survival was the only measure of outcome considered. A later study[69] included the Glasgow Outcome Scale as a measure of functional outcome. Again, there was little variance in outcome among patients classified as BBS-1 and BBS-2, all of whom died. The majority of patients classified as MBS-1 and MBS-2 had a good outcome. However, outcomes in the MBS-3 and MBS-4 groups were highly variable. Review of the data suggests the EEG may be somewhat helpful in clarifying the prognosis of the latter group. However, this question was not subjected to statistical analysis.

Classifications of Electroencephalographic Findings

Improved systems for classifying coma enabled comparison of patients with similar severity of injury and represented a significant advance in the EEG literature related to brain trauma. However, a more difficult problem has been to develop a system of reliably interpreting and categorizing the myriad of potential EEG findings.

In 1965 Hockaday[34] described one of the first EEG classification systems. The scale classifies EEG findings into five grades based on predominant activity (Table 3). Since that time, variations of the scale have been proposed in an attempt to incorporate the various known prognostic indicators in EEG (e.g., sleep spindles).[11,67,68]

Synek[78,79] in 1988 observed that, using existing EEG classification systems, 20% of studied patients were not classifiable. He proposed a system that expanded on Hockaday's original scheme, with subcategories for all known EEG patterns including reactivity, sleep spindles, epileptiform patterns, burst suppression patterns, alpha coma, and theta coma. Essentially, Synek added subdivisions to Hockaday's original five grades, expanding the number of classification grades to 15. He then attempted to establish the prognostic utility of the proposed scale.[79] For each of the 15 grades a judgment was made as to the prognostic significance of the findings. Classification of each grade as malignant (e.g., theta pattern coma), benign (e.g., reactive alpha activity), or uncertain (e.g., predominant delta activity) was based on a review of the literature. The EEGs of 63 anoxic and 104 traumatic coma patients were classified according to the scheme, and outcomes were compared. Patients displaying malignant patterns died or were left with significant disability, whereas all patients with benign patterns survived with little disability. As expected, the "uncertain" group included a wide range of outcomes. Unfortunately, one-half of the posttraumatic EEGs fell into the uncertain category, limiting the prognostic utility of the test.

In 1991 Rae-Grant[65] proposed a markedly different sort of system that converted the EEG interpretation into a single number. Twenty characteristics of the EEG signal were identified, including the majority of favorable and unfavorable prognostic indicators, and each was assigned a numerical weight based on its relative strength as a

TABLE 3.   Electroencephalographic Classification

Grade I	Within normal limits	a.	Alpha rhythm.
		b.	Predominant alpha with rare theta.
Grade II	Mildly abnormal	a.	Predominant theta with rare alpha.
		b.	Predominant theta with some delta.
Grade III	Moderately abnormal	a.	Delta, mixed with theta and rare alpha.
		b.	Predominant delta, with no other activity.
Grade IV	Severely abnormal	a.	Diffuse delta, with brief isoelectric periods.
		b.	Scattered delta in some leads only with absence of activity in other leads.
Grade V	Extremely abnormal	a.	A nearly flat record.
		b.	No EEG at all.

From Hockaday JM, et al: Electroencephalographic changes in acute cerebral anoxia from cardiac or respiratory arrest. Electroencephalogr Clin Neurophysiol 18:575–586, 1965, with permission.

predictor. For example, electrocerebral silence, which is associated with a dismal prognosis, was assigned a score of −10. Normal alpha background activity, a uniformly favorable sign, was assigned a score of +10. Variables were scored as present or absent, and a single numerical score was generated to represent the sum of all characteristics. When compared with the Glasgow Outcome Scale, the EEG score accounted for 27% of the variance in functional outcome. Interrater reliability and intrarater reliability were good. The system has the theoretical advantage of generating a single numerical score and therefore may be useful in incorporating EEG findings into multivariant analysis in the future development of prognostic equations.

Summary of Prognostic Utility of Electroencephalography in Traumatic Coma

EEG displays definite, albeit limited utility in prognostication during traumatic coma. The following observations are generally valid.

1. In acute coma, EEG is a powerful predictor of survival. Some authors[79] report accurate predictions in up to 95% of cases.

2. For patients with coma secondary to an intracranial mass or mass effect (e.g., intracranial hematomas, cerebral edema) classification into stages of rostral-caudal progression provides prognostic information for survival. EEG may be useful in confirming the appropriate clinical classification and may add limited predictive value.

3. To date, few studies have examined the relationship between EEG findings and

functional outcome. Initial work suggests that EEG has a role in functional prognostication. However, it remains to be seen if the predictive value is independent of other clinical prognostic signs (e.g., depth of coma, eye findings).

Brain Death

The importance of prompt and accurate assessment of the absence of cerebral function has been amplified by growing demands for organs for transplantation. Declaration of brain death should be made only by a physician familiar with the procedure. The determination is made based on a combination of physical and electrical findings. On neurologic examination, the pupils must be fixed and a third nerve injury excluded. All movement attributable to the cranial nerves must be absent, and the patient must be apneic. The EEG must confirm the presence of electrocerebral silence on multiple tracings, separated by 6–24 hours, depending on the criteria used. Specific technical standards for recording the EEG signal must be followed carefully.[6]

Conventional Electroencephalography in Mild Traumatic Brain Injury

Documentation of the natural history of EEG changes after mild head injury is sparse, because the majority of studies concentrate on moderate and severe trauma.[9]

Dow[18] used equipment located at the workplace to perform EEGs on injured shipyard workers. Studies were performed within minutes to hours of the initial injury on 197 workers with head trauma and compared with studies of 211 controls. In both groups, equal numbers of EEGs were interpreted as normal, borderline, or abnormal, despite a slightly higher yield of abnormal findings in studies obtained during the first 30 minutes. In an intriguing study,[50] published only in abstract, 72 patients with head trauma had pre- and postinjury EEGs available for comparison. Studies converted from normal to abnormal in 42% of the cases; however, a similar number (31%) converted from abnormal to normal.

More recently, Jacome[36] studied 54 patients with mild brain injury and postconcussive symptoms. All patients had a normal neurologic examination and CT scan of the head. Standard EEGs were obtained as well as 24-hour ambulatory tracings. Participants were instructed to keep a symptom log during the recording period. All studies were normal, and there was no temporal correlation between postconcussive symptoms and EEG abnormalities.

In summary, the limited available data suggest that conventional EEG has little utility in evaluating patients with mild head trauma.[9] A normal study does not exclude the diagnosis of postconcussive syndrome. Conversely, given the variety of findings in normal, noninjured individuals, it is difficult to determine with certainty if an atypical wave form represents true pathology.

QUANTITATIVE ELECTROENCEPHALOGRAPHIC TECHNOLOGIES

When Berger initially recorded a cortical electrical potential in 1924, several years passed before his discovery was accepted by the general neurophysiology community. The debate over the existence of Berger's potentials was often rancorous. His belief that the potentials represented some sort of psychic energy that was transferrable between individuals helped to paint his work as a fringe element and also colored the debate. The current controversy surrounding the clinical utility of various quantitative electroencephalographic (QEEG) technologies bears more than a passing resemblance to issues that initially plagued traditional EEG.

It is beyond the scope of this chapter to provide a comprehensive review of the QEEG literature; several texts have been dedicated to this topic. This section (1) describes the various QEEG technologies, (2) briefly reviews the various methodologic and statistical issues that limit immediate clinical utility, and (3) reviews the QEEG literature that pertains to TBI.

QEEG is a broad term that encompasses a wide variety of techniques, including spectral analysis, compressed spectral array, topographical mapping, and significance probability mapping. A common element in all of these techniques is that they use some means of automated analysis of the traditional EEG signal to establish the frequency of various waveforms. The process is loosely analogous to the separation of white light with a prism. Once a beam of light travels through the prism, it is readily appreciated to be composed of a mixture of the primary colors, red, blue, and yellow.

A traditional EEG recording from a single electrode can likewise be broken down into sinusoidal waves by a mathematical process known as Fourier transformation,[21,84] and the relative amount of alpha, beta, delta and theta activity is determined by an automated process. Although Fourier analysis is not new, its practicality in analyzing electroencephalographs was limited for decades by the excessive numbers of calculations required to process a complex EEG signal. In the mid 1960s analysis of a few seconds of an EEG signal required 6 hours of computer calculation time. The initial breakthrough that made QEEG more practical was not an improvement in computers but the development of the "fast-Fourier transformation," a mathematical algorithm that greatly improved the speed and efficiency of performing Fourier transformation.[23]

Frequency analysis (spectral analysis) represents the fundamental component common to all QEEG technologies. A limited amount of a standard EEG tracing is obtained, commonly 30 seconds. The signal is processed in a manner analogous to the passage of light through a prism. Just as a prism separates white light, revealing the relative amounts of blue, yellow, and red, quantitative analysis of the EEG signal reveals the relative amounts of beta, alpha, theta, and delta activity in the complex EEG signal. The amount of the various waveforms is quantified and displayed in one of several formats, including line graphs and histograms. **Power spectral analysis**, a variation of frequency analysis, is obtained by squaring the frequency.[59]

Topographic mapping is a visual means of displaying frequency or power analyses. Basically, all data obtained from 16–32 individual electrodes are converted to a color or shade of gray in a monochrome system, which is then used to fill in a head-shaped oval. The result is a colorful summary of the data that bears a superficial resemblance to CT or MRI. This display system has the advantage of being easily understood by nonexperts in electroencephalography.

Significance probability mapping takes the process one step further by comparing data points to a normal population. QEEG data are obtained from a population of normal individuals to establish a normative database. Data obtained from each electrode of the patient under evaluation are then compared to the database, and a topographic map is generated that reflects only the data points that vary significantly from normal, usually by two standard deviations.[21] With the advent of inexpensive, powerful personal computers, commercial significance probability mapping systems have become increasing available. Neurometrics[37] and Brain Electrical Activity Mapping (BEAM)[21] are two such systems, both of which use a proprietary normative database.

All QEEG technologies quantify the amount of activity (alpha, beta, delta, and theta) at each recording electrode, whereas traditional EEG generates qualitative data. In addition, QEEG can evaluate data in ways not possible with standard EEG by comparing the relationship of signals received simultaneously from different electrodes.[59] **Phase** or the **phase angle** examines the arrival time of various frequency components of a tracing at different leads.[23] For example, if the cortical generator of a signal lies directly beneath an electrode, it is recorded at that electrode almost immediately but at a more distant electrode after a measurable delay.

Coherence, another interelectrode comparison, measures the tendency of the EEG signal to rise or fall in synchrony at two separate electrodes.[59] Thus, an examiner may evaluate beta activity over both frontal lobes and quantify the degree of coordination between the lobes. Coherence and phase can be measured by using any two EEG electrodes in the montage. Most commonly, any given electrode is compared with a homolog over the opposite hemisphere.

Potential Advantages of Quantitative Electroencephalography

QEEG has several potential advantages. In comparison with advanced imaging technologies such as CT and MRI, QEEG is inexpensive, portable, and free of radiation, and it requires no claustrophobia-inducing confinement of the patient.[60] Therefore, QEEG may prove to be a cost-effective alternative to more traditional imaging, especially in smaller hospitals.

In addition, whereas CT and MRI provide structural information, SPECT evaluates relative blood flow, and PET evaluates cellular metabolism, QEEG is a direct measurement of neurophysiology. It already has demonstrated at least limited utility in intensive care monitoring[60] and may prove useful in other areas such as intraoperative monitoring or in the assessment of drug effects on the central nervous system.

Because QEEG uses computer technology, large amounts of data can be processed and evaluated. Subtle differences in background activity that may not be obvious to the human reader may become apparent after computer analysis.[21] In addition, certain abstract features of the EEG tracing that cannot be visualized may be calculated by the computer.[3] For example, neither phase nor convergence can be appreciated by the human electroencephalographer without the aid of computer analysis.

Finally, in many QEEG techniques, especially topographic and statistical probability mapping, the data are presented in a format that is easily understandable to health care professionals without formal training in electroencephalography. Such ease of understanding may help in communication of results to nonelectroencephalographers.[3] However, at present no existing technology performs a truly automated interpretation of the electroencephalographic signal, and all systems still require the supervision of a trained electroencephalographer to monitor technique, to insure the quality of the tracing, and to provide appropriate interpretation of the results.

Problems with Quantitative Electroencephalography Technologies

Along with the potential advantages of QEEG, certain problems must be addressed before clinical utility can be realized. It is beyond the scope of this chapter to examine in detail all of the issues involved in QEEG, and more complete critiques are available.[49,62,59,67] The basic areas of concern can be organized into five main categories: (1) inherent weaknesses in the technology, (2) lack of standardized techniques, (3) statistical and research issues, (4) inherent problems with a normative database (for statistical probability mapping systems), and (5) inaccessibility of the literature to the medical community at large. Each of these five areas of concern is discussed briefly.

Inherent Weakness in Quantitative Electroencephalography Technologies

The process of fast-Fourier analysis and spectral analysis has the advantage of allowing the rapid, automated evaluation of a complex EEG signal. Such technology, however, involves a tradeoff: whereas regular components of the EEG signal are readily detected and processed, more episodic components are filtered out. As a consequence, sporadically occurring components of the signal, such as epileptiform spikes, may be missed entirely by the computer.[83] In addition, defects and artifacts cannot be reliably detected automatically,[5] and normal variants may be erroneously labeled as abnormal. For these reasons, QEEG is not an "automated EEG," and testing must be conducted by or in collaboration with a qualified electroencephalographer.[4]

Although the technology lacks sensitivity for episodic components, in other ways it is too sensitive. Specifically, QEEG is quite sensitive to changes in the state of the patient. Shifts in attention, changes in level of consciousness, opening of the eyes or a change in the patient's anxiety level may substantially alter the results.[41]

Lack of Standardized Technique

Another problem with the clinical acceptance of QEEG has been the failure of investigators to standardize laboratory procedures so that studies may be repeated and verified. Such concerns are not frivolous, because seemingly minor changes in technique may result in significant changes in results. For example, the choice of a reference electrode has not been standardized. The ear, which is used in many laboratories, may tend to attenuate temporal lobe activity,[41] although this point remains controversial.[49,67] Similarly, there is no consensus about the total numbers of electrodes (typically 16–32) that should be used or the technique for application of the electrodes. In addition, the length of the analyzed EEG signal (epoch) varies among laboratories.[67]

The above methodologic issues affect all QEEG technologies. Additional methodologic issues affect data obtained from systems with a topographic mapping component. As previously mentioned, an advantage of systems that generate color or monochrome maps is the relative ease with which the data can be assimilated by nonexperts. However, such accessibility may result in misinterpretation if the methods by which a map is produced are poorly understood.

The maps produced by topographic mapping systems are reminiscent of CT or MRI images and strongly resemble PET and SPECT images. However, the differences are significant. A CT image is composed of thousands of individual pixels, each of which contains real, measured information. An EEG map also may contain more than 4000 pixels, but all data are obtained by extrapolating from a limited number of true data points.[21] The only points on the map that represent real data are those directly underlying the 16–32 scalp electrodes. Furthermore, the mathematic technique used to perform the extrapolation of data varies in different systems, and such variation may affect results.[14] Novel artifacts unfamiliar to traditional electroencephalographers also may occur.[61]

The addition of color introduces another potential variation among systems and laboratories, because the use of color is not standardized.[41,85] Finally, the nonelectroencephalographer should bear in mind that the head-shaped oval of an EEG mapping system does not represent a slice of the brain at a specific level, as in CT; instead, it is a representation of cortical electrical activity no more than a few millimeters below the scalp.

Such methodologic issues are not serious impediments to the continued use of QEEG, but they help to emphasize two problems that need to be addressed as the technique evolves into a more common clinical tool. First, progress in determining the clinical utility of QEEG would be accelerated if investigators agreed on standardization of methods. Second, professionals in traumatic brain injury, especially those without expertise in electroencephalography, should be aware of the issues discussed above when interpreting the QEEG literature and scrutinize closely the technique of all studies. Unfortunately, many studies fail to provide appropriate detail about specific methods.[60]

Statistical and Research Issues

The greatest current controversy in the QEEG literature is the ongoing debate over the clinical utility of the systems. Whereas most authors believe quantitative EEG is a research tool, others believe it is ready to be used diagnostically.[38] The interested reader is referred to extensive discussions[22,59,61] of the relevant issues, which are reviewed briefly below.

One statistical concern with QEEG research is that it is prone to errors of multiple sampling. A statistical probability mapping system may collect data for 16–20 separate electrodes and 4 different EEG frequencies, as well as perform multiple interelectrode comparisons (phase, coherence). This process may result in hundreds or even thousands of individual data points.[62] If each point that varies by more than two standard deviations from the mean is considered abnormal, each data point has a 5% chance of being labeled abnormal. Therefore, if 1000 data points are investigated, 50 should fall outside the statistical range of normal.[59]

Nuwer,[59] who has written a thoughtful account of problems in the QEEG literature, believes that the vast majority of the research thus far has been exploratory rather than confirmatory in nature; others agree.[22,61] Briefly, in exploratory research a large amount of data is obtained and compared in the hope that some statistically significant relationship will emerge. Variables are not selected with a particular hypothesis in mind, and the data may have no obvious relevance to the problem under study, either intuitively or on the basis of research.[61] This problem is of particular concern, because data about the neurophysiologic significance of the majority of EEG waveforms are scanty.[71] Such research certainly has an important role; it is essentially a "fishing expedition" that may help to identify areas that merit further attention.

Confirmatory research, on the other hand, sets out to confirm a specific hypothesis or set of hypotheses, based on prior research, observation, or theory. A decision is made to limit the collection of data to variables that relate directly to the hypothesis. Errors due to multiple sampling are therefore reduced.[62]

Little work has evaluated the false-positive and false-negative rates of QEEG systems. In addition, few studies have compared the information obtained from EEG studies with information from other available diagnostic tests.[62] Clearly, it is important to establish what information QEEG can add to the clinical picture beyond that provided by physical examination, neuropsychologic testing, and traditional imaging studies. The cost-effectiveness of the various diagnostic procedures also needs to be compared.

Inherent Problems with Normative Data Bases

Statistical probability mapping systems, such as BEAM and Neurometrics, compare QEEG data with a database composed of normal individuals. The use of a normative database introduces additional statistical and methodologic issues of which the reader must be aware.

The quality of a normative database must be tightly controlled. Individuals included must be appropriately screened for neurologic and psychiatric conditions. In addition, age, sex, handedness, and medications may affect the data and should be controlled or matched with the study population.[47] For example, a database composed primarily of male college students is not appropriate for comparison with elderly stroke patients. To perform valid statistical comparisons, data must be collected under identical technical circumstances and from patients with identical characteristics.[47]

Even with careful attention to the quality of the database, error may result from the state sensitivity of the test. Level of arousal, attentiveness, mental activity,[31,63] motor activity,[28] and anxiety may influence the data obtained from QEEG studies. It is certainly possible that an individual who presents to a laboratory as a normal, relaxed healthy volunteer may have a different level of anxiety from a patient referred for a diagnostic test because of known or suspected disease.[59]

Data bases may differ in how tightly subjects are screened and how precisely data are collected. In addition, statistical methods used to process the data may differ. Probability mapping assumes that normal data occupy a bell-shaped curve. However, much of the normative data is non-Gaussian and must be transformed statistically. Different databases use different methods of transformation or fail to transform the data at all.[59]

Finally, because some statistical probability databases are proprietary in nature, their proponents are viewed by the medical community with skepticism because of perceived financial interests.[59]

Inaccessibility of Quantitative Electroencephalography Literature

Three decades ago, Walter[84] made the observation that "the physiologist who finds the computer and probability textbook distasteful, will thereby find himself handicapped in unraveling that most organized complexity, the human brain." A true understanding of QEEG research is also limited by such handicaps, and the complexity of the issues involved limits mastery of the literature by the medical community at large. Some authors question whether the editors of most medical journals possess the necessary degree of technical sophistication to critique accurately much of the QEEG literature.[62] In addition, progress in EEG research is relatively slow, in part because, in stark contrast to the 1940s and 1950s, most electroencephalographers are clinicians rather than basic scientists.[71]

Clinical Utility of Quantitative Encephalography in Other Diagnoses

QEEG has been implicated as possibly useful in the evaluation of cerebrovascular disease,[40,51,54,58] psychiatric disorders,[25,26,30,37,38,45,52,70] dementia,[10,16,20,46] and dyslexia.[1,17,19,24,39,74] The most widely accepted use of QEEG is in the evaluation of acute cerebral ischemia. QEEG has proved more sensitive than traditional EEG in identifying changes in the electrical signature of the brain immediately after an ischemic event.[40,58] In addition, changes in the QEEG signal may precede CT changes[58] and correlate with the severity of neurologic deficits more closely than traditional imaging studies.[51,55]

Utility in other diagnostic areas is less firmly established and mired in controversy, as evidenced by the wealth of point/counterpoint articles in the literature.[1,20,26,38,62,88]

Quantitative Electroencephalography in Traumatic Brain Injury

Investigations into the role of QEEG technologies in the diagnosis and treatment of traumatic brain injury are in their infancy, and the literature is sparse. Most work has used relatively simple frequency and power spectral analyses, and work examining the utility of more sophisticated statistical probability mapping systems is preliminary. Despite the lack of clear consensus in the literature, physicians and other professionals are asked to comment on the significance of QEEG tests with increasing frequency, especially in legal testimony.[48]

To a large degree the evolution of the literature related to QEEG and brain injury mirrors the earlier development of the conventional EEG literature. In both cases, coma research is much more advanced than research in mild brain injury. In addition, both conventional and QEEG literature begins by examining prognosis for survival and later incorporates measures of functional outcome.

Several studies evaluate the role of frequency analysis in the management of coma. In 1978 Bricolo et al.[12] monitored 123 comatose patients, including 87 with traumatic comas, with both frequency and power spectral array. Very poor outcomes were realized in patients with a slow, monotonous pattern in power spectral analysis; 95.6% died. Patients with changeable patterns experienced a mortality rate of only 31.5%.[12] There was also a suggestion that asymmetries of either frequencies or power distributions were indicative of poorer prognoses. Bricolo postulated that the continuous monitoring capability of the compressed spectral array may render it useful in the identification of neurologic deterioration in acute coma, but this hypothesis has not been tested.

Karnaze[44] later obtained similar results in 15 patients with traumatic coma, again using compressed power spectral array. Patients were monitored continuously over 16 hours within 4 days of injury. Functional data were also obtained in the form of the Glasgow Outcome Scale.[44] Again the importance of an alternating, changeable pattern was demonstrated. Of the 12 patients who displayed such a pattern acutely, 10 experienced good or moderately disabled outcomes. Slow, monotonous, unchanging patterns were associated with severe disability, vegetative life, or death. The small number of patients in the study did not permit statistical validation of such trends. Similar results have been obtained by others.[2]

Sironi[73] monitored a larger series of 100 patients with traumatic coma, but collected no data about functional outcome.[73] All patients displayed a high power of slow frequencies and an absence of alpha rhythms. As in previous studies, the best prognosis for survival was associated with changeable, sleeplike tracings (13% mortality rate), whereas patients with slow, monotonous, or silent patterns generally had poor outcomes, with mortality rates of 88% and 100%, respectively. The author believed anecdotally that the technique was useful clinically in identifying the late development of intracranial mass lesions and in monitoring the

neurologic stability of patients being weaned from mechanical ventilation.

Other authors,[52] using spectral analysis measurements, have confirmed the increase in slow activity (i.e., delta and theta waves) and decrease in fast activity (i.e., alpha and beta waves) in patients with acute traumatic coma. However, no study of head trauma to date has compared the information obtained from QEEG with conventional EEG. In addition, when the spectral analysis of various intracerebral diseases is compared, changes are highly nonspecific, limiting the ability to distinguish among different diseases.[52]

The natural history of compressed spectral analysis changes in comatose patients is also beginning to be defined. In one study[13] of 51 comatose patients (32 secondary to trauma), electroencephalographic signals were monitored for 15 hours/day over several days. All patients demonstrated an increase in slow waves, whereas theta and delta activity was noted to be constant, intermittent, or absent. The amount of theta/alpha activity in the first 48 hours was not a valid predictor of ultimate Glasgow Outcome Scale group. However, by the end of day 10, all patients destined for a good recovery displayed constant or intermittent alpha/theta activity, whereas those who died displayed no alpha/theta activity. Once again, the sample size was too small to draw statistically valid conclusions.

Hakkinen et al.[33] reevaluated the prior classification methods of reporting the results of compressed spectral array and devised a schema by which results could be assigned to one of six groups. In testing the prognostic strength of the system, the authors concluded that QEEG may be helpful in separating patients with good or moderate outcomes from patients with poorer outcomes. Once again, this conclusion was not confirmable statistically.

Finally, one study of QEEG in coma merits attention[82] because it provides a good example of exploratory research. Thatcher et al. followed 162 patients with traumatic brain injury and measured outcome with the Disability Rating Scale. The prognostic strength of spectral power array was assessed along with that of CT, brainstem auditory evoked responses, and the Glasgow Coma Scale. Multiple QEEG measurements were obtained from 19 electrodes and 4 frequency bands, including multiple interelectrode comparisons of phase and convergence. The authors concluded that QEEG was useful in the prediction of ultimate functional prognosis. Measures reflective of asymmetry of function, including amplitude asymmetry, coherence and phase, were believed to be most helpful; phase measurements accounted for 44% of the variance in functional outcome. It was suggested that changes in phase and coherence may reflect the severity of diffuse axonal injury, possibly explaining the apparent prognostic power of the measurements.

In summary, QEEG studies in comatose patients have demonstrated the following:

1. Patients with slow, monotonous, unchanging patterns on frequency or power analysis tend to have a poorer prognosis for survival and possibly a poorer functional prognosis as well. Prognostic utility in clinical practice has not been clearly established, but preliminary studies are encouraging.

2. QEEG may have a role in continuous monitoring of comatose patients at risk of neurologic deterioration, although this role has yet to be clearly defined.

3. QEEG measurements that reflect the degree of interelectrode and interhemispheric coordination (i.e., phase and coherence) can be appreciated only by using quantitative techniques and may prove to be useful prognostic tools.

Quantitative Electroencephalography in Mild Head Injury

QEEG in mild brain injury has received minimal attention in the literature, although significant work has been completed. In a pilot study, Tebano et al.[81] performed spectral analysis on 18 patients with post-concussive symptoms within 10 days of their injury. Results were compared to nine uninjured controls. Because only a single occipital electrode was used, measurement of phase and coherence was not possible. The symptomatic patients demonstrated significant increases in slow alpha (8-10 Hz) activity and reductions in fast alpha (10.5-13.5 Hz) and fast beta (20.5-36 Hz) activity. No QEEG differences were detected between symptomatic patients

who did or did not experience loss of consciousness. The authors concluded that this technique could not currently be recommended as a diagnostic test, owing to substantial overlap of results with the control group.

Some authors question[32] the ability of QEEG to discriminate between patients with mild brain injury and normal controls, whereas others[83] believe that the discriminative power is quite good. In an ambitious study, Thatcher et al. performed power spectral analysis of 608 patients with mild brain injury and 108 controls, recording from 19 scalp electrodes.[83] Measurements of coherence and phase were made between all possible pairs of 16 electrodes for each of the 4 frequency bands, generating over 500 potential data points for each patient. The experimental group differed from the controls in three areas: (1) coherence was increased and phase reduced in frontal and frontal-temporal electrodes, (2) power differences between anterior and posterior cortical leads were decreased, and (3) alpha activity was reduced in posterior cortical areas.

The authors report that power spectral analysis discriminated between normal controls and postconcussive patients 90% of the time. This finding should guide future research efforts, but it does not confirm the clinical utility of QEEG in the diagnosis of mild head injury for several reasons. The study was exploratory in nature, and the large number of data points introduces the possibility of errors of multiple measurements, although this possibility was mitigated to an extent by performing the study at multiple sites with validation of the results between sites. In addition, patients were not excluded for comorbidities, such as chronic alcohol abuse, or for the use of potentially psychoactive medications, either of which may affect power spectral analysis.

Although the study demonstrates QEEG differences between a group of normal controls and a group of patients with mild brain injury, the results cannot be extrapolated to confirm the diagnostic utility of the test when applied to a single individual.[62] Prospective, blinded studies are needed; false-negative and false-positive rates must be established before the technology is accepted as a diagnostic tool for mild brain injury.[59]

In summary, QEEG shows promise in the evaluation of mild brain injury and may soon prove to be useful in the assessment of patients. However, the technology currently cannot be recommended for use as a diagnostic tool. Physicians caring for postconcussive patients may find it interesting to monitor electrophysiologic changes over time, or to assess the effect of medication trials,[81] but true clinical validity has yet to be clearly established.

FUTURE TECHNOLOGIES

The wide variety of new and developing technologies no doubt will add to our current understanding of neurophysiologic processes. Initial work using QEEG technologies to study various cognitive functions[28,31,63] may be augmented by the development of high resolution EEG. Methods to enhance the resolution of the EEG signal include placement of larger numbers of electrodes (up to 124), improved anatomic placement of electrodes with MRI, and sophisticated methods to cancel the spread of the cortically generated signal as it passes through cerebrospinal fluid, meninges, bone, and skin.[29] In addition, systems that measure and plot the naturally occurring magnetic field surrounding the cortex, producing a magnetoencephalogram,[8] are under development.

REFERENCES

1. Ahn H, Prichep L, John ER: Developmental equations reflect brain dysfunctions. Science 210:1259–1262, 1980.
2. Alster J, Pratt H, Feinsod M: Density spectral array, evoked potentials and temperature rhythms in the evaluation and prognosis of the comatose patient. Brain Inj 7(3):191–208, 1993.
3. American Academy of Neurology: Assessment: EEG brain mapping. Neurology 39:1100–1101, 1989.
4. American Electroencephalographic Society. Statement on the clinical use of quantitative EEG. J Clin Neurophysiol 4:197, 1987.
5. Barlow JS: Artifact processing (rejection and minimization) in EEG data processing. In Lopes da Silva FH, Storm van Leeuwan W, Remond A (eds): Handbook of Electroencephalography and Neurophysiology. Amsterdam, Elsevier, 1986, p 2.
6. Bauer G: Coma and brain death. In Niedermeyer E, Lopes da Silva F (eds): Electroencephalography: Basic Principles, Clinical Applications and Related Fields. Baltimore, Williams & Wilkins, 1993, pp 453–454.
7. Beaumont JG, Mayes AR, Rugg AD: Asymmetry in EEG alpha coherence and power: effects of task and sex. Electroencephalogr Clin Neurophysiol 45:393–401, 1978.
8. Benzel EC, Lewine JD, Bucholz RD, Orrison WW: Magnetic source imaging: A review of the Magnes system of biomagnetic technologies incorporated. Neurosurgery 33:252–259, 1993.
9. Bernad PG: Neurodiagnostic testing in patients with closed head injury. Clin Electroencephalogr 22:203–210, 1991.
10. Brenner RP, et al: Computerized EEG spectral analysis in elderly normals, demented and depressed subjects. Electroencephalogr Clin Neurophysiol 64:483–492, 1986.
11. Bricolo A, Turella G: Electroencephalographic pattern of acute traumatic coma: Diagnostic and prognostic value. J Neurosurg Sci 17:278–285, 1973.
12. Bricolo A, Turazzi S, Faccioli F, et al.: Clinical application of compressed spectral array in long-term EEG monitoring of comatose patients. Electroencephalogr Clin Neurophysiol 45:211–225, 1978.
13. Cant BR, Shaw NA: Monitoring by compressed spectral array in prolonged coma. Neurology 34:35–39, 1984.
14. Casaglia DC, Pantaleo GG: Brain mapping: A contribution to linear interpolation. Brain Topogr 5:283–288, 1993.
15. Chatrian, GE, White JR, Daly P: Electroencephalographic pattern resembling those of sleep in certain comatose states after injuries to the head. Electroencephalogr Clin Neurophysiol 15:272–280, 1963.
16. Coben LA, Danziger WL, Berg L: Frequency analysis of the resting awake EEG in mild senile dementia of Alzheimer type. Electroencephalogr Clin Neurophysiol 55:372–380, 1983.
17. Colon E, et al: The discriminating role of EEG power spectra in dyslexic children. J Neurol 221:257–262, 1979.
18. Dow RS, Ulett G, Raaf J: Electroencephalographic studies immediately following head injuries. Am J Psychiatry 101:174–183, 1945.
19. Duffy FH, et al: Dyslexia: Regional differences in brain electrical activity by topographic mapping. Ann Neurol 7:412–420, 1980.
20. Duffy FH, Albert MS, McAnulty G: Brain electric activity in patients with presenile and senile dementia of the Alzheimer type. Ann Neurol 16:439–448, 1984.
21. Duffy FH: The BEAM method for neurophysiological diagnosis. Ann NY Acad Sci 457:19–34, 1985.
22. Duffy FH, Bartels PH, Neff R: A response to Oken and Chiappa. Ann Neurol 19:494–497, 1986.
23. Dumermuth G, Fluhler H: Some modern aspects in numerical spectrum analysis of multichannel electroencephalographic data. Med Biol Eng 5:319–331, 1967.
24. Fein G, et al: EEG power spectra in normal and dyslexic children. I. Reliability during passive conditions. Electroencephalogr Clin Neurophysiol 55:399–405, 1983.

25. Fenton GW, et al: EEG spectral analysis in schizophrenia. BR J Psychiatry 136:445–555, 1980.

26. Fisch BJ, Pedley TA: The role of quantitative topographic mapping or "neurometrics" in the diagnosis of psychiatric and neurological disorders: the cons. Electroencephalogr Clin Neurophysiol 73: 5–9, 1989.

27. Gerstenbrand F, Lucking CH: Die akuten traumatischen Hirnstammschaden. Arch Psychiatr Nervenkr 231:264–281, 1970.

28. Gevins AS, et al: Human neuroelectric patterns predict performance accuracy. Science 235:580–585, 1987.

29. Gevins A, Le J, Brickett P, et al.: The future of high resolution EEGs in assessing neurocognitive effects of mild head injury. J Head Trauma Rehabil 7(2): 78–90, 1992.

30. Giannitrapani D, Kayton L: Schizophrenia and EEG spectral analysis. Electroencephalogr Clin Neurophysiol 36:377–386, 1974.

31. Gundel A, Wilson GF: Topographical changes in the ongoing EEG related to the difficulty of mental tasks. Brain Topogr 5(1):17–25, 1992.

32. Haglund Y, Persson HE: Does Swedish amateur boxing lead to chronic brain damage? Acta Neurol Scand 82(6):353–360, 1990.

33. Hakkinen VK, Kaukinen S, Heikkila H: The correlation of EEG compressed spectral array to Glasgow Coma Scale in traumatic coma patients. Int J Clin Monitor Comput 5:97–101, 1988.

34. Hockaday JM, et al: Electroencephalographic changes in acute cerebral anoxia from cardiac or respiratory arrest. Electroencephalogr Clin Neurophysiol 18: 575–586, 1965.

35. Iragui VJ, McCutchen CB: Physiologic and prognostic signatures of "alpha coma." J Neurol Neurosurg Psychiatry 46:632–638, 1983.

36. Jacome DE, Risko M: EEG features in post-traumatic syndrome. Clin Electroencephalogr 15:214–222, 1984.

37. John ER, et al: Neurometrics: Computer-assisted differential diagnosis of brain dysfunctions. Science 239:162–168, 1988.

38. John ER: The role of quantitative EEG topographic mapping or "neurometrics" in the diagnosis of psychiatric and neurological disorders: the pros. Electroencephalogr Clin Neurophysiol 73:2–4, 1989.

39. Johnstone J, et al: Regional brain activity in dyslexic and control children during reading tasks: Visual probe event-related potentials. Brain Lang 21:233–254, 1984.

40. Jonkman EJ, Poortvliet DCJ, Veering MM, et al: The use of neurometrics in the study of patients with cerebral ischemia. Electroencephalogr Clin Neurophysiol 61:333–341, 1985.

41. Kahn EM, et al: Topographic maps of brain electrical activity—pitfalls and precautions. Biol Psychiatry 23:628–361, 1988.

42. Kamp A, Lopes da Silva F: Technological basis of EEG recording. In Niedermeyer E, Lopes da Silva F (eds): Electroencephalography: Basic Principles, Clinical Applications and Related Fields. Baltimore, Williams & Wilkins, 1993, pp 92–103.

43. Karbowski K: Sixty years of clinical electroencephalography. Eur Neurol 30(30):170–175, 1990.

44. Karnaze DS, Marshall LF, Bickford RG: EEG monitoring of clinical coma: The compressed spectral array. Neurology 32:289–292,1982.

45. Karson CN, et al: Computed electroencephalographic activity mapping in schizophrenia. Arch Gen Psychiatry 44:514–517, 1987.

46. Kaszniak AW, et al: Cerebral atrophy, EEG slowing, age, education, and cognitive functioning in suspected dementia. Neurology 29:1273–1279, 1979.

47. Klotz JM: Topographic EEG mapping methods. Cephalagia 13:45–52, 1993.

48. Litvak SB, Amin K, Senf GM: Neurolaw: Update on traumatic head injury. Advocate, Dec. 1993, pp 1, 4, 6, 8, 10.

49. Lopes da Silva FH: A critical review of clinical applications of topographic mapping of brain potentials. J Clin Neurophysiol 7(4):321–326. 1990.

50. Lorenzoni E: Electroencephalographic studies before and after head injuries. Electroencephalogr Clin Neurophysiol 28:216, 1970.

51. Maeshima S, et al: Computed topographic electroencephalographic study in left hemiplegic patients with higher cortical dysfunction. Arch Phys Med Rehabil 75:189–192, 1994.

52. Mies G, Hoppe G, Hossmann KA: Limitations of EEG frequency analysis in the diagnosis of intracerebral diseases. Prog Brain Res 62:85–103, 1984.

53. Murkundan CR: Computed EEG in schizophrenics. Soc Biol Psychiatry 21:1225–1228, 1986.

54. Nagata K, et al: Topographic electroencephalographic study of cerebral infarction using computed mapping of the EEG. J Cereb Blood Flow Metab 2:79–88, 1982.

55. Nagata K: Localization of topographic quantitative EEG in neurological disorders. Brain Topogr 5:413–418, 1993.

56. Niedermeyer E: Historical aspects. In Niedermeyer E, Lopes da Silva F (eds): Electroencephalography: Basic Principles, Clinical Applications and Related Fields. Baltimore, Williams & Wilkins, 1993, p 4.

57. Niedermeyer E: The normal EEG of the waking adult. In Niedermeyer E, Lopes da Silva F (eds): Electroencephalography: Basic Principles, Clinical Applications and Related Fields. Baltimore, Williams & Wilkins, 1993, p 131.

58. Nuwer MR, Jordan SE: The centrifugal effect and other spatial artifacts of topographic EEG mapping. J Clin Neurophysiol 4:321–326, 1989.

59. Nuwer MR, Jordan SE, Ahn SS: Evaluation of stroke using EEG frequency analysis and topographic mapping. Neurology 37:1153–1159, 1987.

60. Nuwer MR: Quantitative EEG: I. Techniques and problems of frequency analysis and topographic mapping. J Clin Neurophysiol 5:1–43, 1988.

61. Nuwer MR: Quantitative EEG: II. Frequency analysis and topographic mapping in clinical settings. J Clin Neurophysiol 5:45–85, 1988.

62. Oken BS, Chiappa KH: Statistical issues concerning computerized analysis of brainwave topography. Ann Neurol 19:493–494, 1986.

63. Petsche H, Pockberger H, Rappelsberger P: EEG topography and mental performance. In Duffy FH (ed): Topographic Mapping of Brain Electrical Activity. Boston, Butterworths, 1986, pp 63–98.

64. Plum F, Posner JB: Diagnostic of Stupor and Coma, Philadelphia, F.A. Davis, 1966.

65. Rae Grant AD, Barbour PJ, Reed J: Development of a novel EEG rating scale for head injury using dichotomous variables. Electroencelphalogr Clin Neurophysiol 79:349–357, 1991.

66. Reilly EL: EEG recording and operation of the apparatus. In Niedermeyer E, Lopes da Silva F (eds): Electroencephalography: Basic Principles, Clinical Applications and Related Fields. Baltimore, Williams & Wilkins, 1993, pp 104–106.

67. Rodin EA: Some problems in the clinical use of topographic EEG analysis. Clin Electroencephalogr 22:23–29, 1991.

68. Rumpl E, Lorenzi E, Hackl JM, et al: The EEG at different stages of acute secondary traumatic midbrain and bulbar brain syndromes. Electroencephalogr Clin Neurophysiol 46:487–479, 1979.

69. Rumpl E, Prugger M, Bauer G, et al: Incidence and prognostic value of spindles in post traumatic coma. Electroencephalogr Clin Neurophysiol 56:420–429, 1983.

70. Schatzberg AF, et al: Topographic mapping in depressed patients. In Duffy FH (eds): Topographic Mapping of Brain Electrical Activity. Boston, Butterworths, 1986, pp 389–391.

71. Schaul N: Pathogenesis and significance of abnormal nonepileptiform rhythms in the EEG. J Clin Neurophysiol 7:229–248, 1990.

72. Silverman D: Retrospective study of EEG in coma. Electroencephalogr Clin Neurophysiol 15:486–503, 1963.

73. Sironi VA, et al: Diagnostic and prognostic value of EEG compressed spectral analysis in post traumatic coma. In Vilans R, et al. (eds): Advance in Neurotraumatology. Amsterdam, Excepta Medica, 1983, pp 329–330.

74. Sklar B, Hanley J, Simmons WW: A computer analysis of EEG spectral signatures from normal and dyslexic children. IEEE Trans Biomed Eng 20:20–26, 1973.

75. Steriade M: Cellular substrates of brain rhythms. In Niedermeyer E, Lopes da Silva F (eds): Electroencephalography: Basic Principles, Clinical Applications and Related Fields. Baltimore, Williams & Wilkins, 1993, pp 27–62.

76. Synek VM, Synek BJL: Theta pattern coma, a variant of alpha pattern coma. Clin Electroencephalogr 15:116–121, 1984.

77. Synek VM, Synek BJL: "Theta pattern coma" occurring in younger adults. Clin Electroencephalogr 18:54–60, 1987.

78. Synek VM: Prognostically important EEG coma patterns in diffuse anoxic and traumatic encephalopathies in adults. J Clin Neurophysiol 5:161–174, 1988.

79. Synek VM: EEG abnormality grades and subdivisions of prognostic importance in traumatic and anoxic coma in adults. Clin Electroencephalogr 19:160–166, 1988.

80. Synek VM: Value of a revised EEG coma scale for prognosis after cerebral anoxia and diffuse head injury. Clin Electroencephalogr 21:25–30, 1990.

81. Tebano MT, Cameroni M, Gallozzi G, et al: EEG spectral analysis after minor head injury in man. Electrocephalogr Clin Neurophysiol 70:185–189, 1988.

82. Thatcher RW, Cantor DS, McAlaster R, et al: Comprehensive predictions of outcome in closed head-injured patients. Ann N Y Acad Sci, 620:82–101, 1991.

83. Thatcher RW, Walker RA, Gerson I, Geisler FH: EEG discriminant analyses of mild head trauma. Electroencephalogr Clin Neurophysiol 73:94–106, 1989.

84. Walter DO: Spectral analysis for electroencephalograms: Mathematical determination of neurophysiologic relationships from records of limited duration. Exp Neurol 8:155–181, 1963.

85. Welch JB: Topographic brain mapping: Uses and abuses. Hosp Pract 27:163–175, 1992.

86. Westmoreland BF, et al: Alpha coma. Arch Neurol 32:713–718, 1975.

87. Williams D: The electroencephalogram in acute head injuries. J Neurol Psychiatry 4:107–130, 1941.

88. Yingling CD, et al: Neurometrics does not detect 'pure' dyslexics. Electroencephalogr Clin Neurophysiol 63:426–430, 1986.

13

Diagnosis and Management of Intracranial Complications in Traumatic Brain Injury Rehabilitation

CONDITIONS INVOLVING RISK OF INFECTION

Certain types of injuries, including depressed skull fractures, basal fractures with dural tears, and gunshot wounds, carry inherent risks of infectious complications. Neurosurgical interventions such as intracranial pressure (ICP) monitors[29] and shunts are also associated with added infection risk.

The rehabilitation physician needs to be aware of the specifics of these injuries and the appropriate interventions. Specific awareness allows both preventive management in some instances and, more importantly, vigilance and monitoring for anticipated complications. For example, a fever in a patient with a known basal skull fracture takes on added significance that would not be appreciated if the injury were characterized simply as "closed head injury." Detailed transfer records and discussion with the referring neurosurgeon help to provide clarification.

Depressed Skull Fractures

Depressed fractures are generally considered significant if the fragment is depressed below the inner table by more than the thickness of the skull. Tangential skull radiographic views show these fractures most effectively. Depressed fractures are called closed or simple when there is no overlying scalp laceration; they are called open or complex when there is an overlying laceration. Compound depressed fractures are much more frequent than simple depressed fractures, accounting for 85% of some series.[34]

Significant cosmetic deformity is generally accepted as a surgical indication. Some neurosurgeons also elevate simple depressed fractures in the hope of preventing epilepsy. Others are discouraged by the hazards of surgery in the absence of substantiating data.

Compound fractures generally are elevated and debrided to reduce the risk of infection. Prophylactic antibiotics are controversial in such patients. One retrospective study showed a lowered infection rate with prophylaxis,[34] but further study is warranted to answer this question definitively.

Cerebrospinal Fluid Fistulas

The base of the skull is comprised of five bones: the sphenoid, ethmoid (including cribriform

333

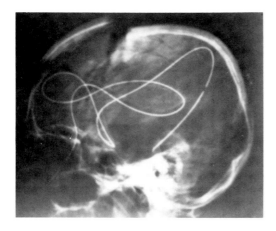

FIGURE 1. Lateral roentgenogram showing massive skull fracture of cranial vault. Basal fractures were not recognized, and a nasogastric tube was introduced intracranially with fatal consequences. (From Cooper PR: Skull fracture and traumatic cerebrospinal fluid fistulas. In Cooper PR (ed): Head Injury, 3rd ed. Baltimore, Williams & Wilkins, 1993, with permission.)

plate), frontal, temporal (petrous and squamous), and occipital bones.[34] Because the dura is closely adherent to the bones of the skull base, basilar fractures are frequently associated with dural tears. The resultant fistulous connection between brain and sinuses or ear provides a possible route of entry for infection; it is this fistula, not a cerebrospinal fluid (CSF) leak or pneumocephalus per se, that creates an increased risk of meningitis. Thus, even if CSF drainage stops, the future risk of meningitis is not necessarily eliminated.

In addition to risk of infection, basal fractures involve the possible loss of structural brain protection. For example, nasogastric tubes should be avoided in patients with frontal fossa fractures to prevent the risk of brain penetration (Fig. 1). Thus, unlike linear skull vault fractures, basal fractures are of clinical consequence and justify efforts to establish their diagnosis.

Of course, CSF leak and pneumocephalus are indications of basal fracture and fistula. Other clues to likely basal fracture include hemotympanum, Battle's sign (ecchymosis in the mastoid region), hearing impairment, peripheral facial nerve weakness, periorbital ecchymosis, fracture of the frontal sinus, or

anosmia.[90] In some patients, computed tomography (CT) or magnetic resonance imaging (MRI) may show evidence of encephalocele (brain protrusion through a skull defect) without clinical signs of basal fractures or CSF leak.

Cerebrospinal Fluid Rhinorrhea

CSF rhinorrhea is a definite indication of a fistulous tract from the intracranial compartment through the dura and skull base. Therefore it is important to determine whether CSF rhinorrhea is present in brain-injured patients with a history of nasal discharge. Direct inquiry about rhinorrhea is important in patients with suspected basilar fracture, because some patients do not report their rhinorrhea spontaneously. CSF rhinorrhea is typically described as a watery discharge with a salty taste.[95] It may increase with manual work or leaning over and may be unilateral. A dull constant headache from low intracranial pressure may be associated.[49,95] Because it is free of mucin, CSF rhinorrhea typically does not cause nasal excoriation and soaks bed linen without stiffening it.[95] In contrast, vasomotor rhinitis is typically bilateral and associated with sneezing and lacrimation; it also contains mucin and eosinophils. More recently, pseudo-CSF rhinorrhea has been described in patients with skull base surgery in the region of the pericarotid sympathetic plexus.[36] Such patients exhibit nasal stuffiness, nasal hypersecretion, facial flushing, absent ipsilateral lacrimation, and exacerbation by warm room temperature.

A traditional test to determine whether fluid is CSF is to check it for glucose. Unfortunately, glucose strips or tape are notoriously unreliable with false-positive rates as high as 75%.[183] However, quantitative glucose determinations of greater than 30 mg/100 ml in clear nasal fluid collected in a test tube are generally reliable. When fluid is difficult to obtain, the yield may be enhanced by asking the patient to lie prone for several hours.[121] The supine position may facilitate spontaneous cessation of CSF rhinorrhea in the first days after trauma but is unlikely to resolve late rhinorrhea such as that which may be encountered during rehabilitation. If bloody nasal discharge contains CSF, a clear rim typically is present when the fluid is spotted onto filter paper.[107] Even quantitative glucose determination is not reliable when fluid is bloody. In these or other questionable cases, the beta-2 transferrin assay is specific for CSF. This form of transferrin is not normally found in serum, tears, saliva, or nasal secretions.

Once CSF rhinorrhea has been recognized, the fistula site must be identified. Common sites include the ethmoid/cribriform plate, posterior frontal sinus, roof of the orbit, and sphenoid sinus regions.[130] Fractures are in fact more common into the ethmoidal air cells just lateral and posterior to the cribriform plate rather than through the plate itself (Fig. 2).[95] Anosmia suggests fracture in the ethmoid region, whereas preservation of smell mitigates strongly against it.[34] In general, dural tears of the anterior cranial fossa do not tend to heal unless there is only a fine linear fracture with good dural approximation. Rhinorrhea into the ethmoid air cells sometimes stimulates fibroblastic proliferation that may grow to close the underlying defect.[95] Persistent rhinorrhea is therefore more often due to a fracture of the posterior wall of the frontal sinus than to a fracture of the cribriform plate or ethmoid region. Signs of frontal sinus fracture include anesthesia of the supraorbital nerves, subconjunctival ecchymosis, air in the orbit, depression over the frontal sinus region, or apparent bone fragments. CSF fistulas are typically associated with fractures in the posterior wall of the orbit or the vicinity of the nasofrontal duct. A leak into the sphenoid sinus is particularly likely to cause profuse rhinorrhea.[107] CSF leaks through the sphenoid sinus are more common when the sinus extends into the greater sphenoid wing as an anatomic variant. Unilateral rhinorrhea accurately predicts the site of the dural tear and fracture in 95% of cases. However, only one-half of patients with bilateral rhinorrhea have bilateral dural tears.[34]

A number of diagnostic tests are used to localize a CSF leak. In radioisotope cisternography, which has been used for many years, radioisotope is injected into the CSF and measured in pledgets placed in the nose. Although this technique can identify and

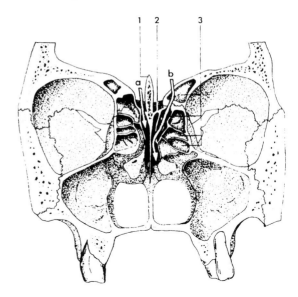

FIGURE 2. (a) Fracture in cribriform plate. (b) Fracture through ethmoidal cells, which is the more usual type. (1) crista galli, (2) cribriform plate, (3) ethmoidal cells. (From MacGee EE: Cerebrospinal fluid fistula. In Vinken PT, Bruyn GW (eds): Handbook of Clinical Neurology, vol. 24. New York, Elsevier, 1976, with permission.)

lateralize a CSF leak, it is not as precise as newer methods for pinpointing the exact location of the leak.

CT cisternography has been particularly useful for fistula localization. The CT scan is obtained after injection of a contrast dye, such as metrizamide, and the actual leak is shown. This method is effective in patients with an active leak but may fail to visualize intermittent leaks that are not active at the time of the study. Seizures are also a possible risk with metrizamide cisternography.

Recently digital subtraction cisternography following C1–C2 puncture has been reported to add further information to that obtained by CT.[183] When this approach is used, both digital subtraction cisternography and CT scan may be obtained following a single cisternal contrast injection.

All of the above approaches are invasive techniques. MRI scan offers a noninvasive way to demonstrate leaks in some patients. Using special MRI techniques, images with heavy T2 weighting may highlight CSF sufficiently to show the leak. Unfortunately, the false-negative rate is higher than with CT

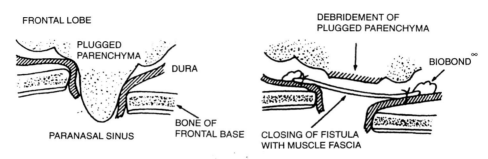

FIGURE 3. Preoperative fistula *(left)* and postoperative state *(right)*. The cerebral herniation (encephalocele) into the fractured bone was confirmed by intradural observation. After debridement of the plugged parenchyma, fascia lata femoralis was patched over the dural opening of the fistula with silk sutures and Biobond from within. (From Okada J, et al: Unusually late onset of cerebrospinal fluid rhinorrhea after head trauma. Surg Neurol 35:215, 1991, with permission.)

cisternography. Therefore, a suggested approach is (1) to determine the presence of a leak, (2) to obtain MRI for attempted localization, and (3) to proceed to invasive approaches such as CT cisternography, if necessary, for definitive localization.[183]

CSF rhinorrhea implies a 10-fold increase in the risk of subsequent meningitis.[175] Although two-thirds of cases of CSF rhinorrhea present immediately[130] and 85% of these cease within 1 week,[158] significant late problems with both rhinorrhea[121] and meningitis[90,130] have been described. A longer duration of CSF leak is associated with a greater risk of meningitis.[175] In addition, meningitis has been reported in 20% or more of patients even when rhinorrhea has been transient.[130] Rhinorrhea persists for over a month in 10% of cases,[175] and multiple cases of rhinorrhea have presented years after the original trauma.[121,130,152] In some late presenting cases brain tissue has been trapped in the dural defect, apparently making a temporary seal but preventing dural closure[121] (Fig. 3). Coughing, sneezing, hard work, or inverted posture may facilitate opening of the leak.

In cases presenting years after the injury the cerebral plug may become inadequate with brain atrophy or change in compliance. In one series of 44 patients with meningitis, over one-half of the episodes occurred more than 1 year after injury.[90] Such late occurrence of meningitis underscores the importance of considering a possible fistula when patients present with meningitis and taking an aggressive approach to ensure closure of dural tears.

Surgical repair of frontobasal dural tears may be performed by either an intracranial or extracranial route. When extracranial repair can be performed, such as via the external ethmoid-sphenoid approach, morbidity and mortality are said to be low and the rate of success high. This approach avoids additional trauma to the brain and is more likely to preserve smell, which is typically lost with the intracranial approach. Intracranial surgery sometimes must be delayed because of edema, but it may have the advantage of addressing other intracranial mass lesions, typically present in 20–25% of such patients. Surgery is strongly recommended for concurrent large mass lesions even if symptoms are minimal, because CSF leakage may help to decrease pressure initially, but acute decompensation may occur, particularly with resolution of rhinorrhea.[130] Lumbar drainage has often been used postoperatively after definitive dural repair, but it is not usually recommended as sole treatment.[113,130,158]

Antibiotic prophylaxis in patients with CSF rhinorrhea remains highly controversial. Although data vary widely for the frequency of meningitis, relative risks in rhinorrhea versus otorrhea, and efficacy of prophylaxis, most authors appear dissatisfied with the current evidence and do not routinely use prophylaxis in patients with CSF leaks.[34,95,175]

Cerebrospinal Fluid Otorrhea

Otorrhea occurs when petrous temporal bone fracture and dural tear are combined with tympanic membrane tear. Approximately 20–25% of patients with temporal bone fractures have otorrhea.[34] Petrous temporal bone fractures are divided into longitudinal and transverse types. Both types are associated with otorrhea. Longitudinal fractures are five times more common. Longitudinal fractures run in the anteroposterior direction and often are associated with torn tympanic membrane, ossicular disruption, delayed transient impairment of the facial nerve, and bloody otorrhea. Transverse fractures run at right angles to the petrous axis and are associated with injury to the labyrinth, cochlea, and eighth nerve, and immediate injury to the facial nerve. Unlike CSF rhinorrhea, CSF otorrhea almost always resolves spontaneously in less than 1 week.[34,121] In the few cases that persist, the reported rate of cessation after a single surgical procedure is 98%.[34]

Pneumocephalus

Pneumocephalus is defined as gas within the cranial cavity. In the posttraumatic setting the gas is usually air. The exception is gas produced by an anaerobic infection, such as an abscess with *Clostridia welchii* after a penetrating missile injury with retained fragments. Air may be present in any of the intracranial compartments. Subdural air, mostly frontal, and intracerebral air were most common in a series of 295 patients.[97] Approximately 15% of patients with a fistula have pneumocephalus,[130] and concurrent rhinorrhea is reported in 30–50% of patients with pneumocephalus.[97]

Two major mechanisms for posttraumatic pneumocephalus have been proposed: the ball-valve mechanism and the inverted bottle mechanism. In the ball-valve mechanism, air is forced into the cranium with pressure, as by a cough or sneeze. Air enters the brain but cannot exit because pia-arachnoid or cerebral tissue tamponades the leak, preventing escape. Pneumocephalus has a peak incidence at 1–3 months after injury; this model is compatible with a delayed build-up of intracranial air from a recurrent one-way valve mechanism. In some cases intracranial air then acts as a mass lesion, compressing the underlying brain and causing focal neurologic deficits. Clinical symptoms may include

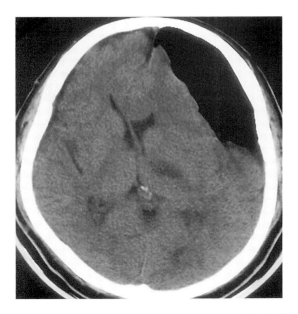

FIGURE 4. CT scan showing sizeable left-sided pneumocephalus with marked midline shift, which occurred as a complication of initial subdural hematoma evacuation.

headache, motor paresis, meningeal signs, and even psychosis. An air collection of this type is sometimes termed a pneumatocele or tension pneumocephalus (Fig. 4).

The inverted bottle mechanism is consistent with relatively early pneumocephalus in patients with rhinorrhea or otorrhea. As CSF escapes from the cranium, eventually air must enter to allow more CSF to exit. The name reflects the fact that this mechanism is similar to what happens when one drinks or pours from a bottle.

Most cases of pneumocephalus are diagnosed radiologically. However, one bedside finding is pathognomonic for pneumocephalus—the "bruit hydro-aerique,"[97] which is essentially a succession splash within the cranium. It is heard by auscultation of the head during head movement and is sometimes also reported subjectively by the patient. Although reported in only approximately 7% of 295 patients with pneumocephalus, the incidence might be higher if cranial auscultation were performed on all patients.

Definitive treatment for pneumocephalus entails repair of the underlying dural tear and fistula. In some obtunded patients with tension pneumocephalus, the air collection was tapped via a burr hole as an initial temporizing measure.[97]

Penetrating Injuries

Gunshot wounds confer a high risk of infection for several reasons. The bullet is retained inside the skull in about 70% of civilian injuries. Although the heat of the bullet may cause local sterilization,[110] it is a nidus for infection. Retained bone fragments are an even greater problem and increase the risk of infection by a factor of 10.[144] Focal necrosis of tissue in the path of the bullet is also believed to be crucial in the possible development of brain abscess. For these reasons, surgical debridement has been emphasized. In contrast to CSF rhinorrhea, in which antibiotic prophylaxis remains controversial, 87% of 966 neurosurgeons reported that they use antibiotic prophylaxis in patients with gunshot wounds.[78] Other types of penetrating injuries include knives in young adults and accidental transorbital accidents in children, such as with pencils or wires.

Cranioplasty

Skull flaps are left out initially in many patients with penetrating or contaminated wounds and in some patients with uncontrollable intracranial pressure. Cranioplasty is eventually required to provide physical protection. Although it is not usually expected to affect neurologic status significantly, occasional mild improvement after cranioplasty has been reported, possibly due to increased cerebral blood flow.[170] Many neurosurgeons delay performance of cranioplasty for 6 months after injury to minimize complications, including infection. In fact, risk of infection has been shown to decrease from almost 20% to less than 4% when cranioplasty is delayed for over 1 year after injury.[139] One concern in such patients is the risk of skull osteomyelitis, a localized process that may present with scalp defect, swelling, or local drainage.[19] In addition to a surgical flap, risk factors include loose bone fragments or comminuted depressed fractures, overlying subgaleal collection, or absent area of scalp.[107] Skull radiographs and bone scan are helpful in diagnosis, whereas systemic blood studies and brain scans usually do not contribute.[19] Infected flaps require removal and at least 6 weeks of antibiotics.

INFECTIOUS COMPLICATIONS

Meningitis

Head injury is the most common cause of meningitis in adults.[61] The classical symptoms of meningitis are well known, including headache, fever, stiff neck, and confusion. However, typical features may be lacking in 20% of patients, particularly the very young, the very old, and the immunosuppressed.[2] Focal signs are typically absent in meningitis, and their presence warrants obtaining a CT scan to rule out abscess, empyema, or other mass lesion. Lumbar puncture characteristically reveals CSF pleocytosis (predominantly polys) with lowered glucose (less than one-third the blood glucose in three-fourths of patients).

Pneumococci are by far the most common causative organisms, accounting for over 80% of some series of posttraumatic meningitis.[61] Hemophilis is, of course, important in young children. Patients with penetrating injuries are more likely to have *Staphylococcus aureus* or gram-negative meningitis.[175] Adult meningitis during the first few days after nonpenetrating injury is almost always pneumococcal and usually is treated with penicillin. Staphylococcal and gram-negative infections usually present later, necessitating broader-spectrum coverage in late presenting meningitis. Shunt-related infections warrant special mention, because they often are indolent clinically and usually caused by *Staphylococcus epidermidis* (see hydrocephalus section for further discussion).

Subdural Empyema

Trauma is an uncommon cause of subdural empyema; paranasal or ear infections are the more common antecedents.[107,175] Subdural empyema is more common in boys and men, and over 50% of cases occur in patients under the age of 20. Presentation is acute and fulminant with fever, headache, and obtundation.[175] Periorbital swelling[12] or tenderness over the sinuses or mastoid may provide

TABLE 1. Infectious Complications

	Meningitis	Subdural Empyema	Brain Abscess
Predisposing condition	Basal fistula	Paranasal sinus/ear injury Penetrating injuries	Depressed fracture Penetrating injuries
Organism	Pneumococci (early) Gram-negatives (late) Staphylococci (late) *Staphylococcus epidermidis* (shunts)	Mixed/streptococci Staphylococci Gram-negative	Polymicrobial/anaerobic Staphylococci
Presentation	Acute (shunt indolent) Headache /nuchal Mental status	Acute/fulminant Periorbital swelling Sinus tenderness Signs of increased ICP Seizures/focal signs	Subacute/progressive Focal signs Signs of increased ICP
Fever	Yes	Yes	Only 50%
WBC, sedimentation rate	Both ↑	Both ↑	Both often normal
CT/MRI scans	Negative or meningeal enhancement	Extraaxial—medial rim enhancement	Intraaxial ring enhance- ment—especially late/ lateral MRI T2 capsule
Lumbar puncture	↑ WBC (polys) ↓ Glucose	Contraindicated (↑ WBC, not ↓ Glucose)	Contraindicated (often negative)
Management options	Antibiotics	Antibiotics Burr hole/craniotomy	Antibiotics Debride Stereotactic aspiration Steroids

WBC = white blood cell count, ICP = intracranial pressure, polys = polymorphonuclear leukocytes.

additional clues. Focal signs and seizures are common.[2,107] CT scan shows an extraaxial collection with medial membrane enhancement.[188] MRI scan typically shows low signal on T1-weighted imaging and high signal on T2-weighted images.[45] Lumbar puncture is contraindicated. Multiple organisms are usually present, including streptococci. When only one organism is cultured, it is most often *Staphylococcus*.[135] In addition to appropriate antibiotics, either burr hole drainage or craniotomy is recommended.[2,12,45,125,175] Although success has frequently been reported with burr holes,[2,12] large size, midline shift, parafalcine or posterior fossa location, and loculation have been identified as factors favoring craniotomy.[125]

Brain Abscess

Risk factors for brain abscess include penetrating injuries, compound depressed skull fractures, and wound complications.[175] Brain abscess is rarely seen as a complication of basal fracture.[110] The presentation of brain abscess peaks at about 2–3 weeks after

injury. Signs of increased intracranial pressure are present in two-thirds of patients, focal signs in 50–75%, and fever in 50–60%.[110,194] In one series headache was present in 90% and vomiting in 65%.[194] Changes in mental status are notable in one-half of patients, and seizures occur in one-third.[110] Table 1 contrasts key features of meningitis, subdural empyema, and brain abscess.

Four stages of abscess formation have been recognized pathologically and correlated with CT scan findings[110]:

1. **Early cerebritis.** At this stage inflammatory cells in a perivascular location are responsible for the term cerebritis. These inflammatory cells also enter the developing necrotic center. Surrounding edema is prominent. CT scan at this stage shows low density with little enhancement, which may be solid, and does not decay on late CT images. Although CT has been reported to have a low false-negative rate in brain abscess,[77] at this stage both radioisotope brain scan[110] and MRI scan[2] are more sensitive. MRI during cerebritis shows uniform signal with indistinct margins.[194]

2. **Late cerebritis.** At this stage the necrotic center reaches maximal size, fibroblasts and macrophages are found at the periphery along with marked vascular proliferation, and surrounding edema also reaches maximal size. CT scan shows increase in the low-density center with a thin rim of enhancement and increasing edema.

3. **Early capsule.** At this point a capsule of collagen and reticulin begins to develop. The capsule forms more slowly on the ventricular side of the abscess. The size of the necrotic center is also decreased. CT scan now shows a ring-enhancing capsule (less medially and with decreased enhancement on delayed films) and decrease in the central lucency.

4. **Late capsule.** At this point the collagenous capsule is prominent, with surrounding gliosis and edema. CT shows prominent ring enhancement and a low-density center. MRI scan shows the capsule as low signal on T2-weighted images.[194]

Most brain abscesses are polymicrobial and include anaerobes. Staphylococci are found in about 10% of brain abscesses and are more frequent after trauma.[110] Lumbar puncture is contraindicated in brain abscess and usually not diagnostically helpful if performed inadvertently. Therefore, choice of antibiotic reflects the anticipated polymicrobial etiology supplemented by information from aspiration of the abscess. Gas on CT scan may help in early differentiation from tumor and suggests anaerobic organisms. As an abscess heals, the capsule becomes more isodense on serial CT scans.

Steroids are frequently used effectively in brain abscess to decrease edema. Unfortunately, they also delay encapsulization of the abscess and containment of the infectious process. They also may decrease ring enhancement on CT scan, necessitating following size rather than enhancement to monitor response to treatment. A corollary is that enhancement on CT in fact may increase when steroids are discontinued, despite ongoing clinical improvement. Surgical management of brain abscess includes CT-guided stereotactic aspiration[106,163] or excision. Indications to the stereotactic approach include surgically inaccessible location, cerebritis stage, or poor neurologic or general medical condition.

Excision is useful for removal of foreign material and necessary for posterior fossa lesions.

Adverse prognostic factors in brain abscess include young or old age; large, deep abscess; coma; or rupture into the ventricular system. Mortality from brain abscess in Vietnam was 54%, and survival was worse with gram-negative organisms. However, considerable improvement may occur; for example, 30% or less of survivors are reported to have significant residual hemiparesis.

HYDROCEPHALUS

Hydrocephalus is the most common treatable neurosurgical complication during rehabilitation of traumatic brain injury (TBI).[35] Identification and treatment of hydrocephalus substantially improves the extent and rate of recovery for some patients. However, differentiation of dynamic hydrocephalus from central atrophy or ex vacuo ventricular dilation remains particularly problematic.[93] Furthermore, the presence of a shunt introduces significant management problems and potential complications that may be troublesome for the rehabilitation physician. Therefore, type, pathophysiology, and clinical presentation of hydrocephalus, noninvasive and invasive diagnostic studies, shunt types, and shunt complications are reviewed in some detail.

Types and Variants

Hydrocephalus is divided into communicating and noncommunicating types.[105] In communicating hydrocephalus, the different portions of the ventricular system are interconnected, and fluid may exit the ventricular system freely to the cisterns and subarachnoid space, whereas noncommunicating hydrocephalus is characterized by obstruction either between the ventricles or in exiting the ventricular system.

Communicating hydrocephalus occurs in the vast majority of posttraumatic cases. Enlargement characteristically involves all components of the ventricular system, although focal porencephalic dilation in areas of tissue loss is often superimposed. Blood products, protein, or fibrosis from TBI typically interfere with circulation of cerebrospinal fluid through the subarachnoid space and its absorption into the bloodstream through the arachnoid granulations.[148]

When only certain portions of the ventricular system are enlarged, noncommunicating hydrocephalus should be considered. For example, large lateral and third ventricles with a small fourth ventricle should raise the possibility of aqueductal stenosis. Although this pattern can be seen in some patients with communicating hydrocephalus,[5] metrizamide ventriculography has demonstrated aqueductal stenosis in the majority of such patients.[94] The distinction has practical significance, because lumbar puncture may be of diagnostic value in communicating hydrocephalus but should be avoided with aqueductal stenosis. Although posttraumatic hydrocephalus is by definition an acquired disorder, trauma may also decompensate a preexisting congenital abnormality. Bedside measurement of increased head circumference may be a clue to developmental hydrocephalus. MRI may provide evidence of associated abnormalities, such as Chiari malformation.

Focal ventricular enlargement frequently occurs on an atrophic or porencephalic basis. Less often, however, trapping of an isolated portion of the ventricular system may produce focal enlargement with signs of increased intracranial pressure or focal deficits.[155] Unilateral hydrocephalus may occur with occlusion of the foramen of Monro. Treatment includes stereotactic fenestration[16] or placement of bifrontal shunt catheters. In patients who already have a shunt, however, the shunted lateral ventricle may be substantially smaller than the unshunted ventricle, without implying obstruction between the two.[114,155] Contrast dye injected via the shunt and MRI flow studies may help to confirm flow through the foramen of Monro in questionable cases.[155] Diverticula of the atrium of the lateral ventricle, which may compress the tectum of the midbrain, are associated with an increase in the suprapineal recess of the third ventricle and may respond to a shunt.[5] Although fourth ventricular prominence is frequently seen after severe TBI as a prognostic factor of injury severity and loss of posterior fossa tissue,[91,178] trapping of the fourth ventricle in a patient with

a lateral ventricular shunt may be associated with headache, ataxia, and vertigo.[5,155] Cavum septum pellucidum, a potential space between the lateral ventricles, is a normal variant in 1% of CT scans[160] and is known to be more common in boxers. However, rare cases of noncommunicating pathologic cava with intermittent postural headache and loss of consciousness when lying down or bending over have been described; patients responded to cyst puncture or shunting.[160]

Occasional cases of multiloculated hydrocephalus are encountered, usually secondary to meningitis, ventriculitis, or intraventricular hemorrhage.[119] CT and MRI scans characteristically show multiple irregular intraventricular septations between dilated cavities in the presence of asymmetrical hydrocephalus (Fig. 5). Septations of fibroglial webs result from intraventricular exudate, along with inflammation of the ependymal surface and glial proliferation. Progressive compartmentalization creates a large multiloculated single cavity and makes it difficult to distinguish normal anatomy in late stages. Treatment includes placement of multiple shunt catheters and fenestration of septations either endoscopically via ventriculostomy or by craniotomy.[43,119]

Pathophysiology of Communicating Hydrocephalus

Communicating hydrocephalus may develop without sustained elevation of intracranial pressure. Several concepts help to explain this counterintuitive development of normal pressure hydrocephalus:

1. Pressure may well be increased early in the clinical course.[50]

2. Intracranial pressure may be intermittently elevated. In fact, so-called B waves of transiently increased pressure are measured in some cases of normal-pressure hydrocephalus, and their presence has been used as an indicator of probable positive response to shunting.[14] Furthermore, CSF flow is also known to be pulsatile. CSF pulse pressure may be increased even when mean pressure is normal.[30,114] Laboratory models of fluid pressure for hydrocephalus have shown a major difference when pulsed flow rather than static fluid pressures are used.[114,115]

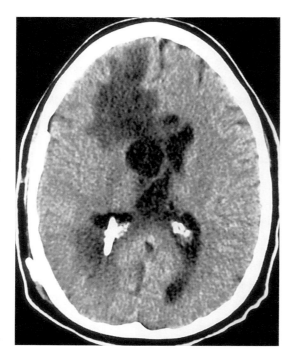

FIGURE 5. Multiloculated hydrocephalus with multiple septations. Right frontal hypodensity is also present.

3. Pascal's law of hydraulic systems states that F = P × A, where F is the force against the ventricular wall, P is the intraventricular pressure, and A is the area of the ventricular wall.[196] This formula implies that when the area of the ventricular wall is large, a substantial expanding force may be generated from within the ventricle without the necessity of high pressure. For example, if a certain degree of ventricular enlargement initially results from increased pressure, ongoing enlargement may take place, even though pressures are no longer elevated.

4. Rather than the absolute intraventricular pressure,[30,196] the so-called transmantle pressure—the difference between the intraventricular pressure and pressure over the convexity—determines ventricular size. This concept may be understood more clearly by considering a balloon. The size of the balloon is determined not only by the pressure inside, but by the pressure of the air inside relative to the air outside the balloon. Changes in the viscoelastic properties of brain parenchyma with related decrease in parenchymal pressure therefore may contribute to the development of hydrocephalus. Of note, decreased cerebral blood flow and altered vascular sympathetic supply have been described in patients with hydrocephalus, particularly in the frontal and periventricular regions, and may contribute to (as well as result from) hydrocephalus development.[22,30]

5. With blockage of absorption through the arachnoid granulations, compensatory mechanisms for CSF absorption and diversion probably are activated only at a certain threshold pressure and therefore may not help to prevent normal-pressure hydrocephalus in some cases.[114]

Clinical Presentation of Communicating Hydrocephalus

Normal-pressure hydrocephalus is well known to present with the clinical triad of dementia, gait ataxia, and urinary incontinence. Of the three, gait impairment is probably the most important diagnostically and is most likely to respond to shunting. The classic gait disturbance has been described qualitatively as a frontal lobe ataxia with short steps, wide base, unsteady turns, "magnetic" difficulty in lifting the feet, and lack of appendicular cerebellar signs.[10] A recent study of the gait pattern in normal-pressure hydrocephalus describes it as a subcortical motor control disorder. Specific features included decreases in cadence, step height, and shoulder counterrotation relative to the pelvis as well as an abnormal tendency to muscle contraction.[168]

In patients with TBI, the presentation of hydrocephalus is not limited to the classic triad of normal-pressure hydrocephalus. Loss of upgaze, characteristic of the pretectal or Sylvian aqueduct syndrome,[81] and akinetic mutism are additional clinical findings that should raise suspicion of hydrocephalus. In fact, hydrocephalus should be considered in any patient with TBI who worsens or fails to progress adequately. Patients with meningitis or intracranial hemorrhage, especially subarachnoid or intraventricular hemorrhage, are particularly at risk for development of hydrocephalus. In contrast, patients with diffuse axonal injury or anoxia are likely to develop ex vacuo ventriculomegaly. Decisions regarding shunting also should consider whether clinical deficits are consistent with known severity (such as severe diffuse axonal injury) or location of injury (aphasia with left posterior temporal contusion) or suggestive of a superimposed process such as hydrocephalus.

Although the usual question during rehabilitation of patients with TBI is whether to shunt for possible normal-pressure hydrocephalus, communicating hydrocephalus also may present with signs of increased intracranial pressure, particularly early after posttraumatic intracranial hemorrhage. Clinical symptoms include headache, nausea, vomiting, and lethargy or decreasing mental status. In patients in whom a skull flap is left out, a consistently bulging flap may indicate increased intracranial pressure, whereas an ingoing skull defect mitigates against increased pressure.

Cushing's triad of hypertension, bradycardia, and hypoventilation is well known to be associated with increased intracranial pressure. Of interest, normal-pressure hydrocephalus also has been correlated with elevated blood pressures.[12,57] Hypertension may be a risk factor for normal-pressure hydrocephalus, possibly through altered ventricular compliance secondary to infarction of deep white matter. Alternatively, normal-pressure hydrocephalus may aggravate hypertension. In one study, a subset of patients with normal-pressure hydrocephalus ran lower blood pressures or needed less antihypertensive medication after shunting, although reduction in blood pressure after shunting was not statistically significant for the overall group.[12]

Computed Tomography

CT scans have been invaluable in providing noninvasive information about ventriculomegaly. However, the distinction between dynamic hydrocephalus and ex vacuo ventricular dilatation remains problematic, and ventricular size alone has not been a reliable predictor of positive response to shunting.[14] Ventricular configuration, indices of enlargement of specific parts of the ventricular system, absence of sulci, presence of periventricular lucency, and time course of ventricular enlargement have provided additional information.

Changes in ventricular configuration that favor dynamic hydrocephalus include enlargement of temporal horns, enlargement of the third ventricle and its recesses, convex shape of the frontal horns with widening of the frontal horn radius and narrowing of the ventricular angle[5] (Fig. 6). The frontal horn index (ratio of the maximal width of the frontal horns to the whole brain at the same level), the lateral ventricular size index (ratio of the lateral ventricular width to whole brain at the level of the cella media), and the third ventricular index (ratio of the maximal width of the third ventricle to the brain at that level) have been used as specific measures of ventricular size.[179] Although such measurements have been useful for research purposes, decisions about shunting have remained largely intuitive in clinical practice.[5]

Ex vacuo ventricular dilatation or cerebral atrophy typically involves sulcal prominence. Small or absent sulci on a CT scan in combination with ventriculomegaly are predictors of a good response to shunting.[14] However, patients with anoxia and diffuse axonal injury are more predisposed to central atrophy in which sulcal prominence is less prominent than ventriculomegaly. In addition, the presence of sulci does not preclude a positive response. In one study 15 of 33 patients with sulci greater than 5 mm showed a positive response to shunting.[14]

Preventricular lucency has been extremely valuable as a predictor of a good response to shunting.[14] In hydrocephalus, fluid seeps across the ependymal lining of the ventricle and causes interstitial edema. This transependymal fluid is seen as lucency on CT. Maximal periventricular lucency is typically anterolateral to the frontal horns (Fig. 7). Of interest, this location mirrors that of expected stress in computer-simulated hydraulics of hydrocephalus.[115] Periventricular lucency is seen most often in patients with subarachnoid hemorrhage[146] and is usually not seen with enlarged sulci.[14] In patients with TBI, transependymal fluid may be confused with the lucency of frontal contusion, although the latter typically appears more irregular and asymmetric.

Ventriculomegaly has been reported in as many as 72% of patients with severe TBI.[91] Early enlargement during the first month

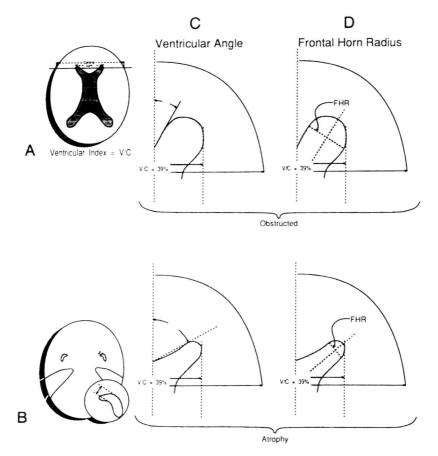

FIGURE 6. Various methods in the radiographic diagnosis of hydrocephalus. *A,* The ventricular index is the ratio of the ventricular diameter at the level of the frontal horns to the diameter of the brain measured at the same level. This is not a very sensitive or specific measurement for the detection of hydrocephalus because the ventricular index is englarged in cerebral atrophy as well as in hydrocephalus. *B,* Enlargement of the temporal horns commensurately with the bodies of the lateral ventricles is probably the most sensitive and reliable sign in the differentation of hydrocephalus from atrophy. In cerebral atrophy the temporal horns are significantly less dilated than the bodies of the lateral ventricles. *C,* The ventricular angle measures the divergence of the frontal horn. In theory the angle made by the anterior or superior margins of the frontal horn at the level of the foramina of Monro is diminished when concentric enlargement of the frontal horns occurs. Compare the illustration of hydrocephalus *(top)* with the illustration of atrophy *(bottom).* The ventricular index in both instances is 39%; however, the ventricular angle is markedly reduced in hydrocephalus. *D,* The frontal horn radius (FHR) measures the widest diameter of the frontal horns taken at a 90° angle to the long axis of the frontal horn. The usefulness of this measurement is demonstrated by the markedly increased frontal horn radius in the patient with hydrocephalus *(top)* as opposed to the patient with atrophy *(bottom).* Overall, no one measurement is completely accurate in the diagnosis of hydrocephalus; the size of the temporal horns, ventricular angle, frontal horn radius, and size of the ventricles compared with the cortical sulci should all be assessed. (From Barkovich A: Hydrocephalus. In Barkovich A (ed): Pediatric Neuroimaging. New York, Raven Press, 1990, pp 205–226, with permission.)

after injury is more likely due to dynamic hydrocephalus. Late enlargement (more than 1 month after injury) is often thought to be related to anoxia or diffuse axonal injury and often correlates with other measures of injury severity.[104,178] Of course, progressive ventricular enlargement on serial CT scans may also indicate an ongoing hydrocephalic process and assist with shunt decisions in equivocal cases.

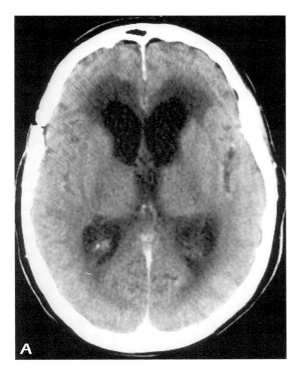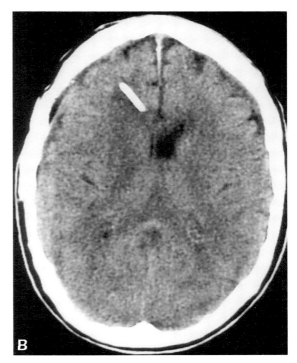

FIGURE 7.   Pre- and postshunt hydrocephalus. *A,* Marked ventricular dilatation is seen along with prominent periventricular lucency anterior to the frontal horns consistent with transependymal fluid. *B,* Following a shunt, both ventriculomegaly and periventricular lucency have resolved in association with marked clinical improvement.

Other Diagnostic Tests

MRI provides more anatomic detail about the configuration of the ventricular system than CT, including imaging of structures such as the Sylvian aqueduct and foramen of Monro. MRI is also more sensitive for transependymal fluid, which appears as an increased periventricular signal on T2-weighted imaging.[53,198] The smooth symmetric periventricular signal is most likely to respond to shunting, whereas a more irregular, asymmetric signal may be seen with demyelination or infarction due to longstanding hydrocephalus or unrelated causes.[53] There is typically no significant periventricular rimming in compensated or arrested hydrocephalus. Although some authorities have questioned the reliability and specificity of ventricular rimming,[166] it is a useful finding in evaluating potential shunt candidates.

   MRI may provide additional information when images are synchronized with the cardiac cycle.[16,154,166] During systole, blood flow

into the choroid plexus within the third ventricles is increased. This pushes cerebrospinal fluid out of the third ventricle into the Sylvian aqueduct. If the ventricular walls are stiffer, more rapid flow through the Sylvian aqueduct is detected as decreased signal or "flow void" in the aqueduct. Such increased pulsatile flow has been described in some cases of normal-pressure hydrocephalus but disappears with shunting.[154] Even more sophisticated assessment of cerebrospinal fluid flow and oscillation can be achieved with two-dimensional phase-contrast cine MRI,[116] which in the future may allow improved noninvasive diagnosis and management of hydrocephalus.

   Changes in cerebral vasculature and blood flow have been found in hydrocephalus.[22] SPECT scans have shown enlarged subcortical regions of low flow in patients with hydrocephalus. In one study, 10 of 11 patients who improved clinically with shunting also showed improved subcortical flow on follow-up SPECT, whereas 3 clinically unimproved patients did not.[184] In contrast, a poor response to shunting has been reported when SPECT shows relatively decreased flow in posterior temporal and parietal regions, a pattern reported in dementia of the Alzheimer's type.[58] PET scanning also may be of value, although results have been inconsistent.[50,52]

Lumbar puncture provides a measure of cerebrospinal fluid pressure. Although a normal pressure reading does not guarantee that pressures may not be elevated intermittently, a pressure under 100 mmHg is less often associated with a successful response to shunting.[10] In addition, the removal of 40–50 ml of CSF has been suggested as a CSF tap test.[54] An improvement in neurologic status after lumbar puncture indicates a good potential for improvement with shunting.[10] However, a lack of response does not preclude positive response to a shunt, because shunting produces more sustained ventricular decompression.[10,148] Therefore, lumbar puncture is most useful in patients who otherwise would not be strong candidates for shunting; a strong candidate would be shunted even in the face of a negative tap test.

Radioisotope cisternography has long been a mainstay in the diagnosis of hydrocephalus. With the advent of newer techniques, however, its use has come into question. Radioisotope is injected via lumbar puncture and its progression assessed at intervals after injection. Pooling in the ventricles rather then progression of uptake over the convexity is characteristic of normal-pressure hydrocephalus. However, a recent study showed that cisternography does not improve the diagnostic accuracy of combined clinical and CT criteria.[181] Cisternography-based predictions were the same in 43% of patients, better in 24%, and worse in 33%.[181]

Placement of a ventricular catheter may add to the diagnostic accuracy in normal-pressure hydrocephalus. Pressure monitoring with the ventricular catheter may identify the presence of repetitive pressure fluctuations called B waves. The presence of B waves for more than 5–10% of the recording time correlates with good outcome from shunting.[14,146]

The infusion of fluid via a lumbar or ventricular catheter with measurement of drainage via a ventricular catheter at a designated pressure gives a measure of the outflow conductance or ease of CSF absorption through the arachnoid granulations and other body compensatory mechanisms.[14] In the equation $V_{abs} = V_{inf} + V_{csf} - V_{out}$, V_{abs} is the volume absorbed, V_{inf} is the volume infused, V_{csf} is the volume of CSF, and V_{out} is the volume that drains out at the set pressure (P). The slope of the regression line dV_{abs}/dP in ml/min/mmHg expresses the conductance to outflow of CSF (C_{out}); in other words, it gives a measure of how readily CSF is absorbed by the body at different levels of intraventricular pressure. If the outflow conductance is high (i.e, significant volumes of CSF can be absorbed), then a shunt is not needed and will not help. If the outflow conductance is low (i.e., CSF is not readily absorbed), the patient is likely to improve with a shunt. Of interest, studies have failed to show a strong correlation between ventricular size and outflow conductance,[15] just as they have failed to show a strong correlation between ventricular size and likelihood of positive response to a shunt.[14]

Infusion studies are not often used in most hospitals. The testing requires a burr hole for the ventricular catheter, considerable time, and skilled staffing; it also involves the risk of infection. On the other hand, the high long-term morbidity of a shunt compared with the relatively low risk of the test, supports the value of infusion studies. The recent suggestion of a one-stage "test and shunt if needed" procedure may make infusion studies more practicable.[94]

Transcranial Doppler (TCD) detects decreases in blood flow or an increased pulsatility index associated with increased intracranial pressure.[151] Although absolute intracranial pressure cannot be identified by TCD, the equivalent of B waves can be identified by simultaneous TCD and recording of intracranial pressure. Thus TCD has been suggested as a screening procedure for normal-pressure hydrocephalus prior to invasive testing with an intraventricular catheter.[41] TCD also has been used with some success in children to identify the increased intracranial pressure associated with shunt malfunction.

Table 2 reviews multiple considerations relevant to identifying dynamic hydrocephalus. Risks of significant complications may

TABLE 2. **Features Distinguishing Dynamic Hydrocephalus from Ex Vacuo Ventricular Dilatation**

Feature or Test	Dynamic Hydrocephalus	Ex Vacuo Ventricular Dilatation
Antecedent history	Hemorrhage, especially IVH or SAH	Anoxia or DAI
Clinical deficits	NPH triad (dementia, gait impairment, and urinary incontinence), Parinaud's syndrome (upgaze paralysis), akinetic mutism	Consistent with location and severity of injury
Skull flap	Bulging (increased ICP)	Depressed
Clinical course	Worsening, intermittent, or static	Chronic slow improvement
Ventriculomegaly pattern	Temporal horns, third ventricle, convex frontal horns	Diffuse enlargement
Ventriculomegaly onset	Early (first month)	Late (after 2 months)
Serial scans	Progressive ventricular enlargement	Stable ventricular size
Sulci, fissures, cisterns	Decreased	Increased
Transependymal fluid	Present (periventricular lucency on CT, smooth periventricular increase on T2 MR)	Absent (or frontal contusions or periventricular infarct/demyelination)
MR acqueductal flow void	Present (decreased signal)	Absent
SPECT	Periventricular low flow	Normal or DAT pattern
LP pressure	Normal or high	Normal or low
CSF tap test	Positive or no response	No response
Radioisotope cisternography	Ventricular pooling	Progression to convexity
ICP recording	Over 5–10% B waves	Absent B waves
Transcranial Doppler	Increased pulsatility index (increased ICP)	Normal
CSF outflow conductance	Decreased (poor CSF absorption)	Increased (good CSF absorption)

IVH = intraventricular hemorrhage, SAH = subarachnoid hemorrhage, DAI = diffuse axonal injury, NPH = normal-pressure hydrocephalus, ICP = intracranial pressure, DAT = dementia of Alzheimer's type, CSF = cerebrospinal fluid.

run as high as 28%.[180] Overall response rates ranging from 29–74% have been described in series of patients with normal-pressure hydrocephalus, but these series have included idiopathic patients with a lower response rate.[179,180] On the other hand, patients with TBI are likely to show only a partial response to shunting, because deficits from hydrocephalus are superimposed on deficits from the original TBI. Final decisions about shunting in patients with TBI are often difficult and depend on clinical judgment.

Treatment

The definitive treatment of hydrocephalus is the placement of a shunt. Treatment with carbonic anhydrase inhibitors, such as acetazolamide or furosemide,[54] or with serial lumbar punctures is only a temporizing measure. Similarly, external ventricular drainage may be used on a temporary basis (particularly for obstructive mass effect or while excessive blood products are likely to clog a shunt), but conversion to a shunt is needed for treatment of persisting hydrocephalus.

Ventriculoperitoneal shunts are used most commonly for posttraumatic hydrocephalus, but ventriculoatrial, ventriculopleural, and lumboperitoneal shunts are useful in certain circumstances. Ventriculoatrial shunts are used more frequently in children with obstructive hydrocephalus. Ventriculopleural shunts, which are useful when CSF protein is very high, characteristically cause a small pleural effusion that disappears with shunt malfunction.[105] Pleural shunts are avoided in younger children because of the likelihood of symptomatic hydrothorax with a smaller pleural cavity.[43] Lumboperitoneal shunts are most often used for pseudotumor cerebri, when ventriculoperitoneal placement may be difficult because of small ventricular size.[105] They also are used for some cases of normal-pressure hydrocephalus, because the ventricles and spinal subarachnoid space should be in continuity. Radiographs of the lumbosacral spine sometimes show shunt displacement or

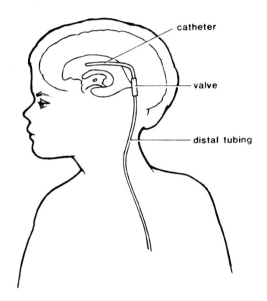

FIGURE 8. The basic tripartite shunt system consists of a ventricular catheter, valve mechanism, and distal tubing. (From Post EM: Currently available shunt systems: A review. Neurosurgery 16:258–259, 1985, with permission.)

disconnection. Placement of lumboperitoneal shunts often obliterates the basal cisterns on CT scan of the head. The return of previously obliterated cisterns is a more reliable indicator of shunt malfunction than ventriculomegaly.[28] Although usually asymptomatic, cerebellar tonsillar herniation (iatrogenic Chiari malformation) has been described in as many as 70% of patients with lumboperitoneal shunts.[27]

The basic components of a ventriculoperitoneal shunt are the ventricular catheter, valve, and distal tubing (Fig. 8). A reservoir may be added proximal to the valve (or even over the burr hole) to facilitate access to the ventricular system. Virtually all shunt systems have some type of one-way valve to allow forward flow down the shunt when the pressure gradient exceeds a threshold range and to prevent back flow from the peritoneum. Therapy staff often ask whether a shunt contraindicates inverted position; because of the one-way valve, this is not a problem.

Although most shunt systems feature a valve mechanism located over the skull, it is also possible to have a slit valve in the distal tubing instead. Types of value mechanisms include slit valves, cruciate valves, ball/

spring valves, diaphragm valves, and mitre valves[128,129] (Figs. 9 and 10). Slit valves open and allow CSF flow when sufficient pressure develops within the tubing; setting is determined by tube thickness. Cruciate valves are similar but have two perpendicular slits instead of one horizontal slit. Sometimes two-slit or cruciate valves are housed in one unit with a pumping chamber between them (e.g., Holter or Holter-Hausner valves, respectively). The Hakim valve also has two valves on either side of a pumping chamber but also features a sapphire ball that pushes against a spring to allow CSF flow. Diaphragm valves allow movement of a diaphragm from its seat or pin as determined by CSF pressure. The leaflets of a mitre valve act as springs to regulate CSF flow.[128]

Reservoirs of flushing chambers are added to many shunt systems. They allow manual pumping of the shunt and potential access to sample CSF or to inject into the shunt system. It is important to know the specifics of a shunt system before injecting into it, because some shunt components (especially older components such as the Spitz-Holter valve, Coe-Schulte second bubble, or Hakim-Cordis valve) may be damaged by needle perforations.[159] Most modern shunts, however, have a portion that can be injected without damage.

Flushing chambers may be of either single-bubble or double-bubble design (Fig. 11). If the chamber is proximal to all valves, compression of a single bubble may send fluid both down the shunt and back into the ventricle. If the chamber is between valves, compression may push fluid only in the forward direction. Compression of the distal bubble of a double-bubble shunt after occluding the proximal bubble may also force fluid in the forward direction. A similar result may be obtained in some single-chamber devices by occlusive digital compression of areas of proximal tubing before compression of the flushing chamber. Alternatively, compression of distal bubble or tubing before digital compression of the proximal chamber may force fluid retrogradely into the ventricle (e.g., intrathecal administration of antibiotics). Of course, access to the ventricle is possible only when a chamber is proximal to all valves.

Shunt valves are also specified by the approximate pressure necessary for opening and forwarding CSF flow. Usual types include low (20–40 mmHg), medium (40–70 mmHg), and high (80–100 mmHg) pressure.[128] Such valve settings are approximate and function differently depending on the compliance of the ventricular system, especially given that CSF flow is pulsatile in nature.[187] In general, because of Pascal's law (F = P × A), larger ventricles require a lower pressure for adequate decompression.[10] When patients do not respond to a shunt, conversion to a shunt of lower pressure occasionally results in clinical improvement.[157]

Because of the obvious undesirability of reoperation to place a valve with a different pressure setting, a valve of variable pressure has been developed and used in Europe. The SOPHY SU8 has a ball-in-cone valve (somewhat similar to the Hakim valve), but the spring position can be rotated with an external magnet, allowing noninvasive adjustment of low-, medium-, or high-pressure

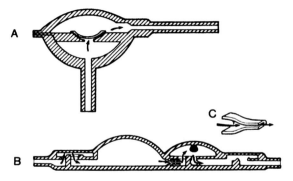

FIGURE 10.   *A,* Diaphragm valve. The proximal end is connected to the ventricular catheter with the valve sitting in the Burr hole. Fluid pressure dislodges the diaphragm and allows CSF flow *(arrow). B,* Miter valve. This device has a horizontal construction with a flush chamber; the miter valve is on the right. On the far right is an on-off device (see text). *C,* Detail of miter valve construction. (From Post EM: Currently available shunt systems: A review. Neurosurgery 16:258–259, 1985, with permission.)

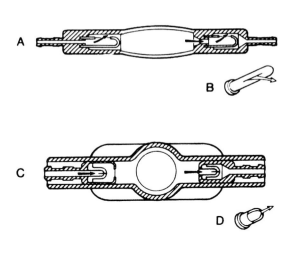

FIGURE 9.   Horizontal valves. All devices illustrated are actually two valves in series. *A,* Holter valve: two single-slit valves connected by a pumping chamber. *B,* Detail of the single-slit valve. *C,* Holter-Hausner valve: two cruciate valves in series connected by a pumping chamber. *D,* Detail of the cruciate valve on the end. *E,* Hakim valve; ball valve. (From Post EM: Currently available shunt systems: A review. Neurosurgery 16:258–259, 1985, with permission.)

settings.[162,169] In a series of 75 cases, the pressure settings were raised 16 times (10 times for subdural hygroma or hematoma, 6 times for symptoms of intracranial hypotension) and lowered 20 times for lack of clinical response or persistent ventricular dilatation.[162] Although MRI is said to be safe in such patients, it is essential to recheck the pressure settings after scanning, and some have placed the valves in the prethoracic region to minimize distortion artifacts.[162,169]

COMPLICATIONS

Shunt complications include shunt failure, infection, seizures, and problems related to overdrainage, including subdural hematoma, low-pressure syndrome, and slit ventricle syndrome. The overall incidence of shunt complications is high. In 356 adult patients over an 18-year interval, the incidence of revision was 29%.[131] In a series of 1,179 patients shunted for hydrocephalus (only 312 patients over age 5 years), the probability of shunt malfunction after 12 years was 81%.[147]

Shunt obstruction, the most common problem, may present with headache unrelieved by position change, irritability, confusion and lethargy. Whereas the original symptoms of hydrocephalus are often quite

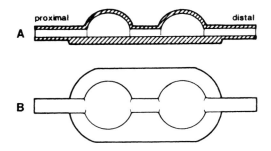

FIGURE 11.   Double-bubble flush chamber. *A,* Side view. *B,* Top view. Each bubble can be depressed individually. Depressing the distal bubble occludes the distal tubing and allows ventricular access. (From Post EM: Currently available shunt systems: A review. Neurosurgery 16:258–259, 1985, with permission.)

gradual, shunt failure may present in a much more fulminant manner; treatment of shunt failure is usually a more urgent matter than placement of the original shunt.[138] Swelling or tenderness along the shunt tract usually indicates tracking of CSF and suboptimal shunt functioning.

Proximal occlusion of the ventricular catheter is the most common source of blockage, usually accounting for at least 30% of cases of shunt dysfunction.[138,155] The ventricular catheter typically becomes obstructed with fibrin, neuroglia, or choroid plexus tissue.[59,147,155] Ventricular overdrainage may predispose to proximal occlusion[147]—for example, by abutting the catheter tip against the ventricular wall.

Distal occlusion is more frequent with distal slit valves than proximal nonslit valves.[147] Early distal occlusion also raises the question of associated infection.[138] One cause of distal shunt obstruction is encystment and loculation of the peritoneal contents around the distal catheter tip.[43,155] Abdominal pain is usual, and the pseudocyst may be palpable on abdominal examination. Ultrasound is diagnostic and also may be used to guide aspiration and culture of peritoneal collections.[155] Treatment may include transplanting the distal shunt to an alternate site.[105]

Valve failure is a less common cause of shunt dysfunction. The ball-in-cone (Hakim) or diaphragm valves are said to be less likely to become occluded with proteinaceous material than the slit valves,[131,138] although a

statistically significant difference has not been demonstrated.[131] Disconnections of shunt components have accounted for as much as 15% of shunt revisions[1] and often are shown by a shunt series of plain radiographs.[135]

Bedside palpation of the shunt sometimes gives a clue to shunt malfunction. Excessive resistance to digital compression of the shunt chamber suggests possible distal occlusion, whereas inadequate refill suggests proximal occlusion. Unfortunately, however, palpation was found to be neither sensitive nor reliable for determining shunt malfunction in a consecutive series of 200 patients.[126]

CT scans, of course, are helpful in demonstrating increase in ventricular size in many cases of shunt malfunction. Definitive information about shunt blockage can be obtained by performing a shuntagram.[5,62,176] Typically a 25-gauge needle is inserted into the safely perforable portion of the shunt, a pressure recording is done, and the progression of isotope is followed down the catheter and into the peritoneum.[62] With distal obstruction, pressure may be elevated with rapid ventricular filling but lack of distal flow. With proximal occlusion, the distal catheter fills, but pressure is low with slow disappearance of tracer and lack of ventricular filling.[176]

Shunt infection has been described in 7–29% of cases.[84] Most infections are acquired at the time of surgery, and 70% present within the first 2 months.[84] *Staphylococcus epidermidis* is most common, accounting for approximately one-half of infections,[153] followed by *Staphylococcus aureus* and gram-negative organisms. Presentation is typically insidious with low-grade fever, malaise, irritability, and nausea.[135,153] Meningeal irritation is usually not present.[135] Erythema over the shunt site, however, is a highly specific sign.[84,135,153]

Tapping the shunt leads to accurate diagnosis in 95% of cases.[84] Diagnosis is based on culture results, because CSF protein and glucose may be normal and cell count may not be much greater with shunt infection than with shunt alone. In contrast to the reliability of a shunt tap, lumbar puncture or ventricular tap is positive in only 7–26% of cases.[84]

Treatment options include shunt removal and replacement after antibiotic treatment, one-stage replacement or partial revision with antibiotics, and antibiotics alone.[24]

Treatment needs to be individualized to the clinical situation, and severe ventriculitis may warrant more aggressive treatment than an infection of external shunt tubing. In general, the highest overall response rate (96%) has been reported with shunt removal or externalization combined with antibiotics.[84] Leukocytes in the vicinity of a shunt lose some of their ability to kill ingested bacteria. Therefore, oral rifampin sometimes is added to intrathecal vancomycin for *Staphylococcal epidermidis* because of its ability to penetrate leukocytes.[24]

The prevalence of seizures after shunting has ranged from 5–48%,[155] but seizures also may result from an accompanying neurologic condition rather than shunting. The risk has been judged insufficient to warrant routine anticonvulsant prophylaxis. A higher incidence of seizures with frontal than occipital shunt insertion has been suggested, but this finding is not consistent. Shunt infection or malfunction also may present with seizure activity.

Chronic subdural hematomas and hygromas, which have been described in 4.5–28% of patients after shunting, sometimes require tying off of the shunt or placement of a higher pressure valve.[10,133,155] Siphoning and low intraventricular pressure are thought to predispose to tearing and leakage from small veins. In addition, leakage from around the catheter may track into the subdural space.[10] Subdural hematomas are particularly likely when ventricles are extremely large preoperatively.[155] Not all subdural collections are clinically significant; with MRI even very small fluid collections can be imaged.[5] Post-shunt meningeal fibrosis, with collagenous material in the subdural space, is distinguished from subdural fluid by its dramatic enhancement with gadolinium.[5,51]

Intraventricular pressure normally becomes slightly subatmospheric when we stand. However, after placement of a shunt, orthostatic intraventricular pressure becomes markedly low,[127] reflecting the additional negative hydrostatic pressure from the distal tubing (Fig. 12). This may cause excessive siphoning of CSF and a low pressure syndrome of orthostatic headache, dizziness, nausea and vomiting, lethargy, and diplopia.[47,133,189]

Small ventricles are a desired result of shunting for hydrocephalus. However, some patients with chronically overdraining shunts develop the slit-ventricle syndrome.[8,47,138,155,189] Such patients develop severe nonpostural

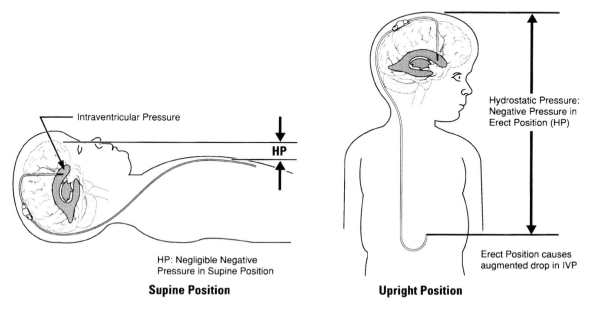

Supine Position

Intraventricular Pressure

HP

HP: Negligible Negative Pressure in Supine Position

Upright Position

Hydrostatic Pressure: Negative Pressure in Erect Position (HP)

Erect Position causes augmented drop in IVP

FIGURE 12. Hydrocephalus of a shunted patient with DP or variable resistance valve. (From Operative Protocol for the Delta Valve in Pediatric Hydrocephalus. Goleta, CA, PS Medical Educational Series, with permission.)

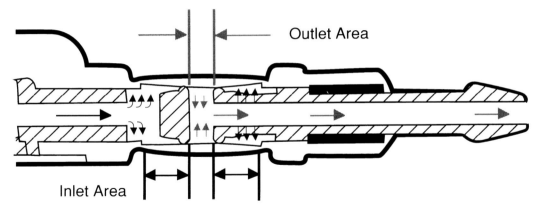

FIGURE 13. Detail of pressure-regulating mechanism of Delta Valve illustrating greater than 20:1 hydrodynamic leverage inlet area to outlet area. (From The Delta Valve: A Physiologic Shunt System. Goleta, CA, PS Medical Educational Series, with permission.)

headaches in the face of persistently small ventricles.[47,138,189] Slight increase in ventricular size at the time of clinical symptoms and sluggish shunt refill suggest intermittent proximal shunt malfunction with ventricular collapse against the catheter. Such symptoms develop an average of 4.5 years after shunting[47] and are analogous to pseudotumor cerebri in the tendency toward elevated pressures with small stiff ventricles.[189]

Problems related to overdrainage have led to the development of several special shunt components. Antisiphon devices have been developed with diaphragms that close to counteract negative standing hydrostatic pressures.[48,127] Successful prevention of the dramatic negative standing intracranial pressure has been documented.[25] A less useful device is the valve with an on/off occluder bubble following the flushing chamber (*see* Fig. 10). Originally designed in hopes of preventing subdural development by transient occlusion, it is not used frequently today. Fortunately palpation or radiographs can determine whether the occluder has inadvertently been compressed.[127,159]

Several newer valves have been designed to assist with CSF overdrainage. The Orbis-sigma valve has variable resistance with three stages of flow. It initially functions like a standard low pressure valve but shows increased resistance with larger flow rates; it also has a decreased resistance safety valve to deal with higher pressures. The Z-flow shunt uses a clever balls-in-cone mechanism

to compensate for adverse gravitational hydrostatic effects.[26] It is similar to an antisiphon device but uses ball position rather than pressure to regulate flow. Finally, the delta valve is similar to an antisiphon device in combination with a standard valve but has been engineered with "hydrodynamic leverage" that allows a much larger inlet than outlet area (Fig. 13). This design allows the valve to increase physiologic resistance to flow in the upright position but to avoid the overshoot sometimes encountered with antisiphon valves.[186]

VASCULAR COMPLICATIONS

Traumatic Aneurysm

Traumatic aneurysms are classified as true, false, mixed, and dissecting types.[6] In true aneurysms, at least the adventitial wall is preserved, whereas in false aneurysms all elements of the vascular wall are disrupted and blood is contained only by the surrounding arachnoid, hematoma, or brain parenchyma. Mixed aneurysms have a combination of true and false elements. In dissecting aneurysms, blood channels within the vessel wall, effectively narrowing or occluding the vessel itself.

Traumatic intracranial aneurysms should be suspected in cases of delayed subarachnoid or intracerebral hemorrhage. They are characteristically sluggish to fill and empty on angiography as well as highly unstable and prone to rupture.[6,46] In fact, although the time interval from injury to rupture varies from days to years, 90% bleed within 3 weeks of injury.[6] Traumatic aneurysms may result from bony fragments or missile injuries or from acceleration-deceleration injuries. The most common locations are the distal middle cerebral branches, anterior cerebral artery, and proximal carotid and vertebral arteries. They are typically false aneurysms[6,46,190] and therefore must be trapped rather than clipped. Because the parent vessel often must be sacrificed, distal revascularization procedures are sometimes helpful. Carotid aneurysms are usually proximal, involving the cervical, petrous, or intracavernous portions. Presentations are known to include pharyngeal mass, hemorrhage, and epistaxis.[102]

Traumatic dissection of the internal carotid and vertebral arteries may be seen after hyperextension and flexion neck injuries, as in motor vehicle accidents. Presentation is typically that of infarction in the distribution of the involved vessel. Revascularization or direct repair is sometimes attempted for carotid dissection, but only if it can be done within 4 hours of onset in a conscious patient.[6] Otherwise management is medical, with consideration of antiplatelet or anticoagulation therapy depending on clinical course and associated injuries.

Carotid Cavernous Fistula

Traumatic carotid cavernous fistulas are typically direct fistulas from the internal carotid with fast flow and high pressure. Classified as type A, they contrast with spontaneous carotid cavernous fistulas (types B, C, and D), which have low pressure and slow flow and typically receive dural blood supply.[13,37] Presenting signs of carotid cavernous fistula include supraorbital bruit, exophthalmus, orbital congestion, oculomotor palsies, trigeminal nerve involvement, and visual impairment.[13,42,108] Pulsatile exophthalmus is seen in carotid cavernous fistula but also has been described in a patient with orbital encephalocele and hydrocephalus.[85] Pulsatile tinnitus may result from arteriovenous fistulas and malformations or from altered jugular venous flow.[18,64,69,143,177] Onset of carotid cavernous fistula is often delayed;

43.5% are diagnosed over 1 month after trauma.[42] Angiography is the definitive diagnostic test.

Spontaneous closure of a carotid cavernous fistula has been described in some patients; it is much more likely with a spontaneous low-flow fistula than with the traumatic high-flow fistula. Patients have been trained in intermittent manual compression of the cervical carotid artery with the contralateral hand. Although the success rate is lower with direct fistulas, 17% of patients had successful closure with this technique.[65] The definitive treatment of traumatic carotid cavernous fistula has become the endovascular placement of detachable balloons.[37] Successful fistula closure was accomplished by the detachable balloon technique in 92 of 95 cases of traumatic carotid cavernous fistula, with preservation of the internal carotid artery in over 70% of cases.[37]

LATE INTRACRANIAL MASS LESIONS

Subdural Hematoma

Subdural hematoma is the most common late-presenting mass lesion. Although acute, subacute (3–20 days), and chronic (3 weeks or more) subdural hematomas are distinguished by time of detection after injury, it is important to recognize that chronic subdural hematoma is a different pathophysiologic process than acute subdural hematoma—not simply an older blood clot.[21,40,80,92,167] As a result, differences are also seen in the epidemiology, clinical presentation, prognosis, and treatment techniques[40,91,156] (Table 3).

The incidence of chronic subdural hematoma peaks in the seventh and eighth decades, and only 60–65% of patients have known TBI.[44,92,156] Male predominance (70–90%) and parietal location (91%) are characteristic.[21,92] Headaches are a cardinal symptom,[33,92] sometimes following a symptom-free interval. Three major clinical presentations include hemiparesis (40%), personality or intellectual change (30%), and signs of increased intracranial pressure, including papilledema (20%).[21] In contrast with acute subdural hematoma, seizures are relatively uncommon with chronic subdural hematoma (4–7%),

TABLE 3. Differences in Acute and Chronic Subdural Hematomas

Feature	Acute Subdural Hematoma	Chronic Subdural Hematoma
Age peak	30–49 yrs	60–70 yrs
Known TBI	Virtually all	60–65%
Clinical presentation	Acute mental status, deterioration, focal signs, seizures, increased ICP	Headache, chronic mental status change (including personality), hemiparesis, increased ICP
Composition	Blood clot	Fluid, membrane
Pathophysiology	Venous bleeding, especially torn bridging veins	Initial venous bleeding, inflammatory process with leaky macrocapillaries, disordered local hemostatic mechanism
Surgery	Craniotomy	Often Burr holes
Seizure risk	High	Low
Mortality	High (57–59%)	Moderate (26%)
Functional recovery	Low (34%)	High (70–90%)

ICP = intracranial pressure.

and ongoing anticonvulsant prophylaxis is not routinely required,[145] although some authorities have recommended it in the immediate postoperative period.[33]

CT scans characteristically show decreased density in chronic subdural hematoma. However, the isodense appearance characteristic of subacute subdural hematoma may last longer than 1 month in some instances.[82] In questionable cases, contrast enhancement helps to identify isodense subdural collections.[174] In other cases, a layer of isodensity or increased density is seen below a hypodense layer; this sedimentation level likely reflects interval rebleeding.[76,174] Isodensity at the medial margin of a fluid collection also may represent fresher bleeding.[174]

Compared with CT scan density, the factors determining signal intensity on MRI are much more complex. Whereas acute subdural hematoma shows increased CT density, subacute and chronic subdural hematoma have increased signal on MRI[33,51,68] (Table 4). Subacute subdural hematoma is seen as a hyperintense collection on T1-weighted images, largely because of the presence of methemoglobin. Chronic subdural hematoma presents with more variable signal intensity on T1-weighted images but consistently shows increased signal intensity on T2-weighted images.[33,51,68] In addition, fluid collections that are homogeneous on CT sometimes show hypointense septations and mixed intensities on MRI. In some instances, a sedimentation level of a hyperintense (fluid) upper layer and hypointense (more cellular) lower layer is seen. Such findings are consistent with the conceptualization of subdural hematoma as an ongoing process with interval rebleeding rather than a static collection of blood. As described below, an outer membrane is characteristic in chronic subdural collections; this membrane enhances significantly with gadolinium on T1-weighted imaging in many cases.[51]

Although CT and MRI are the definitive tests for diagnosing subdural collections, abnormalities also are seen in the electroencephalogram (EEG) and in testing of cerebral

TABLE 4. CT and MRI in Subdural Hematoma

Scan Technique	Acute Subdural Hematoma	Subacute Subdural Hematoma	Chronic Subdural Hematoma
CT (noncontrast)	Hyperdense	Isodense	Hypodense
CT (contrast)	Hyperdense	Enhances	Hypodense
MRI T1	Isointense	Hyperintense	Variable
MRI T2	Hypointense	Hyperintense	Hyperintense
Key MRI factor	Deoxyhemoglobin	Methemoglobin	Protein, methemoglobin

blood flow. In addition to delta slowing on the side of a subdural collection, ipsilateral suppression of voltage is seen in 25% of patients.[44,92] Diffuse reductions in cerebral blood flow preoperatively often show a recovery 1 month postoperatively.[71]

On pathologic examination, the fluid of chronic subdural hematoma shows a range of color and appearance, including brown-black, dark red, amber-brown, and almost clear and watery.[68,92] Coagulated masses of blood and fibrin are sometimes present. A thicker outer membrane attached to the dura and thinner inner membrane bordering on the arachnoid are characteristic.[92] Enlarged ectatic capillaries, often called giant capillaries or sinusoids, are prominent on the outer membrane and associated with inflammatory cells, fibroblasts, and hemosiderin-laden macrophages.[92] With age, the outer membrane also may become calcified.

Although the process by which chronic subdural hematoma develops is incompletely understood, three points are worthy of emphasis:

1. Low intracranial pressure (e.g., after a shunt) and atrophy predispose to development of subdural hematoma.[92]

2. Generation of fluid is ongoing and includes probable leakage of blood from the fragile giant capillaries in the outer membrane induced by the inflammatory process.[40,192,193] Gap junctions in the endothelial cells adjacent to such capillaries probably predispose to blood leakage.[192,193]

3. Probably of greatest importance, a disordered local hemostatic mechanism has been identified in fluid from chronic subdural hematoma.[40,80] Activation of both the clotting system and the fibrinolytic system is excessive with increases in both thrombin and fibrin degradation products. Defective clots are formed and rapidly lysed.[40,80] Removal of degradation products from the subdural space may be important in interrupting the vicious cycle of disordered hemostasis and facilitating the recovery from chronic subdural hematoma. Because of the ratio between the effusion or rebleeding into a chronic subdural collection and resorption of fluid, it is likely that a certain critical mass of fluid cannot be resorbed successfully. Successful surgery, therefore, may reduce the residual volume to a degree that allows further resorption rather than fully removing the blood clot.

In chronic subdural hematoma, fluid often is successfully removed by burr holes.[21,86,92] Occasionally the presence of sizable clots or loculation may necessitate craniotomy, as is commonly done for acute subdural hematoma.[40,109] Postoperative drainage has been advocated to assist with brain reexpansion.[40,86] The hematoma cavity is commonly washed out with saline,[141] and it has been suggested that continuous irrigation (to remove coagulation degradation products) may decrease the duration of drainage or frequency of recurrence.[136] Persisting subdural fluid was described postoperatively in 78% of patients, but had returned to normal by 40 days postoperatively in 27 of 32 cases,[99] leading to the suggestion that reoperation should be avoided until at least 3 weeks postoperatively unless marked clinical deterioration occurs. It also has been suggested that, despite their lack of benefit for acute subdural hematoma, corticosteroids may be helpful for either small or recurrent chronic subdural hematoma in view of its inflammatory nature.[40]

The overall prognosis from subdural hematoma is much more favorable than the prognosis for acute subdural hematoma,[92] although the residual deficits in the areas of personality and memory may be problematic.[141] Patients with even severe neurologic deficits preoperatively may have successful outcomes,[21] although the extent of preoperative deficit has been a useful predictor of outcome in some series.[141]

Subdural Hygroma

The distinction between subdural hygroma and chronic subdural hematoma has often been unclear in the literature. Subdural hygroma or hydroma has been described as a subdural collection of cerebrospinal fluid, often with a modified composition.[171] It has been proposed that a tear in the arachnoid may allow CSF into the subdural space, and rare surgical documentation of this process has been provided.[171] In such cases a one-way flap/valve effect may prevent fluid from escaping from the subdural space, acting as a significant mass lesion.[171]

In fact, a second phenomenon appears to account for a larger number of cases described as hygroma. In such patients, the fluid is xanthochromic and generally believed to have developed from a small hematoma.[171] Here the distinction from chronic subdural hematoma is blurred, because the process by which chronic subdural hematoma develops is known to include an ongoing production of subdural fluid, which may have a relatively watery consistency. Pathophysiologically, some cases of "hygroma" may be classified more accurately as chronic subdural hematomas, particularly if a membrane is present.

Finally, the term hygroma has been used to described other extraaxial collections with low density on CT scan,[171] particularly if such collections are not believed to exert mass effect. In fact, the fluid in such cases is often in the subarachnoid rather than the subdural space. Of note, MRI scan allows more precise localization of fluid in such cases. Cortical veins are displaced medially with subdural fluid but remain peripherally located with subarachnoid fluid or atrophy.[51]

Although both chronic subdural hematoma and subdural hygroma have low CT density, the density of some hygromas has been described as 0 EMI units compared with 4–14 units for chronic subdural hematoma.[171] MRI scans consistently show less intensity for subdural hygroma than for chronic subdural hematoma with both T1 and T2 imaging.[51]

Response to surgical drainage of subdural hygromas is more positive when the intracranial pressure is elevated at the time of surgery. In contrast, many fluid collections do not appear to exert mass effect, can be managed conservatively, and may resolve spontaneously.[80]

Epidural Hematoma

Although epidural hematoma is usually considered the most acute posttraumatic mass lesion, it presents more than 5 days after injury in 10% of cases[73] and may present as late as the second or third week after injury.[70] Although epidural hematoma most often presents in the temporal fossa (57–83% of cases), delayed presentation is more common with extratemporal location, especially frontal or posterior fossa lesions.[66,73]

Clouding or decreased level of consciousness is considered the most important sign of epidural hematoma.[73] Onset is slowest with frontal lesions, and symptoms may be vague. Unilateral exophthalmus is an unusual sign that has been described with subfrontal epidural hematoma.[66]

Posterior fossa epidural hematomas are not common; they are seen in only 0.3% of patients with TBI.[67] However, they have the highest mortality rate[73] and are notoriously difficult to diagnose.[66] An occipital bone fracture is seen in 84.2% of cases and characteristically crosses the venous sinus, causing venous rather than arterial bleeding.[67] A lucid interval is common, and progressive decrease in the level of consciousness is characteristic. Battle's sign is often seen, and neck stiffness, occipital headache, and vomiting may be prominent. Symptoms and signs of increased intracranial pressure as well as brainstem, cranial nerve, and cerebellar dysfunction are common.[67,142]

Intracerebral Hemorrhage

Delayed traumatic intracerebral hemorrhage is defined as an intracerebral hematoma that is not visualized on initial CT but is seen on a follow-up study. Time of onset is typically about 24 hours after original injury;[103] 80% of cases occur within 48 hours of injury.[33] Delayed traumatic intracerebral hemorrhage occurs in 5.6–7.4% of patients with severe TBI.[103] It is often described after evacuation of another mass lesion, such as an epidural or subdural hematoma, which initially may have tamponaded the development of intracerebral hemorrhage. Outcome is worse with temporal lobe location, which shows an increased incidence of herniation.[3]

REFERENCES

1. Aldrich EF, Harmann P: Disconnection as a cause of ventriculoperitoneal shunt malfunction in multicomponent shunt systems. Pediatr Neurosurg 16:309-312, 1990–1991.
2. Anderson M: Management of cerebral infection. Neurol Neurosurg Psychiatry 56:1243-1258, 1993.
3. Andrews BT, Chiles BW, Olsen WL: Pitts LH: The effect of intracerebral hematoma location on the risk of brain stem compression and on clinical outcome. J Neurosurg 69:518–522, 1988.

4. Ashkenazi E, Umansky F, Constantini S, et al: Fever as the initial sign of malfunction in noninfected ventriculoperitoneal shunts. Acta Neurochir 114:131–134, 1992.

5. Barkovich AJ, Edwards MSB: Applications of neuroimaging in hydrocephalus. Pediatr Neurosurg 18:65–83, 1992.

6. Batjer HH, Giller CA, Kopitnik TA, et al: Intracranial and cervical vascular injuries. In Cooper PR (ed): Head Injury, 3rd ed. Baltimore, Williams & Wilkins, 1993, pp 373–404.

7. Batjer HH, Purdy PD, Neiman M, et al: Subtemporal transdural use of detachable balloons for traumatic carotid-cavernous fustulas. Neurosurgery 22:290–296, 1988.

8. Benzel EC, Reeves JD, Kesterson L, et al: Slit ventricle syndrome in children: Clinical presentation and treatment. Acta Neurochir 117:7–14, 1992.

9. Bierbraverks, Storrs BB, McLone DG, et al: A prospective, randomized study of shunt function and infections as a function of shunt placement. Pediatr Neurosurg 16:287-291, 1990–1991.

10. Black PMcL: The normal pressure hydrocephalus syndrome. In Scott RM (ed): Hydrocephalus. Baltimore, Williams & Wilkins, 1990, pp 109–144.

11. Black PMcL, Ojemann RG, Tzouras A et al: CSF shunts for dementia, incontinence, and gait disturbance. Clin Neurosurg 32:632–651, 1985.

12. Bok APL, Peter JC: Subdural empyema: Burrholes or craniectomy? J Neurosurg 78:574-578, 1993.

13. Bonafe A, Manelfe C: Traumatic carotid-cavernous sinus fistulas. In Braakman R (ed): Handbook of Clinical Neurology, vol 13. Amsterdam, Elsevier, 1990, pp 345–366.

14. Borgensen SE, Gjerris F: The predictive value of conductance to outflow of CSF in normal pressure hydrocephalus. Brain 105:65–86, 1982.

15. Borgesen SE, Gjerris F: Relationships between intracranial pressure, ventricular size, and resistance to CSF outflow. J Neurosurg 67:535–539, 1987.

16. Boyar B, Ildan F, Begdatoglv H, et al: Unilateral hydrocephalus resulting from occlusion of foramen of Monro: A new procedure in the treatment: Stereotactic fenestration of the septum pellucidum. Surg Neurol 39:110–114, 1993.

17. Brosnahan D, McFadzean RM, Teasdale E, et al: Neuro-ophthalmic features of carotid cavernous fistulas and their treatment by endoarterial balloon embolization. J Neurol Neurosurg Psychiatry 55:553–556, 1992.

18. Buckwalter JA, Sasaki CT, Virapongse C, et al: Pulsatile tinnitus arising from jugular megabulb deformity: A treatment rationale. Laryngoscope 93:1534–1539, 1983.

19. Bullitt E, Lehman RAW: Osteomyelitis of the skull. Surg Neurol 11:163–166, 1979.

20. Buonanno FS, Moody DM, Ball MR, et al: Computed cranial tomographic findings in cerebral sinovenous occlusion. J Comput Assist Tomogr 2:281–290, 1978.

21. Cameron MM: Chronic subdural hematoma: A review of 114 cases. J Neurol Neurosurg Psychiatry 41:834–839, 1978.

22. Caner H, Ataserer A, Kilinc K, et al: Lipid peroxide level increase in experimental hydrocephalus. Acta Neurochir 121:68–71, 1993.

23. Cervantes LA: Concurrent delayed temporal and posterior fossa epidural hematomas. J Neurosurg 59:351–353, 1983.

24. Chapman PH, Borges LF: Shunt infections: Prevention and treatment. Clin Neurosurg 32:652–664, 1985.

25. Chapman PH, Cosman ER, Arnold MA, et al: The relationship between ventricular fluid pressure and body position in normal subjects and subjects with shunts: A telemetric study. Neurosurgery 26:181–189, 1990.

26. Chabra DK, Agarwal DG, Mittal P, et al: "Z" Flow hydrocephalus shunt: A new approach to the problem of hydrocephalus, the rationale behind its design and the initial results of pressure monitoring after "Z" flow shunt implantation. Acta Neurochir 121:43–47, 1993.

27. Chumas PD, Armstrong DC, Drake JM, et al: Tonsillar herniation: The rule rather than the exception after lumboperitoneal shunting in the pediatric population. J Neurosurg 78:568–573, 1993.

28. Chuang S, Hochhauser L, Fritz C, et al: Lumboperitoneal shunt malfunction. Acta Radiol Suppl 369:645–648, 1986.

29. Clark CW, Muhlbauer MS, Lowrey R, et al: Complications of intracranial pressure monitoring in trauma patients. Neurosurgery 25:20–24, 1989.

30. Conner ES, Foley L, Black PMcl: Experimental normal-pressure hydrocephalus is accompanied by increased transmantle pressure. J Neurosurg 61:322–327, 1984.

31. Connolly MB, Jan JE, Cochrane DD, et al: Rapid recovery from cortical visual impairment following correction of prolonged shunt malfunction in congenital hydrocephalus. Arch Neurol 48:956–957, 1991.

32. Cooper PR: Gunshot wounds of the brain. In Cooper PR (ed): Head Injury, 3rd ed. Baltimore, Williams & Wilkins, 1993, pp 355–372.

33. Cooper PR: Posttraumatic intracranial mass lesions. In Cooper PR (ed): Head Injury, 3rd ed. Baltimore, Williams & Wilkins, 1993, pp 275–330.

34. Cooper PR: Skull fracture and traumatic cerebrospinal fluid fistuals. In Cooper PR (ed): Head Injury, 3rd ed. Baltimore, Williams & Wilkins, 1993, pp 115–136.

35. Cope DN, Date ES, Mar EY: Serial computerized tomographic evaluations in traumatic head injury. Arch Phys Med Rehabil 69:483–486, 1988.

36. Cusimano MD, Sekhar LN: Pseudo-cerebrospinal fluid rhinorrhea. J Neurosurg 8:26–30, 1994.

37. Debrun GM, Vinuela F, Fox AJ, et al: Indications for treatment and classification of 132 carotid-cavernous fistulas. Neurosurgery 22:285– 289, 1988.

38. Dinubile MJ: Infections of the cranial dura and dural sinuses. In Harris AA (ed): Handbook of Clinical Neurology, vol. 8, Amsterdam, Elsevier, 1988, pp 167–183.

39. Dolinskas CA, Bilaniuk LT, Zimmerman RA, et al: Computed tomography of intracerebral hematomas II: Radionoclide and transmission CT studies of the perihematoma region. Am J Roentgenol 129:689–692, 1977.

40. Drapkin AJ: Chronic subdural hematoma: Pathophysiological basis for treatment. Br J Neurosurg 5:467–473, 1991.

41. Droste DW, Krauss JK: Simultaneous recording of cerebrospinal fluid pressure and middle cerebral artery blood flow velucity in patients with suspected symptomatic normal pressure hydrocephalus. J Neurol Neurosurg Psychiatry 56:75–79, 1993.

42. Dubov WE, Bach JR: Delayed presentation of carotid cavernous sinus fistula in a patient with traumatic brain injury. Am J Phys Med Rehabil 70:178–180, 1991.

43. Epstein F: How to keep shunts functioning or "the impossible dream." Clin Neurosurg 32:608–631, 1985.

44. Feldman RG, Pincus JH, McEntee WJ, et al: Cerebrovascular accident or subdural fluid collection? Arch Intern Med 112:204–214, 1963.

45. Feverman T, Wackym PA, Gade GF, et al: Craniotomy improves outcomes in subdural empyema. Surg Neurol 32:105–110, 1989.

46. Flores JS, Vaquero J, Sola RG, et al: Traumatic false aneurysms of the middle meningeal artery. Neurosurgery 18:200–203, 1986.

47. Foltz EL: Hydrocephalus: Slit ventricles, shunt obstructions, and third ventricle shunts: A clinical study. Surg Neurol 40:119–124, 1993.

48. Foltz EL, Blanks J, Meyer R, et al: Shunted hydrocephalus: Normal upright ICP by CSF gravity-flow control. Surg Neurol 39:210–217, 1993.

49. Frederiks JAM: Post-traumatic CSF hypotension. In Vinken PJ, Broyn GW (eds): Handbook of Clinical Neurology, vol. 24. New York, Elsevier, 1976, pp 255–259.

50. Friedland RP: "Normal"-pressure hydrocephalus and the saga of the treatable dementias. JAMA 262:2577–2581, 1989.

51. Gean AD: Imaging of Head Trauma. New York, Raven Press, 1994.

52. George AE, DeLeon MJ, Miller J, et al: Positron emission tomography of hydrocephalus. Acta Radiol Suppl 369:435–439, 1986.

53. Gerard G, Weisberg LA: Magnetic resonance imaging in adult white matter disorders and hydrocephalus. Semin Neurol 6:17–23, 1986.

54. Gilmore HE: Medical treatment of hydrocephalus. In Scott RM (ed): Hydrocephalus. Baltimore, Williams & Wilkins, 1990, pp 37–46.

55. Goh D, Minns RA, Pye SD, et al: Cerebral blood flow velocity changes after ventricular taps and ventriculoperitoneal shunting. Childs Nerv Syst 7:452–457, 1991.

56. Gotok, Hieshima GB, Higashida VV, et al: Treatment of direct carotid cavernous sinus fistulae. Acta Radiol Suppl 369:576–579, 1986.

57. Graff-Radford NR, Godersky JC: Idiopathic normal pressure hydrocephalus and systemic hypertension. Neurology 37:868–871, 1987.

58. Granado JM, Diaz F, Alday R, et al: Evaluation of brain spect in the diagnosis and prognosis of the normal pressure hydrocephalus syndrome. Acta Neurochir 112:88–91, 1991.

59. Gruber R, Jenny P, Herzog B, et al: Experiences with the antisiphon devise (ASD) in shunt therapy of pediatric hydrocephalus. J Neurosurg 61:156–162, 1984.

60. Han JS, Kaufman B, Alfidi RJ, et al: Head trauma evaluated by magnetic resonance and computed tomography: A comparison. Radiology 150:71–77, 1984.

61. Hand WL, Sanford JP: Posttraumatic bacterial meningitis. Ann Intern Med 72:869–874, 1970.

62. Hayden PW, Rudd TG, Shurtleff DB, et al: Combined pressure-radionuclide evaluation of suspected cerebrospinal fluid shunt malfunction: A seven year clinical experience. Pediatrics 66:679–684, 1980.

63. Helmy ES, Koh ML, Bays RA, et al: Management of frontal sinus fractures. Oral Surg Oral Med Oral Pathol 69:137–148, 1990.

64. Hentzer E: Objective tinnitus of the vascular type. Acta Otolaryngol 66:273–281, 1968.

65. Higashida RT, Hieshima GB, Halbach VV, et al: Closure of carotid cavernous sinus fistulae by external compression of the carotid artery and jugular vein. Acta Radiol Suppl 369:580–583, 1986.

66. Hirsh LF: Chronic epidural hematomas. Neurosurgery 6:508–512, 1980.

67. Hooper RS: Extradural hemorrhages of the posterior fossa. Br J Surg 42:19–26, 1954.

68. Hosoda K, Tamaki N, Masumura M, et al: Magnetic resonance images of chronic subdural hematomas. J Neurosurg 67:677–683, 1987.

69. Hvidegaard T, Brask T: Objective venous tinnitus. J Laryngol Otol 98:189–191, 1984.

70. Illingworth R, Shawdon H: Conservative management of intracranial extradural haematoma presenting late. J Neurol Neurosurg Psychiatry 46:558–560, 1983.

71. Ishikawa T, Kawamura SH, et al: Uncoupling between CBF and oxygen metabolism in a patient with chronic subdural hematoma: Case report. J Neurol Neurosurg Psychiatry 55:401–403, 1992.

72. Jamieson KG: Posterior fossa haematoma. In Vinken PJ, Bruyn GW (eds): The Handbook of Clinical Neurology, vol. 24. New York, Elsevier, 1976, pp 343–350.

73. Jamieson KG, Yelland JDN: Extradural hematoma. J Neurosurg 29:13–23, 1968.

74. Jones SR, Luby JP, Sanford JP, et al: Bacterial meningitis complicating cranial–spinal trauma. J Trauma 13:895–900, 1973.

75. Kamiryo T, Fujii Y, Kusaka M, et al: Intracranial pressure monitoring using a programmable pressure valve and a telemetric intracranial pressure sensor in a case of slit ventricle syndrome after multiple shunt revisions. Childs Nerv Syst 7:233–234, 1991.

76. Kao MCK: Sedimentation level in chronic subdural hematoma visible on computerized tomography. J Neurosurg 58:246–251, 1983.

77. Kaufman DM, Leeds NE: Computed tomography (CT) in the diagnosis of intracranial abscesses. Neurology 27:1069–1073, 1977.

78. Kaufman HH: The acute care of patients with gunshot wounds to the head. Neurotrauma Med Rep 4:1–2, 1990.

79. Kaufman HH, Herschberger J, Kopitnik T, et al: Chronic extradural haematomas: Indications for surgery. Br J Neurosurg 6:359–364, 1992.

80. Kawakami Y, Chikama M, Tamiya T, et al: Coagulation and fibrinolysis in chronic subdural hematoma. Neurosurgery 25:25–29, 1989.

81. Keane JR: The pretectal syndrome: 206 patients. Neurology 40:684–690, 1990.

82. Kim KS, Hemmati M, Weinberg PE, et al: Computed tomography in isodense subdural hematoma. Radiology 128:71–74, 1978.

83. Kishore PRS, Lipper MH, Miller JD, et al: Posttraumatic hydrocephalus in patients with severe head injury. Neuroradilogy 16:261–265, 1978.

84. Klein DM: The treatment of shunt infections. In Scott RM (ed): Hydrocephalus. Baltimore, Williams & Wilkins, 1990, pp 87–98.

85. Koehler PJ, Blauw G: Late posttraumatic nonvascular pulsating eye. Acta Neurochir 116:62–64, 1992.

86. Kotwica Z, Brzezinski J: Chronic subdural haematoma treated by burr holes and closed system drainage: Personal experience in 131 patients. Br J Neurosurg 5:461–465, 1991.

87. Landesman S, Cooper PR: Infectious complications of head injury. In Cooper PR (ed): Head Injury, 3rd ed. Baltimore, Williams & Wilkins, 1993, pp 503–524.

88. Larsson A, Jensen CH, Bilting M, et al: Does the shunt opening pressure influence the effect of shunt surgery in normal pressure hydrocephalus? Acta Neurochir 117:15–22, 1992.

89. Las Jaunias P: Angiographic study of carotid cavernous fistulas. In Samii M, Brihaye J (eds): Traumatology of the Skull Base. New York, Springer Verlag, 1983, pp 189–195.

90. Laun A: Traumatic cerebrospinal fluid fistulas in the anterior and middle cranial fossae. Acta Neurochir 60:215–222, 1982.

91. Levin HS, Meyers CA, Grossman RG, et al: Ventricular enlargement after closed head injury. Arch Neurol 38:623–629, 1981.

92. Loew F, Kivelitz R: Chronic subdural hematomas. In Vinken PJ, Bruyn GW (eds): Handbook of Clinical Neurology, vol 24. New York, Elsevier, 1976, pp 297–327.

93. Long D: Issues in behavioral neurology and brain injury. In Ellis DW, Christensen AL (eds): Neuropsychological treatment after brain injury. Boston, Kluwer, 1989, pp 39–90.

94. Lundar T, Nornes H: Determination of ventricular fluid outflow resistance in patients with ventriculomeguly. J Neurol Neurosurg Psychiatry 53:896–898, 1990.

95. MacGee E: Cerebrospinal fluid fistula. In Vinken PJ, Broyn GW (eds): The Handbook of Clinical Neurology, vol 24. Amsterdam, Elsevier, 1976, pp 183–199.

96. Magnaes B: Body position and cerebrospinal fluid pressure. J Neurosurg 44:687–697, 1976.

97. Markham JW: Pneumocephalus. In Vinken PJ, Bruyn GW (eds): Handbook of Clinical Neurology, vol 24, New York, Elsevier, 1976, pp 201–213.

98 Markwalder TM: Chronic subdural hematomas: A review. J Neurosurg 54:637–645, 1981.

99. Markwalder TM, Steinsiepek F, Rohner M, et al: The course of chronic subdural hematomas after burr–hole craniostomy and closed–system drainage. J Neurosurg 55:390–396, 1981.

100. Martinez–Lage J, Poza M, Esteban JA, et al: Mechanical complications of the reservoirs and flushing devices in ventricular shunt systems. Br J Neurosurg 6:321–326, 1992.

101. Martinez–Lage JF, Poza M, Lopez F, et al: Arachnoid cyst as a complication of ventricular shunting. Childs Nerv Syst 7:356–357, 1991.

102. Matricali B: Internal carotid artery aneurisms. In Samii M, Brihaye J (eds): Traumatology of the Skull Base. New York, Springer Verlag, 1983, pp 196–200.

103. Mertol T, Buner M, Acar V, et al: Delayed traumatic intracerebral hematoma. Br J Neurosurg 5:491–498, 1991.

104. Meyers CA, Levin HS, Eisenberg HM, et al: Early versus late lateral ventricular enlargement following closed head injury. J Neurol Neurosurg Psychiatry 46:1092–1097, 1983.

105. Milborat TH: Pediatric Neurosurgery. Philadelphia, F.A. Davis, 1978, pp 91–135.

106. Miller ES, Dias PS, Uttley D, et al: CT scanning in the management of intracranial abscess: A review of 100 cases. Br J Neurosurg 2:439–446, 1988.

107. Miller JD: Infection after head injury. In Vinken PJ, Bruyn GW (eds): Handbook of Clinical Neurology, vol 24. Amsterdam, Elsevier, 1976, pp 215–230.

108. Miyachi S, Negoro M, Handa T, et al: Dural carotid cavernous sinus fistula presenting as isolated oculomotor nerve palsy. Surg Neurol 39:105–109, 1993.

109. Mohamed EEH: Management of chronic subdural haematoma. Br J Neurosurg 5:525–526, 1991.

110. Malavi A, Dinubile MJ: Brain abscess. In Harris AA (ed): Handbook of Clinical Neurology, vol 8. Amsterdam, Elsevier, 1988, pp 143–166.

111. Morgan MK, Johnston IH, Spittaler PJ, et al: A ventricular infusion technique for the evaluation of treated and untreated hydrocephalus. Neurosurgery 29:832–837, 1991.

112. Mysiw WJ, Jackson RD: Relationship of new–onset systemic hypertension and normal pressure hydrocephalus. Brain Inj 4:233–238, 1990.

113. McCormack B, Cooper PR, Perksy M, et al: Extracranial repair of cerebrospinal fluid fistulas: Technique and results in 37 patients. Neurosurgery 27:412–417, 1990.

114. McLone DG, Naidich TP: The investigation of hydrocephalus by computed tomography. Clin Neurosurg 32:527–539, 1985.

115. Nagashima T, Tamaki N, Matsumoto S, et al: Biomechanics of hydrocephalus: A new theoretical model. Neurosurgery 21:898–904, 1987.

116. Naidich TP, Altman NR, Gonzalez–Arias SM: Phase contrast cine magnetic resonance imaging: Normal cerebrospinal fluid oscillation and applications to hydrocephalus. Neurosurg Clin North Am 4:677–705, 1993.

117. Nakstad PH, Hald JK, Sorteberg W: Carotid–cavernous fistula treated with detachable balloon during bilateral transcranial doppler monitoring of middle cerebral arteries. Acta Radiol 33:145–148, 1992.

118. Narayan R, Gokaslan ZL, Bontke CF, et al: Neurologic sequelae of head injury. In Rosenthal M, Band MR, Griffith ER, Miller JD (eds): Rehabilitation of the Adult and Child with Traumatic Brain Injury, 2nd ed. Philadelphia, F.A. Davis, 1990, pp 94–106.

119. Nida TY, Haines SJ: Multiloculated hydrocephalus: Craniotomy and fenestration of intraventricular septations. J Neurosurg 781:70–76, 1993.

120. Noetzel MJ, Baker RP: Shunt fluid examination: Risks and benefits in the evaluation of shunt malfunction and infection. J Neurosurg 61:328–332, 1984.

121. Okada J, Tsuda T, Takasugi S, et al: Unusually late onset of cerebrospinal fluid rhinorrhea after head trauma. Surg Neurol 35:213–217, 1991.

122. Oku Y, Takimoto N, Yamamoto S, et al: Trail of a new operative method of recurrent chronic subdural hematoma. J Neurosurg 61:269–272, 1984.

123. Overgaard J: Traumatic injuries of the planum occipitale and posterior fossa brain parenchyma. In Samii M, Brihaye J (eds): Traumatology of the Skull Base. New York, Springer Verlag, 1983, pp 88–93.

124. Pang D, Horton JA, Herron JM, et al: Nonsurgical management of extradural hematomas in children. J Neurosurg 59:958–971, 1983.

125. Pathak A, Sharma BS, Mathuriya SN, et al: Controversies in the management of subdural empyema. Acta Neurochir (Wien) 102:25–32, 1990.

126. Piatt JH: Physical examination of patients with cerebrospinal fluid shunts: Is there useful information in pumping the shunt? Pediatrics 89:470–473, 1992.

127. Portnoy HD, Schulte RR, Fox JL, et al: Anti-siphon and reversible occlusion valves for shunting in hydrocephalus and preventing post-shunt subdural hematomas. J Neurosurg 38:729–738, 1973.

128. Post EM: Currently available shunt systems: A review. Neurosurgery 16:257–260, 1985.

129. Pozzati E, Frank F, Frank G, et al: Subacute and chronic extradural hematomas: A study of 30 cases. J Trauma 20:795–799, 1980.

130. Probst CH: Neurosurgical treatment of traumatic frontobasal CSF fistulae in 300 patients (1967–1989). Acta Neurochir 106:37–47, 1990.

131. Puca A, Anile C, Maira G, et al: Cerebrospinal fluid shunting for hydrocephalus in the adult: Factors related to shunt revision. Neurosurgery 29:822–826, 1991.

132. Pudenz RH, Foltz EL: Hydrocephalus: Overdrainage by ventricular shunts: A review and recommendations. Surg Neurol 35:200–212, 1991.

133. Pudenz RH: The control of overdrainage in cerebrospinal fluid shunting. PS Med Doc. 10871:3–10, 1990.

134. Quinn MW Pople IK: Middle cerebral artery pulsatility in children with blocked cerebrospinal fluid shunts. J Neurol Neurosurg 55:325–327, 1992.

135. Quintaliani R, Cooper BW: Central nervous system infections due to staphylococci. In Harris AA (ed): Handbook of Clinical Neurology, vol 8. Amsterdam, Elsevier, 1988, pp 71–76.

136. Ram Z, Hadani M, Sahar A, et al: Continuous irrigation–drainage of the subdural space for the treatment of chronic subdural haematoma: A prospective clinical trail. Acta Neurochir 120:40–43, 1993.

137. Reider–Grosswasser I, Loewenstein A, Gafon DD, et al: Spontaneous thrombosis of a traumatic cavernous sinus fistula. Brain Inj 7:547–550, 1993.

138. Rekate HL: Shunt revision: Complications and their prevention. Pediatr Neurosurg 17:155–162, 1991–1992.

139. Rish BL, Dillon JD, Meirowksy AM, et al: Cranioplasty: A review of 1030 cases of penetrating head injury. Neurosurgery 4:381–385, 1979.

140. Roberson FC, Kishore PRS, Miller JD, et al: The valve of serial computerized tomography in the management of severe head injury. Surg Neurol 12:161–167, 1979.

141. Robinson RG: Chronic subdural hematoma: Surgical management in 133 patients. J Neurosurg 61:263–268, 1984.

142. Roda JM, Gimenez D, Perez–Higueras A, et al: Posterior fossa epidural hematomas: A review and synthesis. Surg Neurol 19:419–424, 1983.

143. Rovillard R, Leclerc J, Savary P, et al: Pulsatile tinnitus: A dehiscent jugular vein. Laryngoscope 95:188–189, 1985.

144. Roy R, Cooper PR: Penetrating injuries of the skull and brain. In Broakman R (ed): Handbook of Clinical Neurology, vol 13. Amsterdam, Elsevier, 1990, pp 299–315.

145. Rubin G, Rappaport ZH: Epilepsy in chronic subdural haematoma. Acta Neurochir 123:39–42, 1993.

146. Sahuquillo J, Rubin E, Codina A, et al: Reappraisal of the intracranial pressure and cerebrospinal fluid dynamics in patients with so–called "normal pressure hydrocephalus" syndrome. Acta Neurochir 112:50–61, 1991.

147. Sainte–Rose L, Piatt JH, Renier D, et al: Mechanical complications in shunts. Pediatr Neurosurg 17:2–9, 1991.

148. Salmon JH: Surgical treatment of severe posttraumatic encephalopathy. Surg Gynecol Obstet 133:634–636, 1971.

149. Sampson JH, Cardoso ER: The gravitational shunt: An alternative approach to cerebrospinal fluid shunting. Surg Neurol 40:112–118, 1993.

150. Sandel ME, Abrams PL, Horn LJ, et al: Hypertension after brain injury: Case report. Arch Phys Med Rehabil 67:469–472, 1986.

151. Sanker P, Richard KE, Weigl HC, et al: Transcranial Doppler sonography and intracranial pressure monitoring in children and juveniles with acute brain injuries or hydrocephalus. Childs Nerv Syst 7:391–393, 1991.

152. Schneider RC, Thompson JM: Chronic and delayed traumatic cerebrospinal rhinorrhea as a source of recurrent attacks of meningitis. Ann Surg 145: 517– 529, 1957.

153. Schoenbaum SC, Gardner P, Shillito J, et al: Infections of cerebrospinal fluid shunts: Epidemiology, clinical manifestations, and therapy. J Infect Dis 131:543–552.

154. Schroth G, Klose U: Cerebrospinal fluid flow. III: Pathological cerebrospinal fluid pulsations. Neuroradiology 35:16–24, 1992.

155. Scott RM: The Treatment and prevention of shunt complications. In Scott RM (ed): Hydrocephalus. Baltimore, Williams & Wilkins, 1990, pp 115–122.

156. Seelig GM, Becker DP, Miller JD, et al: Traumatic acute subdural hematoma. N Engl J Med 304: 1511–1518, 1981.

157. Seliger, GM, Katz DI, Seliger M, et al: Late improvement in closed head injury with a low–pressure valve shunt. Brain Inj 6:71–73, 1992.

158. Shapiro SA, Scully T: Closed continuous drainage of cerebrospinal fluid via a lumbar subarachnoid catheter for treatment or prevention of cranial spinal cerebrospinal fluid fistula. Neurosurgery 30:241–245, 1992.

159. Shurtleff DB: Characteristics of the various CSF shunt systems. Clin Pediatr 17:154–160, 1978.

160. Silbert PL, Gubbay SS, Vaughan RJ, et al: Cavum septum pellucidum and obstructive hydrocephalus. J Neurol Neurosurg Psychiatry 56:820–822, 1993.

161. Reference deleted.

162. Sindou M, Guyotat–Pelissou I, Chidiac A, et al: Transcutaneous pressure adjustable valve for the treatment of hydrocephalus and arachnoid cysts in adults. Acta Neurochir 121:135–139, 1993.

163. Stapleton SR, Bell BA, Uttley D, et al: Sterotactic aspiration of brain abscesses: Is this the treatment of choice. Acta Neurochir (Wien) 121:15–19, 1993.

164. Stein SC, Spettell C, Young G, et al: Delayed and progressive brain injury in closed head trauma: Radiological demonstration. Neurosurgery 32:25–31, 1993.

165. Stein SC, Young GS, Talucci RC, et al: Delayed brain injury after head trauma: Significance of coagulopathy. Neurosurgery 30:160–165, 1992.

166. Stollman AL, George AE, Pinto RS, et al: Periventricular high signal lesions and signal void on magnetic resonance imaging in hydrocephalus. Acta Radiol Supp 369:388–391, 1986.

167. Stone JL, Rifai MHS, Lang RGR, et al: Subdural hematomas. Acute subdural hematoma: Progress in definition, clinical pathology and therapy. Surg Neurol 19:216–231, 1983.

168. Sudarsky L, Simon S: Gait disorder in late life hydrocephalus. Arch Neurol 44:263–267, 1987.

169. Sutcliffe JC, Ballersby RDE: Do we need variable pressure shunts? Br J Neurosurg 6:67–70, 1992.

170. Suzuki N, Suzuki SH, Iwabuchi T, et al: Neurological improvement after cranioplasty. Acta Neurochir 122:49–53, 1993.

171. St. John JN, Dila C: Traumatic subdural hygroma in adults. Neurosurgery 9:621–626, 1981.

172. Tans JTJ, Poortvliet DCJ: Relationship between compliance and resistance to outflow of CSF in adult hydrocephalus. J Neurosurg 71:59–62, 1989.

173. Thomsen AM, Borgesen SE, Bruhn P, et al: Prognosis of dementia in normal–pressure hydrocephalus after a shunt operation. Ann Neurol 20:304–310, 1986.

174. Tsai FY, Huprich JE: Further experience with contrast enhanced CT in head trauma. Neuroradiology 16:314–317, 1978.

175. Tunkel AR, Scheld WM: Acute infectious complications of head trauma. In Braakman R (ed): Handbook of Clinical Neurology, vol 13. Amsterdam, Elsevier, 1990, pp 317–326.

176. Uvebrant P, Sixt R, Bjure J, et al: Evaluation of cerebrospinal fluid shunt function in hydrocephalic children using 99m Tc-DTPA. Childs Nerv Syst 8:76–80, 1992.

177. Vallis RC, Martin FW: Extracranial arteriovenous malformation presenting as objective tinnitus. J Laryngol Otol 98:1139–1142, 1984.

178. VanDongen KJ, Braakman R: Late computed tomography in survivors of severe head injury. Neurosurgery 7:14–22, 1980.

179. Vanneste J, Augustijn P, Tan WF, et al: Shunting normal pressure hydrocephalus: The predictive value of combined clinical and CT data. J Neurol Neurosurg Psychiatry 56:251–256, 1993.

180. Vanneste J, Augustijn P, Diruen C, et al: Shunting normal–pressure hydrocephalus: Do the benefits outweigh the risks? Neurology 42:54–59, 1992.

181. Vanneste J, Augustijn P, Davies GAG, et al: Normal–pressure hydrocephalus: Is cisternography still useful in selecting patients for a shunt? Arch Neurol 49:366–370, 1992.

182. Vax R, Duarte F, Oliveira J, et al: Traumatic interhemispheric subdural haematomas. Acta Neurochir 111:128–131, 1991.

183. Wakhloo AK, VanVelthoven V, Schumacher M, et al: Evaluation of MR imaging, digital subtraction cisternography, and CT cisternography in diagnosing CSF fistula. Acta Neurochir 111:119–127, 1991.

184. Waldemar G, Schmidt JF, Delecluse F, et al: High resolution SPECT with 99m Tc-d, 1–HMPAO in normal pressure hydrocephalus before and after shunt operation. J Neurol Neurosurg Psychiatry 56:655–664, 1993.

185. Walter KA, Newman NJ, Lessell S, et al: Oculomotor palsy from minor head trauma: Initial sign of intracranial aneurysm. Neurology 44:148– 150, 1994.

186. Watson DA: The delta valve: A physiologic shunt system. Presented at the Consensus Conference on Pediatrics. Neurosurg, Assisi, Italy, 1992.

187. Watts C, Keith HD: Testing the hydrocephalus shunt valve. Child Brain 10:217–228, 1983.

188. Weisberg L: Subdural empyema. Arch Neurol 43:497–500, 1986.

189. Wisoff JH, Epstein FJ: Diagnosis and treatment of the slit ventricle syndrome. In Scott RM (ed): Hydrocephalus. Baltimore, Williams & Wilkins, 1990, pp 79–86.

190. Wortzman D, Tucker WS, Gershater R, et al: Traumatic aneurysm in the posterior fossa. Surg Neurol 13:329–332, 1980.

191. Wright RL: Traumatic hematomas of the posterior cranial fossa. J Neurosurg 25:402–409, 1966.

192. Yamashima T, Yamamoto S, Friede RL, et al: The rule of endothelial gap junctions in the enlargement of chronic subdural hematomas. J Neurosurg 59:298–303, 1983.

193. Yamoshima T, Yamamoto S: How do vessels proliferate in the capsule of a chronic subdural hematoma. Neurosurgery 15:672–678, 1984.

194. Yang S, Zhao C: Review of 140 patients with brain abscess. Surg Neurol 39:290–296, 1993.

195. Young GB, Bolton CF: The neurology of sepsis. Neurol Chron 2:1–5, 1992.

196. Zander E, Foroglou G: Posttraumatic hydrocephalus. In Vinken PJ, Bruyn GW (eds): Handbook of Clinical Neurology, vol 24. New York, Elsevier, 1976, pp 231–253.

197. Zaret DL, Morrison N, Gulbranson R, et al: Immunofixation to quantity B2–transfer in cerebrospinal fluid to detect leakage of cerebrospinal fluid from skull injury. Clin Chem 38:1909–1912, 1992.

STUART A. YABLON M.D.

14

Posttraumatic Seizures

Traumatic brain injuries (TBIs) inflict a significant toll of morbidity and mortality on the population of westernized nations. In the United States an estimated 422,000 inpatients are treated for TBI annually.[1] A sizable number of survivors have important medical and neurologic sequelae, including seizures.

This chapter focuses on the relationship between TBI and subsequent development of posttraumatic seizure disorders, including incidence, risk factors, prophylaxis, and management. Most of the cited studies address posttraumatic seizures in adults.

CLASSIFICATION OF POSTTRAUMATIC SEIZURES AND EPILEPSY

For purposes of clarification, it is useful to review the terminology used in the discussion of posttraumatic seizure disorders. Seizures have been described as discrete clinical events that reflect a temporary physiologic dysfunction of the brain, characterized by excessive and hypersynchronous discharge of cortical neurons.[196] Epilepsy is a condition characterized by recurrent unprovoked seizures.[96]

Posttraumatic epilepsy is a disorder characterized by recurrent late seizure episodes, not attributable to another obvious cause, in

patients with TBI.[8,21] Although the term posttraumatic epilepsy has commonly been used to designate single or multiple seizures, including early seizures, it should be reserved for recurrent, late posttraumatic seizures. Because many studies of seizures among patients with TBI do not address recurrence, the term posttraumatic seizures (rather than epilepsy) is preferred; a posttraumatic seizure is a single or recurrent seizure episode, not attributable to another obvious cause, in a patient with closed or penetrating TBI.

Posttraumatic seizures have been further classified into early and late categories, primarily because of prevailing opinion that they represent similar manifestations of different pathophysiologic processes.[113] Early posttraumatic seizures refer to episodes that occur within the first week after TBI. Some authors differentiate another category, immediate posttraumatic seizures, which refers to seizures occurring within the first 24 hours after TBI.[124] Late posttraumatic seizures refer to episodes that occur after the first week after TBI.[113]

The exclusion of other obvious causes bears particular relevance to the discussion of seizure disorders in patients with TBI. Seizures may be the result of precipitants unrelated to mechanisms of posttraumatic

363

epileptogenesis. Examples of such precipitants include anoxia,[67] metabolic abnormalities,[149] and mass-occupying lesions, including hemorrhage.[14,70,90,109]

Recreational drugs[11,148] such as alcohol[95,100] and medications such as antipsychotic agents[148] and tricyclic antidepressants[63,106,256] are potential seizure precipitants that warrant special attention by professionals caring for patients with TBI. In a retrospective study, Wroblewski and coworkers concluded that 19% of patients with severe TBI developed seizures largely precipitated by tricyclic antidepressants.[256] Although inhibitors of serotonin reuptake are believed to have lower proconvulsive activity than other antidepressants, fluvoxamine has been implicated in the recurrence of multiple partial seizures in a patient who was free of posttraumatic seizures for 30 years.[51] Bromocriptine and amantadine, dopamine receptor agonists used to treat arousal disorders and expressive aphasias in patients with brain injuries, have been implicated as seizure precipitants.[253] Stimulants used to improve cognitive function, such as methylphenidate and methamphetamine,[84,265] however, do not appear to be associated with increased seizure risk among patients with TBI.[255]

Seizures and seizure disorders have been classified according to their respective clinical and electroencephalographic characteristics, as developed by the Commission on Classification and Terminology of the International League Against Epilepsy.[42] Seizures have been divided into two categories, based primarily on pattern of onset: (1) partial or focal seizures and (2) generalized seizures. Patients with closed head injury frequently have sustained multiple foci of cerebral injury[65,88] and may manifest more than one type of seizure.[112]

Generalized seizures denote convulsions that are bilaterally symmetrical in origin without local onset. The most commonly recognized example of the generalized type is the grand mal or tonic-clonic seizure. The generalized-onset type is seen in slightly less than one-half of the patients with posttraumatic seizures and appears more frequently in patients with nonpenetrating TBI[113,158] and in children.[52,86] Absence (petit mal) seizures, another form of the generalized type, are not

encountered as a manifestation of posttraumatic seizures.[13,44,158,237]

Partial or focal seizures originate in a localized area of one cerebral hemisphere. Partial seizures are subclassified according to whether consciousness is maintained (simple partial) or impaired (complex partial) during the seizure. Characteristics of both simple and complex partial seizures vary, depending on the location of the seizure activity within the brain. Up to 12% of cases of complex partial seizures in the general population may be attributable to TBI.[183] Partial-onset seizures are observed in slightly more than one-half of all patients with posttraumatic seizures and appear more frequently among adults[112] and patients with early seizures,[112,132,158] focal lesions on computed tomography,[47] penetrating traumatic brain injuries,[158,190] and closed head injury of greater severity.[47]

Nonepileptic seizures, also termed pseudoseizures or psychogenic seizures, are episodic behavioral events that superficially resemble epileptic attacks but are not associated with paroxysmal activity within the brain.[102] Nonepileptic seizures are not uncommon in neurologic settings[15,221] and may coexist with epileptic seizures in patients with epilepsy.[67,15,156] Nonstereotypic, asynchronous limb thrashing and head turning,[67,129] particularly of long duration in an awake patient,[119] are associated with nonepileptic seizures. The differentiation between nonepileptic and epileptic seizures cannot be made on the basis of clinical characteristics alone.[67] Electroencephalographic monitoring (particularly with video)[67,221] is often helpful in establishing a diagnosis. Measurement of postictal prolactin[40,46,168] may provide additional diagnostic information if significant elevations are observed, although the utility of this test has recently been questioned, because it does not detect partial seizures of frontal lobe origin.[147]

The prevalence of nonepileptic seizures among patients with TBI has received little attention. Recently, Barry et al. described the characteristics of 16 patients who were thought to have posttraumatic seizures but in fact had nonepileptic seizures, as confirmed on video electroencephalographic monitoring. Patients with nonepileptic seizures had injuries of much milder severity and usually had manifestations of other conversion disorders as well as psychiatric histories that predated the TBI.[12]

Epilepsy has been classified into different syndromes, using two general divisions.[41] One division separates epilepsies characterized by generalized seizures from syndromes characterized by seizures of focal onset (localization-related epilepsies). The other division separates epilepsies of known etiology (secondary or symptomatic) from those that are idiopathic (primary) or cryptogenic. Symptomatic (or secondary) epilepsies are considered the consequence of a known or suspected disorder of the central nervous system, such as trauma,[41] and include syndromes of great individual variability, based mainly on seizure type and anatomic localization.

Temporal lobe and orbitofrontal lobe epilepsies designate specific types of symptomatic, localization-related epilepsies. Both have been described among patients with TBI.[112,133,213] Temporal lobe epilepsy has been described as the sole epileptic manifestation in up to 20% of patients with posttraumatic epilepsy.[112,113] Features of temporal lobe epilepsy include simple partial seizures characterized by autonomic, psychic, and/or sensory phenomena. Orbitofrontal lobe seizures include complex partial seizures characterized by motor arrest followed by buccal automatisms.[41] Transient postictal confusion and amnesia are usually observed after complex partial seizures of temporal lobe origin.[41]

Potential difficulties exist in the recognition of seizures of temporal and frontal lobe origin among patients with severe TBI. Seizure activity in these regions of the brain presents with various manifestations, including behaviors that may not be attributed to an underlying seizure disorder.[247] Frontal lobe epileptic manifestations may include sexual automatisms, such as masturbation,[208,247] or semipurposeful, complex motor automatisms, such as kicking, screaming, and thrashing episodes.[247] The contribution of epileptic phenomena to ictal, periictal, and interictal aggression or violence is controversial.[66] However, it appears that episodes of ictal aggression are quite rare[218,219] and are usually associated with postictal confusion, particularly while the patient is restrained.[54,219] Electrographic manifestations of seizure activity in this region of the brain also may be difficult to recognize.

Interictal scalp electroencephalograms are frequently misleading[247] and may show no abnormality,[41] although specialized basal montages with additional temporal or sphenoidal leads may be of help in clarifying presumed inferomesial temporal discharges.[67]

Unclassified Phenomena

Recent studies describe transient cognitive impairment[1,17] and behavioral symptoms reminiscent of complex partial seizures[182,228,229] among patients without concurrent seizures. In most reports, patients manifest interictal discharges on electroencephalography without the hypersynchronous electroencephalographic activity and stereotyped behaviors that characterize partial seizures and localization-related epilepsies.[228,229] Such episodes are usually reported among patients with mild TBI.[228,229] Many patients respond favorably to anticonvulsants such as carbamazepine.[229] The resemblance of the behaviors to some complex partial seizures of temporal or frontal lobe origin and the favorable response to anticonvulsants tend to confuse clinical diagnosis. Such phenomena appear to support assertions that epileptic disorders represent a spectrum of electrophysiologic abnormality and are not limited to seizures or epilepsy.[182,184]

Nevertheless, the significance of these phenomena and their relationship to currently accepted and classified seizure disorders remain unclear. Some reports describe cognitive dysfunction precisely coinciding with recordings of interictal spike and sharp wave discharges on the electroencephalogram.[1,17] Other reports describe a relationship of abnormal symptoms with paroxysmal theta patterns on the electroencephalogram[228] and do not suggest a simultaneous relationship between symptoms and electroencephalographic abnormalities.[182,228,229] In a number of patients, no electroencephalographic abnormalities are observed.[182,229] Moreover, a broad range of behavioral symptoms is reported, including dysphoric mood, aggressive outbursts, affective lability, and memory impairment, and these frequently occur in the same patient.[182] The heterogeneity of the described behavioral and electrophysiologic abnormalities highlights the need for further study to determine whether such reports describe a distinct class of abnormalities. Given the present controversy, however, the presence of these behavioral abnormalities should not be considered equivalent to a diagnosis of epileptic seizures, particularly for purposes of clinical decision-making and antiepileptic drug therapy. Proper diagnosis remains the first and most important step in the therapeutic approach to the patient with suspected epileptic seizures.

INCIDENCE OF POSTTRAUMATIC SEIZURES

Traumatic brain injuries are an important cause of epilepsy, accounting for 20% of symptomatic epilepsy in the general population and 5% of all epilepsy.[94] Many early studies addressing the relationship between TBI and epilepsy derive from observations of veterans suffering penetrating head injury in battle.[4,10,11,26,34,35,68,165,186,190,237–239,243,250] Studies in civilian settings appeared later[8,9,19,22,37,47–50,52, 65,85,86,98,99,110,112,114,116,122–125,128,134,150,157,192,216,245] and reflect a larger patient population with closed rather than penetrating head injuries. The observed results vary considerably, reflecting differences in inclusion and exclusion criteria, description of seizure phenomena, attention to confounding variables, duration of follow up, and patient population.[55] Nevertheless, these studies (Table 1), particularly those of Jennett[112,114] and Annegers et al.,[8] provide useful information about the incidence, risk factors, and natural history of posttraumatic seizures.

In summary, the overall incidence of late seizures in hospitalized patients with closed head injury is approximately 4–7%, although this figure varies, depending on the injury and patient characteristics.[8,112] Late seizures are observed less frequently among children.[8,86,125] The incidence of posttraumatic seizures among patients with closed head injury in the rehabilitation setting appears substantially higher than the incidence reported in civilian settings.[9,21,37,116,192] This probably reflects the increased severity of injury and multiple risk factors among rehabilitation inpatients.[9] In contrast, the incidence of seizures among adults after mild closed head injury is not significantly greater than the incidence observed in the general population.[8] Posttraumatic seizures are observed in approximately 35–50% of patients with penetrating head injury.[10,34,35,190]

The incidence of early seizures is approximately 5%[112] among all patients with closed head injury and is higher in young children,[8,112,158,86] among whom the incidence is approximately 10%.[8,86] Immediate seizures, which make up 50–80% of early posttraumatic seizures,[112,158,68,125,180] are particularly frequent among children with severe TBI.[8,86] Early posttraumatic seizures are occasionally observed among children with mild TBI[112,86] but are rare among adults with mild TBI. Early seizures among adults with mild TBI warrants investigation for an underlying intracranial hemorrhage. In a recent study of over 4,000 adults with mild TBI, an intracranial hemorrhage was found in almost one-half of the patients suffering early posttraumatic seizures.[128]

NATURAL HISTORY

Recurrence

Approximately one-half to two-thirds of patients who suffer posttraumatic seizures experience seizure onset within the first 12 months; by the end of the second year after injury the proportion increases to 75–80%.[35,47,48,190,237,238] After 5 years, most patients do not appear to have a significantly increased risk relative to the general populations,[8] although some may experience seizure onset after this interval.[8,47,158,190] Approximately one-half of patients experience only a single posttraumatic seizure without recurrence,[49,125] and another quarter suffer a total of 2–3 seizures.[125] Whereas patients with early posttraumatic seizures experience a late seizure in 20–30% of cases, seizure onset after the first week is associated with a much higher likelihood of recurrence.[79,238] Seizure frequency within the first year after injury may be predictive of future recurrence.[190] Persistent posttraumatic seizures may be more common in partial and less common in generalized seizures.[190]

Complications

Potentially significant complications accompany seizure activity in the patient with

TABLE 1.   Studies Addressing the Incidence of Posttraumatic Seizures

Study	No. of Subjects	Subject Population	Trauma Category	Follow-up Duration	Incidence of PTS (%)	Risk Factors Cited*
Military Settings						
Ameen, 1987[4]	NS	Veterans of the Iran-Iraq War	PHI	NS	4.7 (E)	NS
Ascroft et al., 1941[10]	317	Pensioned World War I veterans sustaining PHI	PHI	4 yr	34	Dural penetration, bone/metal fragments, removal of fragments, wound sepsis with dural penetration
Brandvold et al., 1990[26]	113	Israeli, Lebanese, and United Nations soldiers consecutively admitted to a neurosurgical unit	PHI	5.9 yr (mean)	21.7	NS
Caveness and Liss, 1961[34]	407	American soldiers suffering TBI during the Korean War	PHI: 33% CHI: 67%	5 yr	40.3 (PHI) 15.7 (CHI)	"Overt" evidence of brain damage without dural penetration, dural penetration, dural penetration and focal neurologic signs
Caveness et al., 1979[35]	1,030	American soldiers suffering from PHI during the Vietnam War	PHI	6–10 yr	33 4.4 (E); 28 (L)	Multiple lobe lesion
Evans, 1962[68]	422	U.S. servicemen who were wounded during or immediately after the Korean War	PHI: 52.4% CHI: 35.3% "Blast": 12.3%	3–11 yr (most ≥ 7 yr)	32 (L)(PHI) 8 (L)(CHI)	Family history, PHI, DSF (w/CHI only), parietal or temporal lobe sites of injury, ICH, retained bone fragments, PTA > 24 hr
Phillips, 1954[165]	2,000	Soldiers with head injury referred to the Military Hospital for Head Injuries, Oxford, England	CHI	NS	9.5; 2.25 (E)	NS
	500	"Relatively" unselected, acute CHI patients directly admitted to the Military Hospital for Head Injuries	CHI	NS	6	DSF, PTA > 24 hr
Russell and Whitty, 1952[186]	820	British soldiers sustaining PHI in World War II	PHI	5 yr	43	Parietal lobe lesions, lesions of the motor/premotor cortex, focal neurologic deficit
Salazar et al., 1985[190]	421	American soldiers sustaining PHI in the Vietnam War	PHI	15 yr	53 9 (E)	Brain volume loss > 75 ml, aphasia, ICH, retained metal fragments, EEG with epileptiform activity
Walker and Jablon, 1959, 1961[237,238]	739	American soldiers sustaining TBI in World War II	PHI: 62.1% CHI: 37.3%	3–9 yr 99% ≥ 5 yr	28.1 8.2 (E)	PHI, aphasia, hemianopsia, hemiplegia, bone/metal fragments, LOC > 24 hr, parietal and frontal lobe lesions, constipation
Watson, 1952[239]	286	Unselected combat veterans	PHI	3 yr	41.6 (L)	NS
Whitty, 1947[243]	434	Consecutive patients with PHI	PHI	NS	6.7 (E); 6.5 (L)	Family history, prior seizure history, EPTS
	400	Patients with unspecified TBI referred to the hospital	NS	18 mo	5.8 (E); 4 (L)	Parietal lobe injury
Wilson, 1951[250]	953	Pensioned World War II veterans of the Royal New Zealand Armed Forces with TBI	PHI: 20% CHI: 80%	> 5 yr	6.2	PHI, bone/metal fragments

* Not necessarily in order of importance.
CHI = closed head injury, CT = computed tomography, DSF = depressed skull fracture, EEG = electroencephalography, E[PTS] = early posttraumatic seizure, EtOH = alcohol use/abuse, GCS = Glasgow Coma Scale, ICH = intracranial hematoma/hemorrhage, IPTS = immediate posttraumatic seizure (within 24 hr of injury), JFURGPTE = Japan Follow-Up Research Group of Posttraumatic Epilepsy, LOC = loss of consciousness, L[PTS] = late posttraumatic seizure, NS = not specified, PHI = penetrating head injury, PTA = posttraumatic amnesia, PTE = posttraumatic epilepsy, PTS = posttraumatic seizure.   *(Table continued on following page.)*

TABLE 1. **Studies Addressing the Incidence of Posttraumatic Seizures** *(Continued)*

Study	No. of Subjects	Subject Population	Trauma Category	Follow-up Duration	Incidence of PTS (%)	Risk Factors Cited*
Civilian Settings						
Annegers et al., 1980[8]	2,747	Head injured population of Olmsted county, Minnesota	CHI	Until emigrated from region	1.9 (L) 2.1 (L)	ICH, "severe" head injury (documented contusion, ICH, PTA or LOC ≥ 24 hr)
da Silva et al., 1992[47]	154	Consecutive outpatients with PTE at the Hospital de Santo Antonio, Portugal (retrospective)	NS	5 yr	100 (inclusion criteria)	Focal lesions, focal neurologic signs, lower GCS, ICH, diffuse or hemispheric contusions
	152	Consecutive admissions with CHI 1988–1989 at high risk for PTE, due to ICH, PHI, or EPTS (prospective)	NS	1 yr	33	
da Silva et al., 1990[48]	506	Consecutive patients admitted to intensive care unit of the Hospital de Santo Antonio, Portugal	CHI: 88% PHI: 12%	> 3 yr	12.25 4.9 (I)	Focal lesions, focal neurologic signs
De Santis et al., 1979[49]	2,980	Adult patients with TBI admitted to neurosurgery service	NS	NS	2.8 (E)	Operative intervention
De Santis et al., 1992[50]	52	Adult patients with TBI and EPTS, admitted to the neurosurgery service from 1971–1981, without CT	NS	5.6 yr (mean)	23 (L)	Focal lesion requiring surgery
	41	Adult patients with TBI and EPTS, who received CT	NS	1–4 yr	9.4 (L)	Documented focal brain lesions
	85	Children with TBI admitted from 1965–1981, without CT	NS	1–14 yr 5 yr (mean)	23 (L)	EPTS
	60	Patients admitted from 1982–1987 with severe CHI, coma, who received serial CT showing diffuse brain injury	CHI	1–8 yr	0 (L) 1.6 (E); 1/60	Diffuse injury without lesion is not a risk factor
	98	Selected patients admitted with CT-documented focal lesions; and ICH or DSF with surgical treatment	NS	15–55 mo	12.2 (L); 12/98	Documented focal brain lesion
Desai et al., 1983[52]	702	Unselected consecutive series of patients with TBI admitted to Cook County Hospital	CHI	NS	4.1 (E)	PTA/LOC > 30 minutes, ICH, skull fracture, younger age, focal neurological signs, alcohol
Eide and Tysnes, 1992[65]	143	Consecutive admissions with head injury and CT to neurosurgical unit of Haukeland Hospital, Norway	CHI	1–5 yr	13	Multifocal (26%) bilateral > unilateral multifocal (14%) brain contusions
	117	Consecutive admissions with "concussion"	CHI	1–5 yr	7	
Guidice and Berchou, 1987[85]	164	Unselected consecutive patients with severe TBI referred to the author	CHI	≤ 36 mo	25 1.9 (E); 23 (L)	Coma duration > 3 weeks
Heikkinnen et al., 1990[98]	55	Consecutive patients admitted to the Oulu University, Central Hospital, Finland	CHI	5.7 yr (mean) 4.5–6.8 yr	18	ICH, local atrophy on CT scan, EPTS, impaired local cerebral blood flow
JFURGPTE, 1992[110,134]	191	Patients with acute TBI evaluated between 1983–1985	CHI = 89% "Open" = 11%	5 yr	8.3 (L) 16/191	Impaired consciousness >1 mo, abnormal EEG at 1 mo, "open" TBI, surgery, focal/generalized neurological signs, EtOH, ICH
Jennett, 1975[112]	2,000+	Selected groups of patients with TBI at postulated high risk from centers at Oxford, Glasgow, and Rotterdam	CHI	1 yr (minimum)	5 (L) 5 (E)	PTA > 24 hr, DSF, ICH, EPTS, focal neurologic deficit

(Table continued on following page.)

TABLE 1.   Studies Addressing the Incidence of Posttraumatic Seizures (*Continued*)

Study	No. of Subjects	Subject Population	Trauma Category	Follow-up Duration	Incidence of PTS (%)	Risk Factors Cited*
Civilian Settings (*cont.*)						
Jennett and Lewin, 1960[114]	1,000	Consecutive, largely unselected patients admitted to the neurosurgical service of the Radcliffe Infirmary, Oxford	CHI	4–9 yr	3.8 (E)	PTA > 24 hr, DSF, ICH
	275	"Representative" subset of patients from above group	CHI	4–9yr	10.2 (L)	EPTS, ICH, DSF, PTA > 24 hr, DSF + PTA > 24 hr, ICH + PTA > 24 hr
Kollevold, 1976–1979[122–125]	6,723	Unselected patients with TBI admitted to the Department of Neurosurgery, Ulleval Hospital, Oslo	CHI	2–12 yr	2.2 (I), 2.7 (E) 15 (L)	ICH, chronic EtOH, prior TBI, younger age
Lee and Lui, 1992[128]	4,232	Consecutive adult patients with apparently mild TBI treated by the authors in two medical centers in Taiwan	CHI	6 mo	2.36 (E) 1 (I)	ICH, intracerebral parenchymal damage
Locke et al., 1991[132]	321	Consecutive adult patients with TBI admitted to the King-Drew Medical Center	NS	6–18 mo	5.6	Altered mental status on admission, poor verbal GCS score
Paillas et al., 1970[157]	2,331	Patients with TBI treated at the Hopital de la Timone, University of Marseilles, Marseilles, France	CHI: 92% PHI: 8%	3–16 yr	8.7 (CHI) 3.17 (PHI)	ICH, skull fracture
Thomsen, 1984[216]	40	Patients with very severe closed TBI	CHI	10–15 yr	23	Focal lesions: 77% (7/9)
Wiederholt et al., 1989[245]	1,322	Olmsted County residents with brain injury and skull fracture	CHI: >94%	7.4 yr (mean)	"Acute" seizure: 2.1	DSF, basilar skull fracture
Pediatric Settings						
Black et al., 1975[19]	307	Consecutive series of children, with TBI and LOC, skull fracture, IPTS or neurologic abnormality	NS	6 yr	15 (E)	EPTS, febrile seizures, age < 2 yr, linear skull fracture, neurologic deficit, increased coma duration
Hendrick and Harris, 1968[99]	4,465	Consecutive children with TBI, aged < 15 yr, admitted to the Hospital for Sick Children, Toronto	CHI	4–12 yr	7 6.5 (E); 1.3 (L)	NS
Mises et al., 1976[150]	2,500	Children admitted for cranial trauma	CHI	3 yr	1.3 (E) 0.8 (L)	NS
Rehabilitation Settings						
Armstrong et al., 1990[9]	238	Consecutive adult patients admitted to the head injury unit of a free-standing rehabilitation hospital	CHI	NS	37	NS
Bontke et al., 1993[22]	325	Patients with TBI enrolled in the NIDRR Traumatic Brain Injury Model System Program Hospitals	CHI: 92% PHI: 8%	75 days (mean) 8–579 days	16.3 14.2 (E)	NS
Cohen and Grosswasser, 1991[37]	351	Patients with TBI admitted for brain injury rehabilitation	NS	NS	9.4	Locomotor, speech, language, and cognitive disorders
Kalisky et al., 1985[116]	180	Consecutive patients with severe TBI admitted to a free-standing rehabilitation hospital	CHI: 97% PHI: 3%	NS	13 1 (E)	DSF, ICH, shunt placement, PHI
Sazbon and Grosswasser, 1990[192]		Patients in prolonged post-traumatic coma admitted to Loewenstein Rehabilitation Hospital	CHI	NS	33.5 (L) 6.7 (E)	NS

* Not necessarily in order of importance.
CHI = closed head injury, CT = computed tomography, DSF = depressed skull fracture, EEG = electroencephalography, E[PTS] = early posttraumatic seizure, EtOH = alcohol use/abuse, GCS = Glasgow Coma Scale, ICH = intracranial hematoma/hemorrhage, IPTS = immediate posttraumatic seizure (within 24 hr of injury), JFURGPTE = Japan Follow-Up Research Group of Posttraumatic Epilepsy, LOC = loss of consciousness, L[PTS] = late posttraumatic seizure, NS = not specified, PHI = penetrating head injury, PTA = posttraumatic amnesia, PTE = posttraumatic epilepsy, PTS = posttraumatic seizure.

TBI. Obviously, the most noteworthy complications are accompanied by a significant risk of death, as in status epilepticus. Various studies have examined morbidity and mortality in the patient with posttraumatic seizures.[43,181,235,240] An appreciation of potential complications is useful in evaluating risk/benefit relationships in decisions about anticonvulsant treatment.

Status epilepticus is the most clinically significant manifestation of posttraumatic seizures and carries the greatest risk of adverse outcome. Fortunately, status epilepticus is a rare manifestation of posttraumatic seizures.[125] In addition, status epilepticus is usually attributable to another cause, such as withdrawal from anticonvulsant drugs or acute systemic or neurologic injury (e.g., anoxic encephalopathy or stroke).[131] Status epilepticus is more likely to be encountered as a manifestation of posttraumatic seizures in children, although the incidence remains infrequent, even among children with severe TBI.[120] Deaths associated with status epilepticus are usually attributable to the precipitating disorder.[93,130]

Mortality among patients with posttraumatic seizures remains consistently elevated in most reports.[43,235,236,240] However, the contribution of posttraumatic seizures to this increased mortality is unclear. Walker noted that men with posttraumatic seizures have a death rate exceeding that of comparable normal men. But information supplied by relatives suggested that causes of death were not specific for men with TBI but reflected disorders that afflict elderly people.[235] Similarly, Rish et al. noted that among patients with penetrating head injury followed for 15 years, most deaths occurred early in the first year after trauma and were secondary to the direct effects of TBI or sequelae of coma. Posttraumatic seizures appeared unrelated to mortality, and such patients approached the actuarial norm for their peers after only 3 years.[180,181]

Recurrent posttraumatic seizures may exert an adverse effect on functional status and cognition among patients with TBI, independent of the effect attributable to the severity of injury. Among patients with penetrating head injury in the Vietnam Head Injury Study,[35,190] posttraumatic seizures were one of seven impairments that independently and cumulatively predicted employment status.[199] The overall influence of posttraumatic seizures on measures of cognition was largely unclear, although significant deficits in performance IQ were reported.[189] Posttraumatic seizures and increasing loss of brain volume have been noted to exert independent and profound effects on cognitive performance among patients with restricted frontal lobe lesions due to penetrating head injury.[82] Studies among patients with closed head injury also suggest an adverse effect of posttraumatic seizures on functional prognosis[9] and cognition.[56] Unfortunately, indices of injury severity among groups in these studies[9,56] were not well defined; thus the significance of their conclusions may be limited.

In summary, complications associated with isolated posttraumatic seizures are comparable to those found with any seizure. Isolated or infrequent episodes are associated with relatively little risk. Increasing frequency and severity of seizure disorders, including status epilepticus, carry associated risks of increased morbidity or mortality and worsened cognitive and functional prognosis.

POSTTRAUMATIC EPILEPTOGENESIS

Epileptogenesis refers to the dynamic process underlying the appearance and natural history of epilepsy.[67] The pathophysiologic mechanisms involved in posttraumatic epileptogenesis are not well understood. Much of what is known or postulated has been derived from studying various animal models. Complete discussion of the physiologic basis of posttraumatic epilepsy or mechanisms and models relevant to posttraumatic epileptogenesis is beyond the scope of this chapter; the interested reader is referred elsewhere.[170,191,248] Nevertheless, certain models of particular relevance are reviewed briefly.

The kindling model of epilepsy, first described by Goddard,[79] demonstrates particular relevance to posttraumatic epileptogenesis and its prophylactic management.[141,191,232] Brief trains of weak electrical stimulation were applied to susceptible areas of rodent brains until a seizure was observed. When kindling stimulations were continued over a prolonged period of time, progressively less stimulation was required to induce the seizures, and spontaneous seizures eventually appeared. Once the spontaneous seizures appeared, the susceptibility remained essentially permanent. The relevance of kindling to posttraumatic epilepsy derives from the hypothesis that perhaps other forms of stimuli, such as structural brain lesions, may set into motion a similar pattern of epileptic focus development.[32] This model also has been suggested to provide a theoretical basis for assertions that early treatment both suppresses seizures in the short term and prevents the evolution of newly developing seizures into chronic epilepsy.[80,91]

Among anticonvulsant drugs, phenobarbital, valproate, and benzodiazepines consistently inhibit the development of kindled seizures.[198,202] Carbamazepine inconsistently modifies the development but consistently suppresses evocation of previously kindled seizures.[2,234] Phenytoin does not appear to alter the development of kindled seizures.[141,198,232] Drugs that inhibit or prevent the development of epileptic condition, such as valproate and phenobarbital, are said to demonstrate antiepileptic effects.[191]

The original kindling studies were performed on rats. Subsequently, the phenomenon was demonstrated in rabbits, cats, and primates genetically predisposed to seizure.[198] Because neuroanatomic structural differences among species imply functional differences, it is not surprising that animal kindling models demonstrate significant phylogenetic variability in expression.[231] The extent of the relevance of animal models to investigations of human posttraumatic epilepsy, therefore, is controversial.[80]

The iron and ferric chloride models are of theoretical interest because cortical deposits of hemosiderin may be important in the development of recurrent posttraumatic seizures.[249] Patients with cerebral injuries characterized by contact of blood and cortical tissue, such as subdural hematomas[78] and penetrating head injuries,[190] manifest an increased incidence of posttraumatic seizures. Contusion or cortical laceration causes extravasation of red blood cells, with hemolysis and deposition of hemoglobin. Iron liberated from hemoglobin is then sequestered as hemosiderin, a prominent histopathologic feature in patients with posttraumatic seizures.[159] Focal epileptiform discharges have been induced after intracortical injection of blood and blood components.[87] Similarly, Willmore et al. demonstrated that recurrent focal epileptiform discharges may result from cortical injection of ferrous or ferric chloride.[249] The iron salts and hemoglobin in neural tissue may contribute to epileptogenesis by initiating lipid peroxidation, damaging cell membranes, and inhibiting neuronal Na-K adenosine triphosphatase.[248]

Evidence suggests that compensatory collateral axonal sprouting may occur after brain injuries[222] and may be an important mechanism in functional neurologic recovery.[74] Under certain circumstances, however, collateral sprouting may give rise to the development of seizure foci.[170] Axon terminals may be shifted in position from one site (e.g., a dendrite) to another (e.g., a soma) on the neuron. The development of additional excitatory synaptic contacts on cell somata may produce a marked increase in cell excitability, particularly if the new excitatory synapses replace inhibitory ones.[170] If the induced alterations in connectivity increase excitability, neural pathways may become progressively susceptible to epileptiform events and thus contribute to the development of kindled seizures.[209]

ASSESSMENT OF SEIZURE RISK

Methods have been proposed to improve the reliability of identifying patients at risk for development of posttraumatic seizures and therefore most likely to gain from preventive measures. Such methods are based on assessment of the patient's clinical characteristics as well as on information for objective diagnostic modalities (Table 2).

Patient Characteristics

Patients with histories of alcohol abuse, particularly chronic alcoholism, demonstrate an increased risk of seizure development[68,98,110,124,125,134,160] after TBI. In Kollevold's series, chronic alcoholism was the most important predisposing factor for posttraumatic seizures;[123–125] it also was found to be a significant risk factor in other studies.[97,110] It is

TABLE 2. Risk Factors for Posttraumatic Seizure

Risk Factor	References Citing Increased Risk	References Citing No Increased Risk
Patient Characteristics		
Age	19 (LPTS), 52 (EPTS), 99	19 (EPTS), 37, 98, 124, 132
Alcohol	68, 98 (trend), 110, 124, 125, 134, 160	
Family history	35 (slight), 68 (slight), 112 (slight), 243	19, 190, 193, 239
Injury Characteristics		
Bone/metal fragments	10, 68 (bone only), 190, 237, 249	26, 68 (metal only)
Depressed skull fracture	68 (CHI only), 86, 99 (EPTS), 112, 116, 165, 245	19, 134
Focal contusions/injury	48, 47, 50, 65, 78, 98, 216	9
Focal neurologic deficits	37, 48, 47, 52 (EPTS), 110, 112, 134, 186, 190, 238	86, 124
ICH	8, 52 (EPTS), 68, 78, 98, 110, 112, 116, 124, 125, 134, 157	9, 19, 85
ICH-intracerebral	110	157
ICH-SAH	68 (CHI)	
ICH-SDH	68 (CHI), 78, 86, 99 (LPTS), 157	
Lesion location	47, 68, 82, 186, 188, 238, 239, 243	
Penetrating head injury	34, 68, 116, 157, 190, 238, 250	
Severity-GCS	8, 34, 86, 132 (verbal GCS only)	50 (without lesion on CT), 98
Severity-LOC/coma duration	52 (EPTS), 85, 99, 110, 134	37
Severity-PTA	52 (EPTS), 68, 112, 165	
Skull fracture	19, 35, 52 (EPTS)	9, 124
Volume loss	190	
Other Clinical Characteristics		
Electroencephalography	110, 124, 134, 190	98
Early posttraumatic seizures	19, 50 (children), 98, 112, 243	50 (adults)
Multiple risk factors	34, 110, 112, 124, 134	
Operative procedures	10, 19, 110, 134	86

LPTS = late posttraumatic seizures, EPTS = early posttraumatic seizures, ICH = intracranial hematoma/hemorrhage, SAH = subarachnoid hemorrhage, SDH = subdural hematoma, LOC = loss of consciousness, PTA = posttraumatic amnesia, CHI = closed head injury, CT = computed tomograph, GCS = Glasgow Coma Scale.

unclear whether the increased incidence of seizures reflects an independent epileptogenic effect or whether alcohol enhances the epileptic potential of traumatically induced brain lesions. In either case, the incidence of alcohol abuse among patients with TBI is significant,[126,207] and further investigation is warranted to assess the effect of such abuse on complications of TBI, including posttraumatic seizures.

Patients with a family history of epilepsy may have a genetic predisposition for development of posttraumatic seizures. Studies indicate that genetic predisposition influences the appearance of kindled seizures in baboons.[233] Some authors have noted a modestly increased incidence of posttraumatic seizures among patients with closed head injury and a family history of seizures.[33,68,99,112,243] This increase has not been uniformly observed,[193,239] particularly among patients with penetrating head injury,[190] suggesting that the influence of genetic predisposition appears weak compared with the effects of extensive intracranial trauma.[190,193]

As noted earlier, patient age appears to exert a strong influence on risk of posttraumatic seizures.[8,86,125] Children demonstrate markedly lower risk for late posttraumatic seizures but considerably higher risk for immediate and early posttraumatic seizures, compared to adults with similar severity of injury.

Injury Characteristics

Certain traumatic brain injuries demonstrate an increased likelihood of resulting in recurrent, late posttraumatic seizures. Most experts agree about the factors that markedly increase risk of seizure among patients with penetrating head injury.[10,26,34,35,68,190,238,250] Blood appears to have an extremely irritating effect on cortical neurons, as demonstrated by increased incidence of seizures among patients with intracranial hemorrhage, particularly subdural hemorrhage.[8,52,78,86,99,110,112,124,134,190] Penetrating head injuries of greater extent[35,190,236] and closed head injuries of greater severity,[34,86,157,216] as evidenced by prolonged duration of posttraumatic amnesia[8,52,68,85,112,192] or impairment of consciousness,[85,110,134,192] are prominently associated with increased risk of seizure.

Authorities also agree that risk of posttraumatic seizures is increased in patients with TBI characterized by focal neurologic deficits,[34,37,48,110,112,134,186,190,238] depressed skull fractures,[52,68,112,165,245] cerebral contusions,[47,48,50,65,78,98] and retained bone or metal fragments.[10,11,68,238,250] Location of the lesion may affect incidence[47,68,82,186,188,237,238,239,243] and possibly type and frequency[188] of posttraumatic seizures among patients with penetrating head injury. The concurrence of multiple risk factors is consistently associated with increased risk of seizure.[34,110,112,125,134]

Various authors have proposed mathematical methods of estimating the probability of posttraumatic seizures.[72,141,241,242] Feeney and Walker[72] assigned mathematical risk coefficients to clinical characteristics of injury. The coefficients of the four most significant clinical factors were then entered into a formula to predict the subsequent risk of seizure. Remarkable consistency was noted when the formula was applied to later studies of incidence.[241] In some settings this formula is used to determine which patients receive anticonvulsant prophylactic therapy.[6] However, the clinical utility of such assessment has not been demonstrated and is probably limited.

Imaging Studies

Information provided through imaging modalities may help to identify patients at increased risk for development of posttraumatic seizures. Indeed, evidence suggests that contusions observable with computed tomography (CT) may account for the increased risk of seizure among patients with severe closed head injury as opposed to prolonged impairment of consciousness.[47,50] D'Alessandro et al. noted that only intracerebral and extracerebral hemorrhages with satellite intracerebral hematoma were significantly associated with posttraumatic seizures.[45] Posttraumatic porencephaly in patients with closed head

injury[98,263] and increased volume of brain tissue loss in patients with penetrating head injury[190] also have been associated with increased risk of posttraumatic seizures.

Magnetic resonance imaging (MRI) demonstrates advantages over CT in evaluating patients with TBI for evidence of diffuse axonal injury[205,246] and contusions in the mediobasal aspects of the temporal and inferior frontal lobes.[83,205] Imaging characteristics of MRI and CT among patients with posttraumatic seizures include dilatation of the subarachnoid space and the ventricular system, cortical atrophy, porencephalic cysts, and gliotic foci in the frontotemporal region.[16]

Functional imaging techniques may contribute information predictive of increased risk of posttraumatic seizures. Patients with posttraumatic seizures have impaired regional cerebral blood flow in injured brain areas compared with TBI patients without posttraumatic seizures. Differences in regional cerebral blood flow were particularly significant in the postacute stage.[98]

Electroencephalopathy

The usefulness of the interictal electroencephalogram as an objective predictor of posttraumatic seizures appears limited.[44,98,115,157] It is frequently abnormal in patients with TBI, both with and without posttraumatic stress,[20,47,78,195] reflecting the severity of brain damage.[47,115] Sleep-deprivation activation procedures similarly do not appear to differentiate between patients with and without posttraumatic seizures.[215] Localized slow waves, the most frequently observed electroencephalographic abnormality,[44,123] have been noted to persist for long periods without epileptic manifestations.[44] Conversely, a normal electroencephalogram may precede the appearance of posttraumatic seizures,[20,44,115,174] although this finding is associated more frequently with a favorable prognosis.[78,124]

The yield of prognostically significant electroencephalographic findings among patients with TBI is meager.[20,44,115] The rare change of focal slow wave activity to focal spike discharges or persistence of focal spike or sharp wave discharges may be suggestive of increased risk of seizure.[44,124,125,195] Such discharges, however, may be observed on the electroencephalogram of nonepileptic patients[266] and are not always indicative of future seizures,[20,78] particularly in children.[44,150] Such electroencephalographic findings should be evaluated in context with other clinical risk factors in assessing the likelihood of posttraumatic seizures in patients with severe TBI. Greater evidence exists for potential usefulness of electroencephalography in prognostication of focus localization, seizure persistence, and severity once posttraumatic seizures have been observed.[11,44,107]

MANAGEMENT

Asymptomatic Management: Prophylaxis

Prophylaxis has been defined as "specific measures taken to prevent disease in an individual."[104] In the context of posttraumatic seizures, the term applies to anticonvulsant treatment administered to patients who have not manifested seizures. Several justifications can be proposed for prophylaxis of posttraumatic seizures:

1. Anticonvulsants may prevent posttraumatic seizures at a time when they potentially inflict the greatest harm. For example, prevention of early seizures in the acutely injured patient may minimize seizure-induced elevations in intracranial pressure.[53]

2. Seizure prevention may help to avoid loss of employment and driving privileges, or accidental injury.[53] In reference to driving privileges, however, this justification appears tenuous; TBI of sufficient severity to justify prophylaxis is often associated with motor and cognitive dysfunctions that preclude safe driving.[111,227]

3. Prophylaxis mitigates concern over the medicolegal implications of negligent treatment if posttraumatic seizures appear.[212]

4. Administration of anticonvulsants may alter or arrest epileptogenesis. Animal studies suggest experimental evidence that supports a rationale for anticonvulsant prophylaxis.[141,198,223,234]

Clinical Studies: Retrospective, Uncontrolled or Nonrandomized

Encouraged by animal experiments suggesting that anticonvulsants may prevent the development of epileptic foci, retrospective studies and nonrandomized open trials with humans were conducted[35,98,124,152,153,169,180,201,251,259] with generally favorable results[153,169,201,251,259] (Table 3). Young and Rapp evaluated the effectiveness of phenytoin in seizure prophylaxis among selected high-risk (> 15%) patients with severe TBI. Only 6% of patients who received phenytoin developed posttraumatic seizures, despite a low rate of drug compliance.[259] Similarly, Wohns and Wyler noted that among patients followed for at least 1 year, 10% of the phenytoin-treated group developed posttraumatic seizures compared with 50% of patients in the control group.[251] Servit and Musil treated 143 selected patients with a prophylactic of phenytoin and phenobarbital, "sometimes supplemented" with benzodiazepines. The incidence of posttraumatic seizures among the 23 untreated patients was 25% compared with 2.1% in the treatment group.[201]

Uncontrolled prophylaxis studies have used anticonvulsants other than phenytoin or phenytoin-phenobarbital combinations.[98,124,152,153,169] Price retrospectively noted that of 143 high-risk patients treated with valproate, none developed posttraumatic seizures; the author concluded that valproate was highly effective in preventing posttraumatic seizures.[169] Murri et al. reported an incidence of approximately 2% among patients receiving phenobarbital for 2 years.[153] In a larger, recently published, uncontrolled trial with a similar study design, they reported a similar incidence of posttraumatic seizures. In each study, the low incidence of posttraumatic seizures was cited as evidence of prophylaxis efficacy.[152,153]

Clinical Studies of Late Posttraumatic Seizures: Prospective, Randomized and Controlled

Decidedly less impressive results were observed among randomized and controlled prospective studies[18,78,101,134,142,160,164,210,212,261,262] of chronic prophylaxis in late posttraumatic seizures. Young and Rapp randomly assigned 93 high-risk (> 15%) patients with severe TBI to a regimen of phenytoin or phenytoin and phenobarbital. Serum anticonvulsant levels were checked on a regular basis during the 18-month treatment period. Another 74 patients, with roughly equal severity of injury, were assigned randomly to the control group. Patients developing posttraumatic seizures were counted and excluded from further study. No significant difference was observed in the incidence of posttraumatic seizures between patients in the treatment and control groups. However, no patient with serum phenytoin levels in excess of 12 µg/ml developed late posttraumatic seizures, leaving open the possibility that therapeutic levels of phenytoin may have demonstrated a prophylactic effect.[261]

McQueen and associates reported similar findings among 164 patients with severe closed head injury who were treated with phenytoin or placebo. Patients with early posttraumatic seizures were excluded. Attempts were made to maintain therapeutic levels of serum phenytoin among patients in the treatment group. Again, no significant difference in the number of patients developing late posttraumatic seizures was observed between the two groups. The authors concluded that the incidence of late posttraumatic seizures was not high enough to draw conclusions about the effectiveness of phenytoin prophylaxis.[142]

In 1990, Temkin and associates published results of a large, randomized, controlled, double-blind clinical trial that further challenged the potential efficacy of phenytoin in prophylaxis of late posttraumatic seizures. The investigators randomly assigned 404 eligible patients with serious TBI to treatment with phenytoin (n = 208) or placebo (n = 196) for 1 year. Dosages were monitored frequently and adjusted in the phenytoin-treated group, maintaining serum levels in the high therapeutic range. Of the 208 patients randomly assigned to the phenytoin group, 21.5% developed late seizures by the end of the first year and 27.5% by the end of the second year. Such rates were not significantly different from the 15.7% and 21.1% of placebo-treated patients who developed late seizures by the end of the first and second years, respectively. Therapeutic levels of phenytoin were recorded in three-fourths of the patients in whom levels were measured on the day of their first posttraumatic seizures.[210]

Pechadre et al. randomly assigned 86 patients admitted with severe traumatic brain injury into groups receiving phenytoin or placebo. Dose-adjusted phenytoin was administered orally for a minimum of 3 months. After a 2-year follow-up, the difference between treated and untreated patients was significant: only 6% of the treated patients suffered from posttraumatic seizures compared with 42% of the control group.[160] The conflict with earlier studies may be due to important differences in study design. In the study by Pechadre et al., treatment and control groups were not randomized according to risk factors. Patients who manifested early seizures were not excluded from further study and appeared in significantly greater numbers in the control group. Patients with chronic alcoholism and intracranial hemorrhage also were represented in greater proportions in the control group. The cumulative contribution of significant risk factors in the control group is an important confounding factor, limiting the validity of assertions that prophylaxis had a favorable effect.

Carbamazepine also has failed to demonstrate any favorable effect in prophylaxis of late seizures. Glötzner et al. randomly assigned 139 adults at high risk for posttraumatic seizures into groups receiving carbamazepine or placebo. Prophylaxis was initiated immediately after injury and was continued for 1.5–2 years. Dosage was adjusted individually to provide serum levels within therapeutic range. Because nasogastric administration could be attempted no earlier than 12–24 hours after injury, some patients received intravenous phenytoin to suppress early seizures before establishment of therapeutic levels of carbamazepine. No significant difference was noted in late posttraumatic seizures incidence between treatment and control groups.[78]

A multicenter, prospective controlled study using phenobarbital similarly provides no support for prophylactic efficacy in late posttraumatic seizures. The Japan Follow-up Research Group of Posttraumatic Epilepsy randomly assigned patients with acute TBI into one of three groups. Patients with severe TBI were randomized into a group receiving dose-adjusted phenobarbital or a control group receiving no treatment. Patients with mild TBI (n = 76) served as a second control group. There was no significant difference in

TABLE 3. Retrospective, Nonrandomized or Uncontrolled Prophylaxis Studies

Study	No. of Subjects	Subject Population	Trauma Category	(Minimum) Observation
Caveness et al., 1979[35]	1,030	Series of soldiers sustaining PHI during the Vietnam War	PHI: 93%	5 yr
Heikkinnen et al., 1990[98]	55	Consecutive patients with TBI admitted to the Oulu University Central Hospital	CHI	5.7 yr (mean) Range: 4.5–6.8 yr
Kollevold, 1978[124]	149	Series of patients with CHI and EPTS admitted to the Ulleval Hospital in Oslo	CHI	2 yr 91% of patients were followed ≥ 5 yr
Murri et al., 1992[152]	293	Patients admitted within 24 hr of TBI to the Institute of Neurosurgery with ≥ 1 risk factor for PTS	CHI	2 yr (1-yr trial, 1-yr follow-up)
Murri et al., 1980[153]	90	All patients with TBI admitted to the Institute of Neurosurgery over an 18 mo period	CHI	25 mo (2-yr trial, 1-mo follow-up)
Price, 1980[169]	143	Consecutive patients with TBI treated by the author; patients believed to have >15% risk of developing PTS were included	NS	2 yr
Rish and Caveness, 1973[180]	1,614	Series of soldiers sustaining PHI during the Vietnam War	PHI	7 days
Servit and Musil, 1981[201]	167	Patients with TBI under direct care of the principal investigators	CHI: 90% PHI: 10%	3 yr (2 yr trial, minimum of 1-yr follow-up)
Wohns and Wyler, 1979[251]	62	Patient with severe TBI with unequivocal evidence of skull fracture, dural laceration, PTA or LOC > 24 hr, or EEG consistent with focal damage	CHI	18 mo (1-yr trial; ≥ 6-mo follow-up)
Young et al., 1979[259]	84	Patients with severe TBI, believed to have a > 15% chance of developing PTS	CHI: 86% PHI: 14%	12 mo

CHI = closed head injury, EEG = electroencephalography, EPTS = early posttraumatic seizures, LOC = loss of consciousness, NS = not specified, PHI = penetrating head injury, PTA = posttraumatic amnesia, PTS = posttraumatic seizures.

(Columns continued on opposite page.)

the demographic data of the two control groups. Prophylaxis was initiated 1 month after injury, continued for 2 years, and gradually tapered over the third year. Patients were then followed for an additional 2 years. The incidence of late posttraumatic seizures was higher in the phenobarbital-treated group than in either control group, although the difference did not reach statistical significance.[134]

In summary, randomized, controlled prospective studies almost uniformly fail to substantiate evidence of efficacy for anticonvulsant prophylaxis in late posttraumatic seizures.[78,142,164,210,261] In four trials, the incidence of posttraumatic seizures was actually higher among the phenytoin-treated groups.[142,164,210,261] A recent meta-analysis of results in four large, similarly designed randomized trials[142,210,212,261] suggested that phenytoin may be associated with an increased risk of late seizures, although this difference did not reach statistical significance.[212] Most studies that fail to

TABLE 3. **Retrospective, Nonrandomized or Uncontrolled Prophylaxis Studies** *(Cols. cont.)*

Percentage Developing PTS	Anticonvulsant	Comments
PTS: T (continuous): 39% (177/453) T (interrupted): 29% (167/577) C: Incidence NS on patients who received no anticonvulsants	PHT (76%) PHT/PB (20%) PB (4%)	The subjects consisted of the 453 who received continuous anticonvulsant prophylaxis for 3 mo–9 yr (335 for 1 yr), the 524 patients who received intermittent anticonvulsant treatment, and the 53 patients who received no treatment.
PTS: (No control group) T: 18%	CBZ or PHT	All patients routinely received prophylaxis with either CBZ or PHT for 3–6 mo.
LPTS: (≥ 4 wk definition) T: 43% (20/43) C: 18% (18/102)	PHT and/or PB CBZ (n = 1) ETH (n = 1)	Retrospective, nonrandomized study of the patients with IPTS. The treatment group consisted of patients who were treated with anticonvulsants for ≥ 3 mo after IPTS. The control group received no such treatment.
PTS: (No control group) T (low PB level; < 15 µg/ml): (1/106): 1% T (high PB level; 20–28 µg/ml): (5/187): 2.7% Overall: 2.04%	PB*	Nonrandomized, uncontrolled trial of PB in prophylaxis of PTS. Seventy percent were adults (> 16 yr). Patients with EPTS were not excluded and were more frequently represented in the higher level PB prophylaxis group.
PTS: (No control group) T (low dose): 0% T (high dose): 4.7% (2/43) Overall: 2.4%	PB*	Eight percent of the subjects had "mild" TBI, 48% had "severe" TBI, and two subjects had EPTS.
PTS: (No control group) T: 0%	VPA	Specific information regarding injury severity, risk factors, treatment duration, and methods of follow-up were not stated.
EPTS: (only) T: 1.6% (18/1136) C: 3.7% (17/465)	PHT: (93%) PB	The treatment group consisted of the 70% of patients who received anticonvulsant prophylaxis.
PTS: T: 2.1% (3/147) C: 25% (6/24)	PHT/PB	Specific information regarding risk factors among the treatment and control groups was not stated, though the groups were "similar" in severity and locations of injury.
LPTS: T: 10% (5/50) C: 50% (6/12) **EPTS:** 0% (both groups)	PHT*	
PTS: (No control group) T: 6% (5/84)	PHT	

* Denotes dosage adjusted according to serum anticonvulsant level monitoring results.
C = control group, CBZ = carbamazepine, EPTS = early posttraumatic seizures, ETH = ethosuximide, IPTS = immediate posttraumatic seizures, LPTS = late posttraumatic seizures, PB = phenobarbital, PHT = phenytoin, PTS = posttraumatic seizures, T = treatment group, VPA = valproate.

demonstrate significant prophylactic effect use phenytoin as the primary anticonvulsant,[142,164,210,261] although similar disappointment has been encountered in trials primarily administering carbamazepine[78] and phenobarbital.[134]

Failure in the above trials does not necessarily imply that similar results would be encountered with other drugs. Agents with reported antiepileptic properties, such as valproate, have been recommended as suitable candidates in future prophylaxis trials.[91] In fact, such a randomized, controlled trial with valproate is currently ongoing.[7]

Clinical Studies of Early Posttraumatic Seizures: Prospective, Randomized and Controlled

Administration of phenytoin appears to reduce significantly the incidence of early posttraumatic seizures. Temkin et al. noted that 3.6% of the phenytoin-treated group developed early seizures compared with 14.2% of patients in the placebo group.[210] Similarly,

TABLE 4. Prospective, Randomized and Controlled Prophylaxis Studies

Study	No. of Subjects	Subject Population	Trauma Category	(Minimum) Observation
Published				
Birkmayer, 1951[18]	213	Veterans sustaining TBI during World War II	PHI	< 8 yr
Glötzner et al., 1983[78]	139	Adult patients with TBI believed to be at high risk for PTS	CHI: 76% "Open" HI: 24%	1.5 yr (1.5–2-yr trial)
Hoff and Hoff, 1947[101]	100	Veterans sustaining TBI during World War II	PHI	4 yr
Manaka and JFURGPTE, 1992[134]	191	Patients with acute TBI admitted to Japanese medical centers participating in a cooperative multicenter prophylaxis trial	NS	5 yr (3-yr trial, 2-yr follow-up)
McQueen et al., 1983[142]	164	Patients with severe TBI admitted to the neurosurgical services of the 2 study centers	CHI	3 yr (1-yr trial, 2-yr follow-up)
Pechadre et al., 1991[160]	86	Consecutive patients with severe TBI	PHI: 6% "Associated lesions": 19% Remainder: 74%	24 mo (3–12-mo trial, 12-mo follow-up)
Penry et al., 1979[164]	125	Patients admitted with TBI, belonging to one of four high-risk groups	NS	3 yr (18-mo trial, ≥ 18-mo follow-up)
Temkin et al., 1990[210]	404	Consecutive adult patients with severe TBI. Included patients believed to have a ≥ 20% risk of developing LPTS	CHI: 92% PHI: 8%	3 yr (1-yr trial, 2 yr follow-up)
Young et al., 1983[260]	244	Patients with severe TBI believed to have a 10% risk of developing EPTS	CHI: 85% PHI: 15%	7 days
Young et. al., 1983[261]	179	Patients with severe TBI believed to have a >15% risk of developing LPTS	CHI: 87% PHI: 13%	3 yr (18-mo trial, 18-mo follow-up)
Young et al., 1983[262]	41	Children with severe TBI believed to have a 10% risk of developing PTS	CHI: 93% PHI: 7%	18 mo
Unpublished				
Brackett et al. (quoted in Temkin et al., 1991[212])	49	Eligible patients with severe TBI	NS	2 yr (6-mo trial, 18-mo follow-up)
Marshall et al. (quoted in Temkin et al., 1991[212])	154	Eligible adult patients with TBI	NS	2 yr (6-mo trial, 18-mo follow-up
Locke et al. (quoted in Temkin et al., 1991[212])	303	Eligible adult patients with severe TBI	NS	2 yr (6-mo trial, 18-mo follow-up)

* Designates drug regimen in which dosage was adjusted according to results of serum level monitoring.
CHI = closed head injury, EPTS = early posttraumatic seizures, LPTS = late posttraumatic seizure, NS = not specified, PHI = penetrating head injury, PTS = posttraumatic seizures, T = treatment group.

(Columns continued on opposite page.)

TABLE 4.   Prospective, Randomized and Controlled Prophylaxis Studies (*Cols. cont.*)

Percentage Developing PTS	Principal Anticonvulsant	Comments
LPTS: (only) T: 6% (9/150) / C: 51% (32/63)	PHT	Follow-up of patients in the Hoff and Hoff 1947 study.
EPTS: T: 12.5% (8/64) / C: 29.3% (22/75) **LPTS**: T: 21.9% (14/64) / C: 26.7% (20/75)	CBZ* (PHT used for some patients to cover for EPTS until therapeutic CBZ levels were established)	The definition of "seizure activity" included EEG epileptiform activity without clinical manifestations. The drug regimen was found to be effective for EPTS prophylaxis only.
LPTS: (only) T: 4% (2/48) / C: 38% (17/46)	PHT	First prospective randomized study. The author concluded that PHT can prevent or postpone PTS even with relatively small doses.
LPTS: (only) T: 16% 8/50) [12.3% for IA+; 37.5% for IA−] (IA+ = "good compliance") C: 10.5% (8/76) C (II): 0% [0/65] [mild TBI]	PB*	Randomized, multicenter, controlled study investigating the efficacy of phenobarbital as a prophylactic PTS anticonvulsant. The investigators concluded that PB does not have a prophylactic effect on PTE.
LPTS: (only) T: 9.5% (8/84) / C: 8.75% (7/80)	PHT*	
EPTS: T: 6% (2/34) / C: 25% (13/52) **LPTS:** T: 6% (2/34) / C: 42% (22/52)	PHT*	Random assignment into treatment and control groups was based upon the day of admission, not by the presence of important risk factors. Patients manifesting early seizures were not excluded from further study.
PTS: T: 23% @ 36 mo / C: 13% @ 36 mo	PHT/PB	
EPTS: T:3.6% / C: 14.2% **LPTS:** T: 21.5% @ 1 yr, 27.5% @ 2 yr C: 15.7% @ 1 yr, 21.1% @ 2 yr	PHT*	Largest and most comprehensive randomized trial to date. PHT prophylaxis was found to be effective for EPTS only.
EPTS: (only) T: 3.7% (5/137) / C: 3.7% (4/108)	PHT*	No difference was observed in EPTS incidence between treated and control groups, despite PHT levels of > 10 μg/ml in 79% of patients.
LPTS: (only) T: 12.4% (19/92) / C: 10.8% (8/66)	PHT*	
PTS: T: 12% (3/25) / C: 6.2% (1/16)	PHT*	
PTS: T: 14% / C: 39%	PHT/PB*	Randomized, controlled trial of PHT/PB in prophylaxis of PTS. The trial was terminated prematurely due to low accession rate.
PTS: T: 24% / C: 16%	PHT/PB*	Randomized, controlled trial was terminated early because adequate drug levels could not be maintained; 23% of subjects were lost within 48 hr of head injury.
PTS: T: 4% / C: 12%	PHT, PB, PHT/PB	Patients were randomly assigned to one of four treatment groups: PHT, PB, PHT and PB, or placebo. Drug level data were not available.

* Designates drug regimen in which dosage was adjusted according to results of serum level monitoring.
C = control group, CBZ = carbamazepine, EEG = electroencephalography, EPTS = early posttraumatic seizures, LPTS = late posttraumatic seizures, PB = phenobarbital, PHT = phenytoin, PTE = posttraumatic epilepsy, PTS = posttraumatic seizures, T = treatment group.

Pechadre et al. reported that 6% of the phenytoin-treated patients developed early seizures compared with 25% of patients in the control group.[160] Glötzner noted a significantly diminished incidence of early seizures among patients treated with carbamazepine, although some patients also received phenytoin.[78] Young observed no significant difference in the incidence of early posttraumatic seizures[260] among high-risk patients with severe closed head injury.

However, propylene glycol, a diluent used in the intravenous placebo treatment, has been noted to possess potential anticonvulsant activity, which may account for some of the apparent lack of difference in early posttraumatic seizures incidence.[24]

Penetrating Head Injuries

Most of the above studies lack sufficient numbers to exclude the possibility of favorable effect in selected subsets of patients, particularly patients sustaining penetrating TBI. The earliest studies performed among patients with penetrating head injuries suggested that phenytoin, even in small and interrupted doses, can prevent or postpone posttraumatic seizures.[18,101] In contrast, retrospective observation of the incidence of posttraumatic seizures among more than 1,000 veterans in the Vietnam Head Injury Study suggests that evidence for seizure prophylaxis among such patients is not significant.[35,180] Specifically, Caveness monitored the incidence of posttraumatic seizures among subjects with penetrating head injury who received intermittent and continuous antiepileptic drug therapy for 1 year. The incidence of posttraumatic seizures was higher among the patients in the continuous therapy group. Most recent randomized and controlled trials include patients with penetrating head injuries, although they do not analyze separately the incidence of posttraumatic seizures in this group. In summary, the efficacy of anticonvulsants in prophylaxis of posttraumatic seizures among patients with penetrating head injuries is not established.

Symptomatic Management

It is beyond the scope of this chapter to examine critically the breadth of literature pertinent to the treatment of patients with epilepsy, and the reader is referred to textbooks that admirably serve this role.[67,257] However, treatment issues that are particularly germane to discussion of patients with TBI and recurrent posttraumatic seizures are reviewed briefly.

Diagnosis

An initial step in the management of suspected posttraumatic seizures is to establish whether or not a seizure disorder indeed exists. In light of the social, economic, and medical implications that accompany the diagnosis of an epileptic disorder, errors must be avoided. In many cases, a reliable diagnosis can be made from clinical observations of seizure phenomena, particularly those noted by experienced staff in the hospital. Classification of the observed seizures is similarly important, because categorization may have significant prognostic and therapeutic implications.

In certain situations, however, the diverse clinical presentations of posttraumatic seizures may render the diagnosis problematic. As noted earlier, epileptic manifestations (particularly those of complex partial seizures) may not be recognized in patients with significant cognitive and behavioral dysfunction. Alternatively, nonepileptic phenomena such as nonepileptic seizures, myoclonus, or syncopal episodes may be mistaken for posttraumatic seizures. Clinical observations alone may thus be insufficient to render or rule out a diagnosis of posttraumatic seizures, prompting the use of alternative diagnostic options.

Electroencephalography is the single most informative laboratory test for the diagnosis of epileptic disorders[36,67] and should be obtained in any patient with suspected posttraumatic seizures. The electroencephalogram may assist in assessing the likelihood of an underlying epileptic condition when correlated with the clinical diagnosis[226] or in localizing the seizure focus.[67] The diagnostic sensitivity of the standard electroencephalogram has limitations, however, and absence of electroencephalographic abnormalities does not exclude the presence of a seizure disorder.[67] Measurement may be useful in some patients, because significant elevations in levels of serum prolactin reliably occur within 20–40 minutes after generalized tonic-clonic seizures[46] and many complex partial seizures,[46] but not in nonepileptic seizures,[127,168] simple partial seizures,[127] or complex partial seizures of frontal lobe origin.[147] Significant elevation of prolactin after a possible episode of posttraumatic seizure may help to confirm clinical suspicion of an underlying epileptic disorder.[140]

When initial standard evaluations fail to resolve the clinical diagnosis, long-term electroencephalographic monitoring techniques, including ambulatory cassette monitoring[61,62,155] and/or inpatient telemetry,[5] are effective and clinically valuable. Ambulatory cassette monitoring offers an intermediate-level option for recording while the patient conducts normal activities at home, work, or school.[61,62,67] A patient or observer log is maintained to identify the times and descriptions of behavioral episodes suspected of representing seizure activity.[67] A diagnosis of seizure disorder is confirmed by a 2-day recording in a vast majority of epileptic patients,[224] although 24-hour recordings are more common and usually sufficient to yield evidence suggestive of an underlying seizure disorder.[27] Genuine epileptic phenomena may still be missed, however, even during recording.[6,224] A significant incidence of recording artifacts and the lack of video-recorded behavior also limit the diagnostic utility of this technique.[67] Electroencephalographic telemetry with video monitoring provides the best opportunity to obtain an artifact-free ictal electroencephalogram while observing and evaluating associated clinical behavior.[5,67] Definitive diagnosis requires recorded examples of all seizure types experienced by the patient.[67]

Todd's phenomena are a heterogeneous group of focal signs of neurologic dysfunction that may follow a partial[67] or generalized tonic-clonic seizure.[185] Todd's phenomena are recognized as postictal manifestations of posttraumatic seizures.[64] They do not reflect permanent structural damage but rather transient postictal disruption of function that typically resolves within 24–48 hours.[67] The presence of focal motor, sensory, or language deficit of new onset should alert the clinician to the possibility of a recent, unwitnessed posttraumatic seizure.

Treatment and Specific Agents

Despite general agreement that antiepileptic drug treatment is appropriate for patients who manifest two or more seizures, considerable debate remains about the benefits of treatment in reducing the risk of recurrence after a first seizure.[92,217] Of patients with a first documented seizure, 67% have recurrence within 12 months, although seizures that follow an acute precipitant or injury to the brain carry a much lower risk of recurrence.[89] Treatment after a first seizure has been advocated, although few randomized clinical trials have been conducted to establish efficacy. A recent randomized, multicenter clinical trial concluded that treatment of a first seizure with antiepileptic drugs significantly reduces the risk of relapse. The authors added, however, that the decision to start treatment in patients with a first seizure must balance individual risk of relapse, benefits of avoiding the consequences of a second seizure, and risk of antiepileptic drug toxicity.[73]

Once a decision has been reached to initiate pharmacological treatment, an important goal is to attain control of seizures with one medication.[67] The choice of agent should reflect the type of posttraumatic seizure, route and frequency of drug administration, and anticipated and realized adverse effects. Among patients with TBI who manifest seizures of partial onset, carbamazepine is the preferred drug, with phenytoin a second choice.[162] Patients with tonic-clonic seizures of generalized, secondarily generalized, or multifocal onset respond well to valproate.[137,162,196] Carbamazepine[137] and phenytoin are also effective anticonvulsants for generalized tonic-clonic seizures.[28,196] Phenobarbital is effective for control of partial and generalized tonic-clonic seizures,[67,138] although its use is limited by prominent adverse effects on cognition and behavior, which may outlast administration of the drug in children.[69]

Newer Agents. Before the recent release of felbamate and gabapentin, the last antiepileptic drug released for marketing in the United States was valproate in 1978. However, for the 3-year period from 1993 through 1996, it is likely that four anticonvulsants will be approved for use and marketed in the U.S.

Felbamate (Felbatol), a phenyl dicarbamate structurally similar to meprobamate, is approved by the United States Food and Drug Administration (FDA) for use alone or with other drugs in adults with partial seizures with or without secondary generalization. It is also approved for use in children with Lennox-Gastaut syndrome. The mechanism of action is unknown, although in neuronal cultures felbamate blocks sustained repetitive neuronal firing, possibly through an effect on sodium channels. Felbamate is well absorbed from the gastrointestinal tract and circulates primarily as a free drug without significant protein binding. Significant interactions occur with the major antiepileptic drugs.[171]

Uniquely designed, double-blind, controlled studies administering felbamate as monotherapy demonstrate significant reduction in frequency of partial onset seizures.[23,187] Unfortunately, the side effect profile is also significant. Headache, insomnia, anorexia, and fatigue were initially reported to occur in less than 10% of patients and to be mild or moderate in severity.[171] Anecdotal reports of headache and anorexia appear far more prevalent, however, prompting discontinuation of treatment in many cases. Hematologic side effects such as leukopenia, thrombocytopenia, or agranulocytosis are rare, although three cases of fatal aplastic anemia prompted the manufacturer to voluntarily withdraw felbamate from marketing in August 1994.

Gabapentin (Neurontin) is a novel antiepileptic drug with a molecular structure that resembles gamma-aminobutyric acid (GABA), an inhibitory transmitter. Although GABA deficiency has been implicated as a cause of epilepsy, gabapentin appears to demonstrate a unique mechanism of action that does not involve GABA receptors. The primary mechanism of action remains undefined.[171]

Gabapentin demonstrates several advantages, including ease of administration, safety, and efficacy. It is rapidly absorbed after oral administration. It is not bound to plasma proteins and is not metabolized. Gabapentin does not induce hepatic enzymes or interact with other antiepileptic drugs.[171] In placebo-controlled trials, response ratios among patients with refractory partial seizures are significantly better with gabapentin than with placebo and other antiepileptic drugs.[171,225]

Adverse effects are generally mild and transient, occurring at slightly higher frequency among patients receiving gabapentin than among patients receiving placebo in addition to standard antiepileptic drugs. Such effects, which usually include somnolence, dizziness, and ataxia, resolve within 2 weeks of initiation of therapy in most patients.[225] Gabapentin does not affect the serum concentrations of concurrent antiepileptic drugs and is not regularly associated with deviations in laboratory values. Its low inherent toxicity and the lack of drug interactions are likely to make gabapentin useful as add-on therapy in refractory partial epilepsy,[225] particularly for patients with hepatic disease and elderly patients who receive multiple medications.[171]

Lamotrigine (Lamictal), a phenyltriazene, derives from drugs that inhibit dihydrofolate reductase and is chemically unrelated to currently available antiepileptic drugs. It appears to block voltage-specific sodium channels, inhibiting the release of neurotransmitters, principally glutamate.[264] Lamotrigine is absorbed rapidly and completely after oral administration, and binding interactions with other antiepileptic drugs are unlikely. Polytherapy with phenytoin or carbamazepine shortens its half-life, whereas valproate lengthens it. Lamotrigine undergoes hepatic metabolism, and autoinduction does not occur.[171] At least eight randomized, double-blind, placebo-controlled crossover trials have been conducted with lamotrigine, establishing its efficacy in patients with refractory partial epilepsy. Reports suggest that lamotrigine also may be effective in patients with idiopathic generalized epilepsy, including absence seizures.[264] Lamotrigine appears to be well tolerated, with a side effect profile favorable to other antiepileptic drugs. Dosage-related rash has been noted in approximately 3–5% of patients.[171,178] Other notable side effects include ataxia, dizziness, and headache, although they seldom demand discontinuation of therapy.

An advisory committee to the FDA has recommended approval of lamotrigine as add-on therapy for adults with partial seizures, and it has just been released for marketing in the United States. A long half-life and lack of effect on other antiepileptic drugs make lamotrigine easy to dose and to add to a patient's existing regimen.[171]

Vigabatrin (Sabril), a structural analogue of GABA, demonstrates highly specific activity as an enzyme-activated irreversible inhibitor of GABA-transaminase. As a consequence of the diminished GABA transaminase activity, the concentration of brain GABA increases severalfold. Vigabatrin undergoes rapid and complete oral absorption and quickly enters the cerebrospinal fluid. It is not metabolized or bound to plasma proteins, nor does it induce hepatic metabolism. It is rapidly cleared through the kidney.[151] Vigabatrin has been shown to be specifically effective in the management of partial seizures unresponsive to other antiepileptic drugs. In most controlled studies, about 50% of patients with previously uncontrolled seizures have a 50% reduction in frequency,[176,179] and about 4–5% become seizure-free.[151] Clinically, vigabatrin is generally well tolerated; discontinuation most frequently is associated with therapeutic failure.[151] Side effects include weight gain due to increased appetite as well as occasional irritability and restlessness.[252] Rarely, vigabatrin may precipitate reversible depression[179] and schizophrenia-like psychotic reactions.[176] Withdrawal seizures have been observed. Although clinical development of vigabatrin was delayed by concerns about microvacuolization of white matter in dogs and rats, extensive studies have failed to identify this effect in primates or humans.[252] Vigabatrin remains in active development as first-line therapy in patients with newly diagnosed epilepsy and as monotherapy when other antiepileptic drugs have failed.[151]

Adverse Effects

Anticonvulsants commonly used in the treatment of posttraumatic seizures are associated with significant idiosyncratic and dose-related adverse drug reactions[38,39] that require their discontinuation or substitution in as many as 20–30% of patients.[103,203] Adverse reactions include hematologic, dermatologic, hepatologic, neurologic,[177] endocrinologic,[105,172] and teratogenic effects.[9,118,200] Transient or persistent leukopenia and thrombocytopenia may be observed in patients taking phenytoin and carbamazepine, although idiosyncratic

aplastic anemia is extremely rare.[161] Rashes are occasionally encountered with many anticonvulsants.[28,161] Hirsutism and gingival hyperplasia may be problematic in patients treated with phenytoin,[38,161] and weight gain has been significantly associated with valproate.[137] Mild and transient elevations of hepatic enzymes (as high as 2–3 times normal in some cases) are reported in patients receiving anticonvulsant therapy.[167,175] However, frequent and rigorous regimens of laboratory monitoring are unjustified, aside from baseline determination of hematologic and hepatic function, or closer observation of noted abnormalities. Route monitoring does not provide meaningful protection from the rare and potentially life-threatening manifestations of anticonvulsant side effects.[31,163] Appropriate counseling for the patient, family, and/or caregivers about potential complications and symptoms that may herald an adverse event is far more useful and important.[163]

Cognitive effects of anticonvulsant drugs warrant particular attention in patients with TBI. Anticonvulsants, including phenytoin and carbamazepine, significantly impair memory performance in double-blind crossover trials among healthy adults.[143] Patients with severe TBI already have significant cognitive impairment. Anticonvulsant medications may exert independent and additional adverse cognitive effects on patients with TBI who receive chronic therapy.[57,205] Among patients with severe TBI in the prophylaxis trial of Temkin et al.,[210] 78% of those treated with phenytoin demonstrated cognitive impairment of sufficient severity to preclude testing at 1 month after injury. In contrast, such impairment was observed in only 47% of patients treated with placebo.[57]

The comparative profiles of cognitive side effects of various anticonvulsant drug regimens remain controversial.[58,59,60,143–145,203,220] Relevant studies were reviewed recently by Massagli.[136] In summary, comparative studies provide no compelling evidence to assert that carbamazepine, phenytoin, or valproate demonstrates a significant advantage in minimizing cognitive side effects; only two of the studies, however, included patients with TBI.[121,204] Although neither study demonstrated significant differences in cognitive impairment between patients receiving phenytoin and carbamazepine,[121] the design of both studies may limit the significance of their conclusions. For example, Smith et al.[204] found no significant difference in cognitive testing results among patients randomized to withdrawal from phenytoin and carbamazepine. Only 13 of the 82 patients sustained severe TBI; however, the remainder received prophylaxis after craniotomy or mild-to-moderate TBI. Considerable anecdotal evidence suggests that carbamazepine provides a relatively favorable profile of cognitive side effects among patients with severe TBI.[21,77] Such anecdotal evidence is unlikely to be dismissed until randomized comparative studies among patients with severe TBI are conducted.

Although concern for adverse drug effects frequently focuses on observable phenomena such as lethargy or hepatotoxicity, the influence of anticonvulsants on the course of postinjury neurologic recovery also warrants consideration. Specifically, certain drugs, including anticonvulsants, clearly impair recovery after brain injury in laboratory animals.[25,71,81,194] Schallert et al. demonstrated that administration of diazepam to rats with 12 hours of neocortical damage delayed recovery indefinitely, whereas delayed administration resulted in only transient reinstatement of neurologic deficit.[194] Brailowsky observed that phenytoin increased the severity of cannula-induced cortical hemiplegia in rats, although motor impairment was not seen when the drug was administered to the animals after the hemiplegic syndrome had cleared.[25] Such findings suggest that administration of diazepam or phenytoin during certain critical periods after brain injury may have a deleterious effect on subsequent neurologic recovery.

In summary, the above studies serve as a reminder that decisions about chronic anticonvulsant treatment, particularly prophylaxis, cannot be considered solely on the merits of effectiveness. Consideration also must be given to potentially significant adverse effects and toxicities.

Anticonvulsant Substitution

Neurosurgeons have preferred phenobarbital and phenytoin for prophylaxis[173] and symptomatic anticonvulsant treatment, primarily because of their availability in parenteral forms that can be administered in the acute setting, when seizures are most likely to occur. Until quite recently, such patients were maintained on the chosen anticonvulsant until a satisfactory seizure-free duration had passed. Anticonvulsant substitution was usually reserved for failure of seizure control or manifestation of significant drug reactions.[67]

Many authors, however, currently recommend reevaluating the choice of anticonvulsants when the patient is transferred to a rehabilitation unit[21,77,244] because of the potential for adverse cognitive and behavioral side effects, which frequently emerges as a central pharmacologic consideration in patients with TBI. Carbamazepine is suggested as a substitution for phenytoin or phenobarbital when ongoing anticonvulsant treatment is deemed necessary. Such substitution appears to have gained acceptance among institutions specializing in the rehabilitative care of patients with TBI.[77] Wroblewski et al. observed that substitution of carbamazepine enhanced seizure control in most patients with TBI and also appeared safe.[254]

When an anticonvulsant such as carbamazepine is substituted for another anticonvulsant, clinically effective steady state levels of carbamazepine should be attained before any attempt to discontinue the former drug.[67] Carbamazepine therapy should begin gradually, preferably over 1–2 weeks, to minimize side effects.[166] Once the steady state has been achieved, the former drug is tapered gradually, at a rate no faster than 20% of the total daily dose every 5 half-lives.[67]

Duration of Treatment

No clinical studies specifically address the duration of anticonvulsant treatment for patients with recurrent posttraumatic seizures. In general, it is reasonable to consider withdrawal of anticonvulsant medication from patients with epilepsy after 2 years of freedom from seizures.[30] Reported rates of relapse vary considerably and reflect the type of seizure disorder under treatment.[67] The risk of recurrence under a policy of slow anticonvulsant withdrawal is still substantial compared with continued treatment, particularly during the first year of withdrawal.[146] Increased risk of recurrence has been reported among patients with a history of more frequent seizures, treatment with more than one antiepileptic drug, a history of generalized tonic-clonic seizures,[146] and abnormal or epileptiform discharges on prewithdrawal electroencephalograms.[30,75] Among patients for whom the risk of relapse after discontinuation appears low, the psychosocial benefits of discontinuation may be considerable.[108] There is no consensus about the ideal period over which anticonvulsants should be withdrawn in patients with recurrent seizures, although conservative recommendations advise a period of 12 months.[67,197] Worsening of seizures after discontinuation of phenytoin[29,135] or carbamazepine[135] is believed to reflect the loss of therapeutic drug effect rather than a withdrawal phenomenon. In contrast, withdrawal exacerbation of seizures is prominent with barbituates[214] and benzodiazepines[230] and does not indicate that the drug was necessary for maintenance of seizure control.[67]

Few investigations address the duration of prophylactic anticonvulsant treatment. Before publication of the prophylaxis trial by Temkin et al.,[210] a trend toward shorter durations of approximately 1 year had emerged.[21,113,162,206] Serious doubts about the effectiveness of prophylaxis, however, have prompted recommendations to discontinue treatment after 1 week.[211,258] Experience with discontinuation of prophylaxis after such shorter durations is increasing, and a recent preliminary report suggests that no undue seizure or medical risk is incurred and that prophylaxis can be withdrawn safely while patients are treated in the acute rehabilitation setting.[139]

Consultation and Referral

Guidelines for the appropriate level of primary and specialty care of patients with seizures, including recommendations for referral to specialty centers, have been published.[3,154] The first step for patients experiencing an initial seizure or seizures is to consult their primary-care physician, who may choose to begin a treatment program or to refer the patient to a general neurologist for consultation. If seizures continue after 3 months, a referral to a general neurologist certainly is indicated. When the seizures are controlled, many patients appropriately

return to the care of their primary physicians, with follow-up visits to the neurologist as needed. If seizure control is not achieved by the neurologist at the end of the first year of treatment, referral to a center that offers comprehensive diagnostic and treatment services to patients with intractable seizures is indicated.[3,154]

CONCLUSION

The following hypothesis for prophylaxis of late posttraumatic seizures is based on the evidence presented above:

If the patient does not manifest early posttraumatic seizures, routine chronic prophylaxis of late posttraumatic seizures does not appear justified, and no anticonvulsant therapy is provided unless late seizures are reported. If a late posttraumatic seizure is documented, carbamazepine is used for symptomatic management unless toxicity or therapeutic failure supervenes. If the patient is receiving phenytoin, oral or enteral carbamazepine is substituted at the earliest suitable point to minimize adverse side effects, particularly cognitive impairment.

Patients with TBI who are transferred to the rehabilitation setting without reported seizures are gradually tapered from anticonvulsants soon after their admission. This approach facilitates monitoring for the potentially varied manifestations of seizures. Because seizures are more likely to occur in the earlier postinjury period, it also helps to ensure the presence of trained personnel if a seizure is observed during or after anticonvulsant withdrawal. We have observed that marked improvements in cognitive status frequently coincide with termination of anticonvulsant prophylaxis.

If a late posttraumatic seizure is observed, a search for an identifiable precipitant takes place. If no obvious, correctable precipitant is identified, anticonvulsant therapy with carbamazepine may be instituted for approximately 12 months. A diagnosis of seizure disorder should be established before anticonvulsant therapy is initiated.

For most physicians caring for patients with TBI in the rehabilitation setting, the issue of whether to institute prophylaxis of early posttraumatic seizures is moot.

Nevertheless, postinjury prophylaxis of early posttraumatic seizures with phenytoin appears justified in patients with severe TBI who belong to previously identified high-risk groups. Patients are at highest risk at a time when they can least afford to tolerate the complications of a seizure, such as aggravation of increased intracranial pressure. Prophylaxis should be continued for approximately 1 week if seizures are not observed and then tapered gradually.[211] This protocol should take place in a setting in which close observation can be provided. The risks incurred with treatment of such short duration appear minimal and acceptable.

Insufficient data guide antiepileptic drug therapy among patients whose only manifestation of a seizure disorder are early posttraumatic seizures. Most published reports exclude such patients from further study, thereby losing valuable information about the effect of continued antiepileptic drug therapy on the risk of recurrent seizures at a later time. Issues to consider include time of onset (day 1 vs. day 7), severity (particularly status epilepticus), frequency of recurrence, and clinical risk factors for recurrence. Factors favoring continuation of antiepileptic drug therapy include later time of onset, documented episodes of status epilepticus, multiple seizure episodes throughout the first week of injury, and multiple risk factors suggestive of high risk for late posttraumatic seizures, such as penetrating TBI. In contrast, it may be reasonable to consider a closely monitored withdrawal of antiepileptic drug therapy in selected patients with isolated early posttraumatic seizures, particularly if the seizure occurs within the first 24 hours after injury. Our experience suggests that a vast majority of patients with closed TBI and isolated early posttraumatic seizures tolerate discontinuation of antiepileptic drug therapy without recurrence of seizures.[258]

Despite the studies and theories discussed above, important research questions remain, including a broad range of topics pertinent to the diagnosis and treatment of epileptic disorders. Investigation must be directed toward clarifying the natural history of posttraumatic seizures, the prognostic implications of single or isolated seizures, and the effect of anticonvulsant treatment on risk of recurrence. Future studies must address the comparative benefits and adverse effects of anticonvulsant therapy (including newer agents) specifically on patients with TBI and explore the potential effects of such drugs on neurologic recovery. Further research is warranted into the optimal duration of anticonvulsant therapy and the effect of posttraumatic seizures and anticonvulsant therapy on functional outcome.

Finally, each patient's risk and suitability for treatment must be assessed on an individual basis, guidelines or algorithms notwithstanding. Discussion of issues related to posttraumatic seizures with the patient and family members is especially useful and important. The clinician should be aware of the prevailing regional standards for prophylaxis and symptomatic management, and prudence dictates careful documentation of such issues.

REFERENCES

1. Aarts JHP, Binnie CD, Smith AM, Wilkins AJ: Selective cognitive impairment during focal and generalized epileptiform EEG activity. Brain 107:293–308, 1984.
2. Albertson TE, Joy RM, Stark LG: Carbamazepine: A pharmacologic study in the kindling model of epilepsy. Neuropharmacology 23:1117–1123, 1984.
3. Alldredge BK, Lowenstein DH, Simon RP: Seizures associated with recreational drug abuse. Neurology 39:1037–1039, 1989.
4. Ameen AA: Penetrating craniocerebral injuries: Observations in the Iraqi-Iranian war. Milit Med 152:76–79, 1987.
5. American academy of Neurology, Therapeutics and Technology Assessment Subcommittee: Assessment: Intensive EEG/video monitoring for epilepsy. Neurology 39:1101–1102, 1989.
6. Aminoff MJ, Goodin DS, Berg BO, Compton MN: Ambulatory EEG recordings in epileptic and non-epileptic children. Neurology 38:558–562, 1988.
7. Anderson GD, Chabal S, Gidal BE, et al: Effect of valproate on coagulation parameters in a posttraumatic head injury populations [abstract]. Epilepsia 32 (Suppl 3):10, 1991.
8. Annegers JF, Grabow JD, Broover RV, et al: Seizures after head trauma: A population study. Neurology 30:683–689, 1980.
9. Armstrong KK, Saghal V, Block R, et al: Rehabilitation outcomes in patients with posttraumatic epilepsy. Arch Phys Med Rehabil 71:156–160, 1990.
10. Ascroft PB: Traumatic epilepsy after gunshot wounds of the head. BMJ 1:739–744, 1941.
11. Askenasy JJM: Association of intracerebral bone fragments and epilepsy in missile head injuries. Acta Neurol Scanned 79:47–52, 1989.

12. Barry E, Bergey GK, Krumholz A: Nonepileptic posttraumatic seizures [abstract]. Epilepsia 32 (Suppl 3): S54, 1991.

13. Bergamini L, Bergamasco B, Benna P, Gilli M: Acquired etiological factors in 1785 epileptic subjects. Clinical-anamnestic research. Epilepsia 18: 437–444, 1977.

14. Berger AR, Lipton RB, Lesser ML, et al: Early seizures following intracerebral hemorrhage: Implications for therapy. Neurology 38:1363–1365, 1988.

15. Betts T: Pseudoseizures. Seizures that are not epilepsy. Lancet 336:163–164, 1990.

16. Bibileishvili Sh I, Metreveli M Sh: Epileptic syndrome as a remote consequence of a closed craniocerebral injury [abstract]. Epilepsia 32 (Suppl 1): S113–S114, 1991.

17. Binnie CD, Marston D: Cognitive correlates of interictal discharges. Epilepsia 33 (Suppl 6):S11–17, 1992.

18. Birkmayer W: Die behandlung der tramatischen epilepsie. Wien Kiln Wochenschr 63:606–609, 1951.

19. Black P, Shepard RH, Walker AE: Outcome of head trauma: Age and posttraumatic seizures. Ciba Found Symp 34:215–219, 1975.

20. Blackwood D, McQueen JK, Harris P, et al: A clinical trial of phenytoin prophylaxis of epilepsy following head injury: Preliminary report. In Dam M, Gram L, Penry JK (eds): Advances in Epileptology: XIIth Epilepsy International Symposium. New York, Raven Press, 1981 pp 521–525.

21. Bontke CF: Medical complications related to traumatic brain injury. State Art Rev Phys Med Rehabil 3:43–52, 1989.

22. Bontke CF, Lehmkuhl LD, Englander J, et al: Medical complications and associated injuries of patients treated in TBI Model System programs. J Head Trauma Rehabil 8:34–46, 1993.

23. Bourgeois B, Leppik IE, Sackellares JC, et al: Felbamate: A double-blind controlled trial in patients undergoing presurgical evaluation of partial seizures. Neurology 43:693–696, 1993.

24. Bouzarth WF, Goldman HW: Prophylactic phenytoin [letter]. J Neurosurg 59:877, 1984.

25. Brailowsky S, Knight RT, Efron R: Phenytoin increases the severity of cortical hemiplegia in rats. Brain Res 376:71–77, 1986.

26. Brandvold B, Levi L, Feinsod M, George ED: Penetrating craniocerebral injuries in the Israeli involvement in the Lebanese conflict, 1982–1985. Analysis of a less aggressive surgical approach. J Neurosurg 72:15–21, 1990.

27. Bridgers SL, Ebersole JS: Cassette electroencephalography. In Wyllie E (ed): The Treatment of Epilepsy: Principles and Practice. Philadelphia, Lea & Febiger, 1993 pp 278–284.

28. Brodie MJ: Established anticonvulsants and treatment of refractory epilepsy. Lancet 350–354, 1990.

29. Bromfield EB, Dambrosia J, Devinsky O, et al: Phenytoin withdrawal and seizure frequency. Neurology 39:905–909, 1989.

30. Callaghan N, Garrett A, Goggin T: Withdrawal of anticonvulsant drugs in patients free of seizures for two years. A prospective study. N Engl J Med 318:942–946, 1988.

31. Camfield C, Camfield P, Smith E, Tibbles JAR: Asymptomatic children with epilepsy: Little benefit from screening for anticonvulsant-induced liver, blood, or renal damage. Neurology 36:838–841, 1986.

32. Cavalheiro EA, Leite JP, Bortolotto ZA, et al: Long-term effects of pilocarpine in rats: Structural damage of the brain triggers kindling and spontaneous recurrent seizures. Epilepsia 32:778–782, 1991.

33. Caveness WF: Onset and cessation of fits following craniocerebral trauma. J Neurosurg 20:570–583, 1963.

34. Caveness WF, Liss HR: Incidence of posttraumatic epilepsy. Epilepsia 2:123–129, 1961.

35. Caveness, WF, Meirowsky AM, Rish BL, et al: The nature of posttraumatic epilepsy. J Neurosurg 50:545–553, 1979.

36. Chadwick D: Diagnosis of epilepsy. Lancet 336: 291–295, 1990.

37. Cohen M, Groswasser Z: Epilepsy in traumatic brain-injured patients [abstract]. Epilepsia 32 (Suppl 1):S55, 1991.

38. Collaborative Group for Epidemiology of Epilepsy: Adverse reactions to antiepileptic drugs: A follow-up study of 355 patients with chronic antiepileptic drug treatment. Epilepsia 29:787–793, 1988.

39. Collaborative Group for Epidemiology of Epilepsy: Adverse reactions to antiepileptic drugs: A multicenter survey of clinical practice. Epilepsia 27: 323–330, 1986.

40. Collins WCJ, Lanigan O, Callaghan N: Plasma prolactin concentrations following epileptic and pseudoseizures. J Neurol Neurosurg Psychiatry 46: 505–508, 1983.

41. Commission on Classification and Terminology of the International League Against Epilepsy: Proposal for revised classification of epilepsies and epileptic syndromes. Epilepsia 30:389–399, 1989.

42. Commission on Classification and Terminology of the International League Against Epilepsy: Proposal for revised clinical and electroencephalographic classification of epileptic seizures. Epilepsia 22:489–501, 1981.

43. Corkin S, Sullivan EV, Carr FA: Prognostic factors for life expectancy after head injury. Arch Neurol 41:975–977, 1984.

44. Courjon J: A longitudinal electro-clinical study of 80 cases of posttraumatic epilepsy observed from the time of original trauma. Epilepsia 11:29–36, 1970.

45. D'Alessandro R, Ferrara R, Benassi G, et al: Computed tomographic scans in posttraumatic epilepsy. Arch Neurol, 45:42–43, 1988.

46. Dana-Haeri J, Trimble MR, Oxley J: Prolactin and gonadotropin change following generalized and partial seizures. J Neurol Neurosurg Psychiatry 46:331–335, 1983.

47. da Silva AM, Nunes B, Vaz AR, Mendonça D: Posttraumatic epilepsy in civilians: Clinical and electroencephalographic studies. Acta Neurochir Suppl (Wien) 55:56–63, 1992.

48. da Silva AM, Vaz AR, Ribeiro I, et al: Controversies in posttraumatic epilepsy. Acta Neurochir Suppl (Wien) 50:48–51, 1990.

49. De Santis A, Cappricci E, Granata G: Early post-traumatic seizures in adults. J Neurosurg Sci 23:207–210, 1979.

50. De Santis A, Sganzerla E, Spagnoli D, et al: Risk factors for late posttraumatic epilepsy. Acta Neurochir Suppl (Wien) 55:64–67, 1992.

51. Deahl M, Trimble M: Serotonin reuptake inhibitors, epilepsy and myoclonus. Br J Psychiatry 159:433–435, 1991.

52. Desai BT, Whitman S, Coonley-Hoganson R, et al: Seizures and civilian head injuries. Epilepsia 24:289–296, 1983.

53. Deutschmann CS, Haines SJ: Anticonvulsant prophylaxis in neurological surgery. Neurosurgery 17:510–517, 1985.

54. Devinsky O, Luciano D: Psychic phenomena in partial seizures. Semin Neurol 11:100–109, 1991.

55. Deymeer F, Leviton A: Posttraumatic seizures: An assessment of the epidemiologic literature. Cent Nerv Syst Trauma 2:33–43, 1985.

56. Dikmen S, Reitan RM: Neuropsychological performance in posttraumatic epilepsy. Epilepsia 19:177–183, 1978.

57. Dikmen SS, Temkin NR, Miller B, et al: Neurobehavioral effects of phenytoin prophylaxis of posttraumatic seizures. JAMA 265:1271–1217, 1991.

58. Dodrill CB, Troupin AS: Neuropsychological effects of carbamazepine and phenytoin: A reanalysis. Neurology 41:141–143, 1991.

59. Dodrill CB, Troupin AS: Psychotropic effects of carbamazepine in epilepsy: A double-blind comparison with phenytoin. Neurology 27:1023, 1028, 1977.

60. Duncan JS, Shorvon SD, Trimble MR: Effects of removal of phenytoin, carbamazepine, and valproate on cognitive function. Epilepsia 31:584–591, 1990.

61. Ebersole JS, Leroy RF: An evaluation of ambulatory, cassette EEG monitoring: II. Detection of interictal abnormalities. Neurology 33:8–18, 1983.

62. Ebersole JS, Leroy RF: Evaluation of ambulatory cassette EEG monitoring III. Diagnostic accuracy compared to intensive inpatient EEG monitoring. Neurology 33:853–860, 1983.

63. Edwards JG: Antidepressants and convulsive seizures: Clinical, electroencephalographic, and pharmacological aspects. Clin Neuropharmacol 9:329–360, 1986.

64. Efron R: Post-epileptic paralysis: Theoretical critique and report of a case. Brain 84:381–394, 1961.

65. Eide PK, Tysnes OB: Early and late outcome in head injury patients with radiological evidence of brain damage. Acta Neurol Scand 86:194–198, 1992.

66. Engel J Jr: Neurobiology of behavior: Anatomic and physiological implications related to epilepsy. Epilepsia 27 (Suppl 2): S3–S13, 1986.

67. Engel J Jr (ed): Seizures and Epilepsy. Philadelphia, F.A. Davis, 1990.

68. Evans JH: Posttraumatic epilepsy. Neurology (Minneapolis) 12:665–674, 1962.

69. Farwell JR, Lee YJ, Hirtz DG, et al: Phenobarbital for febrile seizures—effects on intelligence and on seizure recurrence. N Engl J Med 322:364–369, 1990.

70. Fraught E, Peters D, Bartolucci A, et al: Seizures after primary intracerebral hemorrhage. Neurology 39:1089–1093, 1989.

71. Feeney DM, Gonzalez A, Law WA: Amphetamine, haloperidol, and experience interact to affect rate of recovery after motor cortex injury. Science 217:855–857, 1982.

72. Feeney DM, Walker AE: The prediction of posttraumatic epilepsy: A mathematical approach. Arch Neurol 36:8–12, 1979.

73. First Seizure Trial Group: Randomized clinical trial on the efficacy of antiepileptic drugs in reducing the risk of relapse after a first unprovoked tonic-clonic seizure. Neurology 43:478–483, 1993.

74. Gage RH, Bjorklund A, Stenevi U: Reinnervation of the partially deafferented hippocampus by compensatory collateral sprouting from spared cholinergic and noradrenergic afferents. Brain Res 268:27–37, 1983.

75. Gherpelli JLD, Kok F, dal Forno S, et al: Discontinuing medication in epileptic children: A study of risk factors related to recurrence. Epilepsia 33:681–686, 1992.

76. Giaquinto S: Traumatic epilepsy: The value of a family study. In Canger R, Angeleri F, Penry JK (eds): Advances in Epileptology: XIth Epilepsy International Symposium. New York, Raven Press, 1980, pp 331–337.

77. Glenn MB, Wroblewski B: Anticonvulsants for prophylaxis of posttraumatic seizures. Head Trauma Rehabil 1:73–74, 1986.

78. Glötzner FL, Haubitz I, Miltner F, et al: Epilepsy prophylaxis with carbamazepine in severe brain injuries. Neurochirurgie 26:66–79, 1983.

79. Goddard BV: Development of epileptic seizures through brain stimulation at low intensity. Nature 214:1020–1021, 1967.

80. Goldensohn ES: The relevance of secondary epileptogenesis to the treatment of epilepsy: Kindling and the mirror focus. Epilepsia 25 (Suppl 2): S156–S173, 1984.

81. Goldstein LB, Davis JN: Restorative neurology. Drugs and recovery following stroke. Stroke 21:1636–1639, 1990.

82. Grafman J, Jonas B, Salazar A: Epilepsy following penetrating head injury to the frontal lobes. Adv Neurol 57:369–378, 1992.

83. Grosswasser Z, Reider-Grosswasser I, Soroker N, Machtey Y: Magnetic resonance imaging in head-injured patients with normal late computed tomography scans. Surg Neurol 27:331–337, 1987.

84. Gualtieri CT: Pharmacotherapy and the neurobehavioral sequelae of traumatic brain injury. Brain Inj 2:101–129, 1988.

85. Guidice MA, Berchou RC: Posttraumatic epilepsy following head injury. Brain Inj 1:61–64, 1987.

86. Hahn YS, Fuchs S, Flannery AM, et al: Factors influencing posttraumatic seizures in children. Neurosurgery 22:864–867, 1988.

87. Hammond EJ, Ramsay RE, Villareal HJ, Wilder BJ: Effects of intracortical injection of blood and blood components on the electrocorticogram. Epilepsia 21:2–14, 1980.

88. Hardman JM: The pathology of traumatic brain injuries. Adv Neurol 22:15–50, 1979.

89. Hart YM, Sander JWAS, Johnson AL, Shorvon SD: National General Practice Study of Epilepsy: Recurrence after a first seizure. Lancet 336:1271–1274, 1990.

90. Hasan D, Schonck RSM, Avezaat CJJ, et al: Epileptic seizures after subarachnoid hemorrhage. Ann Neurol 33:286–291, 1993.

91. Hauser WA: Prevention of posttraumatic epilepsy. N Engl J Med 323:540–542, 1990.

92. Hauser WA: Should people be treated after a first seizure? Arch Neurol 1287–1288, 1986.

93. Hauser WA: Status epilepticus: Epidemiologic considerations. Neurology 40 (Suppl 2): 9–13, 1990.

94. Hauser WA, Annegers JF, Kurland LT: Prevalence of epilepsy in Rochester, Minnesota: 1940–1980. Epilepsia 32:429–445, 1991.

95. Hauser A, Ng SKC, Brust JCM: Alcohol, seizures, and epilepsy. Epilepsia 29 (Suppl 2): S66–S78, 1988.

96. Hauser WA, Rich SS, Annegers JF, Anderson VE: Seizure recurrence after a first unprovoked seizure: An extended follow-up. Neurology 40:1163–1170, 1990.

97. Hauser WA, Tabaddor K, Factor PR, Finer C: Seizures and head injury in an urban community. Neurology (Cleve) 34:746–751, 1984.

98. Heikinnen ER, Ronty HS, Tolonen U, Pyhtinen J: Development of posttraumatic epilepsy. Stereotact Funct Neurosurg 54–55:25–33, 1990.

99. Hendrick E, Harris L: Posttraumatic epilepsy in children. J Trauma 8:547–555, 1968.

100. Hillbom ME: Occurrence of cerebral seizures provoked by alcohol abuse. Epilepsia 21:459–466, 1980.

101. Hoff H, Hoff H: Fortschritte in der behandlung der epilepsie. Monatsschr Psychiatr Neurol 114:105–118, 1947.

102. Holmes GL, Sackellares JC, McKiernan J, et al: Evaluation of childhood pseudoseizures using EEG telemetry and video tape monitoring. J Pediatr 97:554–558, 1980.

103. Homan RW, Miller B: Veterans Administration Epilepsy Cooperative Study Group: Causes of treatment failure with epileptic drugs vary over time. Neurology 37:1620–1623, 1987.

104. International Dictionary of Medicine and Biology. New York, John Wiley & Sons, 1986, p 2316.

105. Isojärvi JIT, Pakarinen AJ, Ylipalosaari PJ, Myllyla VV: Serum hormones in male epileptic patients receiving anticonvulsant medication. Arch Neurol 47:670–676, 1990.

106. Jabbari B, Bryan GE, Marsh EE, Gunderson CH: Incidence of seizures with tricyclic and tetracyclic antidepressants. Arch Neurol 42:480–481, 1985.

107. Jabbari B, Vengrow MI, Salazar AM, et al: Clinical and radiological correlates of EEG in the late phase of head injury: A study of 515 Vietnam veterans. Electroenceph Clin Neurophysiol 64:285–293, 1986.

108. Jacoby A, Johnson A, Chadwick D, Medical Research Council Antiepileptic Drug Withdrawal Study Group: Psychosocial outcomes of antiepileptic drug discontinuation. Epilepsia 33:1123–1131, 1992.

109. Jamjoon AB, Kane N, Sanderman D, Cummins B: Epilepsy related to traumatic extradural hematomas. BMJ 302:448, 1991.

110. Japan Follow-up Group for Posttraumatic Epilepsy: The factors influencing posttraumatic epilepsy: Multicentric cooperative study. No Shinkei Geka 19:1151–1159, 1991.

111. Jennett B: Anticonvulsant drugs and advice about driving after head injury and intracranial surgery. BMJ 28:627–628, 1983.

112. Jennett B: Epilepsy After Non-missile Head Injuries, 2nd ed. Chicago, William Heinemann, 1975.

113. Jennett B: Posttraumatic epilepsy. In Rosenthal M, Griffith ER, Bond MR, Miller JD (eds): Rehabilitation of the Adult and Child with Traumatic Brain Injury, 2nd ed. Philadelphia, F.A. Davis, 1990, pp 89–93.

114. Jennett B, Lewin W: Traumatic epilepsy after closed head injuries. J Neurol Neurosurg Psychiatry 23:295–301, 1960.

115. Jennett B, van de Sande: EEG prediction of posttraumatic epilepsy. Epilepsia 16:251–256, 1975.

116. Kalisky Z, Morrison DP, Meyers CA, Von Laufen AV: Medical problems encountered during rehabilitation of patients with head injury. Arch Phys Med Rehabil 66:25–29, 1985.

117. Kalsbeek WD, McLaurin RL, Harris BSH III, Miller JD: The National Head and Spinal Cord Injury Survey: Major findings. J Neurosurg 53 (Suppl): S19–S31, 1980.

118. Kaneko S, Otani K, Fukushima Y, et al: Teratogenicity of antiepileptic drugs: Analysis of possible risk factors. Epilepsia 29:459–467, 1988.

119. Kanner AM, Morris HH, Lüders H, et al: Supplementary motor seizures mimicking pseudoseizures: Some clinical differences. Neurology 40: 1404–1047, 1990.

120. Kennedy CR, Freeman JM: Posttraumatic seizures and posttraumatic epilepsy in children. J Head Trauma Rehabil 1(4):66–73, 1986.

121. Kirschner KL, Sahgal V, Armstrong KJ, Bloch R: A comparative study of the cognitive effects of phenytoin and carbamazepine in patients with blunt head injury. J Neurol Rehab 5:169–174, 1991.

122. Kollevold T: Immediate and early cerebral seizures after head injuries. Part I. J Oslo City Hosp 26: 99–114, 1976.

123. Kollevold T: Immediate and early cerebral seizures after head injuries. Part II. J Oslo City Hosp 27:89–99, 1977.

124. Kollevold T: Immediate and early cerebral seizures after head injuries. Part III. J Oslo City Hosp 28:78–86, 1978.

125. Kollevold T: Immediate and early cerebral seizures after head injuries. Part IV. J Oslo City Hosp 29:35–47, 1979.

126. Kreutzer JS, Doherty KR, Harris JA, Zasler ND: Alcohol use among persons with traumatic brain injury. J Head Trauma Rehabil 5(3):9–20, 1990.

127. Laxer KD, Mullooly JP, Howell B: Prolactin changes after seizures classified by EEG monitoring. Neurology 35:31–35, 1985.

128. Lee S-T, Lui T-N: Early seizures after mild closed head injury. J Neurosurg 76:435–439, 1992.

129. Leis AA, Ross MA, Summers AK: Psychogenic seizures: Ictal characteristics and diagnostic pitfalls. Neurology 42:95–99, 1992.

130. Leppik I: Status epilepticus: The next decade. Neurology 40 (Suppl 2):4–9, 1990.

131. Leppik IE: Status epilepticus. Neurol Clin 4:633–643, 1986.

132. Locke GE, Molaie M, Biggers S, Leonard E: Risk factors for posttraumatic epilepsy [abstract]. Epilepsia 32 (Suppl 3): S104–S105, 1991.

133. Ludwig B, Marsan DA, Van Buren J: Cerebral seizures of probable orbitofrontal origin. Epilepsia 16:141–158, 1975.

134. Manaka S, Japan Follow-Up Research group of Posttraumatic Epilepsy: Cooperative prospective study on posttraumatic epilepsy risk factors and the effect of prophylactic anticonvulsant. Jpn J Psychiatry Neurol 46:311–315, 1992.

135. Marks DA, Katz A, Scheyer R, Spencer SS: Clinical and electrographic effects of acute anticonvulsant withdrawal in epileptic patients. Neurology 41:508–512, 1991.

136. Masagli TL: Neurobehavioral effects of phenytoin, carbamazepine, and valproic acid: Implications for use in traumatic brain injury. Arch Phys Med Rehabil 72:219–226, 1991.

137. Mattson RH, Cramer JA, Collins JF: Department of Veterans Affairs Epilepsy Cooperative Study No. 264 Group: A comparison of valproate with carbamazepine for the treatment of complex partial seizures and secondarily generalized tonic-clonic seizures in adults. N Engl J Med 327:765–771, 1992.

138. Mattson RH, Cramer JA, Collins JF, et al: Comparison of carbamazepine, phenobarbital, phenytoin, and primidone in partial and secondarily generalized tonic-clonic seizures. N Engl J Med 313:145–151, 1985.

139. McCarthy AD, Barletta AP, Lux WE, Bleiberg J: Withdrawal of anticonvulsants in a head injury rehabilitation setting [abstract]. Arch Phys Med Rehabil 72:81, 1991.

140. McConnell F, Yablon S, Bontke C: The role of serum prolactin measurement in the diagnosis of late posttraumatic seizures [abstract]. Am J Phys Med Rehabil 72:235, 1993.

141. McNamara, JO, Rigsbee LC, Butler LS, Shin C: Intravenous phenytoin is an effective anticonvulsant in the kindling model. Ann Neurol 26:675–578, 1989.

142. McQueen JK, Blackwood DHR, Harris P, et al: Low risk of late posttraumatic seizures following severe head injury: Implications for clinical trials of prophylaxis. J Neurol Neurosurg Psychiatry 46:899–904, 1983.

143. Meador KJ, Loring DW, Abney OL, et al: Epilepsia 34:153–157, 1993.

144. Meador KJ, Loring DW, Allen ME, et al: Comparative cognitive effects of carbamazepine and phenytoin in healthy adults. Neurology 41:1537–1540, 1991.

145. Meador KJ, Loring DW, Huh K, et al: Comparative cognitive effects of anticonvulsants. Neurology 40:391–394, 1990.

146. Medical Research Council Antiepileptic Withdrawal Study Group: Randomized study of antiepileptic drug withdrawal in patients in remission. Lancet 337:1175–1180, 1991.

147. Meierkord H, Shorvon S, Lightman S, Trimble MB: Comparison of the effects of frontal and temporal lobe seizures on prolactin levels. Arch Neurol 49:225–230, 1992.

148. Messing RO, Closson RG, Simon RP: Drug-induced seizures: A 10-year experience. Neurology 34:1582–1586, 1984.

149. Messing RO, Simon RP: Seizures as a manifestation of systemic disease. Neurol Clin 4:563–584, 1986.

150. Mises J, Lerique-Koechlin A, Rimoot BP: Posttraumatic epilepsy in children. Epilepsia 11:37–39, 1976.

151. Mumford JP, Cannon DJ. Vigabatrin. Epilepsia 35 (Suppl 5): S25–S28, 1994.

152. Murri L, Arrigo A, Bonuccelli U, et al: Phenobarbital in the prophylaxis of late posttraumatic seizures. Ital J Neurol Sci 13:755–760, 1992.

153. Murri L, Parenti G, Bonnucelli U: Phenobarbital prophylaxis of posttraumatic epilepsy. Ital J Neurol Sci 1:225–230, 1980.

154. national Association of Epilepsy Centers: Patient referral to specialty epilepsy care. Epilepsia 31 (Suppl 1): S10–S11, 1990.

155. Oxley J, Roberts M: Clinical evaluation of 4-channel ambulatory EEG monitoring in the management of patients with epilepsy. J Neurol Neurosurg Psychiatry 48:930–932, 1985.

156. Özkara C, Dreifuss FE: Differential diagnosis in pseudoepileptic seizures. Epilepsia 34:294–298, 1993.

157. Paillas JE, Paillas N, Bureau M: Posttraumatic epilepsy. Introduction and clinical observations. Epilepsia 5–16, 1970.

158. Pagni CA: Posttraumatic epilepsy. Incidence and prophylaxis. Acta Neurochir Suppl (Wien) 50:38–47, 1990.

159. Payan H, Toga M, Berard-Badier M: The pathology of posttraumatic epilepsies. Epilepsia 11:81–84, 1970.

160. Pechadre JC, Lauxerois M, Colnet G, et al: Prevention de L'epilepsie post-traumatique tardive par phenytoine dans les traumatismes craniens graves. Suivi durant 2 ans. Presse Med 20:841– 845, 1991.

161. Pellock JM: Carbamazepine side effects in children and adults. Epilepsia 28 (Suppl 3): S64–S70, 1987.

162. Pellock JM: Who should receive prophylactic antiepileptic drug following head injury? Brain Inj 3:107–108, 1989.

163. Pellock JM, Willmore LJ: A rational guide to routine blood monitoring in patients receiving antiepileptic drugs. Neurology 41:961–964, 1991.

164. Penry JK, White BG, Brackett CE: A controlled prospective study of the pharmacologic prophylaxis of posttraumatic epilepsy [abstract]. Neurology 29:600–601, 1979.

165. Phillips G: Traumatic epilepsy after closed head injury. J Neurol Neurosurg Psychiatry 17:1–10, 1954.

166. Porter RJ: How to initiate and maintain carbamazepine therapy in children and adults. Epilepsia 28 (Suppl 3): S59–S63, 1987.

167. Porter RJ, Kelley KR: Antiepileptic drugs and mild liver function elevation. JAMA 253:1791–1792, 1985.

168. Pritchard PB III, Wannamaker BB, Sagel J, Daniel CM: Serum prolactin and cortisol levels in evaluation of pseudoepileptic seizures. Ann Neurol 18: 87–89, 1895.

169. Price DJ: The efficiency of sodium valproate as the only anticonvulsant administered to neurosurgical patients. In Parsonage MJ, Caldwell ADS (eds): The Place of Sodium Valproate in the Treatment of Epilepsy. London, Academic Press, 1980, pp 23–34.

170. Prince DA, Connors BW: Mechanisms of epileptogenesis in cortical structures. Ann Neurol 16: (Suppl): S59–S64, 1984.

171. Ramsay RE: Advances in the pharmacotherapy of epilepsy. Epilepsia 34 (Suppl 5): S9–S16, 1993.

172. Ramsay RE, Slater JD: Effects of antiepileptic drugs on hormones. Epilepsia 32: (Suppl 6): S60–S67, 1991.

173. Rapport RL II, Penry JD: A survey of attitudes toward the pharmacological prophylaxis of posttraumatic epilepsy. J Neurosurg 38:159–166, 1973.

174. Reisner T, Zeiler K, Wessely P: The value of CT and EEG in cases of posttraumatic epilepsy. J Neurol 221:93–100, 1979.

175. Reynolds EH: Chronic antiepileptic toxicity. A review. Epilepsia 16:319–352, 1975.

176. Reynolds EH: Vinyl GABA (Vigabatrin): Clinical experience in adult and adolescent patients with intractable epilepsy. Epilepsia 33 (Suppl 5):S30–S35, 1992.

177. Reynolds EH, Trimble MR: Adverse neuropsychiatric effects of anticonvulsant drugs. Drugs 29: 570–581, 1985.

178. Richens A: Safety of lamotrigine. Epilepsia 35 (Suppl 5): S37–S40, 1994.

179. Ring HA, Heller AJ, Farr IN, Reynolds EH: Vigabatrin: Rational treatment for chronic epilepsy. J Neurol Neurosurg Psychiatry 53:1051–1055, 1990.

180. Rish B, Caveness W: Relation of prophylactic medication to the occurrence of early seizures following craniocerebral trauma. J Neurosurg 38: 155–158, 1973.

181. Rish BL, Dillon JD, Weiss GH: Mortality following penetrating craniocerebral injuries. J Neurosurg 59:775–780, 1983.

182. Roberts RJ, Gorman LL, Lee GP, et al: The phenomenology of multiple partial seizure-like symptoms without stereotyped spells: An epilepsy spectrum disorder? Epilepsy Res 13:167–177, 1992.

183. Rocca WA, Sharbrough FW, Hauser WA, et al: Risk factors for complex partial seizures. A population based case-control study. Ann Neurol 21:22–31, 1987.

184. Rodin E: An assessment of current views on epilepsy. Epilepsia 28:261–271, 1987.

185. Rolak LA, Rutecki P, Ashizawa T, Harati Y: Clinical features of Todd's post-epileptic paralysis. J Neurol Neurosurg Psychiatry 55:63–64, 1992.

186. Russell WR, Whitty CWM: Studies in traumatic epilepsy: I. Factors influencing the incidence of epilepsy after brain wounds. J Neurol Neurosurg Psychiatry 15:93–98, 1952.

187. Sachdeo R, Kramer LD, Rosenberg A, Sachdeo S: Felbamate monotherapy: Controlled trial in patients with partial onset seizures. Ann Neurol 32:386–392, 1992.

188. Salazar AM, Amin D, Vance SC, et al: Epilepsy after penetrating head injury: Effects of lesion location. In Wolf P, Dam M, Janz D, Dreifuss FE (eds): Advances in Epilepsy, vol 16, New York, Raven Press, 1987, 753–757.

189. Salazar AM, Grafman J, Jabbari G, et al: Epilepsy and cognitive loss after penetrating head injury. In Wolf P, Dam M, Janz D, Dreifuss FE (eds): Advances in Epilepsy, vol 16. New York, Raven Press, 1987; pp 627–631.

190. Salazar AM, Jabbari B, Vance SC, et al: Epilepsy after penetrating head injury: I. Clinical Correlates. Neurology 35:1406–1414, 1985.

191. Sato M, Racine RJ, McIntyre DC: Kindling Basic mechanisms and clinical validity. Electroencephalogr Clin Neurophysiol 76:459–472, 1990.

192. Sazbon L, Groswasser Z: Outcome in 134 patients with prolonged posttraumatic unawareness. Part 1: Parameters determining late recovery of consciousness. J Neurosurg 72:75–80, 1990.

193. Schaumann BA, Annegers JF, Johnson SB, et al: Family history of seizures in posttraumatic and alcohol-associated seizure disorders. Epilepsia 35: 48–52, 1994.

194. Schallert T, Hernandez TD, Barth TM: Recovery of function after brain damage. Severe and chronic disruption by diazepam. Brain Res 379:104–111, 1986.

195. Scherzer E, Wessely P: EEG in posttraumatic epilepsy. Eur Neurol 17:38–42, 1978.

196. Scheuer ML, Pedley TA: The evaluation and treatment of seizures. N Engl J Med 323:1468–1474, 1990.

197. Schmidt D: Withdrawal of antiepileptic drugs. In Wolf P, Dam M, Janz D, Dreifuss FE (eds): Advances in Epilepsy, vol 16. New York, Raven Press, 1987, pp 373–377.

198. Schmutz M, Klebs K, Baltzer V: Inhibition or enhancement of kindling evolution by antiepileptics. J Neural Transm 72:245–257, 1988.

199. Schwab K, Grafman J, Salazar AM, Kraft J: Residual impairments and work status 15 years after penetrating head injury: Report from the Vietnam Head Injury Study. Neurology 43:95–103, 1993.

200. Scolnik D, Nulman I, Rovet J, et al: Neurodevelopment of children exposed in utero to phenytoin and carbamazepine monotherapy. JAMA 271: 767–770, 1994.

201. Servit Z, Musil F: Prophylactic treatment of posttraumatic epilepsy: Results of a long-term follow-up in Czechoslovakia. Epilepsia 22:315–320, 1981.

202. Silver JM, Shin C, McNamara JO: Antiepileptogenic effects of conventional anticonvulsants in the kindling model of epilepsy. Ann Neurol 29:356–363, 1991.

203. Smith DB, Mattson RH, Cramer JA, et al: Veterans Administration Epilepsy Cooperative Study Group: Results of a nationwide Veterans Administration cooperative study comparing the efficacy and toxicity of carbamazepine, phenobarbital, phenytoin, and primidone. Epilepsia 28 (Suppl 3): S50–S58, 1987.

204. Smith KR Jr, Goulding PM, Wilderman D, et al: neurobehavioral effects of phenytoin and carbamazepine in patients recovering from trauma: A comparative study. Arch Neurol 51:653–660, 1994.

205. Snow RB, Zimmerman RD, Gandy SE: Comparison of magnetic resonance imaging and computed tomography in the evaluation of head injury. Neurosurgery 18:45–52, 1986.

206. Soroker N, Groswasser Z, Costeff H: Practice of prophylactic anticonvulsant treatment in head injury. Brain Inj 3:137–140, 1989.

207. Sparadeo FR, Strauss D, Barth JT: The incidence, impact, and treatment of substance abuse in head trauma rehabilitation. J Head Trauma Rehabil 5(3):1–8, 1990.

208. Spencer SS, Spencer DD, Williamson PD, Mattson RH: Sexual automatisms in complex partial seizures. Neurology 33:527–533, 1983.

209. Sutula T, Xiao-Xian H, Cavazos J, Scott G: Synaptic reorganization in the hippocampus induced by abnormal functional activity. Science 239: 1147–1150, 1988.

210. Temkin NR, Dikmen SS, Wilensky AJ, et al: A randomized double-blind study of phenytoin for the prevention of posttraumatic seizures. N Engl J Med 323:497–502, 1990.

211. Temkin NR, Dikmen SS, Wilensky AJ, et al: Phenytoin for the prevention of posttraumatic seizures [letter]. N Engl J Med 324:341, 1991.

212. Temkin NR, Dikmen SS, Winn HR: Posttraumatic seizures. Neurosurg Clin 2:425–435, 1991.

213. Tharp BR: Orbital frontal seizures. An unique electroencephalographic and clinical syndrome. Epilepsia 13:627–642, 1972.

214. Theodore WH, Porter RJ, Raubertas RF: Seizures during barbiturate withdrawal: Relation to blood level. Ann Neurol 22:644–647, 1987.

215. Thomaides TN, Kerezoudi EP, Chaudhuri KR, Cheropoulos C: Study of EEGs following 24-hour sleep deprivation in patients with posttraumatic epilepsy. Eur Neurol 32:79–82, 1992.

216. Thomsen IV. Late outcome of very severe blunt head trauma: A 10-15 year second follow-up. J Neurol Neurosurg Psychiatry 47:260–268, 1984.

217. Treiman DM: Current treatment strategies in selected situations in epilepsy. Epilepsia 34 (Suppl 5): S17–S23, 1993.

218. Treiman DM: Epilepsy and violence: Medical and legal issues. Epilepsia 27 (Suppl 2): S77–S104, 1986.

219. Psychobiology of ictal aggression. In Smith D, Treiman D, Trimble M (eds): Advances in Neurology, vol 55. New York, Raven Press, pp 341–356, 1991.

220. Trimble MR: Cognitive effects of anticonvulsants [letter]. Neurology 41:326, 1991.

221. Trimble MR: Pseudoseizures. Neurol Clin 4:531–548, 1986.

222. Tsukahara N: Synaptic plasticity in the mammalian central nervous system. Annu Rev Neurosci 4:351–379, 1981.

223. Turner IM, Newman SM, Louis S, Kutt H: Pharmacological prophylaxis against the development of kindled amygdaloid seizures. Ann Neurol 2:221–224, 1977.

224. Tuunainen A, Nousiainen U, Mervaala E, Riekkinen P: Efficacy of a 1- to 3-day ambulatory electroencephalogram in recording epileptic seizures. Arch Neurol 47:799–800, 1990.

225. U.S. Gabapentin Study Group No. 5: Gabapentin as add-on therapy in refractory partial epilepsy: A double-blind, placebo-controlled, parallel-group study. Neurology 43:2292–2298, 1993.

226. van Donselaar CA, Schimsheimer RJ, Geerts AT, Declerck AC: Value of the electroencephalogram in adult patients with untreated idiopathic first seizures. Arch Neurol 49:231–237, 1992.

227. van Zomeren AH: Acquired brain damage and driving: A review. Arch Phys Med Rehabil 68:697–705, 1987.

228. Varney NR, Hines ME, Bailey C, Roberts RJ: Neuropsychiatric correlates of theta bursts in patients with closed head injury. Brain Inj 6:245–260, 1992.

229. Verduyn WH, Hilt J, Roberts MA, Roberts RJ: Multiple partial seizure-like symptoms following 'minor' closed head injury. Brain Inj 6:245–260, 1992.

230. Vining EPG: Use of barbiturates and benzodiazepines in treatment of epilepsy. Neurol Clin 4:617–632, 1986.

231. Wada JA: Erosion of kindled epileptogenesis and kindling-induced long-term seizure suppressive effect in primates. In Wada JA (ed): Kindling 4. New York, Plenum Press, 383–385, 1990.

232. Wada JA: Pharmacological prophylaxis in the kindling model of epilepsy. Arch Neurol 34:389–395, 1977.

233. Wada JA, Osawa T: The generalized convulsive seizure state induced by daily electrical amygdaloid stimulation in Senegalese baboons, Papio papio. Neurology 26:273–286, 1976.

234. Wada JA, Sato M, Wake A, et al: Prophylactic effects of phenytoin, phenobarbital, and carbamazepine examined in kindling cat preparations. Arch Neurol 33:426–434, 1976.

235. Walker AE, Blumer D: The fate of World War II veterans with posttraumatic seizures. Arch Neurol 46:23–26, 1989.

236. Walker AE, Jablon S: A follow-up of head injured men of World War II. J Neurosurg 16:600–610, 1959.

238. Walker AE, Jablon S: A follow-up study of head wounds in World War II (Veterans Administration Medical Monograph). Washington, D.C., U.S. Government Printing Office, 1961.

239. Watson CW: Incidence of epilepsy following cranial cerebral injury. II: Three year follow-up study. Arch Neurol Psychiatry (Chicago) 68:831–834, 1952.

240. Weiss GH, Caveness WF, Eisiedel-Lechtape H, McNeel M: Life expectancy and causes of death in a group of head-injured veterans of World War I. Arch Neurol 39:741–743, 1982.

241. Weiss GH, Feeney DM, Caveness WF, et al: Prognostic factors for the occurrence of posttraumatic epilepsy. Arch Neurol 40:7–10, 1983.

242. Weiss GH, Salazar AM, Vance SC, et al: Predicting epilepsy in penetrating head injury. Arch Neurol 43:771–773, 1986.

243. Whitty CWM: Early traumatic epilepsy. Brain 70:416–439, 1947.

244. Whyte J, Rosenthal M: Rehabilitation of the patient with traumatic brain injury. In DeLisa JA (ed): Rehabilitation Medicine: Principles and Practice, 2nd ed. Philadelphia, J.B. Lippincott, 1993, pp 825–860.

245. Wiederholt WC, Melton LJ III, Anneegers JF, et al: Short-term outcomes of skull fracture: A population-based study of survival and neurologic complications. Neurology 39:96–100, 1989.

246. Wilberger JE, Deeb Z, Rothfus W: Magnetic resonance imaging in cases of severe head injury. Neurosurgery 20:571–576, 1987.

247. Williamson PD, Spencer SS: Clinical and EEG features of complex partial seizures of extratemporal origin. Epilepsia 27 (Suppl 2):S46–S63, 1986.

248. Willmore LJ: Posttraumatic epilepsy: Cellular mechanisms and implications for treatment. Epilepsia 31 (Suppl 3):S67–S73, 1990.

249. Willmore LJ, Sypert GW, Munson JB: Recurrent seizures induced by cortical iron injection: A model of posttraumatic epilepsy. Ann Neurol 4:329–336, 1978.

250. Wilson DM: Head injuries in servicemen of the 1939–1045 war. N Z Med J 50:383–391, 1951.

251. Wohns RNW, Wyler AR: Prophylactic phenytoin in severe head injuries. J Neurosurg 57:507–509, 1979.

252. Wolf P: New antiepileptic drugs already registered. Epilepsia 35 (Suppl 5):S22–S24, 1994.

253. Wroblewski B: Epileptic potential of stimulants, dopaminergics, and antidepressants. J Head Trauma Rehabil 7 (3):109–111, 1992.

254. Wroblewski BA, Glenn MB, Whyte J, Singer WD: Carbamazepine replacement of phenytoin, phenobarbital and primidone in a rehabilitation setting: Effects on seizure control. Brain Inj 3:149–156, 1989.

255. Wroblewski BA, Leary JM, Phelan Am, et al: Methylphenidate and seizure frequency in brain injured patients with seizure disorders. J Clin Psychiatry 53:86–89, 1992.

256. Wroblewski BA, McColgan K, Smith K, et al: The incidence of seizures during tricyclic antidepressant drug treatment in a brain-injured population. J Clin Psychopharmacol 10:124–128, 1990.

257. Wyllie E (ed): The Treatment of Epilepsy: Principles and Practice. Philadelphia, Lea & Febiger, 1993.

258. Yablon SA: Posttraumatic seizures. Arch Phys Med Rehabil 74:983–1001, 1993.

259a. Yablon SA: Unpublished data, 1994.

259. Young B, Rapp R, Brooks W, et al: Posttraumatic epilepsy prophylaxis. Epilepsia 20:671–681, 1979.

260. Young B, Rapp RP, Norton JA, et al: Failure of prophylactically administered phenytoin to prevent early posttraumatic seizures. J Neurosurg 58:231–235, 1983.

261. Young B, Rapp RP, Norton JA, et al: Failure of prophylactically administered phenytoin to prevent late posttraumatic seizures. J Neurosurg 58:236–241, 1983.

262. Young B, Rapp RP, Norton JA, et al: Failure of prophylactically administered phenytoin to prevent posttraumatic seizures in children. Childs Brain 10:185–192, 1983.

263. Yoshii N, Samejima H, Sakiyama R, Mizokami T: Posttraumatic epilepsy and CT scan. Neuroradiology 16:311–313, 1978.

264. Yuen AWC: Lamotrigine: A review of antiepileptic efficacy. Epilepsia 35 (Suppl 5):S33–S36, 1994.

265. Zasler ND: Advances in neuropharmacological rehabilitation for brain dysfunction. Brain Inj 6:1–14, 1992.

266. Zivan L, Ajmone-Marsan C: Incidence and prognostic significance of "epileptiform" activity in the EEG of non-epileptic subjects. Brain 91:751–758, 1968.

CINDY B. IVANHOE M.D.

CATHERINE F. BONTKE M.D.

15

Movement Disorders after Traumatic Brain Injury

DEFINITION

Movement disorders may be defined as neurologic disorders characterized by either an excess or decrease or absence of movement. Brain injury usually is listed as a cause in the assessment of movement disorders, yet the variable nature of these disorders makes the establishment of a causal relationship difficult. Onset of posttraumatic movement disorders may be delayed for variable periods. Just as the onset of presentation is unpredictable, so are the course and response to treatment. Evaluation should include an assessment of quality, rhythmicity, speed, duration, pattern, and inciting event.

The neurochemical disturbances leading to movement disorders are not well understood; the pharmacotherapy, therefore, is based largely on conjecture. Difficult medicolegal considerations may complicate the evaluation process. There is no clear correlation between the severity of the traumatic brain injury and the development or degree of severity of the movement disorder. With the rare exception of nocturnal myoclonus, abnormal movements generally decrease during sleep, although even this rule has its exceptions. Stress or anxiety increase the appearance of the movement disorder, as do the hormonal influences of puberty and menses.

NEUROANATOMIC CORRELATES

Although knowledge of the neuroanatomy of the structures involved in movement disorders has increased over the last few decades, their intricate interactions are not well understood. For a detailed description of anatomy and neurophysiology, the reader is referred elsewhere.[3,81]

The corticospinal and corticobulbar fibers arise from the sensorimotor cortex in and around the precentral and postcentral gyri. Throughout their path through the central nervous system, they remain somatotopically organized.[1] The corticospinal fibers, which connect with the lower motor neurons of the spinal cord, descend in the dorsal area of the posterior limb of the internal capsule. They then decussate and terminate on the lower motor neuron. The corticonuclear fibers, which run from the motor cortex to the lower motor neurons of the cranial nerves, pass through the internal capsule and cerebral peduncles to the motor nuclei of cranial nerves V, VII, IX, X and XII in the pons and medulla.

The basal ganglia are the primary areas of the brain involved in the pathogenesis of movement disorders. This group of periventricular subcortical structures surrounds the thalamus and hypothalamus. They are prone to damage from the effects of increased intracranial pressure and mechanical disruption. The superior cerebellar peduncle (brachium conjunctivum) is particularly susceptible to damage from rotational injury. Basal ganglia and cerebellar inputs to the motor cortex are believed to converge.

The striatum (caudate and putamen) is the main afferent structure of the basal ganglia, receiving projections from all cortical areas. The somatosensory and motor cortices project mainly to the putamen, which is considered the motor portion of the thalamus. Other cortical areas, including the prefrontal cortex, project to the caudate. Normally, this nucleus has a high density of D2 receptors. The striatum also receives input from the ventral midbrain and thalamus.

Direct and indirect pathways back to the cortex have been identified. The direct pathway involves D1 receptors and is excitatory. The indirect pathway involves D2 receptors and is considered inhibitory. Via the indirect pathway the subthalamic nucleus gates output of the medial globus pallidus and substantia nigra, utilizing glutamate as the neurotransmitter. Most of the basal ganglionic and cerebellar fibers ascend through the ventrolateral nucleus of the thalamus, linking the cerebellum with the higher structures. Projections from the cerebellum to the thalamic nuclei regulate motor activity.

Functionally, the cerebellum can be conceived as three areas. The midline area or vermis is predominantly involved in posture and truncal movement. Moving laterally, the paravermal area regulates limb posture. The most lateral portion is the cerebellar cortex and the dentate nuclei, which coordinate fine finger and eye movements. Under normal circumstances, the performance of the basal ganglia and the cerebellum is smoothly integrated, modulating the corticospinal and cortico-brainstem-spinal (pyramidal) system. The superior cerebellar peduncle contains efferents from the dentate nucleus of the cerebellum to the red nucleus in the tegmentum of the midbrain. The red nucleus then relays fibers to the thalamus and spinal cord, making it an integral component of motor control.

Not all neurotransmitters involved in the interactions of the basal ganglia nuclei have been identified. The striatum itself is thought to be inhibitory. Most afferents to the striatum run in the corticostriatal pathway, with glutamate as the neurotransmitter. The striatum is composed of many different cell types[81] with differing roles. Neurotransmitters thought to play a role in motor control include acetylcholine (the most abundant), gamma aminobutyric acid (GABA), somatostatin, and glutamate. Dopamine has an inhibitory effect, whereas acetylcholine is excitatory. These neurons project to the globus pallidus (medial and lateral) and the substantia nigra. The neurons of the globus pallidus utilize GABA as an inhibitory neurotransmitter. The lateral globus pallidus predominantly projects to the subthalamic nucleus, which also receives excitatory input from the motor cortex. Glutamic acid is believed to act as the neurotransmitter. Projections extend from the subthalamic nucleus to the lateral globus pallidus, medial globus pallidus, and substantia nigra pars reticulata. The medial globus pallidus projects to the ventral lateral nucleus of the thalamus. Projections between the subthalamic nucleus and globus pallidus medialis have an established role in parkinsonism in animal models. Dopamine is found in highest concentrations in the substantia nigra and striatum. Stimulation of the substantia nigra elicits further release of dopamine from the striatum, which leads to inhibitory effects on the neostriatal fibers.

GABA is also found in high concentrations in the substantia nigra and striatum. The medial globus pallidus and substantia nigra send inhibitory GABA-ergic projections to the thalamus and brainstem. The thalamus, in turn, projects predominantly to the prefrontal cortex as well as the motor cortex. The neurotransmitter remains unidentified, but glutamate is suspected.

Complex loops and interactions exist among the many nuclei and their ascending and descending tracts. There are at least five corticobasal ganglia-thalamo-cortical circuits: motor, ocular, limbic, dorsolateral, and lateral orbitofrontal.[4] Some degree of dopaminergic interaction exists among these circuits and probably explains the range of movement disorders that can be manifested. In summary, the basal ganglia facilitate movement and inhibit unwanted motor activity. Many hypotheses have been proposed to explain the complex interactions of these structures and the clinical findings associated with their dysfunction.

RIGIDITY

Increased muscle tone with resultant spasticity and rigidity are common findings after traumatic brain injury. Spasticity, which may be defined as velocity-dependent increased resistance to stretch, results from a lowering of the stretch receptor threshold. Rigidity refers to increased resistance to movement, independent of velocity. Muscle tone is increased throughout the entire range of motion. Patients with rigidity are likely to demonstrate slowed movements and loss of postural stability. Rigidity is more common in the flexor muscle groups, although other patterns may be seen.

Patients in coma or a state of minimal responsiveness manifest rigidity as decerebrate or decorticate posturing. In its pure form, decorticate posturing indicates a lesion involving the cortex, internal capsule, basal ganglia, or thalamus. Decerebrate posturing indicates injury to the midportion of the brainstem or above. Because diffuse cerebral damage is incurred after a traumatic brain injury, variable combinations of the two patterns may coexist.

The rehabilitation management of posturing includes multiple modalities, such as positioning techniques to decrease posturing in bed and creation of appropriate seating systems. Creation of a positioning/seating system is often a matter of trial and error. Head straps designed to maintain proper head control and alignment may increase the tendency toward neck flexion. Foam wedges placed appropriately for positioning in bed may encourage knee flexion in patients with lower extremity extensor tone. Passive range of motion and stretching are vital to guard against the loss of future potential range. Serial casting and neurolytic procedures

such as phenol injections and chemodenervation with botulinum toxin should be considered and used judiciously. These procedures are especially useful when deformities are not yet fixed. They also have a role in controlling tone in patients undergoing surgical procedures for contractures, provided tone is still an issue. Consideration must be given to the potential risk of decreasing functional strength.

PARKINSONISM

Definition

Parkinson's disease (PD) is an idiopathic disorder that leads to degeneration of the pars compacta of the substantia nigra with development of Lewy bodies (eosinophilic inclusion bodies). The cardinal features of the disease include bradykinesia, rest tremor, loss of postural reflexes, and rigidity. Parkinsonism describes the clinical manifestations of PD associated with an identified cause. Actual posttraumatic parkinsonism is a rare complication of traumatic brain injury. It is more likely to occur after severe injuries, but other neurologic impairments may mask the signs and symptoms.

Historical Background

The relationship of trauma to the development of Parkinson's disease was ignored until the advent of workmen's compensation legislation in Europe during the late 1800s. The disease was believed to be related to peripheral trauma. In 1911 Kurt Mendel suggested a link between cerebral trauma and Parkinson's disease. During World War I, Guillain and Barré,[1] among other neurologists, associated parkinsonism with mesencephalic injury. However, the first case of posttraumatic parkinsonism with pathologic documentation was reported in 1928. The patient had developed a parkinsonian syndrome after sustaining a gunshot wound to the left temporal area. After 6 years of progressive disease he agreed to have the bullet removed from the left frontal lobe. A chronic subdural hematoma was also found. The patient died after the procedure. Postmortem findings included hemorrhagic lesions in the lenticular and subthalamic nuclei of the basal ganglia.

Crouzon and Justin-Besancon published the first review of posttraumatic parkinsonism, entitled "Le Parkinsonisme traumatique," in 1929. They defined diagnostic criteria to establish the relationship between trauma and the disease: the trauma should be sufficiently violent and lead to a concussion; the interval between the trauma and onset of parkinsonism should be "short"; and the course of the disease should be uninterrupted.

In 1934, Grimberg studied 86 cases of presumed posttraumatic parkinsonism, but only two cases were attributed to trauma after review. He concluded that parkinsonism may result from significant head injury with cerebral injury. Until that time, mild injuries were considered adequate to cause the syndrome. More authors have subsequently reported cases of posttraumatic parkinsonism. Patients present with loss of consciousness, changes in mental status, and evidence of cranial nerve or pyramidal tract dysfunction. Crouzan's criteria should be met to link the traumatic event with the syndrome.[26]

Pugilistic Parkinsonism

Pugilistic parkinsonism with dementia pugilistica is another form of parkinsonism associated with trauma. Unlike the cases described above, this syndrome results from cumulative brain injury due to boxing. Boxers may display varying degrees of symptoms of progressive chronic neurologic injury years after discontinuing their boxing careers. Severity correlates with the length of the career and the number of bouts fought. Multiple subconcussive blows to the head result in neurofibrillary degeneration of the substantia nigra and medial temporal cortex. Accelerated deposition of beta-amyloid plaques, resembling the findings in Alzheimer's disease, also may be responsible for the clinical findings. Widespread damage involving the ventricles, corpus callosum, septum pellucidum, and cerebellum also have been described. Lewy bodies are not found. Maki[56] postulated that shearing forces disrupt branches of the lateral perforator of the middle cerebral artery. Rapid rotation also may contribute to shearing forces in pugilistic parkinsonism.

Hemiparkinsonism with Hemiatrophy

Hemiparkinsonism with hemiatrophy is a disease characterized by hemiatrophy due to birth trauma. Ipsilateral parkinsonism develops in adulthood. Dopaminergic pharmacotherapy has been effective in its management.

Treatment of Parkinsonism

Dopamine precursors such as L-dopa and L-dopa/carbidopa remain the preferred treatment of parkinsonism. Dopamine agonists such as bromocriptine and pergolide are also freely incorporated into treatment. These drugs are less likely to produce the dyskinesias associated with prolonged levodopa therapy. Anticholinergic medications such as trihexyphenidyl may be particularly effective in the treatment of tremor, but patients with brain injury are more susceptible to the side effects. In addition, anticholinergics are not as effective as dopamine agonists for rigidity and bradykinesia.[48] Deprenyl and the antioxidant vitamins C and E may delay disability in the early stages, at least of Parkinson's disease.[27]

Rehabilitation Interventions

All disciplines of rehabilitation have a role in the management of parkinsonism. Therapists address the tendency for contracture formation as well as maintenance of strength and coordination. Relaxation techniques have proved effective in decreasing rigidity. Bradykinesia can be addressed through proprioceptive neuromuscular facilitation, biofeedback, and neurodevelopmental techniques. Adaptive equipment, such as gait aids, needs to be evaluated on an individual basis. Rolling walkers may increase the tendency for festination. Occupational therapy addresses fine motor coordination and adaptive equipment for activities of daily living. Micrographia also may be addressed. Speech therapists may have some success in improving breath support of soft, breathy vocal quality or in the selection of amplification aids.

TREMOR

Classification

Tremor is the most common form of involuntary movement. Movements are rhythmic and oscillatory, produced by contractions of antagonistic muscle groups. Tremors may be divided into resting tremors and intention or action tremors. Action tremors may be further divided into postural, kinetic, position-specific, and isometric. Postural tremors are evident during sustained contraction of antigravity muscles, such as maintaining upper extremities in an outstretched posture. Kinetic tremors may be observed during the initiation, course, or end (terminal tremor) of a movement. They are thought to originate from lesions of the cerebellar outflow pathway (dentate nucleus and superior cerebellar peduncle). Task-specific and position-specific tremors, as their names imply, occur only during specific activities or postures, respectively. Isometric tremors occur during voluntary isometric contractions. In addition, isolated tremors of various body parts have been documented.

Tremor can be assessed through videotaping. Surface electromyography, accelerometer recordings, and frequency analysis provide quantification. The frequency of most tremors is 4–10 Hz. Tremors of 1–3 Hz are designated as slow, whereas tremors of 11–20 Hz are considered fast. Slow tremors usually are associated with brainstem damage. Isolated episodic tongue tremor has been described after traumatic brain injury. The frequency was 3 Hz, and symptoms began within 2–4 months after injury. Brainstem damage was suspected clinically.

Several cases of tremor after brain injury have been reported.[51] Although most were observed in patients following coma, the injury need not be severe. Computerized tomography is often not helpful. Biary et al.[8] described 7 patients who developed tremors after mild brain injury without loss of consciousness. Clonazepam and propranolol were somewhat effective.

Tremor may appear at any time after traumatic brain injury, although the average latency was 10.6 months in one series.[69] It is postulated that the delay in appearance is related to axonal sprouting, changes in receptor sensitivity, or neuronal degeneration. These theories also apply to other disorders mentioned in this chapter.

Pharmacologic Management

Medications found to be of some usefulness in the management of tremors include propranolol, clonazepam, and valproic acid. Peripheral beta adrenergic receptors are believed to play a role in the amplitude of physiologic tremor. Propranolol is the most effective treatment for physiologic tremor. Other beta blockers also may be effective. Although a central mechanism of action has been presumed, the effectiveness of beta blockers that do not penetrate the blood-brain barrier suggests a peripheral mechanism.[34] Side effects of fatigue, sedation, and memory impairment must be weighed against the degree of disability imposed by the particular tremor. Propranolol was demonstrated to be effective in the treatment of action tremor that developed in two children after traumatic brain injury. Although the sample was small, both children served as their own control.[25] Arotinolol was also studied for the treatment of essential tremor.[53] Tremor improved in all 8 patients taking this beta blocker for 8 weeks at a dose of 30 mg/day. Clonidine is effective in desynchronizing tremor by decreasing its amplitude. It has fewer side effects than beta blockers.[18] Primidone, clonazepam, and lorazepam also may have ameliorating effects. Botulinum toxin injections are now being applied to tremor. In an open trial, 61% of patients exhibited at least some improvement in disability.[46] Surgical interventions for tremor are addressed later in this chapter.

Tremor is a frequent manifestation of damage to the cerebellum or its connections. It may be intentional, occurring during voluntary activity, or postural, occurring when posture is maintained against gravity. The pathognomic feature of cerebellar tremor is that it becomes exaggerated during fine, more precise activity. Lesions of the dentate nucleus in the cerebellum or its outflow tract produce tremor of the ipsilateral side. Lesions above the decussation of the cerebral peduncles, in the midbrain around the red nucleus, produce contralateral tremor, also referred to as rubral tremor.

Cerebellar tremors oscillate at a frequency of 4–5 Hz. The presentation of the tremor during movement is related to the severity of the lesion. Milder tremors may not be visible until the end of the movement, such as touching the tip of the nose or the fingertip of the examiner. With increasing severity the tremor affects more proximal musculature and is therefore visible sooner during the action. Like other movement disorders, cerebellar tremors disappear during sleep and worsen with stress. Cerebellar tremors may be difficult to differentiate from essential tremors, which also may increase as a target is approached. Other cerebellar findings, such as nystagmus, ataxia, or dysarthria, suggest a cerebellar origin to the tremor.

As with other tremors, weighting of limbs sometimes reduces their magnitude.[41] Alternatively, resultant muscle fatigue may increase the excursion of the tremor. Pharmacologic treatment of cerebellar tremor is unpredictable and to date unsuccessful. As previously mentioned, botulinum toxin may have a role in the treatment of disabling tremors in patients not amenable to neurosurgical interventions. Thalamic stimulation has been shown to be of benefit in at least one case of posttraumatic tremor.[12] Stereotactic thalamotomy may be effective for tremors that are significantly disabling, but underlying ataxia is not affected. Rubral tremor (midbrain tremor) results from lesions of fibers projecting from the dentate nucleus to the ventrolateral thalamic nucleus in the region of the red nucleus. It shares many features with the parkinsonian rest tremor but is also present with action and postural changes. Levodopa occasionally has been effective in treatment of rubral tremors related to multiple sclerosis that affect the red nucleus of the brainstem.

AKATHISIA

Akathisia is motor restlessness or a sense of inner restlessness. It is associated subjectively with dysphoria and is often misdiagnosed as anxiety or agitation. Patients cannot sit still and frequently pace or fidget. Like tics, akathisia is somewhat relieved by movement. Akathisia may be associated with a sensation of pain or burning. Milder forms may be manifested as toe tapping or other semipurposeful activity. Patients may relate difficulty with concentration or a feeling of uneasiness.

The proposed cause of akathisia is dopamine blockade in the prefrontal area.[76] In psychiatric patients with akathisia secondary to neuroleptic administration, the initial treatment is to reduce or discontinue the inciting drug. Bromocriptine, which acts presynaptically, has been suggested as a treatment, but it may exacerbate psychotic symptoms. Anticholinergics were suggested for use in schizophrenic patients, but aside from their undesirable side effects in patients with traumatic brain injury, they have not proved more effective than placebo.[76] Amantadine also has been suggested, but tolerance may develop.[51] It may be of use in patients who pass through akathisia as a stage of recovery after TBI. Benzodiazepines are of limited value for akathisia. Beta-adrenergic blockers may be more effective in some patients.

ATAXIA

Ataxia, the cardinal feature of cerebellar disease, results in irregular, discoordinated movements. Ataxias may be cerebellar, sensory, labyrinthine, or psychogenic in origin.

Hershkowitz et al. reported a case of ataxic hemiparesis after mild TBI.[39] Symptoms developed within 10 minutes of the injury. The patient's initial work-up was negative, but magnetic resonance imaging (MRI) 18 days after injury revealed abnormal signals in the midbrain. The authors point out that the incidence of isolated midbrain injuries after trauma is unknown. The relatively early onset of symptoms was believed to be compatible with infarction due to axonal injury. Therapeutic interventions for improving function in the face of ataxia include weighting utensils, coordination activities, and beta-adrenergic blockers to decrease the degree of ataxia (see the discussion of tremor). Other medications to consider include acetazolamide, phthalazinol, thyrotropin-releasing hormone, choline, and lecithin.[57] The actual mechanism of action for these agents is unknown.

ATHETOSIS

Athetosis presents as continuous slow, writhing movements (slow form of chorea). It more commonly affects the limbs but also may affect the axial musculature. When associated with chorea, it is referred to as choreoathetosis. Athetotic syndromes are more common in children than adults, with lesions in the basal ganglia. They often are associated with other forms of movement disorders. Surgical treatments include ventrolateral thalamotomy, stereotactic lesioning of the dentate nucleus, and electrical stimulation of the anterior cerebellum. Results vary.

BALLISM

Large-amplitude flinging or flailing movements caused by the proximal musculature describe ballism. Because the disorder is usually unilateral, it is referred to as hemiballism. Hemiballism is due to a lesion in the contralateral subthalamic nucleus or striatum. Biballism may be seen in patients with bilateral lacunes in the basal ganglia[9] and also has been attributed to administration of excessive amounts of levodopa.

Hemiballism is a relatively rare phenomenon but has occurred after TBI.[49] The onset may be weeks to months after injury is sustained, but immediate onset has been reported.[51] Pharmacologic management of hemiballism includes anticonvulsant therapy.[49] Valproic acid has reportedly been somewhat effective. Bullard et al. studied 11 patients with movement disorders secondary to severe traumatic brain injury. Nine patients exhibited hemiballism. Stereotactic thalamotomy yielded variable degrees of improvement.

CHOREA

Choreic movements are rapid, involuntary, irregular, and purposeless. The movements tend to flow from one body part to another. Choreas can be temporarily suppressed or partially incorporated into other movements (parakinesias).

Choreas are attributed to lesions in the contralateral subthalamic nucleus, striatum, and thalamic nuclei. Patients with bilateral lesions in the subthalamic nuclei may develop generalized chorea.[51] A small number of cases of choreoathetosis have been reported after TBI.[1,66] Presentation may be persistent or paroxysmal.

Chandra et al.[21] described a 28-year-old patient who developed delayed-onset choreoathetoid movements on the hemiplegic side many years after a TBI. The disorder responded to valproic acid. Anticonvulsants, particularly valproic acid and phenobarbital, have been found to be of benefit.[49] Approximately 50% of patients who undergo stereotactic destruction of part of the dentate nucleus of the cerebellum experience improvement.[48]

DYSTONIA

Classification

Dystonias are manifested by repetitive twisting movements of variable speed, involving almost any part of the body. They are recognized by their sustained quality. Dystonias related to posttraumatic brain injury may develop within minutes to years after the inciting event. Dyskinesias or varying abnormal movements also may be induced as a side effect of phenytoin.[38] They are sometimes classified according to the speed of movements. Athetotic dystonias are slow, whereas shocklike movements are described as myoclonic dystonia. If the abnormal movement is brief, it may be described as a dystonic spasm. Dystonic movements last for several seconds, whereas dystonic postures may last from minutes to hours.

Dystonias are also classified according to the number of body segments involved. Focal dystonias involve a single body part. Segmental dystonia involves two or more contiguous regions of the body. Finally, dystonias are sometimes classified according to the specific body parts affected. Cranial dystonias may involved the lingual and pharyngeal structures, as with spasmodic dysphonia. Spasmodic dysphonia or laryngeal dystonia is characterized by a strained or breathy vocal quality. Injection of botulinum toxin into the vocalis complex is now considered the first line of treatment.

The underlying pathology in dystonias may be disruption of pathways between the striatum and thalamus with sparing of the corticospinal pathways. Evidence also suggests that dystonias may be related to peripheral trauma and nerve damage.[42]

Clinical Presentation and Management

Muscle tone fluctuates between hypotonia and hypertonia. Voluntary movements aggravate dystonia, whereas sleep provides relief. Superficial sensory stimulation sometimes abolishes the dystonic movements. Dystonic movements may be suppressed using "sensory tricks," which refer to proprioceptive feedback that alters the degree to which the dystonia is manifested. Examples include holding the side of the head to attenuate nuchal dystonia or abducting the thumb to eliminate dystonic movements of the hand. It is sometimes difficult to distinguish the maneuver from the dystonia. Hemiparesis and evidence of striatal damage are risk factors for the development of dystonia. Onset of posttraumatic dystonias is usually delayed.[11,64] They may not develop until months or years after the initial injury and may continue to progress.

Blepharospasm, which is characterized by brief clonic contractions of the orbicularis oculi, is one form of cranial dystonia. When it is accompanied by oromandibular dystonia, it is referred to as Meige's syndrome. Meige's syndrome may be accompanied by dystonic spasms extending to the neck, limbs, or respiratory or abdominal musculature. In additions, tics may be present, mimicking Gilles de la Tourette's syndrome. Patients with blepharospasm may use tricks such as opening their mouths or manually opening their eyelids to initiate eye opening, giving the appearance of apraxia. Voluntary contractions of the frontalis muscle may be observed. Dystonia of the lower facial muscles, called oromandibular dystonia, may be manifested in different ways, including trismus, retraction of the corners of the mouth, tongue protrusion, jaw opening, or jaw tightening. Tics also may be present.

Pharmacologic treatment of oromandibular dystonic syndromes includes clonazepam, lorazepam, baclofen, and trihexiphenidyl. Tetrabenazine was not found to be useful in

the treatment of focal dystonias. Some patients experience symptomatic improvement at the expense of significant side effects.[42] The effectiveness of these medications is limited. Their utility must be weighed against their cognitive side effects, particularly in patients with TBI. In select patients submental injections of botulinum toxin may be preferable to treatment with systemic medications.

Surgical options for the treatment of blepharospasm include myectomy of the orbicularis, facial nerve sectioning, and brow lift.[42] Surgical complications include exposure keratitis, ptosis, and eyelid necrosis. Blepharospasm may recur within months. For these reasons, injection of botulinum toxin is now considered the first line of therapy. Ptosis is the most common side effect.

Cervical dystonia or spasmodic torticollis is a form of nuchal dystonia. The most common form is torticollis (twisting), but head movements may also be directed toward one shoulder (laterocollis), flexion (anterocollis), or extension (retrocollis). Relaxation techniques and physical therapy may help to prevent contractures. Cervical dystonias may cause pain. According to Chan et al., 75% of patients with spasmodic torticollis have pain related to continual contractions.[20]

Pharmacotherapy, although providing little relief for most patients, includes diazepam, lorazepam, clonazepam, cyclobenzaprine, and carbamazepine. Response to these medications is less than ideal. Variable results also have been attained with selective peripheral nerve denervation, but symptoms may recur.

A fair number of studies of hemidystonia have reported head injury as the cause of the dystonia. Maki et al. reported development of hemidystonia and transient athetosis in children with mild or severe traumatic brain injuries, respectively.[56] Pettigrew and Jankovic examined the causes of hemidystonia in 22 patients.[64] The latency of onset for hemidystonia was 14 months to 29 years. Delayed onset may be explained by aberrant neuronal sprouting. Patients have been treated with tetrabenazine, trihexyphenidyl or ethopropazine without success. Thalamotomy has provided mild or transient relief. Sellal et al. described a case of posttraumatic hemidystonia that developed two months after traumatic brain injury. The patient responded to electrical stimulation of the ventroposterolateral nucleus of the thalamus. After 8 months of reduction in dystonic posturing and improved arm swing during gait, the stimulator had to be removed because of scalp complications.[74]

Brett et al.[11] described a young girl who developed clenching of her right hand and difficulty with gait within 1 week after mild traumatic brain injury. She developed right dystonic posturing over the course of 24 months. Her condition improved with time. The cause was a discrete lesion in the contralateral basal ganglia.

Anticholinergic medications such as trihexyphenidyl have been effective in 50% of patients with idiopathic or secondary dystonia, but the side effects are not tolerated in patients with TBI.[49] About 2.5% of patients who receive neuroleptic medications develop acute dystonia within 48 hours. Treatment includes discontinuation of the neuroleptic and addition of an anticholinergic. Evidence suggests that treatment with anticholinergic medications may precipitate tardive dyskinesia[64] in addition to other undesirable side effects.

Posttraumatic hemidystonia may present during nonrapid eye movement sleep. Nocturnal paroxysmal dystonia (NPD) has been described with and without seizure activity. When accompanied by a normal electroencephalogram, such cases are generally refractory to anticonvulsant therapy.[9]

Trauma has been implicated in the onset of dystonia in a patient with a genetic predisposition to the syndrome.[29] Jabbari et al. reported traumatic axial dystonia after closed head injury.[40] The majority of patients fail to improve substantially with pharmacologic management. The most effective medications appear to be muscle relaxants and anticholinergics. In severe cases, dopamine-depleting agents such as tetrabenazine have been suggested. Their use, particularly in patients with TBI, must be weighed against the risk of side effects, such as tardive dyskinesia and other movement disorders. Botulinum toxin injections are now considered the treatment of choice for focal dystonias such as spasmodic dysphonia, torticollis, and blepharospasm, although the results are temporary.

Generally, when dystonic patients require systemic management for widespread involvement, levodopa and anticholinergic agents are instituted. If patients respond to levodopa, they do not usually have the long-term side effects experienced by patients with Parkinson's disease. If patients do not respond to these medications, other suggestions include drugs that are not advocated for use in the brain-injured population, such as clonazepam, baclofen, haloperidol, and diazepam. Intrathecal baclofen has been used to treat a patient with axial dystonia and is recommended for use in select cases of axial or generalized dystonia.[60]

Surgery for treatment of dystonia is reserved for severely disabled patients in whom botulinum toxin injections are not feasible and medications are ineffective. It may provide some relief in cases of severe distal limb dystonia or hemidystonia. Unilateral thalamotomy provides relief in up to 50% of cases. Bilateral thalamotomy increases the risk of creating a disabling dysarthria and is rarely recommended.

PROGRESSIVE SUPRANUCLEAR PALSY

Progressive supranuclear palsy (PSP) is frequently confused with parkinsonism. Like other parkinsonian syndromes, PSP is characterized by bradykinesia, rigidity, postural instability, and hypophonia. However, patients also display severe vertical gaze limitation, hypometric saccades, and dystonic or rigid contraction of the facial muscles. Unlike parkinsonism, patients with PSP do not display a resting tremor and are not responsive to dopaminergic interventions. The presentation is relatively symmetric, and axial rigidity is disproportional to the rigidity of the extremities. The syndrome is associated with atrophy of the midbrain and pontine tegmentum and pallor of the substantia nigra. The substantia nigra and subthalamic nuclei are most consistently involved, whereas the striatum is essentially intact.

Koller et al.[51] described two cases of PSP after closed head injury in men who sustained brain injuries from a fall. Each developed mild dementia. One patient was lost to follow-up, and the other reached a functional plateau.

Pharmacologic interventions for PSP include high-dose levodopa, amitriptyline, and desipramine. Double-blind studies are rare. In one study, fluoxetine, which is serotonergic-specific, decreased postural instability in 30% of cases.

STEREOTYPY

Stereotypy or stereotypic behaviors are purposeless voluntary movements performed repetitively, such as the body-rocking and head-banging in individuals with mental retardation. They can be simple or complex movements. Such behavioral automatisms can be produced by dopamine release due to amphetamine administration. The dopamine antagonist haloperidol has been shown to suppress such behaviors in animal models.[52] In contrast, tardive dyskinesia in patients who have received neuroleptic medication is considered a form of stereotypy. As previously mentioned, this is attributed to dopamine blockade.

It has been suggested that stereotypic behaviors fluctuate according to individual biorhythm; this concept may be incorporated into treatment plans.[14]

TICS

Tics are rarely reported after TBI.[51] They may be simple or complex, motor or phonic. Examples of motor tics include shrugs, head shakes, and grimacing. Phonic tics include sniffing, snorting, or obscene utterances. Tics generally appear paradoxically for brief bursts during normal behaviors. As with akathisia, a preceding uncomfortable sensation is relieved by the tic. Tics usually disappear during sleep and pleasurable activities but worsen in the face of negative experiences. They also have been associated with obsessive-compulsive disorders.

A small number of posttraumatic tics have been described in the literature. Aberrant sprouting of peripheral facial nerves after trauma sometimes leads to the appearance of a tic. Dopamine antagonists have been implicated as a cause. Simple premorbid tics may become more complex after further brain injury.[49] In an effort to move away from the use of neuroleptic medications, clonazepam

(GABA agonist) and clonidine (noradrenergic) have been suggested for management of tics.[51] Their effectiveness is variable. Methylphenidate, frequently used by patients with traumatic brain injury, may exacerbate tics. Psychological interventions may be useful for coping skills but are not recommended as a primary line of treatment.

PSYCHOGENIC MOVEMENT DISORDERS

It may be difficult to differentiate organic from psychogenic movement disorders. Conversion reactions and malingering may play a role in presentations. Imaging studies are not always helpful in distinguishing genuine movement disorders; numerous patients have presented with normal CT scans but abnormal positron emission tomography (PET) scans.[48]

Hyperkinetic forms are more common than bradykinetic forms. Tremors with a large hysterical component may be more likely to change during the course of examination. If the movement disorder is inconsistent over time, one may be suspicious of its origin. Disappearance, as opposed to lessening of a movement disorder with distractions, may suggest a psychiatric diagnosis, as may somatizations and psychiatric disturbances. Movement disorders tend to decrease with appropriate pharmacologic interventions, whereas psychogenic disorders are more likely to resolve completely. Amytal interviews may be helpful in teasing out useful information. However, their usefulness is variable and may only confuse the issue. Organic disorders may improve with amytal administration, whereas psychogenic movement disorders may remain unchanged.[48] In addition, the tendency for emotions to play a role in the presentation of movement disorders may lead clinicians to underestimate the authenticity of a true underlying disorder.

Accurate diagnosis is imperative. In patients with a true psychogenic disorder, psychotherapy is the treatment of choice. Instead, medications may be inappropriately prescribed. If the movement disorder is not of a psychiatric origin, pharmacologic treatment may prove useful. It is possible for a psychogenic disorder to be coupled with an organic disorder. The presence of a conversion disorder does not rule out an underlying neurologic disorder.

DRUG-INDUCED MOVEMENT DISORDERS

In the differential diagnosis and management of movement disorders, one must consider medications as a possible cause. Most drugs that have central effects are capable of producing tremor. Anticonvulsants, tricyclic antidepressants, and neuroleptics are the most frequent culprits administered to patients with brain injury that may predispose to movement disorders. Metoclopromide is frequently administered to patients in acute care and is associated with dystonic reactions. The risk of developing such side effects is probably increased in patients with TBI.

Most of the drugs that cause movement disorders are pre- or postsynaptic dopamine antagonists. Levodopa and central nervous system stimulants also may lead to movement disorders. Because of the risk of tardive dyskinesia, the use of antipsychotic medications (dopamine antagonists), such as haloperidol, fluphenazine, or pimozide, is not recommended in the treatment of movement disorders.[49] Metoclopramide poses the same risk. Tetrabenazine has been advocated for use in patients with hyperkinetic movement disorders, because no case of tardive dyskinesia has been documented with its use.[49] It is also a dopamine antagonist and associated with parkinsonism, sedation, weakness, depression, restlessness, and agitation. However, unlike reserpine, which irreversibly depletes dopamine stores, the effects of tetrabenazines are reversible within 12–24 hours. The concurrent administration of lithium has been suggested to increase the efficacy of tetrabenazine in patients with cranial-cervical dystonia.[49] Dopminergic preparations such as levodopa, bromocriptine, and amantadine are frequently used. A wide range of medications is recommended in the management of movement disorders. Their mechanisms of action are not well understood.

Acute dystonic reactions occur shortly after administration of neuroleptics. They are more common in children, but age less than 30 years and male gender are considered risk factors. Ninety percent of acute dystonic reactions occur within 5 days of initiation of the offending agent. Acute dystonia resolves with withdrawal of the causal agent. The tardive presentations of movement disorders occur after prolonged exposure to dopamine-depleting agents. Such disorders may persist even after the offending agent has been discontinued.

Drug-induced parkinsonism was first recognized in the 1950s. Now all dopamine-depleting agents have been found to cause an akinetic-rigid syndrome. Metoclopramide and most recently clebopride, which are used acutely in brain-injured patients for gastrointestinal disorders, also have been implicated.[35] In drug-induced parkinsonism, bradykinesia predominates over rigidity and tremor, and perioral movements are unique manifestations. Tremor is more likely to be symmetrical. It has been suggested that the tremor of drug-induced parkinsonism can be managed with propranolol. The central and peripheral nervous systems have been proposed as the sites for propranolol's effects.[58] The syndrome begins insidiously, taking weeks to months to manifest fully. Ninety percent of cases are detected within 3 months after initiation of the responsible medication. Risk factors include female gender and advanced age. Drug-induced parkinsonism gradually subsides over months with discontinuation of the offending agent. Rarely do symptoms persist for longer than 1 year.

Dyskinesias are a recognized complication of phenytoin administration. Combination therapy with phenobarbital and valproic acid increases the free fraction of phenytoin and may contribute to the risk of dyskinesias. Static encephalopathy, prior dyskinesias, structural lesions, and neuroleptic treatment predispose to this side effect. Choreoathetosis with and without orofacial dyskinesia is the most common dyskinesia associated with phenytoin.[38] It is postulated that phenytoin disrupts the equilibrium of the basal ganglia receptors. Buspirone, a relatively new nonsedating anxiolytic, has recently been implicated in the development of persistent dystonic and dyskinetic movement disorders.[55] Prior exposure to neuroleptic medications could not be excluded as a contributing factor. Vulnerability to side effects increases when the central nervous system is already disrupted (e.g., after traumatic brain injury).

MYOCLONUS

Myoclonus refers to sudden irregular or rhythmic muscle jerks originating from the central nervous system. Positive myoclonus refers to active contraction of muscle, whereas negative myoclonus is associated with the collapse of muscle tone seen in asterixis. Like the other dyskinesias, myoclonus has variable presentations and may be associated with other movement disorders. It also occurs under normal circumstances such as falling asleep. It is seen in various metabolic, toxic, and hypoxic disturbances.

Myoclonus may be classified according to its distribution, site of origin in the brain, or stimulus eliciting the behavior. Certain types of myoclonus are related to epilepsy. Somatosensory evoked potentials (SEPs) demonstrate giant P25/N33 waveforms in myoclonus of cortical origin. Electromyography (EMG) and electroencephalography (EEG) may be useful in distinguishing epileptic from nonepileptic myoclonus.[37] Different patterns of muscle activity on EMG suggest myoclonus. Back-averaging techniques of EEG are useful, assuming that the EEG was obtained during the episode. Myoclonus may occur in response to sudden stimuli, such as a loud noise.

The dopaminergic system does not appear to play a significant role in the genesis of cortical myoclonus, as it does in other movement disorders. There does not appear to be a myoclonus center in the brain. The brainstem, spinal cord, and cortex have been implicated in its genesis. The cholinergic system has been implicated in essential and palatal myoclonus, and occasional improvement may be seen with anticholinergic medications. The GABA system seems to play the predominant role in cortical myoclonus. Clonazepam facilitates GABA-ergic transmission. Sodium valproate increases levels of GABA at nerve terminals as well as its postsynaptic activity. Increasing the activity of this inhibitory transmitter may assist in the control of pathologic movement.

Palatal myoclonus, which may be unilateral or bilateral, occurs at a rate of 1.5–3 Hz.

Although contractions of the adjacent muscles may be present, palatal myoclonus is rarely associated with contractions of other body parts. A clicking noise is heard by the patient and often by people around the patient. Palatal myoclonus is related to lesions of the cerebello-rubro-olivary tract. PET has demonstrated a role for the inferior olivary nucleus of the medulla.[24] Clonazepam or carbamazepine may provide relief in some cases.

Startle myoclonus produces a crescendo-decrescendo tremor of 4 Hz and is often associated with other cerebellar findings.

Posthypoxic myoclonus is associated with cerebellar ataxia, dementia, postural and gait disturbances, and seizures. Intellect may be spared. Some patients improve with the serotonin precursor 5-hydroxytryptophan, but it can be obtained only by special arrangements. Myoclonus after anoxia or traumatic brain injury may be particularly amenable to treatment with 5-hydroxytryptophan. The principal treatment, however, is clonazepam alone or with combinations of carbamazepine, valproic acid, or primidone.[49] When myoclonus appears with tremor, treatment with propranolol or another beta blocker may prove advantageous.

In one study, patients with severe reflex and action myoclonus were treated with variable regimens of clonazepam, piracetam, sodium valproate, and primidone. Their responses to each drug were monitored through the use of SEPs and EEG. All ten patients showed significant improvement on their respective regimens. The myoclonus arose from a cortical origin and was believed to represent a "fragment of epilepsy."[61]

Myoclonus may be extremely disabling. Cortical myoclonus seems to respond best to sodium valproate in combination with other drugs, such as clonazepam. Clonazepam also may be effective in the management of brainstem myoclonus.

BOTULINUM TOXIN

Injection of botulinum toxin A is the most significant advancement in the management of dystonia and other movement disorders. There are seven immunologically distinct toxins. Botulinum toxin (BTX) is a neuromuscular blocking agent that acts presynaptically by inhibiting release of acetylcholine. It produces chemodenervation and focal muscle atrophy, which in turn decrease contractility and spasms in affected muscles.

Contraindications to BTX injections include myasthenia gravis, myasthenic syndromes, motor neuron disease, aminoglycoside administration, and possibly pregnancy. Complications of botulinum injection resolve within 2–4 weeks and depend on the area of injection. The effects last for approximately 2–4 months until sprouting occurs. No significant systemic side effects have been reported. The injections have been performed under EMG guidance for localization of the targeted muscle. The use of EMG is now less prevalent, depending on the muscles to be injected and the comfort level of the clinician.

Studies of botulinum toxin injection for cervical dystonia have demonstrated improvement in 61–93% of patients.[41] Dysphagia, the most common complication reported after injections about the neck, is managed by altering the consistency of the diet and tends to resolve within a short period.[42,47] Women appear to be at higher risk than men for developing this complication. In addition to local side effects, patients who receive routine injections of botulinum may develop sufficient antibody titers to block the effectiveness of further injections. This response is more the exception than the rule.[47] Botulinum toxin F has been demonstrated to be effective in patients who no longer demonstrate a response to botulinum toxin A.[32] Because the duration of action is shorter, it may prove useful in cases in which only temporary relief is the goal.

BTX diffuses up to 4.5 cm from the site of injection.[10] Multiple injection sites within the targeted muscle are more efficacious than single bolus injections. Local injections of botulinum toxin are associated with increased jitter on single-fiber electromyography 7–12 days after injection. Jitter is seen at the injected muscle as well as distant sites. Systemic distribution by blood flow and retrograde axonal transport within the anterior horn cells have been proposed as possible mechanisms.

Botulinum toxin received Food and Drug Administration (FDA) approval in 1989 for the treatment of strabismus and blepharospasm. It is currently used for other indications, such as spasticity, stiff-person syndrome, and myofascial pain. Insurance carriers are becoming more aware of the potential applications of BTX and often approve treatment for yet unapproved indications.

SURGICAL MANAGEMENT

Neurosurgical procedures alleviate a number of movement disorders, although their primary use has been in the treatment of Parkinson's disease. A strategically placed lesion in the ventrolateral thalamus significantly reduces or eliminates the rigidity and tremor of Parkinson's disease. Most surgeons prefer to lesion the ventralis intermedius of the ventrolateral thalamus. This lesion ameliorates tremor with minimal neurologic deficits. The ideal candidate for thalamotomy is a young patient with unilateral tremor and no speech or gait deficits.[33] For patients with bilateral tremor, a second lesion is more likely to lead to neurologic deficits, such as dysarthria and disequilibrium.

Thalamotomy is usually performed under local anesthetic so that the patient can participate in localization of the site for lesioning and report potential symptoms. The surgical approach is either frontal through a burr hole in the coronal suture or parietooccipital through a posteriorly placed burr hole. Coordinates are determined through the use of ventriculography or CT scan and confirmed physiologically. MRI may have a future role in localization because of its ability to define anatomy. However, evidence suggests that the magnetic field may distort anatomic structures.[33] The site is confirmed physiologically by noting the patient's response as the electrode is advanced to the predetermined coordinates. Because the ventralis intermedius lies immediately anterior to the sensory area for the hands and face, localization is confirmed when the patient reports paresthesias of the contralateral thumb, index finger, and mouth.

The lesion usually is produced through the use of radiofrequency. The patient then is assessed for weakness and residual tremor. The lesion may be extended if necessary. Complications include infection, subdural hematoma, and seizures. Contralateral weakness results if the lesion extends into the corticospinal tracts. Hemiballismus may result from lesions displaced inferiorly, whereas lesions displaced medially may result in memory deficits. Language deficits may result from lesioning of the left thalamus. Bilateral lesions produce speech deficits and decrease vocal volume in 30% of patients.

Ideally, patients spend a few days in the intensive care unit after surgery.[33] Even if the tremor has been obliterated, patients benefit from occupational therapy that instructs them in how to use their newly functional extremity.

Thalamotomy is less specific for hemiballismus and dystonia but may produce significant improvement when considered on a case-by-case basis. In the series of Bullard and Nashold,[15] 11 patients with dyskinesias secondary to severe brain injury underwent thalamotomy. Nine of the patients displayed hemiballism. Five showed marked improvement after surgery, 3 showed moderate improvement, and 1 showed mild improvement.

The best results from surgical treatment of dystonia have been in patients with posttraumatic hemidystonia and a structural lesion on CT or MRI.[5] Unlike patients with Parkinson's disease, the response to surgery increases 1–3 months postoperatively. Surgery is most successful for hand involvement and least successful for truncal dystonia.

Combinations of different procedures are sometimes considered. Stereotactic subthalamotomy carries a great risk of hemiballismus. Experimental evidence suggests that surgical lesioning of this area may limit the bradykinesia, rigidity, and tremor of Parkinson's disease.[6] Stereotactic pallidotomy or sectioning of the globus pallidus carries a risk of homonymous hemianopsia because of proximity to the optic nerve.

Chronic electrical stimulation of the ventralis intermedius has shown some promise in the treatment of tremor due to Parkinson's disease. Results with other movement disorders have been inconsistent. Patients who experience good results are able to reduce pharmacologic therapy. Intrathecal lioresal delivered by pump has been studied extensively for the treatment of spasticity of spinal origin. Fair results also have been achieved in one patient with axial dystonia[60] refractory to other interventions. Its useful-

ness as a routine intervention for movement disorders is limited.

SUMMARY

Movement disorders after traumatic brain injury are not unusual. They are probably underrecognized and underreported. The neurophysiology underlying such disorders is not well understood, and treatments remain largely empiric. Medications likely to be prescribed for movement disorders of other etiologies are less likely to be tolerated in patients with brain injury. Information about long-term outcome remains limited.

Posttraumatic movement disorders may appear after any degree of brain injury. Aside from systemic medications, modalities that may provide relief include relaxation techniques, traditional rehabilitation therapies, botulinum toxin injections, intrathecal lioresal pump implantation, and various surgical procedures.

REFERENCES

1. Adams RD, Victor M: Abnormalities of movement and posture. In Principles of Neurology, 4th ed. New York, McGraw-Hill, 1989.
2. Aisen ML, Holzer M, Rosen M, et al: Glutethimide treatment of disabling action tremor in patients with multiple sclerosis and traumatic brain injury. Arch Neurol 48:513–515, 1991.
3. Alexander GE, DeLong MR, Strick PL: Parallel organization of functionally segregated circuits linking basal ganglia and cortex. Annu Rev Neurosci 9:357–381, 1986.
4. Alexander GE, Crutcher MD: Functional architecture of basal ganglia circuits: Neural substrates of parallel processing. Trends Neurosci 13:266–271, 1990.
5. Andrew J, Fowler CJ, Harrison MJG: Stereotaxic thalamotomy in 55 cases of dystonia. Brain 106: 981–1000, 1983.
6. Aziz TZ, Peggs D, Sambrook MD, et al: Lesion of the subthalamic nucleus for the alleciation of 1-methyl-4-phenyl-1, 2, 3, 6-tetrahydropyridine (MPTP)-induced parkinsonism in the primate. Mov Disord 6:288–292, 1991.
7. Benadid AL, Pollak P, Gervason C, et al: Long-term suppression of tremor by chronic stimulation of the ventral intermediate thalamic nucleus. Lancet 337: 403–406, 1991.
8. Biary N, Cleeves L, Findley L, et al: Post-traumatic tremor. Neurology 39:103–106, 1989.
9. Biary N, Singh B, Bahou Y, et al: Posttraumatic paroxysmal nocturnal hemidystonia. Mov Disord 1:98–99, 1993.

10. Borodic GE, Pearce LB, Smith K, et al: Botulinum toxin for spasmodic torticollis: Multiple vs single injection points per muscle. Head Neck 14:33–37, 1992.

11. Brett BM, Hoare RD, Sheehy MP, Marsden CD: Progressive hemidystonia due to focal basal ganglia lesion after mild head injury. J Neurol Neurosurg Psychiatry 44:460, 1981.

12. Broggi G, Brock S, Franzini A, et al: A case of post-traumatic tremor treated by chronic stimulation of the thalamus. Mov Disord 8:206–208, 1993.

13. Brown P, Steiger OD, Thompson JC, et al: Effectiveness of piracetam in cortical myoclonus. Mov Disord 1:63–68, 1993.

14. Brusca R: Chronobiological aspects of stereotypy. J Ment Def 89:650–652, 1985.

15. Bullard DE, Nashold BS Jr: Stereotactic thalamotomy for treatment of posttraumatic movement disorders. J Neurosurg 61:316–321, 1984.

16. Bullard DE, Nashold BS Jr: Stereotactic thalamotomy for treatment of posttraumatic movement disorders. J Neurosurg 14:316–321, 1984.

17. Burke RE, Fahn S, Gold AP: Delayed onset dystonia in patients with "static" encephalopathy. J Neurol Neurosurg Psychiatry 43:789–797, 1980.

18. Caccia MR, Mangoni A: Clonidine is essential tremor: Preliminary observations from an open trial. J Neurol 232:55–57, 1985.

19. Caparros-Lefebvre D, Deleume JF, Bradai N, Petit H: Biballism caused by bilateral infarction in the substantia nigra. Mov Disord. 9:108–110, 1994.

20. Chan J, Brin MF, Fahn S: Idiopathic cervical dystonia: Clinical characteristics. Mov Disord. 6:119–126, 1991.

21. Chandra V, Spunt AL, Rosinowitz MS: Treatment of posttraumatic choreoathetosis following head injury. Ann Neurol 2:447–448, 1977.

22. Chutarian AM, Root L: Management of spasticity in children with botulinum-A toxin. Intl Pediatr 9:35–43, 1994.

23. David D, Jabbari B: Significant improvement of stiff-person syndrome after paraspinal injection of botulinum toxin A. Mov Disord 3:371–373, 1993.

24. Dubinsky R, Hallett M, Di Chirog, et al: Increased glucose metabolism in the medulla of patients with palatal myoclonus. Neurology 41:557–562, 1991.

25. Ellison PH: Propranolol for severe post-head injury action tremor. Neurology 28:197–199, 1978.

26. Factor SA, Sanchez-Ramos, Weiner WJ: Trauma as an etiology of parkinsonism: A historical review of the concept. Mov Disord 3:30–36, 1988.

27. Fahn S, Cohen G: The oxidant stress hypothesis in Parkinson's disease: Evidence supporting it. Ann Neurol 32:804–812, 1992.

28. Fahn S, Marsden CD, Van Woert MH: Definition and classification of myoclonus. Adv Neurol 43:1–5, 1986.

29. Fletcher NA, Harding AE, Marsden CD: The relationship between trauma and idiopathic torsion dystonia. Mov Disord 6:310–314, 1991.

30. Garner CG, Straube A, Witt TN: Time course of distant effects of local injections of botulinum toxin. Mov Disord 8:33–37, 1993.

31. Golbe LI, Sage JI, Duvoisin RC: Drug treatment of 83 patients with supranuclear palsy. Neurology 40(Suppl):438, 1990.

32. Greene PE, Fahn S: Use of botulinum toxin type F injections to treat torticollis in patients with immunity to botulinum toxin type A. Mov Disord 8:479–483, 1993.

33. Grossman RG, Hamilton WJ: Surgery for movement disorders. In Jankovic J, Tolosa E (eds): Parkinson's Disease and Movement Disorders, 2nd ed. Baltimore, Williams & Wilkins, 1993, pp 531–548.

34. Gaun XM, Peroutka SJ: Basic mechanisms of action of drugs used in the treatment of essential tremor. Clin Neuropharmacol 13:210–223, 1990.

35. Hageman ATM, Horstink MWIM: Parkinsonism due to a subdural hematoma. Mov Disord 9:107–108, 1994.

36. Hallet M: Classification and treatment of tremor. JAMA 266:1115–1117, 1991.

37. Hallett M: Myclonus: Relation to epilepsy. Epilepsia 26 (Suppl 1): S67–S77, 1985.

38. Harrison MB, Lyons GR, Landow ER: Phenytoin and dyskinesias: A report of two cases and review of the literature. Mov Disord 8:19–27, 1993.

39. Hershkowitz N, Bergery GK, Josyin J, Evans DE: Isolated midbrain lesion resulting from closed head injury: A unique presentation of ataxic hemiparesis. Neurology 39:452–453, 1989.

40. Jabbari B, Paul J, Scherokman B, Vandam B: Posttraumatic segmental axial dystonia. Mov Disord 7:78–81, 1992.

41. Jain SS, Kirshblum SC: Movement disorders, including tremors. In DeLisa JA, Gans BM (eds): Rehabilitation Medicine: Principles and Practice. Philadelphia, J.B. Lippincott, 1993, pp 700–715.

42. Jankovic J, Brin MF: Therapeutic uses of botulinum toxin. N Engl J Med 324:1186–1194, 1991.

43. Jankovic J, Fahn S: Physiologic and pathologic tremors. Ann Intern Med 93:460–465, 1980.

44. Jankovic J, Orman J: Tetrabenazine therapy of dystonia, chorea, tics and other dyskinesias. Neurology 38:391–394, 1988.

45. Jankovic J, Pardo R: Segmental myoclonus: Clinical and pharmacologic study. Arch Neurol 43:1025–1033, 1986.

46. Jankovic J, Schwartz K: Botulinum toxin treatment of tremors. Neurology 41:1185–1188, 1991.

47. Jankovic J, Schwartz KS: Clinical correlates of response to botulinum toxin injections. Arch Neurol 48:1253–1256, 1991.

48. Jankovic J, Tolosa E: Parkinson's Disease and Movement Disorders, 2nd ed. Baltimore, Williams & Wilkins, 1993.

49. Katz DI: Movement disorders following traumatic head injury. J Head Trauma Rehabil 5:86–90, 1990.

50. Koller WC, Lang A, Vetere-Overfield B, et al: Psychogenic tremors. Neurology 39:1094–1099.

51. Koller WC, Wong GF, Lang A: Posttraumatic movement disorders: A review. Mov Disord 4:20–36, 1989.

52. Kryzhanovskii GN, Aliev MN: The pathogenesis of stereotypic behavior. Zhurnal Nevropatologiii Psikliatrii Imeni 9:1347–1355, 1979.

53. Kuroda Y, Kakigi R, Shibasaki H: Treatment of essential tremor with arotinolol. Neurology 38:650–652, 1988.

54. Lapresle J: Palatal myoclonus. Adv Neurol 43:265–273, 1986.

55. LeWitt PA, Walters A, Hening W, et al: Persistent movement disorders induced by buspirone. Mov Disord 3:331–334, 1993.

56. Maki Y, Akimoto H, Enomoto T: Injuries of basal ganglia following head trauma in children. Childs Brain 7:113–123, 1980.

57. Manyam BV: Recent advances in the treatment of cerebellar ataxias. Clin Neuropharmacol 6:508–516, 1986.

58. Metzer SW, Paige SR, Newton JEO: Inefficiency of propranolol in attenuation of drug-induced parkinsonian tremor. Mov Disord 8:43–46, 1993.

59. Montagna P, Gabellini AS, Monari L, Lugaresi E: Parkinsonian syndrome after long-term treatment with clebopride. Mov Disord 7:89–90, 1992.

60. Narayan RK, Loubser PJ, Jankovic J, Donovan W: Intrathecal baclofen for the intractable axial dystonia. Neurology 41:1141–1142, 1991.

61. Obeso JA, Artieda J, Rothwell JC, et al: The treatment of severe action myoclonus. Brain 112:765–777, 1989.

62. Obeso JA, Narbona J: Posttraumatic tremor and myoclonic jerking. J Neurol Neurosurg Psychiatry 46:788, 1983.

63. Parker F, Tzourio N, Blond S, et al: Evidence for a common network of brain structures involved in Parkinsonian tremor and voluntary repetitive tremor. Brain Res 584:11–17, 1992.

64. Pettigrew LC, Jankovic J: Hemidystonia: A report of 22 patients and a review of the literature. J Neurol Neurosurg Psychiatry 48:650–657, 1985.

65. Pranzatelli MR, Snodgrass RS: The pharmacology of myoclonus. Clin Neuropharmacol 8:99–130, 1985.

66. Robin JJ: Paroxysmal choreoathetosis following head injury. Ann Neurol 2:447–448, 1977.

67. Rupniak MJ, Jenner P, Marsden CD: Acute dystonia induced by neuroleptic drugs. Psychopharmacology 88:403–419, 1986.

68. Sakai T, Shiraishi S, Murakiami S: Palatal myoclonus responding to carbamazepine. Ann Neurol 9:199–200, 1981.

69. Samie MR, Selhorst JB, Koller WC: Posttraumatic midbrain tremors. Neurology 40:62–66, 1990.

70. Sandel ME, O'Dell MW: Persistent facial myoclonus: A negative prognostic sign in patients with severe brain injury. Arch Phys Med Rehabil 74:411–415, 1993.

71. Sandyk R, Kahn I: Parkinsonism due to subdural hematoma. J Neurosurg 58:298–299, 1983.

72. Sanes JN, LeWitt PA, Mauritz KH: Visual and mechanical control of postural and kinetic tremor in cerebellar system disorders. J Neurol Neurosurg Psychiatry 51:934–943, 1988.

73. Sechi GP, Zuddas M, Piredda M, et al: Treatment of cerebellar tremors with carbamazepine: A controlled trial with long term follow-up. Neurology 39:1113–1115, 1989.

74. Sellal F, Hirsch E, Barth P, et al: A case of symptomatic hemidystonia improved by ventroposterolateral thalamic electrostimulation. Mov Disord 8:515–518, 1993.

75. Sempere AP, Duarte J, Palomares, et al: Parkinsonism and tardive dyskinesia after chronic use of clebopride. Mov Disord 9:114, 1994.

76. Stewart JT: Akathisia following traumatic brain injury: Treatment with bromocriptine [letter]. J Neurol Neurosurg Psychiatry 52:1200–1201, 1989.

77. Strange PG: Dopamine receptors in the basal ganglia: Relevance to Parkinson's disease. Mov Disord 8:263–270, 1993.

78. Szelozynska K, Znamirowski R: Extrapyramidal syndrome in posttraumatic hemiparesisi in children. Clin Pediatr 15:167–174, 1976.

79. Tolosa E, Marti MJ: Blepharospasm-oromandibular dystonia syndrome (Meige's syndrome): Clinical aspects. Adv Neurol 49:73–84, 1988.

80. Turkstra LS: Considerations in pharmacotherapeutic treatment of movement disorders after traumatic brain injury. J Commun Disord 25:143–163, 1992.

81. Weiner WJ, Lang AE: Drug-induced movement disorders. Movement Disord 4:599–644, 1989.

82. Young AB, Penney JB: Biochemical and functional organization of the basal ganglia. In Jankovic J, Tolosa E (eds): Parkinson's Disease and Movement Disorders. Baltimore, Williams & Wilkins, 1993, pp 1–11.

83. Zasler ND: Advances in neuropharmacological rehabilitation for brain dysfunction. Brain Inj 6:1–14, 1992.

NATHANIEL H. MAYER   M.D.

ALBERTO ESQUENAZI   M.D.

MARY ANN E. KEENAN   M.D.

16

Analysis and Management of Spasticity, Contracture, and Impaired Motor Control

Damage to the corticospinal system after traumatic brain injury (TBI) interferes with activities of daily living (ADL), mobility, and communication, by impairing the ability to produce and regulate voluntary movement and inducing spasticity.[64] Spasticity, although variously defined, boils down to a set of mostly unwanted and involuntary motor phenomena when limbs are moved actively by the patient or passively by an examiner. Although the mechanisms underlying spasticity are largely unknown, current theories favor the notion that afferent signals from the limbs and descending signals of supraspinal origin are handled by one or more interneuronal systems at the level of the segmental spinal cord.[32,73] These systems ultimately influence the excitability of the alpha motor neuron pool, which, in the presence of a corticospinal system lesion, becomes excessively excitable. It is not clear whether spasticity is generated by discrete mechanisms that have gone awry (hence allowing the possibility of discrete repairs) or necessarily linked to other kinds of malfunction in the motor control system (hence correctable only as part of repairs to the larger malfunction).

Certainly, from a clinical point of view, functional problems caused by "spastic paresis" usually have more to do with "paretic" motor control of agonist muscles than with spasticity of antagonist muscles.[26] From a treatment perspective, it is much easier to weaken spastic antagonists to a movement than to retrain voluntary production and control of that movement. For example, if the triceps of the arm can voluntarily extend the elbow but a spastic, antagonistic biceps slows the speed of extension, the force of the spastic biceps can be diminished by a motor point block or surgical lengthening.[43] However, if the patient is unable to generate and regulate selective triceps activity and cannot extend the elbow because of "paresis," treatment is much more problematic, given the current state of knowledge. Volitional control over the triceps, including the ability to initiate, develop, adjust and terminate triceps force and speed, may well be influenced by but is generally independent of biceps spasticity.

Everyone complains about spasticity, but few attach the same meaning to the term. A century ago, Sherrington's seminal studies of the cat's myotatic stretch reflex provided strong physiologic underpinnings for later clinical descriptions of spastic signs and symptoms.[65] The central diagnostic role of the stretch reflex is echoed in Nathan's

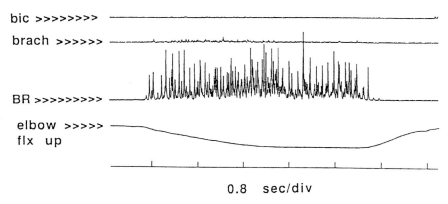

FIGURE 1.   Records of a 23-year old man with spastic hemiparesis of 1 year's duration secondary to TBI. Tonic electromyographic (EMG) activity induced by slow passive extension of the elbow is present in the brachioradialis (BR). Note the paucity of stretch-related activity in the biceps and brachialis.

description of spasticity as "a condition in which stretch reflexes that are normally latent become obvious. The tendon reflexes have a lowered threshold to tap, the response of the tapped muscle is increased, and usually muscles besides the tapped one respond; tonic stretch reflexes are affected in the same way."[54] The short-duration stimulus of a tendon tap resembles an impulse function and, combined with the brief jerk response of the muscle, is often classified as a phasic reflex. In contrast, passive stretch of a muscle induces more sustained tension and reflects underlying stretch reflex activity of the tonic type (Fig. 1). Tonic stretch reflexes have a lowered threshold and an increased response to stretch. In addition to changes in reflex activation, the spastic state is often characterized by increased stiffness and contracture of muscle. Herman has shown that passive tension generated by changes in the rheologic (viscoelastic and plastic) properties of muscle is significantly increased in severe spasticity, especially if contracture already has begun to develop.[31] Changes in the rheologic properties of muscle and other soft tissues play a definite role in hampering motion. Muscle tone—i.e., resistance perceived by an examiner stretching a group of muscles across a joint—is increased in the spastic state because of characteristics of the tonic stretch reflex combined with stiffness changes in the rheologic properties of muscles and other soft tissues of the limb segment.

Signs of spasticity are useful as a diagnostic indicator of an upper motor neuron lesion.

However, rehabilitation clinicians are preoccupied with treating functional problems linked to the consequences of the upper motor neuron lesion. Common terms that reflect their emphasis on practice include "spastic gait," "spastic elbow flexion," "spastic hand," "spastic equinovarus," and even "spastic dysphonia." For rehabilitation clinicians, evaluation and treatment of spasticity takes on broader dimensions, reflecting their interest in clinical patterns of motor dysfunction that produce functional disability. In such a formulation, manifestations of spasticity, muscle stiffness, and contracture, together with the all-important degree of retained motor control, become intertwined factors underlying clinical patterns of motor dysfunction and functional disability.

CONCEPTS OF MOTOR CONTROL AND THEORIES OF SPASTICITY

A century ago, John Hughlings Jackson developed the theory that movements were controlled by a serial hierarchy of motor centers.[2] Command signals were issued from motor centers of the cerebral cortex, received by motor centers lower in the brainstem, and transmitted to neuronal circuits in the spinal cord, where they activated preprogrammed instructions to muscles indicating what movements to perform. Jackson's hierarchical model of motor control, focusing almost exclusively on one-way travel of signals from brain to spinal cord, gave rise to several early theories that emphasized the development of spasticity as a consequence of breakdown in the hierarchical chain of motor control. Pathology affecting higher motor centers could lead to disinhibition of lower centers on the basis of "release of function." Breakdown of control in higher centers also could lead to facilitation of spastic phenomena on the basis of an "influx" phenomenon. After Sherrington described the stretch reflex and devised the first experimental animal model of spasticity, Magoun and Rhines used the cat model to elaborate Jackson's theory of spasticity.[47] They investigated the influence of many different descending motor tracts, both inhibitory and facilitatory, on stretch reflex activity and concluded that spasticity resulted from a net supraspinal imbalance between central inhibition and central facilitation of the stretch reflex. In their view, no homogeneous mechanism for the production of spasticity could be found.

Jackson's model of a hierarchically organized motor control system has been challenged by recent theories that the motor system is organized as a distributed network of neurons. Studies of the control of arm movements by populations of neurons in primate motor cortex found that individual neurons actively fire in association with a wide range of movement directions.[21] Such activity, spread across an entire population of neurons, appears to reflect a code that specifies movement direction. The signal that specifies a particular trajectory of hand movement, for example, is not the firing pattern of a small cluster of "hand" cells but a signal of graded activity produced by a large population of neurons distributed throughout the representation of the arm in the primary motor cortex. Different movements require different patterns of activation within the same population of neurons in the distributed network. Motor cortex cells appear to be able not only to specify the trajectory of a movement but also to compensate for external loads applied against a limb during movement. In addition, for similar hand trajectories, motor cortex cells appear to vary their activity as a function of different postures of the arm, suggesting that motor cortex cells are linked not only to movement selection (indicating which movement to make) but also to movement execution (indicating which muscle to use).

Jacksonian notions of motor control are currently being reexamined. On the basis of perceptive clinical observations of patients with motor seizures, Jackson inferred an orderly representation within the motor cortex of muscle groups from different parts of the body. Extrapolation to the hierarchical model of motor control resulted in the view that the motor cortex functioned as a simple mosaic of cell clusters, each of which controlled a single joint or even a single muscle. Based on recent cell population studies cited above, the concept of population coding is now replacing older Jacksonian views with the idea that clusters of neurons in a distributed network are involved in the control of muscles or movements across more than one joint. Another limitation of the hierarchical model is that it focused almost exclusively on one-way information flow from higher centers to lower ones, whereas, in reality, information also must flow back to higher sites of control to update them about the consequences of the movement that they generated. Motor cortex neurons receive sensory information directly from muscle fibers that they innervate, and feedback coupling between efferent and afferent functions appears to be tight.[3] Muscle spindles may be an important source of such information.[70] Feedback to the cortex has functional utility because it allows direct modulation of motor cortex excitability as a function of applied external loads. From the perspective of motor control, gamma motor neurons regulate the output of muscle spindles, which in turn influence excitability of alpha motor neurons innervating skeletal muscle. Muscle spindles, so-named because of their spindle-shaped connective tissue capsules, are sensors interleaved in parallel between skeletal muscle fibers. They provide information to the central nervous system (CNS) relative to muscle stretch and muscle contraction, including conscious awareness that a muscle has been stretched. In turn, spindles are regulated by the CNS through fusimotor neurons with cell bodies from the ventral horn and innervate the muscular portions of spindle fibers within the spindle capsule itself.

As early as 1925, Wagner pointed out that the stretch reflex serves as a negative feedback loop stabilizing muscle length.[24] We now know that stretching a muscle also stretches spindle fibers. The ensuing barrage of afferent discharges from stretched spindle fibers leads to depolarization of alpha motor neurons. Subsequent contraction of skeletal muscle shortens the stretched muscle and restores its original length. During voluntary concentric contraction, the inverse situation occurs. Contractile shortening of skeletal muscle causes the spindle to become slack, and afferent output from the spindle diminishes. The stronger the extrafusal contraction, the weaker the spindle influence on alpha motor neurons. From an engineering perspective, this loss of influence can be modulated by fusimotor stimulation of intrafusal spindle fibers, even as the alpha motor neurons are causing contraction of extrafusal skeletal muscle fibers. Coactivation of alpha and gamma motor neurons (called alpha-gamma linkage by Granit in 1955) provides an arrangement known in engineering terms as a servomechanism.[25] In most voluntary movements, the effect of a load-opposing movement can be anticipated only approximately. Therefore, it is often necessary to adjust the strength of contraction of a voluntary movement, depending on the opposing load, during the actual course of movement. The servomechanism, operated at the spinal level by means of the gamma loop, may provide automatic adjustment for the effects of changing load. The supraspinal origin and control of gamma motor neurons (emerging from the ventral horn) are not clear. The motor cortex, however, projects particularly to distal musculature, which is generally rich in muscle spindles (especially the hand). Evarts demonstrated that motor cortex is involved in regulating force and directionality of movement.[16] Spindle information may be relevant to such regulation.

In addition to information looped between muscle spindles and motor cortex subserving motor control, recent studies revealed that the motor cortex appears to loop information to the basal ganglia and the cerebellum as well before it transmits a final set of signals to the spinal cord. The function of these loops is poorly understood, but it may enable the CNS to update and modify continually the signals that the motor cortex sends to the spinal cord. The role of the basal ganglia in motor control, particularly the globus pallidus, may be to scale the amplitude of movement[10] (think of micrographia in parkinsonism), but the basal ganglia also may facilitate gating or regulation of perceptual inputs during a motor task.[49]

The cerebellum also plays an important role in motor control, especially in the timing and coordination of movement, motor learning, and regulation of muscle tone.[62] The role of the cerebellum in conditions of increased muscle tone was first established in comparative studies of "decerebrate rigidity" in cats. Sherrington was the first to produce decerebrate rigidity by transecting the brainstem of an animal above the vestibular nuclei.[66] He also demonstrated that he could make the rigidity of one of the limbs disappear by cutting the dorsal roots supplying that limb. Afferent nerve fibers from the muscle spindle were among the dorsal root fibers that were cut. Interruption of afferents from the muscle spindle was considered to be an important factor in this type of preparation because it was assumed that the main factor producing rigidity was excessive firing of fusimotor or gamma motor neurons, which led to an increase in spindle discharges. These discharges subsequently excited the alpha motor neuron pool in the spinal cord, leading to rigid muscular contraction of the limbs. Therefore, the condition was also described as "gamma rigidity."

Another method of producing decerebrate rigidity, introduced by Pollock and Davis, consists of ligating both carotid arteries together with the basilar artery—the so-called method of anemic decerebration.[58] Unlike Sherrington's method of surgically transecting the brainstem, the anemic method destroyed half of the cerebellum and a considerable portion of the pons. The two preparations initially were considered to be neurophysiologically equivalent until it was discovered that cutting the dorsal roots had no effect at all on limb rigidity in the anemic preparation.[57] This observation later led to the theory that hyperexcitability of alpha motor neurons by themselves (i.e. without support from fusimotor neuron and muscle spindle drive) could be responsible for the rigidity. The condition, therefore, was called "alpha rigidity."

These findings, based on two different laboratory methods, suggested to some that at least two different routes led to an increase in alpha motor neuron excitability and that fusimotor system influence may not be as important as was thought.

Of related interest is the idea that descending alpha-adrenergic fibers may play a role in the regulation of fusimotor drive.[48] This theory raises the possibility that alpha-adrenergic blocking agents may be helpful in reducing spasticity.[11,76] Chlorpromazine reduces decerebrate rigidity in cats, probably by means of alpha-adrenergic blockade, but in humans it is sedating. Although human decerebrate posturing is not known to have the same pathophysiology as decerebrate rigidity in cats, phenothiazines and other alpha-adrenergic blockers have been considered for use in persistent, intractable decerebrate posturing after head injury. Other drugs that may influence the fusimotor system include phenytoin and dantrolene sodium, but the real issue is whether the fusimotor system plays a role in spasticity at all. In the early 1960s, Rushworth suggested that increased fusimotor activity contributed to spasticity in humans, because spastic responses were blocked by infiltration of peripheral nerves with a dilute solution of procaine—a technique that presumably blocks small-caliber nerve fibers such as fusimotor fibers.[50,63] Landau disagreed with the fusimotor hypothesis and believed that all instances of clinical hyperreflexia could be attributed solely to hyperexcitability of the alpha motor neuron pool.[45] In the 1970s, Hagbarth, Vallbo, and coworkers recorded from peripheral nerve fibers directly and studied spindle afferent responses to stretch in normal persons and in persons with spasticity associated with stroke and spinal cord injury.[69] They found no clear evidence of increased dynamic or static sensitivity of calve muscle spindles associated with spasticity and clonus. Gilman et al. created lesions in monkeys that became clinically spastic over time.[22] Gilman et al. made direct recordings from peripheral nerves during clinical periods of hypotonia and hypertonia. During the period of spasticity, they found no increase in the afferent discharge from spastic muscles and concluded that no causal relationship

between spasticity and increased fusimotor activity was indicated. At present, the fusimotor hypothesis of spasticity lacks direct evidence.

In contrast to motor cortex, which projects considerably to the distal musculature, the premotor cortex, an area just anterior to the motor cortex, projects mainly to the proximal musculature. Nerve fibers from the premotor cortex innervate primarily motor neurons of the trunk and shoulders.[75] The premotor cortex receives information from the posterior parietal cortex, an area important for spatial orientation. The role of the premotor cortex in motor control appears to relate to orienting the body and preparing the postural muscles for future movements. The supplementary motor cortex, located just above and anterior to the motor cortex, is another site involved in motor control, specifically the planning and production of complex sequences of movements. Computed tomography (CT) scans have shown that the supplementary motor area (SMA) and motor cortex are highly active when people are asked to carry out sequences of finger movements. However, when finger sequences are only imagined, blood flow to the SMA remains high, but blood flow to the motor cortex returns to normal levels.[61] Such findings support the hypothesis that the SMA is a site for high-level planning of movement. The parietal cortex appears to be particularly concerned with the spatial features of movement. Damage to the parietal cortex often results in hemispatial deficits, inability to perform activities requiring spatial information, and deficits in drawing and building three-dimensional structures.[46] Damage to the parietal lobe, particularly the dominant parietal lobe, also has been associated with apraxic breakdown in the retrieval of movement plans or difficulty with enacting such plans once they are retrieved.

The above discussion was concerned largely with supraspinal aspects of motor control. Supraspinal information flows to the spinal cord, which is the final way-station for descending information but the first way-station for incoming information from the limbs. For example, afferent information about stretch of the muscle spindle is signaled to the central nervous system by means of group Ia and group II afferent nerve fibers.[60] The stretch-sensitive annulospiral endings transmit information to the spinal cord by means of the group Ia afferents. When the biceps tendon is tapped, causing a rapid stretch of the biceps muscle, signals pass up the afferent fiber into the spinal cord directly to motor neurons that fire back to the biceps impulses causing contraction.[14] During brief stretch, there is a brief but intense discharge of afferent information to the spinal cord. When a spastic muscle is stretched slowly and stretch is maintained, annulospiral endings continue to discharge impulses tonically and the muscle may develop a sustained, tonic contraction (see Fig. 1). Rapid, sustained stretch may produce combinations of phasic tendon jerklike responses and tonic responses (Fig. 2). The tendon jerk illustrates a simple afferent-efferent reflex arc, but more complicated reflex pathways exist. For example, cutaneous receptors stimulated by pain or pressure on the skin (as in a flexor withdrawal reflex) transmit afferent information to the spinal cord, where a great deal of branching occurs. The pathway to motor neurons is typically by means of interneurons. Enormous numbers of interneurons, many arranged in parallel, some in series, ensure that the reflex will spread widely and that the response of a variety of muscles will be prolonged. Some of this widespreading information is eventually transmitted to conscious awareness. Other information is routed to motor neurons for the purpose of withdrawing the limb from a noxious stimulus even before conscious awareness.[51] In spastic patients, reflex activity generated during everyday sensory exposures ironically may contribute to the development and perpetuation of deformity (Fig. 3).

Sherrington was the first to emphasize the principles of divergence and convergence in the central nervous system.[65] An afferent fiber carrying its own specific signal into the spinal cord may diverge and branch into many lines, activating many nerve cells. In complementary fashion, signal inputs converge from many different lines onto each nerve cell in the central nervous system. For example, many different stretch receptors taking part in a monosynaptic stretch reflex converge onto each of the motor neurons innervating the involved muscle. In addition, however, branch paths from Ia afferent fibers diverge onto interneurons that eventually connect with motor neurons going to antagonist muscles.[59] This arrangement subserves reciprocal inhibition (see below). In a similar manner, polysynaptic reflexes made up of diverging and converging lines send signals not only along the final pathway from motor

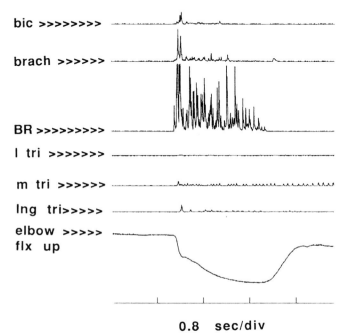

bic >>>>>>>

brach >>>>>>

BR >>>>>>>>

l tri >>>>>>>

m tri >>>>>>

lng tri>>>>>

elbow >>>>>
flx up

0.8 sec/div

FIGURE 2. Rapid passive elbow extension in a patient with spastic hemiparesis produces phasic, tendon jerklike EMG responses in the biceps, brachialis, and brachioradialis, but tonic activity is generated only in the brachioradialis. Stretch-sensitive annulospiral endings in the muscle spindle may be responsible for driving alpha motor neurons of the elbow flexors during stretch, but note the differences in EMG responses across the different flexors. It is common for multiple muscles crossing a joint to vary in spastic reactions.

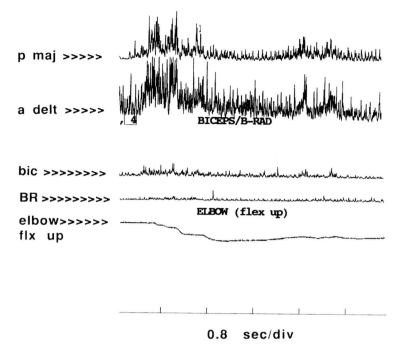

FIGURE 3. Six years after TBI this tracheotomized patient has an adducted/internally rotated shoulder with poor access to the axilla. Dynamic EMG studies revealed that ordinary and necessary tracheal suctioning procedures generated considerable and persistent EMG activity in the pectoralis major and anterior deltoid, two of various muscles that may contribute to such a pattern of motor dysfunction.

neuron to muscle, but also to various interneurons along the way. Because of the many afferent fibers carrying information from many annulospiral endings in skeletal muscle, hundreds of lines in parallel transmit afferent information to the central nervous system and thereby give immense scope for divergence and convergence.

Convergence and divergence of activity may have functional meaning. For example,[14] when a person stands with slightly bent knees, stretching of the quadriceps causes annulospiral stretch receptors to fire signals into the spinal cord that excite the knee extensor motor neurons. Contraction of the quadriceps is augmented by this activity, and the person is able to hold his or her body weight. If for some reason the muscle contraction is inadequate, the knee begins to yield, more stretch of the quadriceps occurs, and an increase in annulospiral receptor activity results. An increased reflex discharge to the quadriceps muscle is brought about through convergence of afferent input onto the many extensor motor neurons innervating the quadriceps. At the same time, anatomic side branches from Ia afferents conduct impulses to inhibitory interneurons that eventually transmit inhibitory information to antagonist motor neurons. This divergent

pathway subserves reciprocal inhibition and prevents antagonist motor neurons, connected to the hamstrings, from firing and opposing contraction of the agonist quadriceps muscle. If the antagonist hamstring flexors contract, the extensor quadriceps muscle is opposed, and support of body weight with a flexed knee by the quadriceps is undermined.

In the damaged central nervous system, supraspinal regulation of divergent and convergent circuitry is impaired. As a result, afferent signals arriving in the spinal cord are mishandled, and relations between agonist and antagonist motor neuron activity is altered.[29] Current knowledge about specific types of alterations or mechanisms is insufficient to deal with clinical problems in highly specific ways. Nevertheless, clinicians may take advantage of the concept that afferent information generated by peripheral receptors may be mishandled in the spinal cord. To reduce unwanted and unpredictable motor activity, clinicians should seek out and eliminate irritative sources of afferent activity.[28] First principles in the treatment of spasticity are to prevent and treat bedsores, skin infection, bladder infection and stones, skin maceration, and nailbed infection. It is important to maintain proper limb positioning and to avoid limb torsion caused by snags and malpositioning in wheelchairs and beds; to unload skin pressures when the patient is seated in a wheelchair or other support system and cannot change position on his or her own; to fit braces and splints properly and to check their fit over an extended period; to control sharp extremes in temperature; to regulate the suddenness of environmental stimuli; and to deal with emotional stressors.

Various theories of spasticity are linked to the concept of signal "mishandling" at the level of the spinal cord. Delwaide points out that the normal mechanism of presynaptic inhibition in the spinal cord is altered in patients with hyperreflexia.[13] Normal adjustment of Ia afferent activity from the muscle spindle at a premotoneuronal level depends on supraspinal facilitatory influences and precedes Ia discharges. In spasticity, according to Delwaide, the interneuron responsible for presynaptic inhibition becomes less active because of reduction of supraspinal facilitatory influences. Accordingly, the stretch reflex of patients with hyperreflexia is no longer subject to tonic inhibitory control by this mechanism of presynaptic inhibition. Instead, all proprioceptive afferent impulses gain direct access to the alpha motor neurons and exert a spastic influence.

In a similar theory involving interneuron neurophysiology, Veale, Rees, and Mark focused on the Renshaw system of cells located in the ventral medial horn of the spinal cord.[71] Renshaw cells are small interneurons that are monosynaptically excited by recurrent collaterals from nearby alpha motor neurons. However, axons of Renshaw cells also form inhibitory synapses with the same motor neurons (and others nearby), thereby causing inhibition of alpha motor neurons. In addition to this inhibitory effect, Renshaw cells also may cause indirect facilitation of motor neurons by a primary action on other interneurons with an inhibitory effect. Consequently, inhibition by Renshaw cells of inhibitory interneurons produces disinhibition or, in effect, facilitation of alpha motor neurons. In studies of human spasticity, Veale, Rees, and Mark found that indirect recurrent effects on inhibitory interneurons, leading to motor neuron facilitation, were stronger than direct recurrent effects that tend toward

inhibition. Thus, recurrent inhibition was largely lost, whereas recurrent facilitation remained strong. The investigators therefore postulated that, in patients with an upper motor neuron lesion, spasticity resulted from abnormal supraspinal regulation of Renshaw cell terminals. An excess of disinhibition resulted in hyperexcitability of the anterior horn cell pool.

Recently Jankowska focused on the spinal cord transmission of group II muscle afferent activity.[33] He also concluded that in patients with an upper motor neuron lesion, alterations in supraspinal regulation of cord interneurons responsible for transmitting activity from group II muscle afferents may produce motor neuron hyperexcitability and spasticity.

At present, clinicians do not have diagnostic tools to establish which of the above mechanisms, if any, contribute to spasticity. Nevertheless, strategies that reduce input to or output from the spinal cord may serve a useful purpose in clinical management. For example, drugs such as baclofen and diazepam may inhibit transmission of widely spreading afferent signals within the spinal cord, thereby influencing excitability of the alpha motor neurons.[12] Similarly, nerve blocks alter spastic signals and reduce the force of muscle contraction and muscle tone. In the future, as definitive mechanisms generating spasticity become identifiable at the clinical level, targeted pharmacological interventions will become more powerful than current options.

Many different types of motor control issues have been identified above. Any given motor act is actualized by the collective effects of distributed networks interacting simultaneously and sequentially. Diffuse neuropathology due to TBI may affect motor control at many different sites in the nervous system and in many different networks. Spasticity is part of the larger set of phenomena unleashed by abnormalities in motor control after head injury. The clinician must be able to see spastic phenomena within the larger context of impaired motor control in order to identify methods of treating functional problems after head injury that are typically caused by spastic phenomena embedded within impaired selective motor control.

GENERAL APPROACH TO EVALUATION

Clinical Aspects. In broad terms, evaluation of spasticity focuses on identification of three factors: (1) the clinical pattern of motor dysfunction, (2) the patient's ability to control muscles involved in the clinical pattern, and (3) the role of muscle stiffness and contracture in relation to the functional problem. For purposes of convenience, we have identified thirteen clinical patterns of motor dysfunction, organized by joint or limb segment, that are typically found in patients with TBI and upper motor neuron lesions (Table 1). Various muscles may contribute to motor dysfunction across joints and limb segments in these clinical patterns. Evaluation focuses on the following characteristics of the involved: (1) voluntary or selective control (2) spastic reactivity, (3) rheologic stiffness, and (4) contracture. Does the patient have voluntary control over a given muscle? Is the muscle spastic to passive stretch? Is the muscle, as an antagonist, activated during active movement generated by an agonist? Does the muscle have increased stiffness when stretched? Does the muscle have fixed shortening (contracture)? When many muscles cross a joint, the characteristics of each muscle may vary. Because each muscle may contribute to motion and movement of the joint, information about each muscle's contribution is useful to the assessment as a whole. Treatment depends on such information. We use dynamic electromyography to identify the voluntary and spastic characteristics of individual muscles in a movement and anesthetic nerve blocks to identify properties of stiffness and contracture in particular muscle groups.

Technology-based Aspects. Laboratory measurement of upper and lower extremity motion is a cornerstone of modern analysis of spasticity and impaired voluntary control of movement.[15] Gait and motor control analysis of spasticity measures the specific contribution of muscles to movement by means of multichannel dynamic electromyography (EMG). Dynamic EMG is correlated to simultaneous measurements of joint motion (kinematics) and ground reaction forces (kinetics).

TABLE 1. Clinical Patterns of Motor Dysfunction

1. Adducted/internally rotated shoulder	7. Excessively flexed hip
2. Bent elbow	8. Scissoring thighs
3. Pronated forearm	9. Stiff knee
4. Bent wrist	10. Bent knee
5. Clenched fist	11. Equinovarus foot with curl toes or claw toes
6. Thumb-in-palm deformity	12. Valgus foot
	13. Hitchhiker's great toe

Force platforms installed flush to the floor of a walkway enable the measurement of ground reaction forces during walking and standing and permit vector analysis of weight-bearing and force. Computer-processed, photo-marker, three-dimensional, quantitative motion data provide information about range, direction, velocity, and acceleration of limb movement during various functional tasks. Clinical correlations and interpretations are enhanced significantly by slow-motion video, which provides frame-by-frame display of walking and other limb and bodily movements. Kinetic, kinematic, and dynamic EMG data from patients performing active movement tasks allow interpretation of capacity for voluntary function, motor control ability, and spastic characteristics. Similar measurements of passive movement responses, combined with pre- and post-nerve block data, allow clinical interpretations of tone and contracture. Clinical examination alone, especially after TBI, is insufficient to identify voluntary and spastic characteristics of the many muscles affected by an upper motoneuron lesion. Combined with clinical information, laboratory measurements provide the degree of detail necessary to generate sensible hypotheses about the patient's pathophysiologic condition. Such hypotheses lead directly to the formulation of rational treatment interventions.

Recovery-based Aspects. Evaluation and treatment also depend on the clinician's expectation for motor recovery. We arbitrarily divide neurologic recovery into two periods: an early period during which motor recovery may be expected and a late period during which, for all practical purposes, motor recovery has ended. In our experience, practical motor recovery most often ceases between

9 and 15 months after head injury. Functional recovery is a different story. Even if many years have elapsed after a head injury, interventions aimed at making functional changes may produce functional results. For example, a patient who cannot ambulate because the base of support is severely compromised by equinovarus deformity during stance phase may regain ambulation through orthopaedic intervention that rebalances muscles crossing the ankle joint, thereby stabilizing the base of support. Functional recovery may occur at any time after head injury, provided that compensatory interventions are feasible and patients have the ability to control the results of such interventions to their advantage.

Clinical Commentary. Before 1975, the cognitive, behavioral, and psychosocial aspects of head injury received little attention. Studies by Bond, Brooks, McKinlay, and others championed the idea that families were much more vulnerable to the burdensome effects of impaired cognition and behavior than to the dysfunctional effects of physical impairment.[5,9] With a relative deemphasis on physical rehabilitation, treatment of spastic limbs was approached less aggressively. Drugs used in spinal cord injury and multiple sclerosis, such as baclofen, dantrolene sodium, and benzodiazepines, were viewed cautiously because of their sedating, fatiguing, and weakening side effects. Typical surgical approaches were based on inferences from physical examination alone and often focused on reducing contracture and deformity rather than increasing functional performance. Empirical procedures were often hit-and-miss, and surgeons virtually ignored cognitive and behavioral factors when making decisions about procedures and postsurgical treatment. Often surgeons, physiatrists, and rehabilitation staff did not work well together, and when a procedure resulted in a different deformity, surgeons backed off and rehabilitationists threw up their hands, vowing to be "less aggressive" next time. Rehabilitation staff with nonmedical backgrounds typically dealt with cognitive and behavioral issues and generally viewed surgery as an aggressive choice of last resort. Many nonsurgical physicians

agreed—especially since the experience of local surgeons with an interest in neurologic problems varied significantly.

This chapter assumes that both conservative and surgical options are applicable to the functional management of patients with spasticity. When TBI produces an upper motor neuron syndrome, the degree of residual voluntary function is highly variable and must be assessed. Spasticity of individual effector muscles is also highly variable. Consequently, interaction among residual voluntary capacity, impaired regulation of that capacity, and coexisting spastic characteristics of effector muscles results in various clinical patterns of motor dysfunction that need sorting. Distinctions need to be made between factors that reflect poor production and regulation of movement and factors that reflect spastic phenomena and changes in muscle stiffness. These distinctions are based not only on physical examination but also on technology-based evaluations, which provide a sound basis for both conservative and surgical interventions. Expectations of variability in the degree of impaired motor control and spasticity after TBI guide the technologic evaluation and may serve as a basis for intervention once voluntary and spastic features have been sorted. The central theme of this chapter is that treatment of motor dysfunction associated with the upper motor neuron syndrome is linked not only to spasticity but, more importantly, to concepts of impaired motor control and changes in the physical properties of muscle and other soft tissues.

PATTERNS OF MOTOR DYSFUNCTION ACROSS UPPER AND LOWER EXTREMITY JOINTS

Focal but variable patterns of muscle dysfunction across upper and lower extremity joints are commonly observed after traumatic brain injury. Characteristics of the upper motor neuron syndrome include spasticity, weakness, and various motor control abnormalities that impair the regulation of voluntary movement. We manage such problems by identifying the muscles that contribute to deformity across a joint, the patient's stage of recovery, and clinically applicable goals.

Common focal patterns of motor dysfunction after head injury are discussed below.

Adducted/Internally Rotated Shoulder

Clinical Description. The humerus is held tightly against the chest wall (Fig. 4). The elbow is often flexed, and the forearm, often pronated, lies against the anterior chest because of shoulder internal rotation. Range of motion into abduction and external rotation are limited, and resistance increases as the examiner attempts to abduct the humerus and/or externally rotate the shoulder. The pectoralis major muscle is typically prominent, but other muscles often contribute as well (see below). Passive abduction and external rotation may be painful as the examiner applies progressive stretch.

Functional Consequences and Penalties. The shoulder functions mechanically like a universal joint, enabling the hand to reach a large variety of locations in three-dimensional space. Spastic adduction and internal rotation of the shoulder severely restricts the reach of the hand, both in space and on the body. A tight shoulder impairs access to the axilla for skin care and hygiene. Reduced motion impairs dressing, washing, and bathing. Painful passive motion compromises passive functions such as being dressed and bathed by a caregiver. The ability to apply upper extremity force at different locations in space for body or object stabilization is also compromised.

Differential Diagnosis and Diagnostic Work Up. Restricted range often results from a combination of dynamic and static deformities, i.e., tone and soft-tissue contracture. Pectoralis major, teres major, latissimus dorsi, subscapularis, and anterior deltoid muscles are important adductors and internal rotators of the shoulder. Clinical examination focuses on the possibility of active shoulder motion, even a small amount. The degree of muscle or tendon prominence during stretch of muscles such as the pectoralis major, latissimus dorsi, and teres major is observed and palpated (Fig. 5). Dynamic (EMG) recordings usually distinguish the

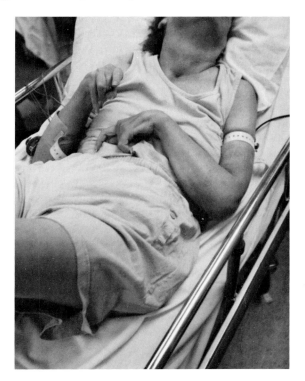

FIGURE 4. A 33-year-old woman sustained severe TBI 7 months earlier and remained in a vegetative state. Nursing home staff could not access the axilla because of an adducted/internally rotated shoulder. Dynamic EMG suggested that the pectoralis major but not the latissimus dorsi contributed to this posture. Phenol blocks to the medial and lateral pectoral nerves were recommended.

voluntary capacity from spastic reaction of adductor muscles during attempted abduction by the patient or passive stretch by the examiner.

In contrast to dynamic patterns of muscle dysfunction, static deformity of the shoulder may be associated with fixed muscle contracture and/or joint capsule contracture (a result of adhesive capsulitis). The examiner inspects and palpates the shoulder for deformity, swelling, tenderness, and pain on motion. Radiographs are obtained to rule out bony deformity, such as a previously missed fracture or dislocation of the shoulder, and heterotopic ossification (HO). HO is seen in approximately 11% of patients with traumatic brain injury, and the shoulder joint is involved in approximately one-fourth of these patients for an overall incidence of shoulder HO of 3%.[19] If a fracture or dislocation is

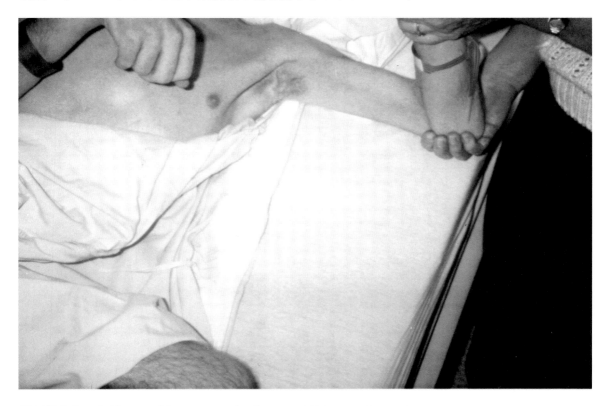

FIGURE 5. A 19-year-old man sustained severe TBI 3 months earlier. Prominence of the pectoralis major is seen. The latissimus dorsi and teres major were also involved.

associated with the brain injury, the incidence of HO rises dramatically. Heterotopic ossification is most commonly located inferior and medial to the humeral head on an anteroposterior radiograph.

If no bony abnormalities such as congenital deformity, missed fractures or heterotopic ossification are found, a supraclavicular diagnostic block of the brachial plexus with a local anesthetic such as lidocaine or bupivacaine may be performed to relax the shoulder muscles. Anesthetic block of the nerves to the various shoulder muscles helps to determine how much of the limited range of shoulder motion is secondary to a fixed myostatic contracture or adhesive capsulitis of the glenohumeral joint. If dynamic EMG studies suggest coactivation of the pectoralis major during attempted abduction of the shoulder, anesthetic block of the medial and lateral pectoral nerves may unmask abduction (Fig.6). Similarly, block of the lower subscapular nerve selectively diminishes activity of the teres major muscle, whereas block

of the upper and lower subscapular nerves selectively diminishes activity of the subscapularis muscle. (These blocks are among the more difficult to do.[27] The frequency with which the subscapularis contributes to the deformity of internal rotation needs further study). Block of the thoracodorsal nerve selectively diminishes activity of the latissimus dorsi. In the potentially functional shoulder, the combination of dynamic EMG with anesthetic blocks of the individual internal rotator muscles (particularly pectoralis major and teres major) is useful for determining whether selective surgical release of one or more muscles will improve movement of the shoulder while preserving function.

Findings and Treatment Options. Usually tone is increased in the pectoralis major with variable activity in the latissimus dorsi and teres major. It is not uncommon to find volitional characteristics in muscles such as the pectoralis major and teres major over and above their spastic reactions during the patient's attempts to abduct the limb. In the early course of recovery, phenol blocks may be applied to reduce spastic reactions during volitional movement as well as mobilization of the shoulder to prevent an impingement syndrome. Passive abduction without concomitant external rotation may produce painful impingement of the greater tuberosity of the humerus against the acromion. Shoulder joint injection may be used for diagnostic and therapeutic purposes in such patients. For the nonfunctional shoulder, 70° of abduction and 45° of external rotation are usually sufficient to allow access to the axilla for washing and sufficient range of motion for dressing. Heterotopic ossification, typically inferomedial, does not interfere with range of motion; restriction of shoulder motion is more likely attributable to other soft-tissue tightness. If HO is present at the shoulder, it is likely to be present at other joints, such as the elbow, hips, or

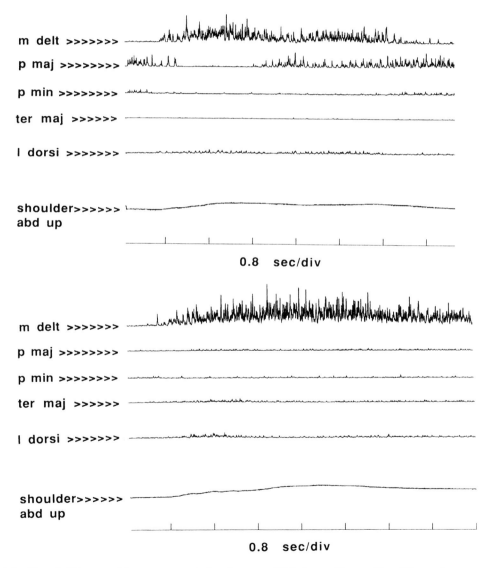

FIGURE 6. *Top*, A 38-year-old woman sustained severe TBI 6 months earlier. When she was asked to abduct her shoulder voluntarily, dynamic EMG revealed that she had voluntary capacity in the middle deltoid, but she also coactivated the pectoralis major, which appeared to restrain motion. *Bottom*, Medial and lateral pectoral nerve blocks with bupivacaine eliminated pectoralis major activity and resulted in an unmasking of abductor strength.

knees; in these locations HO usually causes considerable clinical problems. Treatment options for shoulder HO are considered by some to include disodium etidronate and indomethacin.[44]

Late in the course of recovery, surgical release of offending muscles should be considered. Unfortunately, because of their extensive origins, these muscles do not easily lend themselves to procedures of the slide type, which would diminish pull while preserving function. The distal insertions of the adductor muscles have very short tendons, with minimal overlapping of muscle bellies, and thus do not allow for myotendinous (fractional) or Z-lengthening. However, in patients with functional potential, as determined electromyographically, release of only one or two muscles may be sufficient to improve movement at the shoulder.

In patients with hygiene and dressing problems but no capacity for active functional movement, release from the humerus of the pectoralis major, teres major, subscapularis, and latissimus dorsi muscles may be considered. In such cases the joint capsule, even if tight, should not be released, as subluxation, dislocation, or severe stiffness of the shoulder will result. Once the offending muscles have been released, residual tightness of the joint capsule may be overcome with gentle range of motion.

In patients in whom shoulder motion is severely limited by extensive heterotopic bone, excision should be considered,[18] especially if dynamic EMG studies reveal volitional capacity for the various shoulder muscles. Excision also may be undertaken to improve passive shoulder functions. CT scans of the shoulder, cross-sections, and three-dimensional reconstruction assist with preoperative planning. Radiographic assessment of joints with HO may be severely limited by difficulties with positioning the patient for the necessary view.

Bent Elbow

Clinical Description.   Elbow flexors are usually more spastic than elbow extensors; as a result, typically the patient has a bent elbow or elbow flexion posturing. The patient may have relatively fixed elbow flexion posturing with little volitional motion in flexion or extension, but more often the patient has voluntary flexion and some ability to extend the elbow, although slower extension is asymmetrical with respect to quicker flexion.

Functional Consequences and Penalties. Elbow motion allows the upper limb to be shortened or lengthened, thereby enabling placement of the hand outward in space or towards the face and body. Upper motoneuron lesions affecting elbow flexors and extensors tend to restrict both possibilities. The ability to reach out and exert a stabilizing force against an object as it rests on a surface is also restricted. Severe flexion posturing may cause skin maceration in the antecubital fossa and impair proper hygiene. A markedly bent elbow impedes dressing with the upper extremities.

Differential Diagnosis and Diagnostic Work-Up.   The bent elbow may be a static deformity attributable to soft-tissue contracture or bony ankylosis. Inspection and palpation for deformity and swelling or tenderness should be performed. Range of motion on a passive as well as active basis is also examined. Passive range of motion at slow, intermediate, and rapid velocities of stretch is often helpful in distinguishing among hypertonicity, rigidity, and contracture. The workup should include radiographs to rule out a previously missed fracture or dislocation of the elbow; it is also important to rule out heterotopic ossification.

A dynamic pattern of motor dysfunction is typical, with spastic resistance provided by the elbow flexors during attempted extension movements. The three major elbow flexors are the biceps, brachialis, and brachioradialis. Clinical examination may suggest which of these muscles or combination of muscles contributes to dynamic dysfunction, but dynamic EMG provides definitive evidence. Each of these muscles is accessible to surface electrode recordings. Elbow flexion posturing is often a combination of dynamic and static deformities. The difference in the amount of spasticity and volitional control among the three elbow flexors is often significant[36] (Fig. 7 and 8). Additional work-up may include anesthetic block, which typically is

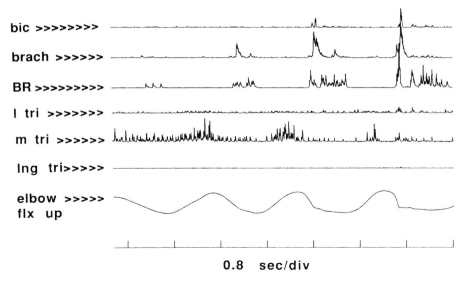

FIGURE 7. A 26-year-old man sustained TBI 3 years earlier and developed left hemiparesis. Passive stretch of the elbow flexors at different velocities revealed that the brachioradialis (BR) was most sensitive to stretch, followed by the brachialis and biceps. The brachialis and biceps demonstrate phasic reactivity, whereas the BR demonstrates phasic and tonic reactivity, especially at higher rates of passive stretch. Differential spasticity across muscles spanning a joint is common after TBI.

done after a dynamic EMG recording. Musculocutaneous nerve block anesthetizes the biceps and brachialis, allowing assessment of the contribution of the brachioradialis to dynamic movement. Similarly, a motor point block to the brachioradialis allows evaluation of the contribution of the biceps and brachialis, and biceps motor point block isolates the biceps from the other two muscles.

Findings and Treatment Options. Many patients show moderate-to-complete EMG interference patterns in the triceps musculature although one or another head of the triceps may be inactive. The biceps commonly demonstrates the presence of volitional activity, but it is frequently active to a variable extent during attempts at elbow extension (Fig. 9). The brachioradialis more often shows a much less volitional pattern during elbow flexion but demonstrates considerable coactivation during attempts at elbow extension. The brachialis may show a complete interference pattern during voluntary flexion, and of the three muscles it is least likely to demonstrate coactivation during attempts at elbow extension.

During the early course of recovery, elbow extension, which is most often impeded by

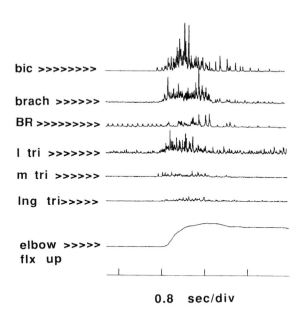

FIGURE 8. The same patient as in Figure 7. Dynamic EMG reveals that he can voluntarily activate biceps and brachialis to flex his elbow, but the EMG interference pattern in the brachioradialis (BR) is very weak. Thus, volition is reduced in the BR, which is also the most spastic of the three elbow flexors (see Fig. 7). Fifteen months or more after TBI, such a muscle may be considered for outright surgical release as opposed to lengthening.

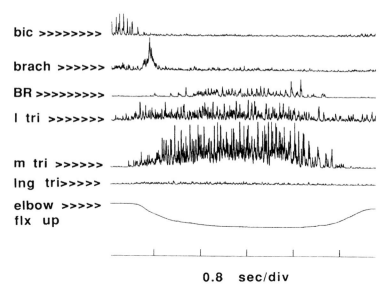

bic >>>>>>>
brach >>>>>>
BR >>>>>>>>
l tri >>>>>>>
m tri >>>>>>
lng tri>>>>
elbow >>>>>
flx up

0.8 sec/div

FIGURE 9. Same patient as in Figures 7 and 8. Dynamic EMG reveals that the brachioradialis is co-activated during voluntary forward reach of the upper extremity towards a target. Biceps and brachialis activity essentially turn off at the beginning of elbow extension, whereas BR activity picks up as elbow extension and flexor stretch proceed. The medial triceps demonstrates a good voluntary interference pattern, whereas lateral triceps pattern is moderate. The long head of the triceps is not activated at all. Thus, the behavior of the agonists and antagonists may show quite a bit of variability in volitional capacity and spastic characteristics.

the brachioradialis, may improve after phenol block to the motor point of the brachioradialis. If the biceps is observed to be the major offender, phenol block to the motor point of the biceps or the musculocutaneous nerve may be considered. Phenol may cause dysesthesia if it is instilled into a mixed sensory and motor peripheral nerve. The musculocutaneous nerve contains a sensory component from the skin. In brain-injured patients with a low level of responsiveness, the clinician may be more inclined to perform a musculocutaneous nerve block with phenol; dysesthesia, if it occurs, often recedes after 3 or 4 weeks. Because the brachialis is least involved as a spastic muscle, motor point block of the biceps with phenol is a common option, especially for persons with higher levels of arousal and cognition.

Because the bent elbow is often a combination of static and dynamic deformities, serial casting is commonly applied after a block. Casts are changed every 3–5 days. A drop-out cast is often useful to allow patients with activation of elbow extensors to attempt to stretch the flexion contracture on their own. In addition, electrical stimulation of the triceps musculature as part of a drop-out cast system also may help to stretch the flexion contracture.

Beyond 12–15 months after head injury, when additional neurologic recovery is not anticipated, surgical lengthening of the elbow

flexors is considered. (Fig. 10). If at that time the brachioradialis shows no volitional capacity on dynamic EMG evaluation, it may be considered for proximal release to improve function of triceps. The biceps and brachialis typically show volition and are therefore lengthened. If the dynamic EMG study demonstrates volitional activation of one or more heads of the triceps, the prognosis for faster and smoother elbow extension is favorable (Fig. 11).

If there is no volitional activity in spastic elbow flexors but positioning and hygiene are problematic, the biceps tendon and brachioradialis muscle are released in conjunction with fractional (myotendinous) lengthening of the brachialis muscle. Leaving the brachialis muscle decreases the amount of dead space in the wound, lessens the incidence of wound hematoma and infection, and prevents the later development of elbow extension contracture from unopposed triceps activity.

If heterotopic ossification (HO) restricts elbow motion, it is surgically excised at maturation. Maturation of HO is determined by the radiographic appearance of a defined cortex and by a normal level of serum alkaline phosphatase. Additional prognostic indicators for successful HO excision are good cognitive recovery (Rancho level VI or greater) and selective motor control in the extremity. Time since onset of brain injury is not an accurate prognosticator when considered

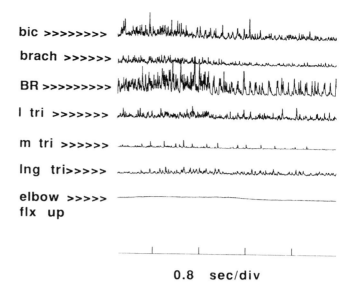

bic >>>>>>>

brach >>>>>>

BR >>>>>>>>

l tri >>>>>>>

m tri >>>>>>

lng tri>>>>>

elbow >>>>>
flx up

0.8 sec/div

FIGURE 10. Same patient as in Figures 7, 8, and 9. During upright ambulation, severe elbow flexion posturing prevented sufficient extension of the elbow for the patient to hold onto a walker. Dynamic EMG during gait revealed that all three elbow flexors were active, especially the brachioradialis (BR), which was also known to have poor volitional characteristics (see Figure 8). The patient underwent lengthening of the biceps and brachialis along with proximal release of the BR. He was able to hold onto a walker for the first time in 3 years.

alone. HO is seen in the elbow in 4% of patients with TBI.[19] However, if fracture or dislocation is associated with brain injury, the incidence of HO rises to 89%. The ulnar nerve may become surrounded by a tunnel of HO, but it can be dissected free with steadfast carefulness. Compression of the ulnar nerve in the cubital canal, unrelated to HO, may be an associated injury in spastic patients with limited elbow control. A bent elbow also may be associated with stretching of the ulnar nerve around a persistently flexed elbow. Surgical transposition of the ulnar nerve may be considered.

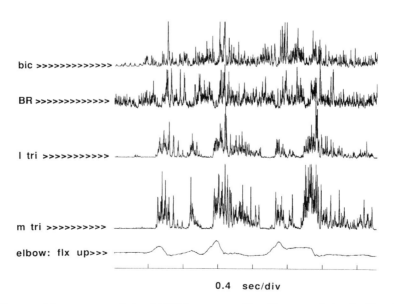

bic >>>>>>>>>>>>

BR >>>>>>>>>>>>

l tri >>>>>>>>>>

m tri >>>>>>>>>>

elbow: flx up>>>

0.4 sec/div

FIGURE 11. A 22-year-old woman sustained TBI 5 years earlier. She complained of having to struggle when she attempted to extend her elbow. During the task of hammering a nail, the patient performed erratically and without smoothness. Dynamic EMG reveals a noisy record, especially for the elbow flexors (biceps and brachioradialis). These flexors coactivate, especially during the extension downstroke of hammering, and clonus appears briefly in both flexors and extensors of the elbow, suggesting loop hyperexcitability of the stretch reflex. Because the patient exhibited voluntary capacity in all elbow flexors and extensors, she underwent lengthening of the three elbow flexors, which resulted in smoother elbow extension.

Pronated Forearm

Clinical Description.   Pronation of the forearm appears to be a more common deformity than supination. Resistance to passive supination is increased, and range of motion usually is restricted to some extent. Many patients show some degree of both active supination and active pronation.

Functional Consequences and Penalties. When the forearm supinates, the hand becomes oriented to the body, whereas pronation orients the hand and objects in it away from the body. Many instrumental activities of daily living depend on supination of the forearm, such as using feeding and grooming utensils and clothing fasteners. Spastic pronators restrict the possibilities of orienting a hand-held object toward the face or body. When supinators are spastic, the possibilities of orienting the palmar surface of the hand toward an object located in space are similarly restricted. A dysfunction of hand orientation can be severely disabling.

Differential Diagnosis and Diagnostic Work-Up.   Pronator dysfunction may have a dynamic basis associated with spasticity of the pronator teres and/or pronator quadratus. Dynamic EMG is helpful in making such a determination (Fig.12). Surface electrodes

are usually sufficient to record EMG from each pronator.

Static deformity may be due to muscle contracture or heterotopic ossification. A radiograph is obtained to rule out previously missed fractures of the radius or ulna, dislocation of the proximal radius, or a bony bridge of heterotopic ossification connecting the radius with the ulna and thereby blocking radioulnar motion. A local anesthetic block to the median nerve above the elbow is useful in assessing contracture. Separate motor point blocks of the pronator teres and pronated quadratus may help to further define this issue.

Dynamic deformity involving supinator muscles may be associated with spasticity of the biceps and/or supinator. Biceps spasticity associated with elbow flexion posturing does not necessarily correlate with biceps-induced supination deformity (flexion deformity at the elbow often is associated with pronation deformity of the forearm). Musculocutaneous nerve block with local anesthetic for biceps motor point block may be useful in assessing the contribution of the supinator muscle to tone and contracture and in making inferences about the contribution of the biceps. Supinator motor point block may be difficult to perform, but radial nerve block above the elbow eliminates supinator spasticity so that

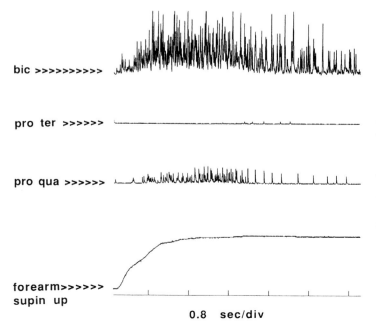

bic >>>>>>>>>>

pro ter >>>>>>

pro qua >>>>>>

forearm>>>>>>
supin up

0.8   sec/div

FIGURE 12.   A 17-year-old man sustained TBI 8 months earlier. Voluntary active supination of the forearm (with elbow flexed) reveals a good voluntary pattern in the supinating biceps but coactivation of pronator quadratus, especially as the limit of supination range is reached. The pronator teres is not stretch-reactive.

FIGURE 13. A 57-year-old man sustained TBI 6 months earlier. The only clinically available movement was a small range of active pronation/supination of the left forearm. The patient used this small range to signal yes/no responses. Dynamic EMG revealed that the pronator quadratus had voluntary capacity for pronation, but the pronator teres did not. However, both pronators were coactivated during supination effort, especially the pronator quadratus. The patient underwent phenol motor point block to the pronator quadratus; considerable improvement in the active range of supination enabled him to communicate more clearly.

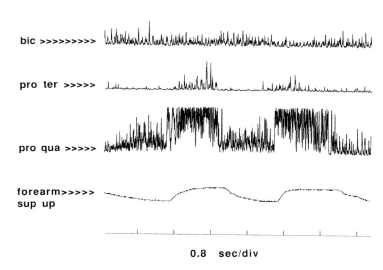

0.8 sec/div

the contribution of the biceps can be isolated and assessed. Dynamic EMG of the biceps can be recorded with a surface electrode, but the supinator muscle requires intramuscular placement of a wire electrode.

Findings and Treatment Options. The pronator quadratus and pronator teres often demonstrate volitional capacity and spastic reaction during attempted supination (Fig. 13). Such findings are often dissociated, that is, one muscle may show volitional capacity or spastic reaction while the other muscle does not. The pronator teres may be a potential muscle for transfer into finger extensors, wrist extensors, the long thumb extensor, or even thumb opposition mechanism. Such transfers are highly dependent on the motor control capabilities of the pronator teres, namely whether there is good control of on/off activity with little or not spasticity.

During the early course of recovery, depending on dynamic EMG findings, phenol block of the pronator teres and/or pronator quadratus may be considered. Aggressive range-of-motion exercises are then carried out. Serial casting may be considered but requires inclusion of the elbow joint into the cast and may result in an elbow flexion contracture. Therefore, serial casting must be combined with progressive stretching of elbow flexors at some point. In late recovery after head injury, release or lengthening of the pronator teres and/or biceps may be considered for their respective deformities.

Release of the pronator quadratus is possible, but the dissection is difficult. We prefer phenol motor point blocks to the pronator quadratus in serial fashion, as needed.

Bent Wrist

Clinical Description. Wrist flexion posturing is more common than wrist extension. Wrist flexors, particularly the flexor carpi radialis, are strong muscles, and the degree of wrist flexion deformity may be great (Fig. 14). Passive motion may be severely restricted, although it is not surprising to find clinical evidence of slight active wrist extension as well as flexion in many patients as they recover.

Functional Consequences and Penalties. The wrist makes small calibration adjustments of hand position as the hand approaches a target variably located in space, and wrist position is an important determinant of grip strength. The wrist also plays an important role in the positioning of objects before their release from the hand and in the release mechanism itself. Spastic flexion deformity of the wrist severely impairs grasp and release functions of the hand. Prepositioning of the hand with respect to objects that need to be manipulated is also impaired by wrist muscle dysfunction.

Differential Diagnosis and Diagnostic Work-Up. Passive stretch of the wrist flexors on physical examination typically reveals the

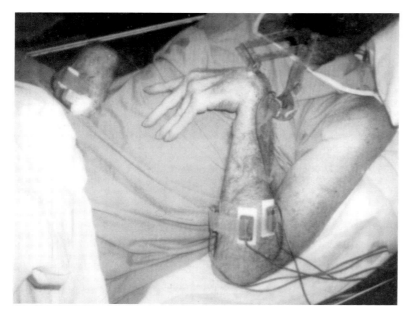

FIGURE 14. A 37-year-old man sustained TBI 7 months earlier. Passive motion of the wrist was severely restricted because of wrist flexor spasticity. Dynamic EMG studies revealed that the patient could activate wrist extensors and flexors voluntarily, but motion was limited (see Fig. 15).

high tension resistance of bent wrist deformity. Because spasticity of the flexor carpi radialis is so obvious, lack of spasticity in the flexor carpi ulnaris may be overlooked. This muscle may not be spastic because of a compression neuropathy of the ulnar nerve in the cubital tunnel. Such a compression neuropathy is not uncommonly caused by repeated trauma on lap boards, wheelchair armrests, and siderails of the patient's bed. In addition, a bent elbow deformity may cause a stretch injury to the ulnar nerve, which is stretched around the bend of the elbow. The examiner should search for signs of intrinsic muscle atrophy in the hand, which may result from ulnar nerve neuropathy at the elbow. Electrodiagnostic studies, including nerve conduction velocities and electromyography, are useful in this context.

Dynamic EMG kinesiology studies of the wrist extensors and flexors is performed to determine whether they have volitional capacity. It is surprising how often wrist extensor activity is present with little or no wrist motion because of the overriding spasticity and contracture problems inherent in the bent wrist deformity (Fig.15). Radiographs of the wrist are useful to rule out subluxation and/or unrecognized fractures. Electrodiagnostic studies of the median nerve in the carpal tunnel should be strongly considered, because severe wrist flexion and pressure on the median nerve against the leading edge of the transverse carpal ligament may result in severe carpal tunnel syndrome.[55]

Findings and Treatment Options. Wrist and finger flexion deformities often coexist. Wrist flexor spasticity may be treated with phenol and motor point blocks.[20] An injection of the nerve proper is undesirable because of the large sensory components of both median and ulnar nerves at the level of the forearm. Surgical dissection of the motor branches of these nerves would be extensive and cause excessive scarring for only temporary relief of spasticity. For these reasons, motor point blocks are performed with needle electrode stimulation.

Because finger flexion deformities are commonly associated with wrist flexion deformities, the fingers must also be treated (see below). If phenol blocks to the motor points of the flexor digitorum sublimis and flexor digitorum profundus are difficult to do, repeated local anesthetic blocks can be performed to the median and ulnar nerves above the elbow to facilitate the application of serial casts. In the late period of motor recovery, wrist and finger flexor lengthenings may be performed and should be considered for functional procedures as well as nonfunctional,

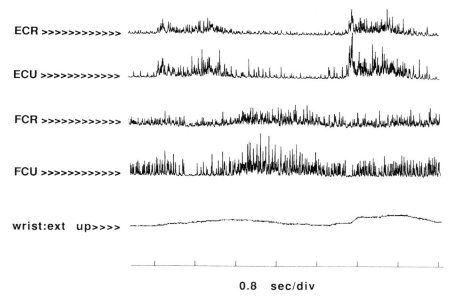

0.8 sec/div

FIGURE 15. Same patient as in Figure 14. Dynamic EMG studies revealed that the patient was able to generate weak but definite EMG activity in the wrist extensors during attempted wrist extension, but these muscles coactivated in a spastic manner during extension effort. Reciprocal inhibition of extensors during flexor effort was fair-to-good; reciprocal inhibition of flexors during extension effort was poor. (ECR, ECU, FCR, FCU = extensor or flexor carpi radialis or ulnaris.)

cosmetic procedures, depending on the findings of dynamic EMG studies.

Clenched Fist

Clinical Description. In the clenched fist deformity, the fingers are typically clasped tightly into the palm (Fig. 16). The metacarpophalangeal and proximal interphalangeal joints are flexed 90°. The distal interphalangeal joints may be extended fully or flexed into the palm. Some relaxation of finger tightness may be obtained if the wrist is positioned in extreme flexion. Finger tightness is enhanced with wrist extension.

Functional Consequences and Penalties. Finger function enables various types of grasp and object manipulations. Release of grasped objects is an equally important function. Impaired motor control, weakness, and spastic reaction cause great difficulty with three-jaw chuck, tip pinch, cylindrical grasp, power grasp, and pail grasp. The clenched fist deformity impairs finger manipulation of objects and selective finger actions in

FIGURE 16. The clenched fist deformity. Extension of the distal interphalangeal (DIP) joints of the long and ring digits suggests that the flexor digitorum sublimis but not profundus was involved for both digits. Flexion of the DIP joints for the index and small fingers suggests involvement of the flexor digitorum profundus.

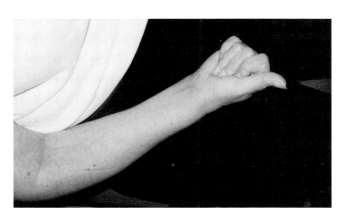

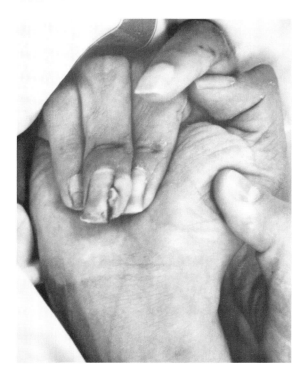

FIGURE 17. Recurrent nailbed infection in a clenched fist deformity.

general. A tightly clenched fist leads to increased skin maceration and breakdown, impaired hygiene, recurrent nailbed infections (Fig. 17), recurrent fingernail laceration of the palmar skin, and poor cosmetic appearance of the hand.

Differential Diagnosis and Diagnostic Work-Up. The extrinsic finger flexors to the four digits of the hand are the flexor digitorum sublimis and flexor digitorum profundus. These muscles—separately, in part, or in their entirety—may show volitional characteristics and spasticity, spasticity with poor volition, or the typical combination of spasticity, contracture, and weakness. In addition, the extrinsic finger extensors are often weak. Hyperactive intrinsic muscles of the hand are commonly associated with hyperactive extrinsic muscles. However, intrinsic spasticity of the hand is often masked by severe spasticity of the extrinsic muscles. Relief of spastic extrinsic muscles may lead to an intrinsic-plus deformity unless intrinsic spasticity of the hand is also relieved. Other potential contributors to the clenched

fist deformity are contracture of the palmar skin and joint capsule and collateral ligament tightness at the various finger joints. Fixed contracture of the intrinsic muscles may also be present.

Physical examination, dynamic EMG, and anesthetic nerve blocks assist in differentiating various pathologies. During physical examination it is helpful to inspect for associated wrist flexion deformity, intrinsic atrophy pattern, absence of normal skinfold markings over the finger joints, tautness of palmar skin maceration, malodor, nailbed infection and nail indentations, or frank breakdown of palmar skin. Passive range of motion of the fingers is tested with the wrists held in extension, neutral position, and flexion. Full extension of the fingers is normally possible while the wrist is maintained in 45° of extension. With the wrist held in different positions and the metacarpophalangeal joint maintained by the examiner in extension, passive range of the flexor digitorum sublimis for each finger may be examined by extending each digit separately at the proximal interphalangeal joint. Greater stretch of the flexor digitorum sublimis occurs when the wrist is held in more extended positions;

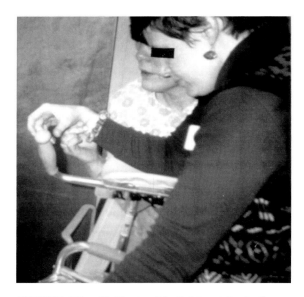

FIGURE 18. Patient with tight extrinsic finger flexors. To open her hand in preparation for grasping the walker, the patient must flex her wrist to place the finger flexors on relative slack. If the wrist remains flexed, power gripping of the walker is diminished.

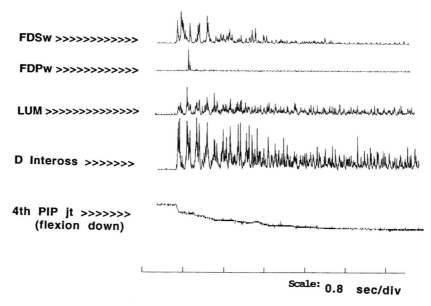

FDSw >>>>>>>>>>>

FDPw >>>>>>>>>>>

LUM >>>>>>>>>>>>>>

D Inteross >>>>>>>

4th PIP jt >>>>>>>
(flexion down)

Scale: 0.8 sec/div

FIGURE 19. In a young man who sustained TBI 3 years earlier, passive metacarpophalangeal joint extension, followed by rapid proximal interphalangeal joint flexion, stretched the intrinsic muscles and produced clonus in the lumbrical and dorsal interossei muscles as well as unsustained clonus in the extrinsic flexor digitorum sublimis (FDSw).

hence, tightness and loss of range are evident as a function of wrist extension (Fig. 19). In similar manner, passive range of motion across the distal interphalangeal joint provides information about flexor digitorum profundus.

Spasticity involving the intrinsic muscles of the hand is common but may be masked by spastic deformities in the extrinsic finger flexors. An adducted thumb, limited extension of the metacarpophalangeal joints, or swan-neck positioning of the fingers should alert the physician to the possibility of underlying intrinsic spasticity. A two-step examination may help to identify intrinsic spasticity and joint contracture.

1. The examiner holds the metacarpophalangeal joint in 90° of flexion while passively flexing the proximal interphalangeal joint. This maneuver causes stretch of the intrinsic muscles across the proximal interphalangeal joint.

2. The examiner passively extends the metacarpophalangeal joint to neutral and then flexes the proximal interphalangeal joint. This maneuver produces additional stretch of the intrinsic muscles across the extended metacarpophalangeal joint (Fig. 19).

If the intrinsic muscles are tight, flexion of the proximal interphalangeal joint is less with the metacarpophalangeal joint held in extension than with the same joint held in flexion. If proximal interphalangeal joint range of motion was found to be equally restricted during each step of the clinical maneuvers, joint capsular contracture should be suspected.

Active motion of the flexor digitorum sublimis is tested with the metacarpophalangeal joint extended. The patient is asked to flex the proximal phalanx. If flexion of the distal interphalangeal joint is observed, the flexor digitorum sublimis may be very weak or absent, with compensation by the flexor digitorum profundus. Combined flexion and extension movements are tested with the metacarpophalangeal joint held first in extension and then in flexion. When the metacarpophalangeal joint is held in extension, extension at the proximal interphalangeal joint is typically accomplished by the extensor digitorum communis and flexion by the flexor digitorum sublimis. When the metacarpophalangeal joint is held at 90° of flexion, extension at the proximal interphalangeal joint may be accomplished by volitional activity in the intrinsic muscles. If the proximal interphalangeal joints are extending, the intrinsic muscles also flex at the metacarpophalangeal joints. According to Basmajian, the lumbrical muscles are active whenever the metacarpophalangeal joints are flexing, no matter what the more distal joints are doing.[4] Thus, in making a complete fist on a voluntary basis, the lumbrical muscles as well as the flexor digitorum sublimis and flexor digitorum profundus are active.

When strong deforming forces play a role in the spastic hand, it may be difficult to sort muscle function on the basis of clinical examination alone. Dynamic EMG enables the study of the extrinsic and intrinsic muscles of the hand. Typically the extrinsic finger flexors, located deep to the wrist flexors in the forearm, are studied with intramuscular wire electrodes. Electrical stimulation of the muscle into which that wire has been inserted demonstrates when the examiner has placed the wire in the desired muscle. An intramuscular wire electrode also may be placed in the extensor digitorum communis when spread of activity from nearby wrist muscles is a concern. We record from the interossei and the lumbrical muscles by using surface electrodes placed between the metacarpals on the dorsal or the volar surface of the hand, respectively. Ulnar and median nerve blocks at the wrist with local anesthetics help to identify contracture of the finger

and thumb intrinsic muscles. Median nerve block at the elbow provides information about extrinsic finger flexor contracture, and ulnar nerve block above the elbow may be necessary to provide information about the flexor digitorum profundus for the fourth and fifth fingers.

Findings and Treatment Options.   In spastic patients the flexor digitorum sublimis often shows little volitional activity but much coactivation during attempted extension (Figs. 20 and 21). The flexor digitorum profundus typically has volitional capacity but is often spastic during attempted finger extension. Although intrinsic muscle spasticity is often present, it is surprising how much volitional capacity the intrinsic muscles often retain. Management during early recovery depends, in part, on the patient's degree of alertness. If the patient has a low level of arousal and appreciation of dysesthesia is not believed to be a consideration, then ulnar and/or median nerve phenol block should be considered. However, in patients functioning at a higher level of arousal with satisfactory sensory awareness, percutaneous motor point blocks to the flexor digitorum sublimis and flexor digitorum profundus with phenol may be considered. Because contracture of extrinsic finger flexors often accompanies spasticity, serial casting also should be considered. Local anesthetic block to the median

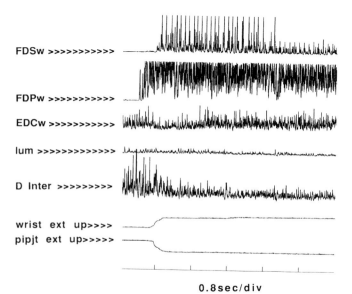

FDSw >>>>>>>>>>

FDPw >>>>>>>>>>

EDCw >>>>>>>>>>

lum >>>>>>>>>>>>

D Inter >>>>>>>>>

wrist ext up>>>>

pipjt ext up>>>>>

0.8sec/div

FIGURE 20.   Patient who sustained TBI 5 years earlier. Intramuscular wire electrodes have been inserted into the flexor digitorum sublimis (FDSw), flexor digitorum profundus (FDPw), and extensor digitorum communis (EDCw). Surface electrodes recorded activity in lumbrical and dorsal interossei muscles. During attempted voluntary flexion of the fingers (i.e., hand closing), FDPw shows an excellent interference pattern, but FDSw is electromyographically weak.

FIGURE 21. Same patient as in Figure 18. This record reveals that during finger extension (i.e., hand opening) the extensor digitorum communis (EDCw) has a good interference pattern consistent with volitional effort, but the flexor digitorum sublimis (FDSw) is coactivated in a spastic manner. The flexor digitorum profundus (FDPw) is largely inactive.

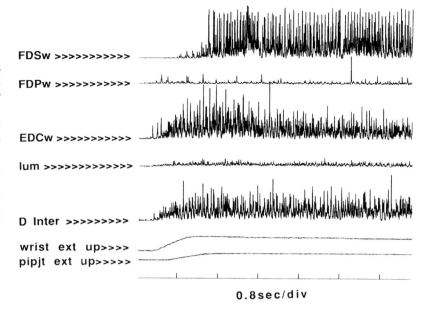

FDSw >>>>>>>>>>>

FDPw >>>>>>>>>>>

EDCw >>>>>>>>>>>

lum >>>>>>>>>>>>

D Inter >>>>>>>>>

wrist ext up>>>>

pipjt ext up>>>>>

0.8sec/div

and ulnar nerves above the elbow may be performed before casting to relax not only the finger flexors but also the wrist flexors. It is often not necessary to reblock when the cast is changed if the clinician does not provoke spasticity by excessive examination of the fingers and wrist after removal of the cast. If necessary, however, it is possible to reblock before recasting. For patients in the late stages of recovery—we consider 9 months after injury as the threshold compared with previous estimations of 12–18 months—more definitive procedures are considered. If the flexor digitorum sublimis and flexor digitorum profundus show volitional capacity along with spastic reaction during extension, lengthening of both muscle groups is recommended.[37] When spasticity is present but volition is absent, a superficialis to profundus transfer is considered to allow the hand to main relatively open and cosmetic in appearance.[38] When the flexor digitorum sublimis is spastic and shows no volitional capacity, this muscle group is considered for release as opposed to lengthening. A temporary anesthetic block to the ulnar nerve in Guyon's canal may be performed to simulate grossly the results of surgery. When the intrinsic muscles of the hand have volitional capacity but also demonstrate spastic reaction, phenol block of the two motor branches of the ulnar nerve in Guyon's canal may be performed

after surgical exposure (i.e., an open phenol block).[39] If the intrinsic muscles are spastic and have no volitional capacity, neurectomy of these motor branches is considered. In patients with contracture of the intrinsic muscles, release is considered. Joint contracture requires capsular release, and skin contracture in the palm may require a Z-plasty or skin grafting. Postsurgical hand rehabilitation emphasizes strengthening of muscles with volitional capacity by means of an active exercise program. Functional electrical stimulation and EMG biofeedback may serve as useful therapeutic adjuncts.

Thumb-in-Palm Deformity

Clinical Description. The thumb is pulled into the palm and unable to function during hand grip or as a post for the fingers. The thumb-in-palm deformity frequently is accompanied by a clenched fist deformity.

Functional Consequences and Penalties. The thumb is key to various grasp patterns, including the prehensile three-jaw chuck, the most common pattern of grasp for the upper extremity. In addition, the thumb plays a major role in lateral pinch or key grasp, and opposition of the thumb combined with distal interphalangeal flexion of the index and long fingers facilitates tip pinch, which allows pick-up of very small objects. The thumb-in-palm deformity essentially impairs various grasp and release patterns, including lateral pinch, three-jaw chuck, tip pinch, cylindrical grasp, and power grasp. Access to the palm for proper hygiene may be impeded, and skin maceration and breakdown may occur.

Differential Diagnosis and Diagnostic Work-Up. The thumb-in-palm deformity is heterogeneous in appearance and may be secondary to spasticity of many different muscles, including the flexor pollicis longus, flexor pollicis brevis, abductor pollicis brevis, opponens pollicis, adductor pollicis, and first dorsal and palmar interossei muscles. Physical examination, selective local anesthetic nerve blocks, and dynamic electromyography are useful in differentiating the contribution from each of these muscles. If physical examination reveals flexion of the interphalangeal joint of the thumb, contribution from the flexor pollicis longus may be confirmed by dynamic electromyography and motor point block. Dynamic EMG provides information about volitional capacity as well as spastic reaction. An alternative approach is to eliminate intrinsic spasticity in the hand through median and ulnar nerve blocks at the wrist.

When the thumb is in a severely adducted position, temporary ulnar nerve block in Guyon's canal at the wrist eliminates spastic contribution of the adductor pollicis and first dorsal interosseus. Adductor pollicis spasticity typically causes flexion at the metacarpophalangeal joint, whereas spasticity of the first dorsal interosseus results in narrowing of the thumb web space. Dynamic EMG studies also help to define the offending muscles.

Persistent thumb metacarpal flexion after ulnar nerve block suggests the possibility of thenar muscle spasticity. The pattern of dysfunction may involve the flexor pollicis brevis, abductor pollicis brevis, and opponens pollicis muscles. Palpable spasm usually reveals their involvement; findings can be confirmed by temporary median nerve block in the carpal tunnel and dynamic EMG testing. After a median nerve block, contracture of the thenar muscles may be observed.

Findings and Treatment Options. Thumb flexion deformity at the interphalangeal joint, particularly when the wrist is also postured in flexion, is often associated with some degree of contracture of the flexor pollicis longus. Nevertheless, even if spasticity is moderate or marked, voluntary characteristics are often present in the flexor pollicis longus as well. This activity may be harnessed for pinch grasp of small objects against the middle or distal phalanx of the index finger in a modified type of lateral pinch. This mechanism may be useful if spastic interphalangeal flexion can be reduced or eliminated. During the early course of recovery, motor point block of flexor pollicis longus with phenol is considered. Stretching of the thumb and the web space with a total contact cast may be considered along with serial bupivacaine blocks at the elbow to include median and ulnar nerves. The ulnar nerve block along with a casting approach is used when web space contracture is present and spastic reactivity needs to be managed to facilitate lateral pinch. Dynamic EMG usually reveals whether there is volitional capacity in the adductor pollicis and first dorsal interosseus that ultimately may be harnessed for lateral pinch. Percutaneous phenol to the ulnar nerve in Guyon's canal is not recommended, because the sensory branch of the ulnar nerve is close by and dysesthesias may result. In patients with a low level of arousal (as in a vegetative state), phenol injection of mixed nerves is sometimes considered.

Thenar muscle control is often problematic, and prognosis for regaining thumb opposition and related hand grasp patterns is unfavorable. Nevertheless, thenar muscle activity may contribute to pinch grasp, although the generation of force is typically weak. Flexion control of fingers and thumb is more important than finger extension, because grasp must be accomplished through flexion grasping by the fingers; crude but usable release may be accomplished by flexor relaxation or passive wrist drop without finger or thumb extension. If extrinsic finger extension can be controlled, a better outcome may be anticipated. During the early course of recovery, motor point blocks to specific thenar muscles with phenol can be performed. A

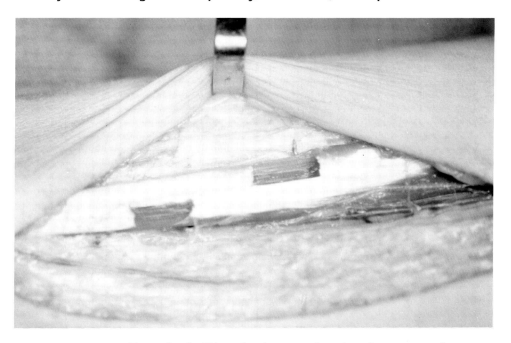

FIGURE 22.   Example of a Z-lengthening procedure in a forearm muscle.

phenol block to the recurrent motor branch of the median nerve is also possible.[35]

During late recovery, spasticity of flexor pollicis longus can be managed by fractional or Z-lengthening (Fig. 22). Excessive flexion contracture of the interphalangeal joint may require stabilization of the joint by arthrodesis. The purpose of such a procedure is to improve grasp and pinch in functional patients. In the late period of recovery, spastic thenar muscles, often associated with contracture, may be released at their origin.[8] Once the origins of the adductor pollicis, flexor pollicis brevis, and abductor pollicis are released and allowed to retract radially, they eventually scar down in a new location, and their function may be preserved while avoiding overcorrection or hyperextension deformity. Web space contracture may be managed with Z-plasty.

Flexed Hip

Clinical Description.   When hip flexors are spastic, they predominate over hip extensors. As a result, severe spasticity of the hip flexors not only causes hip flexor posturing and contractures, but also may contribute to knee flexion deformities. If adductor spasticity is also present, pelvic obliquity often develops.

When the hip is flexed in bed or in a wheelchair, spasticity of the rectus femoris is usually masked. Hip extension during the late stance of gait or knee flexion during early swing may be restricted by spastic hip flexors or the rectus femoris, respectively.

Functional Consequences and Penalties. Much like the shoulder joint, the hip joint functions as a universal joint and enables placement of the foot in a wide variety of locations in space. Restriction of motion at the hip causes a loss of adaptive placement of the leg and foot and, among other consequences, affects step and stride length during gait. Severe hip flexion posturing and contracture interfere with nursing care, prevent proper hygiene, and promote the development of pressure sores over the trochanter by limiting positioning of the patient. Secondary promotion of knee flexion contracture severely impairs the patient's ability to sit in a wheelchair. Patients with an excessively flexed hip and deformity or poor voluntary control of the opposite limb need to be lifted during transfers. When adductor spasticity and/or contracture is also present, the ability to sit in a chair is further compromised and often worsened by pelvic obliquity.

Differential Diagnosis and Work-Up. A number of muscle groups may contribute to an excessively flexed hip, including the iliopsoas, rectus femoris (which also crosses the knee joint), and pectineus (which also adducts the thigh). The adductor longus and brevis also may contribute to hip flexion, and spasticity in these and other adductors often coexists with hip flexor spasticity, thereby exacerbating hip flexion deformity. The Thomas test is used to examine the patient for hip flexor tone and available range of motion. In cases of severe spasticity, the Thomas test may be positive, but a diagnostic motor point block of the iliacus or a lumbar root paravertebral block may eliminate spasticity and helps to assess the presence of contracture more accurately. In addition, if the block leads to improvement, the rectus femoris can be evaluated more easily. The rectus crosses the hip and the knee joint and therefore should be examined by simultaneously extending the hip as much as possible and then flexing the knee. Even with the hip flexed, severe tightness of the rectus femoris restricts flexion at the knee. Tightness of other heads of the quadriceps may confound the examination of knee flexion. Dynamic EMG recording from hip and knee musculature is useful in identifying the contributions of the involved muscles.

Radiographs of the hip rule out heterotopic ossification, hip dislocation (especially if adductor spasticity is also present), and undiagnosed fractures. It is helpful to know whether pelvic fractures are present and whether lumbosacral fractures were sustained during the traumatic incident. Pain can generate spasticity in the hip flexors, and the incidence of heterotopic ossification about the hip joint increases in patients with pelvic or long bone fractures.

Flexor reflexes leading to hip flexion posturing may be triggered by cutaneous sources of stimulation, including nailbed infections, ingrown toenails, skin breakdown, urinary tract infection, bladder stones, rectal problems, and other sources of irritative afferent input. Physical examination and appropriate laboratory tests are revealing.

Findings and Treatment Options. Proning or positioning devices or even the use of a long leg cast with sufficient weight to stretch the hip flexors may be considered in the early period of recovery. If hip flexor spasticity cannot be controlled with positioning and stretching exercises, phenol blocks should be considered. Intramuscular wire electrode studies may reveal spasticity of the iliacus, and phenol motor point block of the iliacus may be considered. Alternatively, paravertebral phenol block of the upper lumbar motor root branches may be performed percutaneously.[23] Depending on dynamic EMG findings, rectus femoris motor point block also may be considered. If severe adduction spasticity complicates hip positioning, phenol block of the obturator nerve may be performed. If no bony deformity is present and spasticity cannot be controlled with blocks, early surgical intervention with lengthening of the iliopsoas and release of the pectineus may be considered.

Episodic flexor spasms are uncommon after head injury, but flexor withdrawal leading to persistent flexion posturing at the hip (and usually at the knee) has been reported. It may be tempting to use baclofen in such a circumstance, but caution is advised in patients who have problems with arousal and attention. Because it allows the use of much smaller doses, intrathecal instillation may be considered when hip flexor spasticity becomes intractable. Intrathecal baclofen has been studied well in patients with spinal cord injury and multiple sclerosis but not in patients with head injury.

Persistent spasticity of hip flexors in late recovery undoubtedly is associated with myostatic flexion contracture. Surgical release of contractured muscles is indicated[43] but corrects only about 50% of the deformity. Postoperative positioning and therapy are extremely important to promote correction of residual deformity. When release of a knee flexion contracture is performed simultaneously with hip flexor surgery, the weight of a long leg cast also provides a correcting force. A lengthening procedure may be undertaken when dynamic electromyography reveals appropriate hip flexor activity during preswing and early swing phases of gait, but inappropriate activity is also observed in other parts of the gait cycle, especially if activity correlates with restricted hip extension during mid to terminal stance.

Severe hip flexion contracture during late recovery should be considered for surgical release. In patients with severe adduction contracture, it may be necessary to perform a percutaneous release of the adductor longus tendon in the groin to allow proper positioning for hip flexor surgery. Muscle groups usually involved in this surgery include the rectus femoris, iliopsoas, pectineus, and sartorius. The tensor fascia lata and the anterior portion of the gluteus medius may be released from the iliac crest if they appear to contribute to the hip flexion deformity when the patient is under general anesthesia. Because the iliopsoas has capsular insertions, release of the associated tendon from the lesser trochanter of the femur does not provide complete release. Postoperative placement of the patient in a prone position 3 times/day for increasing periods of time, along with gentle stretching exercises, assists in correcting residual deformity. When a knee flexion contracture is released simultaneously, the weight of the long leg cast also provides a correcting force.

Scissoring Thighs

Clinical Description. The patient with adductor spasticity sits with "kissing" thighs or walks with a scissoring pattern characterized by medial thigh contact throughout the gait cycle or by a crossover pattern of the scissoring limb during swing phase with ultimate placement of one foot in front of or even lateral to the stance-phase foot. When adductor spasticity is also associated with hip flexor spasticity, the thigh of the involved side practically "sits atop" the opposite thigh.

Functional Consequences and Penalties. Adductor spasticity with scissor thighs leads to a narrow base of support, poor standing balance, unstable gait, and poor position during sitting. Limb advancement and limb clearance are impaired during gait. Patients often have a genu valgus thrust and impairment of contralateral limb advancement. Severe adductor spasticity promotes hip subluxation or dislocation, and often an apparent or functional leg-length discrepancy is associated with pelvic obliquity. Pressure sores over the contralateral knee may develop, transfers are made more difficult, and access to the perineum for hygiene and management of bowel and bladder functions is problematic. Positioning in bed and wheelchair is difficult.

Differential Diagnosis and Work-Up. Various muscles may contribute to limb scissoring, including the adductor longus and brevis, adductor magnus, and gracilis. Physical examination may suggest volitional capacity in the adductors as well as possible weakness in the abductors. Local anesthetic block to the obturator nerve helps to rule out myostatic contracture. Hip adductors may cause involuntary scissoring during the swing phase of gait; in the presence of weak hip flexors, however, the adductors also may function to advance the limb. Gait analysis includes dynamic EMG of hip adductors (Fig. 23), abductors, gluteus maximus, iliopsoas, and medial hamstrings. Three-dimensional motion analysis may be helpful to quantify the amount of hip adduction. Analysis of ground reaction forces helps to quantify mediolateral shear forces during stance phase.

Radiographic examination rules out bony deformities about the hip, including fracture, subluxation, dislocation, or heterotopic ossification. Absolute leg-length discrepancy may be secondary to limb shortening associated with fracture. Relative leg-length discrepancy may be associated with adductor contracture or severe spasticity. In such patients, measurements from the anterior superior iliac spine to the medial malleolus are symmetrical for both lower limbs, but measurements from the umbilicus to the medial malleolus of each side are not. When the examiner attempts to abduct the thigh passively with an adductor contracture, the whole pelvis moves, the anterosuperior iliac spine on the same side appears to "move up," and the pelvis appears oblique (that is, the anterior spine does not fall on a line parallel to the floor or the foot of the bed).

Findings and Treatment Options. When scissoring thighs are noted during gait, dynamic EMG demonstrates adductors with inappropriate activation during swing phase or even throughout the gait cycle. Analysis of

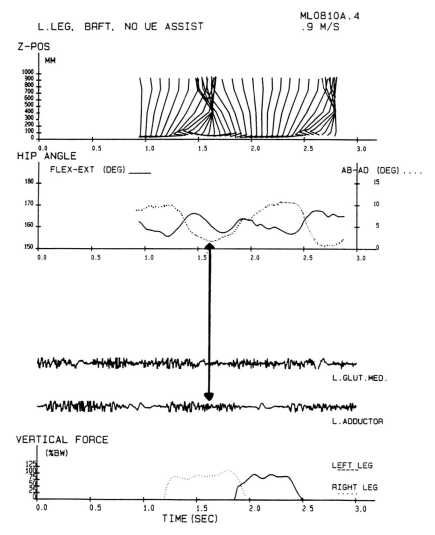

FIGURE 23. Data collected from a person with increased hip adduction. Note the abnormal peak adduction during swing phase, which correlates with the out-of-phase adductor EMG (see arrows).

ground reaction force demonstrates an increase in medial shear forces and a reduction in lateral shear forces. A temporary percutaneous obturator nerve block may reveal a static deformity (contracture) when no significant change in range of motion is noted after the block. However, if range of motion, especially active hip abduction, improves after the block, a dynamic deformity associated with spasticity is present. During the early course of recovery, obturator nerve block with phenol helps to decrease the dynamic deformity and facilitates strengthening of active hip abductors. If the hip adductors rather than hip flexors are used to

produce limb advancement, the obturator nerve block increases difficulty with limb advancement. Under these conditions, it may be better to avoid a phenol block of the obturator nerve; assistance devices, gait training, and orthotic control may serve the needs of advancement during gait.

In late recovery, diagnostic obturator nerve block is performed to distinguish between contracture and spasticity. If no myostatic contracture is present after the block, an isolated neurectomy may be performed to eliminate spasticity. When fixed contracture is present, release of the offending adductor muscles is necessary.[34] The adductor longus is usually released by proximal myotomy. The gracilis and adductor brevis are released close to their pelvic origin. The adductor magnus muscle is usually not included because it functions more as a hip extensor than as an adductor.

Stiff Knee

Clinical Description. Patients with a stiff knee are unable to flex the knee during the swing phase of gait. Usually the knee is maintained in extension throughout the gait cycle. Toe drag, which is likely in the early swing phase, may cause the patient to trip; thus balance and stability also are affected. The limb appears to be functionally longer. Circumduction of the involved limb, hiking of the pelvis, and/or contralateral limb vaulting may occur as compensatory maneuvers.

Functional Consequences and Penalties. Limb clearance and advancement may be impaired. Stability may be compromised by an early swing-phase toe drag. Balance may be impaired secondarily. Additional penalties include interference with the smooth forward progression of the center of gravity and a necessary increase in vertical displacement of the center of gravity as the functionally longer limb is cleared. This may lead to increased energy consumption or to a very slow gait. Gait on uneven surfaces and in cluttered environments becomes highly problematic. A stiff knee may interfere with transfers and wheelchair positioning. Step lengths may be asymmetrical, with the contralateral step length shortened.

Differential Diagnosis and Work-Up. Various factors may cause a stiff knee. Bony deformity must be ruled out, including fracture, subluxation, dislocation, and ossification, which often is found between layers of the quadriceps muscle. Soft-tissue contracture may be present, especially if the patient was in a long leg cast for a prolonged period. A dynamic deformity may be superimposed on soft-tissue contracture. Specific muscles that may contribute to the stiff knee gait include the rectus femoris, vastus medialis, vastus lateralis, vastus intermedius, and hamstrings. If the quadriceps group is overactive

during swing phase, the knee remains extended. If the hamstrings are overactive, the patient may guard against the possibility of sudden knee flexion and attempt to maintain the knee in extension throughout the gait cycle to ward off the possibility of knee collapse. Hip flexor weakness with decreased forward momentum of the thigh during swing phase may give rise to a stiff knee. In addition, patients who use hip adductors to advance the limb may not produce the necessary momentum for knee flexion. If the adductors are used for advancement, the limb is often kept in considerable external rotation. Thus the knee remains extended, because during stance phase the medial collateral ligament serves to prevent flexion of the knee in the line of progression. Patients who select a slow walking velocity may appear to have a stiff knee because walking slowly does not produce the necessary momentum for knee flexion to occur. Calf muscle spasticity with equinus during stance phase may lead to hyperextension of the knee and subsequent carryover during swing phase. Guarding against a weak calf (especially a weak soleus) muscle also may lead to compensatory behavior that results in knee extension or hyperextension during stance phase and subsequent carryover during swing phase.

Diagnostic work-up includes dynamic EMG of the rectus femoris, vastus medialis, vastus lateralis, vastus intermedius, and hamstrings. Three-dimensional motion analysis is helpful to quantify velocity, knee flexion and its timing, hip flexion and its timing, and ankle motion. Analysis of ground reaction forces helps to quantify anteroposterior shear forces. Physical examination includes passive and active range of motion of the knee, hip, and ankle while the patient is in bed, sitting, and standing. The rectus femoris should be tested with the hip in neutral position, and then the knee is passively flexed. Radiographs rule out bony abnormalities.

Findings and Treatment Options. Dynamic EMG may demonstrate activity in one or more heads of the quadriceps (Fig.24). Abnormal, out-of-phase EMG activity may be present in the rectus femoris from preswing through terminal swing or throughout the gait cycle. The rectus femoris and vastus intermedius

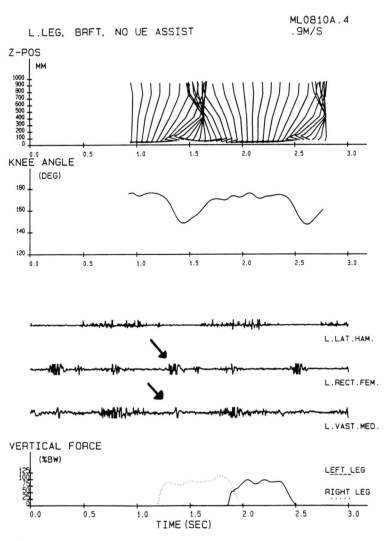

FIGURE 24. Data collected from a person with a stiff knee gait. Note the limited knee flexion during swing (approximately 30° compared with 60° for a normal knee), along with slightly decreased walking velocity (0.9 m/s compared with 1.2 m/s). Both the rectus femoris and vastus medialis show atypical bursts of activity (see arrows). The stick figure at the top is plotted on the same time base as the kinetic and kinematic data.

may demonstrate a similar pattern, or all four heads of the quadriceps may demonstrate out-of-phase activation. If all four heads of the quadriceps are involved in a dynamic deformity, percutaneus motor blocks with phenol are indicated. After the blocks, aggressive quadriceps stretching and strengthening of hip and knee flexors are indicated. In late recovery, selective surgical release of the rectus femoris or of the rectus femoris and vastus intermedius is considered[72] if they are the only muscles dynamically active on EMG study. Surgical release of all four heads of the quadriceps would result in postoperative knee instability. Before surgical correction with selective releases, local anesthetic motor point blocks of the rectus femoris and vastus intermedius may be performed to simulate the effect of surgical weakening. If knee flexion improves with the blocks, the rationale for surgical intervention is strengthened. To augment weak hip flexion, transfer of the rectus femoris to the sartorius or gracilis may be considered.

Bent Knee

Description, Functional Consequences, and Penalties.

When spasticity of the hamstrings is severe, a persistent bent knee posture is observed, and knee flexor contractures may develop quite rapidly. Knee flexion greatly hampers transferring because the weight line of the body causes the knees to flex even more and the patient collapses. Severe flexion deformity of the knees also hampers sitting. Stretching of spastic hamstrings can be quite painful.

Differential Diagnosis and Diagnostic Work-Up.

Physical examination is performed to establish passive and active range of motion. The hamstrings are a two-joint muscle, and spastic hamstrings can either flex the knee or act posterior to the hip joint, causing the trunk to extend. This is a common cause for patient slippage in wheelchairs. Heterotopic ossification in and around the knee and at the hip should be ruled out with appropriate radiographs. In some patients, spasticity may be a part of the early picture but gradually improves. Nevertheless, severe flexion deformity is due to the development of contracture. Dynamic electromyography helps to distinguish between dynamic and static deformity. Alternatively, sciatic nerve block with local anesthetic may be used.

Findings and Treatment Options.

Because of the large sensory component of the sciatic nerve, direct injection with phenol is undesirable. Anatomically, the multiple motor branches to the various hamstring muscles complicate both motor point injections and surgical dissection. If dynamic electromyography suggests spasticity of selected hamstring groups (i.e., medial vs. lateral hamstrings), motor point injections with phenol may be attempted. An alternative approach is to perform repeated local anesthetic blocks of the sciatic nerve before each cast change as part of the serial casting program. A sciatic nerve block also temporarily eliminates calf spasticity and allows serial casting of an equinus contracture of the foot.

In late recovery or early recovery when serial casting and sciatic nerve blocks fail to correct knee flexion deformity or posterior subluxation of the tibia develops as a result of tight hamstrings, the hamstring muscles may be lengthened.[40] The biceps femoris, gracilis, and semimembranous muscles have myotendinous junctions that permit fractional lengthening. The semitendinous muscle is either divided or undergoes Z-lengthening. Casting is still commonly used after lengthening of the hamstrings to correct residual flexion deformity. Postoperative gait and transfer training may be started as soon as the patient can be mobilized with the long leg cast. A walker is commonly used for patients with use of both upper extremities. When upper extremity deformity that inhibits the use of an assistive device can be corrected by surgical intervention, the upper extremity procedure is usually done first so that the patient can use an assistive device for gait training after the lower extremity intervention.

Equinovarus Foot with Curled or Clawed Toes

Description, Functional Consequences, and Penalties.

Patients demonstrate equinovarus posturing in terminal swing and stance. Weight bearing in stance phase is applied to the lateral border of the foot. Increased pressure over this region causes pain, decreased weight acceptance, ankle instability, impaired total body weight bearing on the involved limb, and shortened weight-bearing duration (antalgic pattern). Other findings include hyperextension at the knee with recurvatum thrust, genu varum, interference with smooth forward progression of the center of gravity, relative leg-length discrepancy with resulting clearance and advancement difficulties, and possible increase of energy consumption. Typically the contralateral step is shortened. Equinovarus deformity interferes with transfers.

Differential Diagnosis and Diagnostic Work-Up.

Muscles that may contribute to the equinovarus deformity include both heads of the gastrocnemius, the soleus, tibialis anterior, tibialis posterior, extensor hallucis longus, extensor digitorum, flexor digitorum, foot intrinsics, and peroneus longus (which, on occasion, contributes to equinus). Ankle

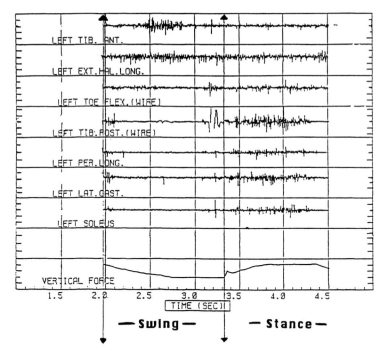

FIGURE   25. Dynamic   EMG recording taken from a patient with equinovarus foot posture during gait. Note continuous activity in the extensor hallucis longus throughout swing and stance and premature activation of the toe flexors, tibialis posterior, and gastrocsoleus muscles before and during early stance. Also note tibialis anterior activity in stance and premature reduction of activity before the swing phase is completed.

range of motion should be examined with the knee extended and the knee flexed. The inversion pull of the tibialis anterior is often noted by inspection. Hind-foot inversion is often generated by a spastic tibialis posterior. Dynamic electromyography is helpful in clarifying the role of various muscles, especially ankle invertors such as the tibialis posterior (Fig. 25). Radiographs rule out bony deformity at the ankle. Tibial nerve block in the popliteal fossa with local anesthetic helps to distinguish between spasticity and contracture. An improved base of support after the block helps to determine ambulatory potential. Alternatively, the tibialis anterior may contribute a strong component of inversion of the foot, which will not improve with a tibial nerve block.

Curled toes may be associated with the equinovarus deformity. During stance phase, curled toes often grip the shoe or floor and may be quite painful. Flexor digitorum is typically active, but contracture of the long toe flexors invariably occurs if the ankle has had prolonged plantarflexion contracture. Claw toes may be a combination of exaggerated activity in the toe extensors and flexors. The intrinsic muscles of the foot also may make a contribution. If a tibial nerve

block is performed to assess the calf musculature, the extrinsic flexors of the toes as well as the intrinsic muscles of the foot will be blocked, and the role of the toe deformity can be evaluated.

Findings and Treatment Options.   A temporary percutaneous tibial nerve block that results in increased ankle dorsiflexion indicates a dynamic deformity attributable to spasticity without contracture. If varus persists in swing phase, the most likely cause is the tibialis anterior and/or extensor hallucis longus. No significant change in the range of motion after a tibial nerve block indicates a static deformity, i.e., contracture.

In the early period of recovery, orthotic management is considered to control equinus, especially with appropriate components to control inversion and toe flexion. A rigid orthosis rather than an articulated type of brace is used if ankle clonus is present. If EMG studies demonstrate dynamic origin of the deformity, percutaneous motor point blocks with phenol should be considered in the offending muscles. After the block, the ankle plantar flexors should be stretched, and the ankle dorsiflexors should be strengthened. The tibial nerve has sensory as well as motor components and is not generally phenolized, although this option may be considered in patients with low level of arousal.

In late recovery, a tendo Achillis lengthening (TAL) or intramuscular lengthening is considered for static deformity.[41] This procedure is usually accompanied by toe flexor release with transfer of the toe flexor tendon into the os calcis to reinforce plantarflexion (now weakened by the TAL) and also to avoid persistent toe flexion. A split anterior tibialis tendon transfer (SPLATT) is considered if inversion, especially during swing phase, is caused by the tibialis anterior. If inversion is caused preferentially by the tibialis posterior, surgical release is indicated. If the tibialis posterior is found to be active in swing phase, tendon transfer to produce ankle dorsiflexion may be considered. Depending on gait and EMG analysis, lengthening and transfer of the extensor hallucis longus and transfer of the peroneus longus may be necessary.

Valgus Foot

Description, Functional Consequences, and Penalties. Valgus foot in stance phase promotes an abnormal base of support that impairs standing balance; promotes a valgus force on the knee during stance phase, which eventually leads to genuvalgum deformity; and causes hind-foot valgus or pronation deformity, which over time may become fixed.

Differential Diagnosis and Diagnostic Work-Up. An overactive peroneus longus muscle pulls the forefoot into pronated or valgus posture. A contributing factor may be a preexisting pes planus or congenital flexible flat feet. In hemiplegic patients, the other foot should be checked for this preexisting condition. Other family members also may be examined. In patients with a rigid pronation deformity, a preexisting tarsal coalition should be ruled out. Although uncommon in patients with head injury, rupture of the tibialis posterior tendon may result in loss of support for the medial longitudinal arch of the foot and thus contribute to valgus deformity. Weakness of the gastrocsoleus muscle may aggravate a tendency to pronation. If the calf is too weak to allow body weight to roll forward over the forefoot, the windlass effect

of the plantar structure that causes supination during terminal stance is lost. Other factors that may contribute to valgus foot include leg-length discrepancy, contralateral hip abductor weakness, and contralateral knee valgus deformity. A contralateral ankle valgus deformity also should be investigated.

On physical examination the position of the legs and both feet is inspected while the patient is standing. The position of the foot during sitting is compared with the position during standing to determine whether the deformity is fixed or rigid. Passive range of motion of the ankle or tibiotalar joint is examined while inverting the hind foot (i.e., the heel is in varus) to lock the subtalar joint. An equinus contracture may lead to pronation deformity by causing the subtalar joint to sublux medially to compensate for the equinus position of the foot. Equinus deformity during stance also may result from severe gastrocnemius tone. Examination should determine leg lengths and whether an adduction contracture is present at the hip. The knee is examined for valgus posture or instability of the medial collateral ligament, and strength and function of the gastrocsoleus group, tibialis posterior, and peroneal musculature are assessed.

Radiographs of the foot and ankle (while the patient is standing, if possible) rule out bony deformity, such as ankle valgus or old fracture, and determine the degree of valgus deformity. Local anesthetic block to the posterior tibial nerve can be considered to rule out dynamic equinus deformity as a cause of pronation. Similarly, local anesthetic block of the common peroneal nerve should be considered to rule out hyperactivity of the peroneus longus. Dynamic EMG during gait analysis often shows overactivity of the peroneus longus muscle as a cause of pronation deformity. This finding may be seen in combination with equinovarus foot during swing phase.

Findings and Treatment Options. Continuous activity of the peroneus longus muscle during swing and stance may cause valgus posture of the foot during swing and stance. Some patients demonstrate inappropriate EMG activity in the peroneus longus muscle during stance phase. This finding may be associated with equinovarus foot during swing and caused by the combination of increased EMG activity in the gastrocsoleus group, flexor hallucis longus, flexor digitorum, and tibialis anterior. Activity in the tibialis posterior is variable.

In the early period of recovery, a molded ankle foot orthosis may control the valgus foot in stance phase if the valgus deformity is not overly strong. A phenol block to the peroneus longus may be helpful. Phenol block to the gastrocsoleus group, flexor hallucis longus, flexor digitorum longus, and tibialis anterior depends on dynamic EMG findings and clinical picture. In the late recovery period, transfer of the peroneus longus across the dorsum of the foot to the navicular bone is considered.[77] For a "combination foot" (i.e., equinovarus foot in swing combined with valgus foot during stance), possible procedures include a SPLATT, tendo Achillis lengthening, toe flexor release, lengthening of peroneus brevis, and transfer of the flexor hallucis longus and flexor digitorum into the os calcis. If the tibialis posterior and extensor hallucis longus are hyperactive, they may be lengthened to weaken their pull.

Hitchhiker's Great Toe

Description, Functional Consequences, and Penalties. Persistent extension of the great toe is a peculiar but not uncommon problem. Patients complain a great deal about not being able to wear a shoe on the involved foot. Alternatively, patients present with the toe box of the shoe cut out. Loss of protection afforded by the shoe is the major penalty with this deformity.

Differential Diagnosis and Diagnostic Work-Up. The main offender appears to be a hyperactive extensor hallucis longus muscle. Dynamic EMG helps to confirm this cause.

Findings and Treatment Options. Dynamic EMG demonstrates persistent activity in the extensor hallucis longus. The condition may be treated by phenol motor point block or surgical section of the tendon of the extensor hallucis longus. A motor point block before surgery is helpful in ruling out the possibility of a coactive flexor hallucis longus. If the lateral muscle is also overactive, a deformity

in the opposite direction may develop if only the extensor hallucis longus is treated. Section of the tendons of both muscles may be required if both are coactive.

CONCEPTS IN PHARMACOLOGIC INTERVENTION

Pharmacologic reduction of spasticity may be beneficial in selected patients. However, drug treatment is often a trade-off between a decrement in spasticity and side effects. Three drugs—dantrolene sodium, baclofen, and diazepam—are commonly used to treat spasticity in various conditions. Their use in TBI must be considered carefully because the side effect of sedation, although typically different for each drug, may prove to be quite problematic in patients with arousal or cognitive dysfunction. It is both ironic and sobering that patients with TBI, who often need help for spasticity more than most, are also among the most sensitive to side effects related to attention and cognition. Other pharmacologic interventions include botulinum toxin, which requires further study, and nerve blocks.

Dantrolene Sodium

In contrast to centrally acting drugs such as diazepam and baclofen, dantrolene sodium exerts its effect directly on skeletal muscle fibers.[53] A neural signal to the muscle triggers a motor unit action potential that causes release of calcium from sarcoplasmic storage sites within the muscle fiber. Calcium ions initiate cross-bridging of myofilaments and subsequent build-up of contractile muscle tension. By influencing the release of calcium from the sarcoplasmic reticulum, dantrolene sodium reduces the force of muscle contraction and, thereby, has the potential to reduce tension in spastic muscles. Tendon jerk responses and electrically induced twitch tensions of muscle are reduced much more effectively than tetanic stimulation or sustained volitional contraction.[30] The amount of calcium released into the sarcoplasmic reticulum over the course of continued stimulation of muscle by nerve activity (whether through volition or electrical stimulation) tends to accumulate and overcome the inhibitory effects

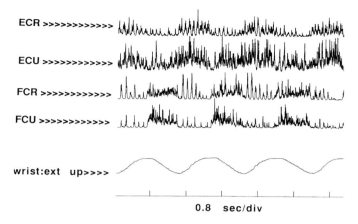

ECR >>>>>>>>>>>

ECU >>>>>>>>>>>

FCR >>>>>>>>>>>

FCU >>>>>>>>>>>

wrist:ext up>>>>

0.8 sec/div

FIGURE 26. A man who sustained a stroke 8 months earlier. Diffuse alternating clonus developed between the wrist flexors (FCR, FCU) and wrist extensors (ECR, ECU) when the patient performed voluntary movement. Clonus in other muscles groups was also observed clinically. Clonic activity of this sort may respond to dantrolene sodium.

of the drug. This observation is important in understanding the clinical utility and limitations of dantrolene sodium as an antispastic agent.

Dantrolene sodium may be useful in treating short-duration, low-frequency spastic phenomena such as clonus or brief spasms[52] (Fig. 26). Phasic small-tension spasticity responds more favorably than tonic large-tension spasticity. Patients with TBI and severe spasticity are not typically responsive to dantrolene sodium. Although its effect on spasticity is peripheral, dantrolene sodium apparently has a number of central effects and may be sedating to patients with arousal dysfunction. Nevertheless, it may be a reasonable choice for mild-to-moderate spasticity, especially for clonus involving many different muscles. Clonus often remits at a dose level of 50 mg 4 times/day, although doses of up to 400 mg/day may be used. Because hepatotoxicity has been reported, liver function tests should be monitored, especially in patients at risk for liver toxicity for other reasons.

Diazepam

Diazepam, which is centrally acting and highly sedating, increases the central inhibitory effects of gamma aminobutyric acid (GABA).[12] It appears to bind to receptors located at GABA-ergic synapses and increases GABA-induced inhibition at those sites. The antispastic characteristics of diazepam appear to arise from GABA-related inhibitory effects on alpha motor neuron activity in the spinal cord. Because diazepam also exerts sedative effects in the brain, some of its muscle-relaxant properties may be due to a more generalized state of sedation. The primary problem with diazepam is sedation at dosages that reduce spasticity of skeletal muscle. In general, diazepam is not a suitable drug for patients with TBI who have attentional or cognitive dysfunction. For patients who have persistent phasic flexor spasms that disturb activities of daily living or nighttime sleep, small doses of diazepam may reduce the frequency and intensity of spasms with tolerable sedation.

Baclofen

Baclofen, a derivative of GABA, appears to act as a GABA agonist, inhibiting transmission at specific synapses within the spinal cord.[74] When used as an antispastic agent, baclofen ultimately appears to have an inhibitory effect on alpha motor neuron activity. It is unclear whether this inhibition is presynaptic (through inhibition of other excitatory neurons that synapse with the alpha motor neuron) or postsynaptic (through action on the alpha motor neuron itself). Nevertheless, the net result of baclofen's action is to inhibit the firing pattern of the alpha motor neuron pool in the spinal cord with subsequent reduction of spasticity in skeletal muscles.

Clinical research studies using baclofen for spasticity have addressed primarily the problems of patients with multiple sclerosis or spinal cord injury.[17,76] Baclofen has been effective in such patients, especially when the clinical problem is related to flexor spasms. Oral baclofen is generally initiated at 10 mg/day in divided doses and increased to 80 mg or more as needed. Such high doses invariably lead to side effects that in many patients overshadow the benefits. In patients with TBI who are in a persistent vegetative state and are not expected to recover, high doses may be considered because cognitive and arousal functions are not an issue. Nevertheless, because of the remote possibility of some degree of recovery, it may be wise to taper the drug periodically and observe the patient.

Baclofen has been little studied in patients with spasticity of cerebral origin. Drowsiness is a common side effect, and confusion and hallucinations have been reported in patients with stroke and in elderly patients with other cerebral disorders. Such side effects would be particularly troublesome in patients with TBI who have cognitive or arousal dysfunction. A possible method for reducing central side effects is intrathecal administration, which has recently been approved by the Food and Drug Administration (FDA) for treating spasticity associated with multiple sclerosis and spinal cord injury.[56] A drug pump is implanted subcutaneously to infuse baclofen into the lumbar subarachnoid space. Compared with oral administration, the pump uses much smaller doses, thereby reducing side effects and enhancing effectiveness in refractory cases. The pump has an 18-ml reservoir, is connected to an intrathecal catheter, and is refilled by percutaneous puncture. The rate of baclofen infusion can be adjusted by an external computer. A marked decrease in muscle tone and associated spasms was found in many patients with multiple sclerosis and spinal cord injury; long-term effectiveness was also reported. Walking capacity appeared to improve in ambulatory patients, but generally patients who were nonambulatory before treatment remained so. No large clinical trials with intrathecal baclofen for head injury have been reported although one recent study reported improvement of spasticity associated with lesions of cerebral palsy. Of concern and interest to clinicians who deal with TBI, side effects from intrathecal baclofen include drowsiness, dizziness, and weakness. Intrathecal overdose may cause seizures, coma, and respiratory depression. Some of these side effects may be associated with pump failure and other technical problems. Sudden withdrawal of the drug (e.g., when pump failure is not recognized) may cause an exaggeration of spasticity along with hallucinations and seizures. The pump system is expensive and potentially hazardous when technical problems occur and "should be reserved for patients who have not responded to or cannot tolerate oral baclofen."[1] However, it may be useful in patients who have diffuse spasticity in the limbs, especially hip flexor and hamstring spasticity. Although the pump also is potentially useful for diffuse involvement of upper extremity muscles, especially large proximal ones, it is not clear how to titrate flow to the cervical cord from the lumbar infusion site without allowing too much drug to flow further to the brainstem respiratory centers.

Botulinum Toxin

Botulinum toxin has strong neuromuscular blocking properties that inhibit the release of acetylcholine and cause flaccid paralysis.[6] The clinical effect of the toxin is thought to be due primarily to its action at the neuromuscular junction. However, after injection of the toxin into a muscle, retrograde axonal transport has been reported with later detection of the toxin in the spinal cord. Of interest, toxin in the spinal cord has been reported to block recurrent inhibition mediated by Renshaw cells (see above for the Renshaw hypothesis of spasticity).

Injection of botulinum toxin is currently approved by FDA for the treatment of blepharospasm, facial spasm, strabismus, and torticollis. Some studies have reported its use in treating spasticity after stroke and multiple sclerosis. Changes in tone, range of motion, and functional activities as measured by Barthel scores and ease of urinary catheterization also have been reported.[67] Because of such initial reports and because the toxin theoretically should relieve spastic muscle contraction regardless of the generating mechanism, research studies are definitely in order to establish the efficacy and safety of the toxin in spastic disorders.

Botulinum toxin is injected directly into the offending muscle. Depending on the size of the muscle injected, therapeutic doses have ranged between 1 and 200 U. Because of the risk of systemic migration, no more than 400 U is administered in a single treatment session. This dose may be sufficient, however, to treat a number of muscles in one session. A delay of 72 hours or more between injection and onset of clinical effect is typical. The technique used in patients with dystonias is injection through a hypodermic needle that also doubles as a recording electrode. When the needle records EMG activity after insertion, the injection is made. This technique is satisfactory for large surface muscles because there is little question about injecting the offending muscle. However, if it is applied to deep-lying spastic muscles (e.g., flexor digitorum sublimis or profundus), other techniques such as electrical stimulation may have to be used. Some physicians aim for the motor endplate and inject after they hear motor endplate potentials. This technique, however, also seems unsuitable for deep-lying muscles.

The major adverse effect is excessive weakness of injected muscles, but nausea, headache, and fatigue also have been reported. Because of the delay between injection of toxin and onset of action, patients may require several sessions to titrate the dose necessary for treatment. This process may increase the frequency of follow-up and expense. Unlike the dystonias, in which voluntary capacity is not an issue, spastic muscles may retain voluntary capacity that the clinician wishes to preserve; therefore, titration of the paralytic effect of the toxin becomes a much more critical factor. Long-term effectiveness of botulinum toxin has been questioned, because antibodies to the toxin appear to develop as successive injections are given. The duration of effectiveness is initially 3–4 months for dystonias, but with the development of antibodies (and perhaps for other unknown reasons), duration and degree of effectiveness of repeated injections decrease. If similar results are found in patients with spasticity, the toxin may not be effective in chronic conditions but may serve as a temporizing measure when spasticity is expected to improve with motor recovery.

The role of botulinum toxin in spasticity needs clarification through clinical studies.

Nerve Blocks

Nerve and motor point blocks are useful in targeting specific muscles or muscle groups for diagnostic and therapeutic maneuvers.[68] The purpose of the nerve or motor point block is to reduce force produced by a contracting spastic muscle or muscle group. Reduction in spastic tension may lead to improvement in passive and active range of motion and allows more successful stretching of tight musculature. More subtly, and more importantly, improved control over movement and posture may allow compensatory behaviors during functional activities. Reduction in spastic activity in one muscle or muscle group may have consequences for tone in other muscle groups of the limb by reducing the overall effort required to perform movement and/or by changing sensory information from the limb to the CNS. Finally, the application of external devices, such as braces, casts, or even shoes, may be facilitated by nerve and motor point blocks.

Blocks may be classified broadly as diagnostic or therapeutic. Diagnostic blocks are typically performed with quick-acting, short-duration local anesthetics such as lidocaine or bupivacaine, which allow the examiner to evaluate factors such as passive range of motion, muscle stiffness unrelated to spasticity, changes in active range of motion when spastic resistance is blocked, and enhanced motor control during functional movements. For example, patients with spastic adductors that cause scissoring during gait may be prone to fall because of the narrow base of support. A temporary block of the obturator nerve with 2% lidocaine allows the examiner to observe whether the base of support widens and stability improves. It is crucial to understand that a diagnostic nerve block is used to test a hypothesis. The hypothesis behind the obturator nerve block is that the base of support is narrowed by excessive adduction of the leg caused by spastic adductors and that a wider base of support leads to greater stability during dynamic gait. After the nerve block is performed with a quick-acting local anesthetic, the patient is ambulated to test the hypothesis. If ambulation improves, more permanent (i.e., less reversible) types of intervention may be contemplated with greater confidence in outcome prediction. Therefore, the prediction of likely outcome is an important feature of temporary nerve or motor point blocks. It is possible, of course, that the base of support will not widen. For example, a severe adductor contracture does not remit after nerve block. However, this information is useful in designing the next step in the treatment program. Similarly, the nerve block may decrease spasticity of the adductors and widen the base of support but lead to only partial improvement in overall gait pattern because of instability from other sources of neuromuscular impairment. Again, this kind of information leads to further diagnostic testing of other hypotheses relevant to understanding the patient's ambulation dysfunction.

Therapeutic nerve and motor point blocks are primarily performed with aqueous solutions of phenol. When it is injected in or near a nerve bundle, phenol denatures protein in the myelin sheath or cell membrane of axons with which it makes contact.[23] When administered in the operating room under direct nerve visualization, phenol is instilled directly into the nerve bundle in a glycerin solution that minimizes leakage. The desired motor nerves are identified by electrical stimulation before injection. Large nerves with mixed sensory and motor fibers are avoided because of consequent dysesthesias, and the effect may last 6 months because the injection of the nerve is so direct. An aqueous solution of phenol, on the other hand, is used for percutaneous injection in the laboratory or at the bedside. The location of the nerve is approximated by an electrical stimulation technique that typically results in variable contact of phenol with axons. In our opinion, contrast variability is a key factor in the duration of effectiveness of a percutaneous phenol nerve or motor point block. As Glenn suggested, a peripheral nerve block is likely to last longer than a block of a motor point (a motor nerve branch located much closer than the peripheral nerve to the muscle).[23] Phenolization of nerve may result in wallerian degeneration; therefore, reinnervation probably takes longer for a peripheral nerve because it

has a longer distance to regrow to the muscle compared with the closer motor point nerve branch. The smaller size of the nerve involved in a motor point block also may make it harder to localize percutaneously. In addition, if a mixed sensory-motor nerve is selected for phenolization (typically in a low-level patient in whom there is less concern about consequent dysesthesia), reduction in afferent drive of spasticity may add to the effectiveness of the block. In our experience, a motor point block with phenol influences spasticity for 3–5 months. Nevertheless, reports of duration of effectiveness have varied from several days to 3 years. In any case, phenol blocks are a temporizing measure, most effective during the period of expectant neurologic recovery. The rationale for the other injectable agents, such as alcohol and botulinum toxin, is essentially the same.

In performing a nerve block, the first step is to locate the selected peripheral nerve or motor point with a surface stimulator. The skin is then prepared with an antiseptic iodine solution, swabbed with alcohol, and subcutaneously anesthetized with lidocaine before insertion of the Teflon-coated, 22-gauge injecting needle. The electrically conductive inner core of the tip of the needle is used to pass current to the tissues. As the needle is advanced closer to the nerve, less current is required to produce similar amounts of muscle contraction. When the minimal current producing a visible or palpable muscle contraction is reached, we typically inject 3–5 ml of aqueous phenol in concentrations of 5–7%. Care should be taken not to inject into a blood vessel. In large quantities, systemically absorbed phenol may cause seizures, central nervous system depression, and cardiovascular collapse. When injecting multiple nerves or motor points, we usually do not exceed a total volume of 15 ml (see Glen[23] for another approach) and are cautious with patients taking anticoagulants, in whom the risk of bleeding associated with needling is greater. The essence of the technique is clinical manipulation of needle advancement toward the nerve. Depth of penetration and directional orientation of the needle tip require a steady hand, competent knowledge of anatomy, and a good assistant. Morbidity is typically benign. Local irritation at the site of the block is treated symptomatically with ice, compression, or mild analgesics. We avoid mixed sensory-motor nerves to prevent painful dysesthesias and substitute motor point blocks that involve motor branches only. The injection technique is a good temporizing measure during the period of expectant neurologic recovery and facilitates serial casting, range-of-motion exercises, passive activities of daily living, active movements, and function.

Borg-Stein et al. reported an initial comparison of phenol and botulinum toxin injections.[6] They indicate that reduction in spasticity due to phenol motor point block tends to diminish after several months but may last as long as several years. The effect of botulinum toxin appears to last for about 3–4 months, with a more complete return to baseline than generally is seen after phenol injection. Clinical resistance to the effects of repeated injections of botulinum toxin has been demonstrated, apparently due to neutralizing antibodies. Botulinum toxin is not associated with dysesthesia, but neither is motor point block with phenol. Only injection of phenol into a mixed sensory-motor nerve may produce such an effect. Although at present experience with botulinum toxin for treatment of spasticity is limited, three major concerns already have been expressed:

1. The cost of the toxin compared with the cost of phenol is enormous and escalates if multiple injections are required to titrate a desired clinical effect.

2. It is not clear how to control the titration process for a spastic muscle that also has volitional capacity. An ideal agent would eliminate the muscle's spastic reaction while preserving its voluntary capacity. Of interest, phenol appears to reduce spasticity more than it affects voluntary activity. It is not yet clear how botulinum toxin behaves in this regard.

3. The technique for identifying deeper muscles that require injection has to be made more explicit and probably involves electrical stimulation to verify identification. Because the toxin appears to be quite liquid, leakage into tissue spaces may become problematic as the needle is advanced toward deeper muscles. Currently, some physicians inject botulinum toxin with a hypodermic type of EMG needle electrode that also picks up endplate potentials. When they are found, the toxin is injected. Although such a technique indicates to the physician that the needle is in a muscle, it does not specify which muscle is being injected. Such a technique may be useful in dystonia but is problematic in spasticity.

The use of botulinum toxin for spasticity needs further research, especially in comparison with aqueous phenol, which is significantly less expensive but has variable duration of effectiveness when performed percutaneously.

CASE EXAMPLE

The following case illustrates our approach to problems of spasticity in the early phase of recovery after severe head injury. Various options are developed and require input from the patient's family, who have their own hopes and beliefs about recovery.

A 19-year-old college student was admitted for acute rehabilitation 3 months after sustaining severe TBI in a high-speed car crash. His acute hospital course was complicated by increased intracranial pressure and a "blown" right pupil, right frontotemporal surgical decompression, multiple facial and mandibular fractures requiring internal fixation and wiring, sacral and pubic fractures, hypertension, percutaneous cholecystostomy, tracheostomy, and feeding via jejunostomy. Several weeks before his transfer to rehabilitation, the patient was noted to mouth words inconsistently. Three days before admission, he spoke a 4-word sentence. He was single and lived with his parents and sister but attended college away from home.

Examination revealed a thin young man supine in bed with elbows, wrists, hips, and knees flexed markedly but asymmetrically. (Fig. 27). He had a soft right frontotemporal craniectomy defect. Passive range of motion of the neck was full, but he was able to turn his head actively only about 30°; there was no nuchal rigidity. On command, he squeezed the examiner's finger with the fingers of his right hand. He mouthed the word "mommy" when his mother telephoned and the receiver was held to his ear. On request, he pursed his lips and perseveratively blew kisses to her while she remained on the line.

The right shoulder was adducted 15° and internally rotated 45°, with increased tone and marked restriction of range into abduction and external rotation. The right elbow was markedly flexed to 120°, with increased tone in the pronators, and lacked at least 30° of supination. The right wrist was flexed 75°, and both the flexor carpi radialis and ulnaris were flexed to the right. The right fingers were flexed into the palm. The right thumb was flexed tightly at the distal interphalangeal joint, but no web space contracture and no intrinsic atrophy were present.

On the left, the shoulder could be passively abducted 75°, with mild but increasing resistance at the end of range; external rotation was possible for about 45°. The left elbow was markedly flexed 90° and resistive to stretching. The left forearm was pronated, with increased tone in the pronators, and lacked at least 30° of supination. The left wrist was flexed 45° with markedly increased tone in the flexor carpi radialis but not the ulnaris. There was intrinsic atrophy of the hand, especially of the first dorsal interosseous muscle, and the fingers were flexed into the palm. The thumb was not adducted into the palm.

The right hip was flexed acutely more than 90° and markedly resisted stretching of only 15°, which also caused immediate eye opening, pupillary widening, vigorous head turning, and facial wincing. The thigh was moderately adducted, the knee was markedly flexed to 135°, and the ankle was plantarflexed 60°. Tone was increased in the adductors, knee flexors, and ankle plantarflexors, with positive Babinski sign of the great toe.

The left hip was flexed 60°, with moderate resistance to stretch, but no facial wincing or vigorous head turning occurred. The knee was flexed 90°, and the ankle was plantarflexed 30°. Tone was increased for the left knee flexors and ankle plantarflexors. The Babinski sign was also positive on the left.

Discussion

The patient presents to the acute rehabilitation hospital with an undoubted mixture of deforming spasticity and contracture 3 months after a severe head injury. As is often the case, such deformities had additional time to

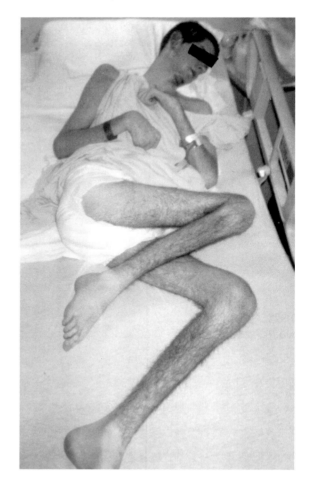

FIGURE 27. A 19-year-old man who sustained severe TBI 3 months earlier had the above limb postures on admission to acute rehabilitation.

develop because of the time needed to handle prolonged complications in acute care (in this case, craniotomy, facial bone surgeries, cholecystitis, pneumonia, and other infections). In addition, the low level of responsiveness for much of the hospital course often casts doubt in the mind of acute care personnel about the patient's suitability for rehabilitation. Aggressive measures to prevent deformities may be given a lesser priority, especially if staff are dealing with complications that have a greater medical priority. The resulting deformities may be quite advanced by the time the patient reaches acute rehabilitation, and intervention becomes more difficult to implement.

At 3 months after injury, families often have high hopes for recovery, especially if certain milestone signs have recently appeared. The patient had recently begun to speak and was clearly following some voluntary commands. Family members were elated at seeing these signs, which gave them hope for future recovery from many other problems. Moreover, because speech seemed to be returning spontaneously, the family could hope for spontaneous remission of deformities.

Expectations tend to color the family's perception and understanding of the limits of recovery, the nature of the various pathologies, and the effects and side effects of medical intervention. For example, spasticity of a muscle may give way to voluntary activity as neurologic recovery unfolds during the first 9–18 months after head injury. Families, therefore, may think that contracture of the same spastic muscle will also disappear when voluntary movement recovers. Aggressive interventions for contracture in the spastic state, therefore, may not make sense to the family. Education of the family is clearly needed, but what they need to know may well depend on drawing out their beliefs, hopes, and expectations. The educational campaign is designed to promote compliance with clinical goals.

In addition to family issues and possibilities of recovery, clinical decisions about treatment of spasticity also depend on the patient's medical risks and functional capacities and needs. For example, in the present case, severe acute flexion with adduction of the right hip raised concerns about the possible development of hip dislocation, which would lead to pelvic obliquity and thus worsen the patient's ability to sit in a chair. Treatment of hip flexor and adductor spasticity was needed to prevent such a complication. From a functional perspective, the patient's ability to sit properly in a chair was also impeded by severe flexion deformity, which impaired the base of sitting support and forced weight bearing on a small surface of skin overlying a thin rump and sacral area. Weight-bearing force distributed over a small surface area leads to painful pressure. Pressure on the sacral fracture, although now 3 months old, may still be a source of pain, generating sensory input to the central nervous system. The resulting spastic "drive"

eventually reaches motoneurons of extremity muscles and may well potentiate a nasty loop in which pain → spasticity → pain → spasticity and so on. The possibility of skin breakdown also must be anticipated.

Given such considerations, what are some of the specific details of the planning process? The case was presented to a combined orthopaedic-physiatric conference about 1 week after admission. This weekly case conference is attended by orthopaedists, physiatrists, allied health therapists, and social workers. Cases are presented to arrive at a management plan that takes into account the patient's recovery pattern, functional capacity and needs, and medical risk factors, as well as family considerations. At a later date, families generally are provided with a series of options that emerge from the conference, and their input is solicited. Such options usually are presented within the framework of a broader, longer-range management plan to give families a sense of how musculoskeletal interventions fit in with and contribute to the overall rehabilitation plan. The attending physiatrist and social worker (and often the patient's psychologist) are responsible for framing the musculoskeletal interventions within the context of the larger plan and its goals. If orthopaedic intervention is planned, the details of the intervention and its purposes are communicated directly to the family and patient by the orthopaedist after the family has been introduced to the global aspects of the management plan by the attending physiatrist and psychosocial team.

In patients with a history of fractures, spasticity, and low-level responsiveness, the detection of restricted motion should trigger the suspicion of heterotopic ossification (HO). In the present patient, severe hip flexor spasticity with marked pain on minimal passive stretch suggested HO at the hip. An active HO process is often painful, and treatment with agents such as disodium etidronate and indomethacin is often effective in reducing the inflammatory aspects of the HO process and quieting the spastic muscles driven by pain. Before the conference, radiographic films were obtained to rule out HO. Right hip films were difficult to read because of the severe flexion posture of the hip with overlapping bone shadows. No HO was evident around the right hip, but it could be definitely ruled out. However, HO was seen under the left quadriceps muscle. There was clinical concern about the medical risk of hip dislocation due to persistent hip flexor and adductor spasticity. The patient's ability to sit in a wheelchair was observed to be functionally compromised. Such issues prompted consideration of early orthopedic intervention to lengthen the iliopsoas and release the pectineus (thereby preserving active hip flexion), to neurectomize the obturator nerve, and to perform distal releases of the hamstrings. Stretching of spastic, powerful hamstrings may result in posterior subluxation of the tibia with respect to the femur. Usually, surgical intervention is not contemplated at the 3-month mark because motor recovery is anticipated during the first 12 months or more after injury. However, the consequences of the deforming forces—risk of hip dislocation, potential for skin pressure, actual pain, and curtailment of biomechanical requirements for tolerance of sitting—appeared to justify early orthopaedic intervention.

The tone of the right hip flexors may be reduced by paravertebral block that anesthetizes nerve branches lying on the psoas major muscle. Phenol, a longer-acting agent, must be used, because severe hip flexor spasticity was already chronic. The block is relatively difficult to perform, and its effectiveness and duration in such a difficult situation are uncertain. An effective block may reveal how much contracture is already present, but the blocking action of phenol is typically incomplete. To determine the extent of contracture not only at the hip but also at many other joints, the suggestion was made to examine passive joint motion under brief general anesthesia. Improved range at the right hip under anesthesia also may allow better hip films to rule out an underlying, painful HO process as contributory to the hip flexor spasticity. Aggressive drug treatment of HO was an option. Serial casting procedures (for the upper extremities and the ankle-foot systems) also may be considered if linked to the relaxation of tone brought on by general anesthesia. A final consideration for the lower extremities was the baclofen pump, which introduces minute amounts of baclofen into spinal fluid and may affect the

upper as well as the lower extremities. Sedation is minimized by the use of small quantities. However, experience with the pump in patients with TBI is limited; it has been used mainly for flexor spasms generated by such conditions as spinal cord injury and multiple sclerosis.

The challenge of the upper extremities is to identify muscle groups that contribute to deformity and to focus intervention on the correct contributors. Although clinical examination may be suggestive, the findings are not necessarily predictive. Passive stretch may generate spasticity in muscles that react differently when the person stretches them during natural actions. Dynamic kinesiologic EMG studies help to distinguish among muscles that are weak, overactive in a spastic manner, or capable of adequate control. In the present patient, tightness of the right shoulder adductor and internal rotator may be a function of the pectoralis major, latissimus dorsi, teres major, anterior deltoid, or possibly subscapularis muscles. Depending on findings, phenol block to the thoracodorsal nerve (for the latissimus dorsi) or motor point block to the pectoralis major or other muscle groups may be considered. Surgical releases are considered infrequently because of the unpredictable results, although a refractory pectoralis major group may be totally released at the shoulder if it restricts abduction and access to the axilla.

On clinical grounds, elbow flexor tightness appeared to be a function of both biceps and brachioradialis spasticity. However, the contribution of the brachialis was more difficult to determine clinically but easy to ascertain electromyographically. Case conference recommended options of musculotaneous nerve block with phenol and motor point blocks of the brachioradialis followed by serial casting. Phenol usually wears off after 2–4 months (sometimes more), and recovery, therefore, is not hindered significantly. During the period of block, spastic and contractured muscle may be progressively stretched. Serial casting, heating of the musculotendinous junction with ultrasound, mechanical stretching, tension splints, and electrical stimulation of antagonist muscle may be considered to achieve range of motion. Phenol applied to the musculocutaneous nerve may produce sensory dysesthesia, because the nerve has sensory fibers that innervate skin on part of the forearm. In low-level patients, dysesthesias may not be problematic (they usually wear off within 1 month), whereas recovery of awareness is generally slow. Biceps motor point block may be effective without dysesthesia. If the brachioradialis is known to be involved from dynamic EMG studies, it too can be blocked at its motor point. In the present patient, the brachioradialis appeared clinically to be stretch-reactive and therefore to require motor point blocking with phenol. Because both sets of elbow flexors were involved, four or more blocks were required to quiet the flexors and to allow serial casting to do its work. The number of required procedures creates difficulty, and other approaches were mentioned. Brachial plexus reservoirs filled with local anesthetic and serving as a kind of continuous anesthesia system have been tried. In the experience of one of the authors (MA Keenan), fibrosis tends to develop. Oral medications such as baclofen, diazepam, or dantrolene sodium have an antispasticity effect, although they do not target offending muscles more than other muscle groups. The main problem with these medications (perhaps dantrolene less so than the others) is that they cause sedation in patients whose arousal level is already low. In cases of severe tightness, they are not particularly effective and were not considered suitable for use in the present case. Because these drugs do not affect contracture, patients require other aggressive modalities. Early orthopaedic intervention at the elbow may be considered if little or no change in range of motion is achieved after a reasonable period of mechanical mobilization with blocks. It is important to check such recalcitrant elbows for heterotopic bone, which blocks motion.

The wrist and fingers present dilemmas in management. On examination, the left wrist demonstrated marked tightness of the flexor carpi radialis, whereas the flexor carpi ulnaris lacked prominence during wrist flexor stretch. Because intrinsic atrophy was evident on the left, it is likely that the flexor carpi ulnaris was affected by peripheral entrapment or compression at the elbow. Such neuropathies are common after head injury

and may be caused by elbow trauma against siderails of beds, hard lapboards, or wheelchair armrests. Elbow pads are useful to blunt such trauma. In addition, persistent elbow flexion posturing may induce traction of the nerve, a finding in the present patient. Traction or stretch injury is not helped by elbow pads. With the flexor carpi ulnaris out of the picture on the left, motor point block of flexor carpi radialis may help to alleviate some of the wrist flexion posturing. However, tightness of the extrinsic finger flexors, flexor digitorum sublimis, and flexor digitorum profundus also contributes to a flexed wrist. It is difficult to block all motor points percutaneously, and both median and ulnar nerves at the elbow must be blocked to anesthetize the fingers fully. Although lidocaine block of median and ulnar nerves is often done to gain information about the range of motion (without spasticity), phenol block of these nerves is highly likely to result in dysesthesias. In low-level patients, dysesthesia may be less problematic, but patients with higher levels of arousal may not tolerate this side effect. Open phenol motor branch blocks may be attempted with an intraoperative stimulator, but the procedure requires extensive dissection. Serial casting may be attempted after lidocaine block of the median and, if necessary, ulnar nerves. The block facilitates application of the cast, especially by reducing pain of stretching as the cast is applied. When the cast is changed, the lidocaine block may be repeated if spasticity is particularly active. When peripheral nerve blocks are deemed too difficult to perform, direct injection of 50% alcohol into muscle bellies may be considered. The effect is to denervate small terminal branches of nerves within the muscle. No sensory dysesthesia results from this procedure, but the effects are relatively short-lasting (2–6 weeks). Botulinum toxin lasts longer and does not result in sensory dysesthesia, but it is currently quite expensive compared with phenol or alcohol, particularly when many spastic muscles require injection.

Treatment of complex cases is highly dependent on analysis of numerous comingled factors, including volitional motor control capacity, spasticity, contracture, and time course of recovery. The patient's cognitive, emotional, and behavioral strengths and weaknesses also play a role in selecting treatment strategies. Technology-based assessments assist the clinician in sorting out many of the factors that affect individual functioning. In the authors' opinion, therapeutic suppression of spastic phenomena is a worthy endeavor only if it enhances function. Accordingly, from a rehabilitation perspective, whether in the clinic or in a laboratory, spastic phenomena are best evaluated by studying functional movements and tasks.

ACKNOWLEDGMENT. We gratefully acknowledge the able professional assistance of Barbara Hirai, BS, Gunilla Wannstedt, MS, PT, and Oliver Woods Jr. in helping to carry out upper and lower extremity studies of spasticity that contributed much valuable information to the present chapter.

REFERENCES

1. Abramowicz M: Intrathecal baclofen for spasticity. Med Lett 36:21–22, 1994.
2. Altman R, Kien J: Many neurons make light work? New Scientist Aug:34–38, 1993.
3. Asanuma H: The pyramidal tract. In Brooks VB (ed): Handbook of Physiology, vol. II. Bethesda, MD, American Physiological Society, 1981 pp 291–295.
4. Basmajian J, DeLuca CJ: Muscles Alive: Their Function Revealed by Electromyography, 5th ed. Baltimore, Williams & Wilkins, 1985, pp 291–295.
5. Bond MR, Brooks DN: Understanding the process of recovery as a basis for the investigation of rehabilitation for the brain injured. Scand J Rehabil Med 8:127, 1976.
6. Borg-Stein J, Stein J: Pharmacology of botulinum toxin and implications for use in disorders of muscle tone. J Head Trauma Rehabil 8(3):103– 106, 1993.
7. Botte MJ, Keenan MA: Percutaneous phenol blocks of the pectoralis major muscle to treat spastic deformities. J Hand Surg 13A:147, 1988.
8. Botte MJ, et al: Surgical management of spastic thumb-in-palm deformity in adults with brain injury. J Hand Surg 14A:174–182, 1989.
9. Brooks DN, et al: The five year outcome of severe blunt head injury—a relative's view. J Neurol Neurosurg Psychiatry 43:525, 1980.
10. Brooks VB: The Neural Basis of Motor Control. New York, Oxford University Press, 1986.
11. Davidoff RA: Pharmacology of spasticity. Neurology 28:46–51, 1978.
12. Davidoff RA: Antispasticity drugs: Mechanisms of action. Ann Neurol 17:107–116.
13. Delwaide PJ: Human monosynaptic reflexes and presynaptic inhibition. An interpretation of spastic hyperreflexia. In Desmedt JE (ed): New Developments in Electromyography and Clinical Neurophysiology, vol. 3. Basel, Karger, 1973, pp 508–522.
14. Eccles JC: The Understanding of the Brain. New York, McGraw-Hill, 1973, pp 66–120.
15. Esquenazi A, Keenan MA: Gait analysis. In DeLisa JA (ed): Rehabilitation Medicine: Principles and Practice, 2nd ed. Philadelphia, J.B. Lippincott, 1991.
16. Evarts EV: Role of motor cortex in voluntary movements in primates. In Brooks VB (ed): Handbook of Physiology, vol. 11. Bethesda, MD, American Physiological Society, 1981, pp 1083–1120.
17. Feldman RG et al: Baclofen for spasticity in multiple sclerosis: Double blind cross-over and three year study. Neurology 28:1094, 1978.
18. Garland DE: Resection of heterotopic ossification in adults with head trauma. J Bone Joint Surg 67A:1261–1269, 1985.
19. Garland DE, Blum CE, Waters RL: Periarticular heterotopic ossification in head-injured adults: incidence and location. J Bone Joint Surg 62A:1143, 1980.
20. Garland DE, Lilling M, Keenan MA: percutaneous phenol blocks to motor points of spastic forearm muscles in head-injured adults. Arch Phys Med Rehabil 65:243–245, 1984.
21. Georgopoulos AP, Schwartz AB, Kettner RE: Neuronal population coding of movement direction. Science 233:1416–1419, 1986.
22. Gilman S, Lieberman JS, Marco LA: Spinal mechanisms underlying the effects of unilateral ablation of areas four and six in monkeys. Brain 97:49–64, 1974.
23. Glenn MB: Nerve blocks. In Glenn MB, Whyte J (eds): The Practical Management of Spasticity in Children and Adults. Philadelphia, Lea & Febiger, 1990, pp 227–258.
24. Granit R: The Basis of Motor Control. London, Academic Press, 1970.
25. Granit R: Receptors and Sensory Perception. New Haven, Yale University Press, 1955.
26. Griffith ER, Mayer NH: Hypertonicity and Movement Disorders. In Rosenthal M, et al (eds): Rehabilitation of the Adult with Head Injury, 2nd ed. Philadelphia, F.A. Davis, 1990, pp 127–146.
27. Hecht (JS): Subscapular nerve block in the painful hemiplegic shoulder. Arch Phys Med Rehabil 73:1036–1039, 1992.
28. Herman RM, Freedman W, Mayer N: Neurophysiologic mechanisms of hemiplegic and paraplegic spasticity: Implications for therapy. Arch Phys Med Rehabil 55:338–343, 1974.
29. Herman R, Freedman W, Meeks SM: Physiological aspects of hemiplegic and paraplegic spasticity. In Desmedt JE (ed): New Developments in Electromyography and Clinical Neural Physiology, vol. 3. Basel, Karger, 1973, pp 579–588.
30. Herman R, Mayer N, Mecomber SA: The pharmacophysiology of dantrolene sodium. Am J Phys Med 51:296–311, 1972.
31. Herman R: The myotatic reflex. Brain 93:273–312, 1970.
32. Herman R, D'Luzansky SC: Pharmacologic management of spinal spasticity. J Neurol Rehab 5 (Suppl 1):515–520, 1991.

33. Jankowska E, Riddell JS: A relay for input from group II muscle afferents in sacral segments of the cat spinal cord. J Physiol (London) 465:561–580, 1993.

34. Jordan C: Current status of functional lower extremity surgery in adult spastic patients. Clin Orthop 233:102, 1988.

35. Keenan MA, Botte MJ: Technique of percutaneous phenol block of the recurrent motor branch of the median nerve. J Hand Surg 12A:806–807, 1987.

36. Keenan MA, Haider TT, Stone LR: Dynamic electromyography to assess elbow spasticity. J Hand Surg 15A:607–614, 1990.

37. Keenan MA, et al: Results of fractional lengthening of the finger flexors in adults with upper extremity spasticity. J Hand Surg 12A:575–581, 1987.

38. Keenan MA, et al: Results of transfer of the flexor digitorum profundus tendons in adults with acquired spasticity of the hand. J Bone Joint Surg 69A:1127–1132, 1987.

39. Keenan MA, et al: Management of intrinsic spasticity in the hand with phenol injection of reurectomy of the motor branch of the ulnar nerve. J Hand Surg 12A:734–739, 1987.

40. Keenan MA, et al: Hamstring release for knee flexion contractures in spastic adults. Clin Orthop 236:221, 1988.

41. Keenan MA, et al: Surgical correction of spastic equinovarus deformity in the adult head trauma patient. Foot Ankle 5:35–41, 1984.

42. Keenan MA, Perry JJ: Evaluation of upper extremity motor control in spastic brain injured patients using dynamic electromyography. J Head Trauma Rehabil 5(4):13–22, 1990.

43. Keenan MA: Surgical decision making for residual limb deformities following traumatic brain injury. Orthop Rev, April 19, 1988.

44. Kolessar DJ, Keenan MA, Berlet AC: Surgical management of upper extremity deformities following traumatic brain injury. Phys Med Rehabil State Art Rev 7:623–636, 1993.

45. Landau WM: Spasticity: What is it? What is it not? In Feldman RG, Young RR, Koela WP (eds): Disordered Motor Control. Chicago, Yearbook, 1980.

46. Luria AR: The Working Brain. New York, Basic Books, 1973.

47. Magoun HW, Rhines R: Spasticity: The Stretch Reflex and Extrapyramidal Systems. Springfield, IL, Charles C Thomas, 1948.

48. Mai J: Depression of spasticity by alpha-adrenergic blockade. Acta Neurol Scand 57:65–76, 1978.

49. Manetto C, Lidsky TI: The effects of movements on caudate sensory responses. Neurosci Lett 96:295–299, 1989.

50. Matthews PBC, Rushworth G: The relative sensitivity of muscle nerve fibers to procaine. J Physiol 135:263–269, 1957.

51. Matthews PBC, Simmons A: Sensations of finger movement elicited by pulling upon flexor tendons in man. J Physiol 239:27–28, 1974.

52. Mayer N, Mecomber SA, Herman R: Treatment of spasticity with dantrolene sodium. Am J Phys Med 52:18–29, 1973.

53. Monster AW, Herman R, Meeks S, et al: Co-operative study for assessing the effects of a pharmacological agent on spasticity. Am J Phys Med 52:163–188, 1973.

54. Nathan P: Some comments on spasticity and rigidity. In Desmedt JE (ed): New Developments in Electromyography and Clinical Neurophysiology, vol 3. Basel, Karger, 1973, pp 13–14.

55. Orcutt SA et al: Carpal tunnel syndrome secondary to wrist and finger flexor spasticity. J Hand Surg 15A:940–944, 1990.

56. Penn RD: Intrathecal baclofen for severe spasticity. Ann NY Acad Sci 531:157–166, 1988.

57. Pollock LJ, Davis L: Studies in decerebration. VI: The effect of deafferentation upon decerebrate rigidity. Am J Physiol 98:47–49, 1931.

58. Pollock LJ, Davis L: The influence of the cerebellum upon the reflex activities of the decerebrate animal. Brain 50:277–312, 1927.

59. Rastad J, et al: Light microscopical study of dendrites and perikarya of interneurones mediating Ia reciprocal inhibition of cat lumbar alpha-motoneurones. Anat Embryol 181:381–388, 1990.

60. Riddell JS, et al: Ascending tract neurones processing information from group II muscle afferents in sacral segments of the feline spinal cord. J Physiol (London) 475:469–481, 1994.

61. Roland PE, et al: Supplementary motor area and other cortical areas in organization of voluntary movements in man. J Neurophysiol 43:118–136, 1980.

62. Rosenbaum DA: Human Motor Control. San Diego, Academic Press, 1991.

63. Rushworth G: Some aspects of the pathophysiology of spasticity and rigidity. Clin Pharmacol Ther 5:828–836, 1964.

64. Sahrmann SA, Norton BJ: The relationship of voluntary movement to spasticity in the upper motor neuron syndrome. Ann Neurol 2:460–465, 1977.

65. Sherrington CS: The Integrative Action of the Nervous System. New Haven, Yale University Press, 1906.

66. Sherrington CS: Decerebrate rigidity and reflex co-ordination of movements. J Physiol 22:319–322, 1898.

67. Snow BJ, et al: Treatment of spasticity with botulinum toxin: a double-blind study. Ann Neurol 28:512–515, 1990.

68. Stone LR, Shin DY: Management of hypertonicity using chemical denervation following traumatic brain injury. In Stone LR (ed): Neurologic and Orthopedic Sequaeli of Traumatic Brain Injury. Phys Med Rehabil State Art Rev 7:527–558, 1993.

69. Vallbo AB, Hagbarth KE, et al: Activity in human peripheral nerves. Physiol Rev 59:919–957, 1979.

70. Vallbo AB: Slowly adapting muscle receptors in man. Acta Physiol Scand 78:315–333, 1970.

71. Veale JL, Rees S, Mark RF: Renshaw cell activity in normal and spastic man. In Desmedt JE (ed): New Developments in Electromyography and Clinical Neurophysiology, vol 3. Basel, Karger, 1973, pp 523–537.

72. Waters RL, et al: Stiff-legged gait in hemiplegia surgical correction. J Bone Joint Surg 61A:927, 1979.

73. Whitlock JA: Neurophysiology of spasticity. In Glenn MB, Whyte J (eds): The Practical Management of Spasticity and Children in Adults. Philadelphia, Lea & Febiger, 1990, pp 8–33.

74. Whyte J, Robinson KM: Pharmacologic management. In Glenn MB, Whyte J (eds): The Practical Management of Spasticity in Children and Adults. Philadelphia, Lea & Febiger, 1990, pp 201–226.

75. Wiesendanger M: Organization of secondary motor areas of cerebral cortex. In Brooks VB (ed): Handbook of Physiology, vol II. Bethesda, MD, American Physiological Society, 1981, pp 1121–1143.

76. Young RR, Delwaide PJ: Spasticity. N Engl J Med 304:28–33, 96–99, 1981.

77. Young S, Keenan MA, Lance R: The treatment of spastic planovalgus foot deformity in the neurologically impaired adult. Foot Ankle 10:317–324, 1990.

17

Management of Musculoskeletal Complications

The high frequency of musculoskeletal injuries associated with traumatic brain injury is well documented.[8,28,32,39] Much of the literature about rehabilitation is devoted to cognitive and behavioral management. However, the speed and extent of successful rehabilitation often correlates with the timely diagnosis and appropriate management of concurrent musculoskeletal injuries.

In the early period after the initial trauma, because of the needs for resuscitation and medical stabilization, the diagnosis of peripheral nerve injuries, fractures, joint dislocations, or compartment syndromes is often missed or delayed.[32] Pain, the usual marker of such injuries, often cannot be elicited from the patient. The index of suspicion for musculoskeletal injuries must be high both in the acute phase and the rehabilitation environment. Missed fractures or nerve injuries invariably exacerbate disability. Therefore, serial examination of limbs and joints is critical, observing evidence of swelling, crepitus, decreased range of motion, or low tone in an otherwise spastic side (e.g., a low-tone arm with a spastic leg on the same side). This need is particularly strong in children. Sobus et al. recently reported on 60 children with traumatic brain injury who underwent bone scan on admission to a rehabilitation facility.[101] Sixteen children had a total of 25 newly detected fracture sites, 19 had previously undetected soft-tissue trauma, and 10 had previously undetected heterotopic ossification. The authors recommend full-body bone scans for children who do not reliably communicate on admission to a rehabilitation program.

Once an appropriate diagnosis is made, treatment usually is influenced by the patient's neurologic status. It is a cardinal error to provide inadequate initial treatment of musculoskeletal injuries because prognosis is assumed to be poor. The progress of patients who recover well may be impeded by the need to reverse the effects of poor initial treatment. However, it is essential to account for the patient's cognitive/behavior status as well as physical factors (i.e., spasticity, hypotonicity) in designing the treatment plan.

During the acute stage the rehabilitation physician should perform a careful examination of all four extremities, looking for signs of injury. Generally, radiographs of the spine, pelvis, and hips should be done once the patient is stabilized during the first 24–48 hours, and further radiographs may be indicated. Initial range of motion, tone status,

459

and pain responses should be recorded. Studies such as computed tomography (CT), magnetic resonance imaging (MRI), or electromyography and nerve conduction studies may need to be considered (electrophysiologic abnormalities may not be evident for several weeks). The peripheral nervous system and musculoskeletal system must be evaluated thoroughly when a patient is transferred to the rehabilitation unit. The results of the examination may indicate the need for further testing to diagnose a previously missed injury (e.g., an occult fracture or peripheral nerve injury not evident until the patient is more cooperative).

Once a diagnosis of soft-tissue or bony injury has been made, generally some form of immobilization is necessary. The difficulty of restraining a confused or agitated patient needs to be taken into account in applying splints or braces. Frequent checks for excessive pressure from immobilizing devices are essential with a patient who has difficulty communicating or impaired sensation. Traction methods are also difficult with restless or agitated patients; in addition, such patients cannot be adequately mobilized.[118] For these reasons, internal fixation on non-stable fractures is generally preferable.[8,28] Internal fixation also promotes early mobilization and allows inspection of joints and early range-of-motion exercises to reduce the possibility of contractures. If internal fixation is not appropriate, specific joint positions are recommended for immobilization. Bottle suggests immobilizing the elbow at 35–45° of flexion, the forearm in supination, the wrist in a neutral position, the metacarpophalangeal joints at 80° of flexion, the proximal interphalangeal joints at 10° of flexion, and the thumb in extension and abduction.[8] In the lower extremity, the hip should be immobilized in neutral position, the knee in extension, and the ankle in neutral position.

Another major issue is the need to promote optimal nutrition. Protein and calorie malnutrition negatively affect wound and fracture healing.[199,113] Severe trauma, fractures, and surgery may need 6000 calories/day. Early control of nausea and avoidance of over-medication with narcotics are important to maintain adequate oral feeding. Nasogastric or gastrostomy feeding may need to be initiated. Such patients often are at high risk for aspiration. If nutritional needs cannot be met by enteral routes, parenteral hyperalimentation may be useful.

FRACTURES

Optimal care of fractures is essential with head-injured patients. Persistent pain, excessive immobilization, and residual deformity are poorly tolerated and increase disability. Injuries to the upper extremity are less common than injuries to the lower extremity.[8] Because a large percentage of traumatic brain injuries result from high-speed motor vehicle accidents, trauma and fractures in the extremities are quite common. Often an early decision needs to be made about limb viability. Various factors determine the chances of survival and successful reconstruction of a severely traumatized limb. In patients with impaired vascular supply, older patients with multiple injuries, patients who have been in shock, and patients with diabetes or other vascular diseases, the chance for limb survival is smaller.[41] The strategy of immediate or early rigid stabilization of the skeleton was developed to protect or enhance blood supply.[40,41] Surgeons often perform early fixation with nailing or intramedullary rods to promote fracture healing, limb survival, and early mobilization. The Ilizarov technique of stabilization and bone transportation may help reconstruction in patients in whom bone loss may lead to possible limb-length discrepancy.[40,41]

Extensive efforts at reconstruction may meet with impressive success; alternatively, they may have tragic complications. Secondary infection may occur in older patients with metabolic disorders and multisystem failure. Several years of hospitalization and surgery may be necessary, with amputation as the ultimate outcome. The expense may be tremendous. Newer prosthetic techniques offer excellent function with lower extremity amputations. The trauma surgeon must weigh such factors when deciding between limb salvage and amputation. The question becomes even more challenging with upper extremities because of the significant loss of function with prosthetics. Bondurant and colleagues have demonstrated that a primary decision to amputate in severe trauma cuts the cost in half compared with delayed amputation.[4]

Botte states that the healing rate of fractures in head-injured patients is essentially the same as the normal population.[8] However, Guanche and Keenan believe that flaccid paralysis in an extremity may result in an increased risk of delayed union or nonunion.[40] Severe brain injury or significant peripheral nerve injuries may lead to a hypotonic limb, thereby limiting the compressive force of the surrounding muscles and complicating fracture healing. In a review of 41 brain-injured patients, Brien et al. described 21 patients with a fracture of the humerus and injury to the ipsilateral brachial plexus.[10] Eleven patients had an associated traumatic brain injury. Seven patients, five of whom were managed nonoperatively, developed nonunions. The authors recommend compression plating for patients with this pattern of injury because it allows anatomic reduction, compression at the site of fracture, and early mobilization.

The difficulties of restraining agitated patients and the complications of immobilization have already been discussed. Furthermore, because spasticity makes it more difficult to control limb position, the risk of malunion is increased. In addition, spasticity often causes joints to assume a flexed position that may lead to flexion contractures. Enhanced osteogenesis may cause heterotopic ossification. For these reasons, Garland states that open reduction and internal fixation are often the treatments of choice; the exception is tibial fractures, in which the outcomes of operative and nonoperative treatment are similar.[27]

Surgery should be delayed until the patient is neurologically and medically stable. Cerebral edema and intracranial pressure are generally at their highest levels within the first 3–5 days but decrease between the seventh and tenth day. The risks of surgery are lessened after this period. On the other hand, early operative fixation (within the first 24 hours) of upper and lower extremity fractures is associated with a decreased risk of adult respiratory distress syndrome (as a result of fat embolism, aspiration, thoracic trauma, or septic shock).[49] Johnson et al. studied 132 patients with multiple musculoskeletal injuries to assess the relationship between the timing of operative stabilization of major fractures and the incidence of adult respiratory distress syndrome (ARDS). Of patients who had early stabilization, 7% developed ARDS compared with 39% of patients with late or no stabilization. In addition, patients who did not have early fracture stabilization also had increased rates of major systems infection and mortality as well as prolonged periods of intensive care, intubation, and hospitalization.[49]

The most common injuries of the upper extremity in head-injured patients involve the shoulder girdle (scapula, clavicle, and acromioclavicular joint).[8] Such fractures are often discovered on routine chest radiographs. Crepitus, deformity, edema, and contusions in the shoulder regions warrant further evaluation. Most of these fractures can be treated with immobilization. Muscle spasticity or further trauma may lead to nonunion or malunion. Open reduction and internal fixation of nonunions may facilitate healing and allow motion.

Methods of closed reduction and external immobilization are difficult with humeral fractures. Traction is problematic, and orthotic devices are hard to maintain. Internal fixation is generally the optimal method of management for head-injured patients. Compression plating or intramedullary rods provide the best fixation, and the limb can be mobilized more quickly. Earlier weightbearing allows earlier wheelchair transfers or crutch-walking. The radial nerve is highly susceptible to injury with humeral shaft fractures.

Garland reported a 3% incidence of elbow fractures in a sample population of patients with head trauma. The incidence of heterotopic ossification with combined head and elbow injury was reported to be close to 90%. Heterotopic ossification is usually seen in the collateral ligaments but may also form anterior or posterior to the joint. Loss of range of motion is related to the amount of heterotopic ossification. Ulnar neuropathy, which may develop with elbow dislocation, prolonged pressure, or heterotopic ossification, can be diagnosed with electrophysiologic testing. Garland noted only two ulnar neuropathies in his series of 548 brain-injured patients.

In one series, open reduction and internal fixation were the preferred treatment for forearm fractures in 47 of 661 head-injured patients.[31] Loss of elbow motion is often a complication of forearm fractures. Synostosis (ossification across the interosseous membrane between the radius and ulna) may lead to loss of function. In Garland's series, 9 of 47 forearm fractures developed complete synostosis.[31] The incidence of synostosis is higher with operative management; nonsurgical treatment, however, often leads to loss of joint motion because of the need for immobilization. Seven of the 9 synostoses occurred in forearms that underwent open reduction with plate fixation.

Forearm fractures may be associated with compartment syndromes due to increased pressure within the fascial compartments of muscle from edema or hemorrhage. A compartment syndrome affects the muscles and associated structures within an osseofascial compartment of the forearm or leg. The most common areas of injury involve the volar compartment of the forearm, anterior compartment of the leg, deep posterior compartment of the leg, or the peroneal compartment. The cause is trauma directly about the compartment or at a proximal level. Edema, which is associated with high intracompartment pressures, may lead to myonecrosis, which in turn leads to fibrous tissue replacement, injury to peripheral nerves, and subsequent muscle contractures. Symptoms include swelling; tenseness over the affected compartment; deep, intractable, poorly localized pain; and distal paresthesias. Immediate diagnosis is imperative and is made by measurement of intracompartment pressures with a wick catheter. Pressures greater than 30 mmHg suggest the need for immediate fasciotomy and debridement of necrotic muscle to protect viable muscle and to prevent further damage. Long-term effects may include contracture, weakness, and pain. Splinting and intensive therapy to maintain or increase range of motion may be indicated.

Fractures of the distal radius are commonly missed in head-injured patients (3 of 10 undetected fractures in a series of 154 head-injured patients involved the distal radius). Malunion may leave residual wrist pain, loss of motion, and instability.[8] Disruption of the distal radioulnar joint may lead to pain and loss of forearm motion[8]; corrective osteotomy is indicated, and the ulnar head may need to be excised. Median, ulnar, and radial nerve lesions with fractures of the distal radius and ulna have been reported.[98,120]

Fractures of the pelvis are often associated with significant blood loss and shock.[8,30] Early diagnosis depends on radiographic evaluation of the pelvis. Pelvic fractures may involve injury to the bladder and urethra. An abnormal urinalysis warrants further evaluation, such as retrograde urethrography. Stable fractures do not require intervention. Unstable fractures, especially when disruption of the pelvic ring is seen, may require traction, external fixation, or internal fixation.

Tile reviewed 494 pelvic fractures and reported a 10% mortality rate.[114] Death may result from hemorrhage, sepsis, renal failure, or other complications. More than 60% of the pelvic injuries were stable. Tile maintains that stable injuries give few major long-term problems and that residual pain is mild to moderate. However, 60% of patients with vertically unstable disruption have pain. Twelve patients (5.5%) had permanent nerve damage, and six (2.5%) had permanent urethral damage.

The stability of the pelvic ring is determined by clinical and radiographic examination. Tile discusses the importance of inlet and outlet views. Clinical signs of instability include severe displacement, marked posterior bruising, severe associated injuries to nerves or vessels, and an open wound. Radiographic evidence of instability includes displacement of the posterior weightbearing sacroiliac complex by greater than 1 cm.[20,107] CT scanning provides the best information to determine stability and the need for operative intervention. The decision about when to operate is reviewed elsewhere.[52,107] Kellan reviewed various methods of fixation, including transition, external fixation, and open reduction and internal fixation. Patients with a stable pelvic ring may be mobilized quickly. Brain-injured patients with unstable fractures may need to be treated more aggressively with surgery because they do not tolerate external fixation and 6–12 weeks of bed rest.

Fractures of the hip occur in approximately 5% of brain-injured patients, and approximately 55% of this group develop traumatic heterotopic ossification.[30] Acetabular fractures are difficult to treat. Open reduction and internal fixation are associated with a higher incidence of heterotopic ossification (5 of 6 hips treated surgically in one series).[30] Botte states that in most cases of acetabular fractures, nonoperative treatment is preferred.[8] Early motion is recommended if traction is used.

Fractures of the femur are quite common after major trauma (68 femoral fractures in a series of 600 patients).[34] Spasticity of the adductor and hamstring is common and may result in angulation and shortening if hemiparesis is present in the ipsilateral extremity. Closed fixation with intramedullary rods is thought to provide the best results.[8,34] Open procedures have a higher incidence of heterotopic ossification (in one series 14% of 43 fractures treated by closed methods developed excessive callous vs. 52% of 25 fractures treated by open reduction and internal fixation).[40] In particular, ossification in the quadriceps muscles may cause loss of knee motion. If the patient is not a candidate for operative fixation, a cast brace may be a suitable alternative that allows quick mobilization. The patient must be closely monitored to ensure that the fixation and alignment are maintained.

Knee ligament injuries may be associated with traumatic brain injury. Primary repair may be indicated for patients who expect to return to full function and can participate actively in postoperative rehabilitation. Botte states that this approach is not necessarily the best option for brain-injured patients.[8] After repair, the knee must be immobilized, generally in flexion; in a spastic patient this often leads to a flexion contracture. Rehabilitation after ligamentous repair requires a cooperative patient. Most brain-injured patients who exhibit cognitive and behavioral problems have difficulty participating effectively. Therefore, reconstructive surgery generally should be postponed until the patient has improved and performed only if the knee remains symptomatic. If pain is an issue, knee stabilization with a cast is usually sufficient.

Tibial fractures are quite common in brain-injured patients (47 tibial fractures in 430 brain-injured patients in one series).[27] The usual treatment is immobilization with a long-leg plaster cast. The knee and ankle should be placed in a neutral position. Garland reported a union rate of 93.5% with an average time of 5.6 months for required union.[27] Casts should be well padded, especially in the region of the fibular neck, to prevent peroneal nerve palsy. Compartment syndromes may occur with tibial fractures, especially closed fractures. Frequent examination is recommended, and compartment pressures may need to be monitored.

Injuries to the ankle and foot are managed as in the normal population. The foot should be positioned in a neutral position, and the cast should be well padded. Displaced or comminuted fractures may require internal fixation, which allows timely rehabilitation efforts.

HETEROTOPIC OSSIFICATION

Dejerine and Ceillier first described heterotopic ossification in 1918 in paraplegic patients injured in World War I. They referred to the process as paraosteoarthropathy. Heterotopic ossification has been defined as the formation of mature lamellar bone in soft tissues.[111] The process involves true osteoblastic activity and bone formation. It has been reported in brain injury, spinal cord injury, stroke, poliomyelitis, myelodysplasia, tabes dorsalis, carbon monoxide poisoning, spinal cord tumors, synringomelia, tetanus, and multiple sclerosis. It has also been reported after burns and total hip replacement.[83,109] Several terms have been used to describe the condition, including heterotopic ossification, ectopic ossification, and myositis ossificans. Three categories of heterotopic ossification have been described:[71,109]

1. Myositis ossificans progressiva is a metabolic bone disease in children with progressive metamorphosis of skeletal muscle to bone. It is a rare autosomal dominant disease.

2. Myositis ossificans circumscripta without trauma is a localized soft-tissue ossification after neurologic injury or burns. This process is also referred to as neurogenic heterotopic ossification.

3. Traumatic myositis ossificans occurs from direct injury to the muscles. Fibrous, cartilaginous, and osseous tissue near bone are affected. The muscle may not be involved.

The reported incidence of heterotopic ossification varies. Garland states that in those patients who suffer severe trauma or insult to the central nervous system, 10–20% develop heterotopic ossification.[24] Mendelson et al. observed heterotopic ossification in 20% of patients with severe brain injury.[67] Other authors have reported an incidence in head-injured patients ranging from 11% to 76%.[109] The incidence is higher in patients who undergo open reduction and internal fixation of a fracture. Garland has extensively studied and reviewed the incidence of heterotopic ossification at different sites after brain injury.[28] With an elbow fracture, dislocation, or fracture-dislocation, the incidence of traumatic heterotopic ossification at the elbow approaches 90%. Traumatic heterotopic ossification of the elbow occurs in 20% of forearm fractures. Fifty-five percent of patients with hip fractures develop heterotopic ossification. The incidence increases to 83% if open reduction and internal fixation are performed. Garland states that the incidence is similar in the upper and lower extremities. The incidence is higher in a spastic extremity; in one series 89 of 100 involved joints in 496 brain-injured patients were in spastic extremities.[24] The incidence in children appears to be lower (3–22.5%).[15,70] In contrast, the incidence of heterotopic ossification after spinal cord injury has been reported at 16–53%.[104]

The specific cause and pathophysiology of heterotopic ossification remain unclear. Major et al. reported that heterotopic ossification is due to an interaction between local factors (pool of available calcium in adjacent skeleton, soft-tissue edema, vascular stasis, tissue hypoxia, mesenchymal cells with osteoblastic activity) and an unknown systemic factor or factors.[66] The basic defect in heterotopic ossification is the inappropriate differentiation of fibroblasts to bone-forming cells.[12] Histologic examination demonstrates that heterotopic ossification is composed of true osseous tissue rather than of calcified soft tissue.[67] Heterotopic bone is metabolically active and exhibits about triple the normal rate of bone formation and double

the normal number of osteoclasts.[83] Rossier et al. studied tissue samples of recent-onset and long-standing disease. They concluded that early edema of connective tissue proceeded to tissue with a foci of calcification and then to maturation of calcification and ossification.

Various authors who reviewed the association of the HLA system and heterotopic ossification have suggested a genetic predisposition to an associated systemic factor;[59,69] thus, an antigenic marker should be available to mark susceptible patients. Garland found no evidence of any association between the HLA system and heterotopic ossification.[25] Minaire et al. found an association between HLA-B 18 and patients with neurologic disorders as well as patients who develop heterotopic ossification.[69] However, 75% of patients with heterotopic ossification lack this marker.

Clinical factors also have been studied. Lal et al. found an increased incidence of heterotopic ossification associated with age greater than 30 years and, in spine-injured patients, with completeness of lesion.[58] In their retrospective study of 100 spinal-injured patients, 92% who were older than 30 years and had a complete lesion, pressure sores, and spasticity developed heterotopic ossification. Sazbon et al. note that the development of heterotopic ossification is independent of sex and age, as well as cause, duration, and outcome of coma, but report a link with occurrence of coma.[95] An association has been cited between spasticity and heterotopic ossification.[24,58] Lal et al. found spasticity in 84% of patients with heterotopic ossification and in 54% of patients without. They also noted that forceful joint manipulation appeared to enhance formation of heterotopic ossification and postulated that the force generated by muscle spasticity may promote its development .

Physical therapy has been thought to be associated with heterotopic ossification as a result of local trauma. In an extensive literature review Stover found that opinion was divided.[104] He noted that patients who received no physical therapy have developed heterotopic ossification.

The earliest sign of heterotopic ossification often is decreased joint range of motion.

Other findings include swelling, erythema, heat, and pain with range-of-motion testing. Fever also may be present. Local pain and a mass may be palpated in the periarticular region. In a retrospective study Sazbon reported onset of heterotopic ossification between 1 and 7 months after severe brain injury in 7 (90%) of 8 comatose patients.[95] Diagnosis was made with plain radiographs. The most common sites are hips, shoulders, elbows, and knees. The proximal interphalangeal joints of the hand, the wrist, and the spine also may be affected.[1,39]

During the acute phase of erythema and swelling, radiographs may be normal. Triple-phase technetium 99 bone scanning detects early increases in vascularity and is a reliable method of diagnosis. The first and second phases of the triple-phase bone scan show increased uptake. Later radiographs (1–2 weeks after onset) often show only soft-tissue swelling. Radiographs show immature ossification and then the appearance of mature bone. Heterotopic ossification may take 8–14 months to reach maturity.[111] Early increases in alkaline phosphatase may be difficult to interpret, because the level rises with other causes such as fractures or hepatotoxicity. Kewalramani reported that the level of alkaline phosphatase paralleled the activity of ossification and that when ossification stopped, the levels returned to normal.[53] He also stated that alkaline phosphatase fractionation studies can distinguish among different reasons for electrical levels. The erythrocyte sedimentation rate is too nonspecific to be of much help in the diagnosis of heterotopic ossification, but an elevated level associated with other clinical features suggests the need for further evaluation.

The differential diagnosis in patients with soft-tissue swelling or loss of range of motion includes thrombophlebitis, cellulitis, septic arthritis, hematoma, fracture, or local trauma.

Heterotopic ossification, once developed, may cause complications through pressure on surrounding anatomic structures. Peripheral nerve compression and vascular compression with subsequent thrombophlebitis and lymphedema may result from heterotopic ossification.[11,58,110] Brooke recommends serial evaluation of deep tendon reflexes to follow peripheral nerve function.[11] The most common complication is decreased range of motion, which in rare cases may progress to joint ankylosis.

Various methods to prevent the formation of heterotopic ossification have been evaluated. Schmidt et al. concluded that indomethacin is highly potent in preventing heterotopic ossification after total hip replacement.[96] The effect is thought to be due to inhibition of the synthesis of prostaglandin. The authors recommend 25 mg 3 times/day. Salicylates and ibuprofen also have been suggested for prophylaxis.[37,110] Schmidt et al. studied the use of indomethacin (25 mg 3 times/day) to prevent heterotopic ossification after hip replacement. Heterotopic ossification occurred in 15% of treated patients compared with 75% of controls.[96]

Low-dose radiation has been used to prevent heterotopic ossification after total hip replacement.[17] Coventry recommended 2000 rads over 12 days, but others have suggested 1000 rads over 5–7 days. Radiation is thought to prevent conversion of mesenchymal cells to bone precursor cells.

The role of etidronate disodium (EHDP) in preventing heterotopic ossification has been studied extensively.[37,102] The literature to date does not adequately support its efficacy in brain-injured patients. EHDP is a diphosphonate that reportedly retards formation, growth, and dissolution of hydroxyapatite crystals; therefore, it is thought to limit ectopic soft-tissue calcification by preventing conversion of calcium phosphate compounds in hydroxyapatite crystals. EHDP is often used to retard heterotopic ossification once it is discovered; it is thought to be more effective if given prophylactically or in the earlier stages of formation.[37] EHDP may provide pain relief because it retards inflammation. It does not dissolve established calcification. Because effect on normal bone healing is questionable, it should be used with caution in patients with long bone fractures. Glenn notes that the manufacturer of EHDP advises delay or interruption of therapy until callus is evident.[37] However, Stover notes that in spine-injured patients vertebral fracture and long bone healing did not appear to be inhibited by EHDP.[104] The side effects are few. Gastrointestinal side effects (diarrhea and nausea) are infrequent and can be minimized by dividing the total daily dose. EHDP should not be given within 2 hours of meals, especially enteral tube feedings. Hyperphosphatemia may be observed early during treatment, but phosphate levels generally return to normal after the drug is stopped.

Spielman et al. looked specifically at heterotopic ossification in brain injury.[102] They believed that early use of EHDP lowered the incidence in patients with severe traumatic brain injury (initial Glasgow Coma Score < 9). Ten patients with severe brain injuries were given EHDP prophylactically and compared with 10 matched controls. Of the 10 treated patients, 2 developed significant heterotopic ossification compared with 7 of the controls. The authors believe that effective prophylactic treatment should be initiated as soon as possible. Dosage guidelines are unclear. Spielman et al. recommended 20 mg/kg/day for 3 months, followed by 10 mg/kg/day for 3 months. Garland recommends 20 mg/kg for 6 months.[33] He notes that dosages less than 20 mg/kg/day are less effective at inhibiting crystal growth. In his study of spinal-injured patients, Stover used 20 mg/kg for 2 weeks, then 10 mg/kg for 10 weeks.[104] The literature to date does not strongly support any particular dosage schedule, nor is efficacy well established.

The treatment of heterotopic ossification often is quite challenging and in many cases unsatisfactory. Garland emphasizes the importance of understanding the natural history of heterotopic ossification in developing treatment strategies.[33] He notes that the majority of heterotopic ossification occurs within 3 months after spinal cord injury. Most roentgenographic evaluation occurs during a 6-month period. Garland concluded that the progress of heterotopic ossification is related to the severity of injury. In patients with severe injuries, roentgenographic progression subsided by 6 months and serum alkaline phosphatase and bone scan activity became normal or significantly decreased . Patients with more severe deficits had larger amounts of bone formation that progressed for more than 1 year, and elevated alkaline phosphatase levels and increased bone scan activity were observed for up to 2 years and in some cases longer.

The role of physical therapy in patients with heterotopic ossification is controversial. The major goal of treatment is to maintain range of motion and thereby preserve function. Range-of-motion exercises, however, are controversial. Several authors have reviewed the literature that compares opposing philosophies.[18,25,33,53,105,116] One theory is that an aggressive regimen of passive range-of-motion exercises may predispose to the development of heterotopic ossification because of microtrauma or local hemorrhage. Several authors suggest that passive stretching and range-of-motion exercises are contraindicated after heterotopic ossification is suspected but recommend active exercise within pain-free range.[18,53]

Other authors[33,67,105,116] stress the importance of range-of-motion exercises to maintain joint mobility and to prevent or retard fibrous ankylosis. They found no evidence for increased heterotopic ossification or decreased range of motion with passive range-of-motion exercises. Garland maintains that forceful manipulation of joints with preexisting heterotopic ossification under anesthesia helps to maintain useful joint range and to prevent ankylosis.[26] He also advocates treatment of underlying spasticity (with medications or nerve or motor point blocks) in the effort to prevent contractures. In Garland's series, 64% of affected joints maintained or gained range of motion with rehabilitation after manipulation. Some required repeated manipulations; none had a detectable increase in heterotopic ossification. The literature generally supports the common use of active and gentle passive range-of-motion exercises to maintain available joint motion and to avoid progressive contractures.

If joint deformity from heterotopic ossification results in significant functional limitations, such as difficulty with hygiene, sitting, or ambulation, surgical resection of heterotopic ossification may be indicated. Surgery also may be appropriate if an underlying bone mass contributes to repeated pressure sores. Various recommendations have been made for the timing of surgery.[53,67,89,35,70,109] A concern with early resection is recurrence of the underlying process. In Sazbon's series of comatose patients, there was no progression of the disease beyond 14 months after the onset of coma.[95] Roberts and Pankratz suggest waiting for the maturation of heterotopic bone before operating and state that the process may take 1–2 years.[89] Kewalramani believes that surgery is contraindicated in patients with clinical, laboratory, or radiographic evidence of active ossification.[53] In the series of Mital et al., heterotopic bone was excised when it significantly restricted joint range of motion and limited function and rehabilitation.[70] Surgery was not performed in patients with an increasing level of serum alkaline phosphatase. The mean period of time from coma to surgery was 7.5 months. Mendelson et al. believed the process stabilized after 6–8 months and that surgery would be of benefit after that time.[67] They operated on 3 of 35 patients with heterotopic ossification. All three showed functional improvement, but the authors do not state whether radiation treatments were given.

Garland believes that, in general, surgery should be delayed for 18 months after brain injury.[35] In his opinion patients with good neurologic recovery, with good motor control, normal or slightly elevated levels of alkaline phosphatase, and a mature lesion may be candidates for surgery before the 18 months. He also believes that such patients show the best progress after surgery. In more severely compromised patients surgery should be delayed longer than 18 months if motor control is still improving and laboratory values are still abnormal. With such patients, the major indication for surgery is limb positioning. The surgical approach to removal of heterotopic ossification is discussed elsewhere.[35]

Surgery is challenging because the ossified mass is highly vascular; postoperative bleeding, hematoma, and infection are common complications. Trauma to nerves also may occur. Preoperative CT scans may guide the surgeon and lower the rate of complications.[9] Various recommendations have been made to prevent recurrence of heterotopic ossification. Low-dose radiation is thought to be effective in the immediate postoperative phase.[35] The use of EHDP and/or nonsteroidal antiinflammatory agents is said to be useful for a 3-month period after surgery.[11,35] Active range-of-motion exercises may be initiated 2–3 days after surgery. More active exercises may begin about 10–14 days after pain and swelling have subsided. Patients with more severe cognitive and motor deficits may require several months of postoperative physical therapy to maintain range of motion. If heterotopic ossification recurs, it becomes evident within 3 months after surgery.[110]

PERIPHERAL NERVE INJURIES

As noted previously, peripheral nerve injuries often go undetected after traumatic brain injury. The actual incidence of peripheral nerve injuries, therefore, has probably been underreported. Garland found that of 254 patients admitted to the head trauma service at Rancho Los Amigos Hospital, 29 (11%) had previously undetected peripheral nerve injuries.[32] The diagnostic delay ranged from 6 to 80 days. In a prospective study, Cosgrove et al. performed electromyographic studies on any patient with flaccidity, areflexia, or abnormal motor patterns.[16] Positive findings were reported in 1%. Thirteen of 132 patients (10%) had 16 distinct nerve lesions. Thirteen lesions occurred at the time of trauma, and pressure palsies occurred in the posttraumatic period. Stone and Keenan screened 50 brain-injured patients and found peripheral nerve injuries in 17 (34%).[103] The majority of patients were injured in motor vehicle accidents. Of note, none of the injuries had been detected before admission to a rehabilitation center. Ulnar nerve entrapment at the elbow was seen most frequently (10)%. Two of 6 cases were associated with heterotopic ossification; the other 4 were associated with compression and traction on the nerve secondary to severe elbow flexion spasticity. Keenan et al. found an incidence of tardy ulnar palsy of 2.5%.[51]

As stated previously, examination of the peripheral nervous system, followed by repeated serial evaluations, is critical in detecting peripheral nerve injuries and thereby avoiding progressive loss of function. Examination is often challenging because of poor patient cooperation, and weakness secondary to concurrent central brain injury. Cosgrove recommended further evaluation when flaccidity, areflexia, and abnormal movement patterns are observed.[16] The presence of long bone fractures should alert the clinician to the possibility of traumatic nerve injuries. In particular, a brachial plexus injury should be suspected in patients with brain injury as a result of a motorcycle accident, a flail upper extremity, and a fracture about the shoulder girdle.

Once a peripheral nerve injury is suspected, electrodiagnostic studies should be considered. Studies are often limited and technically difficult. Poor pain tolerance, altered mental status, and the presence of an upper motor neuron lesion may limit cooperation.

Peripheral nerve injuries often can be explained by the initial trauma. Humeral fractures may be associated with radial nerve injury: radial and ulnar fractures, with medial and ulnar nerve lesions; and pelvic fractures, with femoral nerve injuries and acetabular injuries that lead to lumbosacral plexopathy.[16] The association of heterotopic ossification and peripheral nerve injuries has already been discussed. Brachial plexus lesions are often seen as a result of stretch injuries. Other posttraumatic lesions, often at the elbow or knee, can be explained on the basis of poor bed positioning and pressure. Patients placed in a cast are also at risk.

Stone and Keenan found brachial plexus injuries in 5 (10%) of 50 patients. Four patients had complete spontaneous recovery, whereas one patient did not recover.[103] Garland reported no neurologic recovery in 2 of 3 patients with brachial plexus injuries[32]; in the third patient, surgical exploration was followed by good neurologic recovery. It is important to distinguish between preganglionic injury involving avulsion of the nerve root from the spinal cord and postganglionic injury distal to the intervertebral foramen. Nerve root avulsion cannot be surgically repaired, and the prognosis is poor. Manual muscle testing and electomyography (EMG) help to localize the lesion. A traumatic meningocele or pseudomengocele, a characteristic sign of an avulsed root, can be seen with myelography.

The axon reflex test reflects the integrity of sensory axons and may provide useful information if brachial plexus lesion is suspected.[84] Histamine is injected into the involved dermatome. A positive response of vasodilation, wheal, and flare indicates an intact sensory axon and therefore a preganglionic lesion. The absence of a flare response indicates a postganglionic lesion secondary to distal sensory fiber degeneration. EMG and nerve conduction studies also should be performed. Sensory conduction studies are normal in preganglionic lesions, whereas absent or reduced conductions indicate postganglionic lesions. In addition, if EMG studies indicate normal innervation of the cervical paravertebral muscles but denervation of the more distal plexus muscles, a postganglionic lesion is suspected. Denervation of cervical paravertebrals, shoulder girdle, and limb musculature indicates preganglionic root avulsion.

The diagnosis and management of brachial plexus injuries are discussed in more detail elsewhere.[61,80] The most common mechanism of injury is a stretch lesion during a high-velocity injury. Stress is placed on the lower roots if the patient has sustained a fall with the arm extended and hyperabducted and the head hyperextended and rotated to the opposite side. Stress is greater on the upper roots if the arm is held down at the side or adducted. Penetrating injuries such as a knife or gunshot wound may cause plexus injuries.

Three degrees of nerve injuries have been described. Neuropraxia, the least severe, involves a transient physiologic injury to the axons that blocks neural conduction. Axonotmesis occurs when axonal continuity is interrupted. The connective tissue sheath remains intact, but wallerian degeneration occurs. If recovery occurs, it may take months. The most severe injury is neurotmesis, which involves transection of the nerve with disruption of the axon and neural tubule. Surgery may be the only therapeutic alternative.

The prognosis with brachial plexus injuries is generally determined by the proximity of the lesion to the spinal cord. The pattern of weakness and the subsequent level of function are determined by which portion of the plexus is injured. Upper trunk injuries (C5–C6) or Erb-Duchenne palsy results in an adducted, medially rotated humerus with inability to abduct or laterally rotate the arm, to flex the elbow, or to supinate the forearm. Sensory deficits are seen in the C5–C6 dermatomes. A C8–T1 (Klumpke) or lower trunk injury presents with weakness in the median- and ulnar-innervated muscles of the hand. A total plexus injury with nerve root avulsion at all levels of the plexus results in a flail anesthetic arm and hand with Horner's syndrome. The prognosis is poor.

Surgery may be indicated to repair brachial plexus lesions. The surgical approach is discussed elsewhere.[19,54,55,56] Maximal spontaneous recovery may take up to 2 years. Relatively acute repair of sharp brachial plexus is generally recommended, whereas surgery for traction or stretch injuries may be delayed. Outcome is variable and depends largely on the location of the lesion. Dubuisson and Kline[19] state that 60% of cases are successful, but they do not define success clearly. Outcome is better if the injury is at an intraclavicular level and if surgery is performed within 6 months of injury.

Reconstructive surgical procedures may improve function. A latissimus dorsi muscle transfer may restore elbow flexion, as may a pectoralis major-to-biceps transfer. Initial therapy measures include strengthening and range-of-motion exercises. It is critical to avoid contractures. Splinting for function or positioning often is indicated. A sling helps to keep the arm supported and out of the way during daily activities. Herbison described the potential benefits and limitations of exercise therapies in peripheral neuropathies.[45] Pain often accompanies such injuries and may be quite refractory to treatment. Medications (tricyclic antidepressants, anticonvulsants), nerve blocks, transcutaneous nerve stimulators, accupuncture, and massage have been used with varying degrees of success. Surgical destruction of the dorsal root entry zone (DREZ lesions) has been used to reduce the intractable pain of nerve root avulsions.[74] Such patients are at risk for reflex sympathetic dystrophy, which is characterized by vasomotor and trophic changes. Raj recently reviewed the comprehensive management of reflex sympathetic dystrophy.[85] With severe plexus injuries, another option may be above-elbow amputation, often accompanied by shoulder fusion. In patients with shoulder and elbow control, a below-elbow amputation with subsequent fitting of a prosthesis may improve function.

Other peripheral nerve injuries are also encountered.[16,48,103] In the upper extremity the radial nerve may be injured in the radial groove by fracture, callus formation,

or pressure. Tardy ulnar palsy may result from compression due to poor bed positioning or from heterotopic ossification.[50,112] Median and ulnar injuries may occur with forearm fractures.[92,98,120]

In the lower extremity, various nerve injuries may occur with pelvic fractures. Patterson and Morton retrospectively reviewed 633 patients with pelvic fractures and dislocations.[81] They found neurologic complications in 22 (3.5%). They concluded that neurologic injuries with pelvic fractures are frequently missed and that the level of neurologic injury is difficult to determine. In addition, they found that recovery is never complete and that disability may be permanent. Potential sites of injury include the lumbosacral plexus, and the femoral, sciatic, obturator, or pudendal nerves. The sciatic nerve may be injured with hip fractures. Peroneal neuropathies may occur with adduction injury of the knee, dislocation of the proximal tibiofibular joint, or injury associated with traction after femoral fracture.[32,48] The peroneal nerve also may be compressed by a cast at the fibular head. Indications for surgery to repair peripheral nerve injuries and operative techniques are discussed by Dubuisson and Kline.[19] Primary repair is generally indicated for a clean, sharp, neural laceration. The repair of blunt nerve injuries is often delayed 2–4 weeks. There is little need for early operations for lesions in continuity unless they are complicated by a mass lesion or acute entrapment. Axons regrow at a rate of 1 inch/month. Patients should be followed with serial clinical and EMG evaluations. Persistent paralysis is generally the indication for surgery; timing between injury and surgery usually varies from 2–6 months. Therapy issues and pain management options are discussed above. The importance of proper bed positioning and serial evaluation of peripheral nerve function cannot be overstated.

CONTRACTURES

Contractures are perhaps the most common musculoskeletal complication after traumatic brain injury. The incidence of contractures has been reported to be high as 84%.[119] Contractures have been defined as loss of range of motion in a joint to a degree that impedes activities of daily living.[119] A similar concept is that a muscle or group of muscles has shortened sufficiently to prevent complete range of motion of the joint or joints it crosses.[13] There are multiple causes for contractures. After orthopedic immobilization, prolonged positioning in a shortened position may be necessary. Poor positioning may cause contractures when weakness due to injury to the central nervous system or a peripheral nerve lesion leads to muscle imbalance. A stronger, poorly opposed muscle may shorten where it is not fully stretched by its weaker antagonist. Injury to the central nervous system also may cause spasticity, leaving muscle groups in predominantly shortened position. The role of heterotopic ossification in causing progressive loss of joint range of motion has already been discussed.[116]

Even temporary immobilization of a joint may result in permanent loss of motion.[82] Joint stiffness occurs more quickly if the joint is surrounded by edema. Mobility around joints depends on the formation of loose or areolar connective tissue. Connective tissue demonstrates plastic elongation when subjected to constant tension and progressively shortens when not opposed by a stretching force.[57] In healthy people connective tissue is constantly removed, replaced, and reorganized. With little motion, collagen is laid down with short distances between points of attachment. With immobility, the areolar connective tissue contracts and reorganizes to become dense connective tissue that further limits motion. This process may begin over several days. Loss of hexosamine and decreased synthesis of proteoglycans are thought to be additional factors.[117] Proteoglycans loosely bind and trap water, lubricate the connective tissue, and interface and minimize the anomalous crosslinking of fibers. A decrease in proteoglycans due to immobility results in less lubrication, decreased flexibility, and therefore more time for anomalous crosslinks to develop.

Frank et al. liken the treatment of contractures to that of pressure sores: "Contractures may best be treated by prevention."[22] They underscore the importance of passive range of motion in "stretching" and "lubricating" connective tissue. Kottke provides an excellent overview of specific key joints at risk as well as recommendations for appropriate methods of stretching.[57] He specifically focuses on lower extremity joints because of the pathologic effect on gait and the potential for significant increase in disability. Relaxed standing requires full extension of the hips and knees. With hip or knee flexion contractures, relaxed standing occurs only with compensatory lordosis of the lumbar spine or with active use of muscles. The patient is at risk for chronic back pain or easy fatigability. Pathological gait patterns also are seen.

The severely traumatized brain-injured patient is at risk for lower extremity contractures (hip and knee flexors and ankle plantarflexors) because of the often encountered combination of weakness, spasticity, and prolonged bed rest. Such contractures also interfere with nursing care (hygiene and wheelchair positioning). Stretching of the key joints should be initiated as soon as possible in the acute care setting, ideally in the intensive care unit. Kottke recommends slow, prolonged stretching, often with the use of weights.[57] The patient's own body weight can be used in the prone position (hip flexors) or with a standing frame (ankle plantarflexors). Prior pain medication and ultrasound may increase the effectiveness of stretching.

Upper extremity joints are also at risk for contractures. Brain-injured patients usually assume a flexed position because of the relative over-activity of the wrist and finger flexors, elbow flexors, shoulder adductors, and internal rotators. The role of spasticity in the development of contractures can be a particularly challenging problem because of the difficulty of putting joints through range of motion. The treatment of spasticity is discussed in a previous chapter. Inhibitive casting, antispasticity medications, lidocaine or marcaine blocks to differentiate spasticity from contracture, and phenol nerve blocks may be helpful.

Cherry reviewed therapy alternatives for reducing muscle contracture.[13] The use of passive motion has already been mentioned.[20] Muscle weakness generally contributes to the development of contractures. The therapist should attempt to strengthen the weak agonist of the shortened antagonist. An important adjunctive approach is to attempt to lessen generalized muscle tone. The techniques of Bobath and Rood focus on inhibiting hypertonicity.[108] If such techniques are effective, the involved joints can be moved through a more complete range of motion.

Various approaches have been tried to provide prolonged passive and active stretching to a joint once contracture has developed. Splinting usually provides effective prevention but is inadequate treatment of spasticity-induced contracture. Serial casting may help with spasticity as well as range-of-motion limitations.[6,14,73,106] It has been reported to be most effective within the first 6 months after injury.[6] The casts need to be well padded, especially around bony prominences, to prevent skin breakdown. Booth et al. recommend that the initial cast remain in place for 7–10 days; then drop-out casts are applied at regular intervals until the desired or maximally obtainable range of motion is achieved. The final cast is bivalved and converted into an anteroposterior splint, which is worn at night to maintain position. Short and long arm casts are often used. In the lower extremity, short- and long-leg casts may be necessary to reverse knee flexion contractures as well as equinovarus deformities. Nerve blocks before applying a cast may improve effectiveness. Serial casting may increase intracranial pressure; it should be done cautiously early after injury. Cognitive and behavioral deficits associated with brain injuries, along with poor tolerance of pain, make it difficult to know when a cast is too tight or when a pressure sore has developed. Experienced, consistently available therapists are critical for correct application of casts and for knowing when they need to be removed. Lehmkuhl et al. summarized the available literature about the efficacy of serial casting in reducing contracture (Table 1).[62]

Another approach is a dynamic splint that uses a spring-tension, low-load, prolonged-stretch device.[44,65,87,88] The amount of force applied across the joint can be altered by varying the tension of the springs. This approach has the advantage of lessening the potential for skin breakdown because the device can be regularly removed to inspect the skin. The patient may still experience discomfort, and splint breakdown may occur.

Despite the treatment team's best efforts, brain-injured patients may develop severe contractures that are refractory to conservative treatment and that limit either function or care. Surgery is the only effective alternative but should be performed only to achieve a specific goal. In severely injured patients, the usual indications for surgery are relief of joint pain, improved hygiene or nursing care, and prevention or relief of skin breakdown (e.g., severe elbow flexion contracture that causes breakdown in the antecubital space). In the patient with good recovery, surgery is usually designed to improve function (e.g., reduction of plantarflexion contracture to improve gait pattern). The preoperative evaluation includes examination for heterotopic ossification. Nerve blocks often are used to differentiate spasticity from soft-tissue contracture.[77] Differentiation between muscle tightness and joint contracture is necessary for muscles spanning two joints, as in the hand, wrist, and ankle. The proximal joint is flexed, and the effect on the distal joint is noted. Joint contracture is not affected by change imposition of the proximal joint.

Ough et al. give a comprehensive review of surgical approaches to joint contracture.[77] Surgery is directed towards decreasing muscular activity or releasing myostatic contracture and may involve myotomy, tenotomy, or tendon-lengthening. Neurectomy also may be necessary. The shoulder commonly is contracted in an adducted, internally rotated position. The pectoralis major, subscapulares, teres major, and latissimus dorsi may need to be released. Elbow flexion contractures may require soft-tissue release as well as musculotaneous neuroectomy if spasticity is significant.

Wrist and finger flexion deformities often occur concurrently, leading to difficulties with pain, hygiene, and skin breakdown. Sublimis-to-profundus transfer may improve exposure of the palm.

Wrist and finger flexors may be either released or lengthened with Z-plasty. Postoperative splinting may be necessary to maintain desirable positioning. To avoid overcorrection and possible extension deformities, the surgeon may do fractional lengthening of the finger flexors.

TABLE 1. Summary of Published Studies Documenting the Effects of Serial/Inhibitive Casting on Reducing Contractures of the Elbow, Knee, and Ankle Joints of Brain Injury Survivors (1980–1989)

Investigators/ Publications	Year	Types of Patients	No. of Patients	Joints	Therapeutic Intervention
King Am J Occup Ther 36:671–673	1982	Intracranial hemorrhage Female 46 yrs	1	L elbow	Plaster cast 45 days postinjury
Zachazewski et al. Phys Ther 62:453–455	1982	TBI—MCA Male 25 yrs	1	R ankle L ankle	Plaster casts with tone-inhibiting footplate R, L 4 mos postinjury
Booth et al. Phys Ther 63:1960–1966	1983	Head injury a) Cortical 19 male/5 female x = 23 yrs	24	Ankle 14 unilateral 10 bilateral	Short-leg casts 78 days postinjury
		b) Brainstem 9 male/6 female x = 20 yrs	15	Ankle 10 unilateral 5 bilateral	Short-leg casts
		c) Cortical x = 25 yrs	5	Knee Unilateral	Long-leg casts 114 days postinjury
		d) Brainstem 4 male x = 24 yrs	4	Knee	Long-leg casts 111 days postinjury
Barnard et al. Phys Ther 64:1540–1542	1984	TBI—Fall Male 11 yrs	1	R ankle L ankle	Plaster cast 10 days postinjury
Bronkhorst and Lamb Orthot Prosthet 42:23–20	1987	TBI—MVA Male 28 yrs	1	R ankle L ankle	AFOs with apostic inhibitive bars > 3 mos postinjury
Sullivan et al. Physiother Can 40:346–350	1988	TBI	10	Ankle	Eight of 10 required bilateral casts to 18 ankles 14 days postinjury
		TBI	10	Ankle	Fifteen ankles of 10 untreated controls
MacKay-Lyons Phys Ther 69:292–296	1989	TBI–MVA (pedestrian) Male 20 yrs	1	L elbow	a) Inhibitive cast 1.5 mos post-trauma b) Manual stretching and ice packs 5 mos posttrauma c) Dynasplint 13 mos postinjury
Moore et al. J Head Trauma Rehabil 4(2):63–65	1989	TBI–MVA Male 12 yrs	1	R ankle L ankle	Plaster casts 2 days postinjury

TBI = traumatic brain injury, MVA = motor vehicle accident, MCA = motorcycle accident, R = right, L = left, AFO = ankle-foot orthosis, ROM = range of motion. *(Columns continued on opposite page.)*

TABLE 1. **Summary of Published Studies Documenting the Effects of Serial/Inhibitive Casting on Reducing Contractures of the Elbow, Knee, and Ankle Joints of Brain Injury Survivors (1980–1989)** *(Columns continued)*

Initial Measurement	Final Measurement	Duration of Treatment	Follow-up	Comments
−90°	−15°	16 days 6 casts 3 wks bivalved cast at night	2 mos Gain retained	Full functional use of wrist and hand following onset. Cerebral aneurysm clipped.
During gait scissoring heelstrike, incomplete extension of knee; R > L	During gait heel-strike on L and foot flat on R, less scissoring, complete extension of knee	4 wks molded AFO worn on R for 6 mos and still wearing at last contact	At 6 mos cranioplasty followed by dramatic improvement; at 7 mos walking with minimal assist but still needs AFO (tone inhibiting)	Hypertonicity greater in lower extremities than in upper; all attempted medications produced too much drowsiness.
−16° (−50 to 0)	0.7° (−15 to 20)	28 (7 to 88) days		As compared with those with cortical lesions, patients with brainstem lesions started with worse contractures, received casts later from onset, and took longer to make ROM gains. Nearly 40% of those with excessive muscle tone had less tone after casting.
−24° (−60 to to −5)	2° (−25 to 20)	39 (7 to 92) days		
−32° (−90 to −10)	−5° (−20 to 0)	22 (8 to 66) days		
−25° (−90 to −5)	−10° (−30 to 0)	31 (7 to 58) days		
−25° −20°	5° 0°	10 days	42 days	Partial control Full control Attempted more conservative techniques first.
0° 0°	+10° to +15° +10° to +15°	4 wks	3 mos	Active dorsiflex to +5° Active dorsiflex to +15°
−17° average	+3° average			Average of 5 serial casts to each limb, for a total of 190 casts; 2 had to be removed because of persistent skin discoloration.
Untreated	−15°			
−74°	−74°	4 days		Developed pressure sore over lateral epicondyle.
−80°	−70°	4 mos		
−68°	−15°	6 mos	7 mos	Active and passive ROM remained at −15° 2 mos after discontinuation.
(Decerebrate posturing)	No change	2 days		L diaphysial femur fracture and a R tibial fracture. Two days postinjury, operative stabilization of L femur fracture. Casts bivalved because of swelling. During 2nd postoperative day fasciotomy performed on L leg to relieve pressure; on 6th postoperative day a L below-knee amputation was performed. Patient remained in a vegetative state.

In the lower extremity hip flexion and adduction deformities are common. Improved perineal hygiene and/or improved bed positioning may be the goal of surgery. Anterior obturator neurectomy and iliopsoas release are indicated if it is difficult to care for the patient. If adduction deformity is mild, adductor tenotomy may be an alternative. The prone position is encouraged postoperatively.

Knee flexion contracture may be managed with release of the hamstring as well as the iliotibial band. Postoperative casting often is necessary to maximize range of motion. Knee and ankle contractures often inhibit transferring and/or walking. Improving specific functions is generally the goal of surgery. However, with more severely injured patients, the goal may be simply to promote standing to achieve some weightbearing activities. At the ankle, correction of equinus deformity may be necessary to facilitate wheelchair positioning, transfer, standing, or ambulation. The Achilles tendon may be lengthened in an open or percutaneous procedure. Usually release of the long toe flexor is also required. The ankle is placed in a cast postoperatively for 6 weeks, followed by at least 6 weeks in an ankle-foot orthosis. After surgery, it is necessary to maintain range of motion. Because contracture may occur, the treatment team should consider postoperative splinting, appropriate positioning, and range-of-motion exercises to maintain joint mobility.

SUMMARY

The challenge of brain injury rehabilitation is highlighted by the complex interrelationship among physical, medical, cognitive, behavioral, social, and economic factors that potentially affect both patient and family. Early medical and physical management greatly influences the extent and duration of future disability. This concept is particularly relevant in the management of musculoskeletal complications after traumatic brain injury. The initial primary need is accurate and timely diagnosis of the particular complication. Early comprehensive physical examination of the musculoskeletal system is imperative. Serial evaluations are necessary to monitor the progress of injuries and to diagnose late complications.

Initially occult fractures and peripheral nerve injuries are easily missed. Once they are diagnosed, management strategies must take into account the global clinical picture. Cognitive and behavioral status, other medical complications, and nutritional status may influence clinical decision making. In an increasingly managed-care environment, with trends toward shorter institutional stays and earlier transition to home or long-term care facilities, management strategies must consider cost-effectiveness and outcome data. The physician needs to have a good sense of expected patient outcomes as well as available resources. Often one handles a patient who is expected to remain in a vegetative state differently from a rapidly recovering patient in an agitated state.

The clinician needs to be aware of the natural history of musculoskeletal issues in brain injured patients. Patients should be monitored for development of heterotopic ossification, late neuropathies, and joint contractures. Prevention of potentially late developing musculoskeletal complications is always the best strategy. Once a complication occurs, conservative treatment is generally preferred. However, if contracture or heterotopic bone formation decreases function or makes nursing care more difficult, surgical correction should be considered.

Management of musculoskeletal injuries must begin immediately after the initial trauma. Optimal management invariably improves rehabilitation outcomes. The rehabilitation team and the patient then can focus on other equally challenging issues.

REFERENCES

1. Asselmeier M, Light T: Heterotopic para-articular ossification of the proximal interphalangeal joint. Hand Surg 17A:154–157, 1992.
2. Ayers DC, Pellegrin VD, Evarts CM: Prevention of heterotopic ossification in high risk patients by radiation therapy. Clin Orthop 263:87–93, 1991.
3. Bellamy R, Brower T: Management of skeletal trauma in the patient with head injury. Trauma 14:2032–1028, 1974.
4. Bondurant F, Cotler H, Browner B, et al: The medical and economic impact of severely injured lower extremities. J Trauma 28:1270, 1988.
5. Bone L, Johnson K., Weigett J: Early versus delayed stabilization of femoral fractures. J Bone Joint Surg 71:336–340, 1989.

6. Booth BJ, Doyle M, Montgomery J: Serial casting for the management of spasticity in the head injured adult. Phys Ther 63:1960–1966, 1983.

7. Booth D, Westers B: The management of athletes with myositis ossificans traumatica. Can J Sport Sci 14:10–16, 1989.

8. Botte M, Moore T: The orthopedic management of extremity injuries in head trauma. J Head Trauma Rehabil 2:13–27, 1987.

9. Bressler E, Marn C, Gore R, Hendrix R: Evaluation ectopic bone by CT. AJR 148:931–935, 1987.

10. Brien W, Gellman H, Becker V: Management of fractures of the humerus in patients who have injury of the ipsilateral brachial plexus. J Bone Joint Surg 72:1208–1210, 1990.

11. Brooke M, Heard D, Delateur B: Heterotopic ossification and peripheral nerve entrapment: early diagnosis and excision. Arch Phys Med Rehabil 72:425–429, 1991.

12. Buring K: On the origin of cells in heterotopic bone formation. Clin Orthop Rel Res 110:293–301, 1975.

13. Cherry D: Review of physical therapy alternatives for reducing muscle contracture. Phys Ther 60:877–881, 1980.

14. Cherry D, Weigard G: Plaster drop-out casts as a dynamic means to reduce muscle contracture. Phys Ther 61:1601–1603, 1983.

15. Citta-Pietrolungo T, Alexander M, Steg N: Early detection of heterotopic ossification in young patients with traumatic brain injury. Arch Phys Med Rehabil 73:258–262, 1992.

16. Cosgrove J, Vargo M, Reidy M: A prospective study of peripheral nerve lesions occurring in traumatic brain injured patients. Am J Phys Med Rehabil 68:15–17, 1989.

17. Coventry M, Scanlon P: The use of radiation to discourage ectopic bone. J Bone Joint Surg 63A:201–208, 1981.

18. Crawford C, Varghese G, Mani M: Heterotopic ossification: Are range of motion exercises contraindicated? J Burn Care 7:323–326, 1986.

19. Dubuisson A, Kline D: Indications for peripheral nerve and brachial plexus surgery. Neurol Clin North Am 10:935–952, 1992.

20. Edeiken-Monroe B, Browner B, Jackson H: The role of standard roentgenograms in the evaluation of instability of pelvic ring disruptions. Clin Orthop Rel Res 240, 63–76, 1989.

21. Ellis M, Frank H: Myositis ossificans traumatica: With special reference to the quadriceps femoris muscle. J Trauma 6:724–738, 1966.

22. Frank C, Akeson W, Woo L, et al: Physiology and therapeutic value of passive joint motion. Clin Orthop Rel Res 185:113–125, 1984.

23. Garland D: Surgical approaches for resection of heterotopic ossification in traumatic brain injured adults. Clin Orthop 263:59–70, 1991.

24. Garland D, Blum C Waters R: Periarticular heterotopic ossification in head injured adults. J Bone Joint Surg 62A:1143–1146, 1980.

25. Garland D, Alday B, Venos K: Heterotopic ossification and HLA antigens. Arch Phys Med Rehab 65:531–5323, 1984.

26. Garland D, Razza B, Waters R: Forceful joint manipulation in head injured adults with heterotopic ossification. Clin Orthop 169:133–138, 1982.

27. Garland D, Toder L: Fractures of the tibial diaphysis in adults with head injuries. Clin Orthop Rel Res 150:198–202, 1980.

28. Garland D: Clinical observations on fractures and heterotopic ossification in the spinal cord and traumatic brain injured populations. Clin Orthop Rel Res 233:86–101, 1988.

29. Garland D, O'Hallaren R: Fractures and dislocations about the elbow in the head injured adult. Clin Orthop Rel Res 168:38–41, 1982.

30. Garland D, Miller G: Fractures and dislocations about the hip in head injured adults. Clin Orthop Rel Res 186:154–158, 1984.

31. Garland D, Dowling V: Forearm fractures in the head injured adults. Clin Orthop Rel Res 176:190–196, 1983.

32. Garland D, Baily S: Undetected Injuries in head injured adults. Clin Orthop Rel Res 155:162–165, 1981.

33. Garland D: A clinical perspective on common forms of acquired heterotopic ossification. Clin Orthop 263:13–28, 1991.

34. Garland D, Rothi B, Waters R: Femoral fractures in head injured adults. Clin Orthop Rel Res 166:219–225, 1982.

35. Garland D, Hanscom D, Keenan M, et al: Resection of heterotopic ossification in the adult with head trauma. J Bone Joint Surg 67A:1261–1269, 1985.

36. Gill K, Bucholz R: The role of computerized tomographic scanning in the evaluation of major pelvic fractures. Bone Joint Surg 66A:34–49, 1984.

37. Glenn M: Update on pharmacology:pharmacological treatment of heterotopic ossification. J Head Trauma Rehabil 3:86–89, 1988.

38. Goldman AB: Myositis ossificans circumscripta: a benign lesion with a malignant differential diagnosis. Am J Roentgenol 126:32–40, 1976.

39. Groswasser Z, Cohen M, Blandstein E: Polytrauma associated with traumatic brain injury: Incidence, nature and impact on rehabilitation outcome. Brain Inj 4:161–166, 1990.

40. Guanche C, Keenan M: Principles of orthopedic rehabilitation. Phys Med Rehabil Clin North Am 3:417–425, 1992.

41. Hansen S: Overview of the severely traumatized lower limb. Clin Orthop Rel Res 243:17–19, 1989.

42. Hardy A, Dickson J: Pathological ossification in traumatic paraplegia. J Bone Joint Surg 45B:76–87, 1963.

43. Hepburn G: Case studies: contracture and stiff joint management dynasplint. Orthop Sports Phys Ther 8:498–504, 1987.

44. Hepburn, G, Crivelli K: Use of elbow dynasplint for reduction of elbow flexion contractures: a case study. Orthop Sports Phys Ther 5: 269–274, 1984.

45. Herbison G, Jaweed M, Ditunno J: Exercise therapies in peripheral neurotherapies. Arch Phys Med Rehabil 64:201–205, 1983.

46. Hurvitz E, Mandac B, Davidoff G: Risk factors for heterotopic ossification in children and adolescents with severe traumatic brain injury. Arch Phys Med Rehabil 73:459–462, 1992.

47. Irving J, Brun H: Myositis ossificans in hemiplegia. J Bone Joint Surg 36B:440–441, 1954.

48. Jewell M: Peripheral nerve injuries:mechanisms and locations. Top Acute Care Trauma Rehabil 3:1–9, 1988.

49. Johnson K, Cadams A, Seibert G: Incidence of adult respiratory distress syndrome in patients with multiple musculoskeletal injuries: effect of early operative stabilization of fractures. Trauma 25: 375–384, 1985.

50. Jones B, Ward M: Myositis ossificans in the biceps femoris muscles causing sciatic nerve palsy. J Bone Joint Surg 62B:506–507, 1980.

51. Keenan M, Kauffman D, Garland D: Late ulnar neuropathy in the brain injured adult. Hand Surg 13A:120–124, 1988.

52. Kellan J, McMurtry R, Paley D, Tile M: The unstable pelvic fracture. Orthop Clin North Am 18, 25–41, 1987.

53. Kewalramani L, Orth M: Ectopic ossification. Am Phys Med 56:99–121, 1977.

54. Kline DG, Lusk MD: Management of athletic brachial plexus injuries. In Schneider RC, Kennedy JC, Plant ML (eds): Sports Injuries: Mechanisms, Prevention, and Treatment. Baltimore, Williams & Wilkins, 1985.

55. Kline DG, Hackett ER, Happel LH: Surgery for lesions of the brachial plexus. Arch Neurol 43:170–181, 1986.

56. Kline DG: Operative management of selected brachial plexus injuries. J Neurosurg Psychiatry 42:107–116, 1979.

57. Kottke F, Pauley D, Ptak R: The rationale for prolonged stretching or correction of shortening of connective tissue. Arch Phys Med Rehabil 345–352, 1966.

58. Lal S, Hamilton B, Heinemann A, Betts H: Risk factors for heterotopic ossification in spinal cord injury. Arch Phys Med Rehabil 70:387–389, 1989.

59. Larson J, Michalski J, Collacott E, et al: Increased prevalence of HLA-B27 in patients with ectopic ossification following traumatic spinal cord injury. Rheumatol Rehabil 20:193–197, 1981.

60. Leberte M, Dabezies E: Pelvic fractures. Orthopedics I, 120–123, 1985.

61. Leffert RD: Brachial plexus injuries. N Engl J Med 291:1059–1067, 1974.

62. Lehmkuhl LD, Thoi L, Baize C, et al: Multimodality treatment of joint contractures in patients with severe brain injury: Cost, effectiveness and integration of therapies in the application of serial/inhibitive costs. J Head Trauma Rehabil 5:23–42, 1990.

63. Light K, Nuzik S, Personius W, Barstrom A: Low-load prolonged stretch vs. high load brief stretch in treating knee contractures. Phys Ther 64:330–333, 1984.

64. Lipscomb A, Thomas F, Johnston R: Treatment of myositis ossificans traumatica in athletes. Sports Med 4:111–120, 1976.

65. Mackay-Lyons M: Lowload, prolonged stretch in treatment of elbow flexion contractures secondary to head trauma: A case report. Phys Ther 69:292–296, 1989.

66. Major P, Resnick D, Grenway G: Heterotopic ossification in paraplegia: A possible disturbance of the paravertebral venous plexus. Radiology 136:797–799, 1980.

67. Mendelson L, Grasswasser Z, Najenson T: Periarticular new bone formation in patients suffering from severe head injuries. Scand J Rehabil Med 7:141–145, 1975.

68. Mielants H, Vanhove E, deNeels J, Veys E: Clinical survey of and pathogenic approach to para-articular ossifications in long term coma. Acta Orthop Scand 46 46:190–198, 1975.

69. Minaire P. Betuel H, Girard R, Pilonchery G: Neurologic injuries, paraosteoarthropathies and human leukocyte antigens. Arch Phys Med Rehabil 61:214–215: 1980.

70. Mital M, Garber J, Stinson J: Ectopic bone formation in children and adolescents with head injuries: Its management. J Pediatr Orthop 7:83–90, 1987.

71. Molloy J, McGuirk R: Treatment of traumatic myositis ossificans circumscripta; use of aspiration and steroids. J Trauma 16:851–857, 1976.

72. Moneim MS, Omer GE: Latissimus dorsi muscle transfer for restoration of elbow flexion after brachial plexus disruption. J Hand Surg 11:135–139, 1986.

73. Moore T, Barron J, Modlin P, Bean S: The use of tone reducing casts to prevent joint contractures following severe closed head injury. J Head Trauma Rehabil 4:63–65, 1989.

74. Nashold BS Jr, Ostdahl RH: Dorsal root entry zone lesions for pain relief. J Neurosurg 51:1:59–69, 1979.

75. Noble T: Myositis ossificans. Surg Gynecol Obstet 39:795–802, 1924.

76. Orzel J, Rudd T: Heterotopic bone formation: clinical, laboratory and imaging correlation. J Nucl Med 26:125–132, 1985.

77. Ough J, Garland D, Jordan C, Waters R: Treatment of spastic joint contractures in mentally disabled adults. Orthop Clin North Am 12:143–151, 1981.

78. Parkash S, Kumar K: Fibrodysphasia ossificans traumatica. J Bone Joint Surg 54A:1306–1308, 1972.

79. Parry G. Electrodiagnostic studies in the evaluation of peripheral nerve and brachial plexus injuries. Neurol Clin North Am 10:921–934, 1992.

80. Parry CBW: The management of traumatic lesions of the brachial plexus and peripheral nerve injuries in the upper limb. Injury 1979,11:265–285.

81. Patterson F, Morton K: Neurologic complications of fractures and dislocations of the pelvis. Trauma 12:1013–1023, 1973.

82. Peacock E: Some biochemical and biophysical aspects of joint stiffness: role of collagen synthesis as opposed to altered molecular bonding. Ann Surg 164:1–12, 1966.

83. Pittinger DE: Heterotopic ossification. Orthop Rev 20:33–39, 1991.

84. Remien J: Traumatic injury to the brachial plexus: An overview. Top Acute Care Trauma Rehabil 3: 38–47, 1988.

85. Raj P, Kelly J, Cannella J, McConn K: Multidisciplinary management of reflex sympathetic dystrophy. Pain Digest 2:267–273, 1992.

86. Rhoades M, Garland D: Orthopedic prognosis of brain injured adults. Part I. Clin Orthop Rel Res 131:104–110, 1978.

87. Richard R: Use of the dynasplint to correct elbow flexion burn contracture: A case report. J Bone Joint Surg 7:151–152, 1986.

88. Richard R, Jones L, Miller S: Treatment of exposed bilateral achilles tendons with use of the dynasplint. Phys Ther 68:989–991, 1988.

89. Roberts J, Pankratz D: The surgical treatment of heterotopic ossification at the elbow following long term coma. J Bone Joint Surg 61A:760–763, 1979.

90. Rosin A: Ectopic calcification around joints of paralyzed in hemiplegia, diffuse brain damage and other neurological diseases. Ann Rheum Dis 34: 499–505, 1975

91. Rossier A, Bussat P, Infante F, et al: Current facts on para-osteo-arthropathy. Paraplegia 11:36–78, 1973.

92. Rychak J, Kalenak A: Injury to the median and ulnar nerves secondary to fracture of the radius. J Bone Joint Surg 59:414–415, 1977.

93. Sapega A, Quedenfield T, Moyer R, Butler R: Biophysical factors in range of motion exercise. Physician Sports Med 9:57–65, 1981.

94. Sapega A: Advances in the nonsurgical treatment of joint contracture: A biophysical perspective. Postgrad Adv Sports Med 3–9, 1988.

95. Sazbon L, Najenson T, Tartakovsky M, et al: Widespread periarticular new bone formation in long term comatose patients. J Bone Joint Surg 63B:120–125, 1981.

96. Schmidt S, Kjaersgard-Anderson P, Petersen N, et al: The use of indomethacin to prevent the formation of heterotopic bone after total hip replacement. J Bone Joint Surg 70A:834–838, 1988.

97. Schwartman R: Reflex sympathetic dystrophy and causalgia. Neurol Clin North Am 10:953–974, 1992.

98. Siegel R, Weiden I: Combined median and ulnar nerve lesions complicating fractures of the distal radius and ulna. Trauma 8:1114–1118, 1968.

99. Silver K: Concurrent existence of heterotopic ossification and thrombophlebitis [letter]. Am J Med 88:318, 1990.

100. Smith T: Prevention of complications in orthopedic surgery secondary to nutritional depletion. Clin Orthop Rel Res 222:91–97, 1987.

101. Sobus K, Alexander M, Harcke T: Undetected musculoskeletal trauma in children with traumatic brain injury or spinal cord injury. Arch Phys Rehabil 74:902–904, 1993.

102. Spielman G. Gennarelli T, Rogers C: Disodium etidronate: Its role in preventing heterotopic ossification in severe head injury. Arch Phys Med Rehabil 64:539–542, 1983.

103. Stone L, Keenan M: Peripheral nerve injuries in the adult with traumatic brain injury. Clin Orthop Rel Res 233:136–144, 1988.

104. Stover SL, Hahn H, J. Disodrum etidronate in the prevention of heterotopic ossification following spinal cord injury. Paraplegia 14:146–156, 1976.

105. Stover S, Hataway C Zeiger H: Heterotopic ossification in spinal cord injured patients. Arch Phys Med Rehabil 56:199–404, 1975.

106. Sullivan T, Conine T, Goodman M, Mackie T: Serial casting to prevent equinus in acute traumatic head injury. Physiother Can 40:346–350, 1988.

107. Tile M: Pelvic ring fractures: should they be fixed. J Bone Joint Surg 70B:1–12, 1988.

108. Umphred D, McCormack G: Classification of common facilitatory and inhibitory treatment techniques in neurological rehabilitation. St. Louis, Mosby, 1990, pp 111–161.

109. Varghese G: Heterotopic ossification. Phys Rehabil Clin North Am 3:407–415, 1992.

110. Varghese G, Williams K, Desmet A et al: Nonarticular complications of heterotopic ossification: a clinical review. Arch Phys Med Rehabil 72:1009–1013, 1991.

111. Vernier L, Ditunno J: Heterotopic ossification in the paraplegic patient. Arch Phys Med Rehabil 475–479, 19791.

112. Wainapel S, Rao V, Schepsis A: Ulnar nerve compression by heterotopic ossification in a head injured patient. Arch Phys Med Rehabil 66:512–514, 1985.

113. Warnold I, Lundholm K: Clinical significance of preoperative nutritional status in 215 noncancer patients. Ann Surg 199:299–305, 1984.

114. Warren G, Lehmann J, Koblanski J: Elongation of rat tail tendon: Effect of load and temperature. Arch Phys Med Rehabil 465–473, 1971.

115. Weintraub A, Opat C: Motor and sensory dysfunction in the brain injured adult. Phys Med Rehabil State Art Rev 3:59–84, 1984.

116. Wharton, GW, Morgan TH: Ankylosis in the paralyzed patient. J Bone Joint Surg 52A:105–112, 1970.

117. Woo S, Mathews J, Akeson W: Connective tissue response to immobility. Arthritis Rheum 18:257–254, 1975.

118. Wray J, Davis C: The management of skeletal fractures in the patient with a head injury. South Med J 53:748–753, 1960.

119. Yarkony G, Sahgal V: Contractures a major complication of craniocerebral trauma. Clin Orthop Rel Res 219:93–96, 1987.

120. Zoega H: Fracture of the lower end of the radius with ulnar nerve palsy. J Bone Joint Surg 48:514–516, 1966.

122. Spielman G, Gennarelli T, Rogers C: Disodium etidronate: Its role in preventing heterotopic ossification in severe head injury. Arch Phys Med Rehabil 64:539–542, 1983.

123. Stone L, Keenan M: Peripheral nerve injuries in the adult with traumatic brain injury. Clin Orthop Rel Res 233:136–144, 1988.

NANCY R. MANN M.D.

KERTIA L. BLACK M.D.

18

Balance and Vestibular Dysfunction

Balance dysfunction is one of the most difficult deficits to treat in brain-injured patients. Long after muscle weakness has subsided, mobility may remain problematic because of impaired balance. Thus, functional recovery is slowed despite good motor recovery—a clinical reality that is difficult for patients to accept. The intractability of balance deficits is due in part to the multiple structures involved in maintaining balance and in part to the inadequacy of current treatment techniques. The pervasiveness of this problem makes it a major public health concern.[47]

The true incidence and prevalence of posttraumatic dizziness and balance disorders are unclear, varying with severity and mechanism of injury. Diagnosis and treatment of posttraumatic vestibular symptoms are complex, because such injuries often result from combined peripheral and central lesions.

Dizziness is commonly reported as a feature of mild traumatic brain injury (TBI) and postconcussive disorders. Patients with persisting postconcussive dizziness often have associated psychological symptoms, including anxiety and depression.[4]

Causes of persisting vestibular deficits after moderate and severe TBI include peripheral as well as central nervous system lesions. Associated injuries may include temporal bone fractures. Direct trauma to the bony and membranous labyrinth is most common with transverse fractures, which occur in approximately 20% of temporal bone fractures. Acceleration-deceleration injuries may cause displacement of the mobile inner-ear sense organ.[20]

Positional vertigo with symptoms elicited by head movement is the most common persisting vestibular symptom after TBI. In a study of 240 patients presenting with persisting symptoms of benign positional vertigo, trauma was the cause in 18%.[1]

For full understanding of balance dysfunction, a basic definition of balance is necessary. Oates defines it as "a dynamic process involving the ability to direct or sense body motion, integrate and correctly perceive the sensory information, and coordinate an appropriate motor response."[39] Shepard and Telian outline the three primary goals of balance:

1. To prevent falls by correcting rapidly any inadvertent displacement of the body's center of mass from its equilibrium position over the base of support;

2. To provide accurate perceptions of the position of the body in its environment and direction and speed of movement; and

3. To control eye movements in order to maintain a clear visual image of the external world while the individual, the environment, or both are in motion.[41]

Shumway-Cook[47] straightforwardly equates "balance" with "stability" and defines it as the ability to control the body's center of mass relative to specified limits often referred to as "stability limits." Such limits are task-specific[4] (e.g., a person may fall while walking but not while standing) and also depend on the environment in which the task is performed (e.g., uneven vs. even terrain).

PATHOGENESIS OF BALANCE DYSFUNCTION

Once balance is defined, it is important to analyze how it is achieved. Shumway-Cook proposes a "systems model" or "distributed control model" based on the work of Bernstein. According to this model, balance and stability result from a complex interaction of the musculoskeletal and neural systems (the postural control system) organized around a task (walking, standing) and modified by environmental constraints (various surfaces, darkness, bright light). This interaction allows the body to control its center of mass within the stability limits.[45]

Motor Control

Among the most common impairments after traumatic brain injury are weakness and paralysis. Weakness compromises stability because adequate force to correct for shifts in the center of gravity cannot be generated. When normal people are in danger of falling forward, gastrocnemii, hamstrings, and trunk muscles begin to contract to prevent movement beyond the stable base of support. In the hemiparetic patient, normal synergy cannot occur.

Moreover, loss of balance is not always due to the absolute absence of such postural responses; it is often due to delays in their initiation because of decreased strength. For example, a mildly hemiparetic patient may be able to move the trunk or lower extremity but not with sufficient speed to prevent a fall.

Despite its importance for balance, strength is of reduced value without motor

coordination. Postural control (good balance) also depends on motor coordination processes that organize the action of trunk and leg muscles into movement strategies. Poor coordination may lead to poor aim when adjustments in balance are attempted. In cerebellar brain injury, the typical error of coordination is overshooting of voluntary movements in approaching a target. Overshooting results in misplacement of the center of mass over the base of support— sometimes to such an extent that balance is lost. In brain injury to the basal ganglia, rigidity or movement disorders (e.g., tic, chorea, athetosis) may lead to misalignments that are difficult to correct.

Sensory Processes

In the normal person, three sensory systems work together in a seamless, automatic fashion: vestibular, visual, and somatosensory. After TBI, balance may become precarious, either from dysfunction in individual components of the system or its ability to centrally integrate the information.

The vestibular system, with its multiple afferents and efferents from periphery to cortex, is a major corrective force in the modulation of balance. In a classic 1952 article in *The New England Journal of Medicine*, a physician described in graphic detail the consequence of destruction of the vestibular fibers of his eighth nerve by streptomycin:

> Imagine the result of a sequence taken by pointing the camera straight ahead, holding it against the chest and walking at a normal pace down a city street. In a sequence thus taken and thus viewed on the screen, the street seems to careen crazily in all directions, faces of approaching persons become blurred and unrecognizable and the viewer may even experience a feeling of dizziness or nausea. Our vestibular system normally acts like the tripod and the smoothly moving carriage on which the professional motion picture camera is mounted. Without these steadying influences, the moving picture is jangled and blurred. Similarly, when the vestibular influences are removed from the biologic cinema system, the projection on the visual cortex becomes unsteady.[6]

Such disconcerting symptoms are experienced by more than seven million people per year. Approximately 30% of the U.S. population has experienced episodes of dizziness by age 65 years.

Complementing the vestibular system is the visual system—a fairly obvious aid to balance maintenance. Observation of any patient with a visual deficit attempting to negotiate uneven terrain without assistance will confirm the importance of sight to postural control.

Accurate processing of somatosensory information is an essential ingredient in stability. Poor joint position sense can sabotage the most heroic efforts to ambulate or to perform other gross motor tasks. For example, the motorically intact patient with TBI may demonstrate a steppage gait in an effort to find the correct placement for strong but somatosensory-impaired lower extremities. Maximal assistance from at least one person is often required to keep the patient upright during gait trials. Likewise, in the frequently falling diabetic or alcoholic patient proprioceptive loss prevents normal mobility.

Central Integrative Mechanisms

Ideally, the vestibular, visual, and somatosensory systems work harmoniously to integrate the cacophony of sensory input into a compound signal that is transmitted throughout the nervous system and allows us to remain upright even when challenged. The multiple complex reflex pathways with and between these systems are beyond the scope of this chapter, which focuses only on the vestibuloocular, the vestibulocollic, and cervicocollic reflexes, all of which help to orient the head and body in the environment to maintain central placement of a visual image on the retina. These reflexes are supplemented by such phenomena as optokinetic nystagmus and after-nystagmus mechanisms, which culminate in ocular movements such as smooth pursuit (slow movements used to follow a predictable target) and saccadic movements (fast movements used to track unpredictable targets).[18]

The important point about sensory input is that all three systems must be operational to optimize sensory integration and balance. As the number of avenues of input declines, postural stability suffers proportionately.

Adaptive Processes

Adaptive processes modify sensory and motor systems in response to changing environment and task demands. Such processes also may play a role in functional recovery from balance deficits.

The balance of brain-injured patients often improves sufficiently to allow safe, independent ambulation, even if extreme weakness and incoordination initially precluded ambulation of any kind. The mechanisms underlying this change are not fully understood. They may involve phenomena at axonal level, including resolution of acute factors, collateral sprouting, and use of spare capacity. Changes may occur at the environmental level based on repetition of previously encoded movement patterns, incorporation or suppression of primitive reflex patterns during motor learning, and practice of movements associated with previously encoded movements. Postural adjustments are refined through a process of fine tuning analogous to a 12-month old's progression from the wide-based, forward lurching gait of infancy to the more mature and more stable gait of early childhood.

Musculoskeletal Components

Musculoskeletal injuries often occur in association with TBI. These injuries can result in various biomechanical constraints.[45] Range of motion and weight-bearing are often affected. Limitations in these areas can often lead to the inability to perform corrective movements necessary to maintain postural stability during a challenge.[39] Contractures can cause a person's center of gravity to be shifted toward the stability limits, further increasing the strength required to maintain balance.

Instability results from the disruption of one or more of the components of balance. The degree of functional impairment depends on the extent of compensation by the intact components. Instability after TBI usually involves multiple factors; it is rarely due to dysfunction of an isolated component. Many studies report the presence of balance deficits, but the frequency of specific neuropathologic subtypes is still unclear.

DIAGNOSTIC EVALUATION

As with any pathologic process, the history and physical examination are the cornerstones of diagnosis. They direct evaluation and treatment and can suggest prognosis. Disorders of balance are no different. The patients' descriptions of their symptoms and their past medical history can be essential to unravelling the mystery of their complaints of "dizziness" or "balance problems."[11,41]

The rather vague symptom of dizziness may be associated with disorders of almost every system. A history, for instance, of syncopal episodes, motion sickness, or otologic problems may be a telling clue to the underlying cause of the patient's complaints. Hypertension, diabetes mellitus, valvular or coronary artery disease, endocrine dysfunction, and alcoholism or drug abuse also suggest possible causes.[11,41]

Patients may describe sensations of vertigo, dizziness, lightheadedness, or unsteadiness as troublesome symptoms. The first step is to get patients to accurately describe their symptoms. For example, patients who say that they are dizzy may mean unsteady rather than vertiginous. One helpful means of specifying the exact nature of the complaint is to ask patients whether they experience a sensation of "the room spinning around them" or feel as if they were going to faint. Vertigo, the sense of spinning or rotating, is a strong indicator of a vestibular system disorder. On the other hand, lightheadedness may indicate a vascular problem.[11] It is important to establish the approximate date and character (gradual vs. sudden) of onset, because it is sometimes possible to identify a temporal relationship between some event (trauma, new medication) and the first occurrence of the symptom.

The patient's description of symptoms may help to differentiate between peripheral and central lesions. Oscillopsia, the illusion that stationary objects are moving back and forth, indicates loss of the vestibular ocular reflex and tends to be more severe in central lesions. Patients with severe balance deficits, associated with other neurologic deficits, are more likely to have central lesions. Lightheadedness and syncope may be due to vascular lesions. Severe nausea and vomiting are usually related to peripheral lesions.

Associated hearing loss and tinnitus are more common in peripheral lesions. It is important to monitor the course of recovery. Pure peripheral vestibular lesions tend to compensate rapidly, whereas recovery from central lesions is likely to be much slower.[30,39]

A careful history should include stimuli that provoke or relieve the symptoms. Dizziness that increases with changes in position is consistent with vestibular disorders. Symptoms that increase only in specific positions may indicate otolith dysfunction. Patients who depend on visual input will have an increase in symptoms with eyes closed. Dizziness brought on by eating may be due to fluctuations in blood pressure, whereas dizziness precipitated by fasting may be due to hypoglycemia.[11,39]

Medications

It is well known that the central nervous system of the brain-injured patient can be exquisitely sensitive to a wide variety of medications. It is important to take a detailed medication history with relationship to vestibular symptoms. Many medications can cause vestibular symptoms. Sedating medications can diminish a patient's ability to compensate for vestibular deficits in addition to adversely affecting cognitive and motor skills in brain-injured patients.[47]

The anxiolytics, especially benzodiazepines and even the new less sedating drugs, such as buspirone, may cause sensations of dizziness. Antidepressants, including tricyclics, monamine oxidase inhibitors, and even some of the serotonergic antidepressants such as trazodone, may cause sedation and vestibular deficits. Similarly, anticonvulsants (phenytoin, carbamazepine, and valproate are used most commonly in brain-injured patients) are notoriously sedating. Phenytoin and carbamazepine may precipitate movement disorders (akathisia, tremors) and ataxia, all of which may impair balance. Anticonvulsant-induced nystagmus can impact visual input. Symptoms resulting from the use of these medications tend to be dose-related and, although worse when serum contentrations are at toxic levels, can be seen as an idiosyncratic reaction at therapeutic or even subtherapeutic levels.[8,17,39]

Aminoglycoside antibiotics, including gentamicin and streptomycin, are ototoxic at high serum concentrations and cause hearing loss. They also may damage hair cells in the labyrinth and cochlea, resulting in severe vestibular deficits.

Ironically, dizziness often is brought on by the very drugs designed to alleviate vestibular symptoms such as nausea, vomiting, and headaches; such drugs should probably be avoided if possible. Compazine, often prescribed as an antiemetic, is a phenothiazine with significant sedative properties. The same is true of scopolamine, an anticholinergic drug used to suppress nausea and vomiting associated with motion sickness. Phenergan and meclizine, both of which are used to treat nausea and vomiting related to vestibular disorders, can cause dizziness.

Vestibular symptoms related to these medications appear to occur as a result of a change in the vestibular receptor firing pattern leading to sensory conflicting information. These medications can influence receptor information and interfere with nervous system response, thereby preventing the natural adaptive process from occurring within the central nervous system to reset the receptor firing pattern. The end result is that the supposed "cure" becomes an obstacle to a true cure.[39]

Past Medical History

The key to understanding the cause of balance impairment may be found in the past medical history. Syncopal episodes suggest the possibility of an undiagnosed aortic stenosis or other valvular disorder or vertebrobasilar insufficiency. Motion sickness suggests a vestibular disorder. With concomitant hearing loss or tinnitus, Meniere's disease must be included in the differential diagnosis.

Severe anemia may be associated with a certain lightheadedness related to postural change and exertion. Similarly, in emphysematous patients or hypertensive patients with an unstable adjustment of cerebral blood flow, physical effort may result in giddiness and feelings of faintness. And, of course, formerly bedridden, deconditioned patients often experience a swaying sort of dizziness on abruptly rising from a recumbent or sitting position.[11]

Other useful positive points of past medical history include diabetes, which, with its often fluctuating serum glucose levels, can induce lightheadedness. In longstanding cases, peripheral neuropathy may be responsible for sensations of precarious balance. Coronary artery disease and dysrhythmias also can underlie such symptoms, and psychiatric disorders (e.g., anxiety states) may cause frequent hyperventilation. Finally, a history of adrenal insufficiency, hypothyroidism, and other endocrine disorders or long-term alcohol abuse may help to solve the puzzle.

Current Functional History

As rehabilitation medicine specialists, it is important to assess the impact of balance impairment on function. In brain-injured patients, it is sometimes difficult to differentiate functional impairments that are secondary to balance deficits from those based on cognitive and neurologic deficits. Balance deficits may not be apparent, or their full impact on function identified, until the patient reaches a certain level of recovery from TBI. Vestibular symptoms may not appear until the patient is able to change positions independently or to perform higher level motor skills. An ongoing assessment of balance and vestibular function is an important aspect of TBI management.

Physical Evaluation

Musculoskeletal Evaluation

An intact musculoskeletal system provides the dynamic and structural components that allow us to remain upright in an unpredictable environment. Limitations of range of motion, strength, and flexibility can diminish the ability to perform corrective movements in response to environmental changes. The initial physical examination needs to include a detailed musculoskeletal evaluation that focuses on range of motion, strength, and postural alignment.[39]

Musculoskeletal injuries are commonly associated with TBI. Inadequate control of spasticity secondary to neurologic deficits may lead to the development of contractures. Limitations in range of motion may shift the center of gravity, increasing the strength necessary to maintain balance. Evaluation of strength should focus on the trunk as well as the lower extremities. A patient must be able to generate enough force in the trunk and lower extremities to control the movement of the center of mass.

Postural alignment will help to determine strength necessary to maintain balance in different environments. If the center of mass is aligned appropriately over the center of the foot, only infrequent corrective movements with muscle activity in the gastrocnemius and soleus are necessary to maintain balance. If the center of mass is maintained near the limits of stability because of contractures or poor postural alignment, frequent and rapid corrections with muscle activity in larger muscle groups are necessary to maintain balance. Risk of falling is significantly increased. Physical examination should assess for any asymmetries which displace the center of mass laterally, forward, or backward in relation to the malleoli.[39]

Patients with vestibular deficits often minimize the movement of their head and trunk as a way of controlling symptoms. This can lead to muscular splinting, resulting in increased muscle tension, fatigue, and pain that further limit a patient's ability to move. A careful assessment of cervical and trunk strength and range of motion can aid with early identification of these problems and treatment planning to disrupt this cycle of increasing impairment.

Vision

Orienting ourselves to our environments through the use of visual input is an important part of preserving postural stability. If the examination reveals decreased visual acuity or weakness of extraocular muscles, balance dysfunction can be expected. Optic nerve damage often accompanies TBI. Also commonly seen are peripheral nerve injuries that lead to diplopia or at least blurred vision.

Vestibuloocular Function

Because the visual and vestibular systems work together so intimately in the service of balance, it is important, on physical evaluation, to be cognizant of certain facts regarding their function. The eye movements themselves, the vestibuloocular reflex, and vestibuloocular reflex cancellation are three fundamental aspects of this integrated system that must be understood.

Eye movements may be classified roughly as either smooth or saccadic pursuit. The smooth pursuit system maintains the visual image on the fovea of the retina during a tracking movement of the eyes. For this system to function, the target motion must be predictable and of fairly slow-to-moderate speed.[19,14] Smooth pursuit can be tested by having the patient visually track an object while the head is kept stationary. Smooth pursuit should be evaluated in all visual fields.

Smooth pursuit characterized by rapid, short movements (like the saccades described below) is an abnormal finding often associated with central lesions. Age-related trends, however, suggest that increased saccades are not necessarily a sign of pathology in the elderly.[27]

The functional goal of the saccadic system is to provide for rapid replacement of a visual image onto the fovea. When the head is stationary and the target speed exceeds the limits of the smooth pursuit system, saccadic movements begin to appear. They are rapid eye movements that reposition the target on the fovea in situations where the target movement is unpredictable or target speed exceeds the limits of the smooth pursuit system.[41]

Saccadic movements are tested by having the patient look rapidly between two objects with the head held stationary. Saccades should be tested in both horizontal and vertical planes. When rapid eye movements are used to shift focus from one object to another, the shift normally is made in 1–2 saccades. If three or more eye movements are required or if the patient under- or overshoots the targets, an abnormality of eye movements exists.[5,18]

Optokinetics requires a combination of saccades and smooth pursuit. This combination maintains a steady image on the retina during sustained head rotation. It can be tested by moving repetitive objects or patterns across a stationary visual field.

Vestibuloocular Reflex (VOR).   An extremely important but complex contribution of the visual system to balance is the vestibuloocular reflex, which generates compensatory eye movements in response to head movement. Interacting with the saccades and smooth pursuits, it maintains gaze stability in its effort to ensure that a visual image remains focused on the fovea, regardless of the position of the head.[18,41]

For example, in order to look straight ahead while the head rotates to the right at 10°/second, the vestibuloocular reflex produces a compensatory rotation of the eyes to the left at 10°/second. Thus, the effective direction of gaze is straight ahead.[9]

As part of the physical evaluation, the examiner should move the patient's head vertically and horizontally as the patient fixates on a target. Fixation should be maintained without saccade if the vestibuloocular reflex is functioning normally. If not, a unilateral or severe bilateral vestibular lesion is suspected.

Vestibuloocular Reflex Cancellation (VORC).

As part of the smooth pursuit system, vestibuloocular reflex cancellation allows the head and the target to move together. When the eyes are fixated on a target that is moving (but not too fast), smooth pursuit should be the pattern of eye movement. Clinicians test vestibuloocular reflex cancellation by observing the patient's eyes while head and eye movement occur together. Abnormality is signalled by saccadic movements.[46]

Nystagmus

Nystagmus consists of involuntary, rhythmic oscillations of the eyes and reflects disruption of brainstem oculomotor systems. Often nystagmus secondary to vestibular lesions is accompanied by nausea, vertigo, and oscillopsia.[12] The four basic types of nystagmus are horizontal, vertical, rotary, and mixed. "Jerk" nystagmus includes both fast and slow components and is usually associated with vestibular lesions, whereas "pendular" nystagmus is characterized by excursions of equal velocity. Table 1 identifies components of vestibular nystagmus; Table 2 differentiates between peripheral and central etiologies.[12]

Abnormal nystagmus is a classic sign of cerebellar or vestibular dysfunction. Nystagmus on lateral gaze is normal and should not be considered indicative of pathology. Although abnormal nystagmus is easily elicited in the office or clinic, it is probably best evaluated with electronystagmography.

Patients with unilateral vestibular loss initially have spontaneous nystagmus and complain of vertigo and disequilibrium that increase with head movement. The spontaneous nystagmus is caused by an imbalance between the right and left vestibular nuclei

TABLE 1. Vestibular Nystagmus

Symptoms or Sign	Peripheral (End-Organ)	Central (Nuclear)
Direction of nystagmus	Unidirectional; fast phase opposite lesion	Bidirectional or unidirectional
Purely horizontal nystagmus without torsional component	Uncommon	Common
Vertical or purely torsional nystagmus	Never present	May be present
Visual fixation	Inhibits nystagmus and vertigo	No inhibition
Severity of vertigo	Marked	Mild
Direction of spin	Toward fast phase	Variable
Direction of pastpointing	Toward slow phase	Variable
Direction of Romberg fall	Toward slow phase	Variable
Effect of head-turning	Changes Romberg fall	No effect
Duration of symptoms	Finite (minutes, days, weeks) but recurrent	May be chronic
Tinnitus or deafness	Often present	Usually absent
Common causes	Infection (labyrinthitis), Meniere's disease neuronitis, vascular disorders, trauma toxicity	Vascular, demyelinating, and neoplastic disorders

From DeMyer W: Technique of the Neurologic Examination. New York, McGraw-Hill, 1994, with permission.

TABLE 2. Differences between Peripheral and Central Positional Nystagmus

	Peripheral (Extraaxial)	Central (Intraaxial)
Latency	2–20 seconds	None
Persistence	Disappears within 50 seconds	Lasts longer than 1 minute
Fatigability	Disappears on repetition	Repeatable
Positions	Present in one position	Present in multiple positions
Vertigo	Always present	Occasionally absent, with only nystagmus present
Direction of nystagmus	One direction	Changing directions in different positions
Incidence	Common (85% of all cases)	Uncommon (10–15% of all cases)

From DeMyer W: Technique of the Neurologic Examination. New York, McGraw-Hill, 1994, with permission.

but resolves within a few days when the patient moves in a lit environment. In the dark, however, spontaneous nystagmus may still be present. Although it may be delayed, resolution always occurs after unilateral vestibular loss.[19]

A very low-tech method of assessing the integrity of the vestibuloocular pathways is to try to elicit nystagmus by using the "head-shaking nystagmus" test. This is done by having the patient move his or her head back and forth as fast as possible for about 10 cycles (or alternatively, the examiner can lay hands on the patient's head and move it back and forth). If "head-shaking" nystagmus occurs, it is likely that a unilateral as opposed to bilateral lesion has short-circuited the vestibuloocular pathway. To prevent involuntary fixation of the patient's eyes on random targets in the examining room, Freznel lenses must be worn.[39]

Numerous other provocative maneuvers elicit nystagmus in affected patients. As the patient's head is moved quickly into various positions, the examiner watches for nystagmus and classifies it on the basis of direction, latency, intensity, and duration. These "positional" tests can often be used to differentiate between peripheral and central lesions. For example, benign paroxysmal positional vertigo can be elicited by placing the patient

into the right or left head-hanging or Hallpike position. In this maneuver, the patient's head is laterally rotated to one side and then the patient is lowered rapidly onto his or her back by the examiner, who allows the patient's head to hang over the edge of the examining table so that the downward ear, which is the ear being tested, is 30–45° below the horizontal. This movement stimulates the posterior semicircular canal, which in benign paroxysmal positional vertigo is abnormal. This stimulation causes vertigo and nystagmus.[39]

In benign paroxysmal positional vertigo, as in most peripheral deficits, the latency of nystagmus is 2–20 seconds (usually 2–5 seconds). Moreover, the nystagmus will be in a specific direction (torsional when the eyes are directed toward the affected ear and vertical [upbeating] when the eyes are directed away from the affected ear). Also, the nystagmus will extinguish on repeated testing. In fact, the total duration of nystagmus should not be more than 60 seconds.[15,22]

Benign paroxysmal positional vertigo is the most common peripheral vestibular disorder causing positional vertigo. The signs and symptoms are due to pathologic changes in the posterior semicircular canal that cause the canal to respond abnormally to head position. Normally, only movement of the head in the plane of the canal leads to a response. In benign paroxysmal positional vertigo, however, it is believed that debris adhering to the cupula of the canal causes hypersensitivity to the pull of gravity; as a result, the neurons of the posterior canal discharge when the head is in a tilted position, even though it is not moving. As a consequence, head tilts give a distorted sensation of movement. For this reason the Hallpike maneuver provokes vertigo. The abnormal signal from the canal is sent to the extraocular muscles, which perform torsional nystagmus, another sign elicitable by the Hallpike maneuver. Thus, if a patient with benign paroxysmal positional vertigo tilts the head backward—a movement that stimulates the posterior semicircular canal—vertigo and nystagmus occur.[15,22,39]

In a patient with benign paroxysmal positional vertigo, symptoms are not precipitated by head shaking, a maneuver that stimulates the horizontal canals, or by movements that stimulate the anterior canals, such as learning forward.

In central deficits, on the other hand, vertigo may or may not be present. Nystagmus (usually of the upbeating variety, although it may be variable) characteristically occurs as soon as the patient is moved into the precipitation position (no latency) and continues for as long as the patient remains in that position (no extinction). Of interest, patients with central lesions may or may not complain of vertigo before clinical assessment.[23,39]

Nystagmus that does not extinguish is also seen with compression of the vestibular nerve, a condition that requires surgical intervention, and perilymphatic fistula, a tear in the membranes that separates the middle and inner ear. Patients with perilymphatic fistula, which sometimes is seen after head trauma, complain of sudden hearing loss, disequilibrium, and nausea. Pressure changes in the middle ear affect the vestibular receptors in the inner ear, resulting in torsional nystagmus and, in certain instances, positional vertigo. Like vestibular nerve compression, fistulas must be treated surgically.[31]

Neurologic Assessment

Deficits in coordination, strength, sensation, muscle tone, and reflexes may derail the normal systems responsible for stability and compensation for loss of balance. A thorough neurologic assessment helps to identify impairment in these areas.

Coordination tests include finger-to-nose and heel-to-shin testing to assess for dysmetria and rapid alternating movements to provoke dysdiadochokinesis. Movement disorders such as tics, tremors, athetosis, ballismus, and chorea are usually detectable on inspection or through observation of volitional movement. Strength is assessed by manual muscle testing.[26]

Sensation, a critical substitute for lost vestibular function, is tested in all of its pathways, including light touch, pinprick, and proprioception. Of the three, proprioception is the most important substitution for vestibular function. If it too is impaired, balance becomes at least twice as problematic. The great toes should not be used for

proprioceptive testing because, among the toes, they have the least sensitivity. In the somatosensory homunculus, the great toes have the largest representative area. Unless a lesion is large enough to obliterate a substantial part of that area, proprioceptive loss may not be detectable on examination. On the other hand, the smaller toes have a smaller area of representation in the cortex; thus, even a small lesion in the area will be detected if, for example, the second or third toe is tested.

Other considerations increase the yield of sensory testing. For instance, light touch and pinprick tests on overused areas (palmar surfaces of the hands or plantar surfaces of the feet) are not reliable because of thickened, insensitive skin. In addition, it is much better to test the patient with eyes closed rather than wide open. In an effort to "please the physician," patients often use visual cues to answer questions about sensation instead of letting their other senses speak for themselves.

Testing vibration with a tuning fork on the metatarsal head is a good way to assess posterior column function. It is not enough, however, to note that the patient does or does not sense vibration. The crucial test is the perceived duration of the vibratory stimulus: the difference between the time at which the patient reports cessation of perception and the time at which the vibration in fact stops. A difference less than 15 seconds suggests that the patient's vibratory sense is normal, whereas a difference greater than 25 seconds suggests abnormal function of the dorsal column.

Assessment of spasticity is also essential for complete understanding of the patient's ability to maintain postural control. Spasticity assessment can be performed with a multitude of scales and maneuvers. The 5-point Ashworth scale and the Brunstrom classification are commonly used to describe the presence or absence of velocity-dependent resistance to passive stretch. Increased muscle tone, however, is not the only abnormality that presents difficulties for the brain-injured patient. In fact, sometimes increased tone can be used to facilitate ambulation. Decreased tone (e.g., in cerebellar disease) also may be of concern. Through observation of gait or resistance to passive stretch, deficient muscle tone can be detected (normal subjects have some degree of resistance; patients with cerebellar dysfunction have little or none).

Of similar import is examination of reflexes to determine abnormalities that may interfere with stability or coordination during static positions or gait. Such abnormalities may include either hyperreflexia or hyporeflexia. Of interest, pendular reflexes may be seen in both states. Finally, the presence of pathologic reflexes, including the Babinski, Hoffman's, snout, rooting, glabellar, or tonic neck reflexes, may indicate nervous system abnormalities.

Balance Assessment

A wide variety of testing techniques may identify the overall condition of the systems that modulate balance. Among the best known is the Romberg test, which is taught as a means of evaluating cerebellar function but in fact evaluates the somatosensory system, particularly the dorsal columns. The confusion is understandable, because a number of proprioceptive tracts project through the cerebellum; thus, the Romberg test assesses, at least in part, a certain kind of cerebellar function. The patient stands with feet together (some examiners begin with feet apart and then narrow the base of support as the test continues) and arms folded (or outstretched in front) and then closes the eyes for 50–60 seconds. Excessive sway, loss of balance, or falling toward the affected side constitutes a positive test.

The "sharpened" or "challenged" Romberg test, a more difficult version, involves standing with eyes closed and feet in tandem. This task relies on a "hip strategy" more than the "ankle strategy," and, with the diminution of reliable distal input from ankle proprioception, the patient's task is more daunting.[2]

Yet another traditional balance test is the stand-on-one-leg-eyes-closed (SOLEC) test, in which the patient is required to stand for 30 seconds on one leg with the arms folded across the chest without falling. This is much like the tandem walking or walk-on-floor-eyes-closed (WOFEC) test, in which the patient begins with the feet in tandem, eyes closed, and arms folded across the chest. The patient then attempts to take 10 steps at normal speed (closing the eyes when the first step is taken). This test is scored by counting the number of steps the patient is able to take before sidestepping, stopping, opening the eyes, or unfolding the arms. The final score is a sum of the scores of three trials; the norm for three trials is 10 steps.[16,39]

The Fukada stepping test is a more elaborate technique for identification of a labyrinthine deficit at the level of the middle ear or higher. Two concentric circles are drawn on the floor with diameters of 1 and 2 meters. These circles are divided into 30° increments. The patient starts out in the middle of the circles, then places the arms out in front, closes the eyes, and lifts the legs in a marching fashion for 100 steps. The examiner notes how far the patient turns and how far from the starting point he or she has traveled. If the patient progresses further forward than 1 meter and has an angle of rotation greater than 45°, the performance is considered abnormal.[36]

The Singleton test is useful to identify unilateral vestibular deficits. The patient is asked to walk toward the examiner, turn quickly 180°, and then cross the arms across the chest. The test is performed twice, once to each side, with the expectation of a small amount of normal sway. If a unilateral lesion is present, the patient shows more instability when turning toward the affected side.[39]

Sensory Organization

Without accurate sensory input from the visual, somatosensory, and vestibular systems, even the patient with intact motor function is at risk for postural dysfunction. Moreover, without integration of the various kinds of input from individual pathways, confusion would result—a veritable Babel of stimulation from the environment. Certain central processes are at constant work to mesh and meld information that assists in receiving reports of self-motion. This clearinghouse, the central processing entity, guarantees maintenance of spatial orientation even when inaccurate or conflicting bits of data are received from the environment or data are lacking because a particular sense is absent. The central processing entity includes both the vestibular nuclear complex and the cerebellum. The vestibular nuclear complex, which is located in the pons and the medulla, includes the descending vestibular nucleus, the lateral vestibular nucleus, the medial vestibular nucleus, and the vestibular nucleus as well as several minor nuclei (Fig 1).[18]

The vestibular nuclear complex participates in the vestibuloocular reflex, especially the superior and medial reflexes. The medial and lateral nuclei participate in the vestibulospinal reflexes and coordinate movements of the head with movements of the eyes. The lateral vestibular nucleus is the principal nucleus for the vestibulospinal reflex.[18]

The vestibuloocular reflex is a circuit that includes the inner ear, the vestibular nerve, the vestibular nuclei, the oculomotor nuclei, and the extraocular muscles. This reflex enables perception of a steady image even when the position of the head is not steady; that is, the eye actually remains still in space while the head moves. Hain and Hillman[18] outline the following sequence of events after lateral head rotation to the right:

1. When the head turns to the right, endolymphatic flow deflects the cupulae to the left (Fig 2).

2. The discharge rate from cells in the right crista increases in proportion to the velocity of the head motion, whereas the discharge rate from hair cells in the left lateral crista decreases (see Fig. 2).

3. The changes in firing rate are transmitted along the vestibular nerve and influence the discharge of the neurons of the medial vestibular nucleus.

4. Excitatory impulses are transmitted via white matter tracts in the brainstem to the oculomotor nuclei that activate the right (ipsilateral) medial rectus and the left (contralateral) lateral rectus. Inhibitory impulses are also transmitted to their antagonists.

5. Simultaneous contraction of the left lateral rectus and right medial rectus muscles and relaxation of the left medial rectus and right lateral rectus result in lateral compensatory eye movements toward the left.

Equally well described by Hain and Hillman is the vestibulospinal reflex (VSR), a circuit that is more diffusely located than the vestibuloocular reflex (VOR). Its purpose is to stabilize the head and body. Its components

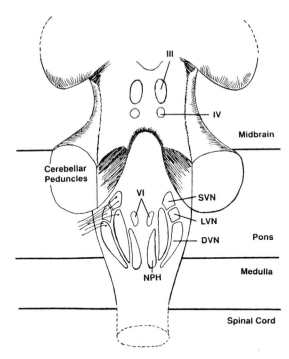

FIGURE 1. The vestibular nuclear complex. This section shows the brainstem with the cerebellum removed. DVN = descending vestibular nucleus, LVN = lateral vestibular nucleus, NPH = nucleus prepositus hypoglossi, III = oculomotor nucleus (inferior oblique muscle and medial, superior, and inferior rectus muscles), IV = trochlear nucleus (superior oblique muscle), VI = abducens nucleus (lateral rectus). The medial vestibular nucleus (MVN), not shown, lies between the NPH and the DVN. (From Herdman S: Anatomy and physiology of the normal vestibular system. In Hain T, Hillman M (eds): Vestibular Rehabilitation. Philadelphia, F.A. Davis, 1994, with permission.)

include several reflexes, the most important of which is the vestibulocollic reflex (VCR). The vestibulocollic reflex connects the vestibular labyrinths, the vestibular nuclear complex, and the muscles in the neck responsible for head turning. It aligns the head with respect to gravity. For example, a patient leaning forward over a walker uses the vestibulocollic reflex to lift the head as he or she ambulates so that the gaze is stabilized and oriented to the vertical position in space. Damage to the labyrinth impairs the vestibulocollic reflex and causes an unstable, oscillating head.[9]

An example of the sequence of events in the vestibulospinal reflex is as follows:

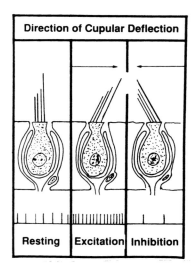
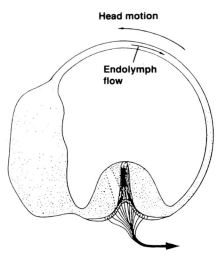

FIGURE 2. Effects of head rotation on the semicircular canals. *Left*, The direction from which hair cells are deflected determines whether or not hair-cell discharge frequency increases or decreases. *Right*, Endolymph flow and cupular deflection in response to head motion. (From Herdman S: Anatomy and physiology of the normal vestibular system. In Hain T, Hillman M (eds): Vestibular Rehabilitation. Philadelphia, F.A. Davis, 1994, with permission.)

1. When the head is tilted to one side, both the canals and otoliths (utricles and saccules) are stimulated.

2. The vestibular nerve and vestibular nucleus are activated as described for the vestibuloocular reflex.

3. Impulses are transmitted via the vestibulospinal tracts to the spinal cord.

4. Extensor activity is induced on the side to which the head is inclined, and flexor activity is induced on the opposite side.

5. The maintained limb position is derived from the otoliths.[18]

Although normal adults usually prefer using somatosensory information as their first database, the flexibility of the central nervous system allows substitution of other modalities.

Motor Coordination

Normal adults should be able to generate, scale, and coordinate inertial and muscular forces to control the center of mass relative to their limits of stability, regardless of the type of surface on which they are positioned. They also should be able to make adjustments to maintain balance in the face of expected and unexpected perturbations. Furthermore, postural adjustments should be accomplished at an automatic, reflexive stage before any voluntary gross limb movements are needed.

This ability depends on processes that organize the action of trunk and leg muscles into movement strategies. A continuum of three types of movement strategies for controlling anterior-posterior postural sway has been described. This continuum includes ankle, hip, and stepping strategies.

The ankle strategy involves making postural adjustments primarily with the ankle joints, rotating the body about these joints so as to reposition the center of mass for maintenance of stable alignment. Most commonly, this strategy is used when the challenge to maintaining position is small and the support surface is firm. It is important when climbing steps, walking on irregular surfaces, and standing on one leg while dressing.[46]

The hip strategy is needed for correction of larger postural perturbations or when the support surface is either not firm or smaller than the feet. It is a bridge between the ankle and stepping strategy when insufficient force is generated at the ankle to prevent taking a step. It requires large, accurately coordinated movements of the hip, trunk, and neck to stabilize the head in space. Standing sideways on a balance beam or performing tandem gait requires use of the hip strategy. Assessment is based on whether it is used prematurely or appropriately at the limits of stability.

Stepping strategies are used to recover the center of mass when it has been displaced outside the base of support. This strategy involves a series of steps or hops designed to bring the support base back into alignment under the center of mass.[45]

A patient may have a particular strategy in his or her repertoire but lack sufficient coordination to use it effectively. Thus, assessment of coordination gives clues to the patient's ability to execute one strategy or another. The examiner must also assess whether the patient appropriately adapts strategies to the changes in postural task, such as standing on one foot or on a balance beam.

The examiner must assess whether the strategies are normally coordinated and whether an appropriate number of strategies is used in varied situations. Normal strategies may be used in an inappropriate environmental context.

Motion-Provoked Symptoms

It is important to observe patients for motion-provoked symptoms by having them assume positions that by history generate vestibular symptoms. It is helpful to leave this part of the assessment until the end, because severe symptoms may preclude further physical examination.

Vestibular Function Tests

Vestibular function tests can be useful in diagnosis and assessment of etiology and site of lesion. This is very important when there is potential for associated peripheral injuries.[26] Many of these studies are difficult to perform in brain-injured patients because they require a significant degree of patient cooperation. One advantage of electronystagmography and rotary chair testing is that both are physiologic rather than functional tests and therefore do not rely on patient report of symptoms; they evaluate the integrity of the horizontal semicircular canals. Electronystagmography and rotary chair testing may be difficult for patients

with behavioral and cognitive deficits to tolerate. In patients with TBI who are likely to have central lesions, the clinician needs to assess carefully whether the potential information from the studies will significantly affect treatment decisions. Dynamic posturography may provide a more functionally oriented assessment of balance deficits.

Electronystagmography

Electronystagmography can assess site and side of peripheral lesions. The technique provides a means of tracking eye movements behind closed lids or in the dark. Changes in eye position are indicated by the polarity of the natural corneal retinal potential relative to each electrode.[50]

Eye movements are assessed in several different clinical conditions. Unprovoked eye movements are observed with eyes closed to look for spontaneous nystagmus. Positional nystagmus is assessed by recording eye movements provoked by changes in the orientation of the semicircular canals relative to gravity. A Hallpike-Dix maneuver[13]—rapid change of position from sitting to supine with head turned to right or left and hanging over the edge of the examination table—is commonly used for diagnosis of benign paroxysmal positional vertigo. Caloric testing, using water-induced temperature gradients to provide a low-frequency stimulus, can measure the responsiveness of one horizontal semicircular canal relative to the other.[21] This can help to identify the involved ear in peripheral lesions.[25]

Rotary Chair Testing

Rotary chair testing measures the response of the vestibular system to high-frequency stimuli and helps to identify site and side of the lesion. It is useful in patients with bilateral vestibular deficits or patients in whom the difference between sides may be quite small and therefore not detectable with caloric testing or low-velocity rotation.

Rotary chair testing is performed in a dark room with the head restrained in a fixed position. There is a constant rate of acceleration and deceleration. The chair can rotate in both vertical and tilted positions. Electrodes monitor eye movements. Patient actions are monitored through an infrared camera. Patients with significant behavioral deficits may be unable to tolerate testing.

Abnormal findings with rotary chair testing usually relate to peripheral vestibular system function. Rotary chair testing is most likely to be useful in patients with potential peripheral vestibular lesions in whom caloric tests are uncertain or unobtainable.[41,51]

Dynamic Posturography

Dynamic posturography is a functional test that allows separate evaluation of sensory organization and motor coordination components of balance. Identification of the integral components of the functional balance deficit may help the rehabilitation team in planning treatment. This technique also may be useful in monitoring neurologic recovery in patients with TBI and balance deficits.

The Sensory Organization Test (SOT)[35] evaluates the patient's ability to make effective use of visual, vestibular, and somatosensory information for maintaining balance in progressively more challenging task conditions. The sensory conflict portions of the test evaluate a patient's ability to screen out inappropriate conflicting sensory information. Two independent forceplates are used with transducers to measure vertical forces and

horizontal shear forces. A computer model of body dynamics calculates center-of-gravity sway angle from vertical force movements when height and weight information are added. Horizontal shear forces are used to measure anteroposterior and lateral acceleration of the center of gravity. They provide information about the pattern of body motion that is used to produce sway. Patients must be able to stand unassisted with eyes open for at least 1 minute in order to undergo testing (Fig. 3).

The SOT has six components representing six sensory conditions (Fig. 4). In conditions 1–3, the platform is stationary. The first condition assesses static balance with eyes open. The second condition is a Romberg test with eyes closed. In the third condition, the visual surround is sway-referenced, tilting about an axis colinear with the ankle joint to follow the movement of the patient's center of gravity. This condition, which results in conflicting visual input, assesses for preferential reliance on visual input, even when it is inaccurate.

In conditions 4–6, the support surface is sway-referenced. Abnormalities in the fourth condition with eyes open identify patients who rely on somatosensory input. The fifth

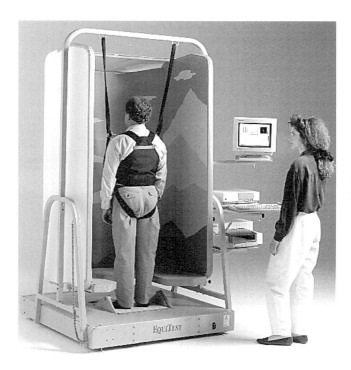

FIGURE 3. Equitest for dynamic posturography. (Photograph courtesy of NeuroCom International, Inc.)

condition removes visual input, and the sixth provides conflicting visual information; both isolate function of the vestibular system.

Inconsistent performance on multiple trials or performance that improves on the more difficult sway-referenced conditions can help to identify nonphysiologic problems, such as anxiety, exaggeration of deficits, or conversion reactions.

Dynamic posturography testing is not available in all settings and may be difficult to access for monitoring of clinical progress. Shumway-Cook and Horak developed a clinical test based on Nashner's model for the SOT. In their version, called the Clinical Test for Sensory Interaction in Balance, a modified Japanese lantern is placed over the head to provide inaccurate visual information for the third and sixth conditions. A dense, compliant foam is used as the support surface for conditions 4–6 to decrease somatosensory information. Each condition is performed for 30 seconds while the examiner assesses the amount of sway and motor strategies used by the patient to maintain balance.[24,46-48]

The Motor Control Test (MCT)[35] evaluates the patient's ability to maintain balance in reaction to brief displacements of the support surface. The support surface is moved horizontally either backward or forward (Fig. 5). The type of motor strategy (ankle, hip, or stepping) and the characteristics of the motor response are quantified. Posture-evoked responses are also assessed by rapidly rotating the support surface in a toes-up or toes-down position (Fig. 6). The results of the MCT are relatively unaffected by patient motivation and effort, because they assess reflexive balance responses that are not consciously mediated. One disadvantage of the MCT is that it does not assess the patient's ability to compensate functionally under more complex task conditions.[34]

Lehmann and colleagues[29] also used a quantitative measurement of sway to assess balance function in patients with TBI. Measurements were performed with eyes open and closed and in comfortable, narrow, and tandem stances. The investigators concluded that increased sway combined with increased failure to perform more difficult test positions may indicate the severity of the functional balance deficit. A correlation was

FIGURE 4. The sensory organization test protocol showing the six sensory test conditions. (Courtesy of NeuroCom International, Inc.)

established between sway and self-selected comfortable walking speed. All patients with a tendency to fall had sway values in the upper distribution.

TREATMENT STRATEGIES

Treatment of vestibular deficits in patients with TBI is complex. Patients are more likely

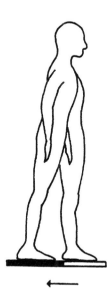

FIGURE 5. Stimulus paradigm for the motor control test. The support surface is translated backward (or forward) while the position of the upper body remains initially stationary. Note that the amplitude of the translation is exaggerated for purposes of illustration. (Courtesy of NeuroCom International, Inc.)

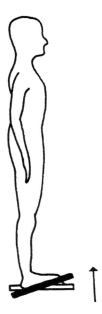

FIGURE 6. Stimulus paradigm for the posture-evoked response tests. The support surface is rapidly rotated toes-up (or toes-down) while the body remains initially stationary. Note that the amplitude of the support surface rotation is exaggerated for purposes of illustration. (Courtesy of NeuroCom International, Inc.)

to have mixed central and peripheral etiologies for their vestibular symptoms. Multiple lesions, both peripheral and central, may decrease the ability of the central nervous system to compensate, thus leading to prolonged symptoms without full recovery.[3,30,39,40]

Functional disability secondary to vestibular deficits may be greater after traumatic injuries. Patients with vestibular lesions often must use conscious effort to maintain spatial orientation in situations where it normally occurs on an automatic, subconscious basis.[49] Such effort may be extremely difficult for patients with cognitive deficits, especially in the areas of attention and executive control.

A basic understanding of mechanisms of recovery from vestibular deficits is important for development of treatment protocols. Such mechanisms are best understood for unilateral peripheral lesions.[7] A degree of spontaneous recovery is often seen in the first 6–12 months after TBI. The vestibular system has the ability to adapt to asymmetries in vestibular input, in part because of active neuronal changes in the cerebellum and brainstem in response to sensory conflicts caused by peripheral vestibular pathology.[43] This mechanism of recovery is most effective in relieving symptoms of stable peripheral lesions. This plasticity is the physiologic basis for habituation exercises. Central damage to the brain after TBI may interfere with this recovery mechanism.

A patient's ability to substitute other sensory input to compensate for deficits has a major impact on functional outcome. Substitution and avoidance of sensory conflict situations are the major compensatory strategies for patients with bilateral peripheral lesions or central involvement.[42]

Patients with posttraumatic vestibular deficits often have mixed central and peripheral lesions complicated by other coexisting motor, sensory, and cognitive deficits. Treatment programs must stimulate functional recovery through vestibular adaptation, substitution, and spontaneous recovery while also focusing on compensatory strategies for functional deficits.

The use of pharmacologic suppressants such as meclizine (Antivert) may delay the recovery process. Such medications depress the central nervous system, influencing sensory receptor input and delaying or preventing central vestibular compensation. Medications such as diazepam, Compazine, Phenergan, meclizine, and scopolamine are often used to suppress vestibular symptoms, inlcuding nausea, vomiting, and headaches. Their use should be avoided if possible, because they often produce serious side effects that exacerbate the offending symptoms of vestibular dysfunction.[43] For example, the benzodiazepine class of drugs (sometimes used to control anxiety related to disturbing sensations of vestibular problems) inhibits GABA synapses located in the reticular activating system, causing sedation. Sedation has a dampening effect on balance, because the reticular activating system—along with the vestibular nuclear complex, the cerebellum, and the oculomotor nuclei—is required to formulate appropriate efferent signals to the extraocular and skeletal muscles, the effector organs of the vestibuloocular and vestibulospinal reflexes.[8,18]

Compazine (a phenothiazine) blocks dopamine receptors. Dopamine is an important neurotransmitter in motor receptors. Because the effector organs of the vestibular system are skeletal muscles, drugs of this class are clearly detrimental to recovery in patients with vestibular dysfunction.[8]

Meclizine is an antihistamine also used to prevent nausea, vomiting, and vertigo. Histamine blockers have a benzodiazepinelike effect on GABA receptors in the reticular activating system and thus adversely affect the balance mechanism. They also have an anticholinergic effect that, given the role of acetylcholine in motor function, can only retard recovery.[17,32]

The use of high-dose aminoglycoside antibiotics should be avoided. Their ototoxic effects can damage hair cells in the labyrinth and cochlea, causing vestibular deficits in addition to hearing loss. Anticonvulsants, tricyclic antidepressants, and tranquilizers can all cause dizziness. These effects are usually dose-related.

Education of patient and family to avoid specific sensory conflict situations can be useful in management of major symptoms. Timing of performance of exercise programs before bedtime or rest periods can be helpful.

The goals of a vestibular rehabilitation program must relate to the overall rehabilitation goals of functional improvement and community reintegration:[49]

1. Independent community level mobility;

2. Functional balance in increasingly more challenging context-specific situations;

3. Improved safety for gait and mobility;

4. Improved general physical condition, endurance, and activity level;

5. Decrease in motion-provoked symptoms; and

6. Patient and family education about the causes of symptoms, mechanisms of recovery, and coping strategies.

Exercise is the stimulus that facilitates the compensatory process. Central nervous system compensation requires exposure to motor activities and sensory conflict situations that provoke the patient's symptoms. Inactivity and restriction of head movement to control symptoms may delay the central compensatory process. Restriction of movement also may exacerbate coexisting musculoskeletal problems, which are common in

the posttraumatic patient, further complicating therapeutic intervention.

Education for patient and family about etiology and goals of treatment is essential. They must understand that initially symptoms will be exacerbated. Patients with TBI often need a great deal of family support and assistance to carry through with a vestibular exercise program.

Cawthorne and Cooksey developed a structured approach to vestibular exercises in the 1940s.[7,10] The exercises utilize head movements coordinated with eye movements. They also include total body movements and balance tasks. The exercises are performed in progressively more difficult positions. They are initially done slowly. Speed is increased as tolerated. Exercises are done with eyes closed to decrease reliance on visual information. Cawthorne and Cooksey stressed a functional approach. They advocated for training to progress to community settings in noisy and crowded environments, where patients with vestibular deficits have more difficulty.[21]

Norre and De Weerdt expanded the work of Cawthorne and Cooksey to include maneuvers that provoke vestibular symptoms. They advocated the use of habituation exercises for vestibular system adaptation, relaxation exercises, and patient education.[37,38]

Shepard and Telian prospectively studied 152 patients using a home exercise regimen of habituation and balance-retraining exercises. After therapy, 80–85% of their patients showed a reduction in symptoms and disability score. Among patients with TBI, symptoms were reduced in 62% and disability scores in 53%.[51] Patients with TBI-related cognitive and motor deficits may need a more structured exercise program approach to achieve compliance. Patients with central lesions secondary to diffuse axonal injury may be more likely to have persisting vestibular symptoms, despite compliance with habituation exercises.[43]

Vestibular exercise programs often must be modified for patients with TBI. Increased time may be needed to learn vestibular exercises. Patients need more physical assistance to compensate for motor deficits. Families often must assist with performance of home exercise programs. Physical therapists need to introduce exercises slowly, with progression based on functional improvement and tolerance of vestibular symptoms. Patients with cognitive deficits have a greater need for structure, cues, and ongoing education.

Exercise programs should be individually designed for each patient based on deficits identified in the initial evaluation. Habituation exercises for positional vertigo and motion perception deficits should be based on repetition of positions and movements of the head and body that cause vertigo. Traditional physical therapy approaches to improve strength, range of motion, and postural alignment should be used in patients with musculoskeletal deficits.

As a patient's musculoskeletal status improves, a generalized conditioning program should be introduced to improve endurance and decrease sedentary behavior. A graduated walking program is often a good starting point. Gradually, other types of recreational sports activities can be included, such as golf and bowling, which involve coordinated hand, eye, and body movements. Swimming should be initiated only in a closely supervised setting, because many patients with vestibular deficits experience disorientation in the relative weightlessness of water.[43] In brain-injured patients, such a program often initially requires structure and close supervision, which, along with community reintegration, may be provided in a recreational therapy group. Family and patient education are extremely important for successful continuation of the conditioning program after discharge from a structured therapy program.

Exercises to improve visual tracking, gaze stabilization during head movement, and visual modulation of vestibuloocular responses are added for patients with vestibuloocular deficits. These exercises can be incorporated into functional tasks—for example, scanning tasks during shopping.

Musculoskeletal deficits should be addressed through a traditional physical therapy program. Goals should include improving strength and endurance and normalizing range of motion and postural alignment. Aggressive treatment of contractures is essential for improvement in functional skills. Patients must have adequate range of motion to maintain postural alignment within limits of stability.

Therapy program planning to address sensory organization deficits must be tailored to individual patients and their specific pattern of deficits. An SOT performed during dynamic posturography testing or the Clinical Test for Sensory Interaction in Balance can provide an excellent basis for program planning. Repeat testing also can be helpful for monitoring of progress. Close monitoring of functional improvement and decrease in frequency and intensity of symptoms is essential. Graphs of results may improve patient motivation and cooperation.

Most patients with TBI have incomplete vestibular lesions but may tend to rely solely on visual and somatosensory information. The therapy program should focus on maintaining balance while both visual and somatosensory cues are varied gradually and systematically. Reliance on visual and somatosensory cues will decrease with increased vestibular compensation.

When sensory compensation is inappropriate, patients incorrectly use visual or somatosensory information in situations where the information is inaccurate. They need to be conditioned not to rely solely on one sensory system, especially in sensory conflict situations. Exercises should involve maintenance of balance in progressively more difficult situations while the therapist systematically varies the availability and accuracy of sensory information. Patients who lose balance only when visual and somatosensory data are distorted simultaneously compensate well and become functional in most situations. They may require only education about which situations to avoid.

Sensory organization deficits may not resolve completely in all patients. Education is a key component of vestibular therapy. Patients must be able to identify which situations are likely to be difficult and when compensatory techniques are likely to be helpful.

Intervention for motor coordination deficits should be guided by the patients' ability to coordinate and use appropriately a variety of movement strategies during functional activities. Practice and repetition of motor skills in progressively more difficult environments can improve both the range and coordination of movement strategies for maintaining balance.

Patients must be strongly encouraged to continue their exercise program after symptoms have resolved. Central nervous system compensation is plastic and fragile; it depends on continued vestibular input. Symptoms may return after periods of inactivity, such as bedrest imposed by viral illness.[43]

The recovery of functional balance after TBI is complex and requires a multifaceted approach, including careful diagnostic assessment and treatment of deficits in multiple realms: the musculoskeletal and vestibuloocular systems, motion perception, sensory organization, and motor coordination. Neurologic recovery may not be complete. Patient education is a key factor in control of symptoms and compensation for persisting deficits.

REFERENCES

1. Baloh RW, Honrubia V, Jacobson K: Benign positional vertigo: Clinical and oculographic features in 240 cases. Neurology 37:3731–378, 1987.
2. Baloh R, Honrubia V: Clinical Neurophysiology of the Vestibular System. Philadelphia, FA Davis, 1990.
3. Berman J, Frederickson J: Vertigo after head injury—A five year follow-up. J Otolaryngol 7:237, 1978.
4. Binder LM: Persisting symptoms after mild head injury: A review of the postconcussive syndrome. J Clin Exp Neuropsychol 8:434–46, 1986.
5. Borello-France D, Whitney S, Herdman S: Assessment of vestibular hypofunction. In Herdman, S, Wolf SL (eds): Vestibular Rehabilitation. Philadelphia, F.A. Davis, 1994, p 253.
6. CJ: Medical intelligence: Living without a balancing mechanism. N Engl J Med 246:458–460, 1952.
7. Cawthorne T: The physiologic basis for head exercises. J Chartered Soc Physiother 30:106, 1944.
8. Ciccone, CD: Pharmacology in Rehabilitation. Philadelphia, F.A. Davis, 1990.
9. Cohen H, Keshner E: Current concepts of the vestibular system reviewed: II Visual/vestibular interaction and spatial orientation. Occup Ther 43: 331–333, 1989.
10. Cooksey FS: Rehabilitation in vestibular injuries. Proc R Soc Med 39:273, 1946
11. Daroff RA: Dizziness and vertigo. In Wilson JD, Brunwald E, Issellbacher K, et al. (eds): Medicine. New York, McGraw-Hill, 1991, pp 140–142.
12. DeMyer WE: Technique of the Neurologic Examination. New York, McGraw-Hill, 1994, pp 165–169.
13. Dix M, Hallpike C: The pathology symptomatology and diagnosis of certain common disorders of the vestibular system. Ann Otol Laryngol 61:987, 1952.
14. Farber S, Zoltan B: Vestibular systems interaction: Therapeutic implications. Head Trauma Rehabil 4(2):10, 1989.
15. Fetter M: Vestibular system disorders. In Herdman SJ, Wolf S (eds): Vestibular Rehabilitation. Philadelphia, F.A. Davis, 1994, pp 90–109.
16. Fregley A, Graybiel A: An ataxia test battery not requiring rails. Aerospace Med 3:277–282, 1968.
17. Gualtieri, CT: Neuropsychiatry and Behavioral Pharmacology. New York, Springer-Verlag, 1991, pp 111–123.
18. Hain TC, Hillman MA: Anatomy and Physiology of the normal vestibular system. In Herdman S: Vestibular Rehabilitation. Philadelphia, FA Davis, 1994, p. 15.
19. Halmagyi GM, Curthorp JS: Clinical changes in vestibular function over time after lesions: The consequences of unilateral vestibular deafferentation. In Herdman S (ed): Vestibular Rehabilitation. Philadelphia, F.A. Davis, 1994, pp 90–109.
20. Healy GB: Hearing loss and vertigo secondary to head injury. N Engl Med 306:1029–1031, 1982.
21. Herdman S: Vestibular Rehabilitation. Philadelphia, F.A. Davis, 1994, pp 128–134.
22. Herdman S: Assessment and management of benign paroxysmal positional vertigo. In Herdman S (ed): Vestibular Rehabilitation. Philadelphia, F.A. Davis, 1994, p 331.
23. Honrubia V: Quantitative vestibular function tests and the clinical examination. In Herdman S (ed): Vestibular Rehabilitation. Philadelphia, F.A. Davis, 1994, pp 115–126.
24. Horak F: Clinical measurement of postural control in adults. Phys Ther 67:1881, 1987.
25. Jacobson GP, Newman GW, Peterson EL: Interpretation and usefulness of caloric testing. In Jacobson GP, Newman CW, Kartush JM(eds): Handbook of Balance Function Testing. St. Louis, Mosby, 1993, pp 193–233.
26. Kendall FP, McCreary EK: Muscle Testing and Function. Baltimore, Williams & Wilkins, 1983.
27. Keshner E: Postural abnormalities in vestibular disorders. In Herdman S (ed): Vestibular Rehabilitation. Philadelphia, F.A. Davis, 1994, p 63.
28. Legg AT: Physical therapy in infantile paralysis. In Mock (ed): Principles and Practice of Physical Therapy, vol II. Hagerstown, MD, W.F. Prior, 1932, p 45.
29. Lehmann JF, Boswell S, Price R, et al: Quantitative evaluation of sway as and indicator of functional balance in posttraumatic brain injury. Arch Phys Med Rehabil 71:955–962, 1990.
30. Leigh J: Pharmacologic and optical methods of treating vestibular disorders and nystagmus. In Herdman S (ed): Vestibular Rehabilitation. Philadelphia, F.A. Davis, 1994, pp 185–193.
31. Mattox DE: Surgical Management of vestibular disorders. In Herdman S (ed): Vestibular Rehabilitation. Philadelphia, F.A. Davis, 1994, pp 202–203.
32. McEvoy G: Drug Information. Bethesda, MD, American Society of Hospital Pharmacists, 1994, p 2.
33. Medical Research Council: Aids to the Investigation of Peripheral Nerve Injuries. War Memorandum No.7, 2nd ed (rev). London, His Majesty's Stationery Office, 1943.

34. Nashner L: Peters JF: Dynamic posturography. In Jacobson GP, Newman CW, Kartush JM: Handbook of Balance Function Testing. St. Louis, Mosby, 1993, pp 280–334.

35. Nashner LM, Peters JF: Dynamic posturography in the diagnosis and management of dizziness and balance disorders. Neurol Clin 8:331–347, 1990.

36. Newton R: Review of tests of standing balance abilities. Brain Inj 3:335–343, 1989.

37. Norre ME, DeWeerdt W: Treatment of vertigo based on habituation. I: Physio-pathological basis. J Laryngol Otol 94: 689, 1980.

38. Norre ME, De Weerdt W: Treatment of vertigo based on habituation. II: Technique and results of habituation training. J Laryngol Otol 94:971, 1980.

39. Oates J: Postconcussive balance dysfunction: A physical therapy approach. State Art Rev Phys Med Rehabil 6:89–108, 1992.

40. Pearson BW, Barber Ho: Head injury: some otoneurologic sequelae. Arch Otolaryngol 97:81, 1973.

41. Shepard NT, Telian SA: Balance disorders ("the dizzy patient"). In Jacobson JT, Northern JL (eds): Diagnostic Audiology. Austin, TX, Pro-ed, 1990, pp 267–294.

42. Shepard NT, Telian S: Habituation and balance retraining therapy. Neurol Clin 8:2, 1940.

43. Shepard NT, Telian SA: Physical therapy rehabilitation in treatment of vestibular disorders. In Proceedings of Clinical Applications of Vestibular Science, February 12–13, 1994, Los Angeles.

44. Shepard NT, Telian SA, Smith-Wheelock M, Raj A: Vestibular and balance rehabilitation therapy. Ann Otol Rhinol Laryngol 102:198–205, 1993.

45. Shumway-Cook A, Olmscheid R: A systems analysis of postural dyscontrol in traumatically brain injured patients. Head Trauma Rehabil 5(4):51–62, 1990.

46. Shumway-Cook A, Horak F: Rehabilitation of vestibular dysfunction and traumatic brain injury. Phys Med Rehabil Clin North Am 8:441–457, 1990.

47. Shumway-Cook A: Rehabilitation of vestibular dysfunction and traumatic brain injury. Phys Med Rehabil Clin North Am 3:355–369, 1992.

48. Shumway-Cook A, Horak F: Assessing the influence of sensory interaction on balance rehabilitation. Am J Otol 12:218–225, 1991.

50. Stockwell CW: ENG Workbook. Baltimore, University Park Press, 1983.

51. Stockwell CW, Bojrab DI: Interpretation and usefulness of caloric testing. In Jacobson GP, Newman CW, Kartush JM (eds): Handbook of Balance Function Testing. St. Louis, Mosby, 1993, pp 249–257.

MILTON D. THOMAS M.D.

NATHAN D. ZASLER M.D.

19

Sensory-Perceptual Disorders after Traumatic Brain Injury

CRANIAL NERVE DYSFUNCTION

Olfactory Nerve and Olfactory Pathway (Cranial Nerve I)

Olfaction, perhaps the most primitive of all senses, warns of coming danger or invites to a pleasant encounter. From airborne molecules that dissolve in the olfactory mucosa, chemical interactions trigger electrical patterns in primary sensory neurons that travel along the neurofibrils passing through the cribriform ethmoid plate. The neurofibrils enter the olfactory bulb and synapse with mitral and tufted cells (secondary neurons). These secondary neurons extend via the olfactory tract along the floor of the frontal cranium through the olfactory stria to the inferomedial aspect of the temporal lobe, where the smell is perceived, although it remains nonlocalizable.

The first report of loss of smell following trauma, quoted by Sumner et al.,[58] was made in 1864 by Hughlings Jackson. Ogle followed three years later with a report of three cases of anosmia following occipital blows, and in the same year (1870) Notta noted that loss of consciousness was not necessary to produce anosmia after head trauma. Since then,

numerous additional accounts have been reported.[38,58,64]

The incidence of traumatic anosmia varies by report, but several large studies report that an average of 7.5% of all patients with blows to the head or face suffer either permanent or temporary complete anosmia.[40,58] Other studies report slightly lower results, but methodologic flaws, including the timing of initial referral after injury, tend to reduce the accuracy of their numbers. Such reports also do not accurately reflect partial loss of the sense of smell, which is quite widespread, but usually of shorter duration.

The pathophysiology of traumatic anosmia is fourfold: (1) injury to the neurofibrils as they pass through the cribriform plate, (2) compression of the olfactory bulbs by hemorrhage and edema or contusion and abrasion of the olfactory bulbs by the cribriform plate, (3) injury to the central pathways of olfaction, and/or (4) injury to the nasal passages themselves. Any of these mechanisms also may cause hyposmia (a decreased sense of smell), parosmia (perversion of the sense of smell), or cacosmia (awareness of a disagreeable or unusually offensive odor that does not exist). Cacosmia may be part of an aura prior to the onset of seizure activity. Late onset (longer than 3–4 weeks after injury) of loss of smell may occur with scarring or gliosis of the tissues in the cribriform plate.

Nontraumatic causes of transient alterations in the sense of smell must also be considered, including acute viral upper respiratory infections, rhinitis sicca, allergic sinusitis, chronic polyposis, depression, and medications.

Testing of the olfactory system involves the use of pure odors, such as floral odors and musk, and the avoidance of irritant substances, such as peppermint or ammonia, which test the trigeminal nerve (cranial nerve V) rather than the olfactory nerve. Bedside testing with pure odors should be done early in the course of recovery to determine any olfactory impairment. Serial testing is important in the patient with loss of smell. Tests that attempt to quantify the loss of smell have been described.[13,21,35] Before quantitative testing, the patient must be at least at level V of the Rancho Los Amigos Cognitive Functioning Scale, although occasionally a comatose patient may evidence change in respiratory pattern or other generalized response when presented with a pure, familiar odor such as coffee.

After the nontraumatic causes of loss of smell and nasal passage trauma have been ruled out and seizure activity (if present) has been treated, any remaining loss of smell is attributable to olfactory neurofibril or central injury. These latter types of injury are highly resistant to treatment.[40,64,38] Some recovery may occur in the initial 4–6 weeks after injury, presumably from resolution of edema or of pressure after hematoma liquefaction and resorption. Later recovery may be due to regrowth of neurofibrils through the cribriform plate. This process, which usually is only partial, may be slowed or stopped by scarring and gliosis.[13] Recovery of function after the first 4–6 weeks may also be due to central adaptation of the perceived odor.

The loss of the sense of smell may have significant consequences for the patient in daily function, avocational interests, and return to work. It also may affect the sense of taste. Patients frequently describe this effect as similar to loss of taste with a severe "head cold." The reader is referred to the excellent review by Costanzo and Zasler[13] for further discussion.

Optic Nerve and Optic Pathway (Cranial Nerve II)

The optic nerve, which in fact is a direct extension of the diencephalon rather than a true cranial nerve, begins in the ganglion cell layer of the retina (secondary sensory neurons). The long axons of the ganglion cells penetrate the lamina cribrosa as the optic nerve, which passes posteriorly through the optic canal. At the optic chiasma, where the fibers from the nasal halves of the retina decussate, the optic tract is formed and continues posteriorly to the lateral geniculate bodies, where a third synaptic relay occurs. At this point, a small number of axons leave the optic tract and project to the pretectal midbrain to form the afferent loop of the Edinger-Westphal nucleus. From the lateral geniculate body, the optic tract continues posteriorly as the optic radiations, which project to the occipital lobe. Throughout their projection to the occipital lobe the neurons maintain a highly topographic orientation of the retinal image.

Injury to the optic nerve typically occurs in one of two ways: (1) from loss of blood supply to the nerve through the small nutrient arteries that feed the nerve itself or (2) from direct injury related to the trauma. Unfortunately, because the optic nerve is a direct extension of the brain, any injury to the axons of the optic nerve, which do not regenerate after injury, is permanent. Loss of vision immediately after injury may be due to ischemia, edema, or shearing or contusion of the nerve. Delayed loss of vision usually is caused by infarction of the optic nerve or, less frequently, by hematoma surrounding the nerve in the canal.

Injury to the optic nerve occurs most frequently in the intracanalicular portion of the nerve, although it also may occur in the intrabulbar, intraorbital, and intracranial portions.[10] In the intracanalicular portion, the nerve is tethered at both ends of the bony canal. Crompton[14] postulates that movement of the contents of the orbit and cranium about the tethered portion of the nerve results in ischemic necrosis and shearing injuries. Ischemic necrosis and shearing injuries also are common in the intracranial portion of the nerve.

Immediate monocular blindness occurs with great frequency in optic nerve injuries, especially in the intracanalicular portion of the nerve. Monocular blindness may be partial, and the extent of partial blindness should be documented immediately and followed closely for deterioration. Surgical decompression of the nerve in the intracanalicular portion is generally of little benefit in patients with no light perception, but the deterioration of partial visual function may be an indication for decompression; certainly it is an indication for prompt action. Anderson et al.[2] reported that in patients with no light perception, the use of megadose steroids (dexamethasone 3–5 mg/kg/day) is of equal or greater benefit than surgical decompression in terms of visual recovery. They believed that surgical decompression should be reserved for patients with delayed visual loss unresponsive to 12 hours of megadose dexamethasone or patients in whom return of vision with megadose steroids treatment was followed by visual decrease, either during treatment or when steroids were tapered. Recent research suggests that such intervention may not be of clinical benefit.[55]

Complete monocular blindness with preservation of normal pupillary reflexes is usually a sign of malingering or other types of functional (nonorganic) disorders.

Visual field deficits are due to injury to the optic nerve or its tracts posterior to the bulbar portion. When such deficits are due to causes other than direct pressure from a mass lesion, surgical intervention is rarely helpful. Some visual field deficits may be helped by special optics that allow the patient to "see" in the affected field.[46,47] Careful evaluation by a neuroophthalmologist or neurooptometrist is warranted, and training in the use of such lenses is often necessary. It is also important for the clinician to recognize nonphysiologic visual field deficits.

Non–nerve-related injury also may affect visual function. Trauma to the cornea may cause visual blurring and scotomata. Visual blurring may be caused by vitreous tears, traumatically induced cataracts, retinal hemorrhage, or retinal detachment. Injury to the cornea or contents of the anterior chamber (including the lens) may cause monocular diplopia.[37] If eyeglasses are of no benefit, surgery may be necessary to correct blurring caused by either corneal or lens problems. Visual blurring also may be caused by Torsion's syndrome (intrabulbar hemorrhage). Such hemorrhage may spontaneously resorb over time or require surgical removal for complete restoration of vision. Patients with intracranial subarachnoid hemorrhage also may have Torsion's syndrome, probably as a result of hemorrhage due to increased intraocular vascular pressure rather than extension of the subarachnoid hemorrhage into the globe.

Ocular Motor Nerves (Cranial Nerves III, IV, and VI)

Oculomotor Nerve (Cranial Nerve III)

The nucleus of the oculomotor nerve arises in the paramedian midbrain ventral to the aqueduct of Sylvius near the superior colliculus. Its fibers course anteriorly through the red nucleus and cerebral peduncle, emerging near the pontomedullary junction at the midline and penetrating the dura at the cavernous sinus. It travels along the lateral wall of the cavernous sinus, adjacent to the trochlear nerve, and superior to the abducens. Parasympathetic fibers from the Edinger-Westphal nucleus, which lies superior and dorsal to the oculomotor nucleus, course in close proximity to the oculomotor nerve through the cavernous sinus. The oculomotor nerve emerges through the superior orbital fissure to innervate its effector organs.

The oculomotor nerve innervates the superior rectus, medial rectus, inferior rectus, and inferior oblique extraocular muscles and the striated muscle of the levator palpebrae superioris. The parasympathetic nerve fibers that travel with the oculomotor nerve innervate the constrictor pupillae and ciliary muscles.

Oculomotor nerve palsy causes a characteristic clinical picture: outward and downward deviation of the eye, ptosis of the eyelid, and, in cases of complete palsy, dilation of the ipsilateral pupil. Isolated oculomotor nerve palsies due solely to traumatic brain injury are not unusual, occurring in 17% of patients in one study of neuroophthalmic findings after closed head injuries.[53] Of interest, bilateral oculomotor nerve palsies also occurred in 17% of patients in the same study. Parinaud syndrome, the paralysis of upward gaze, is caused by injury to the dorsal midbrain, not to the peripheral oculomotor nerves. It often is accompanied by mydriasis, loss of convergence, and loss of pupillary light reflexes. Presumed oculomotor nerve palsy may result from an orbital blowout fracture. The simultaneous finding of infraorbital numbness argues against an oculomotor palsy[38] and suggests the diagnosis of orbital blowout fracture. Rare reports of internuclear ophthalmoplegia caused by head trauma have been summarized by Baker.[4]

Clinical testing of oculomotor function in the conscious patient is not difficult. In the unconscious patient, information is gathered during the performance of other tests, such as the doll's eye maneuver or pupillary light testing. Such tests must be performed serially, especially in the acutely injured patient, to ensure that an expanding lesion, uncal herniation, and/or hemorrhage is not overlooked. Return of function may begin within 2–3 months of injury but remains incomplete; aberrant regeneration of the nerve has been reported.[50]

Trochlear Nerve (Cranial Nerve IV)

The nucleus of the trochlear nerve lies anterior to the central gray matter in the area of the inferior colliculus, immediately caudal to the third nerve nucleus, near the midline. Axons from the nucleus loop posteriorly to decussate in the tectum of the lower midbrain. They emerge from the superior medullary velum, coursing around the cerebral peduncle, and penetrate between the superior cerebellar and posterior cerebral arteries lateral to the third nerve. The trochlear nerve pierces the dura of the cavernous sinus and courses along its superior margin to the superior orbital fissure. It innervates the superior oblique muscle, which turns the eye downward and outward.

Although the trochlear nerve is traumatically injured less frequently than other ocular nerves, trauma accounts for a greater percentage of trochlear injuries (compared with oculomotor and abducens injuries) than any other cause.[8,38] Injury to the trochlear nerve

may be subtle. The patient may complain of vertical diplopia on looking downward. When the patient is tested with gaze downward and inward, contralateral head tilt improves the diplopia, whereas ipsilateral head tilt worsens it.[37] Disruption or dislocation of the orbital pulley, which acts as the fulcrum for the action of the superior oblique muscle, must be considered as a cause for an apparent trochlear nerve injury.

Abducens Nerve (Cranial Nerve VI)

The nucleus of the abducens nerve lies beneath the fourth ventricle in the pons. Nerve fibers extend anteriorly, coursing through the corticospinal tract and exiting from the pontomedullary junction. The nerve travels along the floor of the posterior fossa to the lateral wall of the cavernous sinus, where it travels medial to the oculomotor and trochlear nerves along the ventral aspect, through the superior orbital fissure to the lateral rectus muscle. The lateral rectus muscle turns the eye outward.

In a complete injury to the abducens nerve, the affected eye is turned medially, whereas in an incomplete injury the eye is seen in midline at rest, but the patient is unable to deviate the eye laterally. The patient may tend to hold her or his head turned toward the affected side and, on testing, may be unable to abduct the affected eye.

Combined Traumatic Injuries

Combined traumatic injuries to the ocular motor nerves are quite common in patients with cranial nerve injury.[27,31,48,52,53,57] Concurrent involvement of the sixth and fourth cranial nerves is frequent, as are bilateral abducens and/or bilateral trochlear palsies. Concomitant injury to the abducens and trochlear nerves in the same eye may present quite a diagnostic puzzle, especially in the patient who is comatose or just emerging from coma. The presence of ocular motor injury is best followed by serial diplopia fields. Of course, with any significant blow to the head, a computed tomography (CT) scan of the brain should be done emergently. CT or magnetic resonance (MRI) scan also may help to delineate causes of delayed dysconjugate gaze in the comatose patient. Frequently, periorbital edema and orbital wall fractures, which may entrap extraocular muscles and limit their ability to move the globe, confuse the diagnosis of ocular motor nerve injury. Cavernous sinus thrombosis, which is rarely reported, merits emergent surgical correction.

Other causes of ocular motor nerve palsy include congenital disorders, multiple sclerosis, myasthenia gravis, diabetes mellitus, neoplasm, aneurysm,[48] and tumor.[21] Although these causes are not likely in a patient with traumatic brain injury, their absence should not be assumed if clinical findings of other disease processes are present or difficult to exclude.

Treatment

Treatment depends on the cause of the dysfunction. Monocular diplopia may result from a refractive error, cataract, or dry eye state,[31] and treatment should be directed to the cause. In patients with binocular diplopia, an eyepatch is an easy and inexpensive, although not functionally optimal, means of correction while the patient waits for spontaneous recovery. Current physiatric practice should emphasize preservation of binocular vision in such patients when possible; fresnel prisms may be required for correction of mild-to-moderate diplopia.[47] Botulinum toxin injection should also be considered as a treatment option for neurogenic diplopia.

The loss of depth perception, particularly in the presence of associated balance disorders, may cause significant difficulties with mobility and ambulation because of altered perception of midline. Reading and visual scanning abilities are also likely to be affected. Frequent reevaluations by a neuroophthalmologist or neurooptometrist to change the lenses may be necessary during the early phases of recovery.[46,47] Most cases of binocular diplopia respond to the "tincture of time"[53]; only a small percentage require surgical correction. Surgical intervention usually should be postponed for at least 9–12 months after injury to allow sufficient spontaneous recovery and accommodation.

Surgery, usually nonemergent, may be needed to repair an orbital wall fracture with entrapment of an extraocular muscle or dislocation of the trochlear pulley mechanism. Steroids often are used initially in comatose patients to reduce cerebral edema and

certainly may help to reduce swelling in periorbital tissues and nerves. Daily evaluation of ocular motor function after a severe head injury is necessary to protect remaining function and to diagnose deterioration in status.

Trigeminal Nerve (Cranial Nerve V)

The trigeminal nerve has both motor and sensory function. The motor fibers supply innervation to the muscles of mastication - the masseter, temporalis, and medial and lateral pterygoid muscles. The motor fibers also innervate several smaller muscles - the tensor tympani, tensor veli palatini, mylohyoid, and anterior belly of the digastric.

The sensory fibers mediate light touch and proprioception (principal sensory nucleus), pain and temperature (nucleus of the trigeminal spinal tract), and primary sensation from the mandibular nerve (mesencephalic nucleus). The trigeminal nerve supplies sensation to the skin of the face from the angle of the jaw to the vertex of the scalp anteriorly; the mucous membranes of the mouth and anterior two-thirds of the tongue (not taste); the mucous membranes of the sinuses, the cornea, conjunctiva, and iris; and the dura mater of all three cranial fossae (through its three divisions, the mandibular, maxillary, and ophthalmic nerves).

Clinical testing of the trigeminal nerve involves testing of all three divisions for light touch, pinprick, and vibratory and temperature sensations along all of the peripheral pathways. The cornea can be tested for sensation with a wisp of cotton. Corneal sensation is a crossed reflex and involves motor nerve responses from the facial nerve (cranial nerve VII). Thus, touching one cornea lightly normally evokes prompt closure of both eyelids. Trigeminal and facial nerve palsies can be distinguished with careful testing (Table 1).

The presence of either trigeminal or facial nerve paresis may cause corneal drying and/or corneal abrasions in association with marked scleral injections. Pain may be present in patients who are alert and have intact trigeminal function. Treatment may be as simple as providing copious eye irrigation with a normal saline solution and lubricant gel with patching of the affected eye,

TABLE 1. Eyelid Response to Corneal Testing

	Ipsilateral	Contralateral
Normal response	Closed	Closed
Trigeminal paresis	Open	Open
Facial paresis	Open	Closed

especially at night. If irritation continues, lateral or complete tarsorrhaphy becomes the treatment of choice to avoid corneal ulceration and development of corneal opacities.

Some patients develop decreased salivation as a result of trigeminal injury. Frequent consumption of water or use of sugarless chewing gum often helps. Although synthetic saliva is marketed (e.g., Orex, Xero-lube, Moi-stir, Mouthkote), it is poorly accepted by most patients, who prefer throat lozenges.

The most common injuries to the trigeminal nerve occur with trauma to the superior orbital rim and result in anesthesia of the forehead, eyebrow, and/or nose. Such injuries tend to occur in motor vehicle accidents, unprotected falls, and golfing and baseball injuries. The peripheral branches of the trigeminal nerve may be injured with any type of superficial blow to the face. Numbness typically follows the distribution of the peripheral branch, but numbness or dysesthesias in the mucous membranes also may occur.

Injuries of the gasserian ganglion are rare in patients with blunt head trauma.[38] Although fractures through the petrous bone occur with modest frequency, the ganglion often escapes injury. Penetrating wounds involving the gasserian ganglion also are rare but may cause severe dysesthesias. As with other causes of trigeminal dysesthesias, patients may respond well to the use of carbamazepine, valproic acid, or some of the less sedating tricyclic antidepressants.[54] An inability to look upward, coupled with infraorbital numbness, should raise suspicion of an orbital floor fracture with entrapment of the inferior rectus muscle.

Facial Nerve (Cranial Nerve VII)

The facial nerve is also a mixed motor and sensory nerve. The facial nerve exits the cranium through the stylomastoid foramen,

passes through the parotid gland, and innervates the muscles of facial expression, the posterior belly of the digastric muscle, the stylohyoid, and platysma muscles. It also provides sensory fibers to the tongue, lacrimal gland, submandibular and sublingual salivary glands, and a small portion of skin near the external ear.[39]

Cranial trauma resulting in fracture of the base of the skull frequently injures the facial nerve. Longitudinal fractures account for up to 90% of temporal bone fractures,[32] whereas transverse fractures account for 10–30%.[60] Injury to the facial nerve may result in complete or partial paralysis; onset of paralysis is immediate with tears of the nerve or bony impingement but delayed (longer than 4–6 days) with formation of edema within the epineurium or hematoma. Fisch[23] described surgical findings in 40 patients with facial paralysis and found that more than 90% of injuries due to either transverse or longitudinal fractures occurred in the labyrinthine segment of the facial nerve. Other investigators[11] have found smaller percentages in the labyrinthine segment. Electromyography and nerve conduction studies that compare ipsilateral to contralateral facial nerves are useful to document the severity of axonal loss and to help to determine the need and timing of any surgical procedure.[23]

Depending on the site of injury, hearing may be affected by paralysis of the stapedial reflex, which results in hyperacusis. The sense of taste also may be affected on the ipsilateral tongue, although this abnormality may be difficult to perceive for the patient with only a unilateral facial nerve injury. An unusual or impaired sense of taste may be due to injury of either the facial or olfactory nerve.

Although many traumatic facial nerve injuries resolve without surgery, surgical intervention is indicated in certain cases, which usually involve suspected complete transection of the nerve or delayed onset due to swelling with loss of greater than 90% of the evoked motor unit action potential.[23] In patients with delayed onset due to swelling, decompression of the nerve is usually satisfactory, whereas in patients with complete transection surgical revision and reanastomosis may be required. The recent advent of cable nerve grafts (from the sural or other nerves) for patients in whom anastomosis cannot be accomplished holds the promise of at least partial return of facial nerve function. Other procedures include anastomosing the ipsilateral accessory or hypoglossal nerves to the distal portion of the affected facial nerve, with extensive therapy and reeducation to train the patient to use the substituted nerve for new "facial nerve" function.

When surgery is not indicated or must be delayed, treatment includes the generous use of sterile eye drops and ointments to maintain the integrity of the cornea of the involved side. Taping the eye closed at night is helpful. Occasionally, a lateral lid tarsorrhaphy is needed for adequate protection of the cornea in complete paralysis. In some instances, the use of transcutaneous facial muscle stimulation to retard atrophy of the affected muscles may be of benefit until recovery occurs spontaneously, although this technique is often poorly tolerated unless the ipsilateral trigeminal nerve also has been injured. Transcutaneous stimulation in patients with complete and prolonged paralysis without surgery is generally not recommended because of the poor prognosis for recovery of nerve function. With recovery of function, exercises in front of a mirror may help with muscle strengthening and symmetry of use. Procedures for facial reanimation, such as seven-to-seven reanastomosis and seven-to-twelve nerve grafts, should be considered in patients with significant peripheral involvement of cranial nerve VII. In addition, gold weights may be surgically placed in the eyelid to help with upper lid closure and to minimize risk for corneal abrasion and exposure keratitis.

Vestibulocochlear Nerve (Cranial Nerve VIII)

The vestibulocochlear nerve, which is purely sensory, serves two different functions: (1) audition and (2) linear and angular acceleration of the head. Because the facial nerve and vestibulocochlear nerve travel together through the internal auditory canal, injuries that damage the facial nerve also may injure the vestibulocochlear nerve. Because of the positioning of the cochlear and labyrinthine structures within the temporal bone, the auditory and vestibular end organs may be concussed or disrupted. Longitudinal fractures, which occur in 70–80% of cases, may disrupt the tympanic membrane, among other injuries, but rarely injure the inner ear because of the extreme hardness of the labyrinthine capsular bone.[32] Cochlear concussion, however, may cause mild-to-moderate sensorineural hearing loss. Transverse fractures frequently extend across the petrous pyramid and fracture the labyrinthine capsule, thus involving the semicircular canal, vestibule, and cochlea.

Hearing is commonly tested clinically with tuning forks via the Weber and Rinne tests; in the nonresponsive patient more obvious physical signs, such as otorrhea due to cerebrospinal fluid, hemotympanum, or Battle's sign (bruising over the mastoid), must be sought. In the comatose patient, brainstem auditory evoked responses (BAERs) may be used to determine the relative intactness of the auditory pathway. In the conscious patient, BAERs may be helpful in assessing hearing acuity, vertigo and balance disturbances, nausea, dizziness, and tinnitus. Full audiologic testing may be necessary to determine the presence and extent of hearing loss. In more significant posttraumatic sensorineural deafness, a hearing aid may help to understand verbal information and to respond more appropriately in social situations.

Clearly, the most common problem related to the vestibulocochlear nerve after traumatic injury is positional vertigo, which occurs with sudden changes in position, most commonly from lying to sitting or from sitting to standing. The vertigo usually lasts about 30 seconds and generally requires no treatment other than to warn the patient to halt at the new position until the sensation has passed. Medications should be evaluated to ensure that the sensation is not worsened as a side effect of one or more medications. Positional vertigo usually resolves with time and requires no specific treatment, although positional exercises may facilitate accommodation to the problem.[7] Most forms of vestibular habituation training attempt to overstimulate the vestibular response, thereby promoting habituation. Such therapy may cause the patient to become quite nauseated during exercise by induction of the movements that cause vertigo. Continued therapy should result in decreased vestibular responses to triggering movements and thus to a decrease in functionally significant vertigo.

In patients with extreme symptoms (e.g., travel-induced emesis), meclizine, scopolamine patches, or other vestibular suppressant medications may be tried. Travel-induced emesis usually resolves rather quickly, with or without treatment. Although the patient's family may be highly disturbed by the disorder, surprisingly the patient often is not, because no sense of nausea or vertigo may precede the episode of emesis. The goal, however, should be to use vestibular suppressant medications only for short periods of time and only if they are absolutely necessary; according to theory, based on available animal studies, such medications may slow habituation.

In the patient with hearing loss or traumatic deafness, ossicular chain disruption must be considered.[32] Any patient with abnormal findings on clinical hearing tests should be referred for more extensive evaluations. Surgical repair of ossicular chain disruption is usually successful, although in some patients the disorder will "self-correct."

A perilymph fistula should be considered in a patient who complains of dizziness, hearing loss and/or tinnitus, and other unusual auditory sensations.[38,63] Accurate diagnosis and treatment for this disorder remain controversial. Ultimately, if the patient is unresponsive to conservative management, surgical intervention to seal the leak in the round or oval window is typically recommended.[63]

Glossopharyngeal Nerve (Cranial Nerve IX), Vagus Nerve (Cranial Nerve X), and Spinal Accessory Nerve (Cranial Nerve XI)

The glossopharyngeal nerve provides (1) general cutaneous function and taste to the posterior one-third of the tongue and (2) sensation to the soft palate, pharynx, faucial tonsils, tragus of the ear, and nasopharynx. Its tympanic branch supplies sensation to the tympanic membrane, eustachian tube, and mastoid area. Chemo- and baroreceptors are also carried by the glossopharyngeal nerve from the carotid body and carotid

sinus. Its motor fibers innervate the stylopharyngeus muscle and, along with the vagus nerve, the pharyngeal constrictor muscles. Parasympathetic secretory and vasodilatory fibers travel to the parotid gland.

The vagus nerve also contains motor, sensory, and parasympathetic nerve fibers. Its rootlets emerge from the lateral medulla and pass with the glossopharyngeal and accessory nerves through the jugular foramen. The vagus nerve supplies motor fibers to the striated muscles of the pharynx and soft palate (excepting the tensor veli palatini and stylopharyngeus). Through the superior laryngeal and recurrent laryngeal nerves, the vagus nerve supplies all of the striated muscles of the larynx and also innervates all of the smooth muscle of the pharynx, larynx, and thoracoabdominal viscera. Sensory fibers innervate the skin of the concha of the external ear, the dura mater of the posterior fossa, the pharyngeal plexus, larynx, and thoracoabdominal viscera. Parasympathetic fibers innervate the cardiac plexus and thoracoabdominal viscera.

The accessory nerve is a purely motor nerve that has two parts: (1) the cranial part arises from the caudal medulla to emerge from the lateral medulla, and (2) the spinal part arises from the accessory nucleus located in the dorsolateral part of the spinal cord from the first through the sixth cervical cord segments. After emerging from the spinal cord and ascending through the foramen magnum, the spinal part joins with the cranial part to pass through the jugular foramen with the glossopharyngeal and vagus nerves. The cranial part, in conjunction with the vagus nerve, innervates the pharynx and larynx, whereas the spinal part penetrates and supplies the sternocleidomastoid muscle and terminates in the trapezius muscle.

Injury to any of these nerves causes weakness on the ipsilateral side. Injury to the brainstem by contusion or infarction may injure only the nuclei of the glossopharyngeal and vagus nerves, resulting in dysphagia and dysarthria. Injury to the vagus nerve, especially the recurrent laryngeal nerve, may result in aphonia or weak or hoarse voice with unilateral paralysis of the vocal fold. Except for stab wounds to the neck, which may injure only one or two of these cranial nerves, injury to one is generally accompanied by injury to all. This is especially true of basilar skull fractures that pass through the jugular foramen (Vernet's syndrome) and, on rare occasions, applies to cervical hyperextension (whiplash) injuries.[31] The Collet-Sicard syndrome, characterized by unilateral involvement of the last four cranial nerves, occurs rarely in traumatic brain injury[62] and usually is associated with fractures of the occipital bone. Other causes of lower cranial nerve injury include cervical fractures,[28] cranial bullet wounds,[45] stab wounds, and other cranial fractures.

Treatment of glossopharyngeal and vagal injuries is largely symptomatic, although palatal and pharyngeal exercises may improve dysarthria.[15,49] Exercises for incomplete accessory nerve injury to improve strength and rapidity of contraction of the trapezius may be quite helpful. Surgical repair of the accessory nerve after sectioning may be possible for cosmetic purposes in some patients.

Hypoglossal Nerve (Cranial Nerve XII)

The hypoglossal nerve innervates the intrinsic tongue musculature as well as the hypoglossus, styloglossus, genioglossus, and geniohyoid muscles.

Injury to the hypoglossal nerve causes dysarthria and swallowing difficulties. Testing shows weakness on the ipsilateral side, with protrusion of the tongue toward the side of injury by the unopposed, contralateral muscles. Injury to the hypoglossal nerve alone most often occurs with penetrating wounds to the neck and submental region. With blunt trauma, injury to the hypoglossal nerve most often is associated with other cranial nerve injuries. Exercises, as discussed above, for treatment of dysarthria help to improve tongue coordination and strength. Treatment of hypoglossal nerve injuries due to penetrating wounds is surgical, and the nerve tends to recover quite well.[1]

CENTRAL PAIN SYNDROMES

Pain and the perception of pain may be affected by traumatic brain injury. The mechanisms of pain and pain perception have undergone considerable redefinition in the past several years. No longer is all pain considered to be of peripheral causes, with central mechanisms relegated only to processing and switching functions. Even the widely accepted model proposed by Melzack and Wall[44] in 1965 allowed for "central control" over pain impulses, but this control was exercised in the dorsal column of the spinal cord, in the medial lemniscus, or, at its highest levels, in the brainstem and thalamus. Although researchers recognized that descending efferent fibers from the brain could influence afferent conduction, they believed that this influence played a role only in inhibiting input of painful impulses from peripheral nerves.

One occasionally encounters patients who develop central pain syndromes after traumatic brain injury. This condition is much more poorly understood than peripheral neuropathic pain syndromes, probably because of its lesser incidence and greater degree of heterogeneity in terms of pathophysiologic and pathoanatomic correlates. The bulk of current knowledge about central pain stems from animal studies and, to a lesser extent, psychophysical experimentation in humans.

Behavioral Neurology: Neuropathologic and Clinical Correlates

The major supratentorial structures that are potential generators of central pain after neurotrauma are thalamic and suprathalamic. Lesions affecting the thalamic sensory nuclei cause a relatively complete loss of all forms of general somatic afferent sensation in the contralateral face, trunk and limbs. Such lesions may cause severe dysesthetic pain in the area of sensory loss. Thalamic lesions are by far the most commonly reported cause of posttraumatic central pain syndromes. Such lesions produce severe superficial and deep hemianesthesia, sensory ataxia, and intractable pain; typically they are associated with mild hemiplegia, sometimes in the presence of a movement disorder, most frequently choreoathetosis. Thalamic infarction most often occurs after occlusion of the posteroinferior cerebellar artery secondary to herniation. Vascular insults typically produce the predominant injury to the ventroposterolateral and ventroposteromedial nuclei with relative sparing of the medial nuclei.[34] An interesting clinical sign sometimes observed in thalamic infarction, with or without thalamic pain, is the so-called thalamic hand.[17]

Suprathalamic syndromes typically involve thalamocortical pathways or the end fields of this system. In addition, recent research in humans suggests a role for both the retroinsular and anterior cingulate cortices in the conscious appreciation of pain.[6] Suprathalamic lesions causing pain are exceptionally rare but have been reported after trauma. In contrast to the dense loss of sensation found with thalamic lesions, suprathalamic lesions tend to be characterized by only minimal involvement of pain, temperature, touch, and vibratory sensibility and a severe deficit in the discriminative sensations that require cortical participation. The discriminative sensations include proprioception, two-point discrimination, localization of touch, and stereognosis. In such situations the primary modalities of superficial sensation are perceived and integrated at the thalamic level. Such sensory findings are often seen in patients with parietal lobe insult, and the deficit is typically termed cortical sensory deficit.

Irritative lesions located in the region of the post central gyrus may initiate seizures that manifest clinically as contralateral paresthesias. Lesions confined to the midbrain have not been reported to cause central pain. Vascular lesions affecting the pons and medulla may produce central pain and occasionally result from rotational shear injury and/or vascular shear injury after trauma.

As with neuropathic pain arising from damage to the primary sensory neuron, the pain may be accompanied by no clinically detectable sensory loss. In general there is no correlation between neurologic deficit and severity of pain. Thalamic pain usually involves some degree of early sensory loss, but this abnormality often improves and may resolve. Onset of pain is usually delayed by weeks or months.

Neurophysiology of Central Pain

Some of the theorized mechanisms by which central pain is generated include altered sensitivity of cells, changes in receptive fields, neurochemical alterations, morphologic changes associated with brain injury as well as central nervous system plasticity, and disinhibition of neural function at various levels. Not all plasticity that occurs within the brain is "good" plasticity; in fact, much of the recovery that occurs on a neuroplastic basis may be maladaptive, resulting in such negative clinical behaviors as spasticity, movement disorders, and central pain phenomena.

Multiple suprasegmental mechanisms mediate central pain perception. Several reciprocally connected brain regions form a central pain-controlling network. Some of the structures integral to this network include the cerebral cortex, thalamus, hypothalamus, brainstem, and dorsal horn. Particularly important components include the periacquaductal gray matter of the midbrain; the rostral ventromedial medulla, particularly the raphe nucleus, which produces serotonin; locus ceruleus; and adjacent medullary neurons that produce norepinephrine. All of these components contain significant amounts of opioid-containing structures that mediate analgesic effects and receive input from indirect, ascending nociceptive pathways. Such structures provide feedback inhibition of pain transmission and, when stimulated, produce analgesia and selectively affect pain transmission but do not affect transmission of nonnociceptive information.[59] Newer theories about central pain propose that reverberating localized corticothalamic loops may result in altered processing and production of persistent pain.[5,10]

Neurorehabilitative Treatment

Pharmacologic Management

Multiple therapeutic considerations must be kept in mind with regard to treatment of central pain. Pharmacologic management that includes use of tricyclic antidepressants and/or selective inhibitors of serotonergic reuptake, as well as anticonvulsants, should be considered. Probably the most appropriate medications for central pain states are the anticonvulsants. A trial of phenytoin (100 mg 3 times/day) may be advisable. Carbamazepine appears to be the most effective agent in pain states characterized by episodes of spasmodic pain. No therapeutic levels have been established for the antiepileptic drugs in this application. Dysesthetic pain, which tends to be more constant and relentless, generally resists treatment and may persist for years; patients may benefit from fluphenazine (1–8 mg/day), although this treatment is controversial.[41] Often fluphenazine is given synergistically with tricyclic or other traditional serotonergic agonist antidepressants to augment the clinical antinociceptive effect. Tricyclic antidepressants and related compounds, including newer agents such as selective serotonin reuptake inhibitors (SSRIs) and venlafaxine (with both catecholaminergic and serotonergic agonism), also may be used alone to treat central pain, including dysesthetic states. Mexiletine (a sodium channel blocker) has been found to modulate thalamic pain with minimal side effects.[3]

Other more controversial treatment strategies have been used in an attempt to control central pain states, including intravenous administration of lidocaine and calcitonin. Intravenous lidocaine infusions have been shown to provide good temporary relief in central pain states, particularly phantom pain.[20] Calcitonin appears to have a significant analgesic potential, possibly involving the modulation of descending pain perception control. It may be administered either as an injection or as a nasal spray (the latter is not available in the United States), but its relatively high cost may limit widespread use.[33]

Nonpharmacological Procedures

Neuroablative procedures such as neurectomy, rhizotomy, dorsal root entry zone lesions, anterolateral cordotomy, mesencephalotomy, thalamotomy, and leukotomy may be considered, although all have obvious risks. Probably the most commonly used neuroablative procedure for posttraumatic central pain disorders is thalamotomy; this procedure, however, which typically involves lesions of the ventroposteromedial and ventroposterolateral nuclei of the thalamus, may produce analgesia but often with loss of tactile and proprioceptive sensation. Lesions in the intralamellar group of nuclei may produce impressive selective analgesia; unfortunately, the effect often lasts only a few months. The

incidence of dysesthesias is lower with intralamellar lesions than with other types of neuroablative procedures, such as anterolateral cordotomy and mesencephalotomy.[6] More recent research regarding corticothalamic reverberatory loops suggests that selective stereotactic lesions of the deep frontoparietal corona radiata sensorimotor strip may achieve a permanent cure in central pain states.[10]

Multiple stimulation procedures also have been used for control of central pain, including transcutaneous electric nerve stimulation, acupuncture, and stimulation of the dorsal column, periaqueductal and periventricular gray matter, or thalamus. Recent work also has examined the beneficial effects of chronic motor cortex stimulation for the treatment of central pain.[61]

In general, ablative procedures in either the peripheral or central nervous system have a better effect on central than on neuropathic pain. Even with neuroablative procedures, analgesic effects tend to be short-lived and are commonly associated with dysesthesias, more so in some cases than in others. Stimulation procedures in general have not been found to work as well for central pain as for neuropathic pain. Central nervous system alterations secondary to sensory pathway lesions occur at levels far rostral to the original site of damage. The most significant of these changes in regard to pain is a shifting sensation, evoked by activity in many cells, from nonpainful to painful sensation. This change is typically combined with reduction in the number of normal inhibitory actions.

PERCEPTUAL DEFICITS

Agnosias

The Greek word agnosia, which means absence of knowledge, was introduced by Freud in 1891 to designate impaired recognition of a stimulus. This specific defect in object recognition is said to occur without associated disturbance in the primary sensory system. Agnosia classically has been divided into two main forms: apperceptive and associative. Apperceptive agnosia refers to a recognition impairment that was caused by disturbed integration of otherwise normally perceived components of a stimulus, whereas associative agnosia refers to defective recognition of normally perceived and normally integrated percepts. Associative agnosia is deemed the purer form of recognition impairment.[18] Theoretically, agnosia may occur in relation to any sensory modality, including visual, tactile, and auditory. Several specific types of agnosia are seen more commonly in association with particular types of focal brain injury; examples include prosopagnosia and finger agnosia.[16]

Tactile agnosia, the most common form of agnosia, is associated with lesions of the parietal post-rolandic cortex, which result in deficits of the contralateral upper extremity. Tactile agnosia is manifested clinically by astereognosis (inability to identify objects placed in the affected hand). Auditory agnosia rarely occurs alone and is typically seen in conjunction with other auditory processing disorders. The primary clinical characteristic is the patient's inability to differentiate between various nonverbal sounds despite the concurrent ability to perceive the same sounds. Although it has not been definitively proved, bilateral temporal lobe lesions are probably required to produce this neurobehavioral abnormality.[22]

Visual agnosia occurs when normal visual perception is accompanied by the inability to recognize visual stimuli. Like auditory agnosia, visual agnosia is relatively rare, but it has been better established clinically. Apperceptive visual agnosia has been theorized to be neuropathologically correlated with dysfunction of the bilateral visual association cortices. Associative visual agnosia is a type of disconnection syndrome between the visual and language systems. The patient recognizes the object in question but is unable to name it. The neuropathologic basis presumed responsible for this condition has been theorized to result from occlusion of the left posterior cerebral artery and subsequent infarction of the left occipital lobe and the posterior corpus callosum.

Prosopagnosia is the neurobehavioral syndrome associated with nondominant parietal lobe involvement and manifests clinically as the inability to recognize familiar faces and/or objects. Patients can perform generic recognition but are unable to recognize specific members within the generic class. Problems with color agnosia and alexia are not uncommon in this subgroup. Whereas common parlance assumes that the neuropathologic correlate for prosopagnosia is in the nondominant parietal lobe, research has shown that enduring prosopagnosia is typically associated with bilateral lesions in the inferomesial visual association cortices or their adjacent white matter. The most common cause for the condition is embolization of the posterior cerebral artery circulation. On rare occasions, it may be seen as an ictal phenomenon related to bilateral foci.

Finger agnosia occurs both within and outside the patient's frame of reference. It is most commonly noted during testing of the middle, index, and ring fingers, but all 5 digits may be involved. The responsible lesion is most often in the angular gyrus of the dominant parietal lobe.

Neglect and Hemiinattention

Neglect is a neurobehavioral phenomenon associated with normal sensorimotor function and the inability to report, respond, or orient to novel or meaningful stimuli presented to the side opposite a brain lesion.[30] The basic mechanism accounting for neglect is faulty mediation of both sensory and motor intention. Attention and intention deficits may occur in both spatial and personal domains. Unilateral neglect has been found to be correlated with lesions in the posterior parietal cortex (generally, nondominant), lateral prefrontal cortex, cingulate gyrus, striatum, and thalamus. Various degrees of neglect occur along a neurobehavioral spectrum from extreme neglect to extinction only with double simultaneous stimulation. Somewhere in the middle of this spectrum is the phenomenon of hemiinattention. Patients with unilateral neglect are most inattentive to contralateral stimuli but typically display a lesser degree of ipsilateral inattention. Commonly associated with neglect are other neurobehavioral traits, including anosognosia or explicit verbal denial of illness or deficit. Verbal acknowledgement of the problem but lack of associated concern is termed anosodiaphoria. Patients with alloesthesia misplace the location of the stimulus to the normal side when the side contralateral to a lesion is stimulated.[30]

When testing for neglect, the examiner should assess at least three sensory modalities, preferably touch, vision, and audition. Delaying response time and using distractors aid in amplification of the deficits if they are present. Stimuli should be presented bilaterally and randomly as well as simultaneously. Whereas normal subjects may extinguish to bilateral heterologously applied stimuli (application of bilateral simultaneous stimuli to two different body parts), they should not extinguish to bilateral homologously applied stimuli. Simultaneous bilateral heterologous stimulation sometimes is used to assess for milder forms of extinction.

A clinical caveat in the assessment of auditory inattention is that unilateral hearing loss is almost always due to peripheral dysfunction rather than hemiinattention secondary to the manner in which auditory pathways ascend bilaterally from the brainstem to the cortex (implying that each ear projects to both hemispheres). Thus, a unilateral central nervous system lesion is expected to produce bilateral, *not* unilateral, hearing loss.

In general, neglect and hemiinattention tend to improve over time whether related to traumatic brain injury or cerebrovascular accidents. The exact neuroplastic event responsible for this recovery is unclear. Several rehabilitative interventions have been used to improve the functional disability produced by neglect and its associated syndromes. Such traditional rehabilitation approaches as "anchoring" and "scanning" may be attempted[25]; however, the degree to which these skills generalize to real-world function is probably suboptimal. Neuropharmacologic remediation with dopamine agonists also may be attempted.[24,42] Most of the studies examining drug treatment for neglect have focused on bromocriptine. One group also demonstrated the beneficial effects of vestibular stimulation in treatment of neglect.[51]

Visuoperceptual Disorders

Bilateral visual cortex damage may produce so-called cortical blindness. A type of visual agnosia involving denial of blindness has been associated with this condition and eponymously named Anton's syndrome. Not uncommonly, both denial and blindness are transitory. Such patients often make excuses for their "misperceptions" and may be quite confabulatory. Anton's syndrome may occur with syndromes of posterior fossa herniation, which result in occlusion of the posterior cerebral artery.[26]

One of the classic disorders of spatial analysis is Balint's syndrome, which is marked by the clinical triad of visual disorientation, optic ataxia evidenced as deficient visual reaching, and ocular apraxia, which takes the form of visual scanning deficits. The visual disorientation, also termed simultanagnosia, may or may not be associated with concurrent visual field deficits. Balint's syndrome is hallmarked by the inability to perceive the visual field in its entirety, which produces unpredictable perception and recognition of field components. Associated symptoms include the inability to shift gaze at will toward new visual stimuli and impaired target pointing under visual guidance. Bilateral parietooccipital damage is usually necessary to generate the full neurobehavioral syndrome. Such lesions are probably most commonly generated from ischemic brain injury secondary to hypoperfusion and watershed infarctions of the posterior circulation.[29]

Other perceptual disorders that may be seen after brain injury include pure alexia, topographic disorientation, disordered color perception, and disturbances of stereopsis. Clinicians in the field of brain injury rehabilitation must be familiar with the assessment, treatment, and prognostic implications of these varied perceptual disorders.

Alexia, also called alexia without agraphia or "word-blindness," is a neurobehavioral disorder characterized by recognition of disordered visual patterns. Of interest, patients with alexia can copy what they are unable to read. Lesions that cause a disconnection syndrome between visual association areas and the dominant temporoparietal-based language centers produce pure alexia. Typically, both intrahemispheric and interhemispheric disconnections are responsible for the production of pure alexia.[43]

Topographic disorientation is likely to result from deficits in visuospatial memory.

This disorder may manifest clinically as difficulty with driving from one place to another, inability to find one's way back to one's room, and impairment in giving directions verbally. This condition must be differentiated from the more common condition of geographic disorientation, which denotes the inability to identify cities on a map or to draw a state or other map.[56]

Several disorders involving color perception may be observed after brain injury. Achromatopsias are acquired disorders of color perception that involve all or part of the visual field but preserve the vision of form. Typically, such disorders are caused by damage to the visual association areas. Fullfield achromatopsia is generally seen in association with visual agnosia; however, hemiachromatopsias also may be observed, often related to the contralateral inferior occipitotemporal cortex. Other disorders of color perception and processing include impaired color naming (also called color agnosia) in the absence of color perception defects or language-based dysfunction and impaired color association (i.e., the color of grass is ?).

Stereopsis, the ability to discriminate depth on the basis of binocular vision, is distinct from depth perception that depends on monocular information. In contrast to early research, the current theory is that both hemispheres have stereoptic ability. The exact neuroanatomic correlates of disturbances of stereopsis are not well understood.

Another interesting neurobehavioral manifestation that may take the form of visuoperceptual disturbance is the phenomenon of visual hallucinations in patients with occipital epileptic foci. Such visual hallucinations can be "seen" even in the blind hemifield when the function of visual association is preserved more anteriorly. The site of the seizure focus in the occipital lobe tends to be well correlated with the type of visual hallucination; specifically, posterior foci tend to produce fairly formless hallucinations composed of spots or flashes of light, whereas anterior foci tend to produce formed visual hallucinations.[56]

CONCLUSIONS

Sensory perceptual disorders after traumatic brain injury are extremely common. Clinicians involved in the management of patients with traumatic brain injury must have a clear understanding of the array of deficits that may follow such injuries, their underlying pathoanatomy and pathophysiology, appropriate diagnostic measures, and, of course, appropriate neurorehabilitative interventions.

REFERENCES

1. Alrich EM, Baker GS: Injuries of the hypoglossal nerve: Report of ten cases. Milit Surg 103:20–25, 1948.
2. Anderson RL, Panje WR, Gross CE: Optic nerve blindness following blunt forehead trauma. Ophthalmology 89:445–455, 1982.
3. Awerbuch GI, Sandyk R: Mexiletine for thalamic pain syndrome. Int J Neurosci 55:129–133, 1990.
4. Baker RS: Internuclear ophthalmoplegia following head injury. J Neurosurg 51:552–555, 1979.
5. Beric A: Central pain: "New" syndromes and their evaluation. Muscle Nerve 16:1017–1024, 1993.
6. Bowsher D: Pain syndromes and their treatment. Curr Opin Neurol Neurosurg 6:257–263, 1993.
7. Brandt T, Daroff RB: Physical therapy for benign paroxysmal positional vertigo. Arch Otolaryngol 106:484–485, 1980.
8. Burger LJ, Kalvin NH, Smith JL: Acquired lesions of the fourth cranial nerve. Brain 93:567–574, 1970.
9. Cain WS, Gent JF, Goodspeed RB, et al: Evaluation of olfactory dysfunction in the Connecticut Chemosensory Clinical Research Center. Laryngoscope 98:83–88, 1988.
10. Canavero S: Dynamic reverberation. A unified mechanism for central and phantom pain. Neurosurg Clin 42(3):203-207, 1994.
11. Cannon CR, Jahrsdoerfer RA: Temporal bone fractures: Review of 90 cases. Arch Otolaryngol 109:285, 1983
12. Costanzo RM, Heywood PG, Ward JD, et al: Neurosurgical application of clinical olfactory assessment. N Y Acad Sci 510:242–244, 1987
13. Costanzo RM, Zasler ND: Head trauma. In Getchell, et al (eds): Smell and Taste in Health and Disease. New York, Raven Press, 1991, pp 711–730
14. Crompton MR: Visual lesions in closed head injury. Brain 93:785–792, 1970
15. Daniel-Whitney B: Severe spastic-ataxic dysarthria in a child with traumatic brain injury: Questions for management. In Yorkston KM, Beukelman DR (eds): Recent Advances in Clinical Dysarthria. Boston, Little, Brown, 1989, pp 129–137
16. Damasio AR, Tranel D, Eslinger P: The agnosias. In Asbury, McKhann, McDonald (eds): Diseases of the Nervous System: Clinical Neurobiology, 2nd ed. Philadelphia, W.B. Saunders, 1992, pp 741–750.
17. de Castro-Costa CM, Do Vale OC, Siqueira Neto JI: An association of central post-stroke pain and thalamic hand. Arq Neuropsiquiatr 50:120–122, 1992.
18. de Renzi E, Lucchelli F: The fuzzy boundaries of apperceptive agnosia. Cortex 29:187–215, 1993.

19. Doty RL, Shaman P, Dann M: Development of the University of Pennsylvania smell identification test: A standardized microencapsulated test of olfactory function. Physiol Behav 32:489–502, 1984

20. Edmondson EA, Simpson RK, Stubler DK, Beric A: Systemic lidocaine therapy for post-stroke pain. South Med J 86:1093–1096, 1986.

21. Eyster EF, Hoyt WF, Wilson CB: Oculomotor palsy from minor head trauma. JAMA 220:1083–1086, 1972

22. Farach MJ: Agnosia. Curr Opin Neurobiol 2:162–164, 1992.

23. Fisch U: Facial paralysis in fractures of the petrous bone. Laryngoscope 84:2141–2154, 1974

24. Fleet WS, Valenstein E, Watson RT, et al: Dopamine agonist therapy for neglect in humans. Neurology 37:1765–1771, 1987.

25. Gordon WA, Ruckdeschel-Hibbard M, Egelko S, et al: Perceptual remediation in patients with right brain damage: a comprehensive program. Arch Phys Med Rehabil 66:353–359, 1985.

26. Gouvier WD, Cubic B: Behavioral assessment and treatment of acquired visuoperceptual disorders. Neuropsychol Rev 2:3–28, 1991.

27. Grundy DJ, McSweeney T, Jones HW: Cranial nerve palsies in cervical injuries. Spine 9:339–343, 1984.

28. Hammer AJ: Lower cranial nerve palsies: Potentially lethal in association with upper cervical fracture-dislocations. Clin Orthop Rel Res 266:64–69, 1991.

29. Hausser CO, Robert F, Giard N: Balint's Syndrome. Can J Neurol Sci 7:157–161, 1980.

30. Heilman KM, Valenstein E, Watson RT: Neglect. In Asbury, McKhann, McDonald (eds): Diseases of the Nervous System: Clinical Neurobiology, 2nd ed. Philadelphia, W.B. Saunders, 1992, pp 768–779.

31. Helliwell M, Robertson JC, Todd GB, et al: Bilateral vocal cord paralysis due to whiplash injury. BMJ 288:1876–1877, 1984.

32. Hough JVD, Stuart WD: Middle ear injuries in skull trauma. Laryngoscope 78:899–937, 1968

33. Jaeger H, Maier C: Calcitonin in phantom limb pain: A double blind study. Pain 48:21, 1992.

34. Jeanmonod D, Magnin M, Morel A: Thalamus and neurogenic pain: Physiological, anatomical and clinical data. Neuroreport 4:475–478, 1993.

35. Jefferson G, Schorstein J: Injuries of the trigeminal nerve, its ganglion and its divisions. Br J Surg 42:561–581, 1955.

36. Kase CS, Troncoso JF, Court JE, Tapia JF, Mohr JP: Global spatial disorientation. Clinicopathologic correlates. J Neurol Sci 34:267–278, 1977.

37. Keane JR: Neuro-ophthalmic signs and symptoms of hysteria. Neurology 32:757–762, 1982.

38. Keane JR, Baloh RW: Post-traumatic cranial neuropathies. Neurol Clin 10:849–867, 1992.

39. Kelly WM: Functional anatomy and cranial neuropathy. Neuroimaging Clin North Am 3: 29, 1993.

40. Leigh AD: Defects of smell after head injury. Lancet 1: 38–40, 1943.

41. Loeser JD: Herpes zoster and postherpetic neuralgia. Pain 25:149, 1986.

42. McNeny R, Zasler ND: Neuropharmacologic remediation of hemi-inattention following brain injury. NeuroRehabil Interdisc J 1:72–78, 1991.

43. Mani SS, Fine EJ, Mayberry Z: Alexia without agraphia: Localization of the lesion by computerized tomography. Comput Tomogr 5:95–97, 1981.

44. Melzack R, Wall PD: Pain mechanisms: A new theory. Science 150:971, 1965.

45. Mohanty SK, Barrios M, Fishbone H, et al: Irreversible injury of cranial nerves 9 through 12 (Collet-Sicard syndrome): Case report. J Neurosurg 38: 86–88, 1973.

46. Padula WV: Neuro-optometric rehabilitation for persons with a TBI or CVA. J Optometric Vision Develop 23:4–8, 1992.

47. Padula WV, Shapiro JB: Head injury and the post-trauma vision syndrome. RE:view 24:153–158, 1993.

48. Richards BW, Jones FR, Younge BR: Causes and prognosis in 4,278 cases of paralysis of the oculomotor, trochlear, and abducens cranial nerves. Am J Ophthalmol 113:489–496, 1992

49. Rosenbek JC, LaPointe LL: The dysarthrias: Description, diagnosis and treatment. In Johns DF (ed): Clinical Management of Neurogenic Communicative Disorders, 2nd ed. Boston, Little, Brown, 1985, pp 97–152

50. Rovit RL, Murali R: Injuries of the cranial nerves. In Cooper PR (ed): Head Injury, 3rd ed. Baltimore, Williams & Wilkins, 1993, pp 183–202

51. Rubens A: Caloric stimulation and unilateral visual neglect. Neurology 35:1019–1024, 1985.

52. Rush JA: Causes and prognosis in 4,278 cases of paralysis of the oculomotor, trochlear, and abducens cranial nerves [letter]. Am J Ophthal 114:777, 1992.

53. Sabates NR, Gonce MA, Farris BK: Neuro-ophthalmological findings in closed head trauma. J Clin Neuro-ophthalmol 11:273–277, 1991

54. Solomon S, Lipton RB: Facial pain. Neurol Clin 8:913–928, 1990.

55. Steinsapir KD, Goldberg RA: Traumatic optic neuropathy. Surv Ophthalmol 38:487–518, 1994.

56. Strub RL, Black FW: Neurobehavioral Disorders: A Clinical Approach. Philadelphia, F.A. Davis, 1988.

57. Summers CG, Wirtschafter JD: Bilateral trigeminal and abducens neuropathies following low-velocity, crushing head injury. J Neurosurg 50:508–511, 1979.

58. Sumner D: Post-traumatic anosmia. Brain 87:107–120, 1964.

59. Sweet WH: Deafferentation pain in man. Appl Neurophysiol 51:117–127, 1988.

60. Tos M: Fractures of the temporal bone: The course and sequelae of 248 fractures of the petrous temporal bone. Ugeskr Laeger 133:1449–1456, 1971

61. Tsubokawa T, Katayama Y, Yamamoto T, et al: Chronic motor cortex stimulation for the treatment of central pain. Acta Neurochir Suppl 52:137–139, 1991.

62. Wani MA, Tandon PN, Banerji AK, et al: Collet-Sicard syndrome resulting from closed head injury: Case report. J Trauma 31:1437–1439, 1991.

63. Zasler ND: Neuromedical diagnosis and treatment of post-concussive disorders. In Horn LJ, Zasler ND (eds): Rehabilitation of Post-Concussive Disorders. Philadelphia, Hanley & Belfus, 1992.

64. Zusho H: Posttraumatic anosmia. Arch Otolaryngol 108:90–92, 1982.

20

Gastrointestinal Complications of Traumatic Brain Injury

Of the approximately 400,000 new cases of head injury reported in the United States annually, gastrointestinal problems complicate about 50%, with impaired liver function at the top of the list.[127] Other frequently encountered difficulties include esophagitis, gastritis, duodenitis, peptic ulcer disease, decreased motility, malnutrition, dysphagia, vomiting, and diarrhea. As the push increases to move patients more rapidly from the acute care setting to rehabilitation facilities, much of the burden of diagnostic workups, as well as the design of appropriate treatment plans, necessarily becomes the responsibility of physiatrists. Kalisky et al.[127] reported that 6 of 11 patients with esophagitis, gastritis, or ulcer disease developed their problems on the rehabilitation unit. Therefore, it is important to understand fully the intricacies of the gastrointestinal system. The following sections address the issues of trauma associated with head injuries, normal and dysfunctional metabolism, methods of nutritional provision, and assessment techniques. Also discussed are dysphagia, posttraumatic vomiting, increased and altered bowel motility, ulceration and hemorrhage, and impaired function of the liver and pancreas.

NUTRITION

Traumatic brain injury creates multiple concerns about proper nutrition. Initially, during the acute phase of hypermetabolism and hypercatabolism, weight loss is a major issue. Brooke and Barbour[25,108] reported a mean weight loss of 29 pounds in a group of 57 head-injured patients. As the tissue breakdown continues, muscle wasting and atrophy become evident, and family members may become quite anxious. The most important reason to provide proper nutrition is to improve the clinical outcome of brain-injured patients. Young et al.[299] showed that neurologic recovery from brain injury occurs more effectively and more expediently in patients with better early nutritional support.

Complications of malnutrition are many. Generalized weakness becomes obvious as muscles deteriorate and endurance drops to almost nil. Protein depletion impairs fibroplasia and contributes to impaired or delayed wound-healing, a frequent finding in patients with decubitus ulcers.[6,238] As a result of decreased energy levels, patients become less active, with the potential complications of atelectasis, contractures, deep venous thromboses, and pulmonary emboli.

515

Malnutrition is the most common cause of decreased immunocompetence, especially involving the complement system, cell-mediated immunity, and diminished intracellular killing of ingested bacteria,[6,32,142,265] and, therefore, is related directly to the exaggerated risk of infection. In undernourished patients, the pulmonary system shows signs of impairment with decreases in vital capacity, surfactant production, and repletion of respiratory epithelium;[6,232] such patients are difficult to wean from ventilators. Gastrointestinal effects of inadequate dietary intake include loss of intestinal brush border, decreased enzymes of the brush border, flattened microvilli, and frequent development of diarrhea secondary to malabsorption.[6,129,133] Proper dosages and scheduling of medications are also influenced by poor nutrition because levels of bound and unbound medications vary widely with altered protein availability.

Mechanisms for Nutritional Supply

As previously discussed, trauma patients lose muscle mass secondary to hypermetabolism and resultant gluconeogenesis. Therefore, adequate calories and protein must be supplied if the patient is to recover and rebuild his or her tissues. If the self-destructive process of breakdown is not treated early, the mortality rate may be as high as 70–90%.[18] Bloomfield[18] recommended starting nutritional provisions either parenterally or enterally no later than the second day after injury. Controversy continues as to whether the optimal route for nutrition provision is parenteral or enteral.

The most obvious indication for total parenteral nutrition (TPN) is disruption of the gastrointestinal tract, which makes enteral delivery impossible.[97] In some studies,[37,67,117,278] 35–50% of brain-injured patients could not tolerate enteral nutrition by the first week after injury. Norton et al.[67,203] demonstrated that intolerance of enteral nutrition correlated with increased intracranial pressure and severity of traumatic brain injury. Even if the gut is anatomically intact, function is likely to be reduced in patients with severe traumatic brain injury.[18] Young et al.[299] supported the theory that more calories

can be provided via TPN, although he found no significant difference in neurologic outcome between parenterally and enterally fed patients at 6 months or 1 year after injury. Rapp et al.[226] disagreed, suggesting that outcome was better with TPN than with enteral feeding, although his work was not verified in the literature. Laboratory parameters showed a quicker rise in retinol-binding protein[6,165] in patients fed parenterally. TPN also was found to be safe, with no effect on intracranial pressure after brain injury.[297] Perhaps a reasonable approach to management was proposed by Ott et al.,[67,211] who suggested the initial use of TPN, with slow addition of enteral feedings and a gradual switch to provision of all nutrition via the gastrointestinal system. By studying the effects of TPN on hypoglycemia and hyperosmolality, Combs et al. found no increase in vasogenic edema in cold-injured rats. Their findings were disputed by Waters et al.,[284,297] whose work in cats suggested an increase in vasogenic edema with the administration of 35% dextrose immediately after cold injury to the brain. Several authors[193,251,297] suggested that hyperglycemia as a result of parenteral nutrition supply may lead to an accumulation of lactic acid. Other issues to be considered in TPN include the risks of both iatrogenic pneumothorax and sepsis secondary to contamination of the lines and the inadvertent administration of too much water, which may complicate the edema associated with increased intracranial pressure.

In support of using the gastrointestinal system for provision of nutrition in patients with brain injury, Hadley et al.[97] used the enteral route as their first choice. They reported lower cost, decreased complication rate, and adequate provision of calories and amino acids in support of their choice. If the patient's gastric function is still limited, Turner[275] and others[67] proposed that feeding into the small bowel is usually tolerated and provides a mechanism for moving the patient to enteral nutrition earlier.

Several methods are available for the provision of enteral nutrition. If the patient can tolerate oral feeding, certainly it is the best method, because it is more physiologic and the patient can ingest varying consistencies of food. However, oral feeding requires a higher level of cognitive functioning for safety. Alternative methods include nasogastric and nasojejunal feeding.[37,67] Complications to nasogastric and nasojejunal feeding include intracranial penetration by the tube, especially in patients with comminuted fractures involving the floor of the anterior cranial fossa or of the thin cribriform plate.[41,68,71,92,137,191,248] Severe maxillofacial trauma is a relative contraindication.[41,52,68,71,92,95,130–136,137,180,191] Alternate methods of gastric tube placement include orogastric intubation, fluoroscopically guided nasogastric intubation, and direct laryngoscopic visualization as the tube traverses the posterior pharynx.[41,71,92,248] Pharyngotomy provides an alternate to the usual placement, but it is not used frequently.[61] A critical concern in patients fed by a nasogastric tube is the possibility of aspiration. A few simple principles can help to minimize such risks, including continuous drip infusion; elevating the head of the bed to 30–45°; assessing proper tube placement, preferably by radiograph; checking residual volumes; and considering the use of nasojejunal tubes.[5,77] The use of nasojejunal feeding tubes provides the patient with adequate caloric provision, no aspiration, no problems with high gastric residuals or diarrhea, and less frequent dislodgement of the feeding tube.[67,89] On the other hand, nasojejunal feeding involves discomfort for the patient and is cosmetically less appealing to family members. More acceptable treatments include surgical insertion of a gastrostomy tube or percutaneous endoscopic placement by a gastroenterologist. A less common but also feasible possibility includes insertion of a feeding tube into the jejunum, although bolus feeds are more difficult with this method than with a stomach tube. The advantage, however, is reduced risk of aspiration.

Enteral feeding, however, involves certain risks. Bloomfield[18] reported a higher mortality rate at 18 days after injury in enterally fed patients than in parenterally fed patients. Sneed and Morgan[255] reported greater difficulty in maintaining levels of medication, particularly phenytoin, and in determining proper dosage requirements in patients on enteral feeding. Anderson[5] suggested that it is slightly more difficult to maintain a hyperosmolar state (> 295 mOsm)

in the plasma, which is desirable in brain-injured patients to help to control vasogenic edema. The clinician must determine the proper mechanism for provision of nutrition in each individual case, taking into account all of the applicable variables.

Normal Metabolism

To prepare for the discussion of altered metabolism secondary to traumatic brain injury, it is necessary to review the principles of normal metabolism. The human body is a watery structure (55%), anchored by organic material (40%) and minerals (5%).[133,232] The organic substances include carbohydrates in minimal reserve, proteins in moderate reserve, and fats in large reserve (larger in some than in others). According to Kaufman et al.[133] and Rowlands et al.,[237] an average man weighing 70 kg requires 7560 kJ/day of energy to meet his metabolic demands, including 100 gm of fats, 300 gm of carbohydrates, and 80 gm of proteins. His brain consumes about 25% of the energy and relies almost exclusively on glucose as its energy source. When oxygen is readily available, oxidation is the process by which glucose releases its power. In the event of restricted oxygen delivery, lactate accumulates and the system functions inefficiently.[133,237]

Dysfunctional Metabolism

Cuthbertson[45] first described the physiologic demands induced by injury in his classic studies of patients with fractures. Since that time, similar work has been completed by many other investigators.[53,135,187,291] In the discussion of metabolic changes after brain injury, hypermetabolism refers to the increased energy expenditure and caloric needs of the body, whereas hypercatabolism refers to increased urinary nitrogen and negative nitrogen balance secondary to tissue breakdown. These two processes, along with glucose intolerance, are the hallmarks of serious insult[77] in traumatic brain injury. In the earliest phase after injury, the local response is inflammatory, causing edema and depression of local metabolism (the ebb phase). The ebb phase does not persist for long, but moves into the flow phase, which results in generalized accelerated metabolism. A sympathetic rush results from the hyperactive autonomic state that follows traumatic brain injury.[36,38,77,108,132] This rush is reported to be twice as great as in other trauma and to persist 3 times longer.[108] The sympathetic activity stimulates mobilization of carbohydrate and fat stores and then rouses the protein reserves to release the amino acids, alanine and glutamine (the substrates necessary for liver gluconeogenesis to satisfy the needs of glucose-dependent tissues, such as the brain). Kaufman et al.[133] found that protein breakdown is an essential process and cannot be avoided even by massive intakes of calories and/or proteins. Acting in turn with the sympathetically mediated forces, the catabolic hormones (including epinephrine, norepinephrine, cortisol, glucagon, and growth hormone) increase in activity, and the storage hormones (such as insulin) diminish, resulting in further protein breakdown. The interaction of the catabolic hormones with interleukin-1 may be the impetus for the dramatic metabolic changes in head-injured patients. Ott et al.[209] reported increased levels of interleukin-1 in the cerebrospinal fluid of affected individuals. Numerous studies[57,278] indicate that protein may be the preferred energy source under severe stress such as brain injury.

Multiple factors are responsible for the increased metabolic demands in patients with traumatic brain injury. Decerebrate and decorticate posturing may consume up to 5,000 kcals/day[230,276] in energy requirements. Fever elevates the demand for energy by 13% for each degree Celsius above normal.[132,133,237,290] Other energy-expensive factors include hypoxia, shock, infection, seizures, burn fractures, steroids, and even fear.[10,20,31,97,132,192,207,226,230,237,244,290] Dehydration also leads to increased stimulation that increases metabolism. On the other hand, paralysis, sedation, and mechanical ventilation may decrease energy requirements.[133,277] As a general rule, Dempsey et al.[53] predicted an increased energy need of greater than 26% above the normal expected value in brain-traumatized patients with hypermetabolism. Early supplemental nutrition, therefore, is not only recommended but absolutely necessary.

Of all measures studied by Fruin et al.,[74] only motor activity correlated with the caloric needs of the patient. Equation 1 of the Harris-Benedict formula is frequently used to predict energy expenditure. Basal energy expenditure (BEE) is determined from specific dynamic action of food, activity, and "trauma factor":

$$BEE = 66.473 + 13.7516 \, W + 5.0033 \, HG - 6{,}755 \, A,$$

where W = weight in kg, H = height in cm, and A = age in years.[80,101,103,119,165,239,278] Although this system looks useful at first glance, it is difficult to apply, because the trauma factor has not been well characterized for brain injuries.

Further estimations of metabolic demands are also possible and necessary when planning the nutritional management of a patient with traumatic brain injury, including the required percentage of proteins, fats, and carbohydrates for complete fulfillment of metabolic needs as well as other constituents, such as vitamins, minerals, and water. To determine protein requirements, three methods are commonly used:

1. Established tables are available (for example, 1.3–3.0 gm of protein per kg body weight per day are required for adults with traumatic brain injury compared with 1 gm in unimpaired individuals).[18,276]

2. A ratio of protein to caloric intake may be applied with 1 gm nitrogen needed for every 630 kJ of energy expenditure.

3. The excretion of nitrogen or urea can be monitored.[18,37,176,278]

Supporting the idea that protein is the energy source of choice in patients with brain injury, Bivens et al.[17] showed that an excess of nonprotein calories did not prevent nitrogen wasting. Clifton et al.[38,57] reported the need for protein calories to be about 24% of the total intake for traumatic brain-injured patients. Piek et al.[219,220] showed that early feedings with 2,500–3,000 kcal/day and provisions of 1.5 mg/kg/day of amino acids can reduce the nitrogen deficit and improve the levels of serum proteins necessary for the manufacture of voluntary muscle and organ proteins. Twyman et al.[278] showed significantly higher daily and total nitrogen balances, despite higher levels of nitrogen excretion, in patients receiving at least 2.2 gm/kg/day of protein. Although nitrogen equilibrium is seldom reached, Clifton et al.[37] agreed that increasing the nitrogen content of feeding from 14% to 22% may somewhat improve nitrogen retention.

In addition to the preferred energy substrate protein, traumatically brain-injured patients also require approximately 1,800–2,500 nonprotein calories/day, which may be divided between carbohydrates and fats. Bloomfield,[18] Robertson et al.,[229] and Twyman and Bivins[276] suggested that this requirement translates to 30–35 nonprotein kcals/kg/day. As an example, a 70-kg patient requires at least 105 gm of protein (see above) and 2,100 kcals/day. Caution must be used, however, in providing nonprotein calories, because excessive carbohydrate calories may increase lipogenesis, especially in the liver. In turn, the increased fat deposition in the liver leads to changes in liver function that eventually may lead to liver failure if they are not monitored. Therefore, liver function tests should be performed every few days in patients receiving either parenteral or enteral support. Elevated liver function tests imply excessive carbohydrate calories. An alternative method is to monitor respiratory quotients (RQs), the ratio of carbon dioxide produced to oxygen consumed. The RQ of fats is equal to 0.7, whereas the RQ of carbohydrates is 1.0. An RQ approaching 1 signifies that the patient is burning fuel composed largely of carbohydrates. Through the work of Bloomfield[18] we are reminded that the RQ is approximately equal to 0.8 with a normal diet of mixed substrates.

Fat, the other component of nonprotein calories, provides approximately 40% of normal dietary intake.[18] Fat should provide 20–40% percent of nonprotein calories in a patient with traumatic brain injury. However, caution must be used in patients suffering from pancreatitis, in whom fat must be eliminated totally from the diet. In such patients a dietary consultation is helpful to determine a balance of nutrients in the nonfat diet to make up for the void.

Other nonorganic constituents must be included in the feeding of a patient with traumatic brain injury, including sodium, potassium (which has a larger reserve than sodium), manganese, zinc, iron, calcium, magnesium, and phosphorus. It is not uncommon to see low levels of zinc in the serum with associated high levels of zinc in the urine in patients with severe brain injury. Multivitamins, folic acid, vitamin B12, and vitamin K (aqua, mephyton) are usually added to the feedings once a week.[18] Yoshida et al.[296] suggested that vitamin E also may be helpful to stabilize membranes in patients with traumatic brain injury through physiochemical interaction with phospholipids. This theory came from his work with vasogenic edema in rats.

In an effort to prevent dehydration and to assist in maintaining adequate blood pressure and profusion, water is necessary for recovery in brain-injured patients. However, sodium-free water has to be limited to less than 75% of normal (30–35 cc/kg/day) so that the osmotic gradient does not push fluids into the extravascular space and increase cortical edema.[18] This safer intake should be limited to 20–25 ml/kg/day in brain-injured patients.

Attempts have been made to look at the advantage of supplying precursors and to examine their influence on neurotransmitter production in brain-injured patients in whom neurotransmitter deficiencies are suspected. The administration of precursors such as tyrosine, tryptophan, and choline is thought to influence the production of catecholamines, serotonin, and acetylcholine, respectively, in the central nervous system, because their production is largely substrate-dependent. It is hypothesized that if more neurotransmitters are produced, then more will be available for improving transmission across the synapse. Although the results of tyrosine administration have been less than exciting, numerous studies[77] have shown positive effects from supplying tryptophan and choline (or lecithin). For example, Gadisseux et al.[77] reported on the use of tryptophan for prevention of headache in patients with a history of migraines or for suppression of intention myoclonus in posthypoxic patients. They stated that choline is one of the most successful treatments of tardive dyskinesia. Much work still needs to be done, but the opportunities for improving outcome after traumatic brain injury remain promising.

The possible use of steroids in traumatized patients with brain injuries also merits consideration. Data compiled by Robertson et al.,[18,229] Ford et al.,[69] and Deutschman et al.[54,55] suggest that the use of corticosteroids in patients with traumatic brain injury has a negative effect on nitrogen balance and markedly prolongs the initial metabolic abnormalities. The work by Ford et al.[69] stated that the effects are even more pronounced in children. These authors advised against the use of steroids in patients with brain injury. According to Dickerson et al.,[57] glucocorticosteroid therapy is probably the most important reason why protein oxidation is the main fuel for patients with traumatic brain injury, because steroids increase urinary excretion of nitrogen by as much as 40–50%. On the other hand, Ott et al.[210,276] and Young et al.[298] found no difference in the nitrogen excretion and energy requirements among non–steroid-treated patients compared with steroid-treated counterparts. They theorized that the hypermetabolism in such patients is secondary to the head injury alone and not related to the use of steroids. Nonetheless, clinicians should be cautioned to consider the metabolic effect of steroids in patients with traumatic brain injury.

Assessment

Several parameters are available to determine the adequacy of nutritional supplementation in patients with traumatic brain injury. During the first 2 weeks after head injury, however, when metabolism is accelerated, traditional parameters are not applicable. Weight should be monitored initially and regularly. In the study by Hadley et al.,[97] weight loss of 9.0 kg occurred over the 14-day study period and was associated with a 13% fall in the serum albumin level in both the TPN and enteral nutrition subgroups. A similar state of catabolism secondary to traumatic brain injury was seen in both groups, as evidenced by creatinine excretion. Serum albumin levels have been one of the commonly used indicators of nutritional status. Because serum albumin has a half-life of approximately 21 days, however, it is less sensitive for reflecting acute changes in nutritional status. Starker et al.[264] and Young et al.[299] observed that positive nitrogen balance is not always associated with increases in serum albumin and suggest that changes in body water compartments alone may cause changes in serum albumin levels (regardless of nutritional status) in critically ill brain-injured patients. Because the half-life of albumin is relatively long, perhaps a better measure to evaluate acute changes in severely injured patients is retinol-binding protein, which has a shorter half-life of 12 hours.[6,165] Additional tests sometimes used to evaluate the nutritional status of patients include total protein, total lymphocyte count, transferrin (half-life of 8 days),[133,299] and thyroxin-binding prealbumin (half-life of 12 days). In addition, skinfold thickness at the area of the triceps or limb circumference in the mid-arm region (anthropometry) at days 1, 7, and 14 after injury have been followed by Young et al.[299]

Eventually, during recovery after traumatic brain injury, the affected body tissues restore themselves and usually overcompensate for their deficits by accumulating extra stores of fat. This process is complicated by well-meaning loved ones who supply "extra goodies" as gestures of kindness; meanwhile, the patient develops a more and more spherical shape.[127] Evidence also indicates that traumatic brain-injured patients may have impaired ability to regulate their intake of food during the chronic phase.[108] Reactive depression (particularly in patients with frontal lobe injuries,[108] which leads to increased impulsivity and impaired judgment) as well as psychosocial deficits[269] and alterations in social opportunities[62] influence the patterns of food intake. Generally speaking, an increase in caloric intake by 14%/day was seen in patients with chronic traumatic brain injury.[85,108]

Dysphagia

Dysphagia is defined as "a swallowing disorder characterized by difficulty in oral preparation for the swallow, or in moving material from the mouth to the stomach."[262,300] According to Field and Weiss,[64] patients with swallowing dysfunctions required more than twice as much inpatient rehabilitation as those without, at 126.7 days vs. 62.3 days after injury. By definition, damage to the central nervous system results in neurogenic dysphagia.[236,292] This deficit may be secondary to a number of problems, including decreased cognition because of cortical involvement; impaired reflexes secondary to brainstem lesions; damage to peripheral, sensory, motor nerves or nuclei; and damage to the receptors that act in a coordinated fashion to control this simple action, which normally lasts approximately 750 msec.[192,198,292]

Weinstein[292] reported that about one-fourth of patients with traumatic brain injury had neurogenic dysphagia. Decreased cognition was the most common reason for impaired swallowing, and the second most common was motor control deficits. This finding was supported clinically among patients with traumatic brain injury; 82% with cerebral problems also had swallowing disorders. Outcome studies are promising, however, as 94% of 201 patients in Weinstein's study eventually became successful oral eaters; the average time for return to oral feeding was about 3 months. As expected, associated improvements in cognition, reflexes, and clinical swallowing skills were observed.

Effects of Impairments on the Mechanisms of Swallowing

After traumatic brain injury dysphagia probably results from both decreased cognition and neurologic impairment of the structures involved in the swallowing process.[64] Certainly decreased ability to follow directions, impaired judgment as to the amount and rate of intake, and limited control of impulsivity are related to cognitive status and affect the success of therapy. Although the swallowing reflex is located in the reticular formation of the brainstem,[112,153] cognitive input controlling the voluntary movement of the tongue to initiate the swallow also plays a role. However, the neurologic substrate transferred from the cortex to the brainstem during the swallow reflex is not well understood.[124,153] The act of swallowing or deglutition can be studied in four separate phases that combine to make one coordinated swallow: (1) oral preparatory phase, (2) oral phase, (3) pharyngeal phase, and (4) esophageal phase.[64] Dysfunction in the system at any phase in the process may result in dysphagia

and thus lead to aspiration of food into the airway.

During the **oral preparatory phase**, food is placed into the mouth, moved about by actions of the tongue, lips, and cheeks, and masticated or chewed by the appropriate teeth. During this phase the food substances are mixed with saliva and formed into a cohesive bolus before swallowing.

During the **oral phase**, the tongue moves the food bolus from the anterior to the posterior aspects of the mouth until the swallow reflex is initiated at the anterior faucial arches. This phase generally takes 1 second at the most.[153,163] At the precise point when the bolus passes the back of the tongue, the swallowing reflex should trigger.[153] According to Lazarus and Logemann,[153] deficits are termed as mild (1–5 second increase in oral transit), moderate (5–10 second increase), and severe (> 10 seconds for completion of oral movement).

During the **pharyngeal phase** food is moved through the pharynx after the triggering of the swallowing reflex. Physiologically this phase includes elevation and retraction of the velum (thus closing the nasal pharyngeal passage), initiation of peristalsis through the pharynx, elevation and closure of the larynx, downward tilting of the epiglottis, cessation of respiration, and relaxation of the cricopharyngeal sphincter. The muscles of the pharynx and hypopharyngeal sphincter, which are striated and innervated by motor neurons primarily involving cranial nerves V, VII, IX, and X,[48,64] are involved in involuntary contractions that move the ingested material through the pharynx, past the hypopharyngeal sphincter, and into the esophagus. The pharyngeal transit time, which is usually 1 second,[153,168] is measured from the time the bolus passes from the back of the tongue until it passes the upper esophageal segment and enters the esophagus at the level of the cricopharyngeal junction. According to Lazarus and Logemann,[153] a delay in the triggering of the swallowing reflexes is also graded as mild (0–5 second delay), moderate (5–10 second delay), and severe (> 10 second delay).

During the **esophageal phase** the food is moved by peristaltic waves through the esophagus to the stomach. The upper third of the esophagus is skeletal muscle innervated by motor neurons. The muscle of the lower two-thirds of the esophagus and of the lower esophageal sphincter is smooth muscle, receiving its nerve supply via vagal cholinergic preganglionic fibers that synapse with short postganglionic fibers embedded in the wall of the lower esophagus.[48]

Clinical and Radiographic Tools to Assess Function and Impairment of Swallowing

The clinical bedside examination first described by Logemann[163,164] in 1983 is discussed in this section. Several other evaluations also are considered, including the most common instrumentation techniques—videofluoroscopy (modified barium swallow study), ultrasound, manometry, and manofluorography—as well as scintigraphy, fiberoptic endoscopic examinations, electroglottography, and electrography.

The components of the clinical bedside evaluation are multiple. Initially, the patient's chart must be reviewed, looking at such factors as medical diagnosis, presence or absence of pulmonary disease, vital signs (including respiratory rate), presence or absence of tracheostomy (if present, is it cuffed or uncuffed?), dietary habits, and laboratory reports. If possible, the next step is to interview the patient or the significant other (if the patient is aphasic or cognitively impaired). The interviewer should ask questions related to choking, coughing, gurgling sounds while eating or drinking, and any changes noted in speech or voice quality. Observation is another part of the clinical examination, in which the clinician evaluates the palate at rest and the larynx on dry swallows to see if it elevates as it should. The health of the mucosa and dentition as well as the amount of mucosal moisture also should be evaluated. The language and mental status should be assessed for breathiness, intensity, hoarseness, hypernasality, and efficiency of articulation. A detailed orofascial sensory and motor examination should follow, with particular attention to cranial nerves V, VII, IX, X, and XII. A cursory speech and voice analysis should be performed with a formal visualized laryngeal and acoustic analysis of voice,

if the equipment and facilities are available. Furthermore, mealtime observation with positioning so that the neck is not extended and with the patient sitting upright in bed is desirable, if at all possible. The skilled clinician, generally a speech pathologist, provides valuable information about the likelihood of swallowing pathology.[163,164,256]

A modified barium swallow study or video fluoroscopy, completed in the radiology department with the assistance of the speech-language pathologist, is the second study used to diagnose dysphagia.[116] Such studies can be reviewed both in slow motion and at normal speeds. Field and Weiss,[64] used the following eight abnormalities of swallowing function to evaluate the video fluoroscopy study, both qualitatively and quantitatively:

1. Prolonged swallowing reflex (>1 second) was seen in 88% of control patients, whereas reduced tongue control was seen in about 50% of patients studied by Field and Weiss and in about 85% of the 53 patients with head trauma studied by Lazarus and Logemann.[153]

2. Delayed or absent swallowing reflex was seen in 88% of Field and Weiss's patients[64] and 81% of Lazarus and Logemann's patients.[153]

3. Bolus entering the hypopharynx before initiation of swallow was seen in 38% of Field and Weiss's patients.

4. Pooling in the valleculae was seen in 63% of patients.

5. The swallowing mechanism was triggered at the piriform sinus in 50%.

6. Pooling in the piriform sinus was seen in 63%.

7. Aspiration of barium was noted in 38% of patients in both series.[64,153] The most common cause of aspiration in both groups was delayed or absent swallowing reflex. Unfortunately, many of the patients were "silent aspirators"; that is, although food was aspirated into the airway, they did not cough during or after aspiration. To avoid missing silent aspiration, video fluoroscopy is recommended in addition to the bedside clinical evaluation.[153] In the study by Lazarus and Logemann,[153] aspiration was defined as the entry of material into the airway below the level of the true vocal folds; it may occur before, during, or after the swallow. If aspiration occurs before the swallow, it is secondary

to reduced tongue control and/or impaired (either delayed or absent) swallowing reflex. Reduced laryngeal closure leads to aspiration during the swallow. Aspiration after the swallow occurs secondary to reduced peristalsis in the pharynx, unilateral paralysis of the pharynx, reduced laryngeal elevation, or cricopharyngeal dysfunction. In aspiration after the swallow, particles of food are left in the pharynx and may be inhaled into the airway. Aspiration is rated as mild (trace or less than 20%), moderate (20–30% aspirated), and severe (> 30% aspirated).[153] Clinicians also should be alerted to the possibility that tracheoesophageal fistula is the cause of aspiration, especially in patients who have been on the ventilator for prolonged periods or who suffered chest wounds in combination with brain injury.[153]

8. Reduced pharyngeal peristalsis is diagnosed when food is left in the valleculae bilaterally after the swallow. When residue remains in one side only, unilateral pharyngeal paralysis is diagnosed. When residual food is left in the piriform sinus, the diagnosis is cricopharyngeal dysfunction.

If a patient demonstrates at least one rating of severe swallowing problems in any of the three categories (increase in oral transit time, length of delay in triggering the swallow reflex, or severity of aspiration), the swallowing problem is labeled severe.[153] If two of the three categories are rated as moderate, the swallowing problem is moderate. And, if two or all three categories are rated as mild, the patient has a mild swallowing problem.[153] Moderate-to-severe swallowing problems were demonstrated primarily in patients who had increased intracranial pressure after trauma—a factor related to poor prognosis.[53,148,162,182] Patients with diffuse brain injury showed similar severity of dysphagia after trauma. The average patient with head trauma exhibited more than one swallowing difficulty.

Ultrasound was first used to visualize swallowing in the 1980s.[249,257,258,267] It has the obvious advantage of being totally noninvasive and can gather images from coronal, sagittal, parasagittal, and transverse planes. Such flexibility provides a method for evaluation of patients who are comatose or otherwise unable to cooperate. Normal foods and liquids may be used without adding contrast or radioactive materials, and studies may be repeated as often as necessary because the study itself is harmless. Ultrasound provides patients with safe and direct visualization of swallows and may be used as a biofeedback technique to assist in oral positioning during swallowing.

Manometry is used to assess pressure dynamics of the pharynx and upper esophageal sphincter during swallowing. Drawbacks include the requirement for transnasal insertion of a catheter that houses transducers for recording pressure changes and the need for precise placement and positioning to avoid measurement error. The manometric studies should be performed by a gastroenterologist or otolaryngologist and require special training to insert the catheter, to apply anesthetic to the nasopharynx, and to interpret the results. Manometry adds useful information about pharyngeal and esophageal pressure or tone, contractions of pharyngeal constrictor muscles, contraction or relaxation of the upper esophageal sphincter, and the relationships between these events.[256] Because the corresponding anatomic components are not seen, manometry is incomplete when used alone. This deficit, however, can be overcome by pairing the study with videofluoroscopy, a process termed manofluorography. This procedure, however, exposes the patient to radiation and cannot be used easily with children or with agitated, demented, or severely impaired adults.

Scintigraphy is a special procedure that requires a physician trained in nuclear medicine. This technique[116] uses radionuclide scanning during and after the ingestion of a radioactive bolus (e.g., technetium sulphur colloid 99). Scintigraphy quantifies the amount of radioactive tracer in tissues or structures such as the pharynx or lungs. This procedure is highly accurate in determining the amount and location of the bolus during any specific point of the swallow or thereafter. It is the only technique that can study aspiration precisely, because the half-life of the radioactive material is long enough that it remains in the system for several hours. It is not widely used, however, because of its cost, requirement for specialized nuclear medicine expertise, and unavailability in many facilities.

Fiberoptic endoscopic evaluation (FEES) uses a flexible fiberoptic endoscope with video camera and light source to gather images that can be stored and reviewed as needed. The endoscope is passed transnasally through the nasopharynx and hypopharynx and positioned in the laryngopharynx above the false vocal cords, superior to the epiglottis.[149] Blue-green dye is added to food and liquid so that residue in the pharyngeal sinuses or larynx can be easily identified. One problem with this procedure is that it can evaluate only part of the swallow, because the view is obscured entirely when the vocal cords adduct and the epiglottis descends. FEES, however, shows premature spillage into the hypopharynx and laryngeal vestibule, and residue is evident after the swallow if aspiration has occurred. Some patients report that the tube interferes with normal swallowing. According to Langmore et al.,[149] FEES is contraindicated in patients with cardiac arrhythmias (passing the endoscope into the pharynx may lead to increased reactivity of the vagus nerve), respiratory distress, bleeding disorders, or agitation.

Electroglottography is sometimes used by speech scientists to measure frequency of vocal fold vibration during phonation for speech. It provides a noninvasive method for describing laryngeal motion during swallowing.[214] This type of information may be helpful in determining whether a patient can be taught the Mendelsohn maneuver, to extend duration of laryngeal elevation. It is usually paired with videofluoroscopy and/or manometry in the evaluation of swallowing.

Electromyography provides information about the onset and duration of motor activity as well as the recruitment patterns of the motor units. It is useful in evaluating paralyzed muscles and in determining whether or not various nonswallowing pharyngeal motions can be used therapeutically for dysphagia.[215] The study is invasive and somewhat uncomfortable; it is not done routinely in the work-up of dysphagia.

Therapeutic Techniques

Most rehabilitation programs use a multi-disciplinary management program for neurologically impaired patients with swallowing difficulties.[171] Team members include physiatrists, otolaryngologists, occupational therapists, speech-language pathologists, nurses, and dieticians as well as the patient and his or her family. A successful program improves the patients weight and caloric intake while preserving the integrity of the airway.

In 1983 Logemann[163] described "direct therapy" as the use of food and liquids during treatment with the primary goal of "safe swallowing" (swallowing without jeopardizing the integrity of the airway). Direct therapy uses both facilitation and compensation. Examples of facilitation include small volumes of food or drink per swallow, use of straw, ingestion of puddinglike consistencies to decrease the risk of aspiration, neck flexion to help in closing off the airway, supraglottic swallow, and Mendelsohn maneuver (having the patient volitionally elevate the larynx prior to the swallow). In indirect therapy no food or liquid is used, but the goal is to improve functioning of impaired structures of the oropharynx through exercise. This approach also was described by Logemann in 1983.[163]

Occupational and speech therapists also use oral desensitization through sensory stimulation and thermal stimulation, although definitive data are lacking in these areas. Rosenbeck's work failed to show convincing evidence that thermal application improved swallowing in stroke patients.[234] Muscle reeducation, cognitive perceptual retraining, proper positioning, structuring of the feeding environment, prescription and fabrication of adapted feeding devices, or a combination of these procedures[300] is useful in managing the dysphagia of brain-injured patients.

POSTTRAUMATIC VOMITING

In the study by Ando et al.[7] approximately one-sixth of hospitalized brain-injured patients developed posttraumatic vomiting, which is defined as having its onset within the first 3 days after injury. The investigators found no correlation with age, site of impact, associated fractures, findings on CT or MR scans of the head, severity of brain injury, or loss of consciousness. None of these factors were significantly different in patients who developed posttraumatic vomiting and patients who did not. The only positive correlation appeared to be a history of febrile convulsions and/or previous posttraumatic vomiting. The study also suggested that patients who developed posttraumatic emesis may have had a lower vomiting threshold. Several studies[27,30,114,145,151,271,283] reported that the vomiting center is located in the reticular formation of the lateral medulla and receives its stimulation through the area postrema and nucleus of the tractus solitarius of the medulla, through which the chemical and sensory stimuli are mediated.[30,114,151,176,283] It also seems likely that vomiting secondary to a stimulus of dizziness or other vestibular-mediated sensations also is conducted through the lateral medulla. In addition, the vomiting center of Hess, a site in the hypothalamus adjacent to the mammillary body, causes recurrent vomiting when stimulated.[76,295] This center is likely to cause vomiting secondary to increased intracranial pressure, intracranial hematoma, cerebral edema, or subarachnoid hemorrhage, which leads to irritation of the meninges.[295]

A rare cause of posttraumatic vomiting, with only 3 cases reported in the literature,[111,195,216] is the superior mesenteric artery syndrome in which the third part of the duodenum is compressed against the aorta by the superior mesenteric artery, causing high intestinal obstruction.[195,216] Although the syndrome was first labeled by Rokitinsky in 1942, Wilke gave the first detailed account in 1921. Bouzarth provided the only known description of its occurrence in a patient with severe brain injury in 1973.[22] The syndrome is also known by various other clinical names, such as Wilke's syndrome, Cast syndrome, chronic duodenal ileus, and arteriomesenteric duodenal compression. Classic symptoms include postprandial epigastric pain, vomiting, nausea, and weight loss; symptoms improve with a change to the left lateral position or knee-elbow position.[170,216] Contributing factors in brain-injured children include prolonged supine position; spasticity; hip flexion contractures, which produce increased lumbar lordosis; significant recent weight loss with associated loss of fat in the mesenteric and retroperitoneal region; and abnormally high

fixation of the duodenal fixture of the ligament of Treitz.[111,126] Conservative management includes gastric decompression, perineural feeding or feeding through a tube distal to the obstruction, and positioning with the patient prone or in the left lateral position. If conservative approaches fail, surgery is required. Lee and Mangla,[154] and Philip[216] recommend duodenojejunostomy as the preferred procedure, although some of their colleagues recommend gastrojejunostomy, ligation of the ligament of Treitz, or derotation of the small bowel and right colon. This rare cause of posttraumatic vomiting should be kept in mind if no other source can be discovered.

ULCERATION AND HEMORRHAGE

One of the more frequent complications of traumatic brain injury—and the most commonly diagnosed complication on the rehabilitation unit—is formation of stress ulcers and gastrointestinal bleeding. Kamada et al.[128] reviewed 433 cases that showed a high correlation between severity of brain injury and incidence of bleeding. A relationship was later established between gastrointestinal bleeding and erosive gastritis.[18,120] The most common pathology is multiple erosions and submucosal bleeding, particularly in the fundus in the body of the stomach, although lesions occasionally are seen in the esophagus and duodenum. Animal studies[47,87,105,178] show the appearance of lesions within minutes to hours after brain injury, and Brown et al.[26] showed stress gastritis in humans within 12 hours after severe head injury. A relationship also was established between increased intracranial pressure and increased acid secretion in brain-injured patients. In 1932 Cushing[44] suggested that parasympathetic centers in the hypothalamus and vagal nuclei in the medulla were stimulated by intracranial lesions that led to increased vagal output, which in turn resulted in increased secretion of gastric acid and hypermotility. Larson et al.[150] evaluated 32 patients with severe brain injury endoscopically and found that 22 (69%) had gastritis or duodenitis. They also found that traumatic brain-injured patients have marked output of pancreatic polypeptide, which is probably secondary to affected mid-brain autonomic centers. Their data suggest that head injury leads to increased vagal activity, because the cephalic phase of pancreatic polypeptide release is known to be vagal-cholinergic.

Treatment for peptic ulcer disease should be focused on both prevention and treatment of acute disease. Caution must be used in dispensing medications such as nonsteroidal anti-inflammatory drugs, anticoagulants, steroids, or aspirin, all of which may increase susceptibility to mucosal damage. Because such lesions are associated with high acidity,[18,66] treatment with histamine-2 blockers or antacids may help to prevent stress ulcerations. The antacids can be added through a feeding tube if the patient can ingest nothing by mouth. By making the stomach more alkaline and less acidic, however, bacterial overgrowth may occur,[18,42,60,133] increasing the risk of pneumonia in patients who are aspirating gastric flora; therefore, sucralfates, a nonantacid form of prophylaxis, may have a clinical advantage.[18,133,273]

A mainstay in the prevention and treatment of peptic ulcer disease includes the H2 receptor blockers, such as ranitidine (Zantac), nizatidine (Axid), or famotidine (Pepcid). Currently all of these medications, except nizatidine, are available in intravenous form. Although the study by Halloran et al.[99] showed that cimetidine (another H2 receptor blocker) suppressed hypersecretion of gastric acid in head-injured patients, most physiatrists think it should not be used because of its cognitive side effects. The two studies[282,287] that address this issue suggest that cimetidine penetrates the blood-brain barrier and passes into the cerebrospinal fluid after a single intravenous dose, thereby presumably exerting its effect upon mentation. Blumer et al.[19] showed that ranitidine is safe and effective for the treatment of ulcer disease in children. Because Axid and Pepcid are newer agents, their safety and efficacy in children have not been well studied to date. Sucralfate (Carafate) exerts its gastrointestinal protective effects by coating the mucosa of the stomach and thereby providing a barrier to the harmful effects of hyperacidity, although the acidic content is not decreased. Omeprazole (Prilosec) belongs to a new class of antiulcer medications that act by suppressing secretion of gastric acid through specific inhibition of the H^+/K^+ adenosine triphosphatase enzyme system at the secretory surface of the gastric parietal cell, thus blocking the final step of acid production. Omeprazole is effective in the short-term treatment of active duodenal ulcer disease but should not be used as maintenance therapy. Its safety and effectiveness in children have not been established.

DECREASED GUT MOTILITY

Gastroesophageal reflux, defined as distal esophageal dysfunction that leads to frequent return of stomach contents to the esophagus, is often associated with vomiting.[109,233] In patients with traumatic brain injury, gastroesophageal reflux is a fairly common complication that is exacerbated by decreased consciousness, which leads to decreased protective cough and gag. When such protective mechanisms are impaired, the obvious risk is aspiration. Patients fed with gastrostomy tubes or nasogastric tubes[29,125,179,185,223] are also at risk for reflux and may have better outcomes if they are fed by total parenteral nutrition[1,103,104,277] or by jejunostomy tubes. Good nursing care ensures that the patient is positioned upright at least 30° to help to prevent reflux. Studies[136,223] have shown no significant difference in incidence of aspiration between continuous or intermittent feedings if the patient is positioned properly. According to the proposed pathophysiology of gastroesophageal reflux, the damaged cerebrum loses control of the lower motor nucleus of cranial nerve X, resulting in decreased vagal tone and loss of pressure gradient toward the stomach. This theory has been verified in studies showing that children with traumatic cerebral insult are much more likely to have gastroesophageal reflux than children exposed only to hypoxic brain injury.[235]

Medications are widely used to assist patients affected by gastroesophageal reflux. Metzclopramide (Reglan) has indirect cholinergic effects that increase peristalsis and decrease reflux at the gastroesophageal sphincter. Cisapride (Propulsid), a new medication, also acts in an indirect cholinergic manner; unlike metaclopramide, however, it has direct antiemetic properties and, more importantly, no effect on the dopaminergic system. Because dopamine generally exerts a slow inhibitory action on central nervous system neurons, cisapride is probably the better choice for treatment of gastroesophageal reflux in patients with brain injury.

Gastroparesis is the clinical manifestation of delayed gastric emptying. The study by Power et al.[225] showed no significant difference in gastric emptying time in patients with head injury vs. control groups. However, in the study by Ott et al.[211] a majority of patients with brain injury (Glasgow Coma Scores: 4–10) showed delayed emptying at 1 week. By the third week gastric emptying had improved in a majority of patients, and by day 16 after injury, 83% of patients were tolerating full-strength, full-rate feedings. Gastroparesis has been treated by both metaclopramide and cisapride,[12,32,213,246] but the dopaminergic effects of metaclopramide should be avoided if possible. Erythromycin has been advocated by some clinicians for treatment of decreased stomach emptying[242,285,301]; it may, however, induce symptoms of upper abdominal pain, bloating, nausea, or diarrhea.

The causes of delayed gastric emptying are multiple. Koo[140] suggested that stress adversely affects the upper gastrointestinal tract by way of the sympathetic system; thus drugs that modulate parasympathetic tone may be helpful. Garrick et al.[79,211] showed that increased intracranial pressure decreased both gastric and duodenal contractions. Rapp et al.[226,211] suggested that cytokines are strong inhibitors of gastric emptying. Nompleggi et al.[201,211] implicated interleukin-1 as the causative agent in delayed gastric emptying, and Ott et al.[211] showed that brain-injured patients have significantly elevated levels of interleukin-1 in their cerebrospinal fluid. Other influences to slow gastric emptying include corticotropin-releasing factors,[211] opioid medications,[28,196,211] and certain other drugs, such as phenytoin and antacids.[199,211] The work by Ott et al.,[211] however, found no relationship between antacid administration and delayed gastric emptying. Other studies[35,133,211] have provided further evidence that after brain injury the vagus nerve may be paralyzed, which also may lead to decreased peristalsis and gastric emptying.

Constipation and impaction also are seen occasionally in patients with brain injury. The basic components of a good bowel program are frequently overlooked, including proper diet, adequate fluids, and upright positioning during defecation. Immobilization has a deleterious effect on peristalsis of the bowel. Medications such as stool softeners, natural laxatives, and suppositories may be effective in patients with constipation.

INCREASED MOTILITY

Although less common than slowed bowel function, increased gastrointestinal motility is also an occasional problem for patients with traumatic brain injury. Diarrhea is defined as a large amount of liquid fecal material as opposed to the normal soft, semi-formed stools. Brain-injured patients on enteral or parenteral feedings do not have hard-formed stool; they do not need to be manipulated to produce daily stools. The most common diarrhea in patients on supplemental feedings is osmotic diarrhea, especially at the initiation of feeding. Although osmotic diarrhea may be seen in normal gut mucosa, it is seen more commonly in a malnourished gut. A practical suggestion for reducing symptoms is the initiation of half-strength formula, provided at a constant rate. Then the patient is moved gradually to a bolus feeding program (scheduled "meal" times increase the likelihood of scheduled bowel movements). From a practical point of view, it is much easier for the patient maintained on bolus feeds to participate in a busy day of rehabilitation; additional apparatus (intravenous pole and pump) do not accompany the patient to each therapy session. Increasing the fiber content of the feeding, with a product such as Jevity, may be helpful in controlling osmotic diarrhea.[70]

Other causes of loose stool include medication side effects, especially with antibiotics. Liquid bowel movements also may be seen in patients with bacterial, viral, parasitic, or protozoan infections. Persistent diarrhea, particularly in patients who have been treated with antibiotics, should be evaluated for infection with *Clostridium difficile*, and stool should be sent for culture, sensitivity testing, and assessment for ova and parasites if diarrhea persists. It also may be necessary to rule out an impaction, because the patient may present with diarrhea when, in fact, liquid stool is passing around a blockage of hard stool in the colon.

If the diarrhea begins soon after increasing the rate or the concentration of tube feeding, it is advisable to return to the previous tolerated level for a period of 24 hours before again attempting an increase. If diarrhea has not stopped within 24 hours, tube feeding should be stopped for 24 hours and the protocol reinitiated at the beginning.[5] Once the specimen has been sent to the laboratory for evaluation, the patient can be given medication to help control the liquid stool; options include codeine, deodorized tincture of opium, or Lomotid. It also is necessary to correct for fluid level loss, electrolyte imbalances, or malabsorption syndromes secondary to decreased digestion. If the diarrhea is accompanied by an abdominal distention greater than 2 inches from baseline in measurement and associated with a tense abdomen, a further work-up is indicated[5] to rule out a surgical abdomen (e.g., bowel perforation).

HICCUPS

Hiccups are a phenomenon quite common in most people. They are generally benign and resolve fairly rapidly. On rare occasions, hiccups (singultus) are persistent and do not terminate with the usual methods. In such patients, medications such as antipsychotics, anticonvulsants, or beta blockers may be used. Other unique considerations may be necessary in brain-injured patients.

Many have attempted to explain the anatomy and physiology of hiccups, but no one knows the exact mechanisms involved. It has been postulated that the afferent loop of the hiccup reflex involves the phrenic and vagus nerves as well as the sympathetic chain from thoracic nerve 6 to thoracic nerve 12.[241,272] Components of the efferent arc include the phrenic nerves C3–C5, the anterior scalene muscles C5–C7, and the external intercostal muscles T1–T11. The glottic nerve (the recurrent laryngeal component of the

vagus) also plays a role.[197,250] Hiccups are frequently described in complications of the pulmonary system. However, Davis[49] showed that hiccups had only minimal effect on ventilation as the duration of glottic closure is quite limited and occurs only 35 ms after the onset of activation of the inspiratory muscles. Of note, normal esophageal contractile tone and pressure in the lower esophageal sphincter are decreased during hiccupping, further showing the relationship between hiccupping and the gastrointestinal system.[138] Intra-abdominal stimuli, such as gastric distention, often initiate the hiccup process, suggesting that hiccups in fact fall under the large umbrella of gastrointestinal phenomena.

As noted above, hiccups are generally self-limited and of minimal consequence. They may be caused by ingestion of excessive amounts of food or alcohol as well as by swallowing large amounts of air. Sudden changes in ambient or gastrointestinal temperatures such as those caused by the environment, or extremely hot or cold temperatures of food stuffs also may lead to hiccups. Tobacco nicotine also has been implicated as a source of irritation that initiates the hiccup reaction.

Of greater concern are the causes of persistent hiccups, which may be divided into three main groups: organic, psychogenic, and idiopathic. Organic hiccups may be subdivided into central, peripheral, toxic, metabolic, or pharmacologic origin.[43,83,197,266,272,281] Examples of centrally induced persistent hiccups include diffuse axonal injury, hydrocephalus, vascular changes, contusion, hematoma, and infection. Phrenic or vagus nerve irritation are examples of peripheral involvement, and electrolyte imbalances (e.g., uremia, hypocalcemia, and hyponatremia) or alcohol intoxication are examples of toxic, metabolic, or pharmacologic disturbances. Several pharmacologic compounds are thought to induce hiccups, including intravenous steroids, barbiturates, various benzodiazepines, and alpha-methyldopa. Psychogenic factors leading to hiccups may include stress, excitement, anorexia, or grief.[158,200,204,260] Idiopathic causes may include iatrogenic factors such as intraoperative exploration of thoracic cavity organs, as during a modified barium swallow study, or endoscopy for evaluation of gastrointestinal bleeding.

Persistent hiccups may lead to dehydration, weight loss,[131,241] exhaustion, and insomnia;[115] polydipsia, either as a complication or as an attempted cure, may lead to hyponatremia;[43,158] and esophagitis may result secondary to gastroesophageal reflux.[83,131] Because of the possibility of further complication of hiccups in patients with traumatic brain injury, as well as their discomfort and annoyance, every effort should be taken to provide relief.

Both pharmacologic and nonpharmacologic therapies should be considered for persistent hiccups. Nonpharmacologic interventions include time-honored home remedies, such as swallowing granulated sugar,[16,268,371] biting on a lemon,[43,268] and drinking 10 consecutive sips of water while holding one's breath. In patients who are dysphagic and on modified diets, such methods may not be advisable, and an alternative treatment, such as acupuncture, may be preferable.[166] Another nonpharmacologic treatment is the surgical resection of one of the anatomic components of the hiccup reflex arc. Relief from hiccups also has been obtained from endoscopic maneuvers[15] and digital rectal massage (done gently).[206]

The antipsychotic agent chlorpromazine is the most widely accepted pharmacologic treatment for persistent and intractable hiccups.[50,146,158,197,281,289] Haloperidol, an antipsychotic agent of the butyrophenone class, also has been thought to be an effective medication for treatment of hiccups.[121,146] Such medicines, however, are not the first choice in patients with traumatic brain injury, because they may decrease neurologic recovery or lead to increased sedation. Perhaps a better pharmacologic treatment is carbamazepine or amitriptyline.[75,146] Phenytoin has been suggested by some physicians,[158] but it may lead to slowed mentation in a traumatic brain-injured patient with compromised cognition. Probably the best management is first to attempt to treat the hiccups with nonpharmacologic methods; if they fail, pharmacologic therapies should be tried on a highly selective basis.

INTESTINAL INFARCTION AFTER NON-ABDOMINAL TRAUMA

An infrequent but often deadly complication of severe head injury (92% mortality rate in patients with cerebral trauma) is bowel necrosis without abdominal trauma.[72] The cause appears to be related to decreased mesenteric blood flow, which can be seen in a number of conditions, including hypoperfusion (possibly due to dehydration or use of diuretics), local vasoconstriction, hypovolemia, venous congestion, medications such as epinephrine or digitalis, or disseminated intravascular coagulation. Although the mesenteric vessels remain patent, the most common site for infarctions secondary to decreased blood flow is the left colonic flexure, possibly secondary to the watershed area between the superior and inferior mesenteric arterial supply at a point two-thirds of the distance across the transverse colon. One reason for the high mortality rate is that the patient with traumatic brain injury may have difficulty in expressing pain because of mechanical ventilation or decreased cognition. Pain is the main presenting symptom, in combination with sepsis, multiple organ failure, and abdominal distention. Steroids may influence the outcome favorably by increasing the circulation to the bowel wall,[71] but they cannot be effective if the diagnosis is delayed. Most commonly seen in patients who are in a coma at the time of admission, bowel necrosis is rare but extremely dangerous.

HEPATIC COMPLICATIONS

Increased values on liver function tests represent the most common gastrointestinal complication after traumatic brain injury; in 92% of cases, this increase is drug-induced, especially by anticonvulsant or antispasticity medications.[127] Of epileptic children treated with phenytoin or phenobarbital for longer than 1 year, 88% showed an increase in gamma glutamyl transpeptidase.[2,127] However, no liver cell damage or inflammatory reactions were seen on biopsy,[2] suggesting that a benign enzyme caused the elevated levels. Antispasticity medications also may lead to an increase in liver function tests.[127]

Pharmacokinetics may be described in two phases: phase 1 is characterized by microsomal oxidative metabolism and phase 2 by conjunctive metabolism in the liver. After traumatic brain injury, phase 1 is the more likely to be influenced and may be either induced or inhibited by a wide spectrum of factors, including age, genetics, nutrition, medication, and certain diseases.[21,224] Conjunctive metabolism generally is thought to be less susceptible to changes after injury.[21,144] The increase in hepatic conjunctive metabolism due to severe neurotrauma is most evident at 7–14 days after injury.[21]

Infection, especially after blood transfusions, also may lead to increased values on liver function tests. Hepatitis is the most common infection responsible for the increase; active hepatitis causes 8% of the elevations and chronic hepatitis 3%.[127] Premorbid history of alcohol and drug ingestion also may contribute to elevated liver function values in a patient with brain injury. A careful history from the patient or family may shed light on possible causes. Once the correct cause has been determined, appropriate management (e.g., treatment of infection or discontinuance of the offending medication) should lead to normalization of the values.

PANCREATITIS

Pancreatitis may arise secondary to blunt abdominal trauma.[18] Affected patients are best managed by total parenteral nutrition to allow the gastrointestinal tract to rest and the pancreas to recover. Fat most certainly must be eliminated from the diet. Greenlee et al.[91] suggested the breaking down of amylase levels into pancreatic versus salivary gland fractions. Their work showed that the salivary gland fraction normally is greater than the pancreatic fraction, but in patients sustaining abdominal injury, the pancreatic fraction is greater. Therefore, determination of the amylase isoenzyme is certainly beneficial if the issue is in doubt.[91,133]

CONCLUSION

Gastrointestinal complications are seen in approximately half of the 400,000 cases of head injury reported annually in the United States. Trauma, including cranial injuries, abdominal injuries, and facial or oral injuries, complicate the situation already created by the injured neurologic computer center of the brain. This chapter reviewed the posttraumatic complications of malnutrition as well

as the basic principles of normal metabolism and metabolism pushed into the catabolic and hypermetabolic states, measures for assessing nutritional status, and delivery of adequate nutrition. Dysphagia, including the anatomy and physiology of deglutition, tools for assessment, and therapies to treat deficits were outlined. The review of gastrointestinal complications included discussion of posttraumatic vomiting, ulceration and hemorrhage, and increased and decreased gut motility. Abdominal infarction and decreased hepatic and pancreatic function also complicate the functioning of the gastrointestinal system after traumatic brain injury, and their implications for management and treatment were outlined. It is hoped that such information will be applicable to clinical practice and helpful in managing the gastrointestinal complications of traumatically brain-injured patients.

REFERENCES

1. Adams S, Simonowitz D, Orescovic M, et al: Hyperalimentation of severely injured patients: Parenteral versus enteral nutrition. Presented at the 7th Clinical Congress of the American Society of Parenteral and Enteral Nutrition, Washington, DC.
2. Aiges HW, Daum F, Olso M, et al: Effects of phenobarbital and diphenylhydantoin on liver function and morphology. J Pediatr 97:22–26, 1980.
3. Anand BK, Brobeck JR: Hypothalamic control of food intake in rats and cats. Yale J Biol Med 24:123–140, 1951.
4. Anderson BJ, Marmarou A: Post-traumatic selective stimulation of glycolysis. Brain Res 585:184–189, 1992.
5. Anderson BJ: A theoretical protocol for nutritional maintenance in head-injured patients. J Neurosurg Nurs 16:50–53, 1984.
6. Anderson BJ: The metabolic needs of head trauma victims. J Neurosci Nurs 19:211–215, 1987.
7. Ando S, Otani M, Moritake K: Clinical analysis of post-traumatic vomiting. Acta Neurochir (Wien) 119:97–100, 1992.
8. Andreasen PB, Lyngbye J, Trolle E: Abnormalities in liver function tests during long-term diphenylhydantoin therapy in epileptic out-patients. Acta Med Scand 194:261–264, 1973.
9. Arseni C, Oprescu: Digestive hemorrhages induced by traumatic cerebral lesions. Appl Neurophysiol 38:206–215, 1975.
10. Askanazi J, Carpentier YA, Elwyn DH, et al: Influence of total parenteral nutrition on fuel utilization in injury and sepsis. Ann Surg 191:40–46, 1979.
11. Baigelman W, O'Brien JC: Pulmonary effects of head trauma. Neurosurgery 9:729–740, 1981.

12. Balzola F, Boggio Bertinet D, Solerio A, et al: Dietetic treatment with hypercaloric and hyperprotein intake in patients following severe brain injury. J Neurosurg Sci 24:131–140, 1980.

13. Beaver BL, Colombani PM, Fal A, et al: The efficacy of computed tomography in evaluating abdominal injuries in children with major head trauma. J Pediatr Surg 22:1117–1122, 1987.

14. Becker E, Saxbon L, Najenson T: Gastrointestinal hemorrhage in long-lasting traumatic coma. Scand J Rehabil Med 10:23–26, 1978.

15. Beda BY, Niamkey EK, Ouattara D, et al: Stopping persistent hiccups in the adult by endoscopic maneuver. Ann Gastroenterol Hepatol 29:11–13, 1993.

16. Bhargava R, Datta S, Badgaiya R: A simple technique to stop hiccups [letter]. Indian J Physiol Pharmacol 29:57–58, 1985.

17. Bivins BA, Twyman DL, Young AB: Failure of nonprotein calories to mediate protein conservation in brain-injured patients. J Trauma 26:980–986, 1986.

18. Bloomfield EL: Extracerebral complications of head injury. Neurol Crit Care Clin 5:881–902, 1986.

19. Blumer JL, et al: Pharmacokinetic determination of ranitidine pharmacodynamics in pediatric ulcer disease. J Pediatr 107:301–306, 1985.

20. Border JR, Chenier R, McMenamy RH, et al: Multiple systems organ failure: Muscle fuel deficit with visceral protein malnutrition. Surg Clin North Am 56:1147–1167, 1976.

21. Boucher BA, Kuhl DA, Fabian TC, Robertson JT: Effect of neurotrauma on hepatic drug clearance. Clin Pharmacol Ther 50:487–497, 1991.

22. Bouzarth WF, Crowley JN, Clearfield HR: Vascular compression of the duodenum following severe brain injury. Case report. J Neurosurg 39:405–407, 1973.

23. Bracard S, Marchal J-C, Auque J, et al: Craniofacial fractures and brain injuries. J Neuroradiol 13:265–277, 1986.

24. Britt RH, Herrick MK, Mason RT, Dorfman LJ: Traumatic lesions of ponto-medullary junction. Neurosurgery 6:623–631, 1980.

25. Brooke MM, Barbour PC: Assessment of nutritional status during rehabilitation after brain injury. Arch Phys Med Rehabil 67:634, 1986.

26. Brown TH, Davidson PF, Larson GM: Acute gastritis occurring within 24 hours of severe head injury. Gastrointest Endosc 35:37–40, 1989.

27. Bruce A, Shut L: Concussion and contusion following pediatric head trauma. In McLaurin RL (ed): Pediatric Neurosurgery. New York, Grune & Stratton, 1982, pp 301–308.

28. Burks TF, Galligan JJ, Hirning LD: Brain, spinal cord and peripheral sites of action of enkephalins and other endogenous opioids on gastrointestinal motility. Gastroenterol Clin Biol 11:44–51, 1987.

29. Canal DF, Vane DW, Goto S, et al: Reduction of lower esophageal sphincter pressure with Stamm gastrostomy. J Pediatr Surg 22:54–57, 1987.

30. Carpenter DO: Neural mechanisms of emesis. Can J Physiol Pharmacol 68:230–236, 1990.

31. Cerra FB, Siegel JH, Coleman B, et al: Septic autocatabolism: A failure of exogenous nutritional support. Ann Surg 192:570–580, 1980.

32. Chandra RK: Nutrition and immune responses. Can J Physiol Pharmacol 61:290–294, 1983.

33. Childs A: Naltrexone in organic bulimia: A preliminary report. Brain Inj 1:49–56, 1987.

34. Chiolero R, Schutz Y, Lemarchand TH, et al: Hormonal and metabolic changes following severe head injury or noncranial injury. JPEN 13:5–12, 1989.

35. Clarke RJ, Alexander-Williams J: The effect of preserving antral innervation and of a pyloroplasty on gastric emptying after vagotomy in man. Gut 14:300–307, 1973.

36. Clifton GL, Robertson CS, Chol SC: Assessment of nutritional requirements of head-injured patients. J Neurosurg 64:895–901, 1986.

37. Clifton GL, Robertson CS, Contant CF: Enteral hyperalimentation in head injury. J Neurosurg 62:186–193, 1985.

38. Clifton GL, Robertson CS, Grossman RG, et al: The metabolic response to severe head injury. J Neurosurg 60:687–696, 1984.

39. Cohen LB, Field SP, Sachar DB: The superior mesenteric artery syndrome—the disease that isn't, or is it? J Clin Gastroenterol 7:113–116, 1985.

40. Combs DJ, Ott L, McAninch PS, et al: The effect of total parenteral nutrition on vasogenic edema development following cold injury in rats. J Neurosurg 70:623–627, 1989.

41. Cornett MA, Paris A, Huang T-Y: Case report: Intracranial penetration of a nasogastric tube. Am J Emerg Med 11:94–96, 1993.

42. Craven DE, Kunches LM, Kilinsky V, et al: Risk factors for pneumonia and fatality in patients receiving continuous mechanical ventilation. Am Rev Respir Dis 133:792–796, 1986.

43. Cronin R: Psychogenic polydipsia with hyponatremia: Report of eleven cases. Am J Kidney Dis 9:410–416, 1987.

44. Cushing H: Peptic ulcers and the interbrain. Surg Gynecol Obstet 55:1–34, 1932.

45. Cuthbertson DP: Observations on the disturbance of metabolism produced by injury to the limbs. Quart J Med 21:233–246, 1932.

46. Dahlberg PJ, Cogbill TH, Annis BL, Deering WM: Malignant posttraumatic hypermetabolic syndrome associated with brain injury. Wis Med J 84:15–18, 1985.

47. Dai S, Ogle CW: Gastritis induced by acid accumulation and by stress in pylorus occluded rats. Eur J Pharmacol 26:15–21, 1974.

48. Davenport HW: A Digest of Digestion, 2nd ed. Chicago, Year Book, 1978.

49. Davis J: An experimental study of hiccup. Brain 93:851–872, 1970.

50. Davignon A, Laurieux G, Genest J: Chlorpromazine in the treatment of persistent hiccough. Union Med Can 84:282, 1955.

51. De Castro JM: Circadian rhythms of the spontaneous meal pattern, macronutrient intake, and mood of humans. Physiol Behav 40:437–446, 1987.

52. Dees G: Difficult nasogastric tube insertions. Emerg Med Clin North Am 7:177–182, 1989.

53. Dempsey DT, Guenter P, Mullen JL, et al: Energy expenditure in acute trauma to the head with and without barbiturate therapy. Surg Gynecol Obstet 160:128–134, 1985.

54. Deutschman CS, Konstantinides FN, Raup S, Cerra FB: Physiological and metabolic response to isolated closed-head injury. J Neurosurg 66:388–395, 1987.

55. Deutschman CS, Konstantinides FN, Raup S: Steroids potentiate the metabolic abnormalities and malnutrition of isolated closed-head injury. Surg Forum 36:46, 1985.

56. Deutschman CS: Physiology and metabolism in closed head injury. World J Surg 11:182–193, 1987.

57. Dickerson RN, Guenter PA, Gennarelli TA, et al: Brief communication: Increased contribution of protein oxidation to energy expenditure in head-injured patients. J Am Coll Nutr 9:86–88, 1990.

58. Dminioni L, Trocki O, Mochizuki H, et al: Prevention of severe postburn hypermetabolism and catabolism by immediate intragastric feeding. J Burn Care Rehabil 5:106–112, 1984.

59. Donner MW: Swallowing mechanism and neuromuscular disorders. Semin Roentgenol 9:273–282, 1974.

60. Driks MR, Craven DE, Celli BR, et al: Nosocomial pneumonia in intubated patients given sucralfate as compared with antacids or histamine type 2 blockers. N Engl J Med 317:1376–1382, 1987.

61. du Plessis JJ: Percutaneous pharyngostomy versus gastric tube placement in head injured patients. Acta Neurochir (Wien) 119:94–96, 1992.

62. Elsass L, Kinella G: Social interaction following severe closed head injury. Psychol Med 17:67–78, 1987.

63. Fell D, Benner B, Billings A, et al: Metabolic profiles in patients with acute neurosurgical injuries. Crit Care Med 12:649–652, 1984.

64. Field LH, Weiss CJ: Dysphagia with head injury. Brain Inj 3:19–26, 1989.

65. Fisher DF Jr, Fry WJ: Collateral mesenteric circulation. Surg Gynecol Obstet 164:487–492, 1987.

66. Fitts CT, Cathcart RS III, Artz CP: Acute gastrointestinal tract ulceration: Cushing's ulcer, steroid ulcer, Curling's ulcer and stress ulcer. Am Surg 37:218–223, 1971.

67. Fitzpatrick BC, Harrington TR: Nutrition in head-injured patients. J Neurosurg 76:170–171, 1992.

68. Fletcher SA, Henderson LT, Miner ME, Jones JM: The successful surgical removal of intracranial nasogastric tubes. J Trauma 27:948–952, 1987.

69. Ford EG, Jennings LM, Andrassy RJ: Steroid treatment of head injuries in children: The nutritional consequences. Curr Surg 44:311–313, 1987.

70. Frankenfield DC, Beyer PL: Soy-polysaccharide fiber: Effect on diarrhea in tube-fed, head-injured patients. Am J Clin Nutr 50:533–538, 1989.

71. Fremstad JD, Martin SH: Lethal complication from insertion of nasogastric tube after severe basilar skull fracture. J Trauma 18:820–822, 1978.

72. Frick TW, Kach K, Sulser H, et al: Intestinal infarction after nonabdominal trauma: Association with cerebral trauma. J Trauma 33:870–875, 1992.

73. Frowein RA, Terhaag D, auf der Haar K, et al: Rehabiliation after severe head injury. Acta Neurochir (Suppl)55:72–74, 1992.

74. Fruin AH, Taylon C, Pettis MS: Caloric requirements in patients with severe head injuries. Surg Neurol 25:25–28, 1986.

75. Fry E: Management of intractable hiccup. BMJ 2:704, 1977.

76. Fukuyama Y, Kitahara H: Vomiting in newborn, infants, and children. Neurol Surg (Tokyo) 4:1143–1147, 1976.

77. Gadisseux P, Ward JD, Young HF, Becker DP: Nutrition and the neurosurgical patient. J Neurosurg 60:219–232, 1984.

78. Galloway DC, Grudis J: Inadvertent intracranial placement of a nasogastric tube through a basal skull fracture. South Med J 72:240–241, 1979.

79. Garrick T, Mulvihill S, Buack M, et al: Intracerebroventricular pressure inhibits gastric antral and duodenal contractility but not acid secretion in conscious rabbits. Gastroenterology 95:26–31, 1988.

80. Gazzaniga AB, Polachek JR, Wilson AF, Day AT: Indirect calorimetry as a guide to caloric replacement during total parenteral nutrition. Am J Surg 136:128, 1978.

81. Gentleman D: Causes and effects of systemic complications among severely head injured patients transferred to a neurosurgical unit. Int Surg 77:297–302, 1992.

82. Gentry LR: Facial trauma and associated brain damage. Radiol Clin North Am 27:435–446, 1989.

83. Gluck M, Pope C: Chronic hiccups and gastroesophageal reflux disease: The acid perfusion test as a provocative maneuver. Ann Intern Med 105:219–220, 1986.

84. Godbole KB, Berbiglia VA, Goddard L: A head-injured patient: Caloric needs, clinical progress and nursing care priorities. J Neurosci Nurs 23:290–294, 1991.

85. Gold RM: Hypothalamic obesity: The myth of the ventromedial nucleus. Science 182:488–490, 1973.

86. Gold RM, Jones AP, Sawchenko PE, Kapatos G: Paraventricular area: Critical focus of a longitudinal neurocircuitry mediating food intake. Physiol Behav 18:1111–1119, 1977.

87. Goodman AA, Osbourne MP: An experimental model and clinical definition of stress ulceration. Surg Gynecol Obstet 134:563–571, 1972.

88. Grabow JD, Offord KP, Reider ME: The cost of head trauma in Olmsted County, Minnesota, 1970–1974. Am J Public Health 74:710–712, 1984.

89. Grahm TW, Zadrozny DB, Harrington T: The benefits of early jejunal hyperalimentation in the head-injured patient. Neurosurg 25:729–735, 1989.

90. Granger DN, Richardson PDI, Kvietys PR, Mortillaro NA: Intestinal blood flow. Gastroenterology 78:837–863, 1980.

91. Greenlee T, Murphy K, Ram MD: Amylase isoenzymes in the evaluation of trauma patients. Am Surg 50:637–640, 1984.

92. Gregory JA, Turner PT, Reynolds AF: A complication of nasogastric intubation: Intracranial penetration. J Trauma 18:823–824, 1978.

93. Grinvalsky HT, Bowerman CI: Stercoraceous ulcers of the colon. JAMA 171:1941, 1959.

94. Gurney JG, Rivara FP, Mueller BA, et al: The effects of alcohol intoxication on the initial treatment and hospital course of patients with acute brain injury. J Trauma 33:709–713, 1992.

95. Gustavsson S, Albert J, Forsberg H, Ryrberg C-H: The accidental introduction of a nasogastric tube into the brain. Acta Chir Scand 144:55–56, 1978.

96. Haase J: Social-economic impact of head injury. Acta Neurochir 55(Suppls):47–79, 1992.

97. Hadley MN, Grahm TW, Harrington T, et al: Nutritional support and neurotrauma: A critical review of early nutrition in forty-five acute head injury patients. Neurosurgery 19:367–373, 1986.

98. Hall DMB, Johnson SLJ, Middleton J: Rehabilitation of head injured children. Arch Dis Child 65:553–556, 1990.

99. Halloran LG, Gayle WE, Zfass AM, et al: Cimetidine prevention of gastrointestinal bleeding in severe head injury: A controlled clinical trial. Surg Forum 29:428–430, 1978.

100. Harkins SJ, Marteney JL: Extrinsic trauma: A significant precipitating factor in temporomandibular dysfunction. J Prosthet Dent 54:271–272, 1985.

101. Harris JA, Benedict FG: Biometric Studies of Basal Metabolism in Man. Carnegie Institute, Washington, DC, 1919.

102. Hashimoto I, Nemoto S, Sano K: Hyperexcitable state of the brainstem in children with post-traumatic vomiting as evidenced by brainstem auditory-evoked potentials. Neurol Res 6:81–84, 1984.

103. Hausmann D, Mosebach KO, Caspari R, Rommelsheim K: Combined enteral-parenteral nutrition versus total parenteral nutrition in brain-injured patients. Intens Care Med 11:80–84, 1985.

104. Hausmann D, Rommelsheim K, Josten KU, et al: Brain injured patients—The outcome one week after accident. Intens Care Med 9:239, 1983.

105. Hayase M, Takeuchi K: Gastric acid secretion and lesion formation in rats under water immersion stress. Dig Dis Sci 31:166–171, 1986.

106. Heiskanen O, Torma T: Gastrointestinal ulceration and hemorrhage associated with severe brain injury. Acta Chir Scand 134:562–566, 1968.,

107. Halling TS, Evans LL, Fowler DL, et al: Infectious complications in patients with severe head injury. J Trauma 28:1575–1577, 1988.

108. Henson MB, de Castro JM, STringer AY, Johnson C: Food intake by brain-injured humans who are in the chronic phase of recovery. Brain Inj 7:169–178, 1993.

109. Herbst JJ: Gastroesophageal reflux. J Pediatr 98:859–870, 1981.

110. Hill DJ: Lower oesophageal contractility as an indicator of brain death in paralysed and mechanically ventilated patients with head injury. BMJ 294:1488–1489, 1987.

111. Hines JR, Gore RM, Ballantyne GH: Superior mesenteric artery syndrome: Diagnostic criteria and therapeutic approaches. Am J Surg 148:630–632, 1984.

112. Holstege G, Graveland G, Bijker-Biemond C, Schuddeboom I: Location of motoneurons innervating soft palate, pharynx and upper esophagus: Anatomical evidence for possible swallowing center in pontine reticular formation: HRP and autoradiographical tracing study. Brain Behav Evol 23:47–62, 1983.

113. Houeh W, Gonzalez-Crussi F, Arroyave JL: Platelet-activating-factor-induced ischemic bowel necrosis. Am J Pathol 122:231, 1986.

114. Hugenholz H, Izukawa D, Shear P, et al: Vomiting in children following head injury. Childs Nerv Syst 3:266–270, 1987.

115. Hulbert H: Hiccoughing. Practitioner 167:286–289, 1951.

116. Humphries B, Mathog R, Miller P: Videofluoroscopic and scintigraphic analysis of dysphagia in the head and neck cancer patients. Laryngoscope 97:25–32, 1987.

117. Hunt D, Rowlands B, Allen S: The inadequacy of enteral post-injured period. JPEN 9:121, 1985.

118. Hutchinson DT, Bassett GS: Superior mesenteric artery syndrome in pediatric orthopedic patients. Clin Orthop 250:250–257, 1990.

119. Iapichino G, Gattinoni L, Solca M, et al: Protein sparing and protein replacement in acutely injured patients during TPN with and without amino acid supply. Intens Care Med 8:25, 1982.

120. Innes D, Sevitt S: Coagulation and fibrinolysis in injured patients. J Clin pathol 17:1–13, 1964.

121. Ives T, Fleming M, Weart C: Treatment of intractable hiccups with intramuscular haloperidol. Am J Psychiatry 142:1368–1369, 1985.

122. Jackson MD, Davidoff G: Gastroparesis following traumatic brain injury and response to metoclopramide therapy. Arch Phys Med Rehabil 70:553–555, 1989.

123. Jacobi G, Ritz A, Emrich R: Cranial nerve damage after paediatric head trauma: A long-term follow-up study of 741 cases. Acta Paediatr Hung 27:173–187, 1986.

124. Jean A, Car A: Inputs to swallowing medullary neurons from peripheral afferent fibers and swallowing cortical area. Brain Res 178:567–572, 1979.

125. Jolley SG, Tunell WP, Hoelzer DJ, et al: Lower esophageal pressure changes with tube gastrostomy: A causative factor of gastroesophageal reflux in children? J Pediatr Surg 21:624, 1986.

126. Kakos GS, Grosfeld JL, Morse TS: Small bowel injuries in children after blunt abdominal trauma. Ann Surg 174:238–241, 1971.

127. Kalisky Z, Morrison DP, Meyers CA, Von Laufen A: Medical problems encountered during rehabilitation of patients with head injury. Arch Phys Med Rehabil 66:25–29, 1985.

128. Kamada T, Fusamoto H, Kawano S, et al: Gastrointestinal bleeding following head injury: A clinical study of 433 cases. J Trauma 17:44–47, 1977.

129. Kaminski MV, Freed BA: Enteral hyperalimentation: Prevention and treatment of complications. Nutr Supp Serv 1:29–40, 1981.

130. Kaminski DL, Keltner RM, Willman VL: Ischemic colitis. Arch Surg 106:558, 1973.

131. Kaufmann HH: Hiccups: An occasional sign of esophageal obstruction. Gastroenterology 82: 1443–1445, 1982.

132. Kaufmann HH, Bretaudiere J-P, Rowlands BJ, et al: General metabolism in head injury. Med Clin North Am 77:43–60, 1993.

134. Kilman WJ, Goyal RK: Disorders of pharyngeal and upper esophageal sphincter motor function. Arch Intern Med 136:592–601, 1976.

135. Kinney JM: Consideration of energy exchange in human trauma. Bull NY Acad Med 36:617–631, 1960.

136. Kocan MJ, Hicklish SM: A comparison of continuous and intermittent enteral nutrition in NICU patients. J Neurosci Nurs 18:333–337, 1986.

137. Koch KJ, Becker GJ, Edwards MK: Intracranial placement of a nasogastric tube. AJNR 10:443–444, 1989.

138. Kolodzik PW, Eilers MA: Hiccups (singultus): Review and approach to management. Ann Emerg Med 20:565–573, 1991.

139. Kolpek JH, Ott LG, Record KE, et al: Comparison of urinary urea nitrogen excretion and measured energy expenditure in spinal cord injury and non-steroid-treated severe head trauma patients. JPEN 13:277–280, 1989.

140. Koo MWL, Ogle CW, Cho CH: The effect of cold-restraint stress on gastric emptying in rats. Pharmacol Biochem Behav 23:969–972, 1985.

141. Koretz R, Young B, Rapp R: Nutritional support in acute head injuries. J Neurosurg 60:1334–1335, 1984.

142. Kotra C: Infection in the compromised host—An overview. Heart Lung 12:10–22, 1983.

143. Kotwica Z, Brzezinski J: Head injuries complicated by chest trauma: A review of 50 consecutive patients. Acta Neurochir (Wien) 103:109–111, 1990.

144. Kraus JW, Desmond PV, Marshall JP, et al: Effects of aging and liver disease on disposition of lorazepam. Clin Pharmacol Ther 24:411–419, 1978.

145. Kucharczyk J, Harding RK: Regulatory peptides and the onset of nausea and vomiting. Can J Physiol Pharmacol 68:289–293, 1990.

146. Lamphier T: Methods of management of persistent hiccup (singultus). Md Med J 11:80–81, 1977.

147. Landreneau RJ, Fry WJ: The right colon as a target organ of nonocclusive mesenteric ischemia. Arch Surg 125:591, 1990.

148. Langfirtt TW, Gennarelli TA: Can outcome from head injury be improved? J Neurosurg 56:19–25, 1982.

149. Langmore SE, Schatz K, Olsen N: Fiberoptic endoscopic examination of swallowing safety: A new procedure. Dysphagia 2:209–215, 1988.

150. Larson GM, Koch S, O'Dorisio TM, et al: Gastric response to severe head injury. Am J Surg 147: 97–105, 1984.

151. Lawes INC: The origin of the vomiting response: A neuroanatomical hypothesis. Can J Physiol Pharmacol 68:254–259, 1990.

152. Lazarus CL: Diagnosis and management of swallowing disorders in traumatic brain injury. In Beukelman DR, Yorkston KM (eds): Communication Disorders Following Traumatic Brain Injury: Management of Cognitive, Language, and Motor Impairments. Austin, Tx, Pro-ed, 1991, pp 367–417.

153. Lazarus C, Logemann JA: Swallowing disorders in closed head trauma patients. Arch Phys Med Rehabil 68:79–84, 1987.

154. Lee C, Mangla JC: Superior mesenteric artery compression syndrome. Am J Gastroenterol 70: 141–150, 1978.

155. Lehmkuhl LD, Bontke CF: Rehabilitation of patients with severe traumatic brain injury. Crit Rev Phys Med Rehabil 1:247–286, 1990.

156. Levin HS: Head injury and its rehabilitation. Curr Opin Neurol Neurosurg 5:673–676, 1992.

157. Levin HS, High WM, Eisenberg HM: Impairment of olfactory recognition after closed head injury. Brain 108:579–591, 1985.

158. Lewis J: Hiccups: Causes and cures. J Clin Gastroenterol 7:539–552, 1985.

159. Lind L, Wallace D: Submucosal passage of a nasogastric tube complicating attempted intubation during anesthesia. Anesthesiology 49:2, 1978.

160. Linden P, Siebens AA: Dysphagia: Predicting laryngeal penetration. Arch Phys Med Rehabil 64:281–284, 1983.

161. Lloyd CW, Martin WJ, Taylor BD, Hauser AR: Pharmacokinetics and pharmacodynamics of cimetidine and metabolites in critically ill children. J Pediatr 107:295–300, 1985.

162. Lobato RD, Rivas JJ, Portillo JM, et al: Prognostic value of intracranial pressure levels during acute phase of severe head injuries. Acta Neurochir 28(Suppl):70–73, 1979.

163. Logemann JA: Evaluation and Treatment of Swallowing Disorders. San Diego, College-Hill Press, 1983.

164. Logemann JA: Manual for the Videofluorographic Study of Swallowing. San Diego, College-Hill Press, 1986.

165. Long CL, Schaffel N, Geiger JW, et al: Metabolic response to injury and illness: Estimation of energy and protein needs from indirect calorimetry and nitrogen balance. JPEN 3:452–456, 1979.

166. Lu R, Liu M: Clinical application of single acupoint for treatment. J Tradit Chin Med 11:284–285, 1991.

167. Luce JM: Medical management of head injury. Chest 89:864–872, 1986.

168. Mandelstam P, Lieber A: Cineradiographic evaluation of esophagus in normal adults. Gastroenterology 58:32–39, 1970.

169. Marston A, Pheils MT, Thomas ML, Morson BC: Ischemic colitis. Gut 7:1–15, 1966.

170. Martinez N, Khan AH, Pacis A, Lekas C: Arteriomesenteric duodenal compression syndrome: A study of 24 cases. Vasc Surg 13:1–10, 1979.

171. Martens L, Cameron T, Simonsen M: Effects of a multidisciplinary management program of neurologically impaired patients with dysphagia. Dysphagia 5:147–151, 1990.

172. Masuzawa H: Post-traumatic vomiting in children [letter]. Childs Nerv Syst 4:198, 1988.

173. McCallum RW: Pathophysiology of gastric emptying in humans. Del Med J 56:453–462, 1984.

174. McClain CJ, Cohen D, Ott L, et al: Ventricular fluid interleukin-1 activity in head-injured patients. J Lab Clin Med 110:48–54, 1987.

175. McClain CJ, Hennig B, Ott LG, et al: Hypoalbuminemia in head-injured patients. J Neurosurg 69:386–392, 1988.

176. McLaurin RL, McLennan JE: Diagnosis and treatment of head injury in children. In Youmans JR (ed): Neurological Surgery, vol 4, 2nd ed. Philadelphia, W.B. Saunders, 1982, pp 2084–2136.

177. Meadows JC: Dysphagia in unilateral cerebral lesions. J Neurol Neurosurg Psychiatry 36:853–860, 1973.

178. Menguy R, Masters YF: Gastric mucosal energy metabolism and "stress ulceration." Ann Surg 180:538–548, 1974.

179. Methany NA, Eisenberg P, Spies M: Aspiration pneumonia in patients fed through nasoenteral tubes. Heart Lung 15:256, 1986.

180. Meyers MA: Giffiths' point: Critical anastomosis at the splenic flexure. AJR 126:77, 1976.

181. Miller JD: Changing patterns in acute management of head injury. J Neurol Sci 103(Suppl): S33–S37, 1991.

182. Miller JD, Gudeman SK, Kisore PRS, Becker DP: CT scan, ICP and early neurological evaluation in prognosis of severe head injury. Acta Neurochir 28(Suppl):86–88, 1979.

183. Minami H, McCallum RW: The physiology and pathophysiology of gastric emptying in humans. Gastroenterology 86:1592–1610, 1984.

184. Mochizuki H, Trocki O, Dominioni L, et al: Mechanism of prevention of postburn hypermetabolism and catabolism by early enteral feeding. Ann Surg 200:297–310, 1984.

185. Mollitt DL, Golladay ES, Seibert JJ: Symptomatic gastroesophageal reflux following gastrostomy in neurologically impaired patients. Pediatrics 75: 1124–1126, 1985.

186. Moore FA, Haenel JB, Moore EE, Read RA: Percutaneous tracheostomy/gastrostomy in brain-injured patients—A minimally invasive alternative. J Trauma 33:435–439, 1992.

187. Moore FD, Brennan MF: Surgical injury: Body composition, protein metabolism, and neuroendocrinology. In Ballinger WF, Collins JA, Drucker WR, et al (eds): Manual of Surgical Nutrition. Philadelphia, W.B. Saunders, 1975, p 169.

188. Moore R, Najarian MP, Konvolinka CW: Measured energy expenditure in severe head trauma. J Trauma 29:1633–1636, 1989.

189. Morris SE: Development of oral-motor skills in the neurologically impaired child receiving non-oral feedings. Dysphagia 3:135–154, 1989.

190. Mouawad E, Deloof T, Genette F, Vandesteene A: Open trial of cimetidine in the prevention of upper gastrointestinal haemorrhage in patients with severe intracranial injury. Acta Neurochir 67:239–244, 1983.

191. Moustoukas N, Litwin MS: Intracranial placement of nasogastric tube: An unusual complication. South Med J 76:816–817, 1983.

192. Mullen JL, Buzby GP, Matthews DC, et al: Reduction of operative morbidity and mortality by combined preoperative and postoperative nutritional support. Ann Surg 192:604–613, 1980.

193. Myers RE, Yamaguchi S: Nervous system effects of cardiac arrest in monkeys: Preservation of vision. Arch Neurol 34:65–74, 1977.

194. Nahum AM, Harris JP, Davidson TM: The patient who aspirates—Diagnosis and management. J Otolaryngol 10:10–16, 1981.

195. Naraynsingh V, Adam RU: Arteriomesenteric duodenal compression following head injury. West Indian Med J 32:251–253, 1983.

196. Narducci F, Bassotti E, Granata MT, et al: Functional dyspepsia and chronic idiopathic gastric stasis: Role of endogenous opiates. Arch Intern Med 146:716–720, 1986.

197. Nathan M, Leshner R, Keller A: Intractable hiccups. Laryngoscope 90:1612–1618, 1980.

198. Netter FH: Digestive System. Part 1: Upper Digestive Tract. The CIBA Collection of Medical Illustrations, vol 3. New York, 1966, pp 72–75, 78–79.

199. Nimmo WS: Drugs, diseases and altered gastric emptying. Clin Pharmacokinet 1:189–203, 1976.

200. Noble E: Hiccup. Can Med Assoc 31:38–41, 1934.

201. Nompleggi D, Teo TC, Blackburn GL, Bistrian BR: Human recombinant interleukin-1 decreases gastric emptying in the rat [abstract]. Gastroenterology 94:326, 1988.

202. Norton L, Greer J, Eiseman B: Gastric secretory response to head injury. Arch Surg 101:200–204, 1970.

203. Norton JA, Ott LG, McClain C, et al: Intolerance to enteral feeding in the brain-injured patient. J Neurosurg 68:62–66, 1988.

204. Obis P: Remedies for hiccups. Nursing 4:88, 1974.

205. Obrist WD, Langfitt TW, Jaggi JL, et al: Cerebral blood flow and metabolism in comatose patients with acute head injury. J Neurosurg 61:241–253, 1984.

206. Odeh M, Bassan H, Oliven A: Termination of intractable hiccups with digital rectal massage. J Intern Med 227:145–146, 1990.

207. O'Mahony JB, Palder SB, Wood JJ, et al: Depression of cellular immunity after multiple trauma in the absence of sepsis. J Trauma 24:869–875, 1984.

208. Ott L, McClain C, Young B: Nutrition and severe brain injury. Nutrition 5:75–79, 1989.

209. Ott L, Young B, McClain C: The metabolic response to brain injury. JPEN 11:488–493, 1987.

210. Ott L, Young B, Norton J, et al: The metabolic and nutritional sequelae of non-steroid treated head-injured patients [abstract]. JPEN 9:110, 1985.

211. Ott L, Young B, Phillips R, et al: Altered gastric emptying in the head-injured patient: Relationship to feeding intolerance. J Neurosurg 74:738–742, 1991.

212. Parkerson JB Jr, Tylor Z, Flynn JP: Brain injured patients: Comorbidities and ancillary medical requirements. Md Med J 39:259–262, 1990.

213. Perkel MS, Moore C, Herse T, Davidson EP: Metoclopramide therapy in patients with delayed gastric emptying; randomized, double-blind study. Dig Dis Sci 24:662–666, 1979.

214. Perlman AL, Grayhack JP: Use of electroglottograph for measurement of temporal aspects of the swallow: Preliminary observations. Dysphagia 6:1–6, 1991.

215. Perlman AL, Luschei ES, Du Mond CE: Electrical activity in the superior pharyngeal constrictor muscle during reflexive and non-reflexive tasks. J Speech Hear Res 32:749–754, 1989.

216. Philip PA: Superior mesenteric artery syndrome in a child with brain injury: Case report. Am J Phys Med Rehabil 70:280–282, 1991.

217. Phillips R, Ott L, Young B, Walsh J: Nutritional support and measured energy expenditure of the child and adolescent with head injury. J Neurosurg 67:846–851, 1987.

218. Piek J, Robertson CS: Alimentation of head-injured patients. J Neurosurgery 64:984, 1986.

219. Piek J, Gadisseux P, Ward JD, et al: Parenteral nutrition in head injury. J Neurosurg 60:874–876, 1984.

220. Piek J, Lumenta CB, Bock WJ: Protein and amino acid metabolism after severe cerebral trauma. Intens Care Med 11:192–198, 1985.

221. Piek J, Chesnut RM, Marshall LF, et al: Extracranial complications of severe head injury. J Neurosurg 77:901–907, 1992.

222. Pitts LH, Martin N: Head injuries. Surg Clin North Am 62:47–60, 1982.

223. Podell SK: Intermittent tube feedings and gastroesophageal reflux control in head-injured patients. J Am Diet Assoc 89:102–103, 1989.

224. Powell JR, Cate EW: Induction and inhibition of drug metabolism. In Evans WE, Schentag JJ, Jusko WJ (eds): Applied Pharmacokinetics: Principles of Therapeutic Drug Monitoring. Spokane, WA, Applied Therapeutics, 1986, p 139–186.

225. Power I, Easton JC, Todd JG, Nimmo WS: Gastric emptying after head injury. Anaesthesia 44:563–566, 1989.

226. Rapp RP, Young B, Twyman D, et al: The favorable effect of early parenteral feeding on survival in head-injured patients. J Neurosurg 58:906–912, 1983.

227. Read NW, Hougton LA: Physiology of gastric emptying and pathophysiology of gastroparesis. Gastroenterol Clin North Am 18:359–363, 1989.

228. Renton CJC: Massive intestinal infarction following multiple injury. Br J Surg 54:399, 1967.

229. Robertson CS, Clifton GL, Goodman JC: Steroid administration and nitrogen excretion in the head-injured patient. J Neurosurg 63:714–718, 1985.

230. Robertson CS, Clifton GL, Grossman RG: Oxygen utilization and cardiovascular function in head-injured patients. Neurosurgery 15:307–314, 1984.

231. Robertson CS, Goodman JC, Grossman RG: Blood flow and metabolic therapy in CNS injury. J Neurotrauma 9(Suppl 2):579–594, 1992.

232. Rochester DF, Esau SA: Malnutrition and the respiratory system. Chest 85:411–414, 1984.

233. Rosalki SB, Tarlow D, Rau D: Plasma gamma-glutamyl transpeptidase elevation in patients receiving enzyme-inducing drugs. Lancet 2:376–377, 1971.

234. Rosenbek JC, Robbins J, Fishback B, Levine RL: Effects of thermal application on dysphagia after stroke. J Speech Hear Res 34:1257–1268, 1991.

235. Ross MN, Haase GM, Reiley TT, Meagher DP Jr: The importance of acid reflux patterns in neurologically damaged children detected by four-channel esophageal pH monitoring. J Pediatr Surg 23:573–576, 1988.

236. Roueche JR: Dysphagia: An Assessment and Management Program for the Adult. Minneapolis, Sister Kenny Institute, 1980, pp 341, 349–351.

237. Rowlands BJ, Litofsky NS, Kaufman HH: Metabolic physiology, pathophysiology, and, management. In Wirth FP, Ratcheson RA (eds): Neurosurgical Critical Care. Baltimore, Williams & Wilkins, 1987, pp 81–108.

238. Ruberg RL: Role of nutrition in wound healing. Surg Clin North Am 64:705–714, 1984.

239. Rutten P, Blackburn GL, Flatt JP, et al: Determination of optimal hyperalimentation infusion rate. J Surg Res 18:477, 1975.

240. Sacks BA, Vine HS, Palestrant AM, et al: A nonoperative technique for establishment of a gastrostomy in the dog. Invest Radiol 18:485–487, 1983.

241. Samuels L: Hiccup: A ten year review of anatomy, etiology, and treatment. Can Med Assoc J 67:315–322, 1952.

242. Sarna SK, Soergel KH, Koch TR, et al: Gastrointestinal motor effects of erythromycin in humans. Gastroenterology 101:1488–1496, 1991.

243. Sathyavagiswaran L, Sherwin RP: Acute and chronic pericholangiolitis—an association with multifocal hepatic lymphangiomatosis. Hum Pathol 20:601–603, 1989.

244. Schiller WR, Long CL, Blakemore WS: Creatinine and nitrogen excretion in seriously ill and injured patients. Surg Gynecol Obstet 149:561–566, 1979.

245. Schima W, Stacher G, Pokieser P, et al: Esophageal motor disorders: Videofluoroscopic and manometric evaluation—Prospective study in 88 symptomatic patients. Radiology 185:487–491, 1992.

246. Schulze-Delrieu K: Metoclopramide. Gastroenterology 77:768–779, 1979.

247. Sedman AJ: Cimetidine-drug interactions. Am J Med 76:109, 1984.

248. Seebacher J, Nozik D, Mathieu A: Inadvertent intracranial introduction of a nasogastric tube, a complication of severe maxillofacial trauma. Anesthesiology 42:100–102, 1975.

249. Shawker TH, Sonies BC, Stone M: Sonography of speech and swallowing. In Sanders RC, Hill M (eds): Ultrasound Annual. New York, Raven Press, 1984, pp 237–260.

250. Shim C: Motor disturbances of the diaphragm. Clin Chest Med 1:125–129, 1980.

251. Siemkowicz E, Hansen AJ: Clinical restitution following cerebral ischemia in hypo-, normo-, and hyperglycemia rats. Acta Neurol Scand 58:1–8, 1978.

252. Silver KH, Van Nostrand D, Kuhlemeier KV, Siebens AA: Subglottic aspiration: Preliminary observations. Arch Phys Med Rehabil 72:902–910, 1991.

253. Sinclair ME: Lower oesophageal contractility as an indicator of brain death in paralysed and mechanically ventilated patients with head injury. BMJ 294:1488–1489, 1987.

254. Sinclair ME, Suter PM: Lower oesophageal contractility as an indicator of brain death in paralysed and mechanically ventilated patients with head injury. BMJ 294:935–936, 1987.

255. Sneed RC, Morgan WT: Interference of oral phenytoin absorption by enteral tube feedings. Arch Phys Med Rehabil 69:682–684, 1988.

256. Sonies BC: Instrumental procedures for dysphagia diagnosis, swallowing disorders. Semin Speech Lang 12:171–261, 1991.

257. Sonies BC, Baum BJ: Evaluation of swallowing pathophysiology. Otolaryngol Clin North Am 638–648, 1988.

258. Sonies BC, Parent LJ, Morrish K, Baum BJ: Durational aspects of the oral pharyngeal phase of swallowing in normal adults. Dysphagia 3:1–10, 1988.

259. Sorkin EM, Darvey DL: Review of cimetidine drug interactions. Drug Intell Clin Pharm 17:110, 1983.

260. Souadjian J, Cain J: Intractable hiccups: Etiological factors in 220 cases. Postgrad Med 43:72–77, 1983.

261. Splaingard ML, Gaebler D, Havens P, Kalichman M: Brain injury: Functional outcome in children with tracheostomies and gastrostomies. Arch Phys Med Rehabil 70:318–321, 1989.

262. Staff: Report of the Ad Hoc Committee on Dysphagia. Am Speech Lang Hear Assoc 29:57–58, 1987.

263. Stanghellini V, Malagelada JR, Zinsmeister AR, et al: Stress-induced gastroduodenal motor disturbances in humans: Possible humoral mechanisms. Gastroenterology 85:83–91, 1983.

264. Starker PM, Gump FE, Askanzai J, et al: Serum albumin levels as an index of nutritional support. Surgery 91:194–199, 1982.

265. Steffee WP: Malnutrition in hospitalized patients. JAMA 244:2630–2635, 1980.

266. Stine R, Trued S: Hiccups: An unusual manifestation of an abdominal aortic aneurysm. JACEP 8:368–370, 1979.

267. Stone M, Shawker T: An ultrasound examination of tongue movement during swallowing. Dysphagia 1:78–83, 1986.

268. Stromberg B: The hiccup. Ear Nose Throat J 58:354–357, 1979.

269. Tate RL: Issues in the management of behavior disturbances as a consequence of severe head injury. Scand J Rehabil Med 19:13–18, 1987.

270. Tomaselli P, Massei R, Ferrari Da Passano C, et al: Nutritional support in head-injured patients. Agressologie 29:419–421, 1988.

271. Torrealba G, Villar SD, Arriagada P: Protracted vomiting as the presenting sign of posterior fossa mass lesions. J Neurol Neurosurg Psychiatry 50:1539–1541, 1987.

272. Travell J: A trigger point for hiccup. J Am Osteopath Assoc 77:308–312, 1977.

273. Tryba M: Risk of acute stress bleeding and nosocomial pneumonia in ventilated intensive care unit patients: Sucralfate versus antacids. Am J Med 83(Suppl):117–124, 1987.

274. Turner E, Hilfiker O, Braun U, et al: Metabolic and hemodynamic response to hyperventilation in patients with head injuries. Intens Care Med 10:127–132, 1984.

275. Turner WW Jr: Nutritional considerations in the patient with disabling brain disease. Neurosurgery 16:707–713, 1985.

276. Twyman DL, Bivins BA: Nutritional support of the brain injured patient. Five years of clinical study in perspective. Henry Ford Hosp Med J 34:41–47, 1986.

277. Twyman DL, Rapp RP, Young AB: Parenteral vs enteral feedings in severe head injury patients. Presented at the 6th Clinical Congress of the American Society of Parenteral and Enteral Nutrition, San Francisco.

278. Twyman D, Young AB, Ott L, et al: High protein enteral feedings: A means of achieving positive nitrogen balance in head injured patients. JPEN 9:679–684, 1985.

279. Van Miert ASJ, De La Parra DA: Inhibition of gastric emptying by endotoxin (bacterial lipopolysaccharide) in conscious rats and modification of this response by drugs affecting the autonomic nervous system. Arch Int Pharmacodyn Ther 184:27–33, 1970.

280. Veis SL, Logemann JA: Swallowing disorders in persons with cerebrovascular accident. Arch Phys Med Rehabil 66:372–375, 1985.

281. Wagner M, Stapczynski J: Persistent hiccups. Ann Emerg Med 11:24–26, 1985.

282. Walan A: Cimetidine, but not oxmetidine, penetrates into the cerebrospinal fluid after a single intravenous dose. Br J Clin Pharmacol 14:815–819, 1982.

283. Wang SC, Borison HL: A new concept of the organization of the central emetic mechanism: Recent studies on the site of action of apomorphine, copper sulphage and cardiac glycosides. Gastroenterology 22:1–12, 1952.

284. Waters DC, Hoff JT, Black KL: Effect of parenteral nutrition on cold-induced vasogenic edema in cats. J Neurosurg 64:460–465, 1986.

285. Weber FH Jr, Richards RD, McCallum RW: Erythromycin: A motilin agonist and gastrointestinal prokinetic agent [review]. Am J Gastroenterol 88:485–490, 1993.

286. Weinand ME: Medical management in head injury. Kans Med 89:43–45, 1988.

287. White JM, Rumbold GR: Behavioral effects of histamine and its antagonists: A review. Psychopharmacology 95:1–14, 1988.

288. Williams LF, Wittenberg J: Ischemic colitis: A useful clinical diagnosis, but is it ischemic? Ann Surg 182:439, 1975.

289. Williamson B, Macintyre I: Management of intractable hiccup. BMJ 2:501–503, 1977.

290. Wilmore DW: Catabolic illness: Strategies for enhancing recovery. N Engl J Med 325:695–702, 1991.

291. Wilmore DW: The Metabolic Management of the Critically Ill. New York, Plenum, 1977.

292. Winstein CJ: Neurogenic dysphagia. Phys Ther 63:1992–1997, 1983.

293. Wyler AR, Reynolds AF: An intracranial complication of nasogastric intubation. J Neurosurg 47:297–298, 1977.

294. Yadav YR, Khosla VK: Isolated 5th to 10th cranial nerve palsy in closed head trauma. Clin Neurol Neurosurg 93:61–63, 1991.

295. Yamamoto T, Ogata M: The mechanism of recurrent vomiting after mild head injury in children. Arch Jpn Chir 53:106–116, 1984.

296. Yoshida S, Busto R, Abe K, et al: Compression-induced brain edema in rats: Effect of dietary vitamin E on membrane damage in the brain. Neurology 35:126–130, 1985.

297. Young B, Ott L, Haack D, et al: Effect of total parenteral nutrition upon intracranial pressure in severe head injury. J Neurosurg 67:76–80, 1987.

298. Young B, Ott L, Norton J, et al: Metabolic and nutritional sequelae in the nonsteroid treated head injury patient. Neurosurgery 17:784–791, 1985.

299. Young B, Ott L, Twyman D, et al: The effect of nutritional support on outcome from severe head injury. J Neurosurg 67:668–676, 1987.

300. Yuen HK, Hartwick JA: Diet manipulation to resume regular food consumption for an adult with traumatic brain injury. Am J Occup Ther 46:943–945, 1992.

301. Yurkowski PJ, Calis KA: Erythromycin, motilin, and gastroparesis [review]. Clin Pharmacol Ther 11:917–918, 1992.

MARIA L.C. LABI M.D., Ph.D.

21

Neuroendocrine Disorders after Traumatic Brain Injury

Neuroendocrine dysfunction is not an un-common consequence of traumatic brain injury. Its manifestation varies in severity, time of onset, duration, and clinical expression, which may include abnormalities of appetite regulation or control, lability of temperature, hypertension and other cardiovascular abnormalities, thyroid dysfunction, difficulties in fluid regulation, reproductive and/or sexual dysfunction, and immunosuppression. This chapter focuses primarily on hypertension, temperature dysregulation, alterations of appetite, disorders of fluid regulation, and depression of the immune response after TBI.

That such a wide range of clinical disorders may result from TBI is remarkable but not surprising, because the brain is intimately involved in regulating the internal milieu of the body through its control of the endocrine and autonomic nervous systems. To understand this intricate and complex neural control requires an understanding of the relevant anatomic and neurochemical substrates.

The hypothalamus and its related structures play a key role in the regulation and integration of a wide range of sensory information about the internal milieu of the body and in the subsequent mediation of autonomic and metabolic efferent responses that maintain homeostasis. To understand how and why neuroendocrine dysfunction results from brain trauma requires an understanding of the anatomic, neural, and functional organization of the hypothalamic–pituitary axis.

The pituitary gland (hypophysis) lies in the sella turcica and is connected to the hypothalamus via the pituitary (hypophyseal) stalk. The pituitary has two distinct physiologic sections: the **anterior portion** (adenohypophysis) and the **posterior section** (neurohypophysis), which are separated by an avascular zone called the **pars intermedia**. The pituitary secretes humoral factors that act on target organs. Pituitary secretion, in turn, is controlled by the hypothalamus via stimulating hormones or nerve fibers. The anterior pituitary is a highly vascular organ. Blood entering the pituitary passes first through a capillary bed, then through the median eminence of the hypothalamus, and finally through an intricate vascular network of the hypothalamic–hypophyseal portal system. Neurons in the hypothalamus synthesize and secrete various releasing or inhibitory factors, which in turn control the secretion of anterior pituitary hormones. Such neurons originate in various parts of the hypothalamus and project fibers into the median eminence and tuber cinereum, which extends into the pituitary stalk. Anterior pituitary hormones include thyrotropin-releasing hormone, corticotropin-releasing hormone, gonadotropin hormone-releasing hormone, somatostatin, luteinizing hormone-releasing hormone, and prolactin-inhibiting factor. Dopamine is a prolactin-inhibiting factor.

Posterior pituitary cells, on the other hand, do not secrete hormones. Hormones are secreted in the supraoptic nucleus (arginine dihydrolase [ADH]) and paraventricular nucleus (oxytocin) of the hypothalamus. They are subsequently transported by carrier proteins along nerve fibers that pass to the posterior pituitary through the pituitary stalk; the nerve endings lie on capillary surfaces onto which they secrete ADH and oxytocin. Both hormones are then released with appropriate transmission of impulses via exocytosis.[54]

The hypothalamus extends from the region of the optic chiasma to the caudal tip of the mammillary bodies, comprises the ventral wall of the third ventricle below the hypothalamic sulci, and includes the structures of the optic chiasma, tuber cinereum with the infundibulum, and mammillary bodies. Anteriorly, it passes into the basal olfactory area; caudally, it is contiguous with the central gray matter and tegmentum of the mid brain.[126]

Several nuclei and regions are of special interest for the understanding of the neural regulation of endocrine function: (1) the anterior or supraoptic region, which contains the supraoptic and paraventricular nuclei; (2) the middle or tuberal region, which contains the ventromedial and dorsomedial nuclei; and (3) the caudal/mammillary region, which is continuous with the central gray matter of the cerebral aqueduct. The hypothalamus has extensive and complex fiber connections, including afferent connections to the basal forebrain, hippocampus, cortex, frontal lobe, and thalamus as well as efferent descending fibers connecting the hypothalamus with lower autonomic centers that innervate and control visceral structures.[54,126,130] Connections with the pituitary also have been discussed. Functionally, the hypothalamus and adjacent areas constitute the main subcortical center for the regulation of sympathetic and parasympathetic activities.

POSTTRAUMATIC HYPERTENSION

Persistent elevation of blood pressure that is significant enough to warrant treatment is one of the more common disorders after TBI. It usually occurs during the early or acute phase when the cardiovascular profile typically includes signs of a hyperdynamic state secondary to catecholaminergic surge: hypertension, tachycardia, and increased cardiac output.[26–28,53,89,105,117] Cardiac arrhythmias are not infrequent, particularly during the acute period. Occasionally, however, cardiac dysfunction persists well into the subacute phase long after the hyperdynamic state has resolved. Although its true incidence is not clearly established, 10–15% of patients admitted to rehabilitation facilities have been found to have posttraumatic hypertension.[72,79] Risk factors for posttraumatic hypertension include severe injury and focal insult to selective areas. Injury to the hypothalamus makes the patient vulnerable to disruption of normal regulation of autonomic activity, including regulation of blood pressure. The periventricular nucleus has extensive descending fibers to the spinal cord and plays an important role in regulation of blood pressure.[85] Furthermore, focal insult to the orbitofrontal cortex, which facilitates vagal activity and inhibits sympathetic tone of the cardiovascular system, may result in posttraumatic hypertension.[79] Because of its anatomic location the basal forebrain is frequently involved in TBI.

The natural history of posttraumatic hypertension is rather difficult to establish, given that most clinicians choose to treat the disorder. Indeed, some data suggest that prolonged exposure to increased catecholamine activity may predispose to cardiomyopathy in the long term.[101] Evidence suggests, however, that posttraumatic hypertension tends to be a transient phenomenon and merits close monitoring and frequent reassessment of the continuing need for therapeutic intervention. Most patients in a prospective series with posttraumatic hypertension were successfully weaned from hypertensive medications before discharge from the rehabilitation program.[79] Preliminary unpublished data from a current prospective study by the author seem to support this observation.

Because the neurophysiology of posttraumatic hypertension implicates an increased level of catecholaminergic activity, beta blockers appear to be a rational choice (and probably the first line) of treatment for most patients. Beta blockers have direct cardiac effects as well as effects on presynaptic beta receptors in the sympathetic ganglia. Although propranolol was one of the first beta blockers used to treat posttraumatic hypertension, longer-acting alternatives with greater cardioselectivity and possibly fewer side effects on the central nervous system are available. Calcium channel blockers, especially the newer ones, and angiotensin-converting enzymes also have been used. Vasodilators, although effective antihypertensive agents, are rarely necessary. Concurrent use of beta blockers often is required to control reflex tachycardia,[65,66] and during the acute period the potential for decreasing cerebral perfusion through peripheral vasodilation needs to be taken into consideration.

The specific choice of hypertensive medication, if needed, should take into account noncardiac side effects. For the patient with TBI side effects on the central nervous system, specifically those that may affect cognition, are especially important. In general, lipophilic drugs are more likely to have side effects on the central nervous system because of the greater ease with which they cross the blood-brain barrier. Propranolol, one of the earliest beta blockers, is frequently associated with lethargy, attention problems, and decreased memory. For the patient with significant chronic obstructive pulmonary disease, choice of beta blockers should take into account the respiratory side effects of the less selective agents. Such effects on the central nervous system appear to be less with atenolol and metoprolol, which are more hydrophilic as well as more cardioselective. Alpha-adrenergic agonists (e.g., clonidine) are a rational alternative. Long-acting transdermal patches, which offer the convenience of once-a-week dosing and bypass the oral route in patients with significant dysphagia, warrant at least a trial.

Before starting long-term hypertensive medication in a patient with TBI, a baseline diagnostic work-up is recommended to evaluate associated pathology that may exacerbate the hypertension. A baseline electrocardiogram and echocardiography should be considered if they have not yet been done. In the appropriate clinical setting, other underlying causes such as pheochromocytoma should be ruled out before starting a definitive pharmacologic regimen. Patients with multiple trauma may have an associated undiagnosed cardiac contusion; this possibility needs to be taken into consideration when choosing hypertensive medication.

NEUROIMMUNOLOGY

Infections are a common cause of morbidity in patients after severe trauma, especially to the head. Advances in prehospital care and early aggressive diagnostic and therapeutic management have led to the survival of increasing numbers of victims of severe head trauma. Such patients are at risk for prolonged hospitalizations and subsequent infectious complications. Many studies[8,51,59,106] estimate that about half of such patients develop an infectious complication, usually during the acute phase of hospitalization.

That infections are common is not surprising, because many patients have associated injuries (e.g, fractures, open wounds) that increase susceptibility to infection and frequently require surgical intervention that compounds the risk. Patients also may be at increased risk after head trauma as a direct result of injury to the central nervous system.[46]

An increasing number of clinical and experimental studies suggest that severe head trauma may result in suppression of the immune response, which in part would explain the high risk for infectious complications in this population, particularly during the early course of hospitalization. The precise nature of immunosuppression is not clear at this time, but mounting evidence points to a greater vulnerability of the cellular arm of the immune response after head trauma.[33,67,91,85,110,138] Although the mechanism is not well-understood, depression of the cellular response results in suppression of lymphocyte activation and cytokine production. Furthermore, cellular immunity tends to be maximally depressed during the first 24 hours after injury,[110,138] but the depression may persist for several weeks. In contrast, the humoral response does not appear to be directly affected.[91]

Depression of the immune response after severe trauma has been linked to the neuroendocrine system, which mediates the hormonal and neural response to stress. Glucocorticoids and epinephrine are the most critical hormones released during the response to stress. Hormonal secretion, however, is only the final step in a cascade of events that begin in the brain,[118] which has to perceive the stress before it can set into motion the appropriate hormonal responses via the appropriate neural centers. The end result is a whole series of metabolic, cardiovascular, gastrointestinal, reproductive, and immunologic events aimed at maximizing the potential for immediate survival. Such adaptive responses favor catabolic processes, blunting of pain perception, and suppression of reproductive function. Clinicians who treat patients with severe trauma are well aware of this clinical picture, particularly in the early phases. Paradoxically, this response also results in depression of the immune function during stress. To understand how this occurs, a brief description of the immune system is helpful.

The primary task of the immune system is to defend the body against infectious challenges. The basic cell types that make up the circulating immune system are lymphocytes and monocytes. Lymphocytes consist of two classes, T-cells and B-cells. Although both originate in the bone marrow, T-cells migrate to and mature in the thymus, whereas B-cells mature in the bone marrow. Both have subpopulations with some functional specialization. B-cells and T-cells mediate different forms of immunity. B-cells are involved in antibody-mediated immune response, whereas T-cells play a major role in cell-mediated immunity. However, the two immune compartments are intricately related, and proper functioning of the immune system depends on T-cells collaborating with B-cells for normal production of antibodies.[4,118]

A functional immune system depends on a complex system of activation of cascades involving the different cellular types and subtypes that are scattered in circulation. Communication among different cell types is triggered by chemical messengers; for example, cytokine interleukin-1 (IL-1) is released by a monocyte (macrophage) upon contact with an infectious agent. IL-1 triggers a T-cell (T-helper) to release interleukin-2 (IL-2), which in turn stimulates T-cell proliferation and thus helps in production and proliferation of cytotoxic killer cells that destroy the pathogen.

On the hormonal side, T-cells secrete B-cell growth factor, which stimulates differentiation and proliferation of B-cells. More and more studies indicate the presence of other interleukins and cytokines that most likely have different functional specializations and thus add to the complexity of the immune system.

The neural regulation of the immune system during stress is mediated primarily by glucocorticoids, the main effect of which appears to be inhibitory. Glucocorticoids inhibit the release of cytokines and the sensitivity of target cells by decreasing the number of receptors for the cytokines. Once activated, glucocorticoids inhibit the action of target cells. Glucocorticoids also inhibit release of IL-1 and production of certain complement components and block maturation of developing lymphocytes. The disruption of the network of chemical signals results in inhibition of the proliferative system that the immune system needs to fight off infectious challenges.

The contribution of the sympathetic nervous system to stress-induced immunosuppression needs further research, but experimental animal data suggest that the sympathetic nervous system sends projections into immune tissues such as the spleen, thymus, and bone marrow during stress and that immune activity apparently is enhanced after destruction of such projections. Mice with tumors show a decrease in natural killer cells and reduced survival time after foot-shock stress, but the effect is blocked by the opiate receptor blocker, naltrexone. Furthermore, opiate injection into the periaqueductal gray area suppresses natural killer cell activity, strengthening the hypothesis that opiate-induced immunosuppression may be relayed by the brain.[118] The hypothalamus, either directly or through its complex interactions with other regions, is implicated in this stress-induced depression of natural killer cell activity. Hypothalamic lesions in mice result in total abrogation of natural killer cell activity that is due not to cell-mediated suppressor mechanisms but rather to interference with natural killer cell maturation and activity. It is postulated that hypothalamic lesions, directly or indirectly, block the basal production of neuroendocrine or immune system hormones, (e.g., endorphin, interferon, or IL-2) that may be essential in the maturation and activation of natural killer cells.[46]

The rationale for why immune function is suppressed during stress is not clear at this time. Regardless of the reason, the regulation of the immune system by the neuroendocrine system is well-accepted, although recent evidence suggests that the immune system in turn regulates neuroendocrine function through stimulation of glucocorticoid secretion and adrenocorticotropic hormone from the pituitary by IL-1. Whatever the rationale, a better understanding of the mechanisms of neuroendocrine regulation of the immune system and vice versa raises the possibility of manipulating the immune system to reverse the immunologic deficits noted after severe trauma, thereby decreasing the morbidity and mortality from infection.

TEMPERATURE DYSREGULATION

Fever is the most common complication encountered by the clinician involved in the care of patients who sustain significant TBI, especially during the acute phase and, not infrequently, the subacute phase. Management and treatment initially differ little from the protocol in patients without TBI. Temperature elevations usually trigger a search for a specific, inciting etiology, and treatment is based on the presumed cause. Because fever is the most common physiologic indicator of an underlying infectious or inflammatory process, the search for a specific etiology can be costly, protracted, and sometimes invasive. In the case of true central fever, the work-up is frequently unproductive.

Because the patient with significant brain trauma frequently has other associated conditions, as a result either of multiple trauma or of direct trauma to the central nervous system, a complete and thorough work-up to establish the cause and to rule out an infectious process is necessary, especially early during hospitalization. Such patients may have had surgical interventions—orthopedic, neurosurgical, or abdominal explorations; neurogenic bladders with or without indwelling catheters; tracheostomies—that place them at increased risk for urinary tract infections or respiratory insufficiency. In addition, prolonged immobilization because of fractures, weakness, or poor arousal puts them at increased risk for deep venous thrombosis, an early manifestation of which may be recurrent fever. Other common complications of severe TBI that may be associated with fever include heterotopic ossification and drug fever.

In a small—but probably not insignificant—proportion of patients with severe TBI, the work-up for fever yields no treatable complication, or fever may persist despite adequate treatment or withdrawal of the presumed cause. Thus the clinician is led to conclude that the temperature elevation is most likely due to central fever. Central fever may consist of mild to modest elevations that respond to common symptomatic treatments such as acetaminophen, aspirin, or cooling blankets or resolve with no treatment at all. On the other hand, it may manifest as severe and labile fluctuations of temperature, from severe hypothermia that may or may not respond to cooling or warming blankets and over-the-counter antipyretic medications. In such instances, iced gastric lavage may be helpful in controlling temperatures, although one needs to be careful that the rate of rewarming is not excessively rapid in order to minimize complications. Clifton et al. note that a rate of rewarming of 1.5° C/hr with gastric lavage is well-tolerated.[24]

Occasionally, severe temperature elevations occur as part of a more dramatic constellation of clinical signs referred to as a diencephalic storm: Increased temperatures precede or accompany other signs of severe autonomic dysfunction (e.g., hypertension, diaphoresis, flushing, tachycardia, hyperventilation) that may represent a release phenomenon at the level of the brainstem and diencephalon as a result of loss of cortical and subcortical control.[15]

To understand such clinical manifestations requires an understanding of the neural regulation of temperature. In the normal individual, core body temperature remains constant despite a wide range of external temperature fluctuations to which the body may be exposed. Thus, the body may be exposed to extremes of 60–130° F and still maintain a body core temperature between 98°–100° F. The maintenance of core body temperature within this narrow range depends on an intricate and exquisitely balanced neural circuitry, the central control of which resides in the hypothalamus.[39,54]

Control of body temperature depends on a sensitive balance and interplay of heat-dissipating and heat-producing mechanisms. When body temperature drops, heat-producing mechanisms are triggered primarily through vasoconstriction, piloerection (more significant in nonhumans), and increased shivering by skeletal muscles. Conversely, when body temperature is too great, three important mechanisms come into play to decrease body heat: (1) increased vasodilation through inhibition of sympathetic centers; (2) stimulation of sweating; and (3) inhibition of shivering.[54]

The neural circuitry for the central regulation of body temperature resides in the hypothalamus, where thermoregulatory neurons are most abundant. Thermoregulatory neurons are also found in the cerebral cortex, mesencephalon, medulla, and spinal cord. However, the coordination of the autonomic responses with the appropriate neuroendocrine and behavioral changes to regulate temperature resides in the hypothalamus. The regulation of body temperature is mediated by two hypothalamic areas. The anterior hypothalamus, especially the preoptic area, is sensitive to increases in temperature. When this area is stimulated, thermal information is integrated and relayed through neuronal effectors (probably through the medial forebrain) of heat generation and dissipation located in the posterior hypothalamus. Profuse sweating, due to activation of sweat glands innervated by cholinergic fibers

but also stimulated by circulating epinephrine or norepinephrine, and cutaneous vasodilation result in rapid heat elimination. The posterior hypothalamus is sensitive to conditions of decreasing body temperature. Stimulation of this area sets into motion mechanisms that result in vasoconstriction, piloerection, and increased muscle tone. In the dorsomedial portion of the hypothalamus near the wall of the third ventricle lies an area believed to contain the primary motor center for shivering.[49] Normally this area is inhibited by heat signals from the preoptic area but stimulated by cold signals from peripheral receptors in the skin. In response to cold, the center is activated, and impulses are then transmitted through bilateral tracts down the brainstem to the lateral spinal cord and the anterior motor neurons. Such impulses result in increased tone of the skeletal muscles and shivering. Through this mechanism production of body heat may increase as much as 4–5 times above normal.[54] Bilateral posterior hypothalamic damage results in poikilothermia.[11] In general, destructive lesions of the preoptic and anterior hypothalamus are believed to result in hyperthermia.

Body temperature is believed to be normally regulated around a set point, departure from which sets into motion processes and behavior mediated by the autonomic and endocrine systems that attempt to correct and reestablish body temperature. However, this set point may be altered in disease states. In addition to the neural network centered in the hypothalamic thermoregulatory center, fever appears to be mediated by neurotransmitters and immunologic factors with pyrogenic properties.[39] Endogenous pyrogens are believed to exert their effect by inducing increases in arachidonic acid metabolites. Experimentally, increases in these metabolites are associated with increases in the hypothalamic thermostat to febrile levels. Furthermore, experimental studies show that injection of arachidonic acid into the hypothalamus produces fever. Of these metabolites, prostaglandin E2 appears to be the major metabolite with pyrogenic property. Pyrogens reach the hypothalamus via the arterial circulation and have their major effect on the vascular networks close to the cluster of neurons in the preoptic and anterior hypothalamus. This site, called the organum vasculosum laminae terminalis, appears to have little blood-brain barrier. Removal of this area prevents fever after a peripheral injection of an endogenous pyrogen but has no effect when the endogenous pyrogen is injected directly into brain tissue. Other substances that appear to have endogenous pyrogenic properties include interleukin-1 (IL-1) and tumor necrosis factor. Both are produced by astrocytes and microglia within the central nervous system; thus endogenous pyrogens may be produced near the hypothalamus and therefore reach the hypothalamus by a route other than the carotid circulation.[39] The hypothalamic thermostat normally appears to be set and reset with varying concentrations of such pyrogens. In the presence of hypothalamic dysfunction— as may be the case in patients with severe TBI—the triggered thermogenic response in the presence of circulating pyrogens may be exaggerated and thus explain the not uncommon clinical presentation of markedly disproportionate temperature elevations in the presence of mild infection. In the patient with significant head trauma, such elevations may be further exacerbated by increased levels of circulating catecholamines; epinephrine and norepinephrine may have thermogenic effects through their ability to uncouple the oxidative–phosphorylative process and thus increase oxidation, rate of cellular metabolism, and temperature.[54]

Whether or not central fever needs to be treated depends partly on the degree of temperature elevation as well as the time from onset of injury during which fever occurs. Experimental evidence suggests, however, that treatment is the more prudent course, especially during the early period after the injury for four major reasons:

1. Small variations in brain temperature may critically determine the extent of histopathologic injury.[17,21,38,71]

2. Core body temperature and brain temperature may differ significantly, especially in ischemic areas of the brain, which may have much higher temperatures than the core temperatures.[71]

3. Disruption of the blood-brain barrier increases with temperature after brain injury.[36–38]

4. Elevated temperature may exacerbate the excitotoxic effects of substances released after an acute injury.[16,22–23,48,74,87]

Although the beneficial effects of hypothermia are still a matter of debate, the minimal complications of systemic hypothermia (at or above 30° C) and the potential for improving outcomes after severe TBI[24–25,38,40,119] warrant careful attention to minimizing significant temperature fluctuations, particularly in the early period of management. As in any patient population, recurrent fever in head-injured patients warrants a complete and exhaustive work-up to rule out an occult etiology. Because many head-injured patients may have severely depressed cognitive status, they may not be able to provide a clue or specific complaint; thus work-up is frequently and unavoidably prolonged and expensive. In the author's personal experience, fevers assumed by many house officers to be central in origin are often due to occult etiologies that require vastly different treatments. Other intracranial pathologies, such as acute hydrocephalus[122] or increased intracranial pressure,[43] may manifest as fever that also is classified as central, but treatment obviously addresses the ventricular enlargement and obstructed flow of cerebrospinal fluids.

Thus, the decision to treat or not to treat central fever should take into consideration the total clinical picture, including not only the acuity and severity of the fever but also the vulnerability of the patient to the increased metabolic demands associated with elevated temperatures. During the early period, the need to minimize the negative effects of the initial injury favors treatment of febrile episodes. Furthermore, older or more compromised patients are more likely to require intervention, because they tend to be more vulnerable to increased levels of metabolism.

Treatment of central fever includes the use of cooling blankets and the more common antipyretics (e.g., acetaminophen, aspirin, and other nonsteroidal anti-inflammatory drugs) that block the production of prostaglandins. Less commonly iced gastric lavage is used, usually in the very acute period. A few patients, however, continue to have significant and persistent temperature elevations despite cooling blankets and medications. Controlled clinical studies of pharmacologic management of patients with TBI and central fever are understandably difficult; most published guidelines for treatment of central fever in TBI are based on case reports with limited numbers of patients. Such reports suggest the efficacy of dopaminergic agents with or without the use of opiate agonists,[15] chlorpromazine,[120] and dantrolene sodium, which is effective in the treatment of malignant hyperthermia. In experimental animals, nonopiate sedatives such as chloral hydrate have been shown to have hypothermic effects.[109] The author has successfully reduced excessively high temperatures (up to 108° F) and arrested further progression of fever in a comatose patient with clonidine, a centrally acting alpha agonist. This treatment was selected after observing through serial laboratory measurements that noradrenergic metabolites were significantly elevated during febrile episodes but decreased with resolution of fever. The use of the clonidine transdermal patch offers theoretical advantage in patients whose temperature elevations are more persistent and long-lasting.

The *apparent* effectiveness of a wide variety of drugs with broad (even antagonistic) pharmacologic activity in the treatment of central fever points to the extreme complexity of the neural regulation of temperature, the multiplicity of mediating neurotransmitters, and the wide overlap of various receptor areas in key neuroanatomic regions of the brain. Because dopaminergic and opioid receptor areas overlap in the nigrostriatal, mesolimbic, and tuberoinfundibular systems,[15] lesions may affect multiple systems and multiple neurotransmitters. Neuroleptics are generally avoided in the patient with TBI because of their known antidopaminergic effects and their adverse effect on motor and cognitive function.

ANTERIOR AND POSTERIOR PITUITARY DYSFUNCTION

The regulation of body fluids is mediated primarily through vasopressin or antidiuretic hormone (ADH), a neurotransmitter secreted by neurons in the supraoptic and paraventricular nuclei of the hypothalamus. ADH is subsequently transported along nerve fibers through the pituitary stalk, the nerve terminals of which lie in the posterior pituitary gland.

The supraoptic nucleus appears to be the most vulnerable area of the hypothalamus,[125] and disturbances of fluid regulation are not uncommon after severe TBI. Although they are more likely to occur during the acute period, they may not become manifest until months later.[65,120] Clinically, posterior pituitary dysfunction manifests as syndrome of inappropriate secretion of antidiuretic hormone (SIADH), in which secretion of ADH is excessive, or diabetes insipidus, in which secretion of ADH is absent or inadequate.

Release of ADH is regulated primarily by plasma osmotic pressure and circulating blood volume. ADH acts mainly on the distal tubules of the nephron. In its presence, the tubules are permeable to water and water reabsorption is increased. In its absence, the distal tubules and collecting duct are virtually impermeable to water, resulting in increased loss of free water.[54,97] Under normal circumstances, plasma osmolality is maintained within a narrow range, and secretion or inhibition of ADH is triggered in response to small changes in plasma osmolality. In some circumstances, however, osmotic and volume influences may be competitive; thus defense of plasma volume may override plasma osmolality in stimulating further release of ADH.[97]

Clinical signs and symptoms of hypothalamic–pituitary dysfunction are easily recognized. Patients with diabetes insipidus usually exhibit polydipsia and polyuria, associated with hypernatremia, normal or high serum osmolality, and disproportionately diluted urine. These signs may be accompanied by symptoms of fatigue and—not uncommonly—changes in mental status that may not be easily assessed in the acute or intensive care setting. SIADH, on the other hand, is associated with hyponatremia, lethargy, nausea, and even seizures.

Although diabetes insipidus and SIADH are considered to be relatively rare after TBI,[107] their true incidence is probably greater than current estimates. Autopsy series of patients dying after acute TBI indicate that a large proportion have significant hypothalamic–pituitary lesions[32,57] and suggest that the true frequencies are higher.

Such patients, however, frequently do not survive long enough to manifest clinical signs of pituitary dysfunction because of the severity of brain injury. In patients who survive and manifest pituitary dysfunction, the association with markers of severity of TBI—skull and facial fractures, cranial nerve damage, and significant period of unconsciousness[11–12,35,40,42,47,52,55–56,70,76,82,97–98,107,120,129,134]—is rather compelling. However, diabetes insipidus has been reported even in a patient with head trauma but no direct injury to the head.[121]

The severity of fluid disturbance and course of recovery over time depend on the degree of injury to the supraoptic nucleus, paraventricular nucleus, and neurohypophyseal stalk. Experimental studies indicate that pituitary stalk transection alone does not produce permanent diabetes insipidus in the absence of more proximal lesions in the median eminence. The degree of recovery in diabetes insipidus is related to the number of vasopressin-secreting magnocellular neurons that remain viable after the injury. If less than 10%–20% of the neurons remain viable, diabetes insipidus is more likely to be permanent.[129]

The mechanism of diabetes insipidus may involve transection of the pituitary stalk at various levels with traction, spasm, or occlusion followed by cerebral ischemia, infarction, carotid–cavernous sinus fistulas, laceration, hemorrhage, and necrosis.[32,77,82,126] Fat embolism also has been reported.[56] The mechanism for SIADH after TBI is not as well understood, but it may result from stimulation or irritation of the hypothalamic hypophyseal system.[11,97] Traumatic lesions of the suprasellar region, including fracture and infarction, are now demonstrable with magnetic resonance imaging.[55,86]

Diabetes insipidus is suspected in the presence of polyuria (without concomitant hyperglycemia) with increased (or normal) serum osmolality and dilute urine. The diagnosis is easily and reliably established when urine osmolality reaches a plateau after 12–18 hours of fluid deprivation and then increases after a subcutaneous injection of aqueous vasopressin.[97] This procedure facilitates recognition of even mild cases of diabetes insipidus in which endogenous vasopressin

after dehydration may be sufficient to raise urine osmolality.

Diagnosis of SIADH requires the exclusion of adrenal insufficiency (glucocorticoid deficiency may mimic SIADH[97]) and drug-related SIADH. Many of the medications used in patients with TBI, acutely or otherwise (e.g., carbamazepine), may induce SIADH. The diagnosis of SIADH is usually established—once other confounding variables are ruled out—by an oral water load of 20 ml/kg body weight given over 15–20 minutes. Urine is collected hourly for the next 5 hours with the patient in a recumbent position. In normal individuals, greater than 80% of the water is usually excreted by the end of the fifth hour with a corresponding decrease in urine osmolality to less than 100 mosm/kg. Patients with SIADH, in contrast, usually excrete less than 40% of the water and fail to dilute urine maximally and urine osmolality is hypertonic compared with plasma osmolality. The water-loading test, however, can be dangerous unless serum sodium is above 125 mEq/L.[97]

The drug of choice for treatment of diabetes insipidus is l-d-amino-8-D-arginine-vasopressin (DDAVP). It is available as a nasal spray, has a prolonged antidiuretic action (13–22 hr), and is usually effective in a once or twice daily dose. Carbamazepine at 400 mg/day also has been reported to be effective.[81]

SIADH usually is treated through fluid restriction. The role of pharmacologic agents in treatment of SIADH has been limited, although oxilorphan, a narcotic antagonist, has been reported to improve SIADH due to trauma from a cavernous sinus internal carotid fistula. Other drugs, such as the anticonvulsant diphenylhydantoin (Dilantin), inhibit release of ADH acutely but not in the long-term.[97] Alcohol is known to suppress the release of ADH but its potential usefulness is obviously limited in patients after TBI. When fluid restriction is difficult to maintain, demethylchlortetracycline has been used with minimal adverse consequences in some patients with SIADH due to lung malignancy.[97] Its usefulness in trauma-related SIADH is unclear. Although drugs (such as chlorpromazine) have been noted to have diuretic properties secondary to their inhibition of

ADH release or action, their use in patients with TBI is probably limited by the potential adverse effects of their antidopaminergic action on cognitive and motor function. Needless to say, if SIADH is iatrogenic or drug-related, treatment should focus on the inciting drug.

Compared with posterior pituitary dysfunction, disorders of anterior pituitary function are less frequent after head trauma. In addition, they become clinically evident much later. Because the anterior pituitary is involved in regulating the activities of different organs, clinical manifestations tend to reflect dysfunction in the affected target organ. The anterior pituitary secretes thyroid-stimulating hormone, growth hormone, adrenocorticotropin hormone, follicle-stimulating hormone, luteinizing hormone, prolactin, adrenocorticotropic hormone, and melanocyte-stimulating hormone. Secretion of each of these hormones, in turn, is triggered or controlled mainly by their respective releasing factors produced in the hypothalamus. Trauma to the hypothalamic–anterior pituitary axis can disrupt function of target organs selectively. Occasionally, head trauma results in total disruption of the hypothalamic–pituitary axis leading to the classic clinical syndrome of panhypopituitarism.[12,76]

In the adult, clinical manifestations of pituitary insufficiency after TBI usually reflect signs and symptoms of deficient function of the target organ. Hypogonadism is a frequent manifestation of anterior pituitary disorder after head trauma. The usual presenting symptoms include amenorrhea, decreased libido, impotence, and loss of secondary sexual characteristics. Work-up reveals low levels of gonadal hormones. Levels of gonadotropins also are low. Diagnosis of hypothalamic pituitary lesion is established by luteinizing hormone-releasing hormone (LHRH) stimulation test. In hypothalamic lesions, pituitary responsiveness is restored after LHRH stimulation. The luteinizing hormone and follicle-stimulating hormone response should be absent or low in pituitary lesions. However, in some patients with suprasellar tumors, prolonged administration of LHRH may require added phasic stimulation to elicit a response.[58] Whether this is true for patients with traumatic hypothalamic lesions is uncertain.

Selective growth hormone deficiency after trauma is rarely sufficiently problematic in adults to trigger intensive or extensive investigation and intervention. In children, however, selective growth hormone deficiency that leads to stunting of growth and delay in bone maturation becomes more clinically obvious, thereby triggering further work-up. Pituitary dysfunction has been seen after head trauma due to child abuse.[90] However, although deficiencies of growth hormone are not as apparent in the adult with head trauma, they may exacerbate the patient's vulnerability to the systemic effects of severe trauma. Growth hormone plays a critical role in the mobilization of body stores of fat and increases protein synthesis. Lack of growth hormone, therefore, may exacerbate the catabolic state that commonly follows severe trauma. Normally, hypothalamic signals of emotion, stress, and trauma result in secretion of growth hormone. This secretion is stimulated by growth hormone-releasing hormone from the ventromedial hypothalamus. This same area is also sensitive to hypoglycemia.[54] Growth hormone is inhibited by somatostatin or growth hormone-inhibiting hormone. Treatment in children involves replacement of growth hormones.

The hypothalamic–pituitary–adrenal axis is clinically crucial, because deficiencies of glucocorticoid function are potentially fatal. After hypoadrenalism is ruled out dysfunction is diagnosed by the corticotropin-releasing factor stimulation test. The adrenocorticotropic hormone response by the pituitary is exaggerated in hypothalamic hypopituitarism and subnormal in pituitary-dependent hypopituitarism.[97] Treatment involves replacement of glucocorticoids and mineralocorticoids.

Normal thyroid function is necessary to maintain normal metabolic rate and to stimulate growth in children. The amount of circulating thyroid hormones—T4 and T3—is normally under negative feedback control by the pituitary through secretion of thyroid-stimulating hormone (TSH). TSH secretion, in turn, is under hypothalamic regulation: thyrotropin-releasing hormone (TRH) provides the main signal for release, whereas somatostatin inhibits the release of TSH as well as growth hormones.[54,95] Thus, an intact hypothalamic–pituitary axis is essential in maintaining normal thyroid function and overall metabolism.

The thyrotropic region of the hypothalamus is believed to be in the anterior hypothalamus. Although TRH has been found throughout the hypothalamus, concentrations are highest in the ventral area and median eminence. A high concentration also has been found in the preoptic area, where TRH is believed to play an important role in the TSH response to temperature. TRH also has been reported in other areas of the central nervous system, such as the pineal gland, retina, and spinal cord.[95]

Secretion of TSH is affected by many factors. Somatostatin, dopamine, cholecystokinin (which is present in large amounts in the hypothalamus), glucocorticoids, and opiates or endogenous opioids inhibit secretion. Valproic acid, an inhibitor of gamma-aminobutyric acid (GABA), has been noted to decrease secretion, but the role of GABA is still ambiguous. Secretion of TSH is increased by norepinephrine and clonidine (an alpha agonist) as well as systemic stress such as infections or starvation. The effect of serotonin is unclear, although serotonin blockers have been associated with a decrease in TSH response to TRH stimulation.[95] Likewise, the effect of gonadotropic hormones such as testosterone and estrogen is unclear, but evidence suggests a possible role in modulation. Dopamine decreases TSH probably through direct pituitary inhibition.[73] Because dopamine is often used in patients with TBI, in both acute and later stages, its potential impact on thyroid function should be considered.

The importance of ascertaining normal thyroid function in patients after TBI cannot be overemphasized; their risk for pituitary dysfunction in general and thyroid dysfunction in particular is significant, given the usual mechanism of injury associated with TBI. In addition, patients with TBI frequently have other complications secondary to multiple traumatic injuries. Abnormalities of thyroid function tests are common not only in patients with TBI but in other patient populations as well. In a study of patients admitted to a general medical service, the frequency of abnormalities of at least one thyroid parameter was noted to be over 20%.[50]

The frequency of such abnormalities in patients after TBI is probably comparable, although true epidemiologic studies are lacking. However, the degree to which testing abnormalities reflect true thyroid dysfunction is not always clear; confounding variables that spuriously depress thyroid enzymes—such as medication and protein status—are also common in patients with TBI.[89] Accurate diagnosis usually requires TRH stimulation.[10,97]

It is critical to ascertain a functional hypothalamic–pituitary–thyroid axis, because available evidence suggests a poorer prognosis for patients with severe TBI and associated thyroid dysfunction, at least in the acute period.[20,135] Prolonged unresponsiveness has been associated with hypothyroidism and hypogonadism.[44,115] Whether hypothyroidism prolongs or exacerbates the period of unresponsiveness is of clinical importance. If concomitant hypothyroidism is present, patients, especially those with poor arousal, may benefit from treatment of the hypothyroidism.

Diagnosis of hypothalamic or pituitary hypothyroidism is usually made on the basis of TSH response to TRH stimulation. However, whether the TSH response to stimulation in fact distinguishes between hypothalamic and pituitary lesions is somewhat controversial, because some patients with documented hypothalamic hypothyroidism have impaired TSH response to TRH stimulation.[95] In such cases, the role of inhibitory factors may be important. In patients with TBI the TRH stimulation tests is still the most widely used method of diagnosing hypothalamic–pituitary hypothyroidism.

The hypothalamic–pituitary axis must be viewed as a physiologic unit that influences autonomic and endocrine function; its integrity is critical in maintaining normal homeostasis. The clinical manifestations of lesions along the axis depend not only on the degree of severity of the lesion but also on its specific anatomic location. Whereas lesions may involve primarily the posterior or anterior pituitary axis, concomitant dysfunction in the other region needs to be investigated; patients with clinical manifestations of disturbances of posterior pituitary function also may have decreased anterior pituitary reserves.[98] Although complete disruption of total pituitary function is rare, continuous improvements in emergency and acute care of patients with traumatic brain injury probably will result in survival of more patients with more severe pituitary dysfunction. More precise diagnostic tools are now available, combining biochemical testing with better imaging techniques.[10,55,86] The hypothalamic–pituitary axis is vulnerable to injury from traction, laceration, hemorrhage, ischemia or infarction—mechanisms that are common with head trauma. However, different causes of TBI may carry different risks for hypothalamic–pituitary dysfunction.[14]

DISORDERS OF APPETITE CONTROL

Early descriptions of patients with obesity and pituitary lesions—initially by Mohr in 1840 and subsequently by Frohlich in 1901—provided the impetus for research into the central regulation of appetite and resulting eating disorders. Until Erdheim challenged the validity of the supposition, however, obesity was presumed to be a result of pituitary undersecretion. After careful review of cases, Erdheim suggested that the dysfunction results from a neural lesion. Anand's experimental work[5,6] produced diabetes insipidus and obesity in animals after a hypothalamic lesion and thus provided further evidence implicating the hypothalamus in appetite regulation.

Stereotactic instrumentation allowed the introduction of selective hypothalamic lesions without direct pituitary injury and more precise evaluation of the results and clinical manifestations of selectively targeted lesions. These investigations suggested that obesity usually was produced by lesions in the ventromedial hypothalamus[63,122] and resulted from increased eating activity or hyperphagia. Conversely, lesions in the lateral hypothalamus led to a decrease or complete inhibition of eating, resulting in starvation and death, unless animals were force-fed. Such studies have led to the view that the ventromedial hypothalamus is a satiety center. Stimulation of the ventromedial hypothalamus in experimental animals leads to cessation of feeding; its destruction results in excessive eating. Likewise, the lateral hypothalamus has been viewed as a feeding center, the destruction of which results in cessation of eating.

Human analogs of experimental models of feeding disorders associated with lesions in the central nervous system are relatively rare but are seen in a number of well-known clinical entities. Although Kleine-Levin and Kluver-Bucy syndromes are the most dramatic examples of marked abnormalities of ingestive behavior, many patients with marked hyperphagia in association with hypothalamic neoplasms have been reported.[18,103,113] However, whereas in experimental animal models selective stereotactic lesions can produce feeding abnormalities with a minimum of other disorders, in humans hyperphagia tends to be associated with various other abnormalities, including dementia, rage and autonomic dysfunction[113]; hemiparesis and endocrine disturbances[16]; bizarre behavior; and hypersomnolence.[133] Most reported cases have had neoplastic etiologies, but trauma has been associated with similar disorders with increasing frequency.[13,60,132,133] Unlike the experimental models, however, the lesions in humans are seldom precisely localized, although most tend to involve the presumed hypothalamic centers.

The concept of a satiety and a feeding center residing in and controlled by the ventromedial and lateral hypothalamus, respectively, has come under increasing doubt. More and more research suggests that although hypothalamic lesions may be associated with disturbances in eating behavior, lesions restricted to the ventromedial or lateral area were neither sufficient nor necessary to produce hyperphagia and obesity.[49,101] Indeed, in one patient a tumor in the midline of the hypothalamus resulted in anorexia and inanition instead of the hyperphagia and obesity that otherwise may have been expected.[83] Such observations have led to the search for the underlying mechanisms that mediate the neural regulation of appetite and ingestive behavior.

More recent findings indicate that the concept of the ventral hypothalamus as having two distinct internal centers is a gross oversimplification. Hyperphagia and obesity after hypothalamic lesions are associated with hypersecretion of insulin. In rats subdiaphragmatic vagotomy attenuates hyperphagia and obesity after ventromedial lesions;[31,108] furthermore, the lateral hypothalamic syndrome is associated with alterations in parasympathetic and sympathetic activity.[94] Such observations implicate autonomic regulation of endocrine function in the neurophysiology of obesity and hyperphagia.[137]

The role of various neurotransmitters in mediating or modulating behavior in general and eating behavior in particular continues to be the focus of intense research. To date, findings indicate that feeding, like any other behavior, is most likely controlled by many excitatory and inhibitory mechanisms mediated by multiple central neurotransmitters[60,94–96] and modulated by peripheral factors. Destruction of catecholaminergic neurons in the midbrain through selective neurotoxins has resulted in hyperphagia in animal models.[2,61] Furthermore, loss of noradrenergic terminals in the ventral bundle terminating in the hypothalamus was necessary to produce hyperphagia, whereas damage to the dorsal bundle containing dopaminergic projections was not.[2] In addition, the suppressant effect normally noted for d-amphetamine[102] was not effective in reducing hyperphagia in the absence of functional noradrenergic neurons. The total amount of body weight gained after medial hypothalamic lesions has been found to be inversely related with terminal levels of forebrain norepinephrine content.[29,30]

A role for serotonin as a modulator is suggested by research showing that depletion of 5-hydroxytryptophan by injury to the median raphe impairs the ability of animals with medial hypothalamic lesions to regain weight.[29,30] Saller and Stricker[117] reinforce the concept of a reciprocal relationship between catecholaminergic and serotonergic effects on feeding by demonstrating that extensive depletions of 5-hydroxytryptophan in the brain induce hyperphagia and weight gain in rates only when depletions of norepinephrine do not occur. Destruction of the substantia nigra or the nigrostriatal bundle, a system regulating the dopamine content of the neostriatum, results in severe aphagia, adipsia, and disturbance of water regulation associated with the lateral hypothalamic syndrome. These behavioral correlates have been attributed to depletion of norepinephrine but not of serotonin in the telencephalic regions.[100] Dopaminergic tracts in the nigrostriatal bundle also play an important role in the initiation of feeding.[97]

Other neuropeptides have been implicated, although their roles are not well understood. Activation of separate receptors localized in terminals of dopaminergic neurons in the nigrostriatal pathway increases synthesis of dopamine and turnover in the striatum.[95] Gamma-aminobutyric acid may have a dual effect on food intake; it may increase appetite by inhibiting serotonergic activities in the satiety center, and it may depress food intake by inhibiting the lateral hypothalamic dopaminergic system.[95] Gut peptides, notably cholecystokinin, also have been implicated, but their role in feeding needs to be further elucidated. Intrahypothalamic or intraventricular injections of brain-gut peptides appear to inhibit food ingestion selectively.[64] Endogenous opiates appear to have an important role in inducing feeding.[95]

The therapeutic implications for pharmacologic intervention in clinical disorders of appetite regulation are tremendous. Pharmacologic trials and systematic studies of the efficacy of treatment are understandably lacking, because severe disorders of appetite regulation are rare after TBI. Amphetamines have long been observed to have anorectic effects and have been used in various appetite-suppressant preparations. Opiate antagonists (e.g., naltrexone, naloxone) have been somewhat effective in treating organic bulimia after TBI,[19] hyperphagia associated with the Prader-Willi syndrome,[78] and bulimia of presumed hypothalamic etiology.[41] In massively obese patients, food intake can be decreased acutely by large but not small doses of naloxone.[7] The advent of drugs with more selective serotonergic properties opens the possibility of determining the efficacy of serotonergic blockade or stimulation in appetite regulation. To date, no clinical studies are available. Bulimia and anorexia nervosa are far more common among psychiatric patients than among patients with traumatic brain injury. Lithium has been reported to have some efficacy in patients who have failed conventional behavior therapy.[68] Although it is difficult to extrapolate from non-TBI patients to patients with TBI, the infrequency with which certain clinical disorders occur after TBI makes it worthwhile to look to other populations for a better understanding of possible mechanisms of similar behavioral manifestations.

The extensive—sometimes conflicting—literature on appetite regulation underscores the extreme complexity of the neural regulatory systems and the multiplicity of central and peripheral neurotransmitters involved in appetite control. The classic view that the medial and lateral hypothalamus contain the centers of control is vastly oversimplified; the crucial factor in normal regulation is more likely to be the integrity of neural pathways with excitatory, inhibitory, or modulating functions. Such pathways probably converge in the medial and lateral hypothalamus, which may simply be prominent landmarks.

It is abundantly clear that the maintenance of normal physiologic function in humans depends on a complex neural machinery. Central to this neural regulation is the hypothalamus–pituitary complex, which mediates virtually all physiologic activities via its autonomic and endocrine apparatus. Its anatomic location and functional connections make it vulnerable, especially to trauma. Although current estimates of hypothalamic–pituitary dysfunction after TBI are low, they are likely to be underestimates. Recent advances in traumatology, biochemical and immunological assays, and imaging techniques may result in increased survival and better diagnosis of patients with various degrees of hypothalamic–pituitary dysfunction after TBI.

REFERENCES

1. Abrams GM, Schipper HM: Neuroendrocrine syndromes of the hypothalamus. Neurol Clin 4:769–782, 1986.
2. Ahlskog JE, Hoebel BG: Overeating and obesity from damage to a noradrenergic system in the brain. Science 182:166–169, 1973.
3. Altman R, Pruzanski W: Posttraumatic hypopituitarism: Anterior pituitary insufficiency following skull fracture. Ann of Intern Med 55:149–154, 1961.
4. Aiuti F, Pandolfi F: The role of T-lymphocytes in the pathogenesis of primary immunodeficiencies. Thymus 4:257–264, 1983.
5. Anand BK, Brobeck JR: Hypothalamic control of food intake in rats and cats. Yale Biol Med 24:123–140, 1951.
6. Anand BK: Nervous regulation of food intake. Physiol Rev 41:677–708, 1962.
7. Atkinson RL: Naloxone decreases food intake in obese humans. J Clin Endocrinol Metab 55:196–198, 1982.
8. Baker CC, Oppenheimer L, Stephens B, et al: Am J Surg 140:144–150, 1980.
9. Bauer HG: Endocrine and other clinical manifestations of hypothalamic disease. J Clin Endocrinol 14:13–31, 1954.
10. Barreca T, Perria C, Sannia A, et al: Evaluation of anterior pituitary function in patients with posttraumatic diabetes insipidus. J Clin Endocrinol Metab 51:1279–1282, 1980.
11. Becker RM, Daniel RK: Increased antidiuretic hormone production after trauma to the craniofacial complex. Trauma 13:112–115, 1973.
12. Bevilacqua G, Fovnaciari G: Clinicopathological correlations in a case of posttraumatic pan-hypopituitarism. Acta Neuropathol (Berl) 31:171–177, 1975.
13. Bray GA, Gallagher TF: Manifestations of hypothalamic obesity in man: A comprehensive investigation of eight patients and a review of the literature. Medicine 54:301–330, 1975.
14. Boehm T, Salazar AM: Hypothalamic pituitary function in severely head injured Vietnam veterans. Milit Med 151:535–538, 1986.
15. Bullard DE: Diencephalic seizures: Responsiveness to bromocriptine and morphine. Ann Neurol 21:609–611, 1987.
16. Busto R, Globus MYT, Dietrich WD, et al: Effect of mild hypothermia on ischemia-induced release of neurotransmitters and free fatty acids in rat brain. Stroke 20:904–910, 1989.
17. Busto R, Dietrich WD, Globus MYT, et al: Small differences in intraischemic brain temperature critically determine the extent of ischemic neuronal injury. J Cereb Blood Flow Metab 7:729–738, 1987.
18. Celesia GC, Archer CR, Chung HD: Hyperphagia and obesity: Relationship to medial hypothalamic lesions. JAMA 246:151–153, 1981.
19. Childs A: Naltrexone in organic bulimia: A preliminary report. Brain Inj 1:49–55, 1987.
20. Chiolero RL, Lemarchand-Beraud T, Schutz Y, et al: Thyroid function in severely traumatized patients with or without head injury. Acta Endocrinol (Copenh) 117:80–86, 1988.
21. Chopp M, Chen H, Dereski MO, Garcia JH: Mild hypothermic intervention after graded ischemic stress in rats. Stoke 22:37–43, 1991.
22. Chopp M, Knight R, Tidwell CD, et al: The metabolic effects of mild hypothermia on global cerebral ischemia and recirculation in the cat: Comparison to normothermia and hypothermia: J Cereb Blood Flow Metab 9:141–148, 1989.
23. Chopp M, Welch KMA, Tidwell CD, et al: Effect of mild hyperthermia on recovery of metabolic function after global cerebral ischemia in cats. Stroke 19:1521–1525, 1988.
24. Clifton GL, Allen S, Berry J, Koch S: Systemic hypothermia in treatment of brain injury. Neurotrauma 9(Suppl):S487–S495, 1992.

25. Clifton GL, Jiang JY, Lyeth BG, et al: Marked protection by hypothermia after experimental traumatic brain injury. Cereb Blood Flow Metab 11: 114–121, 1991.

26. Clifton GL, Robertson CS, Kuyper K, Taylor AA, Dhekne RD, Grossman RG: Cardiovascular response to severe head injury. J Neurosurg 59: 447–454, 1983.

27. Clifton GL, Zeigler MD, Grossman RG: Circulating catecholamines and sympathetic activity after head injury. Neurosurgery 8:10–14,1981.

28. Clifton GL, Robertson CS, Kuyper K, et al: Cardiovascular response to severe head injury. J Neurosurg 59:447–460, 1983.

29. Coscina DV, Dewan VM: Serotonin-depleting mid brain lesions fail to mitigate hyperphagia and obesity in the Zucker fatty rate. Physiol Behav 34: 107–114, 1985.

30. Coscina DV, Magder RJ: Effects of serotonin-depleting midbrain lesions on the defense of hypothalamic obesity. Physiol Behav 33:575–570, 1984.

31. Cox JE, Powley TL: Prior vagotomy blocks VMH obesity in pair-fed rats. Am Physiol 240:573–583, 1981.

32. Crompton RM: Hypothalamic lesions following closed head injury. Brain 94:165–172, 1971.

33. Czonkowska A, Korlak J: Cell-mediated immunity after head injuries. Neurol-Neurochir-Pol 13:389–393, 1979.

34. Daniel P: Head injuries. J Clin Pathol 23(Suppl): 150–153, 1970.

35. David BP, Matukas VJ: Inappropriate secretion of antidiuretic hormone after cerebral injury. J Oral Surg 34:609–615, 1976.

36. Dietrich WD, Halley M, Valdes I, Busto R: Interrelationships between increased vascular permeability and acute neuronal damage following temperature-controlled brain ischemia in rats. Acta Neuropathol 81:615–625, 1991.

37. Dietrich WD, Busto R, Halley M, Valdes I: The importance of brain temperature in alterations of the blood brain barrier following cerebral ischemia. J Neuropathol Exper Neurol 49:486–497, 1990.

38. Dietrich WD: The importance of brain temperature in cerebral injury. Neurotrauma 9 (Suppl2): S475–S485, 1992.

39. Dinarelli CA, Cannon JG, Wolff SM: New concepts on the pathogenesis of fever. Rev Infect Dis 10: 168–189, 1988.

40. Drake CG, Joy TA: Hypothermia in the treatment of critical head injury. Can Med Assoc J 87:887–891, 1962.

41. Dunger DB, Leonard JV, Preece MA: Effect of naloxone in a previously undescribed hypothalamic syndrome. Lancet 1277–1281, 1980.

42. Edwards OM, Clark JDA: Posttraumatic hypopituitarism: Six cases and a review of the literature. Medicine 65:281–290, 1986.

43. Feuerman T, Gade GF, Reynolds R: Stress induced malignant hyperthermia in a head-injured patient. J Neurosurg 68:297–299, 1988.

44. Fleischer AS, Radioman DR, Payne NS, Tindall GT: Hypothalamic hypothyroidism and hypogonadism in prolonged traumatic coma. Neurosurgery 49: 650–657, 1978.

45. Friedman MI: Effects of alloxan diabetes on hypothalamic hyperphagia and obesity. Am Physiol 222:174–178, 1972.

46. Formi G, Bindeni M, Santoni A, et al: Radiofrequency destruction of the tuberinfundibular region of hypothalamus permanently abrogates NK cell activity in mice. Nature 306:181–184, 1983.

47. Girard J, Marelli R: Posttraumatic hypothalamo-pituitary insufficiency. J Pediatr 90:241–242, 1977.

48. Globus MYT, Busto R, Dietrich WD, et al: Direct evidence for acute and massive norepinephrine release in the hippocampus during transient ischemia. Cerebral Blood Flow Metab 9:892–896, 1989.

49. Gold RM: Hypothalamic obesity: The myth of the ventromedial nucleus. Science 182:488–490, 1973.

50. Gooch BR, Isley WL, Utiger RD: Abnormalities in thyroid function tests in patients admitted to a medical service. Arch Intern Med 142:1801–1805, 1982.

51. Goris RJA, Draaisma J: Causes of death after blunt trauma. Trauma 22:2, 141–146, 1982.

52 Griffin JM, Hartley JH, Crow RW, Shatten WE: Diabetes insipidus caused by craniofacial trauma. Trauma 16:979–984, 1976.

53. Griffith ER, Taylor N, DeLateur B, Lehman JF: Orthostatic hypertension following brain trauma: Report of a case. Arch Phys Med Rehabil: 376–380, 1971.

54. Guyton AC: Textbook of Medical Physiology. Philadelphia, W.B. Saunders, 1981.

55. Halimi P, Sigal R, Dayon D, et al: Posttraumatic diabetes insipidus: MR demonstration of pituitary stalk rupture. J Comput Assist Tomog 12:135–137, 1988.

56. Hansen OH: Fat embolism and posttraumatic diabetes insipidus. Acta Chir Scand 136:161–165, 1969.

57. Harper CG, Doyle D, Adams JH, Graham DI: Analysis of abnormalities in pituitary gland in non-missile head injury: Study of 100 consecutive cases. J Clin Pathol 39:769–772, 1986.

58. Hashimoto T, Miyai K, Uozumi T, et al: Effect of prolonged LH-releasing hormone administration on gonadotropin response in patients with hypothalmic and pituitary tumors. J Clin Endocrinol Metab 41:712–716, 1975.

59. Helling TS, Evans LL, Fowler DL, et al: Infectious complications in patients with severe head injury. Trauma 28:1575,1577, 1988.

60. Hendry J: Case of Frolichs' syndrome following injury to the sella turcica. Glasgow Med J 96:147–150, 1921.

61. Hernandez L, Hoebel BG: Food intake and lateral hypothalamic self-stimulation covary after medial hypothalamic lesions or ventral midbrain 6-hydroxydopamine injections that cause obesity. Behav Neurosci 163:412–422, 1989.

62. Van Hilten JJ, Roos RAC: Posttraumatic hyperthermia: A possible result of frontodiencephalic dysfunction. Clin Neurol Neurosurg 93:223–225, 1991.

63. Hirsch J: Hypothalamic control of appetite. Hosp Prac 131–138, 1984.

64. Hoebel BG: Brain neurotransmitters in food and drug reward. Am J Clin Nutr 42:1133–1150, 1985.

65. Horn LJ, Glenn MB: Pharmacologic interventions in neuroendocrine disorders following traumatic brain injury—Part 1. J Head Trauma Rehabil 3(2): 87–90, 1988.

66. Horn LJ: Pharmacologic interventions in neuro-endocrine disorders following traumatic brain injury—Part 3(3)86–90, 1988.

67. Hoyt DB, Ozkan AN, Hansbrough JF, et al: Head injury: An immunologic deficit in T-cell activation. J Trauma 30:759–767, 1990.

68. Hsu LKG: Treatment of bulimia with lithium. A J Psychiatry 141:1260–1262, 1984.

69. Isern RD: Family violence and the Kluver-Bucy syndrome. South Med J 80:377–376, 1987.

70. Jambart S, Turpin G, Luc de Gemnes J: Panhypopituitarism secondary to head trauma: Evidence for a hypothalamic origin of the deficit. Acta Endocrinol 93:264–270, 1980.

71. Jiang JY, Lyeth BG, Cliften GL, et al: Relationship between body and brain temperature in traumatically brain-injured rodents. J Neurosurg 74:492–496, 1991.

72. Kalisky Z, Morrison DP, Meyers CA, VonLaufen A: Medical problems encountered during rehabilitation of patients with head injury. Arch Phys Med Rehabil 66:25–29, 1985.

73. Kaptein EM, Spencer CA, Kamiel MB, Nicoloff JT: Prolonged dopamine administration and thyroid hormone economy in normal and critically ill subjects. J Clin Endocrinol Metab 51:387–393, 1980.

74. Katayama Y, Becker DP, Tamura T, Hovda DA: Massive increases in extracellular potassium and the indiscriminate release of glutamate following concussive brain injury. J Neurosurg 73:889–900, 1990.

75. Killeffer FA, Stern WE: Chronic effects of hypothalamic injury. Arch Neurol 22:419–429, 1970.

76.. Klinbeil GE, Cline P: Anterior hypopituitarism: A consequence of head injury. Arch Phys Med Rehabil 66:44–46, 1984.

77. Kornblum RN, Fisher RS: Pituitary lesions in craniocerebral injuries. Arch Pathol 88:242–248, 1969.

78. Kyriakides M, Silverstone T, Jeffcoate W, Laurance B: Effect of naloxone on hyperphagia in Prader-Willi syndrome. Lancet i:876–877, 1980.

79. Labi ML, Horn LJ: Hypertension after traumatic brain injury. Brain Inj 4:365–370, 1990.

80. Labi ML: Use of clonidine in central fever after severe traumatic brain injury: A case report. (in preparation)

81. Landau H, Adin I, Spitz IM: Pituitary insufficiency following head injury. Isr J Med Sci 14:785–789, 1978.

82. Leramo OB, Rao AB: Diplopia and diabetes insipidus secondary to type 11 fracture of the sella turcica: A case report. Can J Surg 30:53–521, 1987.

83. Lewin K, Mattingly D, Millis RR: Anorexia nervosa associated with hypothalamic tumor BMJ 2:629–630, 1972.

84. Livingston DH, Appel SH, Wellhausen SR, et al: Depressed centerforon gamma production and monocyte HLA-DR expression after severe injury. Arch Surg 123:1309–1312, 1988.

85. Loewy AD, McKellar S: The neuroanatomical basis of central cardiovascular control. Fed Proc 39: 2495–2503, 1980.

86. Loughhead MG: Brain resuscitation and protection. Med J Austr 148:458–466, 1988.

87. Mark AS, Phister SH, Jackson DE, Kolsky MP: Traumatic lesions of the suprasellar region: MR imaging. Radiology 182:49–52, 1992.

88. Massie R, Baratta P, Mulazzi D, et al: Impairment of cell-mediated immunity in severe head injury. Aggressologie 29:423–426, 1988.

89. McDonald JW, Chen CK, Tresher WH, Johnston MV: The severity of excitotoxic brain injury is dependent on brain temperature in immature rat. Neurosci Lett 126:83–86, 1991.

90. McLeod AA, Neil-Dwyer G, Meyer CHA, Richardson PL, et al: Cardiac sequelae of acute head injury. Br Heart J 47:221–226, 1982.

91. Miller CH, Quathochi KB, Frank EH, et al: Humoral and cellular immunity following severe head injury: Review and current investigations. Neurol Res 13:117–124, 1991.

92. Miller WL, Kaplan SL, Grumbach MM: Child abuse as a cause of posttraumatic hypopituitarism. N Engl J Med 302:724–728, 1982.

93. Morley JE, Levine AS: The central control of appetite. Lancet i:398–401, 1983.

94. Morley JE, Slag MF, Elson MK, Shafer RB: The interpretation of thyroid function tests in hospitalized patients. JAMA 249:2377–2379, 1983.

95. Morley JE, Levine AS: The role of endogenous opiates as regulators of appetite. Am J Clin Nutr 35:757–761, 1982.

96. Morley JE: Neuroendocrine control of thyrotropic secretion. Endocr Rev 2:396–436, 1981.

97. Morley JE: The neuroendocrine control of appetite: The role of endogenous opiates, cholecystokinin, TRH, GABA and the diazepam receptor. Life Sci 27:355–368, 1980.

98. Moses AM, Miller M, Streetin DHP: Pathophysiologic and pharmacologic alternations in the release and action of ADH. Metabolism 25:697–721, 1976.

99. Notman DD, Mortek MA, Moses AM: Permanent diabetes insipidus following head trauma: Observation on ten patients and an approach to diagnosis. J Trauma 20:599–602, 1980.

100. Oppenheimer JH: Thyroid function tests in non-thyroidal disease. J Chron Dis 35:697–701, 1982.

101. Oltmans GA, Harvey JA: LH syndrome and brain catecholamine levels after lesions of the nigrostriatal bundle. Physiol Behav 8:69–78, 1972.

102. Panksepp J: Is satiety mediated by the ventromedial hypothalamus? Physiol Behav 7:381–384, 1971.

103. Paul SM, Giblin BH, Skolnick P: (+)-Amphetamine binding to rat hypothalamus: Relation to anoxic potency of phenylethylamines. Science 218:487–488, 1982.

104. Pisetsky JE, Roswit B: Obesity following cerebral injury. J Nerv Ment Dis 108:129–136, 1948.
105. Pittman JA, Haigler ED, Hershman JM, Pittman CS: Hypothalmic hypothyroidism. N Engl J Med 285:844–845, 1971.
106. Polk HC, George CD, Wellhausen SR, et al: A systematic study of host defense processes in badly injured patients. Ann Surg 204:282–299, 1986.
107. Popp AJ, Gottlieb ME, Paloski WH, et al: Cardiopulmonary hemodynamics in patients with serious head injury. J Surg Res 32:416–421, 1982.
108. Porter RJ, Miller IA: Diabetes insipidus following closed head injury. J Neurosurg Psychol 2:258–262, 1948.
109. Popp AJ, Porter RJ, Powley TL, Opsahl CA: Ventromedial hypothalmic obesity abolished by subdiaphragmatic vagotomy. A J Physiol 226:25–33, 1974.
110. Quattrochi KB, Frank EH, Miller CH, et al: Impairment of helper T-cell function and lymphakine activated killer cytotoxicity following severe head injury. J Neurosurg 75:766–773, 1991.
111. Quattrocho KB, Frank EH, Miller CH, et al: Suppression of cellular immune activity following severe head injury. J Neurotrauma 7(2):77–87, 1990.
112. Quock RM, Panek RW, Kouchich, Rosenthal MA: Nitrous oxide-induced hypothermia in the rat. Life Sci 41:683–690, 1987.
113. Reinchenbach DD, Benditt EP: Catecholamines and cardiomyopathy. Hum Pathol 1:125–150, 1970.
114. Reeves AG, Plum F: Hyperphagia, rage and dementia accompanying a ventromedial hypothalamic neoplasm. Arch Neurol 20:616–624.
115. Rudelli R, Deck JHN: Selective traumatic infarction of the human anterior hypothalamus. J Neurosurg 50:645–654, 1979.
116. Rudman D, Fleisher AS, Kutner MH, Raggio JF: Suprahypophysial hypogonadism and hypothyroidism during prolonged coma after head trauma. J Clin Endocrinol Metab 45:747–754, 1977.
117. Saller CF, Stricker EM: Hyperphagia and increased growth rates after intraventricular injection of 5,7-dihydioxytryptamine. Science 192:385–387, 1926.
118. Sapolsky RM: Neuroendocrinology of the stress-response. In Becker JB, Breedlove SM, Crews D (eds): Behavioral Endocrinology. Cambridge, MA, MIT Press, 1992.
119. Schulte JAM, Esch M, Pfeifer G: Hemodynamic changes in patients with severe head injury. Acta Neurochir 54:243–250, 1980.
120. Segatore M: Fever after traumatic brain injury. Neurosci Nurs 24:104–109, 1992.
121. Soules MR, Sheldon GW: Traumatic hypopituitarism: Hypophysial insufficiency from indirect cranial trauma. South Med J 72:1592–1596, 1979.
122. Strachan RD, Little IR, Miller JD: Hypothermia and severe head injury. Brain Inj 3:51–55, 1989.
123. Stricker EM: Hyperphagia. N Engl J Med 298:1010–1013, 1978.
124. Stricker EM, Zigmond MJ: Recovery of function after damage to central catecholamine containing neurons: A neurochemical model for the lateral hypothalamic syndrome. Prog Psychobiol Physiol Psychol 6:121–188, 1976.
125. Talman WT, Florek GD, Bullard DE: A hyperthermic syndrome in two subjects with acute hydrocephalus. Arch Neurol 45:1037–1040, 1988.
126. Treips CS: Hypothalamic and pituitary injury. J Clin Pathol 23 (Suppl): 178–186, 1970.
127. Truex RC, Carpenter MB: Human Neuroanatomy. Baltimore, Williams & Wilkins, 1969.
128. Valenta LJ, DeFeo DR: Posttraumatic hypopituitarism due to a hypothalamic lesion. Am J Med 68:614–617, 1980.
129. Verbalis JG, Robinson AG, Moses AM: Postoperative and posttraumatic diabetes insipidus. Front Horm Res 13:247–265, 1985.
130. Ward AA, McCulloch WS: The projection of the frontal lobe on the hypothalamus.
131. Wartofsky L: Alterations in thyroid function in patients with systemic illness. Endocr Rev 3:164–217, 1982.
132. Ward AA, Wartofsky L, Von Wovern F: Obesity as a sequel to traumatic injury to the hypothalamus. Dan Med Bull 13:11–13, 1966.
133. Will RG: Kleine-Levin syndrome: Report of two cases with onset of symptoms precipitated by head trauma. Br J Psychiatry 152:410–412, 1988.
134. Winternitz WW, Dzur JA: Pituitary failure secondary to head trauma. J Neurosurg 44:504–505, 1976.
135. Woolf PD, Lee LA, Hamill RW, McDonald JV: Thyroid test abnormalities in traumatic brain injury: Correlation with neurologic impairment and sympathetic nervous system activation. Am J Med 84:201–208, 1988.
136. Woolf PD, Hamill RW, Lee LA, et al: The predictive value of catecholamines in assessing outcome in traumatic brain injury. J Neurosurg 66:875–882, 1987.
137. York DA, Bray GA: Dependence of hypothalamic obesity on insulin, the pituitary and the adrenal gland. Endocrinology 90:855–894, 1972.
138. Young AB, Ott LG, Thompson JS, et al: The cellular immune depression of non-steroid treated severely head-injured patients [abstract]. Neurosurgery 16:725, 1985.

M. ELIZABETH SANDEL M.D.

22

Sexuality and Reproduction after Traumatic Brain Injury

Our understanding of human sexual behavior has been limited by a number of historical and cultural factors. In the early part of the 20th century, the study of human sexual behavior was primarily the domain of psychology and neurobiology, which were dominated by Freudian, psychodynamic approaches. Neurobiologists have contributed to the field more recently, but their approaches are limited by the use of animal models that may or may not have relevance to an understanding of human sexual and reproductive behaviors. Animal behaviorists have been aware for decades that sexual and reproductive behaviors among different species vary widely. Likewise, sociologists and anthropologists have described wide variations in human sexual behavior across cultures; many such behaviors are considered deviant within our own society. The current search for a gene to account for homosexuality is based on an assumption that biology will explain sexual behavior. More likely, sexual behavior is the result of complex interactions of cultural, psychological, and biologic factors. Finally, much of the research on human sexuality has focused on males, leaving many questions about female sexuality unanswered.

For the person with a disabling disease, condition, or injury, questions of sexuality become even more complex. How do we understand the impact of the pathophysiologic processes on the individual, both alone and in relationship with others? What alterations in sexual functions—drive, arousal, responses—are due to organic factors, and what can be attributed to secondary factors, such as cognitive and communication impairments or mobility deficits that result from the disease, condition, or injury? Because of multiple, interrelated impairments that coexist after traumatic brain injury, etiologic questions concerning sexual dysfunction in this population remain unanswered.

Taking into account such limitations, the first section of this chapter focuses on the following areas: (1) a review of sexual and reproductive physiology and pathophysiology, with emphasis on the role of the central nervous system, and (2) a review of studies of sexuality among patients with cerebral injury, including relevant literature about stroke, seizures, and endocrinologic disorders. Because this text focuses on the medical aspects of rehabilitation, the discussion emphasizes the state of current medical knowledge rather than psychological aspects

557

of sexuality and intimacy. However, because medical and psychological factors are always interconnected in the literature as well as in human interactions, a strict segregation is impossible.

The second section addresses evaluation and treatment, including (1) medical assessment and interventions for sexual dysfunction; (2) management strategies for sexually disinhibited patients; and (3) sex therapy and educational and counseling approaches to address the range of difficulties patients face in forming and maintaining intimate relationships after brain injury.

The third section addresses reproductive issues for women and men with brain injuries, including (1) amenorrhea; (2) pregnancy; (3) contraceptive options; and (4) infertility.

For a comprehensive understanding of sexuality, the reader is referred to a number of new and enlightened texts[2,43,73a] that include information on many aspects of sexual relationships in persons with and without disabilities.

NEUROPHYSIOLOGY AND PATHOPHYSIOLOGY

The neuroanatomic systems that assume roles in human sexual responses and behaviors are widespread and complex. The interrelationships among these systems are not completely understood. However, the peripheral nervous system, including motor, sensory, and autonomic neurons, and subcortical and cortical systems contribute to sexual interest and responsiveness through an elaborate network. Lesions at any level may influence this behavior, although the actual effects of such lesions in humans are not fully established.

Peripheral and Sympathetic Systems

Contributions from the peripheral system include sympathetic and parasympathetic neurons. Sympathetic neurons from the thoracic cord, contained in the hypogastric plexus, provide efferent and afferent innervation to the internal genitalia; this system provides the neurologic basis for emission. Parasympathetic innervation originating at the sacral level, organized in the pelvic nerves, supply

the neuronal inputs and outputs responsible for ejaculation. The pudenal nerves contribute to this neuronal system. In women, these neurologic connections serve similar functions in arousal, lubrication, and possible female ejaculation.[2] Psychogenic mechanisms of arousal may be represented by sympathetic pathways.[96]

Injury to the spinal cord, with effects on these pathways, certainly may occur concomitantly with traumatic brain injury, and patients with this dual diagnosis may have sexual dysfunction on the basis of one or both.

Brainstem Centers, Basal Ganglia, and Thalamus

Brainstem centers that contribute to human sexual responses include the reticular activating systems of the pons and midbrain. These pathways, which provide input for initiation and maintenance of arousal and alertness, connect with limbic and other frontal structures, many of which play a role in sexual and related behaviors as well as in affective responses. The same structures connect with diencephalic structures, including the hypothalamus and thalamus, that have important roles in the generation of sexual and reproductive behaviors. The brainstem carries the afferent and efferent messages from sensory and motor systems which then traverse subcortical structures.[10]

Injury to these systems may influence the general level of responsiveness and thus impair sexual functioning at a very basic level. In addition, injury to brainstem motor or sensory systems may alter sexual arousal.

Sensory inputs from the genitalia as well as other erogenous zones relay information to the thalamus. Stimulation of the thalamus produces erection in animals. The role of the basal ganglia in sexual function is not clear, although stimulation may result in species-specific sexual behaviors.[66]

Limbic, Diencephalic, and Cortical Systems

Limbic and paralimbic structures, including the hippocampus, septal complex, amygdala, and hypothalamus, are crucial structures in the production of sexual behaviors.

Stimulation of these structures produces erection and in some cases (the septal complex) preorgasmic sensations of pleasure. Lesions of the piriform cortex, which is interconnected with the olfactory cortex, produce hypersexual responses in animals. Stimulation of the cingulate gyrus, above the corpus callosum, produces genital hallucinations and erection.[44]

The Kluver-Bucy syndrome, produced by ablation of the anterior temporal poles, results in hypersexual and exploratory behaviors with hyperorality.[62,63] Temporal lobe seizures may be manifested by genital sensations and other sexual phenomena, with hypersexual or hyposexual behavior during both ictal and interictal periods. Endocrine disturbances, which are common in both men and women with temporal lobe epilepsy, result in decreased libido, impotence, menstrual disturbances, and reproductive disorders.[45–47]

Injury to the frontal lobes, particularly the orbitofrontal surfaces, may produce hypersexual responses, in which socially inappropriate behaviors are displayed more often than actual sexual behaviors. Such effects may be caused by lesions of the limbic and paralimbic systems. In the case of dorsolateral frontal injury, when attention and initiation impairments are primary, libido or sexual assertiveness may be impaired.[107] The frontal lobes are clearly involved in the regulation of sexual behaviors. Damage to these areas may also lead to an inability to fantasize.[49] The role of the olfactory system is unclear, but recent research indicates that anosmia may not significantly affect sexual function.[40] Stimulation of the hippocampus results in erection in animals, and damage may lead to sexual dysfunction.[66]

The hypothalamus is a crucial structure in the elaboration of the human sexual response. The hypothalamus receives some of its information in the form of neuronal messages, but other information arrives in the form of chemical messages, including gonadal steroids. In addition, the hypothalamus synthesizes and secretes hormones of its own, many of which exert influences over sex and reproduction. Gonadotropin-releasing hormone stimulates the release of follicle-stimulating hormone (FSH) and luteinizing hormone (LH), which regulate the menstrual cycle in women and testosterone secretion in men. In adults, hypothalamic injury may lead to sexual dysfunction or amenorrhea; in children, such injury may lead to precocious puberty.[8,54,93]

The supraoptic nucleus of the hypothalamus synthesizes oxytocin, a hormone involved in lactation, birthing, and orgasm. Naloxone, an opiate antagonist, prevents the release of oxytocin, suggesting that the release at orgasm is controlled, at lease in part, by the endorphin system.[34,41]

Lesions in the medial preoptic area of the hypothalamus reduce or eliminate copulatory behavior, although monkeys with such lesions will masturbate. Stimulation of the medial preoptic area elicits mounting and other sexual behaviors. This area receives neuronal inputs from other brain regions such as the olfactory system and the cerebral cortex, including the visual cortex. The preoptic area has high concentrations of androgen and estrogen receptors as well as the enzyme that converts androgens to estrogens. Manipulating androgens and androgen receptors in this region affects copulatory behavior.

The dorsomedial nucleus of the hypothalamus, when stimulated, generates ejaculation. This nucleus may receive input from the medial preoptic area and probably from other brain and body regions. The ventromedial nucleus of the hypothalamus appears to play a role in female sexual behaviors. In female rats and monkeys, lesioning results in the elimination or reduction of so-called female sexual behaviors, including lordosis and "presenting." This nucleus is also strongly influenced by sex hormones, in particular estrogen and progesterone, at least in the female rat. In female primates androgens secreted by the adrenal gland are more important in the maintenance of libido than behavior but also may be involved in generating sexual behaviors.[60]

SEXUAL DYSFUNCTION AFTER BRAIN INJURY

Although much of the literature about traumatic brain injury focuses on psychosocial consequences, no well-designed studies have established clear links between the various impairments that frequently occur and sexual dysfunction. Are impairments such as communication or cognitive deficits more important than physical deficits in relationships? What role does depression play? What are the effects of medication? What interpersonal issues contribute to sexual dysfunction? What are the anatomic correlates of sexual dysfunction?

This section focuses on several areas of sexual dysfunction, beginning with related studies in patients with cerebrovascular accidents and seizure disorders. The bulk of the literature about traumatic brain injury addresses the decline in sexual function after injury. However, disinhibited behavior, hypersexuality, and changes in sexual orientation have been reported, although in the form of case reports rather than large studies. Thus, even less is understood about such phenomena. Precocious puberty and the effects of seizures on endocrine function also are discussed.

Cerebrovascular Accidents

A number of studies of sexual dysfunction after stroke have addressed some of these questions, but their relevance to the traumatically injured population is unclear. In one study,[52] 70% of hemiplegic men and 44% of women under the age of 60 years (older than the average brain-injured population) experienced decreased sexual activity. Almost one-third experienced a decrease in libido. In another study, only 36% of 85 hemiplegic patients (mean age, under 60 years), were sexually active to the same extent as before stroke; and 26% ceased all sexual activity. In this group of 85 patients, 83% reported that they were sexually active before the onset of disability.

Decreased frequency of intercourse and ceased or reduced foreplay were reported in another population of 51 stroke patients; 15% of the men reported retarded ejaculation.[97] Sjogren attributed this sexual dysfunction and maladjustment to psychogenic causes, because a previous study[98] demonstrated essentially normal endocrinologic evaluations (including gonadotropic stimulation tests). He concluded that important precipitating factors were "performance

orientation" and "sexual stigmatism"[97] and recommended education and counseling.

The two studies[12,74] reported that fewer than one-half of the men who were capable of achieving erection before stroke retained this ability after stroke. Ejaculation was reduced from 86% of men to 35% after stroke. Women reported decreased lubrication, failure to achieve orgasm, and painful coitus as well as amenorrhea. The researchers attributed sexual dysfunction to fear of another stroke or other devastating medical event.[74] Fugl-Meyer suggests that sensory deficits but not motor impairment contribute to sexual dysfunction.[36] Boldrini found a marked decline in sexual activity after stroke, but respondents to a questionnaire survey indicated that psychological and interpersonal factors were largely responsible for the dysfunction; clinical factors, including severity of insult and specific impairments, did not correlate with sexual dysfunction.[9]

There is no clear consensus about site of lesion and sexual function. Various studies have reported a greater decline of function was seen in patients with left hemisphere stroke,[39,52] in women (but not men) with right hemisphere stroke,[74] and in men with right hemisphere stroke.[22] Yet another study reported no difference in women or men with right or left hemisphere strokes.[97,98] In one study, an increase in libido was observed after right hemisphere stroke,[39] and hypersexuality was documented after stroke with temporal lobe lesions.[75] Of related interest, Cohen recorded electroencephalographic activity from right and left hemispheres at the moment of orgasm and found that the right hemisphere showed a greater amount of activation during periods of erection and orgasm, whereas the left hemisphere was relatively inactive.[17]

In summary, the cause of sexual disorders after stroke is still uncertain. Localization of the lesion, severity of the cerebral insult, or other clinical factors may be important. Medication may inhibit responsiveness or affect libido.[31] Role shifts, the stigmatization of disability, and, in particular, dependency may predispose persons who have suffered strokes to problems with intimate relationships.[97] Overprotection is a common response in people close to the patient, and the spouse may be identified as a parental figure rather than an equal marital partner.[53] Communication may affect the relationship and lead to sexual dysfunction. Fear of precipitating another stroke or another medical event may inhibit sexual interest or response.[74]

Seizure Disorders

Temporal lobe seizures usually arise from limbic structures, such as the amygdala, that exert a modulatory influence on the hypothalamic regulation of the pituitary. Limbic and brainstem structures contain neurons with high concentrations of gonadal hormone receptors.[45]

Approximately 20% of patients with post-traumatic epilepsy have temporal lobe seizures.[51] Up to 58% of men with temporal lobe seizure disorders are impotent or hyposexual, and up to 40% of women have menstrual irregularities or reproductive dysfunction, including polycystic ovarian syndrome, premature menopause, hypogonadotropic hypogonadism, and anovulatory cycles.[47] Estrogens lower the seizure threshold, and frequency of seizures often increases in females at the time of menses and during pregnancy. Temporal lobe epilepsy has effects on the hypothalamic–pituitary–gonadal axis through effects on dopamine. Because dopamine is a prolactin-inhibitory hormone within this system, decreases in dopamine result in hyperprolactinemia.

The hypogonadotropic hypogonadism accompanied by amenorrhea in patients with temporal lobe seizures is associated with low levels of luteinizing hormone (LH). Because no hypothalamic disorder has been described, this abnormality may be due to limbic discharges that result in altered secretion of gonadotropin-releasing hormone.[47] Premature menopause also occurs. In polycystic ovarian syndrome, which also is associated with temporal lobe seizures, LH and prolactin are elevated, whereas follicle-stimulating hormone (FSH) is depressed.[47]

Men with temporal lobe epilepsy and hypogonadism, unlike those with isolated hypogonadism, may have no improvement in libido or potency when parenteral testosterone is given; however, initial treatment of the epilepsy, followed by neuroendocrine treatment (bromocriptine or pergolide for hyperprolactinemia and testosterone for hypogonadism), is sometimes effective.[100]

Traumatic Brain Injury

The impact of traumatic brain injury on relationships within the family, including spousal relationships, has been explored in a large number of studies both in the United States and abroad. Thomsen's study[106] of 50 severely injured Danish patients demonstrated that family members were more disturbed by intellectual than physical deficits. The relationships were better between single adult patients and mothers than between patients and spouses. In Rosenbaum and Najenson's study[87] of brain-injured veterans in Israel, wives endorsed with high frequency the statement "dislikes physical contact with husband." The spouse's mood was associated with decreased levels of sexual activity. Lezak[62] emphasized that emotional adjustment for family members, including spouses, occurred only after detachment and acceptance of the permanence of deficits. This adjustment culminated in divorce, separation, and long-term placements for some partners.

Bond[11] noted that the level of sexual activity among partners was not related to severity as measured by the duration of posttraumatic amnesia or level of cognitive or physical impairment. Kosteljanetz, however, noted a correlation between intellectual impairment and sexual dysfunction in a group of 19 mildly injured patients. Although some studies[87] indicate no relationship between locus of lesion and sexual dysfunction, Miller et al.[73] suggest that medial basal-frontal injury or diencephalic injury is associated with hypersexuality and limbic injury with changes in sexual orientation in a population of 8 patients.

Kreutzer and Zasler[56] studied a population of 21 brain-injured men and noted declines in libido, erectile function, and frequency of intercourse. Although the study suggested no association between affect and sexual dysfunction, a larger study[79] using measures of anxiety and depression for both partners found a significant level of psychiatric dysfunction. Age and time since injury were related to measures of psychosexual dysfunction, but severity of injury was not.

A study by Sandel[90] and associates examined sexual functioning in a group of male and female outpatients with severe traumatic brain injuries (average length of post-traumatic amnesia: 54 days). Sexual function was consistently lower than in the normal population but significantly only on the (1) orgasm and (2) drive and desire subscales of the Derogatis Interview of Sexual Function.[27] Location of injury was relevant in that patients with frontal lesions and right hemisphere lesions reported higher sexual satisfaction and higher function. No correlations were found with cognitive measures or clinical examination.

Sexual function and marital adjustment were studied in a small group of married couples (2 men and 4 women with brain injuries) by Garden and associates.[37] Frequency of intercourse declined for all couples, but to a greater degree for couples in which the husband was brain-injured; orgasm in female spouses also showed a significant decline.

Although two earlier studies[33,55] indicated that posttraumatic hypopituitarism with permanent hypogonadotrophic hypogonadism is a rare complication, a more recent study[16] suggests that hypogonadotropic hypogonadism in fact may be frequent after severe brain injury. Of men with severe head injury, 88% had subnormal testosterone levels at 7–10 days after injury; 3–6 months later, 24% of a smaller sample still had low testosterone levels with loss of libido and impotence.

Sexual reproductive effects of brain injury in children can be identified as either hypogonadotropic hypogonadism or precocious puberty. Klachko and associates[54] reported the case of a 39-year-old man with hypopituitarism due to severe brain injury at age 4 years. The epiphyses remained open, but he gained a height of more than 5 feet despite low levels of growth hormone. His genitalia were infantile and the testes small. No pubic hair was present.

There have also been reports of precocious puberty after traumatic brain injury in childhood. In one case,[93] accelerated growth of pubic hair and estrogenization of the vaginal mucosa occurred within 5 months of the accident. Two girls, aged 3 and 5 years, were

described recently[8] as cases of precocious puberty after traumatic brain injury. Both exhibited breast development, pubic hair, and changes in vaginal mucosa consistent with estrogenization. The neuroendocrinologic mechanism is postulated to be destruction of inhibitory neuronal pathways into the hypothalamus, with premature activation of gonadotropin-releasing hormone from the arcuate nucleus.

MEDICAL EVALUATION

History

The crucial aspect of the evaluation of the patient is the interview,[2] which, whenever possible, should be conducted with the partner. This is particularly important if the person has memory deficits but also may be helpful in providing insight into relationship issues. Questions should focus on the following areas of concern: (1) preinjury and postinjury medical and psychiatric problems; (2) medication; (3) preinjury and postinjury sexual functioning and relationships; (4) birth control; and (5) safe sex practices. Education can be provided during the course of the history-taking session but should be reinforced later with further elaboration and written materials.[42,43,57,77] The examiner must be comfortable discussing all aspects of sexuality, including alternative forms of sexual expression and alternative lifestyles.[67] A nonjudgmental style is essential; staff training that focuses on attitudinal issues as well as education is recommended for physicians.[32] Table 1 lists the diagnostic categories for sexual disorders.

A number of questionnaires have been developed to assess sexuality in more detail than the usual history-taking session. The Derogatis Interview of Sexual Functioning[27] collects information by self-report in the five domains of fantasy, arousal, experience, orgasm, and drive and desire. A general sexual satisfaction score is obtained as well as a total score. The Golombok-Rust Inventory of Sexual Satisfaction,[88] also a self-report scale, provides male and female scores (two versions) in the categories of vaginismus, anorgasmia, impotence, premature ejaculation, non-sensuality, avoidance, dissatisfaction, infrequency, and non-communication, as well as a total score.

Physical Examination

A general examination should be completed, with a focused assessment to identify impairments that may influence communication, positioning, movement, oral ability, and sensory awareness. Aphasias, dysarthrias, aprosodias, and deficits in attention and concentration or memory should be noted. Facial scars, oral and facial movement and visual and hearing impairments should be identified. Range of motion, especially in the proximal lower extremities, must be evaluated, along with movement of the limbs and trunk as well as coordination and motor planning ability. Sensation is a crucial aspect of the examination. The genitalia and rectal area must be examined, and women also should receive a breast examination, Papanicolaou smear, and pelvic examination.[116]

Medication Review

A thorough review of all medications is necessary. The most common cause of impotence in the general patient population is medication. Drug-related effects on sexual function are usually reversible after discontinuation of the drug. Frequently implicated are (1) antihypertensive agents, (2) antipsychotic drugs, (3) antidepressants (see below for beneficial effects), (4) anxiolytics, and (5) sedatives (Table 2). An extensive list is provided in other resources.

Laboratory Tests (see Table 1)

Hypopituitarism may be manifested by low levels of growth hormone, thyroxine or cortisol or by hypogonadism. In men, hypogonadism is characterized by low sperm count, low serum levels of testosterone, and inappropriately low levels of LH and FSH. Because protein-bound testosterone may be increased by thyroid hormone therapy or cirrhosis and decreased by hypothyroidism or obesity, free testosterone levels or sex steroid-binding globulin may give a more accurate picture. In women, hypogonadism is characterized by low serum levels of estradiol and

TABLE 1. Sexual Dysfunctions

Contributing factors
    Organic
    Psychologic
Types of dysfunction
    Sexual desire disorders (sexual aversion, hypoactive sexual desire)
    Sexual arousal disorders (poor lubrication, impotence)
    Orgasm disorders (anorgasmia, premature ejaculation)
    Sexual pain disorders (dyspareunia, vaginismus)
Differential diagnosis
    Depression
    Alcohol, drug use
    Age-related changes
    Other diseases
        Neurogenic
        Vascular
        Endocrine
        Debilitating conditions
    Medications (see Table 2)
    Laboratory screen
        Serum prolactin, testosterone, follicle-stimulating hormone, luteinizing hormone, thyroid function studies

From Allgeier WE, Allgeier AR: Sexual Interactions, 4th ed. Lexington, MA, Heath, 1995, with permission.

inappropriate low serum levels of LH and FSH. Of course, hypogonadism may be caused by primary gonadal failure as well as secondary failure at a central level. Klinefelter syndrome, for example, which has an

TABLE 2. Drugs with Sexual Dysfunction as a Possible Side Effect

Antidepressants	Anticholinergic agents
MAO inhibitors	Antispasmodics
Tricyclic antidepressants	Antiparkinsonian agents
Serotonin reuptake inhibitors	Antihistamines
	Muscle relaxants
Tranquilizers	Miscellaneous
Benzodiazepines	Baclofen
Phenothiazines	Cimetidine
Butyrophenones	Clofibrate
Thioxanthenes	Cyproterone
Antihypertensives	Digoxin
Diuretics	Estrogen
Alpha blockers	Fenfluramine
Beta blockers	Indomethacin
Central sympatholytics	Lithium
	Metoclopramide
Antiseizure medications	Naproxen
Phenytoin	Phenoxybenzamine
	Prazosin
	Progestine
	Reserpine

Adapted from Drugs that cause sexual dysfunction. Med Lett 24:73–76, 1983, with permission.

TABLE 3. Potential Drug Therapy for Sexual Dysfunction in Brain Injury

Drug	Indication	Dose/Frequency	Mechanism	Side Effects
Testosterone	↓ Libido ↓ Arousal (?)	200 mg IM biweekly	(?) Central effect	Fluid retention Hypertension Gynecomastia Acne
Yohimbine	Impotence	5.4 mg (1 tablet 3 times/day)	Alpha blocker	Tachycardia Hypertension Nausea Dizziness
Naltrexone	↓ Arousal Impotence	24–50 mg/day	Endorphin antagonist	Nausea, vomiting Liver enzyme elevations Headaches
Buproprion	↓ Libido ↓ Arousal	225–450 mg/day (3 times/day)	↑ Dopamine	Menstrual disturbances Insomnia Seizures (at high doses)

incidence of 1 in 500 men, may be an unrelated cause of low testosterone in a patient with brain injury. The gonadotropin-releasing hormone test is useful in distinguishing hypothalamic from pituitary causes of hypogonadism, although it is not infallible. The clomiphene citrate-provocative test is also used to evaluate the gonadal axis. Single determinations of any of the above levels may not be accurate reflections of function.[1]

INTERVENTIONS FOR SEXUAL DYSFUNCTION

Pharmacotherapy

Because no studies of pharmacologic treatment of hyposexual desire disorders or sexual response disorders in persons with traumatic brain injuries have been reported, the following review of the literature focuses on medications that theoretically *may* have potential benefit. In addition, often the study populations in pharmacologic trials are heterogeneous, including both healthy persons and persons with diseases, such as diabetes, that have systemic effects. Because only one of the following pharmacologic studies included female patients, we can conclude little about female sexuality.

Pharmacologic agents investigated for the treatment of hypoactive sexual dysfunction in non–brain-injured patients include (1) hormonal agents, (2) antidepressants, (3) dopaminergic agents, (4) opiate antagonists, and (5) alpha adrenergic-blocking agents. A number of these agents are included in Table 3. Only testosterone and yohimbine have been officially approved for such use by the Food and Drug Administration.

Testosterone injections biweekly for 6 weeks increased the frequency of sexual thoughts in a group of eugonadal men with low libido compared with placebo. However, no effect was observed in men with inhibited sexual excitement (erectile function).[80] Apparently testosterone increases sexual interest in men with pretreatment levels in the normal range. This study also suggests that men with hyposexual sexual desire disorder may benefit from testosterone injections even if serum levels are within the normal range. Additional research is needed, however, because the study included only 20 men.

Human chorionic gonadotropin was used as a treatment in 45 men with erectile failure and 6 men with lack of sexual desire.[15] The treatment period was 1 month with twice weekly injections of 5,000 IU or placebo in a double-blind design. The investigators reported that 47% of treated patients had a "good result" compared with 12% of the placebo group; however, they did not separate the cases of erectile failure from the cases of low sexual interest or fully define "good result."

Although many antidepressants (tricyclic antidepressants and monamine oxidase inhibitors) have been noted to cause a variety of sexual side effects, others have been noted to improve sexual functioning in patients without brain injuries, including both older serotonin agents and buprorion, which inhibits reuptake of dopamine. Trazodone and fenfluramine (a sympathomimetic amine with effects on serotonergic systems) have been associated with improvement in libido in a number of case reports,[38,68,102,103] although both also have been reported to cause sexual dysfunction.[31] Buprorion has also been shown to improve libido in individuals with hypoactive sexual desire disorders. In a study of 60 female and male outpatients with psychosexual dysfunction (sexual aversion, inhibited sexual desire, inhibited sexual excitement, and/or inhibited orgasm), 12 weeks of double-blind treatment with bupropion (225–450 mg/day) resulted in significantly greater improvements in sexual functioning among treated patients than in the placebo group. Only 3% of placebo-treated patients reported improvement compared with 63% of the medicated group.[23]

Fluoxetine, one of the newer inhibitors of serotonin reuptake, has been associated with orgasm dysfunction. Researchers postulate an excitatory mechanism for adrenergic systems and an inhibitory role for serotonergic systems,[117] but in view of reports of both increased and decreased sexual functioning, the neurochemical effects are unclear.

Dopaminergic agents such as apomorphine may be efficacious in the treatment of erectile dysfunction. L-dopa was investigated in response to the observation that patients with Parkinson's disease who were treated with the drug reported increased sexual activity. In 10 patients with erectile dysfunction, slight-to-moderate increases in spontaneous erections at night were observed, although increase in libido was reported in only 2 patients and erections were not sustainable for sexual intercourse. In this study, however, the decarboxylase inhibitor was given to only 4 patients and only for the first 3 weeks of a 12-week course; in addition, the patient population included both idiopathic and nonidiopathic diagnostic groups, with no attempt to differentiate responses.[3] Apomorphine is a short-acting dopamine receptor agonist that decreases secretion of prolactin, stimulates production of growth hormone, and induces erections; it is widely used in research to establish potential efficacy of longer-acting agents.[58,59] In one study, apomorphine induced erections in 7 of 9 subjects. However, benztropine, a cholinergic agent, had no effect on erection, essentially ruling out a role for cholinergic agents in the modulation of erectile response.[58] In yet another study, apomorphine induced erections in 10 healthy men with impotence.[26] The preliminary studies of both apomorphine and buprorion suggest a crucial role for dopaminergic systems in sexual dysfunction. Because dopaminergic systems may be particularly vulnerable to traumatic brain injury (especially mesocortical and mesolimbic systems), sexual dysfunction may be associated with decreases in their viability.

Opioids also have been implicated in sexual function. Naloxone potentiated apomorphine-induced penile erections in rats, but methyl naloxone, which does not cross the blood-brain barrier, was ineffective.[5] In a small study involving 7 men, 25–50 mg/day led to full return of erectile function as well as nocturnal penile tumescence in 6 patients.[41] In a study of 30 men (age 25–50 years) with idiopathic impotence, naltrexone, an opiate antagonist, increased "sexual performance" (defined simply as intercourse) in 11 of 15 treated patients. There were no significant side effects. LH, FSH, and testosterone were unaffected, suggesting a central effect.[34]

Yohimbine, an alpha-adrenoceptor blocker, has been investigated in a number of studies of sexual dysfunction.[26,76,83,84,99,104] In a study of 100 organically impotent men, 42.6% of the treatment group compared with 27.6% of the placebo group reported improvement, but the values did not reach statistical significance.[76] The modest effects (at 18 mg/day) suggest that, although yohimbine is relatively safe, the expectation for improvement cannot be high. Another study produced less impressive results: 38% reported some subjective improvement, but only 5% were completely satisfied.[99] Other studies, using similar doses, have shown more dramatic results: for example, in one study 62% of the yohimbine-treated group and 16% of the placebo group reported improvement.[183] Identifying the cause of impotence (arterial insufficiency) may also identify potential responders.[105]

O'Carroll reviewed the results of investigations of hypoactive sexual desire disorder in women and described it as "the major female psychosexual dysfunction."[79] However, little evidence suggests that the disorder can be traced to hormonal inadequacies in women without brain injury. Hypogonadal women demonstrate an increase in sexual interest after androgen replacement.[94]

In summary, the literature is preliminary for non–brain-injured populations. The above studies focused exclusively on men, with the exception of the buproprion study. Clearly more research is needed before conclusions can be reached about what mediations may be useful in any population with sexual disorders.

Alternatives For Men

Self-injection of papaverine (a smooth muscle relaxant) or papaverine with phentolamine (an alpha-adrenergic blocker) is a treatment modality for impotence due to neurologic (in particular spinal cord injury) or vasculogenic causes. Nearly all patients with neurogenic impotence and 60–70% of patients with vasculogenic impotence respond to intracavernous injections.[95] Priapism, fibrosis of erectile tissues, hematomas, vasovagal reflex, and chemical hepatitis have been reported.[61] Intracavernous injection of prostaglandin E1 has been recommended more recently, and results are promising, although painful erection occurs in up to 20% of patients, perhaps related to concentration and/or neuropathy.[50,101] Papaverine (with or without phentolamine) and prostaglandin E1 act by increasing arterial inflow through vasodilation and decreasing venous outflow by occluding draining venules, probably through relaxation of smooth muscle in the corpus cavernosum. Unilateral injection results in bilateral effects through cross-circulation.

Prosthetic surgery is less frequently chosen because other alternatives are available for men with erectile disorders. The two major categories of penile prostheses are the semi-rigid and the inflatable prosthesis. Complications include mechanical failure, infection, pain, and perforation, but the rate of complications is now lower because of technologic advances. The patient-partner satisfaction rate is almost 90%. There have been no reports of the use of prostheses in brain-injured men.

Other alternatives include vacuum constriction devices, vascular reconstruction, and arterial and venous surgery, which are reviewed elsewhere.[43]

Other Alternatives for Women

Because women's sexuality has been inadequately addressed in research, both animal and human, little can be offered beyond common sense approaches. If lubrication is a problem, lubricants can be used, although they may prove more satisfactory for the male partner than for the woman. Other components of the sexual response continuum, including engorgement, elevation, and elongation of the vagina and clitoral erection, are not influenced by lubricants alone. Oral-genital stimulation and the use of vibrators may be helpful, but no clinical research has been done to substantiate their effectiveness in women with neurogenically induced sexual arousal disorder. Dyspareunia and vaginismus may be consequences in women with sexual dysfunction after brain injury, but neither has been studied.

Clearly much more research is needed to understand the types of sexual disorders that occur in women with brain injuries as well as women who have no neurologic disorder.

INTERVENTIONS FOR SEXUAL BEHAVIOR DISORDERS

Documentation of sexual behavior disorders after traumatic brain injury exists chiefly as case reports or anecdotal discussions, rather than large-scale studies.[65,108,110] Such descriptions follow research that documents such types of behaviors in animals.[29,66] The term disinhibition, associated with orbitofrontal injury, presents the underlying force leading to so-called deviant, hypersexual, or inappropriate behaviors.[89] Such behaviors are usually described in the context of interpersonal contact but also may manifest as perseverative behaviors, such as excessive masturbation. The extent to which such behaviors represent response to injury, loss of self-esteem, or need to act out psychic conflict has not been investigated. In a recent study, patients with frontal lobe damage on brain imaging reported high degrees of fantasy and experiences compared with patients without frontal lobe injury, again suggesting an organic basis.[90] Social inappropriateness, however, may manifest in many ways, only one of which is sexual behavior.

For inappropriate social behaviors, education of staff is important to encourage consistent responses. Redirection and education are necessary. Addressing issues of self-esteem directly may be helpful.[117] Aggressive sexual behaviors after brain injury are rare, and case reports can be traced to disinhibition. Sexual offenders have been treated with hormonal therapy such as medroxyprogesterone and other antiandrogens (e.g., cyproterone) that are progesterone derivatives,[6,10,35] to decrease levels of serum testosterone. Such interventions have not been thoroughly studied in brain-injured patients, most likely because violent sexual behaviors are rare. Changes in sexual preference may represent release of inhibitions from frontal damage. Exhibitionism also may result from disinhibition. Brain-injured persons are more likely to be victims of sexual abuse by others, as Cole points out in a recent article.[19]

Sexual Therapy

Sexual therapy focuses on various strategies to improve sexual relationships in couples who may have sexual desire or arousal disorders. Techniques range from desensitization, non-demand pleasuring, masturbation, start-stop techniques, the squeeze technique for premature ejaculation, and use of sexual surrogates.[2] Such techniques vary in effectiveness and require intervention of therapists with specific training. The therapist also should have specific experience in treating disabled persons. The techniques of sexual therapy may be useful for persons with brain injury and their partners, as they explore new ways of relating to each other. Their success in this population, however, has not been established.

Education and Counseling

For many individuals and couples, the key issue is education and counseling. Often lack of education results in problems with establishing healthy intimate, sexual relationships. Communication with a physician or counselor and permission to discuss issues of intimacy and sexuality decrease anxiety and promote a greater likelihood that couples will begin to communicate with each other. A number of recent books,[42,43,57] written for the lay community and in some cases by persons with disabilities, open new doors for education, and such resources should be suggested. Emphasis on communication, both verbal and nonverbal, is important in establishing the basis for intimate physical contact.

Of crucial importance is providing information about sexually transmitted diseases, including gonorrhea, chylamydial infections, herpes simplex viral infections, syphilis, parasitic infections, hepatitis, genital warts, urethritis, prostatitis, and acquired immunodeficiency syndrome. Safer sex practices include a careful selection of partners, mutual screening as necessary, and use of condoms and spermicides.

For further discussion the reader is referred to a number of other publications that address education and counseling programs and services for persons with brain injury.[7,37,69,71,78]

REPRODUCTIVE ISSUES FOR WOMEN WITH BRAIN INJURY

A full discussion of reproductive issues for women with brain injury is beyond the scope of this chapter. However, a number of recent articles and books, written in part by disabled women, are useful for persons with brain injury as well as the professionals who care for and advise them.[43,82,85] Although the specific effects of the primary brain injury on pregnancy, labor, and delivery have not been investigated, other relevant literature (mostly about women with spinal cord injury) offers recommendations for addressing mobility issues.

Several issues with particular relevance to women with traumatic brain injury are addressed below, including (1) amenorrhea, (2) seizure disorders and anticonvulsant medications, (3) other drugs with teratogenic potential, (4) management of pregnant women in coma or vegetative state, (5) contraception, and (6) infertility.

Amenorrhea

Although female reproductive dysfunction after brain injury has been largely unstudied, amenorrhea is frequently observed. Hypopituitarism after head trauma results in amenorrhea, among other clinical signs, but many cases of amenorrhea after brain injury are not associated with hypopituitarism (Fig. 1).

Seizures and Pregnancy

A recent article summarizes the risk factors for malformations associated with use of anticonvulsant drugs during pregnancy in epileptic women.[64] The absolute risk of major malformations in neonates exposed to antiepileptic drugs in utero is 7–10%, which is 3–5% higher than for the general population. Barbiturates and phenytoin are associated with congenital heart malformations and craniofacial anomalies. The fetal hydantoin syndrome is further characterized by prenatal and postnatal growth deficiencies, mental retardation, and limb defects; less often microcephaly, ocular defects, hypospadias, and hernias may be caused by other epileptic agents.[14] Valproate and carbamazepine are associated with spina bifida aperta and hypospadias.[14,86] High daily dosage, high serum concentration, low folate levels, and polytherapy are additional risk factors.[64] Infants of epileptic mothers may develop hemorrhagic disorders, apparently due to a deficiency of vitamin K-dependent factors.[113] Despite such risks, 90% of women with seizure disorders deliver normal infants.

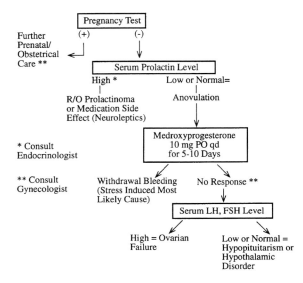

FIGURE 1.   Amenorrhea: diagnostic evaluation.

Because teratogenicity of anticonvulsant medications is associated with elevated levels of oxidative metabolites, an enzymatic marker may be useful in determination of risk. Low enzymatic activity was found in 4 of 19 fetuses, and the predicted high risk for fetal hydantoin syndrome was confirmed postnatally.[14]

The risk of seizures during pregnancy, labor, and delivery is increased in 40% of women who are epileptic, although 50% have no change and 10% have a decrease in seizures.[25] In one study, however, 68% of pregnancies in which seizure frequency increased were associated with noncompliance with treatment recommendations.[91] Pregnancy affects anticonvulsant levels, which decline over time; thus monitoring is necessary. The decrease in levels results from emesis, decreased absorption, and increases in plasma volume, liver metabolism, and renal clearance. In addition, hormone changes may lead to increased seizures, and protein binding may be altered.[91]

The International League Against Epilepsy (ILAE) recently published guidelines for the care of women with epilepsy who may become pregnant. Recommendations include (1) counseling about the risk of seizures, bleeding, and toxemia in pregnant women; (2) counseling about malformations, prematurity, seizures, and developmental disorders in fetus and infant; (3) ultrasound evaluation for neural tube defects, heart malformations, and craniofacial anomalies, and amniotic fluid analysis of alpha-fetoprotein for neural tube defects; (4) counseling about options for termination of pregnancy; (5) careful choice of anticonvulsant and monitoring of anticonvulsant levels, both during pregnancy (when they may decrease) and after delivery (when they may increase); (6) adequate amounts of folate (up to 4 mg is recommended to prevent neural tube defects[24,113]); and (7) adequate sleep.

Anticonvulsant drugs have different rates of transmission in breast milk: 5–10% for valproate, 30% for phenytoin, 40% for phenobarbital, 45% for carbamazepine, 60% for primidone, and 90% for ethosuximide.[21] The ILAE recommends that judgments be based on multiple factors, but clearly sedation and signs of drug withdrawal are not acceptable.[21]

Other Drugs with Teratogenic Potential

Other medications prescribed to persons with traumatic brain injury with relative frequency may have adverse effects on the fetus (Table 4).

Coma and Vegetative State

The treatment of pregnant women with brain injury at trauma centers throughout the country raises medical and ethical issues. Some of the women are in coma, and some emerge from coma during pregnancy; a small percentage, however, evolve into and remain in a vegetative state, and others may be classified as brain dead. Dillon and associates[28] developed a controversial plan of management for pregnancy in the case of maternal brain death. They recommend maternal life-support measures at 24–27 weeks of gestation, followed by cesarean section at 28 weeks, but no extraordinary measures at less than 24 weeks for mother or fetus. Others[48] recommend continued maternal support until 32–34 weeks to increase survival rates. Both maternal survival and emergence from the vegetative state are possible. As evidenced by recent reports in the media, many such cases raise ethical and legal as well as medical questions.

Obviously, for the fetus that does not survive the trauma suffered by the mother, the pregnancy must be terminated to save the mother's life. Experimental evidence suggests that the fetus may be less vulnerable to acute asphyxia than the mother. Redistribution of blood flow to vital organs, anaerobic metabolism, and decreased oxygen consumption may be the essential mechanisms.[18]

Contraception

Options for contraception are generally not limited by medical considerations in patients with brain injury. Poor patient compliance because of memory difficulties may dictate choice; oral contraception may be ill-advised for this reason. Long-acting injectable techniques may be preferable; permanent solutions, if desired, include vasectomy and tubal ligation. Subdermal delivery of the

TABLE 4.   Drug Therapy during Pregnancy

The following medications frequently prescribed to patients with brain injuries may carry some teratogenic risks:

Antipsychotic agents	Anticonvulsants
Antidepressants	Antimigraine agents

synthetic progesin levonorgestrel has a failure rate of 4 or 5/1,000 users/year compared with 20–50/1,000 users for oral contraceptives; for persons taking phenytoin or carbamazepine, pregnancy rates are higher.[33] Oral hormonal contraception may increase the risk of venous thrombosis, and this must be considered in women historically or potentially at risk. Haseltine et al.[43] recently reviewed contraceptive choices for persons with disabilities, and Griffith et al. have provided a helpful manual with an outline of options.[42]

Infertility

Screening tests for men and women with infertility are outlined in a recent monograph.[92] In patients with traumatic brain injury, the first evaluations should include hormonal assays, including LH, FSH, prolactin, thyroid function studies, and total testosterone. Low concentrations of LH, FSH, and testosterone suggest hypopituitary or hypothalamic injury, and a releasing hormone stimulation test should be conducted. Hypothalamic ovulatory dysfunction may be treated with clomiphene citrate, menotropins (human menopausal gonadotropins or LH and FSH), or gonadotropin-releasing hormone. In men, hypothalamic-pituitary failure may be treated with menotropins, human chorionic gonadotropin, or gonadotropin-releasing hormone. Testosterone promotes virilization and may enhance sexual function but has no effect on spermatogenesis. Obviously, assessment and treatment for infertility belong in the hands of a specialist, in consultation with a rehabilitation medicine physician.

CONCLUSION

This chapter reviews the medical literature concerning sexual and reproductive disorders in persons with brain injuries. Much of the scientific research has focused on men or nondisabled persons, with a limited view of sexual functioning. Research methodologies, such as those used by Sjogren[97,98] in studying stroke patients, offer more sophisticated approaches to the questions surrounding intimacy as well as sexual function in patients who are stigmatized by disabilities.

Rehabilitation professionals, especially physicians, must gain experience and comfort in addressing sexual and reproductive issues with patients. If medical professionals do not grant permission for such discussions, they may never occur. Finally, persons with disabilities can provide the able-bodied community with opportunities to learn. They face many challenges in forming relationships and in building and sustaining families. Many have met the challenge and have insights that professionals may not fully appreciate without opening the dialogue.

REFERENCES

1. Abboud CF: Laboratory diagnosis of hypopituitarism. Mayo Clinic Proc 61:35–48, 1986.
2. Allgeier WE, Allgeier AR: Sexual Interactions, 4th ed. Lexington, MA, D.C. Heath, 1995.
3. Benkert O, Crombach G, Kockott G: Effect of L-dopa on sexually impotent patients. Psychopharmacology 23:91–95, 1972.
4. Bensen GS, Boileau MA: The penis: Sexual function and dysfunction. In Gillenwater JY, Grayhack JT, Howards SS, Duckett JW (eds): Adult and Pediatric Urology. Chicago, Year Book, 1987, pp 1407–1447.
5. Berendsen HHG, Gower AJ: Opiate-androgen interactions in drug-induced yawning and penile erections in the rat. Neuroendocrinology 42:185–190, 1986.
6. Berlin FS: Treating sexual disorders with medroxyprogesterone acetate. Curr Affec Illness 6:5015, 1987.
7. Blackerby WF: A treatment model for sexuality disturbance following brain injury. J Head Trauma Rehabil 5(2):73–82, 1990.
8. Blendonohy P, Philip P: Precocious puberty in children after traumatic brain injury. Brain Inj 5:63–68, 1991.
9. Boldrini P, Basaglia N, Calanca MC: Sexual changes in hemiparetic patients. Arch Phys Med Rehabil 72:202–207, 1991.
10. Boller F, Frank E: Sexual Dysfunction in Neurologic Disorders: Diagnosis, Management and Rehabilitation. New York, Raven Press, 1982.
11. Bond MR: Assessment of the psychological outcome of severe head injury. Acta Neurochir 34:57, 1976.
12. Bray GP: Sexual functioning in stroke survivors. Arch Phys Med Rehabil 62:286–288, 1981.
13. Briggs, GG, Freeman RK, Yaffe SJ: Drugs in Pregnancy and Lactation: A Reference Guide to Fetal and Neonatal Risk, 4th ed. Baltimore, Williams & Wilkins, 1994.
14. Buehler BA, Delimont D, van Waes M, et al: Prenatal prediction of risk of the fetal hydantoin syndrome. N Engl J Med 322:1567–1572, 1990.
15. Buvat J, Lemaire A, Buvat-Herbaut M: Human chorionic gonadotropin treatment of nonorganic erectile failure and lack of sexual desire: A double-blind study. Urology 30(3):216–219, 1987.
16. Clark J, Raggatt P, Edwards O: Hypothalamic hypogonadism following major head injury. Clin Endocrinol 29:153–165, 1988.
17. Cohen HD, Rosen RC: Electroencephalographic laterality changes during human sexual orgasm. Arch Sex Behav 5:189–199, 1976.
18. Cohn HE, Sacks EJ, Heymann AA, et al: Cardiovascular responses to hypoxemia and acidemia in fetal lambs. Am J Obstet Gynecol 120:817–824, 1974.
19. Cole S: Facing the challenges of sexual abuse in persons with disabilities. J Sex Disabil 7:77, 1987.
20. Cole TM: Sexual History-Taking: Adults with a Prior History of Sexual Relations with Another Person. Framingham, MA, National Head Injury Foundation, 1965.
21. Commission on Genetics, Pregnancy and the Child, International League against Epilepsy: Guidelines for the care of women of childbearing age with epilepsy. Epilepsia 34:588–589, 1993.
22. Coslett H, Heilman K: Male sexual function: Impairment after right hemisphere stroke. Arch Neurol 43:1036–1039, 1986.
23. Crenshaw T, Goldberg J, Stern W: Pharmacologic modification of psycho-sexual dysfunction. J Sex Marital Ther 13:239–252, 1987.
24. Czeizel AE, Dudas I: Prevention of the first occurrence of neural tube defects by periconceptual vitamin supplementation. N Engl J Med 327:1832–1835, 1992.
25. Dalessio DJ: Seizure disorders and pregnancy. N Engl J Med 312:559–563, 1985.
26. Danjou P, Alexander L, Warot D, et al: Assessment of erectogenic properties of apomorphine and yohimbine in man. Br J Clin Pharmacol 26:733–739, 1988.
27. Derogatis LR: Derogatis Interview for Sexual Function. Baltimore, Clinical Psychometric Research, 1987.
28. Dillon WP, Lee RV, Tronolone MJ, et al: Life support and maternal brain death during pregnancy. JAMA 248:1089–1091, 1982.
29. Doane BK: Doane BK, Livingston KE (eds): Clinical psychiatry and the physiodynamics of the limbic system. In The Limbic System: Functional Organization and Clinical Disorders. New York, Raven Press, 1986, pp 302–304.
30. Donatucci CF, Lue TF: The combined intracavernous injection and stimulation test. J Urol 148:61–62, 1992.
31. Drugs that cause sexual dysfunction: Med Lett 25:73–76, 1983.
32. Ducharme S, Gill KM: Sexual values, training and professional roles. J Head Trauma Rehabil 5:38–45, 1990.
33. Edwards OM, Clark J: Post-traumatic hypogonadism: Six cases and a review of the literature. Medicine 65:281–290, 1986.

34. Fabbri A, et al: Endorphins in male impotence. Evidence for naltrexone stimulation of erectile activity in patient therapy. Psychoneuroendocrinology 14:103–111, 1989.

35. Freund K: Therapeutic sex drive reduction. Acta Psychiatr Scand 62 (Suppl 287):5–37, 1980.

36. Fugl-Meyer AR: Post stroke hemiplegia and sexual intercourse. Scand J Rehabil Med, Suppl 7:158–165, 1980.

37. Garden FH, Bonke CF, Hoffman M: Sexual functioning and marital adjustment after traumatic brain injury. J Head Trauma Rehabil 5:52–59, 1990.

38. Gartrell N: Increased libido in women receiving trazodone. Am J Psychiatry 143:781–728, 1986.

39. Goddess E, Wagner N, Silverman D: Post stroke sexual activity of CVA patients. Med Aspect Hum Sex 13:16-30, 1979.

40. Goldberg RL, Wise TN: The importance of the sense of smell in human sexuality. J Sex Educ Ther 16:236–241, 1990.

41. Goldstein JA: Erectile failure and naltrexone. Ann Intern Med 105:799, 1986.

42. Griffith ER, Lemberg S: Sexuality and the Person with Traumatic Brain Injury: A Guide for Families. Philadelphia, F.A. Davis, 1993.

43. Haseltine F, Cole S, Gray DB: Reproductive Issues for Persons with Physical Disabilities. Baltimore, PH Brookes, 1993.

44. Heath RG: Pleasure response of human subjects to direct stimulation of the brain: Physiologic and psycho-dynamic considerations. In Heath RG, (ed): The Role of Pleasure in Behavior. New York, Harper & Row, 1964.

45. Herzog A, Russell V, Vaitokaitis JL, et al: Neuroendocrine dysfunction in temporal lobe epilepsy. Arch Neurol 39:133–135, 1982.

46. Herzog A, Seibel M, Schomer D, et al: Reproductive endocrine disorders in men with partial seizures of temporal lobe origin. Arch Neurol 43:347–350, 1986.

47. Herzog A, Seibel M, Schomer D, et al: Reproductive endocrine disorders in women with partial seizures of temporal lobe origin. Arch Neurol 43:341–346, 1986.

48. Hill LM: Management of maternal vegetative state during pregnancy. Mayo Clin Proc 60:469–472, 1985.

49. Horn LJ, Zasler ND: Neuroanatomy and neurophysiology of sexual dysfunction. J Head Trauma Rehabil 5:1–13, 1990.

50. Ishii N, Watanabe H, Irisawa Y, et al: Intracavernous injection of prostaglandin E1 for the treatment of erectile impotence. J Urol 141:323–325, 1989.

51. Jennett B, Teasdale G: Management of Head Injuries. Philadelphia, F.A. Davis, 1981.

52. Kalliomaki J, Markkanen T, Mustonen V: Sexual behavior after cerebral vascular accident. Fertil Steril 12:156–159, 1961.

53. Kinsella GJ, Duffy FD: Attitudes toward disability by spouses of stroke patients. Scand J Rehab Med 12:73–76, 1980.

54. Klachko DM, Winer N, Burns TW: Traumatic hypopituitarism occurring before puberty: Survival 35 years untreated. J Clin Endocrinol 28:1768–1772, 1968.

55. Kosteljanetz M, Jensen T: Norgard B, et al: Sexual and hypothalamic dysfunction in the postconcussional syndrome. Acta Neurol Scand 63:169–180, 1981.

56. Kreutzer JS, Zasler ND: Psychosexual consequences of traumatic brain injury: Methodology and preliminary findings. Brain Inj 3:177–186, 1989.

57. Kroll K, Levy Klein E: Enabling Romance: A Guide to Love, Sex, and Relationships for the Disabled. New York, Harmony Books, 1992.

58. Lal S, Ackman D, Thavundayil JX, et al: Effect of apomorphine, a dopamine receptor agonist, on penile tumescence in normal subjects. Prog Neuropsychopharmacol Biol Psychiatry 8:695–699, 1984.

59. Lal S: Apomorphine in the evaluation of dopaminergic function in man. Prog Neuropsychopharmacol Biol Psychiatry 12:117–164, 1988.

60. LeVay S: The Sexual Brain. Boston, MIT Press, 1993, pp 71–81.

61. Levine SB, Althof SE, Turner LA, et al: Side effects of self-administration of intracavernous papaverine and phentolamine for the treatment of impotence. J Urol 141:54–57, 1989.

62. Lezak ML: Living with the characterologically altered brain injured patient. J Clin Psychiatry 39:592–598, 1978.

63. Lilly R: The human Kluver-Bucy syndrome. Neurology 33:1141, 1983.

64. Lindhout D, Omtzigt JG: Pregnancy and teratogenicity. Epilepsia 33:S41–48, 1992.

65. Lusk MD, Kott JA: Effects of head injury on libido. Med Aspects Hum Sex, 16:22–30, 1982.

66. MacLean O: Brain mechanisms of primal sexual functions and related behavior. In Sandler M, Gessa G (eds): Sexual Behavior: Pharmacology and Biochemistry. New York, Raven Press, 1975.

67. Mapou RL: Traumatic brain injury rehabilitation with gay and lesbian individuals. J Head Trauma Rehabil 5:67–72, 1990.

68. Mathews A, Whitehead A, Kellet J: Psychological and hormonal factors in the treatment of female sexual dysfunction. Psychol Med 13:83–92, 1983.

69. McCormick GP, Riffer DJ, Thompson MM: Coital positioning for stroke afflicted couples. Rehabil Nurs 11:17–19, 1986.

70. Medlar TM, Medlar J: Nursing management of sexuality issues. J Head Trauma Rehabil 5:46–51, 1990.

71. Medlar TM: Sexual counseling and traumatic brain injury. Sex Disabil 11:57–71, 1993.

72. Mesulum M: Principles of Behavioral Neurology. Philadelphia, F.A. Davis, 1985.

73. Miller B, Cummings J, McIntyre H, et al: Hypersexuality or altered sexual preference following brain injury. J Neurol Neurosurg Psychiatry 49:867–873, 1986.

73a. Monga TN (ed): Sexuality and Disability. Phys Med Rehabil State Art Rev 9(2):299–569, 1995.

74. Monga TN, Lawson JS, Inglis J: Sexual dysfunction in stroke patients. Arch Phys Med Rehabil 67:19–22, 1986.

75. Monga TN, Monga M, Raina MS, et al: Hypersexuality in stroke. Arch Phys Med Rehabil 67:415–417, 1986.

76. Morales A, Condra M, Owen JA, et al: Is yohimbine effective in the treatment of organic impotence? Results of a controlled trial. J Urol 137:1168–1172, 1987.

77. National Head Injury Foundation: Information Packet on Sexuality. Framingham, MA, National Head Injury Foundation, 1995.

78. Neistadt ME, Freda M: Choices: A Guide to Sex Counseling with Physically Disabled Adults. Malabar, FL, Robert E. Kreiger, 1987.

79. O'Carroll RE: Sexual desire disorders: A review of controlled treatment studies. Sex Res 28:607–624, 1991.

80. O'Carroll RE, Bancroft J: Testosterone therapy for low sexual interest and erectile dysfunction in men: A controlled study. Br J Psychiatry 145:146–151, 1984.

81. O'Carroll RE, Woodrow J, Maroun F: Psychosexual and psychosocial sequelae of closed head injury. Brain Inj 5:303–313, 1991.

82. Patel M, Bonke C: Impact of traumatic brain injury on pregnancy. J Head Trauma Rehabil 5(2):60–66, 1990.

83. Reid K, Morales A, Harris C: Double-blind trial of yohimbine in treatment of psychogenic impotence. Lancet 2:421–423, 1987.

84. Riley AJ, Goodman RE, Kellet JM, et al: Double-blind trial of yohimbine hydrochloride in the treatment of erection inadequacy. Sex Marital Ther 4:17–26, 1989.

85. Rogers JG, Matsumura M: Mother-To Be: A Guide to Pregnancy and Birth for Women with Disabilities. New York, Demos, 1991.

86. Rosa FW: Spina bifida in infants of women treated with carbamazapine in pregnancy. N Engl J Med 324:674–677, 1991.

87. Rosenbaum M, Najenson T: Changes in life patterns and symptoms of low mood as reported by wives of severely brain-injured soldiers. J Consul Clin Psychol 44:881–888, 1976.

88. Rust J, Golombok S: The Glomobok-Rusk Inventory of Sexual Satisfaction (GRISS). Br J Clin Psychol 24:63–64, 1985.

89. Sabhesan S, Natarajan M: Sexual behavior after head injury in Indian men and women. Arch Sex Behav 18(4):349–356, 1989.

90. Sandel ME, Derogatis LR, Williams KS: Sexual functioning following traumatic brain injury (abstract). Arch Phys Med Rehabil 74:1284, 1993.

91. Schmidt D, Canger R, Avanzini G, et al: Change of seizure frequency in pregnant epileptic women. J Neurol Neurosurg Psychiatry 46:751–755, 1983.

92. Shane JM: Evaluation and treatment of infertility. Clin Symp 45:2–32, 1993.

93. Shaul P, Towbin R, Chernausek S: Precocious puberty following severe head trauma. Am J Dis Child 139:467–469, 1985.

94. Sherwin B, Gelfand M: The role of androgen in the maintenance of sexual function in oopherectomized women. Psychosom Med 149:397–409, 1987.

95. Sidi AA, Chen KK: Clinical experience with vasoactive intercavernous pharmacotherapy for treatment of impotence. World J Urol 5:156–159, 1989.

96. Sipski ML, The impact of spinal cord trauma on female sexual function. In Haseltine FP, Cole SS, Gray DB (eds): Reproductive Issues for Persons with Physical Disabilities. Baltimore, PH Brookes, 1993.

97. Sjogren K: Sexuality after stroke with hemiplegia: I. Scand J Rehabil Med 15:55–61, 1983.

98. Sjogren K, Damber JE, Liliequist B: Sexuality after stroke with hemiplegia: II. Scand J Rehabil Med 15:63–69, 1983.

99 Sondra LP, Mazo R, Chancellor MD: The role of yohimbine for the treatment of erectile impotence. J Sex Marital Ther 16:15–21, 1990.

100. Spark RF, Wills CA: Hypogonadism, hyperprolactinaemia, and temporal lobe epilepsy in hyposexual men. Lancet 413–417, 1984.

101. Stakl W, Hasun R, Marberger M: Intracavernous injection of prostaglandin E1 in impotent men. J Urol 141:66–68, 1988.

102. Stevensen RW, Solyom L: The aphrodisiac effect of fenfluramine—Two case reports of a possible side effect to the use of fenfluramine in the treatment of bulimia. J Clin Psychopharmacol 10:69–71, 1990.

103. Subdermal progestin implant for long-term contraception. Med Lett 33:17–20, 1991.

104. Sullivan G: Increased libido with trazodone. Am J Psychiatry 144:967, 1987.

105. Susset JG, Tessier CD, Wincze J, et al: Effect of yohimbine hydrochloride on erectile impotence: A double-blind study. J Urol 141:1360–1363, 1989.

106. Thomsen IV: Late outcome of severe blunt head trauma: A 10-15 year second follow-up. J Neurol Neurosurg Psychiatry 47:260–268, 1984.

107. Walker AE: The neurological basis of sex. Neurol Ind 24:1–13, 1976.

108. Weinstein EA: Effects of brain damage on sexual behavior. Med Aspects Hum Sex 15:162–164, 1981.

109. Weinstein EA: Sexual disturbances after brain injury. Med Aspects Hum Sex 8:10–16, 1974.

110. Weinstein EA, Kahn RL: Patterns of sexual behavior following brain injury. Psychiatry 24:69–78, 1961.

111 Weiss S: Hypopituitarism following head trauma. Am J Obstet Gynecol 127:678–679, 1977.

112. Welner SL: Management approaches to sexually transmitted diseases in women with disabilities. In Haseltine FP, Cole SS, Gray DB (eds): Reproductive Issues for Persons with Disabilities. Baltimore, PH Brookes, 1993.

113. Werler MM, Shapiro S, Mitchell AA: Periconceptual folic acid exposure and risk of neural tube defects. JAMA 269:1292–1293, 1993.

114. Yerby MS: Problems and management of the pregnant woman with epilepsy. Epilepsia 28:S29–S36, 1987.

115. Zajecka J, Fawcett J, Schaff M, et al: The role of serotonin in sexual dysfunction: Fluoxetine-associated orgasm dysfunction. J Clin Psychiatry 52:66–68, 1991.

116. Zasler ND, Horn LJ: Rehabilitative management of sexual dysfunction. J Head Trauma Rehabil 5(2):14–24, 1990.

117. Zencius A, Weslowsky MD, Burke WA, et al: Managing hypersexual disorders in brain injured clients. Brain Inj 4:175–181, 1990.

23

Psychopharmacologic Aspects of Traumatic Brain Injury

TRAUMATIC BRAIN INJURY AS CLINICAL CONDITION

This chapter reviews basic principles and examines the most significant reports on psychopharmaceuticals for traumatic brain injury (TBI) and related conditions. The clinical recognition of TBI as a distinct syndrome worthy of extensive study has come late to rehabilitation. Consequently the psychopharmacologic treatment of TBI has only recently emerged as a specific focus of scientific and clinical investigation. Patients with TBI have a wide spectrum of neurologic, perceptual, motor, cognitive, behavioral, and affective deficits that may be responsive to psychopharmacologic interventions. Although an increasing number of direct studies of psychopharmacologic treatment of head injury are appearing, the data remain inadequate. It is still necessary to also rely on reports of psychopharmacologic use in other, presumably similar, conditions. Most of the uses for these agents in TBI, discussed herein, are generally not FDA "approved indications," but there is no legal prohibition. Therefore, although these drugs may be used in TBI, appropriate caution by the clinician is indicated.

This chapter presupposes a basic clinical familiarity and understanding of the major psychopharmacologic agents and their use. A number of comprehensive texts[35,50,116,117,121,231,269] are available, at least one definitive reference text,[170] as well as an increasing number of journals[33,195] dedicated to various aspects of this subject. Specific reviews of use of psychopharmacologic agents in neuropsychiatric, organic brain conditions are also recently available.[242,280] The clinician is well advised to become familiar, through these general texts, with the basic principles of sound clinical usage, i.e., specifics regarding individual drug actions, dynamics, side effects, etc. The present chapter makes no attempt to recapitulate the information in these more than adequate sources on general psychopharmacology. The author's intent here is to extend the general body of psychopharmacologic information within the context of specific indications and precautions of use in TBI.

This chapter is organized around the treatment of specific target behaviors or symptoms rather than individual drugs and drug classes. However, many classes of drugs have multiple indications in TBI; thus, discussions of the stimulant drugs appear in differing sections on arousal, affect, agitation, and cognition. Because many, perhaps most, symptom complexes following upon TBI have overlapping dimensions, a certain redundancy or arbitrariness in exposition (e.g., whether specific aspects of stimulant use are better discussed under the problem of cognitive impairment or arousal) has been impossible to avoid. The lack of precision which the reader may sense around the discussion of specific indications herein merely reflects the vagueness of our clinical knowledge.

No attempt is made to discuss other important central nervous system (CNS) disorders, such as spasticity or tremor, which might more properly be considered neuroactive rather than psychoactive. A recent review of drug treatment for these indications is available elsewhere.[296] Discussion here is limited to only those aspects germane to drug management of complex behaviors, cognition, and affect.

Traditional TBI Rehabilitation Treatment Options

Over the past 20 years, specific rehabilitation treatment approaches and elaborate systems of rehabilitation care have been developed to manage the various functional problems following significant TBI.[36,96] A comprehensive, multidisciplinary approach has evolved, with specialized rehabilitation teams and vertically integrated continuums of treatment. Historically, rehabilitation of the various TBI personality, behavioral, and cognitive components has been conceptualized as lying within the domains of traditional rehabilitation therapeutic modalities, such as education and counseling. Thus, comprehensive rehabilitation of psychological and personality deficits routinely involves such "classical" rehabilitation technologies as psychotherapy, social skill modeling, peer group experience, behavior modification, and multiple rehearsal. These approaches, more fully addressed elsewhere in this text, have demonstrated a general utility and efficacy in TBI in amelioration of patient deficit, disability, or handicap.[40,148,254]

Current TBI Rehabilitation Treatment Limitations

While these general rehabilitation approaches are accepted and believed to be effective and appropriate for virtually all patients recovering from moderate and severe brain injury, none of these interventions is totally restorative. There are well-recognized limitations in the efficacy of learning, behavioral, and environment-based approaches due to the persistent physiologic deficits characteristic of TBI. Dynamic, insight-oriented, psychotherapeutic interventions, for example, often are impeded by patients' anosognosia, verbal/aphasic deficits, conceptual concreteness, memory impairments, impulse-control deficits, and lack of introspection.[193]

As a practical matter, there are essentially always residual deficits even after the most extensive rehabilitation for severe, moderate, and, to some extent, mild brain injuries. The deficits may be subtle and only apparent in contrast to a patient's premorbid function, but nevertheless clinically quite significant. It is clear that the limitations of current classical rehabilitation call for additional methods of treatment. Psychopharmacologic treatment has become an accepted alternative or complementary intervention to these more classical methods of TBI care.

NEUROPHYSIOLOGY OF PSYCHOACTIVE DRUGS

The brain is a vastly complex, topographically structured organ composed of precise distributions of a very large number of discrete transmitter systems. Further complexity derives from the multiplicity of receptor types and subtypes for each transmitter, e.g., dopaminergic (D_1, D_2, and recently D_3[235] subtypes), adrenergic (α_1, α_2, β_1, and β_2), serotonergic ($_5$-HT_1, $_5$-HT_2, $_5$-HT_3), cholinergic (muscarinic, nicotinic), and opiate (μ [mu], κ [kappa], δ [delta], σ [sigma]). Additional subtypes are continuously being identified. Also, the effects of a specific transmitter depend not only on its specific receptor type and subtype, but also on the pre- or postsynaptic location of the receptor, and the functional system in which the receptor is located. Single neurons may release more than one type of transmitter, as well as a variety of neuromodulators, neuropeptides, etc. A single transmitter may be both excitatory and inhibitory in action. At the behavioral level, neurotransmitters do not have solitary actions. For example, noradrenergic stimulation can be either a rewarding or aversive contingency, depending on the relative levels of transmitter released. A further complexity to the neurophysiology of cognition, affect, and behavior derives from the recently elaborated process of volume transmission, a separate mechanism of brain activity that complements synaptic action. This extrasynaptic transmitter activity is increasingly recognized as important to behavior in its own right.[13,78] Finally, our ignorance of the overall neurochemistry of the brain is vast, and the numbers of known receptors continue to increase.[35,248] As Kolata observes, "Most investigators think that the current picture of how drugs work is a gross oversimplification. It is estimated that only 1 to 5 percent of the brain's neurotransmitters are known."[139] In sum, a precise and detailed theory or understanding of the structure and function of the CNS is beyond our capability, and drugs that affect the CNS are thus significantly indeterminate in their effects.

Despite these difficulties, useful schemas of the basic neurophysiologic mechanisms of the CNS exist. Examples include the work of Mesulum[171] and the model of attention, arousal, and intention offered by Voeller, who conceptualizes three interrelated neural systems: a sensory-attentional, a motor-intentional, and an arousal-attentional.[275] An illustrative structure, modified from Ashton,[8] conceptualizes the complex behaviors of higher organisms, including humans, to be based primarily on the mutual interaction and expression of three major neurologic functional systems: arousal, reward and punishment, and cognition. Disturbances of behavior seen in humans, including those seen following TBI, can be considered as involving relative degrees of dysfunction of these three general systems, and although our knowledge of the roles of specific neurotransmitter roles is rudimentary, certain broad principles are known and are summarized below.

Arousal

Arousal and attention are complex concepts consisting of multiple discrete individual subprocesses. Space is not available to review these concepts in depth. Reviews are

available.[281] Arousal is a multidimensional construct. There are, for example, both general and goal-directed arousal systems. General arousal is subserved by the reticular activating system (RAS), which projects via long axial fibers to the entire cerebrum as well as lower structures and spinal cord. The RAS provides a background excitatory tone for the CNS. In general, sedatives depress while stimulants increase the activity of the RAS. Acetylcholine (ACh), norepinephrine (NE), dopamine (DA), histamine (H), and serotonin (5-HT) are all involved in this system as major transmitters. Sleep-waking cycles are also reflective of activity of these systems, as are the processes of sustained vigilance and resistance to distraction.[128] Goal-directed arousal or focused attention also derives additional valence from the emotional significance attached to an activity, which derives principally from associated inputs from the limbic system. Limbic and reticular systems thus contribute jointly to overall arousal levels and attentional state.

Reward and Punishment

Motivation, goal pursuit, affect, aversion, and drive satiation are major components of the reward-punishment system. Subjective mood states, as well as pain and nociception, are also probably determined in part by activity of this system. The structures principally involved in reward and punishment appear to be extremely diverse and widely distributed; they include: frontal cortex, septal area, amygdala, hypothalamus, and various nuclei in the midbrain, brainstem, and cerebellum, such as the locus coeruleus and ventral tegmental nucleus. Many of the most important of these structures have been grouped under the term "limbic" system. The monoamines NE, DA, and 5-HT have major involvement in this system as well as endogenous opiates and ACh.

Cognition

Cognition involves the general process of learning and memory as well as information processing. Cognition is dependent upon arousal, a necessary prerequisite. There appears to be no specific neurologic structure(s) for general memory function, i.e., every nerve cell evidences basic characteristics that presumably underlie learning such as sensitization, potentiation, habituation, etc., yet there is also significant localization of some aspects of specialized memory: verbal, semantic, procedural, etc. Memory is also conceptualized as having discrete phase components, i.e., acquisition and immediate, short-term and long-term memory as well as a separate process of memory retrieval. These components are all believed to have distinct structural and neurotransmitter analogs. The amygdala, hippocampus, cerebral cortex, cerebellum, and certain diencephalic nuclei are among the most important of these. Physiologically, ACh has a particular significance as a transmitter in learning and memory, but the monoamines are involved as well. Additional interest has focused on the involvement of certain amino acid neurotransmitters (such as gamma aminobutyric acid [GABA], glutamate, and aspartate) and neuropeptides (oxytocin, vasopressin, adrenocorticotropic hormone [ACTH] and ACTH fragments, and opioids) in memory processes. Information processing, a commonly used clinical term, is a somewhat diffuse concept that refers to the general accuracy, facility, and flexibility to which cognitive processes are managed. It appears to have a general relationship to overall cortical functioning but particularly with frontal "executive" processes. DA and NE have been especially associated with information-processing activity.

It is generally believed that the primary effectiveness of most neuroactive agents is based on a particular agonist or antagonist receptor action within specific neurotransmitter system(s). For example, the antipsychotic effectiveness of neuroleptics in schizophrenia and other conditions is best understood as due to their activity as a blocker of postsynaptic dopaminergic transmission. However, the neuroleptics also affect other transmitter systems and so elicit other secondary effects. For example, certain symptoms, such as dry mouth, blurred vision, and urinary retention, are likely caused by the anticholinergic action of the antipsychotic drugs. Sedative and hypotensive effects are related to their blockade of the alpha-adrenergic receptors and their antihistaminic properties.

It must be emphasized that all of these theoretical systems and actions are closely integrated, interactive, and interdependent, and it is only a convenience to discuss the neuropsychologic activity and psychopharmacologic modification of each in isolation. It is the continuous and seamless interplay and variations resulting from these systems' interaction that produce the complexity and subtlety of human psychological life and behavior. Psychoactive drug effects consequently need to be seen as equally subtle and complex and the inclination to apply reductionist terminology to drug action (e.g., antidepressant, antiaggressive, etc.) studiously avoided.

PATHOPHYSIOLOGY OF TBI

TBI pathology involves combinations of generalized axonal shearing and hypoxic lesions as well as more focal contusion, hemorrhage, and infarct. These pathologic changes underlie TBI behavioral and cognitive deficits, e.g., it is believed that generalized shear forces to axial subcortical and cortical structures contribute to problems in memory, attention, emotional regulation, and arousal.[100] Minor head injury, for example, consists primarily of shearing lesions of long axonal tracts.[144,256] It is also important to appreciate that focal injuries themselves have generalized effects. Focal injuries of TBI thus result not only in expected local deficits in neurotransmitter function but also have neurotransmitter effects far beyond the site of injury. Experimental focal brain injury has been shown to produce suppression of activity throughout the entire catecholaminergic system in all its branches, not just in the damaged portions. As Robinson and Bloom stated, "the concept of [focal brain injury] as a local process only . . . is conceptually inadequate."[215] While there are certain typical changes in TBI, in the individual case the pathophysiology of TBI is variable and complex. Pathology is dissimilar in degree of severity as well as topographic distribution from patient to patient. There has been a notable lack of study of the basic neurotransmitter consequences of these various pathologic processes of TBI, particularly in the chronic phase after injury. These neurotransmitter disturbances following traumatic brain injury are intrinsically difficult to characterize since, as noted, TBI is not a single entity and each patient will have his or her own distinct pattern of neurotransmitter function disturbance. Due to the high level of structural organization and complexity of the CNS, measurement of alteration of general levels of neurotransmitter after brain injury (which is essentially what has been technically assayable, via CSF metabolite determination, etc.) may not be as significant in relating to clinical symptomatology as the individual, specific local sites of injury and transmitter disruptions. Psychopharmacologic agents, however, to a great extent affect classes of transmitters or receptors relatively nonselectively throughout the entire CNS and will have, therefore, typically generalized and crude nonspecific effects.

A few general characterizations of pathophysiology may be made with some confidence, however. The shearing axonal injuries characteristic of acceleration/deceleration trauma inevitably include multiple ascending projection systems from lower brainstem areas, e.g., locus coeruleus (noradrenergic), dorsal raphe nucleus (serotonergic), and nucleus basalis of Meynert (cholinergic), etc. These cholinergic, sertonergic, and catecholeminergic projections from brainstem nuclei are probably damaged in many, if not most cases of TBI.[177] It has been reported that there are routine deficiencies of catecholamine and serotonergic metabolites in cerebrospinal fluid of TBI patients which vary depending on the anatomic characteristics of the original brain injury. Studies suggest, for example, "that in the first period of head injury, patients with a frontotemporal-lobe contusion showed a decreased cerebral dopaminergic activity as well as a decreased serotonergic activity. In contrast, patients with a diffuse cerebral contusion, especially in the comatose state, . . . had an increased serotonergic activity only."[274] These data are regrettably few and inadequate, and even a basic understanding of this area awaits further study.

Multiple cognitive, affectual, and behavioral disturbances are found following TBI. These include various deficits in memory, attention, emotional regulation, arousal and mood disorders, etc. A listing of major general syndromes following TBI would include: frontal syndrome (or syndromes), temporohippocampal amnestic and affective syndromes, and general impairment of intellectual-cognitive function.[257,286] (For further discussion see elsewhere in this volume.) Pure forms of these syndromes rarely present in TBI, however. Patients usually demonstrate varying components of each type as well as varying degrees of severity. Each patient has a unique profile of underlying neurophysiologic deficits and clinical symptoms. These deficits, although often improving over time after injury, are usually persistent in nature. Thomsen's long-term follow-up of 40 severely injured TBI patients found personality changes that included childishness, lability, restlessness, loss of spontaneity, and poverty of interests, which persisted 4–5 years in 80% and 10–15 years after injury in 65%.[264]

With any individual TBI patient presenting to some extent a complex and variable mixture of neurophysiologic alterations and a consequently unique behavioral or psychological syndrome, it is very difficult to predict with confidence the effect of any specific drug intervention. Therefore, any general drug indication must be understood to apply only to a certain subpopulation of TBI patients (even if presenting with a similar epiphenomenology of syndromes). The final clinical effect of any neuroactive drug in a specific TBI patient will depend on the complex variable mixture of differing pathology and primary and secondary drug actions in that case. Each TBI patient presents a specific set of physiologic deficits requiring to some greater or lesser degree a unique psychopharmacologic solution. Prescriptive dictums regarding specific TBI syndromes and indicated drugs of first choice are rarely possible, and in any event are absolutely contingent upon empirical confirmation in the individual case.

Notwithstanding these problems, there are clinically identifiable syndromes after head injury[10] and preliminary taxonomies of TBI behavioral and cognitive syndromes have been given.[11,145,154,207,258] Such considerations can provide an empirical and theoretical basis to guide psychopharmacologic interventions in TBI. For example, Gualtieri has remarked:

> Profound deficits in monoaminergic neurotransmission are seen in TBI patients ... presumably as a consequence of shear damage to axial brain structures, where the monoamines are concentrated. The administration of monoaminergic drugs such as stimulants is, in this context, rational pharmacotherapy, that is, drug therapy intended to correct an underlying neurochemical deficit.[100]

PSYCHOPHARMACOLOGIC MANAGEMENT OF TBI

The discovery and development of the various classes of drugs with potent psychoactive properties has been one of the major triumphs of medical science over the past generation. The development of psychopharmacologic treatments has produced a revolution in the conceptualization, management, and prognosis of many of the most severe psychiatric conditions such as schizophrenia, depression, mania, phobias, and obsessive-compulsive disorders. As noted, an adequate taxonomy of cognitive and neurobehavioral TBI syndromes has not yet been developed or verified, contributing to the lack of specificity and sensitivity in current studies of drug effect in TBI. Additionally, even for more generalized signs and symptoms such as irritability or aggression, neuropsychiatry lacks adequate nosologic and conceptual structures.[60] For TBI populations, there has, to date, been very little systematic investigation, and certainly few prospective double-blind and controlled studies done regarding the use (or misuse) of psychoactive drugs. This is not to say, however, there is no scientifically valid information available regarding their use in TBI. The deficiencies of relying solely on controlled clinical trials to identify or establish psychopharmacologic efficacy have been cogently discussed.[45] Astute clinical observation and case study historically have had, and continue to keep, a valuable place in developing valid new indications for psychiatric drug treatment. It is instructive to keep in mind the manner in which clinical advances have principally been achieved in psychopharmacology. The preponderance of such achievements has been based on small clinical trials (really case studies) of drugs in conditions and syndromes for which there was, and is, no basic pathophysiologic understanding. In this sense many of the advances in indications for particular drug usage have been more the result of heuristic intuition (based in most part on surface phenomenologic symptoms or syndrome similarities) rather than on basic understanding of underlying relevant pathophysiology. This, what might appear to be superficial, approach has been both typical and productive throughout the record of psychopharmacologic advance. As we, to date, have little fundamental understanding of the relationship of any particular damaged neurotransmission system and any distinct behavior following TBI, it is more than appropriate to approach the neuropharmacologic treatment of brain injury in a similarly heuristic manner. Specific symptoms may frequently represent a final common pathway event. For example, in a review of the concept of apathy Marin stated:

> Neurobehavioral and neuropsychological analyses of frontal lobe function provide a fertile source of reinterpreting apathy, based on the frontal lobe effect on drive, sequencing, and the so-called executive functions, such as anticipation, goal-setting, planning and monitoring. From a neurochemical standpoint, it may be noteworthy that functional deficiency of dopaminergic systems has been postulated to underlie a number of disorders causing apathy, including neuroleptic-induced akinesia, negative symptoms in schizophrenia, post-psychotic depression, subcortical dementing diseases such as Parkinson's disease, and frontal lobe syndromes. Flat affect, lack of initiative, psychomotor slowing, and other features associated with apathy have been noted in these disorders as well as in depression.[156]

In other words, we should consider that syndromes with similar behavioral characteristics, whether or not arising from varying etiologies (e.g., stroke, TBI, infection, attention deficit disorder, etc.), may, in fact, reflect final common pathway neurophysiologic events—and thus may be responsive to similar neuropharmacologic treatment. Much clinical evidence supports this position. Thus, psychopharmacologic treatment of TBI is guided, principally, not by underlying diagnosis but by manifest "target" symptoms.

Despite our vast ignorance and uncertainty in TBI, the sometimes encountered nihilistic attitude apparent in clinicians to psychopharmacologic treatment seems unwarranted. It should be recalled that these very same methodologic problems and uncertainties attend the drug treatment of virtually all psychiatric syndromes or diagnoses and yet have not prevented major clinical advances in their drug treatment. Certainly, although the empirical base in TBI is small, it is rapidly growing. The theoretical basis for psychopharmacologic intervention in TBI is as good as in any other major psychiatric disorder, and better than in many.

For purposes of exposition, the psychopharmacologic management of TBI will be considered in four general clinical areas: the underaroused or attentionally impaired patient, the agitated or aggressive patient, the affectively disordered patient, and the cognitively impaired patient. It must be understood that in clinical practice there is much overlap among these syndromes, and one should not attempt too rigidly to segregate pharmacologic indications by these pedagogic divisions.

Disorders of Arousal and Attention

The most fundamental disorder following TBI is impairment of arousal. Adequate CNS activation is a prerequisite to all other cognitive and behavioral functions. In regard to arousal disorders, mention must first be made of the high frequency with which patients' arousal levels are inadvertently depressed by prescribed medications. Before venturing to improve arousal with psychopharmacologic agents, all potentially offending medications already being used must be identified, considered, and eliminated if possible.

Many psychotropics, including neuroleptics, antidepressants (particularly the agents with nonactivating profiles such as amitriptyline or doxepin), anticonvulsants (particularly phenytoin and phenobarbital), antianxiety agents (benzodiazepines), and beta blockers, are directly, or through secondary effects, CNS depressants. The neuroleptics are particularly significant offenders in clinical settings because of the common blurring of their beneficial antipsychotic and their generally nontherapeutic sedating effects. The antidepressants also may produce, to varying degrees, sedation and decreased cognition due to both cholinergic and alpha-adrenergic blockade. The anticonvulsants, particularly phenytoin and phenobarbital, are now known to have appreciable negative cognitive (and affective) influence apart from their anticonvulsant action.[249] There is an evident toxic encephalopathy associated with elevated serum levels of these drugs. Reynolds, in a review of this effect, reported that "phenytoin . . . produce[d] a syndrome of . . . encephalopathy, resulting in impairment of intellectual function and/or memory" and that "this syndrome was especially likely to be overlooked in brain-damaged or mentally retarded children."[210] These effects occur with normals and in general populations of patients receiving anticonvulsants. Reduction or removal of the drug has been reported to produce improved mood and cognition.[73] Carbamazepine, in contrast to phenytoin and phenobarbital, alternatively has been shown in some studies to have a minimal or even beneficial effect on cognition. Trimble has reported that many anticonvulsants produce deficits in memory, attention, and concentration and that carbamazepine has less of these effects than other common anticonvulsant drugs.[266] It has been suggested that, due to these beneficial cognitive considerations, carbamazepine may be the anticonvulsant of choice for TBI, although other studies have failed to demonstrate such differential benefit. Comprehensive reviews of these and other psychiatric effects of anticonvulsants have been done by Rivinus[213] and Massagli.[160]

Many other drugs produce deficits in general cognitive function, in addition to their intended primary effect. A recent comprehensive listing of the many prescribed agents (not just psychoactive) that have been associated with psychiatric side effects, including hallucinations, delirium, and mania, is available.[55]

Additionally, a wide variety of clinical conditions, such as metabolic disturbance (including inadequate nutrition), infection, endocrine problems, late cerebral pathology (subdural hematomas, hydrocephalus), etc., also may lead to depressed arousal or prolonged coma. Such medical conditions are frequently not immediately obvious and should be considered, searched for diligently, and ruled out or treated before venturing to pharmacologic attempts at increasing arousal. Once such potentially correctable causes of depresssed alertness are accounted for, one may consider pharmacologic assays at promoting arousal.

Stimulants, Dopaminergics, and Antidepressants

The stimulants, presumably by increasing generalized deficiencies in catecholamine function, are most promising as agents to promote arousal, and are clinically the most utilized. A number of uncontrolled studies suggest such agents as amphetamines, methylphenidate, and L-dopa are able to improve the arousal level of patients in either a low arousal or stuporous state. Experienced TBI clinicians appear to be routinely using these drugs in the rehabilitation setting to promote increased arousal. The somewhat common concern that stimulants may predispose TBI patients to convulsions is probably misfounded, at least for therapeutic dose ranges; these drugs have been reported to be even somewhat protective against seizures in brain-injured patients.[290]

Antidepressants also may have a direct stimulantlike effect. Protriptyline has been reported particularly effective in improving these attentional symptoms in TBI patients via its strongly noradrenergic profile.[288] Also, decreased arousal may be seen as a secondary reflection of depression, when symptoms of apathy and inertia are prominent and thus indirectly benefited by antidepressant treatment.

Levodopamine is a catecholamine precursor and agonist. Clinical reports of the effectiveness of levodopa in elevating consciousness in comatose patients first appeared in 1978. In large series of organic brain impaired patients (encephalitics) with persistent coma or extreme underarousal, L-dopa was associated with improvements in arousal, electroencephalographic (EEG) patterns, and outcome, in a double-blind study.[28] Higashi reported its effect on improving

consciousness in the comatose state after traumatic brain injury[113] and has reported resolution of chronic vegetative state by use of L-dopa.[114] In the U.S. Lal has similarly reported on the successful use of L-dopa/carbidopa (Sinemet) to arouse and increase function in 12 chronic low-level brain-injured patients.[141] In some of these very chronic cases, the return of arousal and function appears truly extraordinary. Similarly Crismon has reported on a series of patients with akinetic mutism due to diffuse brain injury who had similar responses to the dopaminergic agent bromocriptine.[44]

Cholinergic Agents

Cholinergic agents historically had been proposed to promote cognitive recovery of brain-injured patients.[155] Currently, it appears that in the acute injury phase, excessive intrinsic cholinergic activity may lead to further neuronal injury and death.[109] In the chronic phase after injury, however, cholinergic agonists may have a therapeutic effect.[110] Increased alertness and cognition have been demonstrated to occur in a single-case methodology in a stuporous TBI patient after administration of methylphenidate and the anticholinesterase physostigmine.[279]

Before venturing with such pharmacologic trials in the chronically vegetative patient, however, it should be appreciated that serious concerns can exist regarding the clinical appropriateness and ethicality of intervening pharmacologically in these cases. In almost all cases of persistent vegetative state, the result of treatment will be to raise the patient from an unresponsive state, not to a return to normalcy but rather into a highly likely condition of partial or incomplete awareness and severe dependency. An objective view might suggest this result is not in the patient's or in the patient's family's best interests. For example, with such arousal the patient could be felt to experience a heightened sense of discomfort, frustration, and suffering. The grieving process of the family could easily be seriously impeded by such a clinical result. The family might feel increased pressure to bring such a newly "aware" member back into the home setting (with associated increased demands and costs for the family) rather than allowing or continuing placement in a long-term care facility. Therefore, a trial of pharmacologic treatment in the chronically vegetative patient should be made only after a complete review and integration of all such psychological, social, and ethical issues. Conversely, in the acute rehabilitation process or phase, particularly for patients already aware but underaroused, such treatment may very well be indicated. Neglect or hemiinattention is a particular syndrome within general attentional impairment. Of interest, it is appearing that this condition may yield in some cases to pharmacologic treatment. Bromocriptine has been reported successful in single-case trials in significantly reducing clinical neglect.[74,169]

Disorders of Behavior (Aggression/Agitation)

The second and probably the most common problem that elicits psychopharmacologic intervention is the agitated, aggressive, or assaultive patient.

Agitation and aggression cover a wide range of behaviors and are summary terms for a complex construct. The taxonomy of aggressive behaviors has been difficult for researchers; general categorization into basic types such as predatory, autonomic, and nondirected has been based on animal models and seem to have only a modest relationship to human aggression. Cassidy has briefly reviewed these concepts.[27] He proposes that the neuroexcitatory transmitters such as ACh, NE, and DA may be expected to increase aggression, whereas inhibitory transmitters such as GABA should decrease such behaviors. A wide variety of classes of agents have been suggested as having efficacy in reducing aggression, including anticholinergics, beta blockers, alpha$_2$ agonists, and possibly tricyclic antidepressants (via downregulation of NE activity). Others (trazodone, fluoxetine) may act as 5-HT enhancers, whereas lithium, benzodiazepines, and valproic acid may be GABA antagonists.[27] In their milder form the processes that lead to agitation probably underlie initiation and activation and are associated with desirable functional characteristics such as motivation and drive. An appreciation and evaluation of these latter positive contributions to overall behavior need to be considered before a decision to treat agitation pharmacologically is made. In practical terms, agitation and aggression are commonly seen as problematic and attended to when they become disruptive or destructive to clinical or social routines. The hypervigilant, distractible, volatile patient, who erupts into frank violence at little or no provocation, is familiar to all who work with the brain-injured patient. General surveys have revealed that most assaults on hospital staff are by patients who have organic brain impairment, rather than schizophrenia and manic-depressive illness, as might be expected. Some aggressive or violent behavioral syndromes described in psychiatric literature have been suggested as being the result of unappreciated earlier brain trauma. Bach-y-Rita and Lion, for example, reported results of a 2-year study of 130 psychiatric patients with chief complaint of explosive violent behavior. Although not the major focus of the study, they noted that "our patients often described past histories of birth-injury, mental retardation, coma-producing illness such as meningitis, febrile convulsions in infancy, or head injury with prolonged unconsciousness."[14] This problem tends to be not only a very difficult, but a very common one at early stages of recovery from TBI, and while it is difficult to obtain accurate incidence figures, it appears to be very prevalent and is probably by far the most frequent clinical situation that currently elicits psychopharmacologic intervention in clinical practice.

Early after injury, the comatose patient does not present a management problem in terms of behavior; however, with ongoing recovery as the patient regains arousal, behavioral problems emerge. Cognition and judgment characteristically lag behind motor recovery; the patient can be agitated, confused, irritable, frightened, emotionally labile, and impervious to normal explanation, reassurance, or counseling. These patients may manifest such agitation in the acute medical or surgical floor or later in the rehabilitation unit. There certainly is a need to protect the patient him/herself, other patients, and staff from the extremes of behavior that these patients occasionally display. Before pharmacologic approaches are routinely chosen, however, it should be recalled that much agitation in the head-injured is reactive in nature, and occurs in response to overly stimulating or frustrating environments, or in response to painful or frustrating stimuli such as a too vigorous exercise/ joint ranging program or cognitive challenge. It also must be kept in mind that the large majority of such TBI patients exhibit this agitation only transiently. As further recovery proceeds with return of cognitive functions, the behavioral problems tend to recede spontaneously. Thus, a generally accepted principle to follow in the acutely recovering TBI patient is a conservative approach to medication intervention.

Nonpharmacologic behavioral and environmental interventions for agitation are possible (e.g., isolation rooms, soft restraints, etc.) and in most nonemergency situations preferable to immediate reliance on medications. Decreasing performance demands during therapy sessions or providing appropriate analgesia, for example, may be more effective in reducing unwanted agitation or aggression than a tranquilizing drug. Even the most refractory or severe types of aggression have been demonstrated to be frequently responsive to an appropriately structured environment and contingency management.[59] A well-trained and responsive team able to utilize these behavioral and environmental interventions is more appropriate in many situations than immediate reliance on psychoactive drugs. Patients alternatively may find their way to psychiatric facilities for such problems. However, psychiatric units' psychodynamically based "therapeutic milieu" and other traditional psychiatric approaches are routinely ineffective for these "demented" patients. Despite these possibilities for behavioral interventions on the medical/ surgical, rehabilitation, and psychiatric unit, however, if the problems are at all persistent, behaviorally disruptive patients are ultimately almost always managed by psychopharmacologic intervention. Unless a true behavioral emergency exists, the primary approach to disordered activity in most cases should initially be environmental or behavioral in nature. This is true not only because the potential side effects of a behavioral program are less severe than the side effects of drug intervention, but also because this allows the documentation of clear and stable baselines of the behaviors in question.

Agitation and aggressive behavior patterns may, in a relatively small number of cases, not be transient but rather become chronic, longstanding characteristics that may, in fact, persist for years and be severely disabling. These latter are a very challenging and difficult class of patients. In this group an aggressive pharmacologic approach is nearly always indicated either in conjunction with or following formally structured behavioral programs.

Similar to the previous discussion regarding iatrogenic suppression of arousal, it is certain that many cases of disordered behavior are the result of ill-advised medication use. This may be the inadvertent result of medications prescribed for other conditions, but is often the result of ineffectual medications prescribed for the control of agitation itself. It is always possible to suppress agitated disruptive behaviors in any patient through pharmacologic intervention. However, this is often accomplished in practice by means of general sedation with suppression of all behaviors, adaptive as well as agitated. For the acutely recovering TBI patient in delirium, there commonly is no specific agent to reduce agitation; rather, patients must be managed essentially by being reduced to the point of stupor with obvious detrimental effects on their rehabilitation program. Trials of removal of potentially offending drugs should be a first step in these cases. An illustrative report demonstrating resolution of long-standing severe agitation in a brain-injured patient by the expedient appropriate behavioral intervention along with sequential psychotrope withdrawal has been provided by Cantini et al.[26] Not infrequently, however, behavioral management is impractical or ineffective, and psychopharmacologic treatment of agitation is needed. For certain TBI patients such drug treatment can be quite effective. A variety of different classes of drugs have been reported useful for the agitated patient.

Neuroleptics

In standard medical, psychiatric, and neurologic texts, the most commonly recommended class of drug for the agitation of TBI (i.e., dementia, organic brain syndrome, or delirium by DSM-III–R classification) is the neuroleptic.[107,119,133] Although a time-honored choice, reasons exist to doubt the appropriateness of this drug class as a first-line approach in TBI. Massive numbers of prospective, blind, and controlled investigations of these drugs have been performed on traditional psychiatric diagnoses, such as schizophrenia, mania, and paranoia, which clearly document the efficacy and relative safety of neuroleptics in these conditions. However, startlingly little evidence is available regarding neuroleptics' effectiveness in the organic brain conditions (including TBI). A worrisome amount of evidence exists which suggests only a *limited* efficacy in organic brain conditions in general. In 1985 Helms reviewed the entire literature about neuroleptic use in the dementias and found only 21 adequate studies. Reviewing these, he concluded that "results of the studies appear to justify [only] the judicious use of antipsychotic medication in the management of behavioral complications of dementia." He noted the relative scarcity of adequate studies and called for further research.[111]

Another review of adequately controlled studies has indicated that neuroleptics are only somewhat successful in controlling agitation in dementia.[234] Similar conclusions of only moderate effectiveness of antipsychotics in the mentally retarded were given by Rothman, Chusid, et al.[221] Another review of the many currently accepted indications (including aggressive behavior associated with CNS damage) for the use of haloperidol indicates the relative safety of this drug. However, due to the serious toxic effects of this drug (particularly tardive dyskinesia), general restraint in its use is urged.[68] Similar alternatives to neuroleptics are recommended in a thorough review of the general efficacy of pharmacologic approaches to "aggression."[201] A similar review of studies of neuroleptic usage in behavioral disorders of mental deficiency indicated an equally limited specific efficacy (i.e., neuroleptics effective for stereotypic behaviors but little else), but rather an effect through generalized suppression of all behaviors.[21] In a comprehensive meta-analysis of controlled studies of neuroleptic treatment in dementia, it was estimated that only 18 of each 100 patients derived specific benefit from this class of drug.[234] These reviews also conclude that general restraint is appropriate in the use of neuroleptics for organic CNS diagnoses due to increasingly recognized toxicity associated with their use.

There are essentially no controlled studies of the specific effect of neuroleptics in TBI. The probability exists that while possibly controlling behavior, neuroleptic drugs are also exacerbating a number of the principal disabling deficits of TBI. Finally, although neuroleptics have a general reputation of safety, a generation of experience has demonstrated that these drugs are far from benign. The high frequency of adverse effects associated with the use of antipsychotics underscores the need to consider the risks versus the benefits of these agents and emphasizes the need to explore alternative interventions in this population.[17] A solitary retrospective review of haloperidol used to control behavior in TBI patients is in the literature and concluded that neuroleptic use was not associated with apparent adverse toxicity[198] (however, see below). No conclusions regarding efficacy were drawn. A provocative case study of psychosis precipitated by chlorpromazine in an agitated patient with TBI is a clear cautionary note.[229] A presumption of efficacy and safety should not be made for neuroleptic treatment of TBI. What efficacy neuroleptics do possess in reducing agitation may be due in large part to generalized sedation. Despite this general consensus regarding the relatively low specific efficacy of neuroleptics in treatment of organic agitation, it is of interest that *low-dose* neuroleptic use has been reported effective in organic disturbances when higher doses have been ineffective. This may be due to the fact that low-dose neuroleptic use tends to block preferentially the presynaptic dopaminergic autoreceptors, blocking this negative-feedback loop, thus acting as a dopaminergic agonist rather than antagonist.

There are a few specific situations in which antipsychotics may be primarily indicated for TBI. They appear to be particularly effective if the clinical picture after TBI includes symptomatology similar to classic primary signs of schizophrenia, involving such target symptoms as hallucinations, paranoid ideations, loose associations, bizarre ideation, or ideas of reference. In these situations the antipsychotics may have a uniquely focused effect and be the agent of choice. When neuroleptics are utilized, the choice of a high-potency drug such as haloperidol or trifluperazine minimizes but does not eliminate sedation.

Newer neuroleptics, such as clozapine, may not have some of these general problems of neuroleptics and also may have an antiaggressive activity,[202] but to date no reports of their use in TBI or associated conditions are available.

A commonly associated side effect of the antipsychotics (and other classes of psychoactive medications such as the tricyclics) is anticholinergic activity. As discussed earlier, the integrity of the cholinergic system is essential to the encoding component of memory. Anticholinergic drugs reliably produce an amnesiac syndrome that is neuropsychologically difficult to distinguish from the memory defect commonly seen after TBI—an inability to encode ongoing events into long-term memory. Simple episodic information such as names of attending clinicians or of the treating facility cannot be encoded for recall. This blockade of the cholinergic system, among other effects, and even before the predictable toxic psychosis of anticholinergic overdose, reliably prevents the transition of immediate into long-term memory.[225,267] It is of interest that TBI patients treated with haloperidol during their rehabilitation, compared with matched patients who did not receive such medication, were reported to have significantly increased duration of posttraumatic amnesia.[198]

In addition to sedative and anticholinergic side effects, the neuroleptics are epileptogenic. It is fairly well appreciated that the neuroleptics have a high association (0.5–10%) with onset of seizures[151] and for this reason would also be relatively contraindicated in TBI.

Perhaps a more serious concern with neuroleptic use is the real probability that extended use of these agents may lead to development of tardive dyskinesia and associated conditions, such as tardive dystonia and supersensitivity psychosis (a reputed worsening of a patient's underlying psychotic condition upon withdrawal of the neuroleptic due to induced dependency on D_2 blockade). The neuroleptic malignant syndrome, a serious, frequently fatal complication of neuroleptic use, characterized by hyperthermia, muscular rigidity, and changes in mental status and autonomic system function, is also believed to be a substantially higher risk in brain-injured patients. It is of unknown etiology, but probably related to deficient hypothalamic or basal ganglial dopaminergic functioning. It has been suggested that preexisting brain damage significantly increases the risk of developing this syndrome, and that although the basal fatality rate is approximately 10%, it may be up to three times higher in patients with brain damage.[142,237] Parenthetically, nonneuroleptic, antidopaminergic medications commonly used in TBI also may produce neurologic and behavioral deficits. Metoclopramide (Reglan), frequently used to stimulate gastric motility in the acute period, is antidopaminergic, and some clinical suggestions of its negative impact on recovery from TBI have been made.[58] An alternative choice to treat the gastric problems of the acute phase may be cisapride, which acts via serotonergic receptors, causing release of acetylcholine and thus stimulating gastric motility.[32]

Neuroleptics are also less desirable on theoretical grounds in that their clinical efficacy is presumably based on blockade of dopamine receptors, whereas insufficiency of dopamine activity is likely a component of many of the deficits of TBI, as discussed elsewhere in this chapter. In addition, there are animal work and limited human data which suggest that neuroleptics may impair the neurologic recovery of the brain-injured through their anti–alpha-adrenergic effect (see the discussion of plasticity).

In conclusion, it is evident that the widespread belief in the efficacy and safety of neuroleptics in the management of agitation and aggression in the TBI population is not strongly warranted, and while they may be effective in some patients, particularly in low doses, there are substantial demonstrated and theoretical reasons to consider other pharmacologic approaches as alternatives.

Antidepressants

The antidepressants are a heterogeneous group of drugs that includes the tricyclics, heterocyclics, and monamine oxidase inhibitors, among others. A major pharmacologic property of most (but not all) of these drugs is an agonist effect on catecholaminergic transmission systems. The typical primary classification of these heterogeneous agents as antidepressants is heuristically useful in indicating their most common clinical utility; however, many other uses are demonstrated for these drugs, including use in phobia, incontinence, pain syndromes, etc.

A rationale exists, as well as limited clinical studies, suggesting the efficacy of tricyclic antidepressants for agitation in TBI. The rationale is based in part on their demonstrated efficacy as an alternative to CNS stimulants with the attention deficit hyperactivity disorders (ADHD) and associated conditions.[41,283] ADHD conceptually is related to TBI first in that many series of ADHD patients report a subset of patients who have a history of significant brain trauma. Further, the symptomatology onset occasionally dates precisely from the time of a known brain injury. Also, many of the psychological and behavioral symptoms of ADHD appear similar to those of TBI (particularly the milder cases of TBI). Both populations have routinely impaired attention and concentration capabilities and subtle psychomotor impairments. With mild or moderate brain-injured patients, the similarity of the distractibility, impulsivity, and irritability to patients diagnosed with ADHD can be striking. Both have deficits in impulse control. Both have well-known increases in dyssocial and aggressive behaviors. Brain injury, therefore, is likely to be one etiology in the development of an ADHD syndrome. The clinical symptoms of ADHD are variably but clearly ameliorated by antidepressants, which are usually seen as second-tier drugs after stimulants, methylphenidate, and amphetamines. The hypothesis is that both antidepressants and stimulants (see below) may be similarly useful for these ADHD-like symptoms in patients with TBI, as they are for ADHD itself

Several recent studies in TBI lend support to this concept. Effective tricyclic management (with amitriptyline and imipramine) of impulsive, agitated acutely recovering TBI patients has been reported by Mysiw and Jackson. Improvement was also documented for certain formal cognitive measures.[123,180] It was postulated that the catecholaminergic properties of the tricyclic led to increased cortical arousal, thereby decreasing confusion and agitation. Similar efficacy of amitriptyline in the agitation resulting from anoxic encephalopathy has been reported.[260] These are clearly preliminary reports, and it is unclear how frequently the agitation of such patients will respond to this treatment. It also must be kept in mind that antidepressants are conversely reported on occasion to elicit paradoxical rage.[196] Similar to neuroleptics, many tricyclic antidepressants have strong anticholinergic effects, which may interfere with memory, as well as strongly sedating properties. The newer nontricyclic antidepressants may be less problematic in this regard[216] and have antiaggressive activity as well. Fluoxetine in particular has recently been reported to have general antiagitation, mood-lability, and aggression effects[158,212] as well as specific efficacy in this area for brain-injured patients.[236,246]

Tricyclic antidepressants are epileptogenic. Tricyclics also have been shown to induce seizures in approximately 0.5–1.0% of treated patients.[153] The tetracyclic antidepressants may involve an even higher risk (up to 15.6%).[122] A significant incidence of seizures has been reported with use of tricyclics (amitriptyline, desipramine, and protriptyline) in severe TBI patients.[291] Nevertheless, the difficulties in ascertaining the actual incremental risk for epilepsy from available studies are significant, and little can be said with confidence on this matter other than some increased risk is present.[219] However, some of this concern may be spurious and simply the result of a more stringent drug development review process in place at present. Bupropion, although seemingly a very promising antidepressant for TBI based on its benign side-effect profile (i.e., minimal sedation or psychomotor impairment), is believed to be medicolegally risky to use in TBI patients due to its reputed high epileptogenic properties. Extensive recent formal trials, however, have indicated that the actual risk of seizures with bupropion is 0.4%[127]—well within the generally accepted range for the more usual and acceptable tricyclic antidepressants.

Anticonvulsants

The common relevance of anticonvulsants in clinical care of TBI is, of course, their use for seizure management. A great number of traumatic brain injury patients are treated with anticonvulsants, usually with phenytoin, phenobarbital, or carbamazepine. Valproate is being added to this group of preferentially used anticonvulsants. There is probably a cognitive price or deficit associated with the use of this class of medication, certainly with phenobarbital and phenytoin. Phenytoin and phenobarbital have been reported to significantly impair cognition and behavior independent of any influence on seizure frequency,[209] although a recent review of this issue has concluded that only phenobarbital has a significantly increased cognitive impairing profile.[182] Intellectual measures such as Wechsler IQ scores among epileptics are known to be impaired with these drugs, and reliable and reproducible increase in cognitive function results from their decrease or discontinuation. This cognitive impairment is dose-related and occurs even at therapeutic blood levels. Carbamazepine and valproate are believed by some researchers and many clinicians to have substantially different effect on cognition or behavior than phenytoin or phenobarbital, i.e., they produce no substantial impairment. There is evidence that for some patients the use of carbamazepine may improve mood, attention, information processing, and general functioning.[63] After the acute trauma phase of care (where the parenteral route available for phenytoin and phenobarbital gives them significant advantages) when anticonvulsants are indicated for chronic control of established epilepsy, carbamazepine (and probably valproate) may be the anticonvulsant(s) of choice for chronic control of established epilepsy in brain injury.

In contrast with this indication for treatment of established epilepsy, there appears to be no generally accepted approach to the pharmacologic *prophylaxis* of posttraumatic epilepsy. Some reports indicate that prophylactic anticonvulsants decrease the long-term incidence of posttraumatic epilepsy, reducing the incidence in matched patients from 50% to 10%.[284] More recent studies appear to indicate that anticonvulsants are not effective for the prophylaxis of epilepsy.[261,393] Glenn and Yablon have discussed the perplexing issues still current regarding anticonvulsants and

concluded that there is likely to be a benefit to avoidance of phenobarbital, and possibly to avoidance of phenytoin, and that prophylactic anticonvulsant usage is not indicated in TBI and as at this time evidence does not support a prophylactic effect, efforts should be made, when clinically feasible, to carefully remove anticonvulsants used for this purpose in TBI patients.[85,292]

Aside from the antiepileptic treatment and prophylactic usage of these drugs, other indications for anticonvulsants exist. The concept of disordered behavior, particularly aggressive behavior, as a manifestation of or as related to complex-partial (psychomotor) seizure activity in the brain-injured patient is long-standing and complex.[190] It is most so in cases where the presumed epileptic process is less than evident, e.g., when consciousness is not obviously altered, or when integrated and seemingly goal-directed behaviors occur as opposed to purposeless, stereotyped behaviors (albeit of a violent or aggressive nature). In this situation, the diagnosis of complex partial seizures[134,194] is considered but often is difficult to establish. In tightly controlled studies, the actual incidence of paroxysmal aggression due to complex partial seizures appears quite low.[262] Beyond the difficulties concerning diagnosis of complex-partial seizure activity, it also has been proposed that there is an *interictal* syndrome of hyperirritability and aggressiveness associated with, but not representing, seizure activity per se. This concept has been termed temporal or limbic lobe instability or irritability. Although no demonstrable overt seizure disorder is evident, localized dysfunction is postulated in limbic circuits which produces labile mood, irritability, aggression, and rage attacks. Over time, as well, it is believed that a postulated interictal personality may develop. Patients with prolonged seizure disorders thus have been noted to progressively develop distinctive personality disturbances characterized by truculence, irritability, and tendency toward assaultiveness. Anticonvulsants will produce clinical improvement in these symptoms independent of any overt seizure disorder per se. Carbamazepine has been suggested as particularly effective in reducing the symptomatology of this interictal personality process and has been postulated for the analogous behavior following TBI. Carbamazepine has been reported helpful in these behavioral symptoms of psychiatric patients with temporal lobe abnormalities but without evident seizure disorder[181] and has been reported useful in paroxysmal behavior disorders of other organic etiologies.[80] A prospective, blind study reported carbamazepine roughly as effective as propranolol in patients with uncontrolled rage outbursts; diagnoses included attention deficit disorder (residual), intermittent explosive disorder, and organic disorders.[161] This increased aggressiveness has been reported specifically as a consequence of head trauma,[157] and anticonvulsants have been proposed as effective for this condition. Further, many anticonvulsants, particularly carbamazepine, are believed to have a generalized therapeutic effect on aggression and violence.[18] Valproate has been reported successful in the agitation of head injury as well.[191] Anticonvulsants have been reported helpful in treating paroxysmal behavior disorders which may be a residual of childhood ADHD or brain damage[59] and which may or may not be equivalent to complex-partial seizures (limbic or temporal lobe epilepsy).[162] Without definitively resolving the debate in this difficult area, it is clear that the anticonvulsants, particularly carbamazepine, have been frequently found to have beneficial effects on aggression and irritability in populations with brain injury who do not necessarily have seizures, and that they are of potential use in general TBI aggressivity.

Lithium

Lithium is commonly thought of as primarily an antimanic agent, useful principally in the bipolar disorders, but it has been reported effective in a wide variety of clinical conditions. Reviews have listed multiple atypical indications for the use of lithium, including schizophrenia, pathologic impulsive aggressiveness and hypersexuality, affective disorders in organic brain syndromes, pathologic emotional instability in children and adolescents, and various movement disorders. Pharmacologically, lithium's effective action is unknown, and it is hypothesized to affect a number of transmitter systems as well as membrane ionic interactions; among these presumed effects it may act in part by affecting the storage capabilities of central noradrenergic neurons, leading ultimately to a reduction in norepinephrine content.

Lithium is now seen to probably have a basic effect on mood itself, acting to stabilize lability. Lithium-treated manic-depressive patients show less mood variation than other psychiatric patients or control subjects while they are on lithium.[49]

Lithium is a useful but probably rarely considered option for management of agitated or chronically aggressive/irritable TBI patients. It is known that with certain CNS lesions, including neoplasms, cerebrovascular accidents, trauma, etc.,[124] a secondary manic psychosis can occur. This secondary mania is clearly responsive to lithium.[46] Many of these reported studies of secondary mania include patients whose specific diagnosis is TBI.[86,241] Compared with primary mania, in clinical presentation, these organic manias tend to display more irritability than grandiosity and to have a higher likelihood for aggressivity.

Further, lithium appears to have a general mood-stabilizing or antiaggressive effect even in the absence of a specific manic syndrome (primary or secondary). Prospective blind studies in various diagnostic groups, including mental deficients and aggressive or violent prisoners, have demonstrated lithium's ability to reduce the frequency and degree of aggressive and assaultive episodes.[239] Lithium's effectiveness for agitated disturbance in organic brain syndromes of various etiologies has been reported.[25,105,232,282] This has also been demonstrated on incarcerated delinquents,[240] adults,[268] and hyperactive, aggressive mentally retarded.[89] Many individuals within these populations also appear to have suffered TBI. It is reasonable, therefore, to consider lithium as a general mood stabilizer, similar to carbamazepine, and generally indicated for TBI patients who have chronic problems with irritability, aggressivity, etc.

Lithium also has been used with success in a number of patients whose aggression and violence derive specifically from traumatic brain injury.[34,105,187,232] Glenn in particular has published a persuasive series of case analyses describing the use of lithium in TBI.[87] Conversely, lithium is known, in rare cases, to exacerbate intractable aggression.

Lithium has a narrow therapeutic index and is associated with significant neurologic side effects, including tremor, neuroleptic malignant-type syndrome, and a toxic encephalopathy, which have occurred even at therapeutic levels.[147] There is some feeling among clinicians that the brain-injured patient is more susceptible to these toxic effects of lithium. Close monitoring for these effects is essential. However, very rarely do these neurologic sequelae appear to be permanent,[53] and they may be reliably expected to resolve with reduction in dosage or withdrawal of drug.

Stimulants

Many reports document the ability of stimulants (amphetamines and methylphenidate) to decrease the aggression of psychiatric syndromes such as ADHD and aggressive antisocial personality.[211] The rationale for the use of stimulants (amphetamines and methylphenidate) for the irritable, agitated, or aggressive TBI patient is essentially similar to that discussed for the antidepressants in ADHD (see above). Similar to antidepressant effects in ADHD, stimulants may ameliorate such behaviors as irritability, impulsivity, and distractibility. Evans and Gualtieri have recently reviewed the cognitive and behavioral effects of psychostimulants on normal and ADHD patients. They further proposed that ADHD has a basic neural substrate frontal lobe dysfunction and point out the many clinical similarities between ADHD and TBI patients, namely, attention difficulties (both distractibility and perseverance), minor motor abnormalities (clumsiness), and hyperactivity.[65] The use of amphetamines to successfully control agitation in posttraumatic brain syndrome was first reported by Hill in 1944[115] and more recently by Lipper and Tuchman in 1976.[149] A large (n=38) placebo-controlled, blind study of methylphenidate to control TBI-related anger showed statistically significant benefit on formal measures of anger and memory, but not attention. The side-effect profile was also reported as very benign in this study.[176] There is increasing literature about the efficacy of this class of drugs on these disturbances following brain injury.[64,66,76] Clearly, stimulants should have a high priority as a drug class for management of aggression and agitation, particularly when they present as a low-level underlying irritability contrasted to paroxysmal releases of rage.

Antianxiety Agents

Benzodiazepines are the major class of antianxiety drugs, although newer unrelated agents (e.g., buspirone) have recently appeared. The benzodiazepines are well recognized for their safety and efficacy in reducing anxiety and producing calming, sedative, or hypnotic effects. In an acute behavioral emergency (agitation) in which the underlying diagnosis is in doubt, these drugs are usually relied upon to establish quick, reliable sedation. In addition to their straightforward sedative action, benzodiazepines have been reported to have specific beneficial effects on dyssocial and aggressive behaviors. Based on studies, including psychotics, juvenile delinquents, neurotics, and children with attention deficit disorder, they have been reported to have a "taming" effect. It is not clear to all investigators, however, that benzodiazepines are effective in such circumstances by a mechanism other than depression of arousal. Control of agitation may have been achieved at the expense of adaptive as well as dysfunctional behaviors. Thus, while the benzodiazepines have enjoyed a certain reputation as effective "antiaggressive" agents, this is probably not highly deserved, and to the extent such an effect exists it has been shown to be species- and situation-specific. In a comprehensive review of this issue recently, Rodgers and Water conclude that the benzodiazepines have a variety of differing effects on aggression, depending on dosage, setting and species, and type of aggression.[217] Similarly, a comprehensive review of all published information regarding the efficacy of benzodiazepines for the treatment of psychoses concluded that these drugs are not as effective as either the neuroleptics or lithium.[95] Interestingly, animal studies have shown that one major psychological effect of benzodiazepines is to decrease tolerance of reward delay,[263] an intolerance which will be familiar to clinicians who treat TBI patients. They have substantial advantage over other possible choices of drugs in the rarity of serious side effects produced. They have a well-deserved reputation for cardiovascular and respiratory safety (although respiratory depression and arrest is an increased risk in patients with organic brain impairment), even in the large doses required to control the most severely agitated patients. They do not have the anticholinergic potential of the antipsychotics and antidepressants. They are in general antiepileptogenic and will be appropriate in managing withdrawal syndromes from occult alcohol-sedative-hypnotic addiction as well, should this be a consideration. In particular, because of its relative short half-life, absence of active metabolites, and capacity for both oral and parenteral administration, lorazepam is an attractive choice among the benzodiazepines.

Benzodiazepines, however, are GABA agonists and cortical suppressants and therefore impair arousal and cognitive processes in an often unacceptable manner for chronic use. In addition, it should be realized that disordered behavior may result from the use of these or other sedating agents through the process of disinhibition.[81] Benzodiazepines have been reported to exacerbate agitation idiosyncratically.[255] This effect has been reported in up to 10% of the patients treated.[218,228] The benzodiazepines may not all be equivalent in their tendency to cause this response. In one study, chlordiazepoxide was reported to increase hostility, whereas oxazepam had no such effect.[82] Buspirone, a nonbenzodiazepine anxiolytic, has been proposed as an advantageous advance over traditional anxiolytics due to its lack of sedation and psychomotor retardation. In a well-controlled study, it is shown to cause less impairment of acquisition and retention of memory than equivalent doses of alprazolam.[15] It has been used to treat agitation in severe TBI patients with mixed success and in mild TBI patients for postconcussive symptoms.[98] A retrospective series of 20 organic aggressive patients, 14 with TBI, treated with buspirone showed that improvement may require higher than standard doses and long-term administration (up to at least 60 mg/day and for a minimum of 12 weeks).[252] It should be remembered that buspirone is currently believed to have a delayed onset of effect of 4–6 weeks.

In conclusion, anxiolytics generally should not be considered first-line choices in the management of the long-term behavioral disturbances of TBI; however, in emergency situations, when reliable and quick control is critical and when there is a lack of diagnostic certainty regarding the etiology of the disturbance, the antianxiety agents may be an excellent choice for acute management of the agitated TBI patient. They also may have a role in the treatment of generalized anxiety following minor head injury. Buspirone might be considered a first-choice anxiolytic for TBI.

Beta Blockers

In addition to their known antihypertensive effects, beta blockers have been widely reported useful in diverse syndromes, including phobias and panic attacks, the psychoses of schizophrenia, and rage and aggression, and have emerged in the last decade as effective general psychotropes.[52] These drugs inhibit the beta-adrenergic system both centrally and peripherally. Propranolol is the most prominent and frequently used member of this class, although many choices exist, each with unique ratios of effect on beta-1 and beta-2 receptors as well as relative hydrophilic and lipophilic qualities with presumed differential effects. Lipophilic agents have been suggested as being potentially more effective for organic aggressiveness due to their better ability to penetrate the blood-brain barrier. Regardless of this theoretical issue, most studies to date have used propranolol; whether there are more effective choices in this class for this purpose remains to be seen. In a number of recent studies of brain-injured patients, propranolol has been reported effective in the treatment of both acute, episodic rage[61,295] and the longer-term aggressiveness of chronic brain syndrome,[200,294] including that from traumatic head injury. An alternative beta blocker, metoprolol, was reported effective in controlling intermittent explosiveness in patients with brain injury (infection and trauma) after the failure of other drugs, including propranolol.[163] These therapeutic responses have occurred, in most reports, after prior use and failure of multiple other "antiaggressive" agents, such as the antipsychotics, antidepressants, and lithium. It should be noted that the required effective dosages of beta blockers appear at times to be quite high (over 1000 mg/day of propranolol).

The beta blockers appear to be a feasible and perhaps first-order alternative to other more usually considered antiaggressive drugs.

Dopaminergic Agents

L-dopa has also been used with apparent success in relieving symptoms of explosive temper, diminished concentration, depression, hyperactivity, and impulsiveness in adults with attention deficit disorder (residual type). Interestingly, these successes were obtained after failure of amphetamines, methylphenidate, and pemoline.[203] In addition to the well-known agonist precursor L-dopa, other dopaminergic drugs are available, such as bromocriptine and amantadine. These act via distinct and varying actions on pre- and postsynaptic dopaminergic receptors. Thus, the lack of effect of one dopaminergic choice may not rule out a therapeutic effect by another. Bromocriptine, a mixed dopamine agonist-antagonist, is believed to possibly have multiple psychiatric applications, including usage in schizophrenia, depression, mania, and others.[245] Amantadine, with both pre- and postsynaptic dopaminergic activity, has been reported by Gualtieri to be highly successful for the treatment of agitation and irritability as well as for abulia and akinesia in TBI populations.[99] Dopaminergic agonists, however, are frequently associated with increased as well as decreased agitation. The overall place of dopaminergic agents in aggression and agitation following TBI remains unclear. They are probably second-order choices (similar to antidepressants) following the psychotropic anticonvulsants (carbamazepine), beta blockers, and stimulants, although this is clearly a matter of opinion at this point.

Miscellaneous Drugs

Occasionally, inappropriate sexual behavior or sexually driven aggression develops after TBI. This usually reflects an underlying loss of impulse control or social sensibility. Often, with counseling and/or contingency management, such problems resolve or become manageable. On rare occasions, usually in young males, sexually associated behavioral disturbance is severe, persistent, and very difficult to manage. Antiandrogenic agents have been used in psychiatric settings for aggressivity and intractable sexual disturbance in schizophrenics and temporal lobe epileptics.[22,184] Reports indicate that this treatment effectively reduces sexual interest and activity and ultimately sexual offenses. Medroxyprogesterone (Depo-Provera) has been most commonly used for reversible inhibition of androgen effect. There appear to be no published reports of medoxyprogesterone use for the persistently hypersexual TBI patient, but in the author's experience it has been effective in a few cases. For example, this approach was quite effective in our clinic in controlling a TBI male whose sexual behavior was repetitively extreme, nearly to the point of assault. Success was achieved with medroxyprogesterone injections in obtaining control of this sexual aggression (directed toward young females) after the failure (short of inducing stupor) over years of other drugs. In selected cases, this approach is probably indicated. Due to the sensitive personal, social, and legal considerations involved, extreme care must be taken to obtain informed consent from the family and, as best possible, of the patient and to document both need and effect.

Aggressive, agitated behaviors following TBI also have been described as related to unregulated appetitive drive or bulimic states. Such cases have, in a few instances, been reported to respond favorably to the opiate kappa receptor-blocking agent, naltrexone.[30]

Akinetic mutism, aphasias (secondary to stroke), and other CNS-derived communication disorders have been mentioned in a number of reports to have responded significantly to dopaminergic agents. Wroblewski and Glenn have recently discussed the pharmacologic treatment of these conditions.[289]

Disorders of Affect

Traumatic brain injury undoubtedly leads to major affective disorder, i.e., depression and mania. As previously noted, secondary mania and hypomanias have been reported to occur from a variety of organic brain lesions, including trauma.[253] These secondary manias may be difficult to distinguish behaviorally from the manic type of primary bipolar disease, but they have a higher component of aggression and thus were discussed under disorders of behavior (above).

The problem of depression in TBI begins with diagnosis. For example, there is a basic question of whether a patient with significantly impaired cognition is able to manifest true depression. For depression, in brain-injured patients of multiple etiologies, a consistently confounding clinical problem is to distinguish relevant signs and symptoms, such as psychomotor retardation, lack of verbal behaviors, or other vegetative disturbances (e.g., sleep, appetite, or sexual disruption) as reflecting straightforward neurologic deficits or superimposed depressive illness. Ross et al. point out the difficulties in diagnosis of depression in brain-damaged patients due to aphasia, neurologic distortion of emotional sensitivity and output (aprosodias), and neglect.[220] This distinction between true depression and "pseudodepression" may be more theoretical than real. It is possible that the symptoms in question are identical epiphenomena reflecting a common neurotransmitter defect, albeit from differing etiologies. A review of 25 published studies addressing this issue in mentally retarded populations concludes that classic forms of depression are possible, although specific symptoms and signs may be altered or absent.[250] There is also evidence appearing from thorough studies in stroke populations, with similar "depressive-neurologic" symptoms, that a true secondary depression does in fact occur in patients with injury or impairment of the central nervous system.[214] In TBI various studies have given incidences of depression ranging from below 10% for mild injuries[223] to above 50% for severe injuries.[243,270] In a well-designed prospective study of depression following TBI, not only was a significant incidence of depression reported, but interestingly there seemed to be at least two varieties of depression: acute (mainly physiologic in origin) and delayed (with psychodynamic etiology, i.e., loss and grieving), for which there may be presumably differing treatments.[129]

It must be recalled that multiple drugs, particularly antianxiety agents and beta blockers, are notable for their potential as iatrogenic causes of depression, and this possibility must be considered in each patient presenting with depressive symptoms or signs.

Antidepressants

Tricyclics have been used successfully to treat depression after stroke. These patients respond to tricyclics roughly as well as non-neurologically impaired depressives.[150] A variety of new nontricyclic antidepressant drugs, particularly the selective serotonergic reuptake inhibitors (SSRIs; e.g., fluoxetine, sertraline), may have significant advantages over traditional tricyclics due to a better side-effect profile. They seem to have little or no effect on psychomotor performance at therapeutic dosages.[106] Fluoxetine, in particular, is nonanticholinergic.

It has been suggested that depression following focal compared with diffuse TBI may have differing neurophysiologic substrates and be responsive to differing medications. Patients with focal TBI are more responsive to traditional antidepressants, whereas patients with diffuse TBI are more responsive to dopaminergic agents and stimulants.[243] At the moment, however, these are speculative distinctions. It is appropriate for the clinician to consider TBI patients who "look depressed" to be considered so and to be expected to have a similar positive response to standard antidepressants. Pathologic pseudoemotionality, such as laughing and crying (although arguably only a defect of mood), may also be responsive to antidepressants. In 12 patients with pseudoemotionality secondary to bilateral forebrain disease, treated with amitriptyline in a double-blind, crossover design, significant improvement has been reported.[23] Such organic pseudoemotionality also has been successfully treated with L-dopa and anticonvulsants.[271]

Neuroleptics

The common identification for neuroleptics in affective disorders is for the treatment of psychotic features associated with depression or mania (e.g., delusions, hallucinations, etc.). Experience for this indication has not been reported in the literature for TBI specifically, but presumably experience in other conditions suggests that neuroleptics would be an appropriate choice as an adjunct to standard antidepressant treatments in such cases.

Stimulants

Dextroamphetamine and methylphenidate have frequently been believed to be useful in depression following major stroke.[159] Clinical response is more rapid than with conventional tricyclic drugs, and the side-effect profile is not excessive, although stimulants can cause agitation and aggressivity.[126] Such indications may be most commonly indicated for mood disturbances following mild TBI.

Electroconvulsive Therapy

Although not a pharmacologic treatment, electroconvulsive therapy (ECT) is traditionally included in psychopharmacologic discussion as an essentially somatic treatment and hence comparable in some ways to drug treatment. It is indicated primarily for both severe depression and manic excitement. It should be noted that the prohibition against ECT in patients with acute brain pathology is generally based on the danger of inducing increases in intracranial pressure. For the immediate recovery phase of TBI, this is probably a valid consideration. In the chronic rehabilitation phase, however, it seldom applies. A second concern is with ECT's amnesia induction. Unilateral low-voltage ECT may be preferable to bilateral for this reason. There are reports of successful use of ECT after various forms of brain injury, including TBI resulting from gunshot,[222] and it is recommended by experienced clinicians.

Disorders of Cognition

A recently examined area in which medications are considered as possible interventions in TBI is in remediating the basic cognitive deficits of these patients. Cognition is a complex neuropsychological concept, and a number of different formal conceptualizations of the cognitive structure and the deficits following brain injury have been offered.[143] Additionally, cognitive losses inevitably are coincident with or conducive to deficits in the areas of personality and behavior.[23] It is known that these cognitive and personality deficits are the most common and most disabling of all the sequelae of TBI. There is often no restorative treatment and no complete recovery from these TBI cognitive effects. Even "mild" deficits in the cognitive area can be devastating to personal, social, and vocational goals of patients. As Cope pointed out,

> Attention and memory refer to multiple levels of processes ranging from complex social

interaction to basic neuronal or molecular activity. Behavior represents an interrelated hierarchy where . . . psychological activity is a consequence of underlying basic neuronal and biochemical processes. Pharmacologic modification of neurophysiologic processes, intended or *inadvertent*, will have important effects upon higher-order psychological processes.[37]

For a comprehensive review of the cognitive effects of psychotropic medications in general, the reader is referred to the review by Judd, et al.[130] As with other indications, the inadvertent deleterious effects of multiple medications need to be continually kept in mind. Cognitive enhancement or remediation of TBI deficits by pharmacologic agents has to date only a small literature, and one that derives more from study in a variety of associated organic brain syndromes, such as mental deficiency (retardation), senile dementia of Alzheimer's type (SDAT), general cognitive impairment of aging or alcoholic dementia, and attention deficit disorder with hyperactivity (ADHD) than from TBI itself.[94,285] McLean, et al. recently reviewed this area with a particular focus on brain injury.[166]

In theory, TBI should be a clinical area more responsive to the effects of cognitive-enhancing drugs than the more extensively studied progressive conditions (e.g., dementia). TBI has an improving or stable functional cognitive level relative to the declining baseline of SDAT. Thus, for TBI the therapeutic effects of cognitive-enhancing agents will not be eroded or washed out over time with the progression of the disease, as occurs in SDAT. Therefore, the modest therapeutic results of these drugs (as are reported in most positive studies with SDAT) would have a much greater clinical importance in TBI as it would presumably be stably manifest over the many years of expected life span of the typically young TBI patient. A wide variety of agents have been investigated in attempts to improve cognitive function in general and in TBI in particular.

Cholinergic Agents

It is clear from a very large number of studies that cholinergic systems, particularly the basilar forebrain system originating largely from the nucleus basalis of Meynert, play a central role in cognitive processes, particularly the intrinsic memory systems.[20] Korsakoff's and Alzheimer's dementias, although distinct conditions with varying neuropathologic pictures, have as a common feature hippocampal and amygdalar pathology,[42,298] structures also frequently damaged in TBI. Studies in both animals and humans demonstrate that a deficiency of cholinergic transmission is present in these conditions as well as following TBI, which leads to expected cognitive deficits, even following mild injuries.[51] Parenthetically, TBI has been believed to be a possible risk factor for subsequent development of dementia of the Alzheimer's type.[178] Anticholinergic drugs have been shown to impair memory in normals[189] and in organic brain conditions.[225] An overview of neuropharmacologic remediation of these conditions in the aged population[205] has been published. Cholinergic drugs appear to have a beneficial effect on both attentional and memory aspects of information processing.[277] Treatment with cholinergic drugs has ameliorated various cognitive losses, including memory, in both animals and humans.[47] Cholinergic agents have often been reported to be helpful in improving memory, both in normals and various pathologic states.[48,62,72] Specific cholinergic therapeutic effects in organic brain conditions, including posttraumatic memory loss and cognitive deficits, have been reported,[90,91,174,247,276] although some other well-designed studies have shown no such effect.[7,108] Recently, the effectiveness of a combination of cholinergic agonists (i.e., a choline precursor and a cholinesterase inhibitor) in producing an additive enhancement of memory has been reported.[75] Cholinergic (lecithin) and anticholinesterase (physostigmine) agents have been reported in case studies to be effective in remediating cognitive and memory deficits following TBI. Drug withdrawal and reintroduction phases, associated with a decrement and recovery of function, demonstrated treatment effect in a double-blind, placebo-controlled study (A-B-A design) utilizing physostigmine.[296] Goldberg, in a similar placebo-controlled, single-case study of a TBI patient, demonstrated statistically significant improvement in verbal memory with administration of the same drugs.[92] McLean et al. have reported on the significant efficacy of the anticholinesterase physostigmine in managing organic brain-injured patients.[167]

Clinically, however, use of cholinergic agents has been hampered by the short half-lives and narrow therapeutic ranges of available drugs. Beneficial response is tightly related to the specific drug level achieved in the CNS; too little is ineffectual, whereas too much leads to significant cognitive, behavioral, and autonomic toxicity. These problems have so far precluded routine clinical use of these cholinergic strategies. A new agent, tetra-hydro-amino-acridine (THAA), marketed as Tacrine, is a central anticholinesterase with long duration of action and has shown promise in large-scale, double-blind, placebo-controlled studies in SDAT populations.[67,259] It has been approved by the FDA within the past year as effective for the cognitive decline of SDAT, and so should soon be available to clinicians. No studies using this particular cholinergic drug in TBI are available, however, and at present it should be regarded only as a promising agent for investigation in this condition. In summary, there is a great deal of evidence that the cholinergic system is central in human memory and its pathology and that cholinergic drugs may have the potential to improve memory in multiple conditions, including TBI, but no effective agent or treatment protocol has been reliably demonstrated to date. Clinically, it is more critical to avoid use of medications with anticholinergic profiles (side effects) than to attempt to benefit patients with agonists.

Antidepressants

As noted, the antidepressants are believed to be an alternative to stimulants in the treatment of ADHD. Many of the ADHD studies show improvement on formal cognitive measures as well as behavior.[140,283] The cognitive literature in this area (ADHD) is vast, and these referenced studies are meant simply as an introduction to this topic. The tricyclics have been the antidepressant most associated with ADHD treatment. Reports of efficacy of tricyclics in neuropsychiatrically impaired patients, some with frank brain injury, including TBI, have been made. A single-case study of amitriptyline efficacy in TBI has been made by Jackson et al.,[123] in which therapeutic response was imputed to be due to improved cognitive and attentional capability. This same research group reported upon a group study of TBI patients who achieved similar benefit from imipramine.[179] Other reports of successful clinical use of tricyclics for cognitive impairment after TBI are available.[56] Protriptyline, with a strongly noradrenergic profile, has been reported as an effective "stimulant" choice in brain-injured patients after the failure of first-line choices such as levodopa, methylphenidate, and bromocriptine.[288]

Stimulants and Other Catecholamine Agonists

Kety first suggested that catecholamine (CA) neurons were involved in behavioral arousal.[132] CA neurons synthesize, store, and release the catecholamines: epinephrine, norepinephrine, and dopamine. Catecholamines, dopamine, norepinephrine, and epinephrine affect memory processes, but these actions appear to be modulatory in nature rather than intrinsic. It is probably unnecessary to emphasize that a portion of the clinical "memory" deficit that TBI patients manifest is in reality due to defects in underlying attention. Brain-injured patients routinely have impaired arousal, attention, information processing, and memory, and these deficits may be due, in part, to damage to the CA system. Drugs that affect the catecholaminergic systems probably affect memory principally via changes in arousal and attention. The psychostimulants, while probably not directly improving memory processes, have clinically often proved helpful in improving measures of memory, probably through this mechanism of increasing attention, vigilance, motivation, and other cognitive processes.

Aside from memory, catecholamines, particularly dopamine and norepinephrine, have been known for many years to play a central role in arousal and cognitive processes.[9,230,272] Catecholamine agonist activity within the prefrontal cortex is particularly related to higher-level analytic processes, initiative, mental flexibility, and attention. Stimulants are the most studied and widely used drugs in the catecholaminergic category. They consist of amphetamines, methylphenidate (Ritalin), magnesium pemoline (Cylert), and others.

Stimulants can improve cognitive performance of normal subjects under certain conditions.[135] Animal and human work demonstrates that drugs of this class can remediate a wide range of behavioral and cognitive deficits resulting from dysfunction of the frontal and other higher cortical structures.[6,29] The first such use of amphetamines in TBI was reported in 1976.[149] Evans and Gualtieri have made persuasive clinical and theoretical arguments that stimulants are effective in ameliorating the cognitive disturbances of TBI in a manner similar to their action in ADHD,[64] and their methodologically sophisticated analysis demonstrated beneficial effects of both dextroamphetamine and methylphenidate on memory and learning skills, increased attention, and overall behavior in a TBI patient.[66]

They have also demonstrated such an effect in a larger number of TBI patients in a double-blind, single-case methodology.[64] A double-blind cross-over study of 15 chronic TBI patients with problems of attention, memory, impulsiveness, excitability, and other personality-affective symptoms showed a strong clinical response, although statistical findings were less unambiguous.[102] In Norway Klove has similarly reported upon stimulant effectiveness for the cognitive deficits of TBI.[136] Glenn has recently reviewed the indications and use of stimulants in TBI and found them effective for a variety of cognitive and arousal deficits.[88] Conversely, however, a recent well-controlled study of stimulant effect on cognition and behavior in TBI patients failed to show benefit.[251]

The mesolimbic dopaminergic system has been demonstrated to be integrally related to frontal lobe functions and cognition. For example, in Parkinson's disease both cognition and delayed memory have been shown to be positively related to dopaminergic activity in this system.[24,173] Such dopaminergic efficacy has also been reported for the cognitive symptoms in ADHD patients.[203] Sinemet has been successful in remediating locked-in syndrome after unresponsiveness to bromocriptine.[199] Interestingly, aphasia of neurologic origin has also been reported to respond to dopaminergic agents (bromocriptine).[2,103] Bromocriptine has also been reported effective in remediating the frontal syndrome of aneurysmal bleed,[186] and Eames has reported its successful usage in TBI and theoretically contrasted the postsynaptic nature of this drug with the essentially presynaptic actions of L-dopa.[57]

Dihydrogenated Ergot Alkaloids (Hydergine)

Dihydrogenated ergot alkaloids were initially thought to elicit an effect by improving cerebral circulation, a view no longer held. They are partial agonist/antagonists of dopaminergic and serotonergic receptors and appear to antagonize adrenergic receptors. Their major clinically relevant action may be as enhancers of neuronal metabolism (e.g., decreased breakdown of adenosine triphosphate and cyclic adenosine monophosphate). They are demonstrated to have an "activating" effect on electroencephalographs in animals. Placebo-controlled, double-blind studies have consistently shown significant but modest improvements in function and cognition in humans.[118] Only one presented but unpublished paper reporting Hydergine use in TBI is available, a blind, prospective study, which indicated some efficacy in improving certain neuropsychological measures.[79] Hydergine, however, with its demonstrated effect in other conditions and its low toxicity and low side-effect profile, would seem an enticing drug for clinical trials in TBI.

Nootropics

Nootropics are a new putative class of agents that, as their name implies, have a presumed primary effect of improving cognition.[84] Piracetam is the prototype and most studied agent of this class, although newer, apparently more potent cogeners have been developed (e.g., pramiracetam).[183] There are approximately a half-dozen agents of this type currently under investigation for their putative beneficial effects on general cognitive processes.[175]

Most studies of these cognitive-enhancing drugs to date have been done on demented patients. Placebo-controlled, double-blind studies of organically impaired geriatric populations have shown significant improvement on clinical, psychometric, and neuropsychological measures with oxiracetam (a piracetem cogener).[227] Current studies in the U.S. are most actively investigating pramiracetam. McLean has reported upon six brain-injured patients who showed a modest but significant improvement in memory and cognition with pramiracetam—an effect that persisted at 18-month follow-up. The efficacy, however, varied greatly among individual patients. Patients who showed significant psychometric improvement also showed improvement in general measures of function.[168] This class of drugs apparently has a very low toxicity and side-effect profile but is not yet clinically available in the U.S. These are very promising agents, however, and may be available shortly for clinical usage.

Neuropeptides

A variety of neuropeptides have been suggested as having activity in general cognitive and memory processes. Vasopressin and a variety of associated synthetic analogs are the most thoroughly studied. Most work has been on the deficits of the elderly[265] and in ECT-induced amnesia.[188] Vasopressin has been reported helpful in the amnestic syndromes associated with alcoholic dementia, ECT, and head trauma.[185] Specific clinical trials of vasopressin's use in head injury have produced inconclusive results but suggest some effectiveness.[125,138] A review concluded that the putative beneficial effect of vasopressin may reflect not a direct action on memory per se but possibly on reinforcement mechanisms or modulation of arousal.[226] Other neuropeptide agents currently implicated include adenocorticotropic hormone (ACTH) and various ACTH fragments, especially the 6-10 moiety, thyrotropin-releasing hormone (TRH), and oxytocin, all of which have been reported effective in various studies in improving cognitive measures.[285]

Miscellaneous Drugs

Other classes of drugs, including opioid antagonists,[205] have been investigated for general cognitive-enhancing effects, but are even less well defined or studied.

Clonidine, an alpha-adrenergic agonist, has been reported helpful in the memory deficits of Korsakoff's disease.[164] Clonidine has also appeared to be effective in improving the attention and cognition of patients with ADHD, even after the failure of more conventional agents.[120] Clonidine, an alpha-2 adrenergic agonist, has been given to a few TBI patients in attempts to improve memory function with no benefit demonstrable on formal neuropsychologic measures.[165]

The cognitive consequences of mild traumatic brain injury are particularly vexatious for the clinician, tied up as they are with frequently subjective symptomatology, emotional overlay, forensic issues, and secondary gain. Yet in terms of absolute incidence they are by far the most frequent.

These problems are most preeminent in mild TBI. Comprehensive discussions of the approach to the mild brain-injured patient are available.[19,146] A virtual formulary of drugs has been suggested as efficacious in the protean symptomatology of this condition; for psychotropes these include tricyclics, lithium, monoamine oxidase inhibitors, buspirone, sertraline, trazodone, fluoxetine, carbamazepine, valproate, catecholaminergic and cholinergic agents, methylphenidate, stimulants, amantadine, propranolol, and benzodiazepines.[297]

Overall, these recent reports of modestly successful remediation of cognitive dysfunctions in TBI suggest in some cases a real clinical benefit. Although these early reports offer reasonable encouragement, it must be stated that no reliably effective pharmacologic mechanisms exist to improve cognition after TBI. In general, psychopharmacologic enhancement of TBI cognitive deficits is in a very early phase of development. While there are currently 19 different new cognitive-enhancing compounds in phase II or III clinical trials for use in SDAT at the present time, according to the Pharmaceutical Manufacturers Association,[208] the author knows of no such drug in the process of FDA investigation for TBI at present.

In conclusion, it is fair to state that while no reliably effective drug has yet been identified to improve cognition, arousal, or memory, many drugs currently available for clinical use have shown promise in small studies, and intriguing new drug prospects are under development at present for conditions similar to TBI. Individual TBI patients seem, on occasion, to derive real improvement cognitively from a wide variety of these drugs.

PHARMACOLOGIC TREATMENT AND BRAIN RECOVERY/ PLASTICITY

Virtually all of the indications for psychopharmacologic intervention in TBI discussed herein are directed at ameliorating or compensating for symptoms deriving from relatively fixed and static pathologic deficits. This is treatment for symptom relief, not deficit resolution. At a more basic level than symptom relief, however, there are important issues to be considered regarding the use of psychopharmacologic agents in the TBI patient.

Neuropharmacologic treatment is generally utilized to modify existent cognitive or behavioral problems after brain injury. Less often considered is the potential of these agents in the longer, chronic view to improve (or exacerbate) basic neurologic recovery. These drugs may have prolonged effects via influences on brain plasticity. It is possible that many of the psychoactive agents that are commonly in clinical use today are preventing or inhibiting full recovery from the underlying injury. Alternatively, some drugs may be accelerating or enhancing such recovery.

We know quite well that drugs that act on the CNS are not free of long-lasting or even permanent effects. Tardive dyskinesia, the most notorious of this kind of problem and a serious consequence of neuroleptic use, is generally estimated to affect 15–20% of patients who receive long-term treatment. However, its prevalence in populations on long-term maintenance regimens has been estimated to be as high as 40%.[43] Its incidence in TBI has not been documented but should be proportionate to the frequency of use of neuroleptic medications in this group. Tardive dyskinesia is of practical and theoretical importance due to its frequent appearance following the use of neuroleptics and the frequent administration of neuroleptics to TBI patients. Although it appears most clearly related to the total lifetime dose of neuroleptics, tardive dyskinesia can occur shortly after drug initiation. In a large percentage of cases, the syndrome is irreversible, presumably reflecting long-lasting or permanent change in the neurochemical organization of the brain. It is generally accepted that there is no effective treatment to manage this problem. Based on this increasingly recognized risk, the American Psychiatric Association concluded that the use of neuroleptics for organic brain syndromes (e.g., TBI) is indicated only for short-term management (6 months).[3] Neuroleptic drugs are not alone in this characteristic of inducing long-term plastic changes. Antidepressants probably produce their major effect via long-term modulation of the number or sensitivity of pre- and postsynaptic monoamine receptors,[112] and withdrawal signs can occur when these drugs are abruptly discontinued. It has been reported that the stimulant medications may lead to persistent, perhaps permanent, movement disorders (e.g., tics and Tourette's syndrome).[152] Such plastic alterations of the CNS may be a general characteristic and risk of many varying neuroactive drugs.

Another dimension of concern is that neuroleptics (probably based on their anti–alpha-adrenergic action) have been shown to significantly retard recovery of learned motor and discrimination tasks in brain-lesioned animals. In general, drugs that interfere with catecholaminergic action appear to interfere with recovery from CNS damage. Neuroleptics have been demonstrated to elicit the reappearance of neurologic behavioral deficits in experimental animals long after apparent recovery from brain damage. Van Hasselt demonstrated that even after apparently complete motor recovery from experimentally induced cortical sensory-motor deficit in animals, the administration of a single dose of haloperidol would reinstitute hemiplegia. The deficit could be repetitively induced each time the drug was administered.[273] Animal studies by Feeney and associates[70,71] investigated recovery from sensory-motor cortical lesions (both ablation and contusion models) in rats and cats. The rate of motor recovery from hemiplegia following cortical ablation was followed. Amphetamine (a catecholamine agonist), given shortly after the cortical lesion procedure, resulted in significant acceleration of recovery, whereas haloperidol (a catecholaminergic-blocking agent) induced a prolonged delay before recovery occurred. There is some evidence from human work that this negative effect on recovery also occurs in clinical settings. Porch reported on measurement of language recovery in 32 aphasic patients. Patients who received haloperidol or certain antihypertensive medications (primarily catecholamine antagonists) showed significantly poorer recovery from aphasia than patients not receiving these medications.[192] Goldstein showed a significantly poorer motor and functional outcome for matched stroke patients who were exposed to anticatecholaminergic agents during clinical management.[93]

Alternatively, there is also the possibility that certain psychotropic drugs (e.g., stimulants) may have the ability to increase recovery from CNS damage. Chrisostomo demonstrated a beneficial clinical effect to single doses of amphetamines in stroke patients in terms of recovery of motor function.[31]

These naturalistic studies offer some indication that the theoretical risks suggested by the above animal studies may indeed have clinical significance and should give pause to clinicians in their rush to prescribe. Feeney has reviewed this issue.[69]

It is also of interest that evidence suggests that a positive response to drugs in the acute recovery period does not necessarily indicate a chronic requirement for drug treatment. Wright,[287] for example, reported that a patient with akinetic mutism who initially responded to Sinemet was successfully weaned from this agent in the chronic phase. Biochemical assays suggested brain adjustment over time to initial dopaminergic deficiency.[287] Thus, the brain may modulate transmitter systems to make such drug responsiveness only a temporary phenomenon.

The clinical implications for TBI recovery of these and similar studies are not clearly known, but they may be significant. The issue of pharmacologically modifying recovery, as would be expected, is quite complex, with multiple possibilities for improving or impeding recovery, including differing effects from the same drug(s).[83] The methodology required in demonstrating these potentially beneficial or harmful effects on recovery is difficult and not yet adequately developed to allow convincing human studies. In conclusion, there is evidence that suggests that the use of agents which affect neurotransmitter activity in the CNS may be inducing an unperceived additional neuropathologic benefit or burden in patients with brain injury. This possibility also suggests caution in the use of these agents.

METHODOLOGIC CONSIDERATIONS IN PSYCHOPHARMACOLOGIC TREATMENT

A number of methodologic issues exist in the area of psychopharmacologic treatment of TBI. Given that there is a wide variety of agents that may be reasonably expected to produce benefits in the various arousal, affective-behavioral, and cognitive deficits of at least a subset of the general head-injured population, and yet also acknowledging the current inadequacy of the nosology of head injury syndromes and the inability to predict accurately which particular patient will respond to any specific agent, how then should the clinician proceed when pharmacologic control appears to be indicated? Some guidelines on the proper integration of psychopharmacologic treatment in the TBI rehabilitation process are appropriate.

Behavioral and cognitive deficits are ubiquitous problems following TBI. If the efficacy and indication for traditional rehabilitation and psychotherapeutic interventions are clearly established for these patients, what should be the role of psychopharmacologic treatment? The sum of the effects of the use of these mediations may produce unexpected and perhaps subtle losses, damages, and complications. As reviewed in this chapter, while many of these TBI deficits have at least a reasonable potential to be ameliorated by psychopharmacologic treatments, there is little certainty about the likelihood of success in the individual case. Uncertainty exists regarding many aspects of these approaches. A generally negative attitude toward the use of psychotropic medications has characterized rehabilitation approaches historically. Negative side effects and toxicities are usually well respected by clinicians. How should the clinician integrate pharmacologic treatment of the TBI patient with other interventions? This dilemma is particularly vexatious given the current health care environment (i.e., the increasing level of technical, fiscal, administrative, and regulatory restrictions applied to clinical practice and research) as well as the medicolegal perils evident.

Traditional rehabilitation approaches are usually considered the "primary" intervention. For example, the appropriate standard treatment for a depressed TBI patient is to address and rectify, to the extent possible, the disabilities and handicaps that restrict function and diminish life choices; for an agitated patient, the basic approach might be simplification of the patient's environment and reduction of frustrating performance demands through increased environmental structure, etc. It is often only after these methods have been fully applied that resort to psychopharmacologic treatment is believed to be justified by many. In some of the most sophisticated neurobehavioral units, it is acceptable to work with contingency-based interventions for many months before considering a pharmacologic approach. For cognitive loss, the most frequent TBI impairment, the reliance on psychologically based "cognitive-retraining" methods at the expense of pharmacologic treatment is even more pronounced in clinical practice. In essence, for cognitive, affective, and behavioral deficits psychological treatment has been considered integral and pharmacologic treatment a secondary or back-up option; pharmacologic treatment rarely has been integrated into rehabilitation planning.

This tradition is oddly illogical given the fundamentally organic nature of the underlying deficits in TBI. The consequences of TBI are obviously fundamentally expressed in large part by disturbances of neurotransmitter function. It is plain that pharmacologic intervention in other psychiatric (psychobehavioral) conditions (e.g., schizophrenia, bipolar disease, depression) with much less demonstrated underlying neurotransmitter pathology is routine, even mandatory by current clinical standards. Failure to initiate appropriate pharmacologic intervention in these conditions might be considered a major deviation from standards of care.

In the most rigorous sense, data available to support drug use in TBI are incomplete and noncompelling. Virtually no randomized, prospective, double-blind studies exist for TBI. Physicians operate in a vastly more litigious environment than prior eras. Most psychotropic drug indications and early experience were gained in a more benign legal environment.

Rehabilitation physicians in general lack training and expertise in use of psychotropic medications. There is also fundamental discord between medical and psychological models of neuropsychological dysfunction. Psychologists have, in general, been the most prominent in describing and developing interventions for the cognitive and behavioral deficits of TBI, yet they have little background or expertise with, or ability to utilize, pharmacologic treatments. Rehabilitation physicians historically have been much more concerned with musculoskeletal and other traditionally "medical" concerns. From this perspective it may not be too surprising that psychopharmacologic treatments have lagged behind psychological ones.

Disregard of pharmacologic treatments for cognitive deficits is a special case of neglect. While cognitive loss is the most frequent and disabling of all TBI sequelae, it has suffered from the most medical oversight. Cognitive impairment is most evident in moderately and severely injured patients, but a substantial portion of patients with mild TBI also have disabling cognitive limitation, either transiently or permanently. As noted, it appears that even these more mildly injured TBI patients may benefit from appropriate pharmacologic intervention. As Gualtieri states:

> Research has not advanced to the point where it is possible to predict *which* TBI patients should be treated with stimulant drugs. It is the authors' clinical impression, however, that the best response occurs in relatively high-level, mild to moderately impaired patients, with relatively circumscribed deficits in attention, memory, organization or initiative, and stimulants are currently indicated for TBI patients who have prominent symptoms of: (1) attention deficit/hyperactivity . . . (2) anergia/apathy . . . (3) the frontal lobe syndrome.[100]

Behavioral and affective disturbances are usually given high valence by treating physicians, but they tend to underestimate the significance of cognitive deficits in TBI, particularly when they are of a subtle degree.

While they are not as dramatic as those of the assaultive or abulic patient, and cognitive disturbance is less disruptive to family, society, and the treating team, based on incidence and prevalence such cognitive deficits are the *core problems* of TBI rehabilitation and affect virtually every TBI survivor. Undoubtedly, cognitive loss causes more disability than all other problems combined. Pharmacologic treatment of cognitive loss in the routine case of TBI is nevertheless rare today.

What does a positive response to psychoactive medication mean in patients with TBI? Irritability or agitation may be decreased, but important additional questions should include the effects on adaptive behaviors, motivation, and mood.

How is the clinician to proceed? In practice it must also be acknowledge that the decision to use medications in clinical settings is increasingly not solely a clinical one. There are significant nonmedical influences on such use. In nursing home and institution settings, patients with significant organic impairment tend to be chronically and inappropriately maintained on psychotropic medications,[278] almost certainly because of administrative and economic pressures that favor the use of medications by treating physicians. Strong economic incentives exist to manage disruptive patient behavior by non–labor-intensive (i.e., pharmacologic) means. While clinical guidelines increasingly recommend trial of a strict contingency management behavioral protocol to manage the majority of behaviorally disturbed patients before recourse is made to long-term psychopharmacologic approaches, in practice this rarely occurs. This is almost certainly due to the expense in time and staffing levels of such behavioral intervention. A prescription is less expensive than the organization and training of a team for behavioral management.

It may be considered appropriate, given the current level of uncertainty, to follow the dictum first to do no harm through unnecessary or ill-considered drug interventions, but this disregards the harm done when a potentially effective pharmacologic treatment is denied to a patient. Psychopharmacologic intervention should not take the place of appropriate, established rehabilitation protocols, but psychopharmacologic intervention should in many cases be considered an integral component of the rehabilitation process.

Single-Case Methodology

Because the effects of psychotropic drugs are complex and difficult to predict with certainty and because there are significant real and potential side effects, some of which may be difficult to monitor or discern, it is essential that each TBI patient treated with psychopharmacologic agents be considered an empirical experiment. Diligent observation and quantification of both putative positive responses and side effects must be made using adequate single-case design methodology.[16]

It is most appropriate to follow a course of sequential evaluations of multiple drugs at varying dosages, using this single-case methodology. The patient is used as his or her own control. An adequate baseline of significant behaviors must first be obtained. Positive as well as negative behaviors should be assessed, as in almost all cases there will be a trade-off between the dampening or elimination of unwanted behavior and suppression of desirable or adaptive behavior. Frequently implicit in this approach is an adequate initial trial of behavioral techniques to optimize the patient's level of function. Any further increase or improvement in behavior is then more clearly presumed to be due to the drug in question. Such an approach has been described for management of TBI.[66,104] Placebo use is an ideal component of this approach but clinically may be difficult to achieve if the target behavior is extreme or if drug side effects are highly perceptible. Whether or not a placebo is used, it is nearly always a good idea to perform a subsequent medication-withdrawal phase. It is far too often the case that head-injured patients receive potent medications for years with little documented justification and with significant adverse effects on performance, alertness, and cognition. A common error is to institute a drug treatment phase immediately, measure only the target behavior, and do no drug-withdrawal challenge.

There are problems (at least in the U.S.) in following this idealized treatment scheme. With increasingly limited willingness by payors to fund health care, restrictions on rehabilitation benefits are emerging. Utilization review and length-of-stay constraints have a limiting effect on clinicians' ability to strictly apply this methodology. Increasing utilization review pressures make maintenance of patients in a treatment program for sufficient time to use methods of the single-case approach problematic. In this very practical sense, consideration of the relative *cost-effectiveness* of various rehabilitation interventions is increasingly critical. The rehabilitation physician must decide the relatively optimal allocation of available health care dollars, and such a process may lead to early and more aggressive use of psychopharmacologic treatment than strict scientific considerations would indicate.[39]

The aggressiveness of psychopharmacologic intervention should depend on the three general phases of recovery: emergent or acute care, active rehabilitation, and chronic fixed-deficit treatment.

Emergent Care

In the immediate (hours and days) postinjury period, there are promising neuropharmacologic approaches to minimize primary or secondary CNS injury.[224] These specific interventions, however, are generally within the purview of neurologists, neurosurgeons, and intensivists rather than rehabilitationists. Thus, during this period, pharmacologic intervention is not routinely a rehabilitation issue. Promising agents include gangliosides, anticholinergics, lazeroids, and alpha-adrenergic agonists. While encouraging results with animal models have been obtained, human trials are just beginning. A full discussion of such interventions is not the focus of this chapter.

Nevertheless, the rehabilitation physician is occasionally involved in the emergent care of patients with TBI. The major problem leading to consideration of psychopharmacologic treatment is the coma-emerging patient with agitation and aggression. Guidelines given previously for aggression apply in this situation, but particularly in light of potential interference with active ongoing neurologic recovery, drugs currently believed to inhibit recovery should be relatively contraindicated; drugs that appear to stimulate recovery are relatively more indicated.

Active Rehabilitation

This is the period after medical stabilization that generally encompasses the active rehabilitation process. It extends from a number of days or weeks after injury throughout the duration of active recovery, which may last from months to several years. Progressive improvement is normally seen during this phase, and while underway a modified restraint should be the guiding principle regarding pharmacologic intervention. As long as the patient's progress is satisfactory (admittedly at present a largely subjective determination), drug treatments probably should be deferred, except for specific indications (e.g., obvious depression, seizure, uncontrollable disruptive behaviors, etc.). While the use of drugs in these obvious situations is fairly accepted practice, another potentially significant indication is the physician's considered judgment, even in the face of clinical progress, that drugs have a reasonable likelihood of increasing the rate of recovery or improving the patient's ability to cooperate with the rehabilitation process. Because virtually all patients have limited resources and a limited amount of time to achieve maximal benefit from rehabilitation, an increasingly appropriate indication for psychopharmacologic treatment is to make the rehabilitation process more efficient. Psychopharmacologic treatment in this instance is not reserved for patients in whom traditional rehabilitation has failed or reached an impasse. There are few objective standards to assist in making such a judgment, and it calls for the physician to use all of his or her previous experience with TBI and to integrate the medical, functional, psychologic, and social-financial elements of each patient's situation to arrive at the proper conclusion. It is a difficult decision with clear risks to such use, as discussed herein, such as unintended primary effects, toxic side effects, and plasticity concerns that may impede recovery. Current attitudes toward drug intervention in this phase are often strongly conservative for this reason. However, absolute conservatism is not acceptable, and it is increasingly appropriate to use as a first-stage intervention a combination of traditional rehabilitation and psychopharmacologic treatments with a goal of increasing relative rehabilitation response.

Examples of such situations might include patients who are agitated or aggressive to a degree that, while not totally uncontrollable, nevertheless impairs full participation in therapy and who do not indicate a quick response to simple and behavioral environmental interventions. It is not reasonable to delay such pharmacologic intervention by weeks or months while waiting for behavioral approaches to take effect when a limit on total rehabilitation expenditures is usually present for that patient. Another example is the "depressed" or apathetic patient who is "unmotivated" to participate fully in treatment or the abulic patient with strong psychomotor retardation. Current evidence indicates that all these patients may benefit from a trial of early and aggressive pharmacologic interventions. Kneale et al. gave several case examples of such appropriate and effective early psychopharmacologic interventions, including (1) a male patient with severe TBI and secondary bipolar disorder and (2) a patient with minor TBI, seizures, and abulia. These patients were treated concurrently with traditional therapies and (1) carbamazepine or (2) carbamazepine and bromocriptine; both had improved outcomes.[137]

Chronic Fixed-Deficit Treatment

At some point months or years after injury, it becomes clinically evident that further significant resolution of deficits is unlikely. Long-term disability and handicap, whether of major or minor degree, are evident and relatively fixed. This typically signals an end to active rehabilitation interventions (if they have continued this long) and the beginning of maintenance care. Rehabilitation physicians frequently do not stay actively involved in cases at this point, but in many cases further significant medical contribution may be made.

A number of points about chronic TBI patients should first be made before discussing these possibilities. As noted, many survivors have significant and major ongoing deficits in cognition and behavior in this chronic phase. For many other TBI patients the residual deficits and handicaps are subtle and less obvious. Given the total prevalence of TBI and the extended postinjury life expectancy of the typical brain-injured patient, the absolute magnitude of these residual disabilities is immense. These patients and their problems do not represent a small or insignificant health care issue. Silver et al. pointed out:

> Traumatic brain injury . . . has . . . a rate that is at least three times greater than that of schizophrenia, and a prevalence that is greater than that for . . . schizophrenia, mania, and panic disorder. Disorders arising from traumatic injuries to the brain are more common than any other neurological disease, with the exception of headaches.[244]

These disabilities are essentially life-long in effect, and although in many instances they may be subtle and, in fact, termed "minor" by clinicians, they are, in fact, anything but trivial to the patients and their families. These deficits interfere with and in many cases prevent the patient from resuming a meaningful and satisfying independent life. The effects of these "minor" deficits in cognition, emotional control, and behavior can be catastrophic for that patient's life. Simply projecting how similar deficits would affect the treating physician in personal and professional terms should illustrate the point. Finally, these deficits are not terminal problems. Whereas improving the cognition of a patient with Alzheimer's disease has a limited period over which to impact quality of life, for a TBI patient there is an entire lifetime of potential benefits if deficit amelioration can be achieved.

Thus, a strong case can be made that there is an additional role for psychopharmacologic treatment in this chronic "fixed-deficit" phase. Although prospective, double-blind studies are only beginning to emerge in the area of late treatment of personality changes, cognition, and behavior, a growing body of single-case design studies is demonstrating that selected individual patients obtain significant, sometimes dramatic, benefit from appropriate pharmacologic intervention. Most drugs to be considered are well-understood and have been used for many years in associated conditions. They mainly have low or acceptable toxicity and side effects. No long-term exposure to such medications would normally be indicated in such cases unless there were clearcut clinical benefits demonstrated, thus limiting concerns around issues of long-term toxicity, negative "plasticity," and cost. Even modest

symptom resolution with these drugs may have a major effect on the patient's and family's quality of life.

Thus, although these pharmacologic interventions are shown only variably effective, they may be seen as having both relatively low risk and high therapeutic potential. It seems evident that the risk/benefit ratio of such trials is acceptable. Lack of definitive studies of efficacy thus should not discourage appropriate clinical trials in individual TBI patients. Patients who are educated in the potential risks and benefits of these drugs should be allowed the opportunity to give informed consent to such trials. It should be emphasized that this chronic-phase treatment is an additional clinical rehabilitation intervention to what is now commonly offered, but one that is overdue.

In our current state of knowledge it seems at times as if any drug may be used for any symptom, and it is true that there are multiple choices and one can make no conclusive prescriptions in TBI. An empirical approach is appropriate, in which differing agents are sequentially evaluated. One chooses specific agents based on relative evidence of efficacy; for example, paroxysmal, seizurelike dysfunction might call for a psychotropic anticonvulsant or depressive, apathetic symptoms for an antidepressant. A second principle is to choose drugs with lower toxicity and fewer side effects. A third principle is to choose drugs that can be expected to manifest potential therapeutic responses quickly, i.e., a stimulant rather than an antidepressant.

A traditional piece of wisdom from psychiatry is applicable. The number of possible psychopharmacologic agents is very large—and growing. One clinician cannot gain clinical experience with all; therefore, the clinician should choose a few representative drugs from each psychoactive class and learn them well. This has been good advice for general psychopharmacologists; it is good advice for rehabilitation physicians.

Legal Considerations

Significant legal dimensions exist in regard to use of psychotropic medications in the brain-injured. A review of such issues is available.[38] Many issues of informed consent for treatment in general by the cognitively impaired, head-injured patient are problematic. What is certain is that society, via legislatures and courts, has been quite aggressive in defining specific safeguards for the mentally impaired in regard to psychopharmacologic treatment. Many rather elaborate administrative and judicial procedures are often necessary (in the legal sense) before psychopharmacologic treatments can be provided legally and ethically to mentally impaired patients. In theory, consistency would indicate that the same considerations apply with equal force for the impaired brain-injured patient as to the prototypically mentally ill patient (schizophrenia, dementia, etc.). Nevertheless, as a practical matter, uninformed and often involuntary treatment occurs with high frequency in general medical and rehabilitation populations with organic brain syndrome.[4]

This use of medication without informed consent is in some situations both ethical and legal when used as a temporary management intervention only. The danger lies in this temporary response to behavioral emergency becoming a chronic solution to a persistent behavioral problem. This risk is real, as manifested by the many patients who are found to be on long-term regimens of these drugs in surveys of organic populations. Rango, for example, has reported on a survey of 173 nursing homes involving 5,902 residents, many of whom had organic brain syndrome. Seventy-five percent of all patients had a prescription for psychotropic medications, and 43% of all patients were receiving at least one antipsychotic medication.[197] The indication and documentation surrounding such use were seriously deficient. TBI patients frequently end up chronically medicated in a similarly inappropriate manner.

Three major issues exist:

1. It is difficult to ensure competency in a patient who has significant organic deficits. In general, a presumption of competency exists for adult patients; yet the very fact that a patient has suffered brain damage or injury presumably implies the possibility of incompetence and lack of ability to give informed consent to treatment. A good rule is that if a patient is considered to be competent or has

been so determined by an administrative or legal proceeding, then under no circumstances should that patient be treated without obtaining informed consent, unless the situation is an emergency with significant risk to life or health. It is appreciated that this will create many difficult clinical situations, but nevertheless it must be adhered to.

2. Even after competency is determined, *informed* consent is difficult to ensure in an area in which established indications for treatment are so lacking. What type of information should be given to a patient and family about risks and benefits?

3. Extreme care must be used to prevent abusing medical prestige and power by administering medication against legal guidelines or without consent. This proves a great temptation when difficult behaviors occur in apparently unreasonable patients. Physicians who practice in this area need to be aware and understand these legal issues. Reviews of this area exist.[54,77,172]

A further legal issue is that nearly none of the proposed uses of the drugs suggested as useful in this chapter are "indicated" usages according to FDA regulations and determination. The FDA-approved guidelines for many of these drugs list brain injury as a relative contraindication to their use. Thus, treatment of TBI with these drugs is an "off-label" use, which, although not technically prohibited by law, probably does increase the risk of legal action related to a poor result by an unhappy patient and family. Adequate patient and family education and informed (and recorded) consent are essential precautions.

Economic Considerations

Physicians' unrestricted ability to access many of these drugs for their patients is coming under increasing pressure. Increasingly stringent utilization review (UR) methodologies by payment entities are relying on computer lists of "acceptable" or "indicated" drugs. Similarly, hospitals and health maintenance organizations (HMOs) are increasingly attempting to manage costs with such restricted lists. For example, the American Psychiatric Association Committee on Research on Psychiatric Treatments has published

Psychopharmacological Screening Criteria to be used by organizations, research groups, etc., in carrying out drug utilization evaluation, covering the major psychotropic drug classes. Alarmingly, but not surprisingly, the symptomatic indications of TBI discussed in this chapter are not once listed as indications for a single drug in these criteria.[131] And when drug prescription is "off-label" or not "standard," availability or reimbursement is being increasingly denied. The physician who ventures to use uncommon drugs or common drugs in nonstandard ways may increasingly face fiscal, administrative, and clinical review in the future. These practices are eroding physicians' ability to respond to the clinical needs of their patients. For example, in a parallel situation, a discussion of how such restrictions are believed to be constraining physicians in management of oncology patients has recently been presented.[1]

As the ultimate refractoriness of TBI deficits, even with aggressive traditional rehabilitation methods, is becoming more evident, increasing acceptance of psychopharmacologic approaches as a complementary component of a comprehensive treatment plan is emerging. This is augmented by awareness of the increasingly stringent restrictions on the dollars made available for rehabilitation by payors. For this reason, in the late phase of care it may actually be an advantage, in terms of reimbursement, for rehabilitation services to continue to have a clearly indicated "medical" treatment modality (i.e., psychopharmaceuticals) to offer. The Omnibus Budget Reconciliation Act of 1987 increased the Medicare benefit for treatment of "mental, psychoneurotic, or personality disorders" and specifically removed all limits and special co-payments from the "medical management of psychopharmacologic agents" (i.e., it is to be covered no differently from outpatient treatment of all other medical illnesses).[238] Similar to this legislation and recent court decisions that have declared psychopharmacologic management of certain biologic psychiatric conditions (e.g., schizophrenia and bipolar disorder) to be a basic medical benefit and thus not liable to special "mental health" insurance benefit restrictions. Logic and analogy would suggest the same legal standing for pharmacologic treatment of TBI

in the chronic phase (after acute rehabilitation is finished), thus avoiding increasingly strict insurance benefit restrictions on these late-phase rehabilitation services. A consequence of this is that physician pharmacologic interventions in the late, chronic phase of care are significantly less likely to face payment denial on the basis of the "chronicity" of deficits. The perspective that many of the long-term deficits of TBI are physiologic dysfunctions amenable to management by medication is a rationale to obtain long-term rehabilitation access for these patients.

Conclusions

The empirical data guiding psychopharmacologic interventions in TBI continue to be inadequate, but they are growing. Psychopharmacologic drugs may produce tremendous improvements in the survivors of this condition. Increasing and convincing evidence now exists (based principally on numerous, well-designed case studies of single-case design) that multiple effective psychopharmacologic treatments for TBI are available, which for individual TBI patients can be dramatically effective in benefiting a variety of symptomatic areas. These pharmacologic approaches should be considered for every TBI patient to assess their potential contribution to the recovery.

The following conclusions are made:

- Conventionally recommended drugs may not be as appropriate as less familiar choices.
- Traditional rehabilitation procedures should not be separated from psychopharmacologic strategies; both should be considered complementary to other treatments.
- Treatment choices must encompass cost-effective considerations. If all of a patient's resources are expended in ineffective or inefficient nonpharmacologic efforts to address disordered agitation or impaired attention, for example, essential rehabilitation goals could be denied.
- It is clear that this population has lagged far behind other diagnoses in the amount and sophistication of study given it. Firm guidelines are almost nonexistent; the

clinician is rightly perplexed regarding an appropriate approach to these difficult patients. Methods exist to help clarify this situation, and it appears that an increasing effort is being addressed by many treatment centers to look more critically into this topic.

- Although matched, double-blind studies are rare, increasing evidence is being produced demonstrating a major useful role for psychopharmacologic agents in the rehabilitation of TBI. Series of cases, many of them quite acceptable single-case design, are available. Historically, most of the major advances in psychopharmacology were characterized by great methodologic imprecision. Indications for usage of each major class of psychopharmacologic drugs initially came from the observations of astute clinicians in relatively few patients rather than from large controlled studies.[12]

- Rehabilitation physicians must become expert in the use of psychopharmacologic agents if they are to care for TBI patients. Psychopharmacologic interventions will comprise an increasing proportion of the rehabilitation of the TBI patient at all phases of such care. Historically psychopharmacologic treatments have played a secondary role in the management of TBI. In the future, they will be increasingly integral and complementary with older methodologies.

REFERENCES

1. Abeloff MD: Off-label uses of anti-cancer drugs. JAMA 267:2473–2473, 1992.
2. Albert ML, Bachman DL, Morgan A, et al: Pharmacotherapy for aphasia. Neurology 38:877–879, 1988.
3. APA Statement on Tardive Dyskinesia. Hosp Comm Unity Psychiatry 36:902, 1985.
4. Applebaum PS, et al: Involuntary treatment in medicine and psychiatry. Am J Psychiatry 141:202–205, 1984.
5. Appleton WS: The Fifth Psychoactive Drug Usage Guide. Memphis, Physicians Postgraduate Press, 1991.
6. Artsen AFT, Goldman-Rakic PS: Catecholamines and cognitive decline in aged nonhuman primates. Ann NY Acad Sci 444:218–234, 1985.
7. Ashford JW, et al: Physostigmine and its effect on six patients with dementia. Am J Psychiatry 138:829–830, 1981.
8. Ashton H: Brain Function and Psychotropic Drugs. Oxford, Oxford Medical Publications, 1992.
9. Aston-Jones G, Ennis M, Pierbone VA, et al: The brain nucleus locus coeruleus: Restricted afferent control of a broad efferent network. Science 234:734–737, 1986.
10. Auerbach SH: Cognitive rehabilitation in the head injured: A neurobehavioral approach. Semin Neurol 3:152–163, 1983.
11. Auerbach SH: Neuroanatomical correlates of attention and memory disorders in traumatic brain injury: An application of neurobehavioral subtypes. J Head Trauma Rehabil 1:1–12, 1986.
12. Ayd FJ Jr: The early history of modern psychopharmacology. Neuropsychopharmacology 5:71–84, 1991.
13. Bach-y-Rita P: Neurotransmission in the brain by diffusion through the extracellular fluid: A review. NeuroReport 4:343–350, 1993.
14. Bach-Y-Rits, Lion G Jr, et al: Episodic dyscontrol: A study of 130 violent patients. Am J Psychiatry 127:49–54, 1971.
15. Barbee JG, Black FW, Todorov AA: Differential effects of alprazolam and buspirone upon acquisition, retention, and retrieval processes in memory. J Neuropsychiatry Clin Neurosci 4:308–314, 1992.
16. Barlow DH, Heroines M: Single Case Experimental Designs: Strategies for Studying Behavior Change, 2nd ed. New York, Pergamon Press, 1984.
17. Barnes R, et al: Efficacy of antipsychotic medications in behaviorally disturbed dementia patients. Am J Psychiatry 139:1170–1174, 1982.
18. Barratt ES: The use of anticonvulsants in aggression and violence. 29:75–81, 1993.
19. Barth JT, Macciocchi SN (eds): Mild Traumatic Brain Injury [issue]. J Head Trauma Rehabil 8: 1993.
20. Bartus RT, Dean RL, Pontecorvo MJ, et al: The cholinergic hypothesis: A historical overview, current perspective, and future directions. Ann NY Acad Sci 444:332–358, 1985.
21. Baumeister AA, Todd ME, Sevin JA: Review: Efficacy and specificity of pharmacological therapies for behavioral disorders in persons with mental retardation. Clin Neuropharmacol 16: 271–294, 1993.
22. Berlin FS, Meinke CF: Treatment of sex offenders with antiandrogen mediation: Conceptualization, review of treatment modalities and preliminary findings. Am J Psychiatry 138:601–607, 1981.
23. Bleiberg J, Cope DN, Spector J: Cognitive assessment and therapy in traumatic brain injury. Phys Med Rehabil State Art Rev 3:95–121, 1989.
24. Brown RG, Marsden CD, Quinn N, et al: Alterations in cognitive performance and affect-arousal state during fluctuations in motor function in Parkinson's disease. J Neurol Neurosurg Psychiatry 47:454–465, 1984.
25. Campbell M, et al: Behavioral efficacy of haloperidol and lithium carbonate. Arch Gen Psychiatry 41:650–656, 1984.
26. Cantini E, Gluck M, McLean A: Psychotropic-absent behavioral improvement following severe traumatic brain injury. Brain Inj 6:193–197, 1992.

27. Cassidy JW. Neurochemical substrates of aggression: Toward a model for improved intervention. Part 1. J Head Trauma Rehabil 5:83–86, 1990.

28. Chandra B. Treatment of disturbances of consciousness caused by measles encephalitis with Levodopa. Eur Neurol 17:265–270, 1978.

29. Chiarello RJ, Cole JO: The use of psychostimulants in general psychiatry. Arch Gen Psychiatry 44:286–295, 1987.

30. Childs A: Naltrexone in organic bulimia: A preliminary report. Brain Inj 1:49–55, 1987.

31. Chrisostoma EA, Duncan PW, Propst M, et al: Evidence that amphetamine with physical therapy promotes recovery of motor function in stroke patients. Ann Neurol 23:94–97, 1988.

32. Cisapride for nocturnal heartburn. Med Lett 36:11–13, 1994.

33. Klawans HL: Clinical Neuropharmacology, vol. II. New York, Raven Press, 1977.

34. Cohen CK, Wright JR, et al: Post head trauma syndrome in an adolescent treated with lithium carbonate—case report. Dis Nerv Syst 38:630–631, 1977.

35. Cooper JR, Bloom FE, Roth RH (eds): The Biochemical Basis of Neuropharmacology. New York, Oxford University Press, 1986.

36. Cope DN: Traumatic closed head injury: Status of rehabilitation treatment. Semin Neurol 5:212–220, 1985.

37. Cope DN: The pharmacology of attention and memory. J Head Trauma Rehabil 1:34–42, 1986.

38. Cope DN: Legal and ethical issues of the psychopharmacologic treatment of traumatic brain injury. J Head Trauma Rehabil 4:13–21, 1989.

39. Cope DN: An integration of psychopharmacologic and rehabilitation approaches. J Head Trauma Rehabil 1994.

40. Cope DN: Traumatic brain injury rehabilitation studies in the United States. In Christensen A, Uzzel B (eds): Perspectives in Neuropsychological Rehabilitation. Hillsdale, NJ, Lawrence Erlbaum Associates, in press.

41. Cox WH: An indication for use of imipramine in attention deficit disorder. Am J Psychiatry 139:1059–1060, 1982.

42. Coyle JT, Price DL, et al: Alzheimer's disease. A disorder of cortical cholinergic innervation. Science 219:1184–1190, 1983.

43. Crane GE: Persistent dyskinesia. Br J Psychiatry 122:395–405, 1973.

44. Crismon LM, Childs A, Wilcox RE, et al: The effect of bromocriptine on speech dysfunction in patients with diffuse brain injury (akinetic mutism). Clin Neuropharmacol 11:462–466, 1988.

45. Cromie BW: The feet of clay of the double-blind trial. Lancet 994–997, 1963.

46. Cummings JL, et al: Secondary mania with focal cerebrovascular lesions. Am J Psychiatry 141:1084–1087, 1984.

47. Davies P: A critical review of the role of the cholinergic system in human memory and cognition. Ann NY Acad Sci 444:212–217, 1985.

48. Davis KL, et al: Enhancement of memory processes in Alzheimer's disease with multiple-dose intravenous physostigmine. Am J Psychiatry 139:1421–1424, 1982.

49. Depaulo JR, Correa EI, et al: Does lithium stabilize mood? Biol Psychiatry 18:1093–1097, 1983.

50. Devane CL: Fundamentals of Monitoring Psychoactive Drug Therapy. Baltimore, Williams & Wilkins, 1990.

51. Dixon CE, Taft WC, Haye RI: Mechanisms of mild traumatic brain injury. J Head Trauma Rehabil 8:1–12, 1993.

52. Dominguez RA, Goldstein BJ: Beta-blockers in psychiatry. Hosp Comm Unity Psychiatry 35:565–566, 1984.

53. Donaldson IM, Cunningham J: Persisting neurologic sequelae of lithium carbonate therapy. Arch Neurol 40:747–751, 1983.

54. Drane JF: Competency to give an informed consent. JAMA 252:925–927, 1984.

55. Drugs that cause psychiatric symptoms. Med Lett 35:65–70, 1993.

56. Ducote C, Moore K, Gandolini J, et al: Imipramine for the treatment of akinetic mutism and arousal-attention deficits after traumatic brain injury. Presented at the 48th Annual Assembly of the American Academy of Physical and Medical Rehabilitation, Baltimore, 1986.

57. Eames P: The use of Sinemet and bromocriptine. Brain Inj 3:319–320, 1989.

58. Eames P: Personal communication, 1991.

59. Eames P, Wood R: Rehabilitation after severe brain injury: A special-unit approach to behavior disorders. Intern Rehabil Med 130–133, 1985.

60. Eichelman B, Hartwig A: The clinical psychopharmacology of violence: Towards a nosology of human aggressive behavior. Psychopharmacol Bull 29:57–63, 1993.

61. Elliott FA: Propanolol for the control of belligerent behavior following acute brain damage. Ann Neurol 1:489–491, 1977.

62. Etienne P, et al: Lecithin in Alzheimer's disease. 1206, 1978.

63. Evans RW, Gualtieri CT: Review: Carbamazepine: A neuropsychological and psychiatric profile. Clin Neuropharmacol 8:221–241, 1985.

64. Evans RW, Gualtieri CT: Psychostimulant pharmacology in traumatic brain injury. J Head Trauma Rehabil 2:29–33, 1987.

65. Evans RW, Gualtieri CT, Hicks RE: A neuropathic substrate for stimulant drug effects in hyperactive children. Clin Neuropharmacol 9:264–281, 1986.

66. Evans RW, Gualtieri CT, Patterson D: Treatment of chronic closed head injury with psychostimulant drugs: A controlled case study and an appropriate evaluation procedure. J Nerv Ment Dis 175:106–110, 1987.

67. Farlow M, Gracon SI, Hershey LS, et al: A controlled trial of Tacrine in Alzheimer's disease. JAMA 268:2523–2529, 1992.

68. Fauman MA: Treatment of the agitated patient with an organic brain disorder. JAMA 240:380–382, 1978.

69. Feeney DM: Pharmacologic modulation of recovery after brain injury: A reconsideration of diaschisis. J Neurol Rehabil 5:113–128, 1991.

70. Feeney DM, Bailey BY, Boyeson MG, et al: The effect of seizures on recovery of function following cortical contusion in the rat. Brain Inj 1:27–32, 1987.

71. Feeney DM, Gonzalez A, Law WA, et al: Amphetamine, haloperidol and experience interact to affect rate of recovery after motor cortex injury. Science 217:855–857, 1982.

72. Ferris SH, et al: Long-term treatment of memory impaired elderly patients. Science 205:1039–1040, 1979.

73. Fischbacher E: Effect of reduction of anticonvulsants on well being. BMJ 285:423–425, 1982.

74. Fleet WS, Valenstein E, Watson RT, Heilman KM: Dopamine agonist therapy for neglect in humans. Neurology 37:I-765–I-770.

75. Flood JF, et al: Memory enhancement: Supra-additive effect of subcutaneous cholinergic drug combinations in mice. Psychopharmacology 86:61–67, 1985.

76. Frances A, Jensen PS: Separating psychological factors from brain trauma in treating a hyperactive child. Hosp Community Psychiatry 36:711–713, 1985.

77. Freishtat HW, et al: Right to refuse treatment issues still far from settled. J Clin Psychopharmacol 1(3):163–164, 1981.

78. Fuxe K, Agnati LF: Volume Transmission in the Brain. New York, Raven Press, 1991.

79. Galski T, Krotenberg R: The usefulness of Hydergine on cognition in patients with traumatic head injury. Arch Phys Med Rehabil 70:A-12, 1989.

80. Garbutt JC, Loosen PT, et al: Is carbamazepine helpful in paroxysmal behavior disorder: Am J Psychiatry 140:1363–1363, 1983.

81. Gardos G: Disinhibition of behavior by antianxiety drugs. Psychosomatics 21:1025–1026, 1980.

82. Gardos G, et al: Differential actions of chlordiazepoxide and oxazepam on hostility. Arch Gen Psychiatry 18:757–760, 1968.

83. Gillman MA, Lichtfield FJ: Recovery after brain injury—some neurotransmitter and clinical implications. Br J Anesthesia 56:1319, 1984.

84. Giurgea C: Piracetam: Nootropic pharmacology of neurointergrative activity. In Essman WB, Valzelli L (eds): Current Developments in Psychopharmacology, vol 3. New York, Spectrum Publications, 1976, pp 223–273.

85. Glenn MB: Anticonvulsants reconsidered. J Head Trauma Rehabil 6:85–88, 1991.

86. Glenn MB, Joseph AB: The use of lithium for behavioral and affective disorders after traumatic brain injury. J Head Trauma Rehabil 2:68–76, 1987.

87. Glenn MB, Wroblewski B, Parziale J, et al: Lithium carbonate for aggressive behavior or affective instability in ten brain-injured patients. Am J Phys Med Rehabil 68:221–226, 1989.

88. Glenn MB. CNS stimulants: Applications for traumatic brain injury. J Head Trauma Rehabil 1:74–76, 1986.

89. Goetzl U, Grunberg F, et al: Lithium carbonate in the management of hyperactive aggressive behavior of the mentally retarded. Compr Psychiatry 18:599–605, 1977.

90. Goldberg E, et al: Effects of cholinergic treatment on posttraumatic anterograde amnesia. Arch Neurol 39:581, 1982.

91. Goldberg E, et al: Selective effects of cholinergic treatment on verbal memory in posttraumatic amnesia. J Clin Neuropharmacol 4:219–234, 1982.

92. Goldberg E, Gerstman LJ, Mattis, S, et al: Selective effects of cholinergic treatment of verbal memory in posttraumatic amnesia. J Clin Neuropsychol 4:219–234, 1982.

93. Goldstein LB, Matchar DB, Morgenlander JC, et al: Influence of drugs on the recovery of sensorimotor function after stroke. J Neurol Rehabil 4:137–144, 1990.

94. Gottfries GC: Review: Pharmacology of mental aging and demential disorders. Clin Neuropharmacol 10:313–329, 1987.

95. Greenblatt DJ, Raskin A: The use of benzodiazepines for psychotic disorders: A literature review and preliminary clinical findings. Psychopharmacol Bull 22:77–87, 1986.

96. Grimm BH, Bleiberg J: Psychological rehabilitation in traumatic brain injury. Handbook of Clinical Neuropsychology, vol. II. New York, John Wiley & Sons, 1986, pp 495–560.

97. Gualtieri CT: Neuropsychiatry and Behavioral Pharmacology. New York, Springer Verlag, 1991.

98. Gualtieri CT: Buspirone: Neuropsychiatric effects. J Head Trauma Rehabil 6:90–92, 1991.

99. Gualtieri CT, Chandler M, Coons TB, et al: Review. Amantadine: A new clinical profile for traumatic brain injury. Clin Neuropharmacol 12:258–270, 1989.

100. Gualtieri CT: Review: Pharmacotherapy and the neurobehavioral sequelae of traumatic brain injury. Brain Inj 2:101–129, 1988.

101. Reference deleted.

102. Gualtieri CT, Evans RW: Stimulant treatment for the neurobehavioral sequelae of traumatic brain injury. Brain Inj 2:273–290, 1988.

103. Gupta SR, Mlcoch AG: Bromocriptine treatment of nonfluent aphasia. Arch Phys Med Rehabil 73: 373–376, 1992.

104. Haas JF, Cope DN: Neuropharmacologic management of behavior sequelae in head injury: A case report. Arch Phys Med Rehabil 66:472–474, 1985.

105. Hale MS, et al: Lithium carbonate in the treatment of organic brain syndrome. J Nerv Ment Dis 170 (6):362–365, 1982.

106. Hale AS: New antidepressants: Use in high-risk patients. J Clin Psychiatry 54 (suppl):61–70, 1993.

107. Hales RE, Yudofsky SC: Textbook of Neuropsychiatry. Washington, DC, American Psychiatric Press, 1987.

108. Harris CM, et al: Effect of lecithin on memory in normal adults. Am J Psychiatry 140:1010–1012, 1983.

109. Hayes RL, Lyeth BG, Jenkins LW: Neurochemical mechanisms of mild and moderate head injury. In Levin H, Eisenberg HM, Benton AL (eds): Mild Head Injury. Oxford, Oxford University Press, 1989.

110. Hayes RL, Lyeth BG: Reply. Brain Inj 1:207–209, 1987.

111. Helms PM: Efficacy of antipsychotics in the treatment of the behavioral complications of dementia: A review of the literature. J Am Geriatr Soc 33: 206–209, 1987.

112. Henninger GR, Charney DS: Mechanisms of antidepressant treatments: implications for the etiology and treatment of depressive disorders. In Meltzer HY (ed): Psychopharmacology: The Third Generation of Progress. New York, Raven Press, 1987, pp 535–544.

113. Higashi K, et al: Clinical analysis of patients recovered from persistent vegetative state, with special emphasis on the therapeutic and prophylactic effects of L-dopa. Brain Nerve 30:27–35. 1978.

114. Higashi K, Hatano M, Abiko S, et al: Five-year follow-up study of patients with persistent vegetative state. J Neurol Neurosurg Psychiatry 44: 552–554, 1981.

115. Hill D: Amphetamine in psychopathic states. Br J Addiction 44:50–54, 1944.

116. Hippius H, Winokur G (eds): Psychopharmacology. Vol 1: A Biennial Critical Survey of the International Literature, Vol 2: Clinical Psychopharmacology. Amsterdam, Excerpta Medica, 1983.

117. Hollister LE, Csenansky JG: Clinical Pharmacology of Psychotherapeutic Drugs, 3rd ed. New York, Churchill Livingstone, 1990.

118. Hollister LE, Ysavage J: Ergoloid mesylates for senile dementias: Unanswered questions. Ann Intern Med 100:894–898, 1984.

119. Horvath TB, Siever LJ, Mohs RC, et al: Organic mental syndromes and disorders. In Kaplan HI, Sadock BJ (eds): Comprehensive Textbook of Psychiatry, 5th ed., vol 1. Baltimore, Williams & Wilkins, 1989.

120. Hunt RD, Minderaa RB, et al: The therapeutic effect of clonidine in attention deficit disorder with hyperactivity. A comparison with placebo and methylphenidate. Psychopharmacol Bull 22:229–236, 1986.

121. Iversen SD (Ed). Psychopharmacology: Recent Advances and Future Prospects. Oxford, Oxford University Press, 1985.

122. Jabbari B, et al: Incidence of seizures with tricyclic and tetracyclic antidepressants. Arch Neurol 42:480–481, 1985.

123. Jackson RD, Corrigan JD, Gribble MW: Amitriptyline for agitation in head injury. Arch Phys Med Rehabil 66:180–181, 1985.

124. Jampala VC, et al: Mania secondary to left and right hemisphere damage. Am J Psychiatry 140: 1197–1199, 1985.

125. Jenkins JS, Mather HM, Couglan AK: Desmopressin and desglycinamide vasopressin in posttraumatic amnesia. Lancet 3:39, 1981.

126. Johnson ML, Roberts MD, Ross AR, et al: Methylphenidate in stroke patients with depression. Am J Phys Med Rehabil 71:239–241, 1992.

127. Johnson JA, Lineberry CG, Ascher JA, et al: A 102-center prospective study of seizure in association with bupropion. J Clin Psychiatry 52:450–456, 1991.

128. Jones BE: The role of noradrenergic locus coeruleus neurons and neighboring cholinergic neurons of the pontomesencephalic tegmentum in sleep. Prog Brain Res 88:533–543, 1991.

129. Jorge RE, Robinson RG, Arndt SV, et al: Comparison between acute and delayed onset depression following traumatic brain injury. J Neuropsychiatry Clin Neurosci 5:43–49, 1993.

130. Judd LL, Squire LR, Butters N, et al: Effects of psychotropic drugs on cognition and memory in normal humans and animals. In Meltzer HY (ed): Psychopharmacology: The Third Generation of Progress. New York, Raven Press, 1987.

131. Kane JM, Evans DL, Fiester SJ, et al: Psychopharmacological screening criteria by APA Committee on Research on Psychiatric Treatments. J Clin Psychiatry 53:184–196, 1992.

132. Kety SS: The central physiological and pharmacological effects of the biogenic amines and their correlations with behavior. In Quarton GC, Melnechuk T, Schmitt FO (eds): The Neurosciences. New York, Rockefeller University Press, 1967, pp 444–451.

133. Klawans HL, Goetz CG, Tanner CM: Textbook of Clinical Neuropharmacology and Therapeutics. New York, Raven Press, 1992, pp 281–282.

134. Kligman D: Goldberg DA: Temporal lobe epilepsy and aggression. J Nerv Ment Dis 160:324–3341, 1975.

135. Klorman R, Bauer LO, Coons HW, et al: Enhancing effects of methylphenidate on normal young adults' cognitive processes. Psychopharmacol Bull 20:3–9, 1984.

136. Klove H: Activation, arousal, and neuropsychological rehabilitation. J Clin Exp Neuropsychol 9: 297–309, 1987.

137. Kneale TA, Eames P: Case study: Pharmacology and flexibility in the rehabilitation of two brain-injured adults. Brain Inj 5:327–330, 1991.

138. Koch-Hendrickson N, Nielsen H: Vasopressin in posttraumatic amnesia. Lancet 3:38–39, 1981.

139. Kolata GB: New drugs and the brain. Science 205:774–776, 1979.

140. Kupietz SS, Balka EB: Alterations in the vigilance performance of children receiving amitriptyline and methylphenidate pharmacotherapy. Psychopharmacology 50:29–33, 1976.

141. Lal S, Merbitz CP, Grip JC. Modification of function in head-injured patients with Sinemet. Brain Inj 2:225–233, 1988.

142. Lazarus A: Neuroleptic malignant syndrome and preexisting brain damage. J Neuropsychiatry 4: 185–187, 1992.

143. Levin HS, Grafman J, Eisenberg HM: Neurobehavioral Recovery from Head Injury. New York, Oxford University Press, 1987.

144. Levin HS, Handel SF, Goldman AM, et al: Magnetic resonance imaging after "diffuse" nonmissile head injury. A neurological study. Arch Neurol 42:963–968, 1985.

145. Levin HS, Benton AL, Grossman RG: Neurobehavioral Consequences of Closed Head Injury. New York, Oxford University Press, 1982.

146. Levin HS, Eisenberg HM, Benton AL (eds): Mild Head Injury. New York, Oxford University Press, 1989.

147. Lewis DA: Unrecognized chronic lithium neurotoxic reactions. JAMA 250:2029–2030, 1983.

148. Lewis L, Athey GI, Eyman J, et al: Psychological treatment of adult psychiatric patients with traumatic frontal lobe injury. J Neuropsychiatry 4:323–330, 1992.

149. Lipper S, Tuchman MM: Treatment of chronic posttraumatic organic brain syndrome with dextroamphetamine: First reported case. J Nerv Ment Dis 162:366–371, 1976.

150. Lipsey JR, Robinson RG, Pearlson GD, et al: Nortriptyline treatment of post-stroke depression: A double-blind study. Lancet 1:297–300, 1984.

151. Logothetis J: Spontaneous epileptic seizures and electroencephalographic changes in the course of phenothiazine treatment. Neurology 17:869–877, 1967.

152. Lowe TL, Cohen DJ, et al: Stimulant medications precipitate Tourette's syndrome. JAMA 247:1729–1731, 1982.

153. Lowry MR, et al: Seizures during tricyclic therapy. Am J Psychiatry 137:1461–1462, 1980.

154. Luria AR: Higher Cortical Functions in Man, 2nd ed. New York, Basic Books, 1980 (originally published in 1962).

155. Luria AR, Naydin VL, Tsvetkova LS, et al: Restoration of higher cortical function following local brain damage. In Vinken PJ, Bruyn GW (eds): Handbook of Clinical Neurology, vol 3. Amsterdam, North Holland, 1969.

156. Marin RS: Apathy: A neuropsychiatric syndrome. J Neuropsychiatry Clin Neurosci 3:243–254, 1991.

157. Mark VH: Epilepsy and episodic aggression [letter]. Arch Neurol 39:384–385, 1982.

158. Markowitz PI: Effect of fluoxetine on self-injurious behavior in the developmentally disabled: A preliminary study. J Clin Psychopharmacol 12:27–31, 1992.

159. Masand P, Murray GB, Pickett: Psychostimulants in post-stroke depression. J Neuropsychiatry Clin Neurosci 3:23–27, 1991.

160. Massagli TL: Neurobehavioral effects of phenytoin, carbamazepine, and valproic acid: Implications for use in traumatic brain injury. Arch Phys Med Rehabil 74:224–225, 1993.

161. Mattes JA, Rosenberg J, et al: Carbamazepine versus propanolol in patients with uncontrolled rage outbursts: A random assignment study. Psychopharmacol Bull 20:98–100, 1984.

162. Mattes JA: Carbamazepine for uncontrolled rage outbursts. Lancet 17:1164–1165, 1984.

163. Mattes JA: Metoprolol for intermittent explosive disorder. Am J Psychiatry 142:1108–1109, 1985.

164. McEntee WJ, Mair RG: Memory enhancement in Korsakoff's psychosis by clonidine: Further evidence for a noradrenergic deficit. Ann Neurol 7:466–469, 1979.

165. McIntyre FL, Gasquoine P: Effect of clonidine on posttraumatic memory deficits. Brain Inj 4:209–211, 1990.

166. McLean A, Cardenas DD, Haselkorn JK, et al: Cognitive psychopharmacology. Neurorehabilitation 3:1–14, 1993.

167. McLean A Jr., Stanton KM, Cardenas DD, et al: Memory training combined with the use of oral physostigmine. Brain Inj 1:145–159, 1987.

168. McLean A, Cardenas D, Bergess D, et al: Placebo-controlled study of pramiracetam in young males with memory and cognitive problems resulting from head injury and anoxia. Brain Inj 5:375–380, 1991.

169. McNeny R, Zasler ND: Neuropharmacologic management of hemi-inattention after brain injury. Neurorehabilitation 1:72–78, 1991.

170. Meltzer HY (ed): Psychopharmacology: The Third Generation of Progress. New York, Raven Press, 1987.

171 Mesulam M (ed): Principles of Behavioral Neurology. Philadelphia, F.A. Davis, 1985.

172. Mills JM, et al: Continuing case law development in the right to refuse treatment. Am J Psychiatry 140:715–719, 1983.

173. Mohr E, Fabbrini G, Ruggieri S, et al: Cognitive concomitants of dopamine system stimulation in Parkinsonian patients. J Neurol Neurosurg Psychiatry 50:1192–1196, 1987.

174. Mohs RC, et al: Choline chloride treatment of memory deficits in the elderly. Am J Psychiatry 136:1275–1277, 1979.

175. Moline K: Cognitive enhancing drugs. Headlines May/June: 22–23, 1992.

176. Mooney GF, Haas LJ: Effect of methylphenidate on brain injury-related anger. Arch Phys Med Rehabil 74:153–160, 1993.

177. Morrison JH, Molliver ME, Grzanna R: Noradrenergic innervation of cerebral cortex: Widespread effects of local cortical lesions. Science 205:313–316, 1979.

178. Mortimer JA, et al: Head injury as a risk factor for Alzheimer's disease. Neurology 35:264–267, 1985.

179. Mysiw WJ, Corrigan JD, Gribble MW: Application of reaction-time monitoring during pharmacologic intervention in traumatic brain injury. Arch Phys Med Rehabil 67:677, 1986.

180. Mysiw WJ, Jackson RD: Tricyclic antidepressant therapy after traumatic brain injury. J Head Trauma Rehabil 2:34–42, 1987.

181. Neppe VM: Carbamazepine as adjunctive treatment in nonepileptic chronic inpatients with EEG temporal lobe abnormalities. J Clin Psychiatry 44:326–331, 1983.

182. Nichols ME, Meador DJ, Loring DW: Review: Neuropsychological effects of antiepileptic drugs: A current perspective. Clin Neuropharmacol 16:471–484, 1993.

183. Nicholson CD: Pharmacology of nootropics and metabolically active compounds in relation to their use in dementia. Psychopharmacology 101:147–159, 1990.

184. O'Connor MO, Baker HWG: Depo-medroxy progesterone acetate as an adjunctive treatment in three aggressive schizophrenic patients. Acta Psychiatr Scand 67:399–403, 1983.

185. Oliveros JC, Jandali MK, Timsit-Berthier M, et al: Vasopressin in amnesia. Lancet 1:42, 1978.

186. Parks RW, Crockett DJ, Husseini KM, et al: Assessment of bromocriptine intervention for the treatment of frontal lobe syndrome: A case study. J Neuropsychiatry 4:109–111, 1992.

187. Parmelee DX, Kowatch RA: The use of lithium carbonate in brain-injured, behaviorally-dysfunctional adolescents. Presented at the Postgraduate Course on Rehabilitation of the Brain-injured Adult and Child, Williamsburg, Va, June 5, 1986.

188. Partap M, et al: Vasopressin-8-lysine in prevention of ECT induced amnesia. Am J Psychiatry 140:946–947, 1983.

189. Petersen DC: Scopolamine-induced learning failures in man. Psychopharmacology 52:283–289, 1977.

190. Pincus JH: Can violence be a manifestation of epilepsy? Neurology 30:304–307, 1980.

191. Pope HR Jr, McElroy SL, Satlin A, et al: Head injury, bipolar disorder, and response to valproate. Comp Psychiatry 29:34–38, 1988.

192. Porch B, Wyckes J, et al: Haloperidol, thiazides and some antihypertensives slow recovery from aphasia [abstract]. Soc Neurosci, May 1, 1985.

193. Prigatano GP, Altman IM, O'Brien KP: Behavioral limitations that traumatic brain-injured patients tend to underestimate. Clin Neuropsychol 4:163–176, 1993.

194. Pritchard PB, Lombroso CT, et al: Psychological complications of temporal lobe epilepsy. Neurology 30:227–232, 1980.

195. Psychopharmacology Bulletin, Washington, DC, National Institute Mental Health Government Printing Office, 1992.

196. Rampling D, et al: Aggression: A paradoxical response to tricyclic antidepressants. Am J Psychiatry 135:117–118, 1978.

197. Rango N: Nursing home care in the United States N Engl J Med 307:883–890, 1982.

198. Rao N, Jellinek HM, Woolston DC: Haloperidol effects on rehabilitation outcome. Arch Phys Med Rehabil 66:30–34, 1985.

199. Rao N, Costa JL: Recovery in non-vascular locked-in syndrome during treatment with Sinemet. Brain Inj 3:207–211, 1989.

200. Ratey JJ, et al: Use of propanolol for provoked and unprovoked episodes of rage. Am J Psychiatry 140:1356–1357, 1983.

201. Ratey JJ, Gordon A: The psychopharmacology of aggression: Toward a new day. Psychopharmacol Bull 29:65–73, 1993.

202. Ratey J, Levoroni C, Kilmer D, et al: The effects of clozapine on severely aggressive psychiatric inpatients in a state hospital. J Clin Psychiatry 54:219–223, 1993.

203. Reimherr FW, Wood DR, et al: An open clinical trial of L-dopa and carbidopa in adults with minimal brain dysfunction. Am J Psychiatry 137:73–75, 1980.

204. Reference deleted.

205. Reisberg B, et al: An overview of pharmacological treatment of cognitive decline in the aged. Am J Psychiatry 138:593–599, 1981.

206. Reisberg B, Ferris SH, Anand R, et al: Effects of Naloxone in senile dementia: A double blind trial. N Engl J Med 308:721–722, 1983.

207. Reintan RM, Wolfson D: Neuroanatomy and Neuropathology: A Clinical Guide for Neuropsychologists. Tucson, Neuropsychological Press, 1985.

208. Report: New Medications in Development for Older Americans. Washington, DC, Pharmaceutical Manufacturers Association, 1993.

209. Reynolds EH, Trimble MR: Adverse neuropsychiatric effects of anticonvulsant drugs. Drugs 29:570–581, 1985.

210. Reynolds EH: Anticonvulsants and mental symptoms. In Sandler M (ed): Psychopharmacology of Anticonvulsants. Oxford, Oxford University Press, 1982.

211. Richmond JS, et al: Violent dyscontrol responsive to d-amphetamine. Am J Psychiatry 135:365–366, 1978.

212. Ricketts R, et al: Fluoxetine treatment of severe self-injury in young adults with mental retardation. J Am Acad Child Adolesc Psychiatry 32:865–869, 1993.

213. Rivinus TM: Psychiatric effects of the anticonvulsant regimens. J Clin Psychopharmacol 2:165–192, 1982.

214. Robinson RG, Starr LB, Lipsey JR, et al: A two-year longitudinal study of post stroke mood disorders. J Nerv Ment Dis 173:221–226, 1985.

215. Robinson RG, Bloom FE: Pharmacological treatment following experimental cerebral infarction: Implications for understanding psychological symptoms of human stroke. Biol Psychiatry 12:669–680, 1977.

216. Robinson DS: Adverse reactions, toxicities and drug interactions of newer antidepressants: Anticholinergic, sedative and other side effects. Psychopharmacol Bull 20:280–290, 1984.

217. Rodgers RJ, Waters AJ: Benzodiazepines and their antagonists: A pharmacoethological analysis with particular reference to effects on "aggression." Neurosci Biobehav Rev 9:21–35, 1985.

218. Rosenbaum JF: Emergence of hostility during alprazolam treatment. Am J Psychiatry 141:792–793, 1984.

219. Rosenstein DL, Nelson JC, Jacobs SC: Seizures associated with antidepressants: A review. J Clin Psychiatry 54:289–299, 1993.

220. Ross ED, Rush J: Diagnosis and neuroanatomical correlates of depression in brain-damaged patients. Arch Gen Psychiatry 38:134–1354, 1981.

221. Rothman CB, Chusid E, et al: Mental retardation: Behavior problems and psychotropic drugs. NY State J Med 79:709–715, 1979.

222. Ruedrich SL, Chu CC, Moore SL: ECT for major depression in a patient with acute brain trauma. Am J Psychiatry 140:928–929, 1983.

223. Rutherford WH, Merrett JD, McDonald JR: Sequelae of concussion caused by minor head injuries. Lancet 1:1–4, 1977.

224. Sabel BA, Stein DG: Pharmacologic treatment of central nervous system injury. Nature 323:493, 1986.

225. Sadeh M, Braham J, Modan M: The effects of anticholinergic drugs on memory in Parkinson's disease. Arch Neurol 39:666–667, 1982.

226. Sahgal A: A critique of the vasopressin-memory hypothesis. Psychopharmacology 83:215–228, 1984.

227. Saletu B, Linzmayer L, Grunberger J, et al: Double-blind, placebo-controlled, clinical, psychometric and neuropsychological investigations with oxiracetam in the organic brain syndrome of late life. Neuropsychobiology 13:44–52, 1985.

228. Salzman C, DiMascio A, et al: Chlordizepoxide, expectation and hostility. Psychopharmacologia 14:38–45, 1969.

229. Sandel EM, Olive DA, Rader MA: Chlorpormazine-induced psychosis after brain injury. Brain Inj 7:77–83, 1993.

230. Sara SJ: Noradrenergic modulation of selective attention: Its role in memory retrieval. Ann NY Acad Sci 444:178–193, 1985.

231. Schatzberg AF, Cole JO: Manual of Psychopharmacology. Washington, DC, American Psychiatric Press, 1986.

232. Schiff HB, et al: Lithium in aggressive behavior. Am J Psychiatry 139:1346–1348, 1982.

233. Schiffer RB, Herndon RM, Rudick RA: Treatment of pathologic laughing and weeping with amitriptyline. N Engl J Med 312:1480–1482, 1985.

234. Schneider LS, Pollock BE, Lyness SA: A metaanalysis of controlled trials of neuroleptic treatment in dementia. J Am Geriatr Soc 38:553–563, 1990.

235. Schwartz J, Levesque D, Martres M, et al: Review: Dopamine D₃ receptor: Basic and clinical aspects. Clin Neuropharmacol 16:295–314, 1993.

236. Seliger GM, Hornstein A, Flax J, et al: Fluoxetine improves emotional incontinence. Brain Inj 6:267–270, 1992.

237. Shalev A, Hermesh H, Munitz H: Mortality from neuroleptic malignant syndrome. J Clin Psychiatry 50:18–25, 1989.

238. Shafstein SS, Goldman H: Financing the medical management of mental disorders. Am J Psychiatry 146:345–349, 1989.

239. Sheard MH, Marini JL, Bridges CI, Wagner E: The effect of lithium on impulsive aggressive behavior in man. Am J Psychiatry 133:1409–1413, 1976.

240. Sheard MG, Marini JL: Treatment of human aggressive behavior. Four case studies of the effect of lithium. Compr Psychiatry 19:37–45, 1978.

241. Shakla S, Cook BL, Mukherjee S, et al: Mania following head trauma. Am J Psychiatry 144:93–96, 1987.

242. Silver JM, Yudofsky SC: Pharmacologic treatment of neuropsychiatric disorders. Neurorehabilitation 3:15–25, 1993.

243. Silver JM, Yudofsky, SC, Hales RE: Depression in traumatic brain injury. Neuropsychiatr Neuropsychol Behav Neurol 4:12–23, 1991.

244. Silver JM, Hales RE, Yudofsky SC: Neuropsychiatric aspects of traumatic brain injury. In Hales RE, Yudofsky SC (eds): The American Psychiatric Press Textbook of Neuropsychiatry. Washington, DC, American Psychiatric Press, 1987, pp 363–395.

245. Sitland-Marken PA, Wells BG, Froemming JH, et al: Psychiatric applications of bromocriptine therapy. J Clin Psychiatry 51:68–82, 1990.

246. Sloan RL, Brown KW, Pentland B: Fluoxetine as a treatment for emotional lability after brain injury. Brain Inj 6:315–319, 1992.

247. Smith CM, et al: Choline therapy in Alzheimer's disease. Lancet 2:318, 1978.

248. Synder D: Drug and neurotransmitter receptors in the brain. Science 224:22–31, 1984.

249. Snyder D: Intellectual and behavioral effects of anticonvulsants. West J Med 142:79–80, 1985.

250. Sovner RS, et al: Do the mentally retarded suffer from affective illness? Arch Gen Psychiatry 40:61–67, 1983.

251. Speech TJ, Rao SM, Osmon DC, et al: A double-blind controlled study of methylphenidate treatment in closed head injury. Brain Inj 7:333–338, 1993.

252. Stanislav S, et al: Buspirone's efficacy in organic-induced aggression. Psychopharmacology 2:126–130, 1994.

253. Starkstein SE, Boston JD, Robinson RG: Mechanisms of mania after brain injury: 12 case reports and review of the literature. J Nerv Ment Dis 176:87–100, 1988.

254. Stern MJ, Stern B: Psychotherapy in cases of brain damage: A possible mission. Brain Inj 4:297–304, 1990.

255. Strahan A, Rosenthal J, Kaswan M, et al: Three case reports of acute paroxysmal excitement associated with alprazolam treatment. Am J Psychiatry 142:859–861, 1985.

256. Stritch SJ: The pathology of brain damage due to blunt head injuries. In Walker AE, Caveness WF, Critchley M (eds): The Late Effects of Head Injury. Springfield, IL, Charles C Thomas, 1969.

257. Stuss DT, Gow CA: "Frontal dysfunction" after traumatic brain injury. Neuropsychiatry Neuropsychol Behav Neurol 5:272–282, 1992.

258. Stuss DT: Contribution of frontal lobe injury to cognitive impairment after closed injury: Methods of assessment and recent findings. In Levin HS, Grafman J, Eisenberg HM (eds): Neurobehavioral Recovery from Closed Head Injury. New York, Oxford University Press, 1987.

259. Summers WK, Majovski LV, Marsh GM, et al: Oral tetrahydroaminoacridine in long-term treatment of senile dementia, Alzheimer type. N Engl J Med 315:1241–1245, 1986.

260. Szlabowicz JW, Stewart JT: Amitriptyline treatment of agitation associated with anoxic encephalopathy. Arch Phys Med Rehabil 71:612–613, 1990.

261. Temkin NR, Dikmen SS, Wilensky AJ, et al: A randomized, double-blind study of phenytoin for the prevention of posttraumatic seizures. N Engl J Med 323:497–502, 1990.

262. Theodore WH, et al: Complex partial seizures: Clinical characteristics and differential diagnosis. Neurology 33:1115–1121, 1983.

263. Thiebot M, et al: Benzopdiazepines reduce the tolerance to reward delay in rats. Psychopharmacology 86:147–152, 1985.

264. Thomsen IV: Late outcome of very severe blunt head trauma: A 10–15 year second follow-up. J Neurol Neurosurg Psychiatry 47:260–268.

265. Tinklenberg JA, et al: Vasopressin effects on cognition and affect in the elderly. In Ordy JM, Sladek JR, Reisberg B (eds): Neuropeptide and Hormone Modulation of Brain Function and Homeostasis. New York, Raven Press, 1981.

266. Trimble MR, Thompson RJ: Anticonvulsant drugs and cognitive function. Arch Phys Med Rehabil 65:618, 1984.

267. Tune LE, Strauss ME, Lew MF, et al: Serum levels of anticholinergic drugs and impaired recent memory in chronic schizophrenic patients. Am J Psychiatry 139:1460–1462, 1982.

268. Tupin JP, Smith DB, et al: The long-term use of lithium in aggressive prisoners. Compr Psychiatry 14:311–317, 1973.

269. Tupin JP, Schader RI, Harnet DS (eds): Handbook of Clinical Psychopharmacology, 2nd ed. Northvale, NJ, Aronson, 1988.

270. Tyerman AL, Humphrey M: Changes in self concept following severe head injury. Int J Rehabil Res 7:11–23, 1984.

271. Udaka F, Yamao S, Nagata H, et al: Pathologic laughing and crying treated with Levodopa. Arch Neurol 41:1095–1096, 1984.

272. Van Dongen P: Human locus coeruleus in neurology and psychiatry. Prog Neurobiol 17:97–139, 1981.

273. VanHasselt P: Effect of butyrophenones on motor function in rats after recovery from brain damage. Neuropharmacology, 12:245–247, 1973.

274. van Woerkom TC, et al: Difference in neurotransmitter metabolism in frontotemporal-lobe contusion and diffuse cerebral contusion. Lancet 1:812–813, 1977.

275. Voeller KKS: What can neurological models of attention, intention, and arousal tell us about attention-deficit hyperactivity disorder? J Neuropsychiatry Clin Neurosci 3:209–216, 1991.

276. Walton R: Lecithin and physostigmine for posttraumatic memory and cognitive deficits. Psychosomatics 23:435–436, 1982.

277. Warburton DM, Wesnes K: Drugs as research tools in psychology: Cholinergic drugs and information processing. Neuropsychobiology 11:121–132, 1984.

278. Waxman HM, Klein M, Carner EA: Drug misuse in nursing homes: An institutional addiction? Hosp Comm Unity Psychiatry 36:886–887, 1985.

279. Weinberg RM, Auerbach SH, Moore S: Pharmacologic treatment of cognitive deficits: A case study. Brain Inj 1:57–59, 1987.

280. Whyte J, Cope DN (eds): Head Trauma Rehabil 9(3):1994.

281. Whyte J: Neurologic disorders of attention and arousal: Assessment and treatment. Arch Phys Med Rehabil 73:1094–1103, 1992.

282. Williams KH, Goldstein G: Cognitive and affective responses to lithium inpatients with organic brain syndrome. Am J Psychiatry 136:800–803, 1979.

283. Winsberg BG, Bialer I, Kupietz S, et al: Effects of imipramine and dextroamphetamine on behavior of neuropsychiatrically impaired children. Am J Psychiatry 128:109–115, 1425–1431, 1972.

284. Wohns RNW, et al: Prophylactic phenytoin in severe head injuries. J Neurosurg 51:507–509, 1979.

285. Wolkowitz OM, Tinklenberg JR, Weingartner H: A psychopharmacological perspective of cognitive function: II. Specific pharmacologic agents. Neuropsychobiology 14:133–156, 1985.

286. Wood RL: Neurobehavioral Sequelae of Traumatic Brain Injury. London, Taylor & Francis, 1990.

287. Wright RB, Costa JL, Brandabur M, et al: A variant of akinetic mutism: Biochemical and physiological studies during successful withdrawal from Sinemet. J Neurol Rehabil 4:163–167, 1990.

288. Wroblewski BA, Glenn MB, Cornblatt R, et al: Protriptyline as an alternative stimulant mediation in patients with brain injury: A series of case reports. Brain Inj 7:353–362, 1993.

289. Wroblewski BA, Glenn MB: Pharmacologic treatment of arousal and cognitive deficits. J Head Trauma Rehabil 9:19–42, 1994.

290. Wroblewski BA, Leary JM, Phelan AM, et al: Methylphenidate and seizure frequency in brain injured patients with seizure disorders. J Clin psychiatry 53:86–89, 1992.

291. Wroblewski BA, McColgan K, Smith K, et al: The incidence of seizures during tricyclic antidepressant drug treatment in a brain injured population. J Clin Psychopharmacol 10:124–128, 1990.

292. Yablon SA: Posttraumatic seizures. Arch Phys Med Rehabil 74:983–1001, 1993.

293. Young B, Rapp RP, Norton JA: Failure of prophylactically administered phenytoin to prevent early posttraumatic seizures. J Neurosurg 58:231–235, 1983.

294. Yudofsky SC, et al: Propanolol in the treatment of rage and violent behavior in patients with chronic brain syndromes. Am J Psychiatry 138:218–220, 1981.

295. Yudofsky SC, et al: Propanolol in the treatment of rage and violent behavior associated with Korsakoff's psychosis. Am J Psychiatry 141:114–115, 1984.

296. Zasler ND: Advances in neuropharmacological rehabilitation for brain dysfunction. Brain Inj 6:1–14, 1992.

297. Zasler ND: Mild traumatic brain injury: Medical assessment and intervention. J Head Trauma Rehabil 8:13–29, 1993.

298. Zola-Morgan S, Squire LR: The neuroanatomy of amnesia: Amygdala-hippocampus versus temporal stem. Science 218:1337–1339, 1982.

Index

Page numbers in **boldface type** indicate complete chapters.